WASHINGTON AND LEAVER'S PRINCIPLES AND PRACTICE OF
Radiation Therapy

FIFTH EDITION

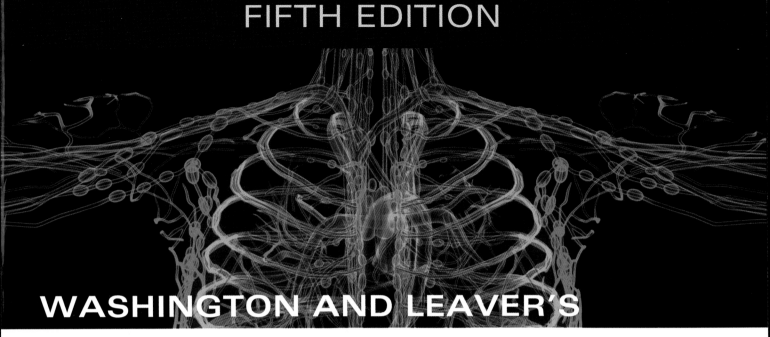

WASHINGTON AND LEAVER'S

PRINCIPLES AND PRACTICE OF
Radiation Therapy

Charles M. Washington,
EdD, MBA, RT(T), FASRT
Senior Director
Radiation Oncology
Memorial Sloan Kettering Cancer Center
New York, New York

Dennis Leaver,
MS, RT(R)(T), FASRT
Professor Emeritus
Department of Biology
Southern Maine Community College
South Portland, Maine

Megan Trad,
PhD, MSRS, RT(T)
Associate Professor
Radiation Therapy
Texas State University
San Marcos, Texas

ELSEVIER

Elsevier
3251 Riverport Lane
St. Louis, Missouri 63043

WASHINGTON AND LEAVER'S PRINCIPLES AND PRACTICE OF
RADIATION THERAPY, FIFTH EDITION   ISBN: 978-0-323-59695-4

Notice

Practitioners and researchers must always rely on their own experience and knowledge in evaluating and
using any information, methods, compounds or experiments described herein. Because of rapid advances
in the medical sciences, in particular, independent verification of diagnoses and drug dosages should be
made. To the fullest extent of the law, no responsibility is assumed by Elsevier, authors, editors or contributors for any injury and/or damage to persons or property as a matter of products liability, negligence or
otherwise, or from any use or operation of any methods, products, instructions, or ideas contained in the
material herein.

Previous editions Copyright © 2016, 2010, 2004, 1996.

Library of Congress Control Number: 2019953768

Executive Content Strategist: Sonya Seigafuse
Senior Content Development Manager: Lisa P. Newton
Senior Content Development Specialist: Tina Kaemmerer
Publishing Services Manager: Deepthi Unni
Project Manager: Haritha Dharmarajan
Designer: Brian Salisbury

Printed in China

Last digit is the print number: 9 8 7 6 5 4 3 2 1

Working together
to grow libraries in
developing countries

www.elsevier.com • www.bookaid.org

To those who have run and continue to run the race against cancer.
We sincerely hope those who read this work will grow in the knowledge
and understanding necessary to provide direction, care,
and compassion to their patients, family, and supportive friends.
Let us not grow tired in running our own race,
but instead encourage those around us.

Robert D. Adams, EdD, MPH, FAAMD, FASRT
Assistant Professor
Radiation Oncology
University of North Carolina
Chapel Hill, North Carolina

Lisa Bartenhagen, MS, RT(R)(T) ARRT
Department Chair and Program Director
Medical Imaging and Therapeutic Sciences
University of Nebraska Medical Center
Omaha, Nebraska

E Richard Bawiec Jr., MS
Senior Medical Physicist, Varian Medical
    Systems. Barling, AR. Palo Alto,
    California

Lior Zvi Braunstein, MD
Assistant Attending
Radiation Oncology
Memorial Sloan Kettering Cancer Center
New York, New York

Leila Bussman Yeakel, MEd, RT(R)(T)
Program Director and Assistant Professor
Radiation Therapy Program
Mayo Clinic School of Health Sciences
Rochester, Minnesota

Jessica Church, MPH, RT(R)(T), CMD
Assistant Professor
School of Health Professions
The University of Texas MD Anderson
    Cancer Center
Houston, Texas

Gil'ad N. Cohen, MS
Senior Physicist
Medical Physics
Memorial Sloan Kettering Cancer Center
New York, New York

Annette M. Coleman, MA, RT(T)
Senior Project Manager
Portfolio Management, Oncology Informatics
    Elekta
Sunnyvale, California

Laura D'Alimonte, MRT(T), BSc, MHSc
Clinical Practice Manager
Radiation Therapy
Windsor Regional Hospital
Windsor, Ontario
Canada

Lawrence T. Dauer, PhD
Associate Attending Physicist
Department of Medical Physics, Department
    of Radiology
Memorial Sloan Kettering Cancer Center
New York, New York

Lisa DiProspero, MRT(T), BSc, MSc
Director, Practice-Based Research and
    Innovation
Director, Education Research Unit
Assistant Professor, Department of Radiation
    Oncology, University of Toronto
Sunnybrook Health Sciences Centre
Toronto, Ontario Canada

Erin Gillespie, MD
Radiation Oncologist
Radiation Oncology
Memorial Sloan Kettering Cancer Center
New York, New York

Amy Heath, MS, RT(T)
Program Manager, Radiation Therapy
Radiation Oncology
UW Health
Madison, Wisconsin
Adjunct Faculty
Radiation Therapy Program
University of Wisconsin – La Crosse
La Crosse, Wisconsin

Jana Koth, MPH
Clinical Education Coordinator
Radiation Therapy Program
University of Nebraska Medical Center
Omaha, Nebraska

Ronnie G. Lozano, BS, MSRS, PhD
Chair and Associate Professor
Radiation Therapy Program
Texas State University
San Marcos, Texas

Mazur Lukasz, PhD
Assistant Professor and Director of Division
    of Healthcare Engineering
Radiation Oncology, School of Medicine
University of North Carolina
Chapel Hill, North Carolina;
Assistant Professor
Carolina Health Informatics Program and
    School of Information and Library Science
University of North Carolina
Chapel Hill, North Carolina

Heather Mallett, MBA, RT(T)
Program Director
Radiation Oncology
Northwestern Memorial Hospital
Chicago, Illinois

James Mechalakos, PhD
Attending Physicist
Medical Physics
Memorial Sloan Kettering Cancer Center
New York, New York

Matthew Palmer, MBA, BA, CMD
President and Chief Operating Officer, Legion
    Healthcare Partners, Houston, Texas

Simon Powell, MD, PhD
Chair
Radiation Oncology
Memorial Sloan Kettering
New York, New York

Kameka Rideaux, MBA, BS(R)(T)
Senior Program Manager
Global Site Solutions VPT
Varian Medical Systems
Palo Alto, California

Narayan Sahoo, PhD
Professor
Radiation Physics
The University of Texas MD Anderson
    Cancer Center
Houston, Texas

Zachary Smith, MBA, RT(R)(T)
Director
Radiation Oncology/Respiratory Care
Baton Rouge General Pennington Cancer
    Center
Baton Rouge, Louisiana

Amanda Sorg, MLS, R(T), (CT)
Program Director
Radiation Therapy
Indiana University Northwest
Gary, Indiana

Maria Thompson, BS, RT(T)
Clinical Coordinator
OHSU Radiation Therapy Program
Oregon Health and Science University
Portland, Oregon

Kristi L. Tonning, BS, MS
Director
Radiation Therapy Program
Oregon Health and Science University
Portland, Oregon;
Assistant Professor
Department of Radiation Medicine
Oregon Health and Science University
Portland, Oregon

Nora Uricchio, MEd, RT(R)(T)
Program Director
Health Careers
Manchester Community College
Manchester, Connecticut

Melissa R. Weege, MS, RT(T), CMD
Radiation Therapy Program Director
Health Professions
University of Wisconsin – La Crosse
La Crosse, Wisconsin

Ana Weeks, MSc
Lead Product Owner
VisionRT
London, United Kingdom

Bettye Wilson, MA Ed. RT(R)(CT), RDMS, FASRT
Associate Professor Emerita
Critical and Diagnostic Care
University of Alabama at Birmingham
    School of Health Professions
Birmingham, Alabama;
Adjunct Faculty
Radiography
Arizona Western College
Yuma, Arizona

Carol Chovanec, MS, RT(T)
Radiation Therapy Program Director
Bergen Community College
Paramus, New Jersey

Laura D'Alimonte, MRT(T), BSc, MHSc
Clinical Practice Manager
Radiation Therapy
Windsor Regional Hospital
Windsor, Ontario
Canada

Becky Dodge, PhD, RT(R)(T)
Assistant Professor/Coordinator
Master of Health Science Program
Washburn University
Topeka, Kansas

Anna Elizabeth Drew, RT(R)(CT)(T)
Radiation Therapist
Radiation Oncology
Northern Light Health
Cancer Center of Maine
Brewer, Maine

Janelle Duquette, BSc, MRT(T)
Faculty Service Officer
Radiation Therapy Program
University of Alberta
Edmonton, Alberta
Canada

Ruth M. Hackworth, MS, RT(R)(T)
Program Director, Radiation Therapy
The Ohio State University
James Cancer Hospital
Columbus, Ohio

Leia Levy, EdD, RT(T)
Program Director and Assistant Professor
University of St. Francis
Joliet, Illinois

Brian Liszewski, MRT(T), BSc
Radiation Therapist
Department of Radiation Oncology
University of Toronto
Toronto, Ontario
Canada

Don McCoy, RT(T)
Associate Professor
Community College of Denver-School of
    Health Sciences
Denver, Colorado

Amy Carson VonKadich, MEd, RT(T)
Department Chair
Diagnostic Medical Imaging
NHTI: Concord's Community College
Concord, New Hampshire

Since the first edition of this text was published in 1996, the field of radiation therapy has experienced tremendous growth. Improvements in conformal treatment planning, intensity-modulated radiation therapy, image-guided radiation therapy, particle therapies, adaptive therapies, brachytherapy, and patient immobilization have all allowed the radiation therapy team to enhance and improve clinical outcomes. More integrated electronic charting has allowed the entire radiation therapy team to improve treatment delivery documentation and quality assurance practices. Although the face of radiation therapy has evolved through these advances, this textbook remains committed to its original purpose. It is still designed to contribute to a comprehensive understanding of cancer management, improve clinical techniques involved in delivering a prescribed dose of radiation therapy, and apply knowledge and complex concepts associated with radiation therapy treatment planning and delivery. As the methods of delivering a prescribed dose of radiation therapy have expanded and improved, so has the effort to localize, plan, and deliver accurate daily treatment.

NEW TO THIS EDITION

Since the fourth edition, a new chapter has been added, and several chapters have been consolidated and additional information included. The infection control chapter has been divided into two to discuss infection as it relates to the person and infection's impact on the radiation oncology department. A new Advanced Procedures chapter has been developed to give further insight into the increasing complexity of radiation-based care delivery. Color images are now used throughout the text to better demonstrate key aspects that are not easily conveyed in grayscale.

LEARNING AIDS

Pedagogical features designed to enhance comprehension and critical thinking are incorporated into each chapter. Elements retained from the previous editions include the following:

- Chapter Outlines
- Key Terms lists
- Spotlight boxes that highlight key information and/or direct readers to more information on important topics
- Bulleted chapter summaries for easier reference
- An updated Glossary that includes significant terms from all chapters
- Review Questions
- Questions to Ponder

Of particular note are the Review Questions and Questions to Ponder at the end of each chapter. Review Questions reinforce the cognitive information presented in the chapter, helping the reader incorporate the information into the basic understanding of radiation therapy concepts. The Questions to Ponder are open-ended, divergent questions intended to stimulate critical thinking and analytic judgment. Answers to the Review Questions are found on the student Evolve website.

In addition, each chapter offers a reference list, giving the reader additional information sources. In each edition, the focus of every chapter has been to present the comprehensive needs of the radiation therapy management team. In fact, dozens of experts in the field have contributed to this new edition, including radiation therapists, medical dosimetrists, physicians, physicists, radiation oncologists, nurses, and radiation therapy students.

ANCILLARIES

For Instructors

A robust instructor ancillary suite is available online on the Evolve website, and includes the following:

- Test Bank of approximately 900 questions in ExamView format
- PowerPoint presentations for each chapter
- Image collection of all figures from the book

For Students

The student site contains the Answer Key to the Review Questions from the text.

Charles M. Washington
Dennis Leaver
Megan Trad

ACKNOWLEDGMENTS

We are grateful to the contributors of the chapters and for the reviewers who offered helpful feedback and suggestions. We also offer special thanks to the editorial staff at Elsevier for their patience and valuable contributions during the preparation and production of this work.

With this edition, we are pleased to introduce our third editor, Dr. Megan Trad, who is an associate professor at Texas State University. Megan serves on several national professional committees and continues to promote the field of radiation therapy. Her attention to detail and knowledge of radiation therapy principles augments the fifth edition of this work.

We would like to acknowledge and thank Dennis Leaver, one of the founding editors of the textbook, for his efforts in shaping radiation therapy education over the last 25 years. His pioneering spirit helped the educational field of radiation therapy transition from resources originally written for physicists and physicians, towards a focused effort of more than 5200 printed pages with over 200 separate contributors through five editions. A majority of that work was contributed by radiation therapists. His impact on the profession is undeniable.

Finally, it is our hope the expanded knowledge and progress in treatment planning, delivery, and patient care outlined in this work will ultimately enrich the patient's quality of life and reduce suffering from the effects of cancer.

Charles M. Washington
Dennis Leaver
Megan Trad

CONTENTS

Cancer: An Overview

Melissa R. Weege

OBJECTIVES

- Discuss how the changing theories of cancer affect treatment choices and outcome.
- Discuss how patient-focused care will provide an optimum treatment environment.
- Differentiate between benign and malignant tumors.
- Differentiate between stage and grade of a tumor.
- Explain what information physicians would need to know about a patient and his or her cancer to decide on an appropriate plan of treatment.
- Design a chart that details the strengths and weaknesses of the three major cancer treatments: radiation therapy, surgery, and chemotherapy.
- Discuss how each member of the radiation oncology team contributes to effective patient care and treatment.

OUTLINE

KEY TERMS

Adenocarcinoma
Adjuvant therapy
Anaplastic
Benign
Biopsy
Carcinomas
Cellular differentiation

Chemotherapeutic agents
Clinical staging
Epidemiology
Etiology
Exophytic
False negative
False positive

Grade
Immunotherapy
In situ
Interferon
Intrathecal
Malignant
Medical dosimetrist

Radiation therapy is the medical specialty that uses ionizing radiation to treat cancer and some benign diseases. The goal of radiation therapy is to deliver the maximum amount of radiation needed to kill the cancer while sparing normal surrounding tissue, also known as the therapeutic ratio.[1] To accomplish this goal, radiation therapy relies heavily on physics and biological sciences, including radiobiology and computer science. The technological and medical advances during the last 30 years have thrust radiation therapy into a new and exciting era in which the highest level of accuracy and the ability to greatly reduce dose to the normal structures is possible. However, it is important to remember that although the technology and equipment are advanced and exciting, the focus of radiation is on the person diagnosed with disease. The focus of the radiation therapist remains the patient, providing quality care, performing the daily radiation therapy treatments, educating, making referrals as needed, and making daily assessments. A meaningful, daily connection with the patient is as important as any other task the therapist accomplishes. Patients and their families should be seen as the most important focus of a radiation therapist's work.

PATIENT PERSPECTIVE

Although cancer is often a curable disease, the diagnosis is a life-changing event. In studying the various aspects of neoplasia, care providers can easily lose sight of the person behind the disease. The patient must be the focal point of all of the radiation therapist's actions. The highest level of quality care results from an in-depth knowledge of the disease process: psychosocial issues, patient care, and principles and practices of cancer management, including knowledge of radiation therapy as a treatment option. This knowledge provides the radiation therapist with the tools necessary for optimal treatment, care, and education of the cancer patient. Care that does not consider the whole person is unacceptable. Patient satisfaction has always been important in healthcare and continues to be a measured outcome in many cancer centers. Famiglietti et al[2] conducted a patient satisfaction survey where data were collected from 8069 patients receiving radiation treatments. Each question was rated on a 10-point Likert scale and analyzed for the patient's overall satisfaction. The results of this study align with other published findings that the most important determinant of patient satisfaction is the patient-provider relationship. In many healthcare settings, the provider is best defined as the physician. However, in this study, which focused on radiation oncology, the radiation therapist's relationship with patients was found to be the most significant contributor to overall patient satisfaction. The two variables with the greatest effect on patient satisfaction were the care provided by radiation therapists and pain management.[2] A significant connection with the patient each day is as important as any other task the therapist accomplishes during the delivery of a prescribed course of radiation therapy.

The Person Behind the Diagnosis

When providing treatment for a large number of people in whom cancer develops, care providers can easily forget that the patient has a life outside of treatment. The patient's concerns and worries continue, adding to the emotional, social, psychological, physical, and financial burdens that accompany a cancer diagnosis. In addition, other medical concerns unrelated to cancer may complicate treatment and further burden the patient. By the time a patient ends up in radiation therapy, they have seen numerous doctors and may have many other appointments scheduled.

Factors such as patient age, culture, religion, support systems, education, and family background play important roles in medical treatment compliance, attitudes toward treatment, and responses to treatment. Knowing as much as possible about the patient and factors that influence treatment outcome can help the radiation therapist provide quality patient care. An example would be the patient who requests a treatment time not convenient for the department schedule. For a radiation therapist who has many patients to accommodate and a very tight schedule, this request may seem unreasonable. It may turn out that a working relative is providing daily transportation to the clinic and does not have a flexible work schedule. An appointment time that interferes with the relative's work schedule may lead to the loss of employment. In this example, there are three possible outcomes. First, the radiation therapist gives the patient an appointment time that fits the treatment schedule and lets the patient work out the transportation issues. Second, the radiation therapist gives the patient the requested appointment time and changes other patient appointments, or third, the radiation therapist refers the patient and relative to community transportation resources and works with all parties to develop a plan for treatment. For reasons such as these, an in-depth knowledge of available patient resources is essential to ensure that all patients receive the care and help they need to deal with the disease and resulting life issues. The actual radiation treatment is only part of the radiation therapist's responsibility. A patient is not an organ with a cancer but a complete individual with a multitude of issues and needs that must be addressed. Because cancer affects the whole family, it is the responsibility of the radiation therapist to provide information and available resources to assist the patient and family in dealing with all the issues and challenges that a diagnosis of cancer brings. It is good to remember that sometimes the smallest act of compassion and connection with the patient and/or his or her family will transform the radiation treatment experience from frightening and overwhelming to comforting and trusting (Fig. 1.1).

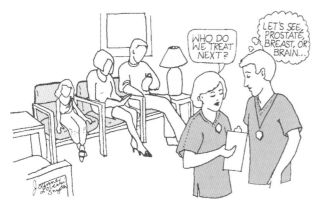

Fig. 1.1 Focus on the whole person, not the disease. (Courtesy Joanne Lobeski-Snyder.)

Cancer Patient Resources

In each medical facility, there is generally a myriad of cancer support services. These services can include general education, cancer site–specific education, support groups, financial aid, transportation to and from treatment, and activity programs. Social work departments are available to assist with the financial, emotional, and logistic issues that arise, and community services through churches and other organizations are available to support individuals and their families. National organizations such as the American Cancer Society have established programs and information hotlines that are available to all patients. Caring for a cancer patient is often a 24-hour-a-day job, and it is essential that resources are available at all hours. Community services are usually available for the caregivers because the caretaking toll can be physical, mental, emotional, and financial. Radiation therapists must become familiar with the services offered in their communities and nationally to better serve the patients and their family member caregivers. This is especially true for radiation therapists working at freestanding clinics not affiliated with a medical center. Educating patients and their families about available programs or services to address specific needs is an important component of quality care provided by the radiation therapist. Now that we have established that the patient is the focus for every member of the radiation therapy healthcare team, a historic look at cancer investigation is in order.

Two excellent national resources are:
American Cancer Society: https://www.cancer.org/
National Cancer Institute: https://www.cancer.gov/

Throughout recorded history, cancer has been a subject of investigation. Lacking current surgical techniques and diagnostic and laboratory equipment, early investigators relied on their senses to determine characteristics of the disease. Investigators were unable to thoroughly examine cells, so infections and other benign conditions were included in their category of cancer. Knowledge about these early observations, including examinations, diagnosis, and treatment, comes in part from Egyptian papyri dating back to 1600 BCE.[3] Initially, investigators believed that an excess of black bile caused cancer. This belief defined cancer as a systemic disease for which local treatment (such as surgery) only made the patient worse. In light of this, cancer was considered to be fatal with little possibility of a cure. When investigators could not prove the existence of black bile, the theory of cancer as an initially localized disease emerged. With this theory came the possibility of treatment with a potential for cure. However, because of the limited information available, few cures were accomplished.

In the fifth century BCE, Hippocrates began the classification of tumors by observation. Later, the discovery of the microscope enabled investigators to classify tumors on the basis of cellular characteristics.[3] Classification of tumors and their stages of growth continue as technology advances.

The cause of this deadly disease remained a mystery, and, for many decades, people even thought that cancer was contagious. This theory brought isolation and shame to cancer victims. Although this belief has long since vanished, less than 30 years ago, patients expressed concern about spreading the disease to loved ones. Unfortunately, today many cancer patients still suffer discrimination in the workplace and when trying to obtain health insurance coverage.

With the ability to examine the genetic makeup of a cancer cell, scientists can now determine many of the mutations that are responsible for a specific cancer initiation. This knowledge leads to earlier diagnosis in higher-risk individuals, improved screening examinations, and ultimately better treatment. It is now possible to develop specific chemotherapy, immunotherapy, and targeted therapy drugs for individual cancers and provide drugs that will be effective in blocking specific cancer initiation in high-risk individuals. This area is still in its infancy but has very exciting possibilities.

BIOLOGIC PERSPECTIVE

Building on the work of early investigators and aided by technologic advances, researchers are able to diagnose many tumors in extremely early stages. In addition, scientists are able to examine the deoxyribonucleic acid (DNA) of cells obtained through biopsy to determine mechanisms causing uncontrolled growth. Although it is true that technology and knowledge about cancer has increased during the past decades, there is still much to be learned.

Theory of Cancer Initiation

Tumors are the result of abnormal cellular proliferation. This can occur because the process by which cellular differentiation takes place is abnormal or because a normally nondividing, mature cell begins to proliferate. Cellular differentiation occurs when a cell undergoes mitosis and divides into daughter cells. These cells continue to divide and differentiate until a mature cell with a specific function results. When this process is disrupted, the daughter cells may continue to divide with no resulting mature cell, thus causing abnormal cellular proliferation.

The cause of this cellular dysfunction has been the subject of research for many years. Researchers now know that cancer is a disease of the genes. Normal somatic cells (nonreproductive cells) contain genes that promote growth and genes that suppress growth, both of which are important to control the growth of a cell. In a tumor cell, this counterbalanced regulation is missing. Mutations occurring in genes that promote or suppress growth are implicated in the deregulation of cellular growth. Mutations in genes that promote growth force the proliferation of cells, whereas mutations to the genes that suppress growth allow unrestrained cellular growth. For many tumors, both mutations may be required for progression to full malignancy.[4–7]

The terms for the genes involved in the cancer process are *proto-oncogenes*, oncogenes, and *antioncogenes*. Proto-oncogenes are the normal genes that play a part in controlling normal growth and differentiation. These genes are the precursors of oncogenes (gene that regulates the development and growth of cancerous tissues), or cancer genes. The conversion of proto-oncogenes to oncogenes can occur through point mutations, translocations, and gene amplification, all of which are DNA mutations. Oncogenes are implicated in the abnormal proliferation of cells. Antioncogenes are also called *tumor-suppressor genes*. These are the genes that tell cells to stop multiplying. Inactivation of antioncogenes allows the malignant process to flourish.[4–7]

> DNA point mutations, amplification, or translocations transform a proto-oncogene into an oncogene, resulting in unrestricted cellular growth.

What causes these mutations to occur? For somatic cells, exposure to carcinogens such as certain viruses, sunlight, radiation, and cigarette smoke is implicated. In some situations, such as the familial form of retinoblastoma, gene mutations are passed down through generations. Random mutations that occur during normal cellular replication can also lead to unregulated cellular growth.

Researchers have identified several gene mutations, including the gene implicated in the familial form of breast cancer. With the use of gene mapping and advanced technology, study in this area will continue. To understand the principles of cancer treatment, a review of the cell cycle and an overview of tumor growth are necessary.

Review of the Cell Cycle

Mammalian cells proliferate through the process of mitosis, or cellular division. The outcome of this process is two daughter cells that have identical chromosomes as the parent. The cell cycle consists of the period of time and the activities that take place between cell divisions. The cell cycle consists of five phases called G0, G1, S, G2, and M (Fig. 1.2).

G0 is depicted outside of the cell cycle continuum because these cells are fully functioning but are not preparing for DNA replication. Most cells making up a tissue or organ are in the G0 phase. Given the proper stimulus, this reserve pool of cells can reenter the cell cycle and replicate.

G1, or the first growth phase, is characterized by rapid growth and active metabolism. The length of time that a cell remains in G1 is variable. Cells that are rapidly dividing spend little time in the first growth phase, whereas cells that are slow growing remain in G1 for a long period. The length of time spent in G1 varies from hours to years. During this time, the cell synthesizes the necessary ribonucleic acid (RNA) and proteins to carry out the function of the cell. Later in the first growth phase, the cell will commit to replication of DNA.

S phase, or synthesis, is the period in which DNA is replicated to ensure that the resulting daughter cells will have identical genetic material. G2, or the second growth phase, is the period in which the cell prepares for actual division. Enzymes and proteins are synthesized and the cell continues to grow and moves relatively quickly into the M, or mitotic, phase.

> Cells are most sensitive to radiation during G2 and M phases of the cell cycle.

Tumor Growth

When all cells are operating normally, there is a balance between cells that are dying and the replication of cells. Although tumor growth is a result of an imbalance between replication and cell death, the rate of growth is influenced by many factors. Malignant cells possess damaged genetic material, resulting in increased cell death. In addition, while the tumor grows larger, the blood, oxygen, and nutrient supply is inadequate, creating areas of necrosis, or dead tissue.[8]

Initially, tumor growth is exponential, but although the tumor enlarges and outgrows the blood and nutrient supply, the rate of cell replication more closely equals the rate of cell death. This is demonstrated by the Gompertzian growth curve (Fig. 1.3). Tumors that are

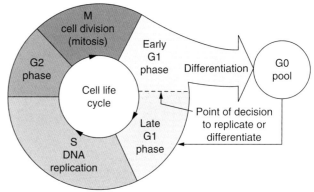

Fig. 1.2 Cell generation cycle. (From Otto SE. *Oncology Nursing*. 2nd ed. St. Louis, MO: Mosby; 1994.)

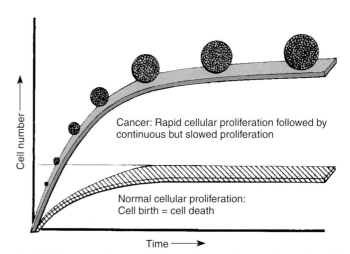

Fig. 1.3 Gompertz function as viewed by growth curve. (From Otto SE. *Oncology Nursing*. 2nd ed. St. Louis, MO: Mosby; 1994.)

clinically detectable are generally in the higher portion of the curve. Treatment reduces the number of cells, thus moving the tumor back down the curve where the growth rate is higher. Tumor cells that were previously in the G0 phase are prompted to reenter the cell cycle. Cells that are rapidly dividing are more sensitive to the effects of radiation and chemotherapy.

> Cancer cells do not die after a programmed number of cell divisions as do normal cells. Hence, cancer cells have the ability to proliferate indefinitely.

Tumor Classification

Tumors are classified by their anatomic site, cell of origin, and biologic behavior. Tumors can originate from any cell; this accounts for the large variety of tumors. Well-differentiated tumors (those that closely resemble the cell of origin) can be easily classified according to their histology. Undifferentiated cells, however, do not resemble normal cells, so classification is more difficult. These tumors are called undifferentiated, or anaplastic, which is a pathologic description of cells, describing a loss of differentiation and more primitive appearance.

Tumors are divided into two categories: benign or malignant (Table 1.1). Benign tumors are generally well differentiated and do not metastasize or invade surrounding normal tissue. Often, benign tumors are encapsulated and slow growing. Although most benign tumors do little harm to the host, some benign tumors of the brain (because of their location) are considered behaviorally malignant because of the adverse

TABLE 1.1	General Characteristics of Benign and Malignant Disease	
Characteristics	**Benign**	**Malignant**
Local spread	Expanding, pushing	Infiltrative and invasive
Distant spread	Rare	Metastasize early or late by lymphatics, blood, or seeding
Differentiation	Well differentiated	Well differentiated to undifferentiated
Mitotic activity	Normal	Normal to increased mitotic rate
Morphology	Normal	Normal to pleomorphic
Effect on host	Little (depending on treatment and location of tumor)	Life-threatening
Doubling time	Normal	Normal to accelerated

TABLE 1.2	Classifications of Neoplasms	
Tissue of Origin	**Benign**	**Malignant**
Glandular epithelium	Adenoma	Adenocarcinoma
Squamous epithelium	Papilloma	Squamous cell carcinoma
Connective tissue smooth muscle	Leiomyoma	Leiomyosarcoma
Hematopoietic	—	Leukemia
Lymphoreticular	—	Lymphoma
Neural	Neuroma	Blastoma

TABLE 1.3	Histologies Associated with Common Anatomic Cancer Sites
Site	**Most Common Histology**
Oral cavity	Squamous cell carcinoma
Pharynx	Squamous cell carcinoma
Lung	Squamous cell carcinoma
Breast	Infiltrating ductal carcinoma
Colon and rectum	Adenocarcinoma
Anus	Squamous cell carcinoma
Cervix	Squamous cell carcinoma
Endometrium	Adenocarcinoma
Prostate	Adenocarcinoma
Brain	Astrocytoma

effect on the host. Benign tumors may be noted by the suffix *-oma*, which is connected to the term indicating the cell of origin. For example, a *chondroma* is a benign tumor of the cartilage. Although this is a general rule, there are malignant tumors, such as melanoma, that end with the same suffix but are malignant.

Malignant tumors often invade and destroy normal surrounding tissue and, if left untreated, can cause the death of the host.

A well or moderately well-differentiated malignant tumor cell will resemble the cell from which it originated. A poorly differentiated cell will have very few of the characteristics of the originating cell, and an undifferentiated cell will have no characteristics of the original cell. They have the ability to metastasize, or spread to a site in the body distant from the primary site.

> Malignant tumors often invade and destroy normal surrounding tissue and, if left untreated, can cause the death of the host.

Tumors arising from mesenchymal cells are known as sarcomas. These cells include connective tissue such as cartilage and bone. An example is a chondrosarcoma or a sarcoma of the cartilage. Although blood and lymphatics are mesenchymal tissues, they are classified separately as leukemias and lymphomas.

Carcinomas are tumors that originate from the epithelium. These include all the tissues that cover a surface or line a cavity. For example, the aerodigestive tract is lined with squamous cell epithelium. Tumors originating from the lining are called *squamous cell carcinoma* of the primary site. An example is squamous cell carcinoma of the lung. Epithelial cells that are glandular are called adenocarcinoma. An example is the tissue lining the stomach. A tumor originating in the cells of this lining is called *adenocarcinoma of the stomach*. Table 1.2 lists examples of nomenclature used in neoplastic classification. As in any classification system, some situations do not follow the rules. Examples include Hodgkin disease, Wilms tumor, and Ewing sarcoma. The system of classification continues to change while more knowledge of the origin and behavior of tumors become available. Table 1.3 lists histologies associated with common anatomic cancer sites.

Cancer Outlook

The American Cancer Society[6] estimates that approximately 1.7 million new cases of cancer will be diagnosed each year. Of those patients, approximately 607,000 will die of their disease.[9] Basal and squamous cell skin cancers and most in situ cancers (an early form of cancer defined by the absence of invasion) are not included in these numbers, except for bladder cancer. The cancer death rate has declined during the last 30 years and varies by age, gender, and race. Excluding carcinoma of the skin, the most common types of invasive cancers in the United States include prostate, lung, and colorectal cancer in men, and breast, lung, and colorectal cancer in women.[9] These statistics are not static and change with environmental, lifestyle, health, technologic, and other societal factors. According to a recent Surveillance, Epidemiology, and End Results Program (SEER) Cancer Statistics Review, the 5-year relative survival rate (from 2008 to 2014) for all primary cancer sites combined is nearly 70% (69.7%).[9] This is largely because of screening, better treatment techniques, and health education. Interestingly, obesity is now a significant risk factor in the development of many cancers.[9] Invasive carcinoma of the cervix has also decreased during the past 20 years as a result of cancer screening with the Papanicolaou (Pap) smear. Currently, more carcinoma in situ, or preinvasive, cancers of the cervix are found than invasive tumors. These in situ carcinomas, which carry a better prognosis, are not recorded in the American Cancer Society statistics.

Depending on the geographic location, the incidence of tumor sites also varies. For example, the incidence of stomach cancer is much greater in Japan than in the United States, and skin cancer is found more frequently in New Zealand than in Iceland. Diet and geographic environmental factors contribute to these tumor incidence differences.

ETIOLOGY AND EPIDEMIOLOGY

A tremendous amount of knowledge exists about factors that influence the development of cancer and the incidence at which it occurs.

Etiology and epidemiology are the two of these areas that have contributed to the growing knowledge in these areas.

Etiology

Etiology is the study of the cause of disease. Although the cause of cancer is unknown, many carcinogenic agents and environmental and genetic factors have been identified and are called risk factors. Experts use this information, as they have done with tobacco use, to establish prevention programs and identify high-risk individuals.

> Etiologic factors may include cigarette smoke, human papillomavirus, alcohol, sun exposure, diet, and obesity.[10]

Etiologic and epidemiologic information is helpful in determining screening tests for early detection, producing patient education programs, and identifying target populations. An example is a set of guidelines from the American Cancer Society for early detection of cancer.[11] These guidelines give recommendations for cancer screening exams for breast, colorectal, cervical, endometrial, lung, and prostate cancers.[11]

Epidemiology

Epidemiology is the study of disease incidence. National databases, such as SEER,[8] provide statistical information about patterns of cancer occurrence and death rates. With this information, researchers can determine the incidence of cancer occurrence in a population for factors such as age, gender, race, and geographic location. Researchers can also determine which specific type of cancer affects which specific group of people. An example is the higher incidence of prostate cancer in African-American males. Epidemiologic studies also help determine trends in disease such as the recent decrease of lung cancer in men, the decline of stomach cancer or the increase in malignant melanoma in the United States, and the increase in obesity-related cancers.[10]

DETECTION AND DIAGNOSIS

Early detection and diagnosis are keys to the successful treatment of cancer. Generally, the earlier a tumor is discovered, the lower the chance of metastasis or spread to other parts of the body and the better the chance for cure. For some tumors, such as carcinoma of the larynx, early symptoms, such as a very hoarse voice, cause the patient to seek medical care early in the course of the disease. As a result, the cure rate for early-stage larynx (glottic) (or true vocal cord) tumors is extremely high. Cancer of the ovary, however, is associated with vague symptoms such as bloating, upset stomach, or abdominal discomfort that could be the result of a number of medical problems. Consequently, a diagnosis is often made late in the course of the disease. Low cure rates for ovarian cancer reflect the results of late diagnosis.

Advances in medical diagnostic imaging, especially the use of computed tomography (CT), magnetic resonance imagining (MRI), and positron emission tomography (PET) imaging, allow physicians to see into the body and even visualize cellular activity. These increased capabilities have played a pivotal role in earlier detection and diagnosis of cancer. These advances have also provided the knowledge needed to reduce treatment volume to spare normal surrounding tissues in radiation therapy.

Screening Examinations

To identify cancer in its earliest stages (before symptoms appear and while the chance of cure is greatest), screening tests are performed. Examples include the Pap smear for cervical cancer, fecal occult blood testing or colonoscopy for colorectal cancer, low-dose CT scans for high-risk people, and mammograms for breast cancer.[11] Unfortunately, for many cancers, screening examinations are not readily available because of the inaccessibility of the tumor or the high cost in relation to the information yield associated with the tests.

To be useful, screening examinations must be sensitive (ability of a test to give a true-positive result) and specific (ability of the test to obtain a true-negative result) for the tumors they identify. If an examination is sensitive, it can identify a tumor in its extremely early stages. A sensitive test will not result in false-negative findings. A false-negative finding would be one where it appears that there is no cancer present when indeed there is cancer. For example, a Pap smear is sensitive because it can help detect carcinoma of the cervix before the disease becomes invasive. If a test is specific, it can identify a particular type of cancer. For example, a prostate-specific antigen (PSA) in the blood is used specifically for prostate cancer. Unfortunately, it results in a number of false-positive readings. Carcinoembryonic antigen may be elevated in a number of benign and malignant conditions. For this reason, the test is not specific, but it is the most sensitive test available for determining recurrences of colorectal cancer.

Screening tests may yield false-positive or false-negative readings. A false-positive reading indicates disease when in reality none is present. In these cases, patients may undergo additional unnecessary, morbid, and costly screening exams or treatments. A false-negative reading is the reverse; the test indicates no disease when in fact the disease is present. In these cases, a patient does not have needed treatment until later in the disease trajectory. The perfect scenario is to have a screening examination that is both very sensitive and specific. The cost of the screening examination often limits its use to all but extremely high-risk populations.

In 2002, the National Cancer Institute (NCI)[1] began a national lung screening trial for high-risk individuals that compared standard chest radiography with spiral CT as a screening tool. By April 2004, more than 53,000 individuals were enrolled in the study, and data were collected. In 2011, the NCI reported the finding of a 24% reduction in lung cancer mortality with low-dose CT screening when compared with conventional x-rays.[12] This program continues to be adopted nationwide to detect lung cancer in its early stages in the identified high-risk populations.

> A false-positive, sensitive but low-specificity screening examination results in the necessity of additional, often costly, diagnostic procedures to determine the diagnosis.

Workup Components

After a tumor is suspected, a workup, or series of diagnostic examinations, begins. The purpose of the workup is to determine the general health status of the patient and to collect as much information about the tumor as possible. To treat the patient effectively, the physician must know the type, location, and size of the tumor; the degree the tumor has invaded normal tissue; the amount of differentiation of the cells; the presence or absence of spread to distant sites; the lymph node involvement, if any; and amenability to specific treatment regimens. These questions are answered in the workup.

The workup depends on the type of cancer suspected and the symptoms experienced by the patient. The workup for a suspected lung tumor is different than that for a suspected prostate tumor. The same questions are answered, but because the two tumors are extremely different, the tests are based on the specific tumor characteristics. Additionally, the workup for an early-stage tumor will be different from later-stage disease. The incidence of bone metastasis in a stage I breast cancer is extremely low, unlike stage IV disease. Therefore, the workup for stage I disease will not include a bone scan but would be ordered for stage IV disease.

> For patients who have lifestyle habits that include carcinogens such as cigarette smoking, moderate to heavy alcohol use, chewing tobacco, and obesity, the workup will include diagnostic procedures to rule out the possibility of second primary cancers.

With advancing technology, more information is available to the physician than ever before. As new technologies emerge and prove useful in the information-gathering process, treatment becomes more effective. Before CT or MRI became available, small tumor extension into normal lung tissues was not visible on chest radiographs. The physician had to make an educated guess about the extent of the tumor invasion and to treat the patient based on the suspected condition. As a result, treatment fields had to be larger to encompass all the suspected disease. Much of the guesswork is eliminated with the use of ultrasound, CT, MRI, and PET, so treatment volumes can include only areas of known disease while limiting dose to the normal tissue, thereby producing a more effective treatment with fewer short-term and chronic treatment side effects.

Today, with the added imaging tool of PET and PET-CT, physicians can identify very small foci of disease that may be active near the primary tumor or located in other parts of the body undetectable to other forms of diagnostic imaging. PET has diagnostic value for tumors of the lung, head and neck, and breast, as well as for colorectal and esophageal tumors, lymphoma, and melanoma. The effectiveness of PET for other tumor types is under investigation. Determination of whether a suspicious posttreatment area is recurrent disease or an expected tissue change is another area in which PET excels.

Staging

Tumor staging is a means of defining the tumor size and extension at the time of diagnosis and is important for many reasons. Tumor staging provides a means of communication about tumors, helps in determining the best treatment, aids in predicting prognosis, and provides a means for continuing research. Staging systems have changed with advancing technologies and increased knowledge and will continue to progress while more information becomes known. For this reason, tumors that occur frequently have detailed staging classifications, whereas those that are rare have primitive or no working staging systems.

According to the American Joint Committee on Cancer (AJCC),[13] there are four types of staging that occur in cancer care. The first is clinical staging, which is based upon physical exam, pertinent imaging exams, and biopsies.[13] Pathologic staging refers to clinical staging with the addition of information from surgical removal of all or part of a tumor.[13] Posttherapy staging is determined after the first course of chemotherapy or hormone therapy and/or radiation therapy to see how treatment has impacted the cancer.[13] Lastly, restaging is performed in the cases of cancer recurrence after treatment.[13]

A common staging system adopted by the International Union Against Cancer and the AJCC is the TNM system. It should be noted that the TNM system for each cancer is different. Complete information on each cancer is available from the AJCC in the form of a Cancer Staging Manual.[13] The T category defines the size or extent of the primary tumor and is assigned numbers 1 through 4 or x. A T1 tumor is small and/or confined to a small area, whereas a T4 tumor is extremely large and/or extends into other tissues. The x indicates that there was an inability to obtain information necessary to make a determination. N designates the status of lymph nodes and the extent of lymph node involvement. A 0 through 4 or x designation exists depending on the extent of involvement, with N0 indicating that no positive nodes are present. N1 indicates positive nodes close to the site of the primary tumor, whereas N4 indicates positive nodes at more distant nodal sites. Nx indicates that the nodal status was not assessed. Not all cancers have the designation of N1 through N4. The natural history of a particular cancer and clinical treatment knowledge will affect the complexity of the staging system. M is the category that defines the presence and extent of metastasis. Again, the M category is generally categorized as 0, 1, or x, depending on the extent of metastatic disease. The designation M0 indicates no evidence of metastatic disease was found, whereas M1 indicates disease distant from the primary tumor. Mx indicates that the presence or absence of metastasis was not assessed. Specific tumors with a detailed staging criteria may have an expanded M designation (Fig. 1.4).

In TNM staging, additional subcategories are used for commonly occurring tumors. Notations are often used to determine whether the staging was accomplished through clinical, surgical, or pathologic methods. Although the TNM system is widely used, numerous staging systems exist that more accurately detail important tumor characteristics for prognostic and treatment information. For example, the International Federation of Gynecology and Obstetrics system is more commonly used in the staging of gynecologic tumors.

Surgical/Pathologic Staging

Surgical/pathologic staging offers the most accurate information about the tumor and the extent of disease spread. Although staging can be performed clinically, or without the use of invasive procedures, the status of the lymph nodes and micrometastatic spread would remain in question. During surgical staging, the physician has the opportunity to perform a biopsy of suspicious-looking tissue, obtain a sample of lymph nodes for microscopic examination, and observe the tumor and surrounding tissues and organs.

Ovarian disease may be staged surgically through the use of an intraoperative examination or surgical exploration of the abdomen because these tumors often spread by seeding into the abdomen. During the procedure, the primary tumor site is identified, the tumor is removed, suspicious areas are biopsied, and fluid is introduced into the abdominal cavity to be removed and examined for cancer cells. The amount of tumor left behind following the surgery provides important treatment and prognostic information. The greater the amount of information obtained about the tumor, the more accurate the staging is likely to be, which results in more effective treatment. Accurate staging is also able to limit aggressive treatment to only those patients who will benefit.

With the ability to look at a tumor's cellular DNA, a physician has even more information available to determine, within a tumor type, which tumor is more sensitive to a particular treatment and which tumor has a greater chance of recurrence. Tumor cell DNA examination is standard practice for a variety of cancers, and the staging has changed to include DNA characteristics, as well as clinical factors. For example, with breast cancer, overexpression of *HER2/neu* proto-oncogene or *BRCA1* or *BRCA2* will influence the overall treatment plan.[1]

Grade

The grade of a tumor provides information about its aggressiveness and is based on the degree of differentiation. Differentiation is divided into four categories: well differentiated, moderately well differentiated, poorly differentiated, and undifferentiated or anaplastic. Cancer cells that have the most characteristics of the original cell are well and moderately well differentiated. Cells in which the original cell is barely or not distinguishable are poorly differentiated or undifferentiated.

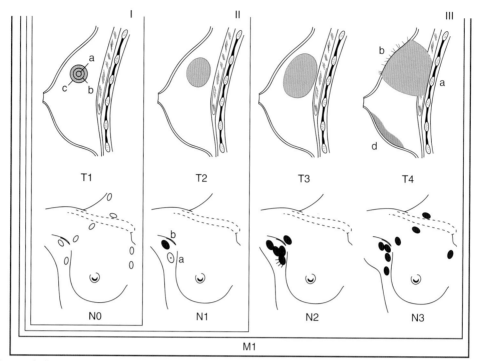

Fig. 1.4 A diagrammatic depiction of the breast cancer staging system. (From Rubin P. *Clinical Oncology.* 7th ed. Philadelphia, PA: WB Saunders; 1993.)

Degree of differentiation is determined only by examination of cells obtained through biopsy under a microscope. For some tumors, such as high-grade astrocytoma, grade is the most important prognostic indicator. Grade is also more important than stage in bone and muscle tumors in determining treatment and prognosis.

Stage and grade offer an accurate picture of the tumor and its behavior. When physicians know the exact types of tumors with which they are dealing, treatment decisions can be made that effectively eradicate the tumors. (A detailed description of cancer detection and diagnosis is provided in Chapter 5.)

> Grade can be determined only by examining tumor cells under a microscope.

TREATMENT OPTIONS

Cancer treatment demands a multidisciplinary approach. Tumor boards were established so that cancer specialists can work together to review information about newly diagnosed tumors and devise effective treatment plans. There are typically cancer-specific types of tumor boards, e.g., head and neck, breast, gastrointestinal, and brain. Participants of a tumor board can include surgeons, radiation oncologists, medical oncologists, radiologists, pathologists, social workers, plastic surgeons, and other medical personnel. All of these individuals play key roles in developing a treatment plan that effectively treats the tumor while helping the patient maintain a high quality of life (Fig. 1.5). Radiation therapists must be knowledgeable about the other modalities of treatment because their patients may have other treatments at the same time as radiation delivery, which will then change the side effects and the treatment plan. There is a difference in the radiation treatment plan when patients have surgery before or after the radiation is delivered or if chemotherapy is to be administered before or during radiation treatment. Radiation therapists, as part of the radiation therapy team, must interact intelligently with all members of the healthcare team.

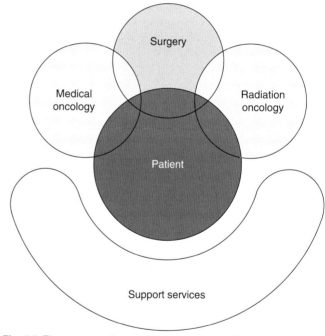

Fig. 1.5 The cancer patient receives treatment and support from multiple sources during disease management.

Surgery

As a local treatment modality, surgery plays a role in diagnosis, staging, primary treatment, palliation (noncurative treatment to relieve pain and suffering), and identification of treatment response. As a tool for diagnosis, surgery is used to perform a biopsy of a suspected mass to determine whether the mass is malignant and, if so, the cellular origin.

Biopsies are the only way to know for sure whether a lump or growth is cancerous. To provide the most effective treatment, the histology and cellular characteristics must be identified. The majority of biopsies that are performed on patients do not end up finding cancer. Many biopsy methods exist, and the characteristics of the suspected mass determine the use of a particular method.

Common biopsy (surgical removal of a small tissue sample from a solid tumor to determine the pathology) methods include fine-needle aspiration, core needle, endoscopic, image guided, incisional, and excisional. The information obtained through a biopsy is essential for appropriate treatment management. A fine-needle aspiration biopsy would be used to determine the histology of a suspicious breast mass or other superficial lesion. During the biopsy, sample cells are collected in the needle from several areas of the suspected tumor (Fig. 1.6). The cells are then transferred to a microscopic slide for further examination. This method of biopsy is relatively quick and easy, with minimal patient discomfort and healing time. The disadvantage is that the collected cells are examined without the benefit of their neighboring cells to provide a glimpse of the tumor architecture. There is also the chance that malignant cells will be seeded along the needle track as the needle is withdrawn from the tumor.

A large-gauge needle (14 or 16 gauge) is used to perform a core-needle biopsy. As the needle is inserted into the suspected tumor, a core of tissue is collected. The tissue obtained can be sectioned and examined under a microscope. Using this method, the tumor architecture is preserved, allowing better identification of the tumor tissue of origin (Fig. 1.7).

During endoscopic procedures, such as a bronchoscopy or colonoscopy, suspicious tissue can be collected with the use of a flexible biopsy tool. The tool is passed through the scope, and tiny pincers are used to gather a small tissue sample. Tissue samples can then be frozen or embedded in paraffin, sectioned, stained, and examined under the microscope.

Image-guided biopsies are often used during needle biopsies to sample the tissue in the correct area. Often these areas are lungs, kidneys, liver, and lymph nodes, and are challenging to safely insert needles. Such imaging modalities that can be used for this include ultrasound, CT, interventional radiology, and MRI. A newer image-guided technique is MRI-guided biopsy of the prostate gland.[14]

A recent study indicates that MRI for prostate cancer can identify patients who are more likely to need a biopsy versus those who are not. The study included 651 men screened for prostate cancer with a PSA blood test and digital rectal exam. Each patient then underwent three procedures: an MRI scan, a biopsy guided by transrectal ultrasound (TRUS), and a biopsy guided by both a TRUS and MRI scan. Of the 651 men scanned, 289 were identified as having intermediate-stage prostate cancer, defined as a Gleason score of 7 or higher. The researchers found that using an MRI scan to determine the need for biopsy could have avoided 38% of biopsies and still identified 89% of clinically significant cancers.[15]

During an incisional biopsy, a sample of the tumor is removed with no attempt to remove the whole tumor. This method is often used with larger tumors or those that are locally advanced (Fig. 1.8). In excisional biopsies, on the other hand, an attempt is made to remove the entire tumor and any possible local spread, as in the case of malignant melanoma. When a nevus, or mole, becomes suspicious by changing colors or growing larger, an excisional biopsy is performed. The nevi and normal surrounding tissue (to include a safe margin of underlying tissue) are removed en bloc, or as one piece.

Surgery plays a major role in the treatment of cancer. With advances in knowledge, equipment, and techniques, procedures that are performed are now less radical and are apt to be part of a multidisciplinary treatment plan. The success of surgical intervention is dependent on the medical condition; wishes of the patient; and size, extent, and the location of the tumor.

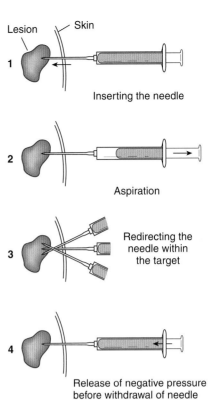

Fig. 1.6 The steps in aspiration of a palpable lesion. Step 3 indicates the way that the needle should be redirected in the target, and step 4 emphasizes the importance of releasing the negative pressure before withdrawing the needle. (From Koss LG. Needle aspiration cytology of tumors at various body sites. In: Silver CE, et al, eds. *Current Problems in Surgery*. Vol. 22. Chicago, IL: Year Book Medical Publishers; 1985.)

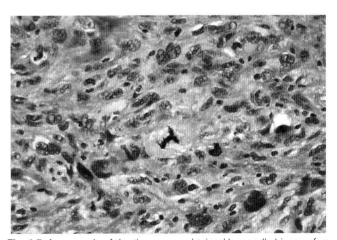

Fig. 1.7 An example of the tissue core obtained by needle biopsy of an anaplastic tumor shows cellular and nuclear variation in size and shape. The prominent cell in the center field has an abnormal appearance. (From Kumar V, Abbas A, Aster J. *Robbins Basic Pathology*. 9th ed. St. Louis, MO: Saunders; 2013.)

Not all patients are surgical candidates. Patients with preexisting medical conditions may have an unacceptable increase in surgical risk. For example, if the patient's pulmonary function is compromised, general anesthesia may be contraindicated, and surgical procedures are impossible. In addition, as with any treatment modality, the patient may decide not to have surgery, in favor of another type of treatment or no treatment at all.

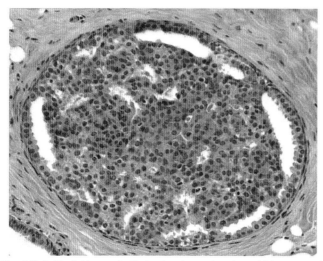

Fig. 1.8 Epithelial hyperplastic benign tumor in a breast biopsy specimen. The duct lumen is filled with a heterogeneous population of cells of differing morphology. Irregular slit-like fenestrations are prominent at the periphery. (From Kumar V, Abbas A, Aster J. *Robbins Basic Pathology*. 9th ed. St. Louis, MO: Saunders; 2013.)

> Risks associated with surgery include adverse reactions to anesthesia, infection, and potential loss of function.

Because surgery is a localized treatment, it is most successful with small tumors that have not spread to neighboring tissues or organs. During surgery, the physician attempts to remove the entire tumor and any microscopic spread, requiring the removal of normal tissue. As the size and/or extent of the tumor increases, more normal tissue must be removed, thus increasing the risk of the procedure. Surgical intervention may be the only treatment necessary if the tumor can be completely removed. If, however, the surgical margins are positive for cancer cells, the tumor has a high recurrence rate, or gross tumor was left, further treatment is necessary.

Before surgery, radiation therapy or chemotherapy may be given to increase the likelihood of a complete resection. This is often referred to as neoadjuvant therapy. The goals of radiation or chemotherapy in this case are to destroy microscopic and subclinical disease and shrink the tumor. Lower doses of radiation and/or chemotherapy are used to prevent complications during and following surgery.

The location of the tumor is an important factor in the success of surgical treatment. If a tumor is located in an area that is inaccessible or close to critical structures or organs at risk (vital organs or normal tissue structures), surgery may not be possible. Damage to critical structures may be incompatible with life or may leave the patient in worse condition than before treatment. A cancer of the nasopharynx, for example, is located in an area in which accessibility is difficult because the cancer is close to the base of the brain and the cranial nerves. For these reasons, patients with cancers of the nasopharynx are not good candidates for surgical intervention. With improved technology and procedures, however, location of the tumor continues to become less of a barrier to successful treatment.

Surgical palliation is used to relieve symptoms the patient may be experiencing as a result of the disease. Removal of an obstruction of the bowel does not have a curative effect on the disease but provides the patient with symptom relief for an improved quality of life. Cutting nerves to reduce or eliminate pain caused by the tumor is another example of palliative surgery.

Radiation Therapy

Radiation therapy is a local treatment that can be used alone or with other treatment modalities. It can be used for a curative intent, as well as for tumor control, or for palliation. When it is used in conjunction with chemotherapy and/or surgery, it is referred to as adjuvant therapy, meaning "in addition to." Benefits of radiation therapy include preservation of function and better cosmetic results. An early-stage laryngeal tumor can be effectively treated by surgery or radiation. Surgery may require removal of the vocal cords, thus leaving the patient without a voice. Radiation therapy, however, can obtain the same results while preserving the patient's voice. In the past, surgery for patients with prostate cancer commonly left the patient impotent with a high chance for incontinence. Radiation therapy can preserve function in a majority of sexually active males while providing effective treatment.

Surgery and radiation therapy combined also obtain an optimal cosmetic result. In the past, breast cancer was usually treated with a radical mastectomy, leaving the patient disfigured. Currently, a common treatment for some types of breast cancer consists of a lumpectomy with sentinel node biopsy followed by adjuvant radiation therapy, and this leaves the patient with minimal disfigurement and an equal chance of cure. Examination of the sentinel node, or the primary drainage lymph node, decreases the extent of an axillary node dissection. As a result, the patient experiences fewer range-of-motion deficits, and the risk of lymphedema is lowered.

Radiation therapy plays a major role in palliation, as in the case of bone metastasis. If the condition is left untreated, the patient may experience a great deal of pain and is at risk for pathologic bone fractures. Radiation therapy to these sites usually eliminates the pain and prevents fractures. If a tumor is pressing on nerves, radiation therapy is given to reduce the size of the tumor, thus eliminating pressure on the nerves and providing pain relief.

Radiation therapy is limited to a local area of treatment. Patients with tumors that are diffuse throughout the body are not candidates for radiation therapy. Radiation therapy is further limited to areas in which a curative dose may be delivered without harming critical structures. Newer radiation therapy techniques of adaptive therapy, conformal therapy, image-guided radiation therapy, intensity-modulated radiation therapy, stereotactic radiosurgery, and proton treatments take advantage of the advances in diagnostic medical imaging and are able to almost "paint the tumor" with radiation, which greatly spares the normal tissues. Patients treated with these techniques experience fewer side effects than those treated with conventional radiation therapy techniques. All factors for a specific treatment plan must be examined to determine the most appropriate technique because one technique will not work for all types of treatments.

As with surgery, the patient's medical condition must be such that the patient can tolerate the treatment. If a patient is suffering from lung cancer and has little pulmonary function, radiation therapy may not be a suitable treatment option because it may further compromise the patient's ability to breathe. Numerous methods to deliver radiation exist. The two broad categories are external beam radiation therapy and brachytherapy.

> Adverse long-term side effects of radiation are minimized by careful treatment planning and the use of appropriate fractionation schedules.

External Beam

Through the use of external beam x-rays, electrons, protons, or gamma rays can be delivered to the tumor. Linear accelerators are capable of producing x-rays within a specific energy range. Some treatment machines can produce multiple x-ray, or photon, energies in addition to a range of electron energies and imaging capabilities. Cyclotrons or similar equipment are needed for proton treatment. Proton treatment is housed in larger cancer centers but is becoming more available even in smaller centers. External beam gamma rays are produced by cobalt 60 machines; although they were the primary treatment machine more than 40 years ago, their use is very limited today to MRI guided linear accelerators, such as ViewRay.[16]

> The difference between x-rays and gamma rays is the mechanism of production. X-rays are produced by the interaction of electrons striking a target, whereas gamma rays are produced through radioactive decay.

High-energy x-rays are used to treat tumors that are deeper in the body, whereas electrons are effective at delivering energy to superficial tumors. For tumors such as pancreatic or breast cancer, electrons can be given at the time of surgery. Intraoperative radiation therapy is delivered directly to the tumor during surgery. This method allows a high dose to be delivered to the tumor while sparing the normal surrounding tissues. Not all tumors are amenable to this type of treatment because of their location, the extent of disease, or the patient's ability to withstand the rigors of surgery.

Treatment today is more precise and accurate than ever before. With the use of advanced treatment–planning computers, sophisticated treatment equipment, and much better imaging technology, a high dose of radiation can be safely delivered to the tumor with minimal damage to surrounding normal tissue. Conformal therapy, intensity-modulated radiation therapy, and adaptive radiation therapy are three examples of recent advances. Very simply explained, these techniques change the treatment field size and/or dose to vary with the shape of the tumor as the treatment machine is positioned or rotates around the body. These more advanced treatment techniques are covered in depth in Chapters 15 and 16.

Brachytherapy

Brachytherapy, or "short-distance therapy," uses radioactive materials such as cesium-137 (^{137}Cs), iridium-192 (^{192}Ir), palladium-103 (^{103}Pd), cesium-131 (^{131}Cs), or iodine-125 (^{125}I). Through the use of brachytherapy, the radioactive sources can be placed next to or directly into the tumor. Because the energy of the radioactive sources is low, a high energy is delivered to the tumor, with the nearby normal tissues receiving a very small dose. Brachytherapy is accomplished by using a multitude of techniques, including interstitial, intracavitary, and oral applications.

During an interstitial (in-tissue) implant, radioactive sources are placed directly into the tumor. The sources may remain in place permanently, or they may be removed once the prescribed dose has been delivered. Treatment of prostate cancer is a good example for both of these methods. For a permanent implant, tiny seeds of ^{103}Pd, ^{131}Cs, or ^{125}I are placed in the prostate. These seeds remain in the prostate, with their radioactivity decreasing with time. Because of the low energy of the radioactive material, the patient poses no threat to his family and friends. Determination of the type of implant offered depends on the skill and preference of the radiation oncologist, the available resources, and the patient's wishes. Cancers of the head and neck and breast are suitable for interstitial implants.

High-dose afterloading equipment is available in many departments, eliminating the need for extended hospitalization. For example, during the lumpectomy for breast cancer, a special balloon or catheter is placed in the tumor bed. The balloon is attached to a catheter that extends outside of the patient's body. Later, when the patient has been discharged from the hospital with the balloon in place, they will go for radiation therapy treatment. Treatment is delivered in a specially designed suite. Once all of the quality assurance tests have been completed to ensure a safe and accurate treatment, the catheter will be connected to the high-dose afterloading machine. The treatment begins when a radioactive source enters the catheter and travels into the balloon. The source will pause at predetermined spots, delivering the dose prescribed to the tumor bed. This technique is referred to as high dose-rate brachytherapy. Recently, this technique has also been used for prostate cancer treatment as well.[17]

Intracavitary implants are performed by placing the radioactive material in a body cavity, as in the case of treatment for cervical or endometrial cancers. Applicators are placed in the body cavity, often at the time of surgery, and later the radioactive sources are inserted and remain until the prescribed dose has been delivered. The prescribed dose can be delivered during several days as an inpatient procedure (low-dose brachytherapy) or, more commonly, in one or more fractions, as an outpatient procedure (high-dose brachytherapy).

Interluminal brachytherapy is used when the radioactive material is placed within a body tube such as the esophagus or bronchial tree. The radioactive material is positioned in the lumen at the tumor site and removed once the prescribed dose is delivered.

Brachytherapy can also be used to treat choroid melanomas of the eye.[18] In this procedure, tiny pellets of radiation are placed on a small carrier called a plaque, which is sewn to the back of the eye.[18] This is very effective treatment and often eliminates the need to have an enucleation or eye removal.[18]

Radioactive drugs called radiopharmaceuticals can be delivered by mouth or by vein. For cancers of the thyroid, bone, or prostate, this can be a very effective treatment method. This can also be known as systemic radiation. Common radioactive sources used in these procedures include radioactive iodine, strontium, and samarium.[19]

> Brachytherapy provides a high dose to a small area, which spares normal surrounding tissue.

The tremendous arsenal of treatment delivery methods and the successful outcomes achieved make radiation therapy a major weapon in the fight against cancer. While the ability to detect and image a tumor improves, the precision of the treatment delivery methods will continue to advance. Treatments that are commonly used today were only dreams 20 years ago.

Chemotherapy

Unlike surgery and radiation therapy, chemotherapy is a systemic treatment (killing cells of the primary tumor and those that may be circulating through the body). With the use of cytotoxic drugs (drugs with the ability to kill cancer cells) and hormones, chemotherapy aims at killing cells of the primary tumor and those that may be circulating through the body. Chemotherapy may be administered as a primary treatment or as part of a multidisciplinary treatment plan as an adjuvant treatment modality. Similar to other major cancer treatments, chemotherapy is most successful when the tumor burden is small. Many chemotherapy agents affect the cell during a specific phase of the cell cycle. Tumors that rapidly divide provide more opportunities for the cytotoxic effects to take place because more cells are in the cell cycle. Today, biologic drugs are developed that are specific to individual treatment. A sample of a tumor is grown and analyzed with the drugs developed to attack the specific cancer mutations or weaknesses.[20]

Administration of chemotherapeutic agents is accomplished through a variety of methods, depending on the drugs prescribed. The route of administration depends on the drugs used, the type of cancer, and patient-related factors. Oral administration is the easiest method, but it requires full patient compliance in taking the drugs and in taking the drugs at the correct times. Injections can be self-administered by the patient or administered by the oncology nurse. Intraarterial administration requires an infusion pump connected to a catheter that has been placed in an artery near the tumor. Heparin, a blood thinner, is added to the cytotoxic agent to prevent clotting at the catheter site. Bladder cancer is often treated with an intracavitary administration, whereby the chemotherapy drugs are instilled directly into the bladder. Cytotoxic drugs are introduced into the abdomen using an intraperitoneal administration through a catheter or implanted port. Intrathecal injection requires drugs to be instilled into the space containing cerebrospinal fluid, as is often the case with leukemia treatment. Although most chemotherapy drugs can be administered by the patient or a nurse, intrathecal administration is done only by a physician. One of the more common methods of drug installation is the intravenous (IV) route. Drugs may be administered by using a syringe entering the vein directly or piggybacked with other fluids. Typically, a patient has a central line called a port-a-cath for access to the venous system.[21] This helps to preserve the veins that can become damaged from repeated injections. Blood can be drawn, injections can be given, and drugs can be administered via the central line (Fig. 1.9).

Chemotherapy agents are very toxic, and safety precautions must be taken during preparation and administration, such as the wearing of gloves, gowns, and face shields. Certain drugs have vesicant or blistering potential and, if spilled on the skin or outside of the vein, will cause ulceration and tissue damage, so extra precautions must be taken. For these reasons, patients coming to radiation therapy with IV lines for chemotherapy must be treated with extra care to preserve the patency of the IV line. Often these individuals have small, weak veins, so finding a site for the IV line is difficult at best. If a problem occurs with an IV line, the therapist should immediately call the nurse charged with the care of that patient to prevent total failure of the site. Precautions must also be taken when treating patients with central lines or port-a-cath to prevent accidental dislodgment of the device.

> Chemotherapy administration methods depend on the types of drugs prescribed.

Chemotherapeutic Agents

Chemotherapeutic agents are classified by their action on the cell or their source and include alkylating agents, antimetabolites, antibiotics, hormonal agents, nitrosoureas, vinca alkaloids, targeted cancer drugs, and miscellaneous agents[5,20,22] (Table 1.4).

Alkylating agents were the first drugs identified to have anticancer activity. This class of drugs is related structurally to mustard gas; they are not cell cycle specific, but rather work throughout the cycle. The mechanism of action is to bond with nucleic acids, thereby interfering with their action. Side effects include bone marrow depression, amenorrhea in women and azoospermia in men, and carcinogenesis. Administration of alkylating agents is associated with an increased risk of acute myelogenous leukemia and is related to the total drug dose. Examples of alkylating agents include cyclophosphamide and chlorambucil.

Antimetabolites act by interfering with the synthesis of new nucleic acids. They are cell cycle specific and are much more toxic to proliferating cells but are not associated with delayed bone marrow suppression or carcinogenesis. Side effects include gastrointestinal toxicity and

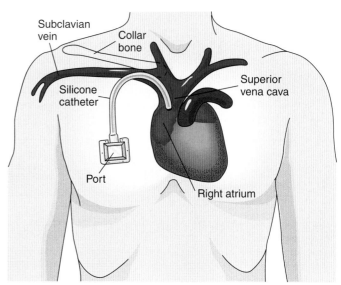

Fig. 1.9 Port-a-cath central line. Commonly used in chemotherapy treatment for access to the venous system. (From Perry AG, Potter PA, Ostendorf WR. *Nursing Interventions and Clinical Skills.* 7th ed. St Louis, MO: Elsevier; 2020.)

acute bone marrow suppression. Examples of antimetabolites include methotrexate, often used with intrathecal administration, gemcitabine, and 5-fluorouracil.

Antitumor antibiotics are derived from microbial fermentation. Antibiotics act on the DNA to disrupt DNA and RNA transcription. Although they are not cell cycle specific, the effects of the antibiotics are more pronounced in the S or G2 phase. Examples of anticancer antibiotics include doxorubicin (Adriamycin), bleomycin, epirubicin, mitomycin C, and actinomycin D. Side effects include cardiac toxicity, skin ulceration with extravasation, pulmonary toxicities, bone marrow suppression, and increased effects of radiation therapy.

Hormonal agents act to eliminate or displace natural hormones. Lupron is an injectable hormone therapy used to treat prostate cancer. Lupron is injected under the skin or into a muscle and can help to slow down cancer growth. Steroid hormones are used to clinically manipulate cells by binding to specific intracellular receptors and interacting with DNA to change cellular function. The most common use is in the treatment of breast cancer when the tumor is positive for estrogen and progesterone receptors. Examples of hormonal agents include tamoxifen, raloxifene (Evista), fulvestrant (Faslodex), anastrozole (Arimidex), and letrozole (Femara).[22] Side effects include hot flashes, depression, loss of libido, deep vein thrombosis, and an increase in endometrial cancers.

Nitrosoureas are not cell cycle specific, but they are lipid soluble and able to cross the blood-brain barrier. Their action is similar to that of alkylating agents in that they interfere with DNA synthesis. Examples include carmustine (bis-chloroethylnitrosourea) and streptozocin. Side effects include delayed myelosuppression, gastrointestinal toxicity, and delayed nephrotoxicity.

Vinca alkaloids are derived from the periwinkle plant. By binding to a substance that is needed for mitosis and solute transport, the vinca alkaloids stop cell replication in metaphase. Neurotoxicity, severe ulceration of the skin (if extravasation occurs), and myelosuppression are the dose-limiting side effects. Examples include vincristine, vinblastine, and etoposide (VP-16). Such drugs are used in the treatment of lymphoma, leukemia, and testicular cancers.

Miscellaneous agents are a class of drugs that have varied action and are from a number of different sources. The platinum

TABLE 1.4   Chemotherapeutic Drug Classifications with Side Effects

Drugs	Major Side Effects
Alkylating Agents	
Carboplatin	Nausea and vomiting, bone marrow suppression, ototoxicity, neurotoxicity, and hyperuricemia
Cisplatin	Neurotoxicity, myelosuppression, nephrotoxicity, nausea and vomiting, hypokalemia, and hypomagnesemia
Cyclophosphamide	Myelosuppression, anorexia, stomatitis, alopecia, gonadal suppression, nail hyperpigmentation, nausea and vomiting, diarrhea, and hemorrhagic cystitis
Dacarbazine	Nausea and vomiting, anorexia, vein irritation, alopecia, myelosuppression, facial flushing, and radiation recall
Melphalan	Hypersensitivity, nausea, myelosuppression, amenorrhea, pulmonary infiltrates, and sterility
Antimetabolites	
Capecitabine	Diarrhea, nausea, vomiting, neurotoxicity, myelosuppression, and sores in mouth
Cytarabine	Myelosuppression, diarrhea, nausea and vomiting, alopecia, rash, fever, conjunctivitis, neurotoxicity, hepatotoxicity, pulmonary edema, and skin desquamation of the palms and soles of the feet
Gemcitabine	Nausea, vomiting, rash, hair loss, bruising, bleeding, and myelosuppression
Methotrexate	Nausea and vomiting, oral ulcers
5-Fluorouracil (5-FU)	Oral and gastrointestinal ulcers, nausea and vomiting, diarrhea, alopecia, vein hyperpigmentation, and radiation recall
Antitumor Antibiotics	
Bleomycin	Anaphylaxis, pneumonitis, pulmonary fibrosis, alopecia, stomatitis, anorexia, radiation recall, skin hyperpigmentation, fever, chills, and nausea and vomiting
Dactinomycin (actinomycin D)	Nausea and vomiting, stomatitis, vesication, alopecia, radiation recall, myelosuppression, and diarrhea
Doxorubicin	Myelosuppression, vesication, cardiotoxicity, stomatitis, alopecia, nausea and vomiting, radiation recall, and diarrhea
Epirubicin	Hair loss, flushing, itching, or rash, sores in mouth, diarrhea, nausea, vomiting
Mitomycin	Myelosuppression, vesication, nausea and vomiting, alopecia, pulmonary fibrosis, hepatotoxicity, stomatitis, and hyperuricemia
Hormonal Agents	
Corticosteroids Dexamethasone Hydrocortisone Prednisone	Nausea, suppression of immune function, weight gain, hyperglycemia, increased appetite, cataracts, impaired wound healing, menstrual irregularity, and interruption in sleep and rest patterns
Antiandrogen Flutamide	Impotence and gynecomastia
Antiestrogen Tamoxifen Goserelin acetate (Zoladex)	Nausea and vomiting, hot flashes, fluid retention, changes in menstrual pattern, increase in bone pain, and hypercalcemia
Gonadotropin-releasing hormone Leuprolide	Impotence, decreased libido, increase in bone and tumor pain, genital atrophy, and gynecomastia
Nitrosoureas	
Carmustine	Nausea and vomiting, vein irritation, myelosuppression, stomatitis, nephrotoxicity, and pulmonary fibrosis
Streptozocin	Nausea and vomiting, fever, chills, nephrotoxicity, diarrhea, myelosuppression, and hypoglycemia
Plant Alkaloid	
Etoposide	Nausea and vomiting, diarrhea, stomatitis, parotitis, anaphylaxis, hypotension, myelosuppression, radiation recall, hepatotoxicity, and alopecia
Paclitaxel (Taxol)	Anaphylaxis, hypotension, nausea and vomiting, cardiotoxicity, myelosuppression, neurotoxicity, alopecia, stomatitis, and diarrhea
Vinblastine	Neurotoxicity, anorexia, myelosuppression, stomatitis, alopecia, gonadal suppression, peripheral neuropathy, and vesication
Vincristine	Neurotoxicity, constipation, myelosuppression, alopecia, vesication, peripheral neuropathy, and paralytic ileus
Miscellaneous Agents	
Asparaginase	Anaphylaxis, nausea and vomiting, fever, chills, myelosuppression, hyperglycemia, abdominal pain, diarrhea, pancreatitis, and anorexia
Hydroxyurea	Nausea and vomiting, alopecia, myelosuppression, allergic reactions, radiation recall, rash, azotemia, and dysuria
Pentostatin	Nausea and vomiting, rash, myelosuppression, vein irritation, nephrotoxicity, and hyperuricemia
Procarbazine	Nausea and vomiting; stomatitis; peripheral neuropathy; and severe gastrointestinal and central nervous system effects if taken with foods containing tyramine, alcohol, or monoamine oxidase inhibitor
Topotecan	Diarrhea, nausea and vomiting, myelosuppression, anorexia, and influenza-like symptoms

compounds such as cisplatin and carboplatin are included in this category, along with the taxanes such as paclitaxel and docetaxel. Cisplatin and carboplatin act similar to the alkylating agents, with nephrotoxicity and myelosuppression as the dose-limiting side effects. The action of the taxanes is opposite of that of the vinca alkaloids and results in a disrupted mitosis, along with other cellular processes. Toxicities include neutropenia, cardiac toxicity, mucositis, alopecia, and neuropathy.

It is important for the radiation therapist to be familiar with the various chemotherapy drugs and how they interact with radiation therapy. For example, the treatment for a breast cancer patient who has taken Adriamycin or bleomycin will be modified to consider the synergistic effects of these drugs. Adriamycin is toxic to the heart and in combination with radiation therapy has a much greater toxic effect. The same is true for bleomycin and radiation therapy treatment to the lungs. Radiation therapy methods to minimize the toxic effects would include shielding or lowering the total dose.

> Some chemotherapy drugs can enhance the effects of radiation by increasing cellular sensitivity.

Chemotherapy Principles

Chemotherapy is used as a primary treatment and in combination with surgery and radiation therapy. Surgery is performed in an attempt to remove as much of the tumor as possible, decreasing the number of tumor cells. Chemotherapy drugs are then administered to eliminate the residual tumor cells at the primary site and those that are circulating throughout the body. In combination with radiation therapy, chemotherapeutic agents, such as doxorubicin, often act as radiosensitizers (chemicals and drugs that help enhance the lethal effects of radiation) and increase the effects of treatment. Radioprotector (certain chemicals and drugs that diminish the response of cells to radiation) chemotherapeutic agents such as amifostine limit the effect of the radiation on the normal cells, decreasing treatment side effects.

Although single-agent chemotherapy is used occasionally, a combination of drugs is more often administered. Each of the drugs selected for a particular treatment will have a known effect on the specific tumor treated. With combination chemotherapy, the physician can select drugs that act on the cell during different phases of the cell cycle, increasing the cell-killing potential. In addition, drugs with different known toxicities are used for maximum effectiveness, resulting in fewer side effects.[23]

Targeted Cancer Therapies

Targeted cancer therapies are drugs or other substances that interfere with specific target molecules in the cancer cell that are responsible for abnormal growth and spread.[24] These drugs work by either blocking the cellular instructions to proliferate or by providing instructions to the cell to die. These drugs focus on specific targets within the cell that have a major role in cellular proliferation. Targeted therapies approved for use in cancer treatment include angiogenesis inhibitors, apoptosis inducers, cancer vaccines and gene therapy, gene expression modulators, hormone therapies, immunotherapies, monoclonal antibodies, and signal transduction inhibitors.[24] Some examples are imatinib mesylate (Gleevec), bevacizumab (Avastin), trastuzumab (Herceptin), rituximab (Rituxan), G-CSF (Neupogen), and erlotinib (Tarceva), pembrolizumab (Keytruda), and nivolumab (Opdivo)[24] (Table 1.5).

PROGNOSIS

A prognosis is an estimation of the life expectancy of a cancer patient based on all the information obtained about the tumor and from clinical trials. A prognosis is, however, only an estimate. The duration of a person's life is a mystery, and thousands of cancer patients have outlived or underlived their estimated life expectancy. A patient's mental attitude plays an important role in the prognosis but is not a factor usually considered.

> Prognostic determination does not consider the patient's mental attitude, which has an enormous impact on disease survivability.

Prognosis plays a role in the treatment plan. If a patient has a prognosis of 2 months, treatment is given in a manner such that the patient has the maximum time allowable to spend with family and friends. In this situation, a treatment lasting 7 weeks would likely be more

TABLE 1.5 Targeted Therapies

Drug	Cancer Treatment	Action
Imatinib mesylate (Gleevec)	Specific types of leukemia and GI cancers	Targets tyrosine kinase enzymes or proteins that lead to uncontrolled growth
Trastuzumab (Herceptin)	Breast cancer and gastroesophageal adenocarcinoma tumors with overexpression of HER2/neu protein	Prevents *HER-2* from sending growth-promoting signals
Rituximab (Rituxan)	B-cell non-Hodgkin lymphoma, chronic myelogenous leukemia (CLL)	Antibody against CD20 antigens on tumor cells causing cell death
Nivolumab (Opdivo)	Colorectal, head and neck, kidney, lymphoma, liver, lung, skin	Induces antitumor immune response when it binds to PD-1 cell receptor
Erlotinib (Tarceva)	Non-small cell lung cancer and pancreatic cancer	Targets tyrosine kinase enzymes associated with epidermal growth factor receptors and inhibits cell growth
Bevacizumab (Avastin)	Breast, cervical, colorectal, kidney, lung, ovarian cancer	Blocks growth of blood vessels to tumors, which reduces tumor growth and spread
Pembrolizumab (Keytruda)	Bladder, cervical, head and neck, lymphoma, skin, and stomach cancer	Induces antitumor immune response when it binds to PD-1 cell receptor
Growth-colony stimulating factor (Neupogen)	Hematopoietic cells, cells of bone marrow	Regulates and stimulates production of neutrophils
Cetuximab (Erbitux)	Squamous cell carcinoma of the head and neck Colorectal cancer	Binds to epidermal growth factor receptor and prevents activation from growth signals

GI, Gastrointestinal; *HER2,* Human epidermal growth factor (Also called HER2/neu); *CD20,* An antigen found on B-Cells; *PD-1,* A protein found on T-Cells.

intrusive than helpful. The goal of treatment is to eradicate the tumor or provide palliation while preserving quality of life for the patient. The prognosis provides the information to ensure that this goal is accomplished. When a patient is labeled terminal, it can also affect friends and caregivers. Friends may suddenly disappear because of the belief that they don't know what to say to the patient, and caregivers may provide care that is more distant. Remember that a person is alive until they die and should be treated with the same compassion, empathy, and care as any other friend or patient.

For patients and their families, this information provides a timeline to accomplish tasks or goals in preparation for impending death. This may include making a will, taking a long-awaited trip, and gathering family members from across the country. Factors specific to each tumor determine the prognosis. The natural history (the normal progression of a tumor without treatment) provides information about the tumor behavior. For example, some tumors grow slowly and cause the host few problems until late in the disease process, whereas other tumors grow rapidly and spread to distant sites at an early stage of tumor development. Generally, slow-growing tumors are associated with better prognoses than are tumors that have already metastasized at the time of presentation. Natural history information is also valuable in determining the most effective treatment for the patient, thus affecting the prognosis. The method of treatment also determines the prognosis based on information obtained through clinical trials. As more effective treatment is delivered, the prognosis improves. As stated earlier, cancer demands a multidisciplinary approach to treatment. Finding the most effective combination of treatments has a profound effect on the prognosis.

Patterns of Spread

Growth characteristics and spread patterns of a tumor have important prognostic implications. Tumors that tend to remain localized are more easily treated and thus generally have a better prognosis than do those that are diffuse or spread to distant sites early in the development of the malignancy.

Tumors that are exophytic, or grow outward, have better prognoses than those that invade and ulcerate underlying tissues. When a tumor is exophytic, it does not communicate with blood vessels and lymphatic vessels until later in the disease process. Blood vessels and lymphatic vessels are the highways of cancer cell transport to distant sites. Multicentric tumors, or tumors that have more than one focus of disease, can be more difficult to treat because the volume of tissue required for treatment is larger to encompass the entire organ or region. In addition, detecting all the tumor foci that may be at different stages in the development process is difficult.

Tumor dissemination, or spread, can be accomplished through the blood, lymphatics, and seeding, or extension into surrounding tissues. Tumor cells invading blood or lymph vessels can be transported to distant sites in the body. The mechanisms responsible for these cells taking root and growing in one area and not another are not clear. However, many tumors have a propensity to spread to specific sites.

Prostate cancer commonly metastasizes to the bones. For this reason, a bone scan is included in the workup if evidence exists that metastasis has already occurred at the time of diagnosis. In addition, when the primary tumor is unknown and the patient presents with metastatic disease, the sites of the metastasis give a clue about the primary tumor's location. Table 1.6 lists metastatic sites associated with common primary sites.

Tumor cells may also disseminate through seeding. Cells break off from the primary tumor and spread to new sites, where they grow. Ovarian cancer cells often spread by way of the peritoneal fluid to the abdominal cavity by this method; thus, the staging intraoperative examination is an important diagnostic and staging tool. Cells from a medulloblastoma of the brain often seed into the spinal canal by means of the cerebrospinal fluid, thus necessitating the treatment of the entire spinal cord and brain.

Tumor cells may also extend past the origin or original organ. This is known as extension or regional spread. It can include invasion through the organ wall into nearby organs or tissues.[25] This can also include tumors extending into the walls of nearby lymphatics. For example, a tumor in the head and neck region can extend into the cervical lymph nodes, known as extracapsular extension.[25] This is generally considered a poor prognosis.

Prognostic Factors

For each tumor, specific prognostic factors are based on the cellular and behavioral characteristics, tumor site, and patient-related factors. Determination of prognostic factors is made through clinical trials in which factors related to the disease and patient are statistically analyzed for a group of patients. With this method, factors that have the greatest influence on prognosis are determined.

Tumor-related factors that are often of prognostic significance include grade, stage, tumor size, status of lymph nodes, depth of invasion, and histology (including molecular information related to genes and cell receptors present). Patient-related prognostic factors include age, gender, race, and medical condition. Each factor displays a different level of importance in specific tumors. For example, the main prognostic indicator for breast cancer is the status of the axillary lymph nodes and molecular receptor status, whereas for a soft tissue sarcoma, it is histologic grade.

CLINICAL TRIALS

Much of the progress made in the management of cancer is the result of carefully planned clinical trials. This type of research can be conducted at a single clinical site or in collaboration with many institutions. The advantage of collaboration is that a greater number of patients can participate in the study, thus increasing the significance of the results. Because cancer management is multidisciplinary, clinical trials are often a collaborative effort among disciplines. Research methodology for clinical trials can be accomplished through retrospective or prospective studies that examine randomized or nonrandomized samples of the population to be studied.

> Clinical trials provide research-based evidence about specific treatment effectiveness. It is through these trials that the most effective treatment with the fewest long-term side effects can be achieved.

TABLE 1.6 Common Metastatic Sites of Primary Tumors

Primary Site	Common Metastatic Sites
Lung	Liver, adrenal glands, bone, and brain
Breast	Lungs, bone, and brain
Stomach	Liver
Anus	Liver and lungs
Bladder	Lungs, bone, and liver
Prostate	Bone, liver, and lungs
Uterine cervix	Lungs, bone, and liver

Retrospective Studies

Studies that review information from a group of patients treated in the past are retrospective. The treatment has already been delivered, and the information is collected (often on a national basis) and analyzed. Retrospective studies have an advantage in that the information can be obtained rather quickly; the investigator does not have to wait years to see the results of a particular treatment. However, a number of drawbacks are apparent with retrospective studies and can lead to errors. Complete information about a treatment is not always easy to obtain and is often incomplete. Outside factors that may have influenced the treatment and results are not controlled and may not be accurately documented.

Prospective Studies

A clinical trial that is planned before treatment, with eligibility criteria for patient selection, is a prospective study. Investigators have the advantage of knowing the information that is essential to the study, thus leading to more complete and accurate documentation. In addition, better control of external factors that might influence the results of the study is possible. A disadvantage of prospective studies is the length of time needed to observe the results of a particular treatment. Depending on the length of the follow-up necessary to accurately assess the results, prospective trials can last 5 years or longer. The lung cancer screening study mentioned at the start of the chapter is an example of a prospective study.

Studies that examine the effectiveness of treatment are classified by the study objectives. Phase I studies are used to determine the maximum tolerance dose for a specific treatment. The end point can be either acute or long-term toxicity. Phase II studies are used to determine whether the Phase I treatment is significantly effective—given the acute and/or long-term side effects—to continue further study. Phase III studies are used to compare the experimental treatment with standard treatment with a randomized sample. Phase IV studies are conducted once treatments are approved by the US Food and Drug Administration. The study entails watching over a longer period of time the effects of the treatment in terms of survival and long-term side effects.[26]

Randomized Studies

Clinical studies often include several methods of treatment to determine which method results in the best outcome. After meeting all eligibility requirements for the study, patients are randomly selected for one of the treatment arms. The purpose of randomization is to eliminate any unintentional "stacking of the deck" and increase the accuracy of results and conclusions. Although patients may have the same type, grade, stage, and extent of cancer, each person responds individually to the disease and treatment. Care providers cannot control these factors, but randomization helps minimize their effects on the end result. With randomization, each arm of the study has approximately equal numbers of individuals with varying reactions.

Survival Reporting

In the planning stages of a clinical trial, an end point or objective must be established; otherwise, the study can continue indefinitely with no data analysis. Rates of survival at a set end point are one type of information used to determine the benefit of one treatment over another. Survival reporting, however, can be accomplished with many methods. With absolute survival reporting, patients alive at the end point and those who have died are counted. Patients lost to follow-up are included, but the fact that patients may have died from other causes is not considered. Adjusted survival reporting includes patients who died from other causes and had no evidence of disease (NED) at the times of their deaths. Relative survival reporting involves the normal mortality rate of a similar group of people based on factors such as age, gender, and race.

In addition, survival reporting at the end point includes information about the status of the disease. At the end point, the patient may be alive with NED, disease free, or alive with disease. Of equal importance is the information about treatment failures. Treatment failures are classified as local, locoregional, or distant and are based on tumor recurrences at the primary or nearby lymph node sites or metastatic disease. This information is valuable for ongoing clinical trials and for determining types of treatment techniques to prevent future failures.

THE RADIATION ONCOLOGY TEAM

The effectiveness of patient care and treatment is dependent on the teamwork of individuals in the entire radiation therapy department, the patient, and related medical professionals. From the receptionist to the physician, each individual has an important role in the goal of treating the person with cancer (Fig. 1.10). The radiation oncologist has the overall responsibility for the patient's care and treatment. The patient is an important member of the team and works in collaboration by complying with treatment requirements and letting team members

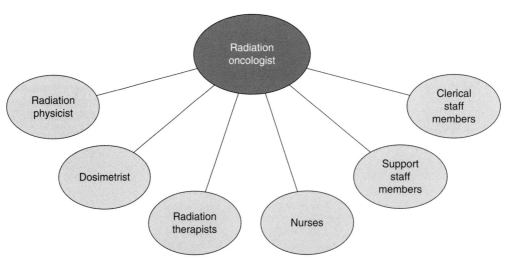

Fig. 1.10 The radiation oncology team.

know the individual effects of treatment. The patient also brings into the treatment their family and support system, who also influence the treatment outcome. Community and national cancer support resources play a role in providing information and possible financial or emotional support following the cancer diagnosis. The support that is provided by these sources is important in the overall emotional and psychosocial wellness of the patient.

Each member of the radiation therapy team, under the direction of the radiation oncologist, is essential in providing the most effective patient care and treatment. Team members work together collaboratively to share their expertise and contribute their abilities to the treatment process. Every day in every department, each of the radiation therapy team members has the opportunity to improve the quality of life for the cancer patient and his or her family. It may be answering a question, referring the patient to a support group, or giving a family member a hug. Each of these small actions has the potential to have a huge positive effect on the patient and his or her family.

When a patient enters the radiation therapy department, the first person he or she interacts with is the administrative assistant. Before the patient's arrival, this individual is involved in obtaining the patient's medical records and diagnostic images. The administrative assistant obtains insurance and the appropriate personal information and informs the other members of the radiation therapy team that the patient has arrived. The patient is taken to the consult/examination room to talk with the radiation oncologist (the physician who reviews the medical findings with the patient and discusses treatment options and the benefits of radiation therapy as well as the possible side effects). By the time the patient is in the examination room, the physician has become very familiar with the patient's medical history by talking with the patient's primary physician and reviewing all of the medical records. The physician reviews the medical findings with the patient and discusses treatment options that are available. The physician and patient will discuss the benefits of radiation therapy and the possible side effects. By the end of the consult and examination, the physician will have a treatment plan in mind, and the patient will be sent on for treatment planning and/or simulation. A medical dosimetrist (radiation therapy practitioner responsible for production of the patient's treatment plan and any associated quality assurance components) is responsible for designing the patient's treatment to accomplish the physician's prescription by using the most effective techniques possible. A medical dosimetrist is often a radiation therapist who has had additional education but may also be an individual with a physics or medical physics background. The medical dosimetrist will work collaboratively with a medical physicist. The medical physicist is responsible for quality assurance of all radiation therapy equipment from acceptance testing and commissioning of new equipment to regularly scheduled calibration and testing of equipment already in the department. The medical physicist oversees all treatment planning and radiation safety programs and is involved with clinical physics procedures. Before treatment, the patient will undergo a simulation or a procedure designed to delineate the treatment fields and construct any necessary immobilization or treatment devices. During a simulation, the radiation therapist (medical practitioner on the radiation oncology team who sees the patient daily and is responsible for treatment delivery and daily assessment of patient tolerance to treatment) is able to explain the simulation and treatment procedures and answer any questions the patient may have. Simulation provides an excellent time to assess the patient's medical condition and educational and support needs. Once the physician has approved of the simulation and treatment plan, the patient goes to the treatment machine. Depending on the purpose of treatment, the patient may be scheduled for 1 to 7 weeks of treatment. During treatment, the radiation oncologist generally sees the patient once a week to ensure that the treatment is progressing as expected. The radiation therapist sees the patient every day and is responsible for assessing the patient's reaction to treatment and the general medical condition. Radiation therapists and department nursing staff educate the patient about skin care, nutrition, and support services and provide appropriate referrals as necessary. Once the radiation therapy prescription has been completed, the patient will be scheduled for a follow-up appointment. The radiation oncologist may see the patient in follow-up for many years, or the primary physician may follow the patient.

Depending on the size of the department, the team may be very small or very large. In a small outpatient facility, the team may consist of a physician, radiation therapist, administrative assistant, and part-time physicist (see Fig. 1.10). The role of the team members in this scenario is vastly different from that of the members in a large department with multiple physicians, treatment and simulation radiation therapists, medical dosimetrists, physicists, nurses, and clerical and support staff. Generally, as the department grows larger, the job descriptions of the team members become more specific. In a large department, a radiation therapist's role may be limited to the actual treatment, and another radiation therapist is responsible for simulations. The role of the radiation therapist in dosimetry might be limited to treatment planning, calculations, and quality assurance procedures. In a large department, the role of the physician may also be limited to one area of expertise. For example, one physician might treat only those patients with head and neck tumors. In a small department, however, the radiation therapist's role will include treatment, simulation, treatment planning, patient care, and quality assurance. For the radiation therapist, there are opportunities for working in a number of different clinical sites, from freestanding comprehensive cancer centers to university medical centers. Each center offers different opportunities and challenges for the radiation therapist who is willing to continue to learn and grow.

For an individual who is interested in joining the radiation therapy team, it is important to learn and understand as much as possible about all aspects of radiation therapy. It is not enough to "study for the exam," because the important examinations do not happen in the classroom but rather in the clinic, with real patients.

SUMMARY

- Remember that the patient has a life outside of the cancer diagnosis. His or her past, cultural mores, religious beliefs, and other factors will influence all aspects of the treatment trajectory.
- Patient support resources are available at local, regional, state, and national levels. Radiation therapists should be aware of these resources to better meet the needs of their patients.
- Cancer has been studied for centuries, and there is still much to learn.
- Cancer occurs when normal cellular proliferation mechanisms break down.
- Cells that are rapidly dividing are more responsive to the effects of radiation and chemotherapy.
- Tumors are classified by their anatomic site, cell of origin, and biologic behavior.
- Benign tumors are generally well differentiated and do not harm the patient.
- Malignant tumors may be well differentiated to undifferentiated, may grow rapidly or very slowly, often metastasize, and invade surrounding tissues.
- Tumors are generally named for the tissue in which they arise.
- The stage of cancer defines the extent of the disease and is determined by the type of tumor.

- The grade of a tumor is determined following examination under a microscope and determines how aggressive a tumor will be.
- A multidisciplinary approach to cancer treatment is essential. Working together, physicians from all disciplines develop treatment plans that best treat the cancer and preserve the quality of life for the patient.
- Clinical trials are important in gaining information regarding the effectiveness of treatment modalities and methods. This research furthers the knowledge base in the treatment of cancer.

- The radiation team encompasses those in the radiotherapy department and those associated with the patient and other healthcare providers. Communication and teamwork are essential in providing the patient the best treatment and treatment experience possible.
- The radiation therapist has the ability to have a monumental and positive impact on each of the patients treated. This opportunity comes through accurate treatment, positive and engaging attitude, and genuine caring for patients.
- The care given by the radiation therapists had the greatest influence on overall patient satisfaction.

REVIEW QUESTIONS

The answers to the Review Questions can be found by logging on to our website at: http://evolve.elsevier.com/Washington+Leaver/principles

1. How would a theory of cancer as an initially diffuse disease affect the treatment and outcome?
2. What are the characteristics of benign and malignant cells?
3. What would a primary tumor of the bone be called?
4. What would a tumor arising from cells lining the oral cavity be called?
5. What are the roles surgery plays in the overall management and treatment of cancer?
6. What is the role of radiation therapy in the treatment of cancer?
7. What is the role of chemotherapy in the treatment of cancer?
8. What is the difference between etiology and epidemiology?
9. What roles does the radiation therapist play in patient care and treatment?

QUESTIONS TO PONDER

1. An 8-year-old child comes to your department for treatment. What factors need to be considered when scheduling an appointment?
2. What cancer patient resources are available in the hospital in which you work? What resources are available in your community?
3. Mr. Jones has a T2 tumor of the larynx, and Mrs. Smith has a T4 tumor of the larynx. What differences would you expect to see in the tumors and in the treatment plans for each of these patients?
4. How are etiology and epidemiology related to cancer screening?
5. Is prostate-specific antigen a specific and sensitive screening exam?
6. Analyze a clinical trial taking place in the hospital in which you work. What type of research is being done?

REFERENCES

1. Beasley M, Driver D, Dobbs HJ. Complications of radiotherapy: improving the therapeutic index. *Cancer Imaging*. 2005;5(1):78–84.
2. Famiglietti FM, Neal EC, Edwards TJ. Determinants of patient satisfaction during receipt of radiation therapy. *Int J Radiat Oncol Biol Phys*. 2013;87:148–152.
3. Sudhakar A. History of cancer, ancient and modern treatment methods. *J Cancer Sci Ther*. 2009;1(2):1–4.
4. Baumann M, Cordes N, Naase M, et al. Molecular cancer and radiation biology. In: Halperin EC, Brady LW, Perez CA, et al, eds. *Perez and Brady's Principles and Practice of Radiation Oncology*. 7th ed. Philadelphia, PA: Lippincott, Williams, and Wilkins; 2019.
5. Solomon E, Borrow J, Goddard AD. Chromosome aberrations and cancer. *Science*. 1991;254(5305):1153–1159.
6. Weinberg RA. Tumor suppressor genes. *Science*. 1991;254(5305):1138–1145.
7. Yunis JJ. The chromosomal basis of human neoplasia. *Science*. 1983;221(4607):227–235.
8. SEER program. National Cancer Institute website. https://seer.cancer.gov/. 2018. Accessed January 23, 2019.
9. Noone AM, Howlader N, Krapcho M, et al, eds. SEER Cancer Statistics Review, 1975–2015. https://seer.cancer.gov/csr/1975_2015/. Accessed February 4, 2019.
10. ACS cancer prevention blueprint targets controllable risk factors. American Cancer Society website. https://www.cancer.org/latest-news/acs-cancer-prevention-blueprint-targets-controllable-risk-factors.html. 2019. Accessed January 23, 2019.
11. American Cancer Society facts and figures 2019. American Cancer Society website. https://www.cancer.org/research/cancer-facts-statistics/all-cancer-facts-figures/cancer-facts-figures-2019.html. 2019. Accessed January 23, 2019.
12. Aberle DR, Adams AM, Berg CD, et al. Reduced lung-cancer mortality with low-dose computed tomographic screening. *N Engl J Med*. 2011;365(5):395–409.
13. Cancer staging system: what is cancer staging? American Joint Committee on Cancer website. https://cancerstaging.org/references-tools/pages/what-is-cancer-staging.aspx. 2019. Accessed January 23, 2019.
14. Moore CM, Robertson NL, Arsanious N, et al. Image-guided prostate biopsy using magnetic resonance imaging-derived targets: a systematic review. *Eur Urol*. 2013;63(1):125–140.
15. MRI may reduce unnecessary prostate biopsies. Harvard Men's Health Watch website. https://www.health.harvard.edu/mens-health/mri-may-reduce-unnecessary-prostate-biopsies. 2018. Accessed February 4, 2019.
16. ViewRay website. https://viewray.com/. Accessed January 25, 2019.
17. Yamada Y, Rogers L, Demanes DJ, et al. American Brachytherapy Society consensus guidelines for high-dose rate prostate brachytherapy. *Brachytherapy*. 2012;11(1):20–32.
18. Radiation therapy for eye cancer. American Cancer Society website. https://www.cancer.org/cancer/eye-cancer/treating/radiation-therapy.html. 2014. Accessed January 23, 2019.
19. Systemic radiation therapy. American Cancer Society website. https://www.cancer.org/treatment/treatments-and-side-effects/treatment-types/radiation/systemic-radiation-therapy.html. 2017. Accessed January 24, 2019.

20. American Joint Committee on Cancer. *Cancer Staging Manual.* 8th ed. New York, NY: Springer; 2018.

21. NCI dictionary of cancer terms. National Cancer Institute website. https://www.cancer.gov/publications/dictionaries/cancer-terms/def/port-a-cath. Accessed January 25, 2019.

22. Skeel RT. *Handbook of Cancer Chemotherapy.* 9th ed. Philadelphia, PA: Lippincott Williams & Wilkins; 2016.

23. How chemotherapy drugs work. American Cancer Society website. https://www.cancer.org/treatment/treatments-and-side-effects/treatment-types/chemotherapy/how-chemotherapy-drugs-work.html. 2016. Accessed January 23, 2019.

24. Targeted cancer therapies. National Cancer Institute website. https://www.cancer.gov/about-cancer/treatment/types/targeted-therapies/targeted-therapies-fact-sheet. 2019. Accessed January 25, 2019.

25. SEER training modules: cancer registration and surveillance modules. National Cancer Institute website. https://training.seer.cancer.gov/staging/systems/summary/regionalized.html. 2018. Accessed January 24, 2019.

26. What are the phases of clinical trials? American Cancer Society website. https://www.cancer.org/treatment/treatments-and-side-effects/clinical-trials/what-you-need-to-know/phases-of-clinical-trials.html. 2016. Accessed January 25, 2019.

27. Jain RK, Kozak KR. Molecular pathophysiology of tumors. In: Halperin EC, Brady LW, Perez CA, et al, eds. *Perez and Brady's Principles and Practice of Radiation Oncology.* 7th ed. Philadelphia, PA: Lippincott, Williams, and Wilkins; 2019.

2

The Ethics and Legal Considerations of Cancer Management

Bettye Wilson

OBJECTIVES

- List and define the terminology associated with the ethics and legal consideration of cancer management.
- Discuss the traditional ethical theories and models.
- Define patient autonomy and informed consent.
- Discuss advance directives.
- Differentiate between the types of living wills.
- Evaluate the patient care partnership to determine the scope of patient rights included therein.
- Explain how informed consent and patient autonomy are related.
- Recognize the role of the healthcare team in patient confidentiality.
- Apply Health Insurance Portability and Accountability Act (HIPAA) compliance standards in the clinical setting.
- Identify the stages of grief.
- Support dying patients and their families.
- Quote the legal doctrines applicable to patient care.
- Examine the role of risk management.
- Discuss medical records, their content, confidentiality of, and electronic record vulnerability.
- Determine the role of the Standards of Ethics and Practice Standards on the practice of radiation therapy.

OUTLINE

KEY TERMS

Advance directives
Analytical model
Assault
Autonomy
Battery
Beneficence
Civil law
Code of ethics
Collegial model
Confidentiality
Consequentialism
Contractual model
Covenant model
Deontology
Doctrine of foreseeability
Doctrine of personal liability
Doctrine of res ipsa loquitur

Doctrine of respondeat superior
Durable power of attorney for healthcare
Emotional intelligence
Engineering model
Ethics
False imprisonment
Incident
Informed consent
Invasion of privacy
Justice
Laws
Legal concepts
Legal ethics
Libel
Living will
Medical record
Moral ethics

Negligence
Nonconsequentialism
Nonmaleficence
Practice standards
Priestly model
Risk management
Role fidelity
Scope of practice
Slander
Teleology
Tort law
Values
Veracity
Virtue ethics

A diagnosis of cancer is one of the most, if not the most, feared diagnoses any patient can receive. Although numerous advancements have been made in the treatment of these diseases and there are many survivors, it is general knowledge that a cancer diagnosis is a life-altering event. Whether surgery, medical oncology, radiation oncology, or any combination of the three is used to treat the disease, patients often feel that they have little real control over the outcome. They are also acutely aware of the potential morbidity associated with treatment measures. One cancer patient may have summed up the experience of being diagnosed with cancer in a newspaper column she wrote about the event: "We cancer patients tend to recall our diagnosis day with the kind of clarity that comes with any catastrophic event. 'I'm sorry, but …,' the oncologist begins. Your heart races… or maybe it seems to stop. Your hands sweat. The noise of blood coursing through your veins deafens you to everything but the doctor's voice: 'You have cancer.' Just as many Americans can tell you where they were when the twin towers fell, so can we recall, in often minute detail, that moment when our world stood still."[1]

Each year in the United States, more than 1.5 million people will receive a cancer diagnosis. More than one-third of those who are diagnosed will succumb to their illness.[2] A diagnosis of cancer changes a person's life in ways many can only imagine. Although the diagnosis does not mean that the disease is terminal, it is certainly bad news and a negative event. Dr. Elisabeth Kübler-Ross is perhaps the best known authority on the subject of dealing with those experiencing forms of grief. In her studies on people with terminal illnesses, she found that the emotional cycle experienced by those with terminal illnesses was not unique to them but is also found in individuals experiencing circumstances they perceive as having a negative effect on their lives.[3] A diagnosis of cancer certainly fits the bill. The quest to beat the disease begins with personal courage and fortitude and with extensive involvement of dedicated healthcare professionals. Those who care for and treat cancer patients must understand their obligations as professionals. Not only must they care for and treat the patients, they must also deal with the emotions of the patients' families and other healthcare professionals. There are also legal issues that must be addressed and sometimes avoided, as will be discussed in the chapter.

THE CASE FOR ETHICS IN RADIATION THERAPY

Every aspect of the world of healthcare is fast paced and ever changing, and radiation therapy is no exception. To provide quality patient care in this fast-paced dynamic world, all healthcare providers must keep abreast of the latest treatment developments and technological advancements. In addition, all must be well versed in the ethical and legal considerations of cancer management. Radiation therapists and radiation therapy students deal with patients who have specific needs related to their attempts to control catastrophic diseases that are taking over their lives and the lives of those close to them. Defining the roles and responsibilities of the radiation therapy student, the practicing radiation therapist, and other members of the radiation oncology team as they care for their patients is extremely important. In addition to developing the technical skills necessary to practice in the profession, members of the radiation oncology team must develop an understanding of the basic theories regarding ethics, patients' rights, and the scope of practice and code of ethics for radiation therapy. The medical-legal aspects of informed consent, record keeping, and confidentiality are also important.

Radiation therapists and medical imaging technologists are credentialed by the American Registry of Radiologic Technologists (ARRT). The ARRT uses the terms Registered Technologists (RTs) and Registered Radiologist Assistants (RRAs) to describe those certified under

---

BOX 2.1 Code of Ethics for Radiation Therapists

- The radiation therapist advances the principal objective of the profession to provide services to humanity with full respect for the dignity of mankind.
- The radiation therapist delivers patient care and service unrestricted by concerns of personal attributes or the nature of the disease or illness and nondiscriminatory with respect to race, color, creed, sex, age, disability, or national origin.
- The radiation therapist assesses situations; exercises care, discretion, and judgment; assumes responsibility for professional decisions; and acts in the best interest of the patient.
- The radiation therapist adheres to the tenets and domains of the scope of practice for radiation therapists.
- The radiation therapist actively engages in lifelong learning to maintain, improve, and enhance professional competence and knowledge.

From the American Society of Radiologic Technologists, 2018.

---

its umbrella. Upon certification, individuals may use the initials RT followed by the initial(s) designating their area(s) of certification. In radiation therapy, these initials would be RT(T) ARRT. The primary professional membership organization for those credentialed by the ARRT is the American Society of Radiologic Technologists (ASRT). The ASRT developed a code of ethics to guide radiation therapy students on elements of the field while they develop their knowledge and skills, and to guide practicing radiation therapists in their professional conduct (Box 2.1). However, the Code of Ethics for Radiation Therapists does not list all principles and rules by which radiation therapists are governed. The ARRT developed a mission-based, more comprehensive document called the "Standards of Ethics."[4] This document is published and enforced by the ARRT. The Standards of Ethics are applicable to individuals who are certified through the ARRT and are either currently registered or were previously. The Standards of Ethics also apply to applicants for ARRT examinations and certifications, as well as students enrolled in radiation therapy educational programs. The document is composed of a preamble and three parts or sections: Section A outlines the Code of Ethics, Section B contains the Rules of Ethics, and Section C describes the administrative procedures followed by the ARRT when an individual is accused of violating the Code as related to the established rules.

The ARRT Code of Ethics contains 10 guiding principles (Box 2.2). As stated at the beginning of the code, "The Code of Ethics shall serve as a guide by which Registered Technologists and Candidates may evaluate their professional conduct as it relates to patients, health care consumers, employers, colleagues, and other members of the health care team."[5] This is quite a powerful and comprehensive statement. It is so inclusive that it seems be a guide to how RTs and candidates should behave around everyone. Isn't everyone a potential consumer? Does this statement mean that professional behaviors extend into off-the-job activities? The answer to both of these questions is yes. But it must be remembered that the Code of Ethics is aspirational, which simply means that the principles of the code are those to which the ARRT hopes RTs and candidates will aspire or will seek to achieve. On the other hand, mandatory rules do exist in the second part or section of the Standards of Ethics. Appropriately, these rules are titled the "Rules of Ethics." The ARRT Board of Trustees recommends modification of the Standards of Ethics when necessary. In 2009 the ARRT Board recommended revision of some of the rules. Rule 2 was expanded to better address examination subversion. Rule 18 was incorporated into Rule 6, and a new Rule 18 was added to better address subversion of the ethical standards for continuing education (CE). In addition, a new

The Code of Ethics forms the first part of the "Standards of Ethics." The Code of Ethics shall serve as a guide by which certificate holders and candidates may evaluate their professional conduct as it relates to patients, healthcare consumers, employers, colleagues, and other members of the healthcare team. The Code of Ethics is intended to assist certificate holders and candidates in maintaining a high level of ethical conduct and in providing for the protection, safety, and comfort of patients. The Code of Ethics is aspirational.

1. The radiologic technologist acts in a professional manner, responds to patient needs, and supports colleagues and associates in providing quality patient care.
2. The radiologic technologist acts to advance the principal objective of the profession to provide services to humanity with full respect for the dignity of mankind.
3. The radiologic technologist delivers patient care and service unrestricted by the concerns of personal attributes or the nature of the disease or illness, and without discrimination on the basis of sex, race, creed, religion, or socioeconomic status.
4. The radiologic technologist practices technology founded upon theoretical knowledge and concepts, uses equipment and accessories consistent with the purposes for which they were designed, and uses procedures and techniques appropriately.
5. The radiologic technologist assesses situations; exercises care, discretion, and judgment; assumes responsibility for professional decisions; and acts in the best interest of the patient.
6. The radiologic technologist acts as an agent through observation and communication to obtain pertinent information for the physician to aid in the diagnosis and treatment of the patient and recognizes that interpretation and diagnosis are outside the scope of practice for the profession.
7. The radiologic technologist uses equipment and accessories, uses techniques and procedures, performs services in accordance with an accepted standard of practice, and demonstrates expertise in minimizing radiation exposure to the patient, self, and other members of the healthcare team.
8. The radiologic technologist practices ethical conduct appropriate to the profession and protects the patient's right to quality radiologic technology care.
9. The radiologic technologist respects confidences entrusted in the course of professional practice, respects the patient's right to privacy, and reveals confidential information only as required by law or to protect the welfare of the individual or the community.
10. The radiologic technologist continually strives to improve knowledge and skills by participating in continuing education and professional activities, sharing knowledge with colleagues, and investigating new aspects of professional practice.

From the American Registry of Radiologic Technologists, 2017.

administrative procedure was incorporated to link ethics infractions to violation of both federal and state laws. After a period of public comment on the changes, they went into effect in August 2009. There are currently 22 Rules of Ethics (Box 2.3). These are rules that truly govern the professional behaviors of RTs, RRAs, and candidates for ARRT certification. The Rules of Ethics are not aspirational; they are enforceable. Those individuals found in violation of the ARRT Rules of Ethics are subject to sanctions ranging from private reprimand to the most dreaded sanction of all—permanent revocation of certification. The rules not only govern activities in which an RT, an RRA, or a candidate might personally engage; they also include instances in which individuals, although not directly involved, are aware of activities that violate ethical standards but permit the activities to occur. A thorough examination and understanding of the ARRT Standards of Ethics must be an integral part of education in radiation therapy and imaging sciences. Students, especially those with questionable criminal

activity in their background, unless the matter was adjudicated in juvenile court, should be encouraged to submit a preapplication for ARRT certification at least 6 months before graduation from their educational program. By doing so, their past criminal activity may be examined by the ARRT Ethics staff and/or the ARRT Ethics Committee in the determination of whether the individual has violated the Rules of Ethics and whether he or she is eligible or ineligible for ARRT certification. The names of individuals sanctioned by the ARRT are published in the "Annual Report to Technologists" and may also be found on the ARRT website.

Any professional code of ethics serves two major functions: education and regulation. It educates persons in the profession who do not reflect on ethical implications of their actions unless something concrete is before them. It also educates other professionals and the general public regarding the ethical standards expected of a given profession.[6] Professional codes of conduct should accomplish several objectives: (1) describe the values held by the profession, (2) impose obligations on practitioners to accept the values and practices included within the code, and (3) hold professionals liable for adherence to those obligations with possible penalties for nonconformance.[7] It is an obligation to society of any profession to assist in the development of social attitudes and policies that govern not only the operation of the profession but also the expectations of the public.[7] Understanding ethical concepts and legal issues and developing interpersonal skills, through the study of the material in this chapter, should enable students and practicing radiation therapists to care for their patients humanely and compassionately while adhering to the professional code of ethics. After all, it is not just the cancer that is being cared for and treated—it is the patient.

ETHICAL ASPECTS OF CANCER MANAGEMENT

Definitions and Terminology

Webster's New Collegiate Dictionary[8] defines ethics as "(1) the discipline dealing with what is good and bad, moral duty, and obligation; (2) a set of moral principles or values; (3) a theory or system of moral values; and (4) the principles of conduct governing an individual or a group." Ethics for an individual derive from the person's values.[9] There are four main sources of values: culture, experience, religion, and science.[6] Individuals gather an understanding of right and wrong from the cumulative experiences of life and develop patterns of approaching situations in which the complexities of right and wrong must be addressed.[10]

Cancer patients experience a variety of emotions, and although radiation therapy students and practitioners are cognitively and intellectually prepared to treat their cancer, they must also be able to treat the emotions they experience. This requires that students, therapists, and other members of the patient care team develop an understanding of their personal level of emotional intelligence (EI).

Although addressed by many individuals in the field of psychology throughout the years, the concept of EI was popularized by Daniel Goleman in his 1995 text *Emotional Intelligence: Why It Can Matter More Than IQ*. Goleman describes EI as the ability to perceive, evaluate, understand, and control emotions in ourselves and others.[11] In earlier work, Peter Salovey and John Mayer described the same ability as "the subset of social intelligence that involves the ability to monitor one's own and others' feelings and emotions, to discriminate among them and to use this information to guide one's thinking and actions."[12] Salovey and Mayer also described four factors that influence EI: perceiving emotions, reasoning with emotions, understanding emotions, and managing emotions.[12] To assess personal EI, individuals need to first determine their own emotional perceptions and how they reason

BOX 2.3 Rules of Ethics

The Rules of Ethics form the second part of the *Standards of Ethics*. They are mandatory standards of minimally acceptable professional conduct for all certificate holders and candidates. Certification and registration are methods of assuring the medical community and the public that an individual is qualified to practice within the profession. Because the public relies on certificates and registrations issued by the American Registry of Radiologic Technologists (ARRT), it is essential that certificate holders and candidates act consistently with these Rules of Ethics. These Rules of Ethics are intended to promote the protection, safety, and comfort of patients. The Rules of Ethics are enforceable. Certificate holders and candidates engaging in any of the following conduct or activities, or who permit the occurrence of the following conduct or activities with respect to them, have violated the Rules of Ethics and are subject to sanctions as described hereunder:

1. Using fraud or deceit in procuring or attempting to procure, maintain, renew, or obtain or reinstate certification or registration as issued by ARRT; employment in radiologic technology; or a state permit, license, or registration certificate to practice radiologic technology. This includes altering in any respect any document issued by the ARRT or any state or federal agency, or by indicating in writing certification or registration with the ARRT when that is not the case.

2. Subverting or attempting to subvert ARRT's examination process, and/or the structured self-assessments that are part of the Continuing Qualifications Requirements (CQR) process. Conduct that subverts or attempts to subvert ARRT's examination and/or CQR assessment process includes, but is not limited to:

    (i) disclosing examination and/or CQR assessment information by using language that is substantially similar to that used in questions and/or answers from ARRT examinations and/or CQR assessments when such information is gained as a direct result of having been an examinee or a participant in a CQR assessment or having communicated with an examinee or a CQR participant; this includes, but is not limited to, disclosures to students in educational programs, graduates of educational programs, educators, anyone else involved in the preparation of candidates to sit for the examinations, or CQR participants; and/or

    (ii) receiving examination and/or CQR assessment information that uses language that is substantially similar to that used in questions and/or answers on ARRT examinations or CQR assessments from an examinee, or a CQR participant, whether requested or not; and/or

    (iii) copying, publishing, reconstructing (whether by memory or otherwise), reproducing, or transmitting any portion of examination and/or CQR assessment materials by any means, verbal or written, electronic or mechanical, without the prior expressed written permission of ARRT or by using professional, paid, or repeat examination takers and/or CQR assessment participants, or any other individual for the purpose of reconstructing any portion of examination and/or CQR assessment materials; and/or

    (iv) using or purporting to use any portion of examination and/or CQR assessment materials that were obtained improperly or without authorization for the purpose of instructing or preparing any candidate for examination or participant for CQR assessment; and/or

    (v) selling or offering to sell, buying or offering to buy, or distributing or offering to distribute any portion of examination and/or CQR assessment materials without authorization; and/or

    (vi) removing or attempting to remove examination and/or CQR assessment materials from an examination or assessment room, or having unauthorized possession of any portion of or information concerning a future, current, or previously administered examination or CQR assessment of ARRT; and/or

    (vii) disclosing what purports to be, or what you claim to be, or under all circumstances is likely to be understood by the recipient as, any portion of "inside" information concerning any portion of a future, current, or previously administered examination or CQR assessment of ARRT; and/or

    (viii) communicating with another individual during administration of the examination or CQR assessment for the purpose of giving or receiving help in answering examination or CQR assessment questions, copying another candidate's, or CQR participants answers, permitting another candidate or a CQR participant to copy one's answers, or possessing unauthorized materials including, but not limited to, notes; and/or

    (ix) impersonating a candidate, or a CQR participant, or permitting an impersonator to take or attempt to take the examination or CQR assessment on one's own behalf; and/or

    (x) use of any other means that potentially alters the results of the examination or CQR assessment such that the results may not accurately represent the professional knowledge base of a candidate, or a CQR participant.

3. Convictions, criminal proceedings, or military court-martials as described below:

    (i) conviction of a crime, including a felony, a gross misdemeanor, or a misdemeanor, with the sole exception of speeding and parking violations. All alcohol and/or drug related violations must be reported; and/or

    (ii) criminal proceeding where a finding or verdict of guilt is made or returned but the adjudication of guilt is either withheld, deferred, or not entered, or the sentence is suspended or stayed; or a criminal proceeding in which the individual enters a plea of guilty or nolo contendere (no contest); or in which the individual enters into a pretrial diversion activity; or

    (iii) military court-martials related to any offense identified in these Rules of Ethics.

4. Violating a rule adopted by a state or federal regulatory authority or certification board resulting in the individual's professional license, permit, registration or certification being denied, revoked, suspended, placed on probation or a consent agreement or order, voluntarily surrendered, subjected to any conditions, or failing to report to ARRT any of the violations or actions identified in this Rule.

5. Performing procedures which the individual is not competent to perform through appropriate training and/or education or experience unless assisted or personally supervised by someone who is competent (through training and/or education or experience).

6. Engaging in unprofessional conduct, including, but not limited to:

    (i) a departure from or failure to conform to applicable federal, state, or local governmental rules regarding radiologic technology practice or scope of practice; or, if no such rule exists, to the minimal standards of acceptable and prevailing radiologic technology practice;

    (ii) any radiologic technology practice that may create unnecessary danger to a patient's life, health, or safety.

Actual injury to a patient or the public need not be established under this clause.

1. Delegating or accepting the delegation of a radiologic technology function or any other prescribed healthcare function when the delegation or acceptance could reasonably be expected to create an unnecessary danger to a patient's life, health, or safety. Actual injury to a patient need not be established under this clause.

2. Actual or potential inability to practice radiologic technology with reasonable skill and safety to patients by reason of illness; use of alcohol, drugs, chemicals, or any other material; or as a result of any mental or physical condition.

BOX 2.3 Rules of Ethics—cont'd

3. Adjudication as mentally incompetent, mentally ill, chemically dependent, or dangerous to the public, by a court of competent jurisdiction.
4. Engaging in any unethical conduct, including, but not limited to, conduct likely to deceive, defraud, or harm the public; or demonstrating a willful or careless disregard for the health, welfare, or safety of a patient. Actual injury need not be established under this clause.
5. Engaging in conduct with a patient that is sexual or may reasonably be interpreted by the patient as sexual, or in any verbal behavior that is seductive or sexually demeaning to a patient; or engaging in sexual exploitation of a patient or former patient. This also applies to any unwanted sexual behavior, verbal or otherwise.
6. Revealing a privileged communication from or relating to a former or current patient, except when otherwise required or permitted by law, or viewing, using, or releasing confidential patient information in violation of HIPAA.
7. Knowingly engaging or assisting any person to engage in, or otherwise participating in, abusive or fraudulent billing practices, including violations of federal Medicare and Medicaid laws or state medical assistance laws.
8. Improper management of patient records, including failure to maintain adequate patient records or to furnish a patient record or report required by law; or making, causing, or permitting anyone to make false, deceptive, or misleading entry in any patient record.
9. Knowingly assisting, advising, or allowing a person without a current and appropriate state permit, license, registration, or an ARRT registered certificate to engage in the practice of radiologic technology, in a jurisdiction that mandates such requirements.
10. Violating a state or federal narcotics or controlled substance law.
11. Knowingly providing false or misleading information that is directly related to the care of a former or current patient.
12. Subverting, attempting to subvert, or aiding others to subvert or attempt to subvert *ARRT's Continuing Education (CE) Requirements for Renewal of Registration,* and/or ARRT's CQR. Conduct that subverts or attempts to subvert ARRT's CE or CQR Requirements includes, but is not limited to:

   (i) providing false, inaccurate, altered, or deceptive information related to CE or CQR activities to ARRT or an ARRT recognized recordkeeper; and/or
   (ii) assisting others to provide false, inaccurate, altered, or deceptive information related to CE or CQR activities to ARRT or an ARRT recognized recordkeeper; and/or
   (iii) conduct that results or could result in a false or deceptive report of CE or CQR completion; and/or
   (iv) conduct that in any way compromises the integrity of the CE or CQR requirements such as sharing answers to the posttests or self-learning activities, providing or using false certificates of participation, or verifying credits that were not earned.
13. Subverting or attempting to subvert the ARRT certification or registration process by:
   (i) making a false statement or knowingly providing false information to ARRT; or
   (ii) failing to cooperate with any investigation by the ARRT.
14. Engaging in false, fraudulent, deceptive, or misleading communications to any person regarding the individual's education, training, credentials, experience, or qualifications, or the status of the individual's state permit, license, or registration certificate in radiologic technology or certificate of registration with ARRT.
15. Knowing of a violation or a probable violation of any Rule of Ethics by any certificate holder or candidate and failing to promptly report in writing the same to the ARRT.
16. Failing to immediately report to his or her supervisor information concerning an error made in connection with imaging, treating, or caring for a patient. For purposes of this rule, errors include any departure from the standard of care that reasonably may be considered to be potentially harmful, unethical, or improper (commission). Errors also include behavior that is negligent or should have occurred in connection with a patient's care, but did not (omission). The duty to report under this rule exists whether or not the patient suffered any injury.

From the American Registry of Radiologic Technologists, 2018.

with them. They may ask themselves what evokes certain feelings within themselves and why they feel certain emotions. Then they must ask themselves how they deal with those feelings. Personal examination of EI will assist in understanding what emotions a patient may be feeling and how those emotions are manifested in the clinical setting. With that understanding, the student or therapist will be better able to empathize and modify, if necessary, patient interaction and treatment.

> Ethics are based on values.

In the study of ethics, a person must distinguish between moral and legal ethics. Morality has to do with conscience. It is a person's concept of right or wrong as it relates to conscience, God, a higher being, or a person's logical rationalization. *Morality* can be defined as fidelity to conscience. Legal concepts are defined as the sum of rules and regulations by which society is governed in any formal and legally binding manner. The law mandates certain acts and forbids other acts under penalties of criminal sanction. Laws, the foundation of which is ethics, are primarily concerned with the good of a society as a functioning unit.[13,14]

> The foundation of law is ethics.

In dealing with ethical issues in cancer treatment, healthcare professionals should consider bioethics. *Miller-Keane Encyclopedia & Dictionary of Medicine, Nursing, & Allied Health, Seventh Edition*[15] defines *bioethics* as the application of ethics to the bioethical sciences, medicine, nursing, and healthcare. The text further states that the practical ethical questions raised in everyday healthcare are generally in the realm of bioethics. There are seven written principles associated with bioethics. Referred to as the *Principles of Biomedical Ethics,* the seven are inclusive of autonomy, beneficence, confidentiality, justice, nonmaleficence, role fidelity, and veracity.[5] It is generally desirable for those who practice in the healthcare setting to innately prescribe to the aforementioned principles. Autonomy emphasizes the right of patients to make decisions for themselves, free of interference by others. It also recognizes that patients are to be respected for their independence and freedom to control their own actions and decision-making capacity. Theoretically, each person should be recognized and respected for his or her social uniqueness and moral worth. In healthcare, this theory means that individuals should and must be respected for their abilities to make their own choices and develop their own plans for their lives.[16] Beneficence is defined as doing good and calls on healthcare professionals to act in the best interest of patients, even when it might be inconvenient or sacrifices must be made. Palliative treatment may be considered a form of beneficence in radiation oncology because it helps relieve pain and suffering, thereby "doing good," but this can be viewed as a problem in some cases. When a patient has expressed no desire for prolongation of her or his life by any means, palliative treatment may not be viewed as a beneficent act. Confidentiality is the principle that relates to the knowledge that information revealed by a patient to a healthcare provider, or information that is learned in the course of a healthcare provider performing her or his duties, is private and should be held in confidence. To hold something in confidence in essence means to keep it secret. A secret is information that a person has a right or an obligation to conceal. In healthcare, confidentiality is based on obligatory secrets, of which there are three types: natural, promised, and professional.[17,18] Natural secrets are those that involve information that is naturally harmful if it were to be revealed. Promised secrets are those that involve information that an individual has promised someone that they will not reveal. The professional secret is the type of secret that is of most importance in healthcare. Professional secrets are knowledge and information learned in the course of professional healthcare practice that, if revealed, would harm the patient while also harming the profession and the society that depends on the profession for important care and services.[16] The obligation of healthcare providers to keep professional secrets is not only recognized within the frame of bioethics but also is seen as a patient right and is protected within the frame of law as well. In 1973, the American Hospital Association (AHA) constructed and adopted what became known as "A Patient's Bill of Rights." This document was further refined, revised, and copyrighted in 1992 and 1998. More recently, the document has again been revised and renamed the "Patient Care Partnership." The document, a patient brochure, is intended to provide patients with an explanation of what to expect during their stay in the hospital, and to explain their rights and responsibilities. The brochure is currently available in eight languages. The translation into multiple languages reflects the patient diversity within the healthcare population of the United States. The brochure contains the tenets of "A Patient's Bill of Rights," with information included on the following patient rights and responsibilities:

- High-quality patient care
- A clean and safe environment
- Patient's involvement in his or her care
- Protection of the patient's privacy
- Help when the patient leaves the hospital
- Help with the patient's billing claim

As noted in the list of brochure topics above, protection of a patient's privacy is considered a patient right. The "Patient Care Partnership" is also related to other topics in ethics and will be discussed further in a later section of this chapter.

In 1996, the federal government became more involved in the regulation of healthcare with the passage of the Health Insurance Portability and Accountability Act (HIPAA), Public Law 104-191. Under this provision of healthcare law, overseen primarily by the U.S. Department of Health and Human Services, healthcare facilities, providers, and employees are mandated under penalty of law to publish rules to ensure (1) standardization of electronic patient administrative, financial, and health data; (2) creation of unique health identifiers for employees, healthcare providers, and health plans; and (3) security standards that protect the confidentiality and integrity of "individually identifiable health information," past, present, and future.[19]

All employees working in healthcare and students in healthcare educational programs are required to be trained in HIPAA regulatory requirements and compliance. At the heart of HIPAA regulations is confidentiality of health information. Confidentiality is the ethical principle that relates to all of the others.

> Confidentiality is the ethical principle that binds all the seven bioethical principles.

Justice is the ethical principle that relates to fairness and equal treatment for all. Essentially, the application of the bioethical principle of justice asks persons to ensure that fairness and equity are maintained among individuals.[20] Treatment of all patients as equals regardless of the nature of their illness, age, gender, sexual preference, socioeconomic status, religious preference, national origin, and similar factors is considered a form of justice. The Patient Protection and Affordable Care Act of 2010 (HR 39620) (Public Law 111-148) is yet another step in ensuring equal treatment of all individuals seeking medical help. Also called "Obama Care," among other things, the Act contains the following provisions:

- Prohibits health insurers from denying a patient coverage because of their medical histories
- Prevents health insurers from charging different premiums based on medical histories and gender
- Provides a subsidy to low- and middle-income Americans to help purchase insurance
- Expands Medicaid to include more low-income Americans

The Act has come under major scrutiny by the current administration, and attempts have been made to rescind the Act, with nothing in line to replace it. Although the Act has flaws, it attempts to bring "Justice" into the realm of American healthcare.[21]

Nonmaleficence directs healthcare professionals to avoid harmful actions to patients. Professionals must avoid mishandling or mistreating patients in any manner that may be construed as harmful. Indeed, most healthcare professionals can recite what has been expressed as the first part of the original Hippocratic Oath: "First, do no harm." Role fidelity is the principle that reminds healthcare professionals that they must be faithful to their role in the healthcare environment. Healthcare professions have defined standards of practice, which will be discussed later in this chapter. The last of the seven principles of biomedical ethics is veracity. Veracity is truthfulness within the realm of healthcare practice. Under certain conditions, it is acceptable for confidentiality to be breached and veracity to be disregarded. These situations include, but are not exclusive to, civil cases, criminal cases, suspected child and elder abuse, and matters of public health and safety.[7] Even under the aforementioned conditions, healthcare professionals should safeguard as much patient information as they can by answering only the questions asked of them and disclosing only subpoenaed information.

Ethical Theories and Models

Ethics is the systematic study of morals (e.g., the rightness or wrongness of human conduct and character as known by natural reason), although many people believe that ethics simply means using common sense. A respectable value system and appropriate ethical behaviors are desirable traits for those serving in any healthcare profession. Ethical problem-solving begins with an awareness of ethical issues in healthcare and is the sum of ethical knowledge, common sense, personal and professional values, practical wisdom, and learned skills.[18] Although an individual's personal system of decision-making may be developed from values and experiences, it generally involves some understanding and application of basic principles common to formal ethical theories.[5]

Ethical theories may be divided into the following three broad groups:

1. Teleology (consequentialism)
2. Deontology (nonconsequentialism)
3. Virtue ethics

Teleological ethical theories assert that the consequences of an act or action should be the major focus when deciding how to solve an ethical problem. Because of this, teleology is also called consequentialism. It has often been stated that teleologists believe that the ends justify the means. Two forms of consequentialism exist: egoism and utilitarianism. In egoism, the best long-term interests of an individual are promoted. Egoists believe that in evaluating an act or action for its moral value, the act or action must produce a greater ratio of good over bad for the individual, for the long term, than any of the possible alternatives. There are essentially two types of egoism: impersonal and personal. Impersonal egoists generally believe that everyone should behave in a fashion that promotes her or his best long-term interests, whereas personal egoists pursue their own best long-term interests and perform in a manner that benefits only themselves. They usually make no attempt to advocate or control what others should do. Because the role of healthcare professionals is to serve others, the practice of egoism in any form is incompatible and undesirable. The ethical theory of utilitarianism holds that people should act to produce the greatest ratio of good to evil for everyone. Attributed to the work of Jeremy Bentham and his student John Mill, this theory is considered most applicable to ethical decision-making in healthcare.[22] Bentham and Mill surmised that behaviors are right if they promote happiness and pleasure for everyone, and wrong to the extent that they do not produce pleasure, only pain. There are two categories or forms of utilitarianism: act and rule. Those who practice act utilitarianism believe that ethical behaviors should be geared toward performing acts that produce the greatest ratio of good to bad. The act itself, and its positive consequences, is their only genuine consideration. Rule utilitarianists believe that individuals should base their ethical choices on the consequences of a rule or rules under which an act or action falls without primary consideration of the consequences. The so-called rules may be those derived from religious belief, such as the Ten Commandments; those offered by professional codes of conduct or ethics, such as the Code of Ethics for Radiation Therapists; those developed by professional organizations in the interest of their clients, such as the AHA's Patient Care Partnership; or those that may be considered an arbitrary set of an individual's personal beliefs.[7]

Deontology, or nonconsequentialism, uses formal rules of right and wrong for reasoning and problem-solving. Developed by Immanuel Kant in its purest form, the ethical theory of deontology seeks to exclude the consideration of consequences when performing ethical acts or making ethical decisions. Kant surmised that morality is based on reason and that the principles derived from reason are universal and should be designated as universal truths. Because there was no definition or explanation of these truths, Kant created what is known as the "categorical imperative." The categorical imperative states that "... we should act in such a way as to will the maxim of our actions to become universal law."[14] A maxim is a statement of general truth, fundamental principle, or rule of conduct.[23] Although there are several maxims attributed to Kant, the one that is most relevant to the healthcare professions is "We must always treat others as ends and not as means only."[14] Application of this maxim to healthcare professionals simply means that those adhering to this principle would never view their positions as just jobs for which they receive financial remuneration, but instead would consider each patient as an individual (autonomy) to whom a professional duty is owed (beneficence, confidentiality, justice, nonmaleficence, role fidelity, and veracity) and to which these principles of biomedical ethics should be applied.

Virtue ethics is the use of practical wisdom for emotional and intellectual problem-solving. Practical reasoning, consideration of consequences, rules established by society, and the effects that actions have on others play important parts in applying the theory of virtue ethics. This approach to problem-solving serves the healthcare professional by integrating intellect, practical reasoning, and individual good.[18] Application of this theory to healthcare may be problematic, because instead of focusing on the acts or actions of individuals, this theory focuses on the individual performing the act or action.[23] Healthcare professionals

work together as a team to provide patients with high-quality care. Promotion or consideration of self, like egoism, has no place in the healthcare professions.

Regardless of which values a person holds and to which ethical theory he or she subscribes, the person will face ethical problems that must be solved. Healthcare professionals, radiation therapists included, will face these types of problems almost daily. Many ethicists have described and identified numerous types of ethical problems. Four categories consistently traditionally emerged from the numerous types identified: ethical dilemmas, ethical dilemmas of justice, ethical distress, and locus of authority issues.[7] *Ethical dilemmas* arise when an individual is faced with an ethical situation to which there is more than one seemingly correct solution. The only problem is that all solutions cannot be applied, and choosing one precludes choosing the other(s). In ethical dilemmas, a choice must be made and implemented. Ethical problems associated with the distribution of benefits and burdens on a societal basis are called *ethical dilemmas of justice*. The most obvious manifestation of ethical dilemmas of justice in healthcare is that of allocation of scarce resources. *Ethical distress* occurs when there is a problem that has an obviously correct solution, but there are institutional constraints prohibiting its application. *Locus of authority* issues occur when there is a problem and there is a question as to whose authority the problem falls under. In other words: Whose job is it to clean up this mess or rectify this situation? No one wants to take the responsibility. In recent years, the past 15 to 20 or so, a new category of ethical problem has surfaced in healthcare—conflict of interest.[13] Conflicts of interest arise when an individual engages in an activity from which he or she could profit in several ways, such as when a conflict exists between a person's obligations to the public and his or her own self-interest. Consider the following example:

Dr. Jones is a radiation oncologist at Intercollegial Medical Center. He also is part owner of a freestanding medical imaging center that has a positron emission tomography-computed tomography scanner (PET/CT). Dr. Jones refers all of his oncology patients to the freestanding center for frequent PET/CT scans. Could this possibly be a conflict of interest? It could be viewed as such, because by sending these patients to the freestanding center, Dr. Jones is increasing the income of the center, thereby increasing the profit margin of the owners, of which he is one. Joint venture and self-referrals are just two of the areas that have been identified as presenting the potential for conflicts of interest.[19]

In addition, oral presentations given at state, regional, and national conferences that provide CE credits for attendees should communicate a conflict of interest statement by the presenter at the beginning of the talk. If the presenter has a conflict of interest, it can compromise the presentation and at times distort the interpretation of clinical research. Disclosure of conflicts of interest is an important step for a speaker, as it usually addresses the issue of potential bias.

Models for ethical decision-making involve different methods of interaction with the patient. The engineering or analytical model identifies the caregiver as a scientist dealing only in facts and does not consider the human aspect of the patient. The engineering model is a dehumanizing approach and is usually ineffective.[18] For example, with the engineering model, the radiation therapist considers the patient only as a lung or brain rather than as an individual who has thoughts, feelings, and emotions. This type of approach in the care of cancer patients is cold, unfeeling, and extremely inappropriate.

The priestly model provides the caregiver with a godlike, paternalist attitude that makes decisions *for* and not *with* the patient. This approach enhances the patient's feeling of loss of control by giving the caregiver not only medical expertise but also authority about moral issues.[24] An example of this model is the therapist or student forcing a patient to comply with planning or treatment procedures regardless of the patient's pain or discomfort because the physician ordered it or because the disease is known to respond to treatment. Patients must be allowed to make their own decisions regarding their treatment (autonomy).

The collegial model presents a more cooperative method of pursuing healthcare for both provider and patient. It involves sharing, trust, and consideration of common goals. The collegial model gives more control to the patient while producing confidence and preserving dignity and respect.[18] For example, the therapist takes the extra time required to get acquainted with patients and listen to their needs. This knowledge enables the therapist to help patients cooperate with the demands of positioning for planning and treatment. Although the collegial model takes time, its application is crucial to the humane treatment of cancer patients.

The contractual model maintains a business relationship between the provider and patient. A contractual arrangement serves as the guideline for decision making and meeting obligations for services. With a contractual arrangement, information and responsibility are shared. This model requires compliance from the patient; however, the patient is in control of the decision making.[18] The contractual model is best represented by the process of informed consent. When provided with comprehensive and thorough information, competent patients will be able make decisions in an informed manner.

The covenant model recognizes areas of healthcare not always covered by a contract. A covenant relationship deals with an understanding between the patient and healthcare provider that is often based on traditional values and goals.[18] The covenant model is demonstrated by a patient trusting the caregiver to do what is right. This trust is often based on previous experience with healthcare, particularly cancer care procedures and treatment.

The role of the radiation therapist in regard to ethical decision-making involves the application of professionalism, the selection of a personal theory of ethics, and the choice of a model for interaction with the patient. The difficulties encountered are the result of constant changes in healthcare, patient awareness, and evolving growth of radiation therapy in a highly technical and extremely impersonal world of healthcare.[24] Additional difficulties may arise when some healthcare professionals realize that they have never selected or examined which ethical theory that they subscribe to or their level of EI. To subscribe to an ethical theory, individuals must first examine their personal values. As mentioned earlier in this chapter, ethics are based on values and are derived from four main sources:

- Culture
- Experience
- Religion
- Science

Although individuals vary in how many and what values they derive from each source, studies show that culture and religion are at the forefront of values development. Many scholars agree that religion, or even the lack of religious beliefs, is a part of culture.[25] Seeking to understand the cultural and religious belief of patients is essential to the understanding of their underlying values.

Values are core beliefs concerning what is desirable and help assess the worth of intangibles.[7] They provide the foundation for decisions individuals make in their personal and professional lives.

It is not especially easy for people to examine and clarify their values. For that reason, several individuals have sought to develop a useful means of doing just that. One of those individuals was the ethicist Louis Rath.[9] In the mid-1960s, Rath developed what he termed *values clarification*. Rath formulated a values clarification exercise to assist individuals in discovering, analyzing, and prioritizing their personal

values. The exercise contains questions that prompt individuals to make choices based on their particular feelings about specific topics and examine the feelings that were associated with their choices. By completing the exercise, Rath hoped that individuals would discover and be able to describe their values. He also sought to encourage these individuals to exhibit their discovered values daily. Discovering personal values will assist in the development of professional values. This will serve radiation therapists well as they provide quality patient care and treatment.

Patients should actively participate in their own care. Patients' awareness of their rights, their needs, and the availability of the many treatment options provides both opportunities and complications. As mentioned earlier, the AHA has published the "Patient Care Partnership: Understanding Expectations, Rights, and Responsibilities" (Box 2.4), and every medical institution has the responsibility to make this document available to its patients. Each patient's responsibility for the treatment process grows with the knowledge provided by patient education.[18]

PATIENT AUTONOMY AND INFORMED CONSENT

Cancer remains one of the most dreaded diseases and often evokes images of death, disfigurement, intolerable pain, and suffering. In the late 1980s, the central ethical issue in caring for the cancer patient was whether to tell the patient that the diagnosis was cancer. Today, advancements in treatment, surgery, chemotherapy, and radiation therapy have resulted in longer periods of remission, improved survival, and even cures. These advances have generated more complex ethical issues.[26] More than half of all cancer patients ultimately need radiation therapy. The physician and patient must weigh the benefits of therapy against possible complications.[2]

The healthcare professional's ability to listen to patients sensitively, grasp the patient's truth, and honor that truth is indispensable, even across religious, social, cultural, and age barriers. To be effective and supportive, physicians and caregivers must, in a sense, be masters of each patient's personal language. This ability to listen and communicate is an extremely important clinical skill that must be learned. There are at least three courses or areas within a radiation therapy program curriculum where these skills can be taught: patient care, ethics, and clinical education. Mastery of listening and communicating should be highly valued.[24]

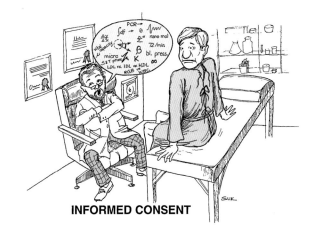

INFORMED CONSENT

Truth telling, which is required for informed consent, is an extremely curious principle. Many people have been taught from

BOX 2.4   The Patient Care Partnership: Understanding Expectations, Rights, and Responsibilities

When you need hospital care, your doctor and the nurses and other professionals at our hospital are committed to working with you and your family to meet your healthcare needs. Our dedicated doctors and staff serve the community in all its ethnic, religious, and economic diversity. Our goal is for you and your family to have the same care and attention we would want for our families and ourselves. The sections in this brochure explain some of the basics about how you can expect to be treated during your hospital stay. They also cover what we will need from you to care for you better. If you have questions at any time, please ask. Unasked or unanswered questions can add to the stress of being in the hospital. Your comfort and confidence in your care are very important to us.

What to expect during your hospital stay:

- **High-quality hospital care.** Our first priority is to provide you the care you need, when you need it, with skill, compassion, and respect. Tell your caregivers if you have concerns about your care or if you have pain. You have the right to know the identity of doctors, nurses, and others involved in your care, in addition to students, residents, or other trainees.
- **A clean and safe environment.** Our hospital works hard to keep you safe. We use special policies and procedures to avoid mistakes in your care and keep you free from abuse or neglect. If anything unexpected and significant happens during your hospital stay, you will be told what happened, and any resulting changes in your care will be discussed with you.
- **Involvement in your care.** You and your doctor often make decisions about your care before you go to the hospital. Other times, especially in emergencies, those decisions are made during your hospital stay. When decision-making takes place, it should include:
- Discussion of your medical condition and information about medically appropriate treatment choices. To make informed decisions with your doctor, you need to understand:
  - a. The benefits and risks of each treatment.
  - b. Whether your treatment is experimental or part of a research study.
  - c. What you can reasonably expect from your treatment and any long-term effects it might have on your quality of life.
  - d. What you and your family will need to do after you leave the hospital.
  - e. The financial consequences of using uncovered services or out-of-network providers.

Please tell your caregivers if you need more information about treatment choices.

1. *Discussing your treatment plan.* When you enter the hospital, you sign a general consent to treatment. In some cases, such as surgery or experimental treatment, you may be asked to confirm in writing that you understand what is planned and agree to it. This process protects your right to consent to or refuse a treatment. Your doctor will explain the medical consequences of refusing recommended treatment. It also protects your right to decide if you want to participate in a research study.
2. *Getting information from you.* Your caregivers need complete and correct information about your health and coverage so that they can make good decisions about your care. That includes:
   - Past illnesses, surgeries, or hospital stays.
   - Past allergic reactions.

- Any medicines or dietary supplements (such as vitamins and herbs) that you are taking.
- Any network or admission requirements under your health plan.

3. *Understanding your healthcare goals and values.* You may have healthcare goals and values or spiritual beliefs that are important to your well-being. They will be taken into account as much as possible throughout your hospital stay. Make sure your doctor, your family, and your healthcare team know your wishes.
4. *Understanding who should make decisions when you cannot.* If you have signed a healthcare power of attorney stating who should speak for you if you become unable to make healthcare decisions for yourself, or a "living will" or "advance directive" that states your wishes about end-of-life care, give copies to your doctor, your family, and your care team. If you or your family need help making difficult decisions, counselors, chaplains, and others are available to help.
5. *Protection of your privacy.* We respect the confidentiality of your relationship with your doctor and other caregivers, and the sensitive information about your health and healthcare that are part of that relationship. State and federal laws and hospital operating policies protect the privacy of your medical information. You will receive a Notice of Privacy Practices that describes the ways that we use, disclose, and safeguard patient information and that explains how you can obtain a copy of information from our records about your care.
6. *Help preparing you and your family for when you leave the hospital.* Your doctor works with hospital staff and professionals in your community. You and your family also play an important role in your care. The success of your treatment often depends on your efforts to follow medication, diet, and therapy plans. Your family may need to help care for you at home. You can expect us to help you identify sources of follow-up care and to let you know if our hospital has a financial interest in any referrals. As long as you agree that we can share information about your care with them, we will coordinate our activities with your caregivers outside the hospital. You can also expect to receive information and, where possible, training about the self-care you will need when you go home.
7. *Help with your bill and filing insurance claims.* Our staff will file claims for you with healthcare insurers or other programs such as Medicare and Medicaid. They will also help your doctor with needed documentation. Hospital bills and insurance coverage are often confusing. If you have questions about your bill, contact our business office. If you need help understanding your insurance coverage or health plan, start with your insurance company or health benefits manager. If you do not have health coverage, we will try to help you and your family find financial help or make other arrangements. We need your help with collecting needed information and other requirements to obtain coverage or assistance.

While you are here, you will receive more detailed notices about some of the rights you have as a hospital patient and how to exercise them. We are always interested in improving. If you have questions, comments, or concerns, please contact _____.

Courtesy, American Hospital Association, 2018.

early childhood to tell the truth, but doing so is often extremely difficult and sometimes even seems wrong. Not long ago, lying to a patient about the cancer diagnosis was the norm. Caregivers believed that telling the truth would be destructive and that patients preferred ignorance of their conditions. Studies over the years, however, have conclusively documented that cancer patients want to know their diagnoses and do not suffer psychological injury as a result of the truth.[26]

As discussed earlier, the claim that each person is free to make life-directing decisions is known as the bioethical *principle of autonomy*. The concept of autonomy, understood in this sense, is crucial to ethics. Without some sense of autonomy, no sense of responsibility exists, and, without responsibility, ethics is not possible.[27] In conventional cancer therapy, patient autonomy is protected further by the practice of consent. The American Medical Association's principles of medical ethics imply the following about informed consent: a

---

BOX 2.5 Informed Consent

To give informed consent, the patient must be informed of the following:
1. The nature of the procedure, treatment, or disease.
2. The expectations of the recommended treatment and the likelihood of success.
3. Reasonable alternatives available and the probable outcome in the absence of treatment.
4. The particular known risks that are material to the informed decision about whether to accept or reject medical recommendations.

From Gurley LT, Callaway WJ. *Introduction to Radiologic Technology.* 7th ed. St. Louis, MO: Mosby; 2011.

---

physician shall be dedicated to providing competent medical service with compassion and respect for human dignity, shall deal honestly with patients and colleagues, and shall make relevant information available to patients. Patients should be informed and educated about their conditions, should understand and approve their treatments, and should participate responsibly in their own care.[28] The basic element of informed consent is the patients' right to understand and participate in their own healthcare. Informed consent is a doctrine that has evolved sociologically and legally with the changing times. Every patient is entitled to receive information about a procedure or treatment before it is performed[17] (Box 2.5). Consent contains three important aspects: communication, ethics, and law.[7] The communication aspect of consent involves physicians or their agent telling the patient what he or she needs to know so that they may make a decision as to what course of action is best for him or her. The aspect of ethics in consent may involve conflict between the beneficent approach of the healthcare professional (doing good by providing the best level of care that they can) and patient autonomy (the patient's right to make his or her own decisions, even those that may be considered bad decisions), regarding his or her care. The law aspect is simply the fact that patients have legal rights that have been established through guidelines and the court system in the consent process. Although there are several types of consent, informed consent is the most critical. Informed consent must be secured in writing for all procedures, treatments, and research considered invasive and/or that pose significant risk(s).

Informed consent must be secured in writing.

Informed consent is considered a procedure in which patients may agree to or refuse treatment based on information provided to them by their physician or designee(s). The patient must be fully informed concerning the nature of the procedure or treatment—the associated risks, including complications; side effects and potential mortality; desired outcome; and possible alternative procedures or treatments. To give consent, a person must have the legal capacity to do so. The capacity is ensured if a person is a competent adult; the legal guardian or representative of an incompetent adult; an emancipated, married, or mature minor; the parent or legal guardian of a child; or an individual obligated by court order.[7]

Competency refers to the minimal mental, cognitive, or behavioral ability or trait required to assume responsibility. In general, the law recognizes only decisions or consents made by competent individuals. Persons older than the age of 18 years are presumed to be competent; however, this may be disputed with evidence of mental illness or deficiency. If the individual's condition prevents the satisfaction of criteria for competency, the person may be deemed incompetent

for the purpose of informed consent. Mental illness does not automatically render a person incompetent in all areas of functioning. Respect for autonomy demands that individuals, even if they are seriously mentally impaired, be allowed to make decisions of which they are capable. Minors are not generally considered legally competent and therefore require the consent of parents or designated guardians.[28] As noted earlier, there are exceptions to this rule. When a minor legally marries, he or she is considered an autonomous adult. The same applies to minors who petition the court and are granted emancipated or mature minor status. These minors generally do not live with their parents nor are they dependent on them for support. In addition, minors serving in the uniformed services are also given autonomous adult status.[23]

A person's competency status may be altered if he or she is under the influence of certain medications, especially those used for pain control. The rule directing that a patient may not sign a document or give informed consent for a procedure after being medicated was established to protect the person going to surgery. Persons who have been premedicated for procedures are considered incompetent. However, persons experiencing intractable pain may be incapable of exercising autonomy until after they are medicated and pain free or experiencing pain control.[20]

The responsibility for obtaining informed consent from a patient clearly remains with the physician and cannot be delegated. However, it is known that many times, other healthcare professionals secure informed consent for certain procedures. The legality of this can be challenged if the facility does not have appropriate written policies and procedures regarding the securing of informed consent by a nonphysician. The courts believe that a physician is in the best position to decide which information should be provided for a patient to make an informed choice. The scope of disclosure in any situation is a physician's responsibility. Some states, however, also have legislative standards or state statutes that define the information that the physician must tell a patient.[6]

Informed consent must be secured by a physician, unless otherwise specified by facility policy and procedure, or state law.

Often, a third person (a healthcare provider) is present during the informed consent session because patients are reluctant to question their physicians but will likely question the witness. The witness can then inform the physician about the patient's lack of understanding. The third-party signature is merely an attestation that the informed consent session took place and that the signature on the document is that of the patient.[28] The patient must be able to understand the information as presented, and no attempt must be made to influence the decision. In the United States today, obtaining true informed consent can present a real challenge because of language barriers (linguistic diversity). Medical interpreters and other services are seeing increased use as those seeking healthcare services in the United States continue to become more diverse. General agreement exists that informed consent is an active, shared decision-making process between the healthcare provider and patient. To give informed consent, patients must understand the information that is provided to them. Communication is key to the process, and, when a patient and his or her healthcare providers cannot communicate because of language barriers, quality healthcare may be compromised. To deliver quality healthcare to everyone, all providers of healthcare must continuously seek better forms and more venues of communication. Medical interpreters and consent forms in a patient's language are two of the current attempts to communicate essential information to patients, establish their understanding, and ensure that they truly are informed before they give consent.

Confidentiality

A struggle exists in medical practice between confidentiality and truthfulness. According to Garrett et al,[16] truthfulness is summarized in two commands: "Do not lie," and "You must communicate with those who have a right to the truth." Truthfulness must not be the only consideration in discussing patients' rights and caregivers' obligations to patients. One of the major restrictions a healthcare profession imposes is strict confidentiality of medical and personal information about a patient. This information cannot be revealed without consent of the patient.

Breach of confidence is one of the major problems encountered in providing patient care and can result in legal problems. Information should not be discussed with other department personnel, except in the direct line of duty if it is requested from one ancillary department to another or with the nursing service to meet specific medical needs. In the radiation therapy setting, staff members must be especially careful not to discuss patients in hallways or around the treatment area unless the discussion is directly related to the treatment. Unless a patient expressly and explicitly forbids such, healthcare professionals have the right to consult other healthcare providers in the effort to help the patient.[16] Staff members should never discuss information with their own families or friends, even in the most general terms, because doing so is a violation of confidentiality and HIPAA. The patient's treatment chart should be kept in a secure area, inaccessible to anyone not involved in the treatment. Electronic patient records should only be accessed by those with a specific need to know the contents of the record, or by those required to document care within the record. Confidentiality issues must be stressed in every educational program at every opportunity.[10] Implementation of HIPAA regulations has provided more strict regulations regarding the confidentiality of patient information contained within standard or electronic forms. All healthcare professionals and others who may be exposed to confidential information while working in the healthcare setting are required to receive HIPAA training. Noncompliance with HIPAA regulations is dealt with harshly. Violation of HIPAA policies can result in institutional sanctions and monetary fines, and individuals may be terminated for their violations. To help ensure HIPAA compliance, all healthcare employees and students undergo mandatory HIPAA training.

> All healthcare employees and students must receive mandatory HIPAA training.

There are some exceptions to confidentiality. These exceptions are generally grouped under four general headings: those commanded by state law, those arising from legal precedent, those resulting from a peculiar patient-provider relationship, and in cases of proportionate reason.[19] Exceptions may include particular types of wounds (e.g., gunshot and knife), certain communicable diseases (e.g., human immunodeficiency virus, hepatitis, and syphilis), acute poisonings (ingestion of caustic substances), automobile accidents, and abuse (especially child, elder, and spousal).[18] Subject to state law, confidentiality may also be overridden when the life or safety of the patient is endangered, such as when knowledgeable intervention can prevent threatened suicide or self-injury. In addition, the moral obligation to prevent substantial and foreseeable harm to an innocent third party usually is greater than the moral obligation to protect confidentiality.[29]

Roles of Other Healthcare Team Members

Patients and families dealing with cancer may be suddenly thrust into a new and potentially threatening world of blood tests, diagnostic procedures, therapeutic procedures, and specialists. A family physician or internist who is familiar with the patient's history and has established a trusting relationship with the patient can be a key member of the cancer management team. This physician can help the patient and his or her family, make appropriate treatment decisions, and can act as a liaison between the patient and others involved in the evaluation and treatment. If a patient does not have a physician to act as an advocate at the time of the cancer diagnosis, a physician should quickly be chosen to serve in this capacity throughout the course of the illness.[24]

In most situations, other healthcare professionals are available to help patients cope with the emotional effects of cancer. Nurses who spend much time at a patient's bedside can provide important information to the patient and physician. Social workers are invaluable in assessing the level of a family's psychological distress and their capacity to cope with the illness.[28] Community resources such as veteran patient programs (e.g., Reach to Recovery) that involve people who have coped with cancer in their own lives can provide valuable information and help reassure patients and their families. The local clergy may be able to provide spiritual guidance based on their knowledge of a particular patient's and family's needs.[25] Ultimately, most cancer patients will be treated by a radiation therapist. The therapists must not only treat the patient's body; they must also help provide emotional support, all within the scope of practice for the profession. The responsibilities and scope of practice of radiation therapists are included in Box 2.6.

DYING PATIENTS AND THEIR FAMILIES

Care for the dying patient and family has changed dramatically over the years with improvements in technology. The evolution of terminal care changed curing to caring, beginning with the publication of Dr. Elisabeth Kübler-Ross's book *On Death and Dying.*[3] Because radiation therapists and their students deal daily with terminally ill patients, they must explore questions concerning patients' rights, refusal of treatment, and quality of life, and must understand the emotional state of cancer patients. A basic fear of dying is present in all humans. Patients fear the diagnosis, the treatment, the disease, and the death associated with it.[20] Dr. Kübler-Ross identified a grief cycle experienced by individuals with terminal illnesses and other catastrophic events that negatively affect their lives.[3] The grief cycle may include the following stages:

1. Shock: The initial reaction to hearing news of the bad event
2. Denial: Pretending that what is, isn't
3. Anger: Outward demonstration of pent-up emotion and frustration
4. Bargaining: Trying to find a way out of the situation
5. Depression: Realization of the facts
6. Testing: Searching for realistic resolutions to the problem
7. Acceptance: Coping with the situation and finding a way forward

Those in the grief cycle obviously experience highs and lows. It is a part of the radiation therapist's job to identify the cycles and to provide whatever type of emotional support is necessary to get the patient through the cycles. As mentioned earlier in the chapter, discovering one's own EI helps to identify and cope with the emotional needs of patients, although a listening ear is often all that patients require.

Although the final stage of a terminal illness is obvious, its beginning is less well-defined. At some point during the treatment of patients who have metastatic cancer, the focus of management shifts

BOX 2.6 Practice Standards for Medical Imaging and Radiation Therapy (Radiation Therapy Practice Standards)

Preface to Practice Standards

A profession's practice standards serve as a guide for appropriate practice. The practice standards define the practice and establish general criteria to determine compliance. Practice standards are authoritative statements established by the profession to judge the quality of practice, service, and education provided by individuals who practice in medical imaging and radiation therapy.

Practice standards can be used by individual facilities to develop job descriptions and practice parameters. Individuals outside the imaging, therapeutic, and radiation science community can use the standards as an overview of the role and responsibilities of the individual as defined by the profession.

The individual must be educationally prepared and clinically competent as a prerequisite to professional practice. Federal and state laws, accreditation standards necessary to participate in government programs, and lawful institutional policies and procedures supersede these standards.

Format

The practice standards are divided into six sections: introduction, scope of practice, clinical performance, quality performance, professional performance, and advisory opinion statements.

Introduction. The introduction provides definitions for the practice and the education and certification for individuals in addition to an overview of the specific practice.

Scope of Practice. The scope of practice delineates the parameters of the specific practice.

Clinical Performance Standards. The clinical performance standards define the activities of the individual in the care of patients and delivery of diagnostic or therapeutic procedures. The section incorporates patient assessment and management with procedural analysis, performance, and evaluation.

Quality Performance Standards. The quality performance standards define the activities of the individual in the technical areas of performance, including equipment and material assessment, safety standards, and total quality management.

Professional Performance Standards. The professional performance standards define the activities of the individual in the areas of education, interpersonal relationships, self-assessment, and ethical behavior.

Advisory Opinion Statements. The advisory opinions are interpretations of the standards intended for clarification and guidance for specific practice issues.

Each performance standards section is subdivided into individual standards. The standards are numbered and followed by a term or set of terms that identify the standards, such as "assessment" or "analysis/determination." The next statement is the expected performance of the individual when performing the procedure or treatment. A rationale statement follows and explains why an individual should adhere to the particular standard of performance.

Criteria. Criteria are used in evaluating an individual's performance. Each set is divided into two parts: the general criteria and the specific criteria. Both criteria should be used when evaluating performance.

General Criteria. General criteria are written in a style that applies to imaging and radiation science individuals. These criteria are the same in all of the practice standards, with the exception of limited x-ray machine operators, and should be used for the appropriate area of practice.

Specific Criteria. Specific criteria meet the needs of the individuals in the various areas of professional performance. Although many areas of performance within imaging and radiation sciences are similar, others are not. The specific criteria are drafted with these differences in mind.

Introduction to Radiation Therapy Practice Standards

Definition

The practice of radiation therapy is performed by healthcare professionals responsible for the administration of ionizing radiation for the purpose of treating diseases, primarily cancer.

The complex nature of cancer frequently requires the use of multiple treatment specialties. Radiation therapy is one such specialty. It requires an interdisciplinary team of radiation oncologists, radiation therapists, medical radiation physicists, medical dosimetrists, and nurses. Typically, the radiation therapist administers the radiation to the patient throughout the course of treatment. Radiation therapy integrates scientific knowledge, technical competency, and patient interaction skills to deliver safe and accurate treatment with compassion.

Radiation therapists must demonstrate an understanding of anatomy, physiology, pathology, and medical terminology. In addition, comprehension of oncology, radiobiology, radiation physics, radiation oncology techniques, radiation safety, and the psychosocial aspects of cancer are required.

Radiation therapists must maintain a high degree of accuracy in positioning and treatment techniques. They must possess, use, and maintain knowledge about radiation protection and safety. Radiation therapists assist the radiation oncologist in localizing the treatment area, participating in treatment planning, and delivering high doses of ionizing radiation as prescribed by the radiation oncologist.

Radiation therapists are the primary liaison between patients and other members of the radiation oncology team. They also provide a link to other healthcare providers, such as social workers and dietitians. Radiation therapists must remain sensitive to the physical and emotional needs of the patient through good communication, patient assessment, patient monitoring, and patient care skills. Radiation therapy often involves daily treatments extending over a period of several weeks utilizing highly sophisticated equipment. It requires a great deal of initial planning, as well as constant patient care and monitoring. As members of the healthcare team, radiation therapists participate in quality improvement processes and continually assess their professional performance.

Radiation therapists think critically and use independent, professional, and ethical judgment in all aspects of their work. They engage in continuing education to include their area of practice and to enhance patient care, radiation safety, public education, knowledge, and technical competence.

Education and Certification

Radiation therapists prepare for their role on the interdisciplinary team by successfully completing an accredited educational program in radiation therapy and attaining appropriate primary certification by American Registry of Radiologic Technologists (ARRT). Those who have passed the radiation therapy examination use the credential R.T.(T).

To maintain ARRT certification, radiation therapists must complete appropriate continuing education requirements to sustain a level of expertise and awareness of changes and advances in practice.

Overview

An interdisciplinary team of radiation oncologists, radiation therapists, dosimetrists, medical physicists, and other support staff plays a critical role in the delivery of health services as new modalities emerge and the need for radiation therapy treatment procedures evolve. A comprehensive procedure list for the radiation therapist is impractical because clinical activities vary by practice needs and expertise of the radiation therapist. Although radiation therapists gain more experience, knowledge, and clinical competence, the clinical activities for the radiation therapist may evolve.

BOX 2.6 **Practice Standards for Medical Imaging and Radiation Therapy (Radiation Therapy Practice Standards)—cont'd**

State statute, regulation, or lawful community custom may dictate practice parameters. Wherever there is a conflict between these standards and state or local statutes or regulations, the state or local statutes or regulations supersede these standards. A radiation therapist should, within the boundaries of all applicable legal requirements and restrictions, exercise individual thought, judgment, and discretion in the performance of the procedure.

Radiation Therapist Scope of Practice

The scope of practice of the medical imaging and radiation therapy professional includes:

- Providing optimal patient care.
- Receiving, relaying, and documenting verbal, written, and electronic orders in the patient's medical record.
- Corroborating patient's clinical history with procedure, ensuring information is documented and available for use by a licensed independent practitioner.
- Verifying informed consent.
- Assuming responsibility for patient needs during procedures.
- Preparing patients for procedures.
- Applying principles of ALARA (as low as reasonably achievable) to minimize exposure to patient, self, and others.
- Performing venipuncture as prescribed by a licensed independent practitioner.
- Starting and maintaining intravenous access as prescribed by a licensed independent practitioner.
- Identifying, preparing, and/or administering medications as prescribed by a licensed independent practitioner.
- Evaluating images for technical quality, ensuring proper identification is recorded.
- Identifying and managing emergency situations.
- Providing education.
- Educating and monitoring students and other healthcare providers.
- Performing ongoing quality assurance activities.
- Applying the principles of patient safety during all aspects of patient care.

The scope of practice of the radiation therapist also includes:

1. Delivering radiation therapy treatments as prescribed by a radiation oncologist.
2. Performing simulation, treatment planning procedures, and dosimetric calculations as prescribed by a radiation oncologist.
3. Utilizing imaging technologies for the explicit purpose of simulation, treatment planning, and treatment delivery as prescribed by a radiation oncologist.
4. Detecting and reporting significant changes in patients' conditions and determining when to withhold treatment until the physician is consulted.
5. Monitoring doses to normal tissues within the irradiated volume to ensure tolerance levels are not exceeded.
6. Constructing/preparing immobilization, beam directional, and beam modification devices.
7. Participating in brachytherapy procedures.

Radiation Therapy Clinical Performance Standards

Standard One—Assessment
  The radiation therapist collects pertinent data about the patient and the procedure.
Standard Two—Analysis/Determination
  The radiation therapist analyzes the information obtained during the assessment phase and develops an action plan to complete the procedure.
Standard Three—Patient Education
  The radiation therapist provides information about the procedure and related health issues according to protocol.

Standard Four—Performance
  The radiation therapist performs the action plan.
Standard Five—Evaluation
  The radiation therapist determines whether the goals of the action plan have been achieved.
Standard Six—Implementation
  The radiation therapist implements the revised action plan.
Standard Seven—Outcomes Measurement
  The radiation therapist reviews and evaluates the outcome of the procedure.
Standard Eight—Documentation
  The radiation therapist documents information about patient care, the procedure, and the final outcome.

Radiation Therapy Quality Performance Standards

Standard One—Assessment
  The radiation therapist collects pertinent information regarding equipment, procedures, and the work environment.
Standard Two—Analysis/Determination
  The radiation therapist analyzes information collected during the assessment phase to determine the need for changes to equipment, procedures, or the work environment.
Standard Three—Education
  The radiation therapist informs the patient, public, and other healthcare providers about procedures, equipment, and facilities.
Standard Four—Performance
  The radiation therapist performs quality assurance activities.
Standard Five—Evaluation
  The radiation therapist evaluates quality assurance results and establishes an appropriate action plan.
Standard Six—Implementation
  The radiation therapist implements the quality assurance action plan for equipment, materials, and processes.
Standard Seven—Outcomes Measurement
  The radiation therapist assesses the outcome of the quality management action plan for equipment, materials, and processes.
Standard Eight—Documentation
  The radiation therapist documents quality assurance activities and results.

Radiation Therapy Professional Performance Standards

Standard One—Quality
  The radiation therapist strives to provide optimal patient care.
Standard Two—Self-Assessment
  The radiation therapist evaluates personal performance.
Standard Three —Education
  The radiation therapist acquires and maintains current knowledge in practice.
Standard Four—Collaboration and Collegiality
  The radiation therapist promotes a positive and collaborative practice atmosphere with other members of the healthcare team.
Standard Five—Ethics
  The radiation therapist adheres to the profession's accepted ethical standards.
Standard Six—Research and Innovation
  The radiation therapist participates in the acquisition and dissemination of knowledge and the advancement of the profession.

Radiation Therapy Advisory Opinion Statements

Injecting medication in peripherally inserted central catheter lines or ports with a power injector is within the scope of practice where federal or state law and/or institutional policy permits.

From the American Society of Radiologic Technologists. *The Practice Standards for Medical Imaging and Radiation Therapy: Radiation Therapy Practice Standards.* Albuquerque, NM: American Society of Radiologic Technologists; 2018.

from aggressive therapy to palliative care, from efforts to suppress tumor growth to attempts to control symptoms. Signals that the goals of treatment must be changed include the recognition of the tumor's progression, the failure of therapy to control the disease, the patient's deteriorating strength, and the patient's loss of interest in pursuing previously important objectives and pleasures. Rarely is this decision difficult; rather, it reflects the natural acceptance of the inevitability of patients' deaths on the part of families, caregivers, and patients themselves.[28] Indeed, Dr. Kübler-Ross identifies this acceptance as the last stage in the grief cycle.

During the past decade, people in many countries have come to accept the notion that aggressive life support (i.e., prolonging life to the bitter end) is often not the right action to take. The ethics of allowing terminally ill patients to die with dignity has evolved. In recent years, the concept of the individual's right of self-determination has been central in the resuscitation issue. The medical and legal communities have recognized that self-determination is no more than an extension of the patient's right to informed consent. In the past, some physicians may have been placed in the extremely uncomfortable position of wanting to comply with a patient's wish to die in peace and dignity but fearing a malpractice suit by family members for failing to do all that should, could, or might have been done to prolong the life of the dying patient. The response to this dilemma, the living will, also called an Advance Directive, was created. The purpose of the living will is to allow the competent adult to provide direction to healthcare providers concerning his or her choice of treatment under certain conditions, should the individual no longer be competent by reason of illness or other infirmity, to make those decisions. The living will also provides the patients' family with knowledge of what a person would or would not want done. The concept of the living will assumes that the individual executing the directive:

1. Demonstrates competency at the time.
2. Directs that no artificial or heroic measures be undertaken to preserve his or her life.
3. Requests that medication be provided to relieve pain.
4. Intends to relieve the hospital and physician of legal responsibility for complying with the directives in the living will.
5. Has the signature witnessed by two disinterested individuals who are not related, are not mentioned in the last will, and have no claim on the estate.[28]

In practice, actions to carry out a living will may involve withholding or discontinuing interventions such as ventilator support, chemotherapy, surgery, radiation therapy, and even assisted nutrition and hydration.[24] The decision to withhold curative therapy is based on the conclusion that the course of the patient's disease is irreversible and extraordinary measures to sustain life are not in the patient's best interest. To nullify the routinely mandatory order for cardiopulmonary resuscitation in the event of a cardiac arrest, many hospitals require the physician in charge of a terminally ill patient to issue a specific do-not-resuscitate (DNR) order. The Joint Commission requires that every hospital have a no-code DNR policy.[16] Plans for the patient's death, including issuance of the DNR order, should be made soon after the issue has been discussed with the patient and family. In most situations, patients and their families are relieved to know that every effort will be made to maintain the patient's comfort and that death will be peaceful.[26] The only problem with this is that often those treating the patient are not aware of the DNR order, and many times a patient may be resuscitated in the diagnostic imaging or radiation therapy department. To comply with a DNR, everyone involved in the patient's care must be made aware of its existence. All hospitals must have written policies and procedures describing the

way that patients' rights are protected at their institutions. The living will is not the only document that can be used by individuals to guide the direction of their medical treatment should they become unable to do so.

POLST, which stands for Physician Orders for Life-Sustaining Treatment, is a national movement that promotes the rights of seriously ill or frail patients to make informed decisions about medical treatments and to have those preferences honored by healthcare professionals. More information is available at: http://polst.org/professionals-page/?pro=1.

The durable power of attorney for healthcare is another such document. The durable power of attorney for healthcare is a legal document that allows an individual to designate any willing individual, 18 years of age or older, to be his or her surrogate and make decisions in matters of healthcare. The designee can be a family member, friend, or another trusted individual. The durable power can be used to accept or refuse treatment; however, the treatments that are desired or not desired must be specified in the document. Both the living will and the durable power of attorney for healthcare are considered advance directives. Both documents are useful in that they clearly describe the wishes of the patient when he or she was considered competent. These documents may also contain instructions for disposal of the body upon death, especially when an individual chooses to donate his or her body to medical science for research. This helps avoid treatment and other conflicts among families and surrogates.[16]

Before treating a patient, always check the healthcare record for do-not-resuscitate orders and advance directives.

Hospice Care

During the Middle Ages, a hospice was a way station for travelers. Today a hospice represents an intermediate station for patients with terminal illnesses. The hospice movement began with programs to provide palliative and supportive care for terminally ill patients and their families, and still provides those services today. Hospice services also include home, respite, and inpatient hospital care and support during bereavement. In addition to providing 24-hour care of the patient, the goal of hospice care is to help the dying patient live a full life and to offer hope, comfort, and a suitable setting for a peaceful, dignified death. The hospice team assists family members in caring for the patient by providing physical, emotional, psychological, and spiritual support. Several types of hospices are available, including free-standing facilities, institutionally based units, and community-based programs.[13]

Patients may enter the hospice on their own or may be referred by family members, physicians, hospital-affiliated continuing care coordinators and social workers, visiting nurses, friends, or clergy. Although admission criteria vary, they usually include the following: a terminal illness with an estimated life expectancy of 6 months or less; residence in a defined geographic area; access to a caregiver from immediate family members, relatives, friends, or neighbors; and the desire for the patient to remain at home during the last stage of the illness. On the initial assessment visit, a member of the hospice team obtains the patient's medical history and emotional and psychosocial histories of the patient and family and discusses nursing concerns. After the program begins, team members meet regularly to review the care plan for each patient and put into effect and supervise services for the patient and family.[26]

Most families prefer home care for dying relatives if they can rely on the supportive environment offered by a hospice. Institutionalization is perceived as impersonal and impractical, and acute care hospitals are not designed for the long-term care of terminal patients. A private home can be transformed to accommodate the level of care required, and nurses can instruct family members in physical care techniques, symptom management, nutrition, and medications. After the patient and family are made to feel confident and capable of managing the physical care, they can begin to address the emotional and spiritual issues surrounding death. During a patient's terminal illness, many problems arise, some of which test the hospice team's ingenuity and endurance. In general, however, simple remedies, common sense, good nursing care, preventive medicine, and the generous use of analgesia should be used to help reduce patient suffering.[20]

MEDICAL-LEGAL ASPECTS OF CANCER MANAGEMENT

Definitions and Terminology

Radiation therapists need to perform their duties with confidence, especially in today's litigious society. They must be aware that consumers are more aware of the standard of care that they should receive and more cognizant about seeking legal compensation. Healthcare professionals must become more knowledgeable about legal definitions concerning the standard of care. Legally, the term "standard of care" means exercising that degree of care, education, knowledge, and skills that is possessed by others in the same profession.[29]

The type of law that governs noncriminal activities is known as civil law. One type of civil law is commonly called "tort law." The word *tort* is an Old French word meaning "wrong."[23] In today's terms, a tort is considered a wrongful act committed against a person or a person's property, the one exception being breach of contract. Tort law is personal injury law. The act may be malicious and intentional or the result of negligence and disregard for the rights of others. Torts include conditions for which the law allows compensation to be paid to an individual damaged or injured by another. This type of law was created to preserve peace among individuals by providing a venue for assessing fault for wrongdoing (culpability), deter those who wrong others, and provide compensation for those injured.[28] Two types of torts exist: unintentional and intentional.[17] Unintentional torts are considered those acts that are not intentionally harmful but still result in damage to property or injury to person. Examples of unintentional torts in the healthcare setting include failure of the healthcare provider to properly provide for the safety of a patient or failure to properly educate a patient, resulting in harm. Intentional torts are defined as willful acts committed against person or property. Healthcare providers incur duties incidental to their professional roles. The law does not consider the professional and patient to be on equal terms; greater legal burdens or duties are imposed on the healthcare provider.[28]

> Tort law is a type of civil law.

Several situations exist in which a tort action can be taken against the healthcare professional because of deliberate action. Intentional torts include assault, battery, false imprisonment, libel, slander, invasion of privacy, and intentional infliction of emotional distress.

Assault is defined as the threat of touching in an injurious way. If patients feel threatened and believe they will be touched in a harmful manner, justification may exist for a charge of assault. To avoid this, professionals must always explain what is going to happen during a procedure and reassure the patient in any situation involving the threat of harm.[17] Radiation therapists must always seek permission to touch and treat a patient.

Battery consists of the actual act of harmful, unconsented, or unwarranted contact with an individual. Again, a clear explanation of what is to be done is essential. If the patient refuses to be touched, that wish must be respected. Battery implies that the touch is a willful act to harm or provoke, but even the most well-intentioned touch may fall into this category if the patient has expressly forbidden it. This should not prevent the therapist from placing a reassuring hand on the patient's shoulder, as long as the patient has not forbidden it and the therapist does not intend to harm or invade the patient's privacy. However, any procedure performed against a patient's will may be construed as battery.[6]

False imprisonment is the intentional confinement without authorization by a person who physically constricts another with force, threat of force, or confining clothing or structures. This becomes an issue if a patient wishes to leave and is not allowed to do so. Inappropriate use of physical restraints may also constitute false imprisonment. The confinement must be intentional and without legal justification. Freedom from unlawful restraint is a right protected by law. If the patient is improperly restrained, the law allows redress in the form of damages. Proof of all elements of false imprisonment must be established to support the claim that an illegal act was performed. False imprisonment requires proof that the alleged victim was really confined, that the confinement was intended by the perpetrator, and that consent was not obtained. If they are dangerous to themselves or others, patients may be restrained. An example of false imprisonment is a therapist using restraints on a patient without the patient's consent or without informing and obtaining consent from the family of a child.[24]

Libel is written defamation of character. Oral defamation is termed slander. These torts affect the reputation and good name of a person. The basic element of the tort of defamation is that the oral or written communication is made to a person other than the one defamed. The law recognizes certain relationships that require an individual to be allowed to speak without fear of being sued for defamation of character. For example, radiation oncology department supervisors who must evaluate employees or give references regarding an employee's work have a qualified privilege. Radiation therapists can protect themselves from this civil tort by using caution while conversing within the hearing of patients and their families.[28]

Invasion of privacy charges may result if confidentiality of information has not been maintained or the patient's body has been improperly and unnecessarily exposed or touched. Protection of the patient's modesty is vital during simulation, planning, and treatment procedures.[24] Healthcare providers must make sure that the patient is covered to the extent that treatment allows. Maintaining privacy is also extremely important in regard to video monitors in treatment areas. No one should ever be in the viewing area except authorized and necessary staff members.

Negligence refers to neglect or omission of reasonable care or caution. An unintentional injury to a patient may be negligence. The standard of reasonable care is based on the doctrine of the reasonably prudent person. This standard requires that a person perform as would any reasonable individual of ordinary prudence with comparable education and skill and under similar circumstances. In the relationship between a professional person and a patient, an implied contract exists to provide reasonable care. An act of negligence in the context of such a relationship is called *malpractice*. Negligence, as used in malpractice law, is not necessarily the same as carelessness. A person's conduct can be considered negligent in the legal sense even if the individual acts carefully. For example, if a therapist without prior education and training on a specific procedure attempts the procedure and does it carefully, the conduct can be deemed negligent if harm results to the patient.[13]

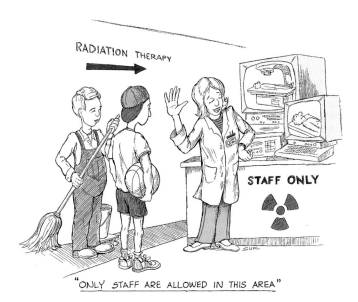

RADIATION THERAPY

STAFF ONLY

"ONLY STAFF ARE ALLOWED IN THIS AREA"

LEGAL DOCTRINES

Doctrine of Personal Liability

Radiation therapists should be concerned about the risk of being named as defendants in medical malpractice suits. Things can go wrong, and mistakes can be made. The legal responsibility of the radiation therapist is to give safe care to the patient.

The fundamental rule of law is that persons are liable for their own negligent conduct. This is known as the doctrine of personal liability and means that the law does not permit wrongdoers to avoid liability for their own actions, even though someone else may also be held legally liable for the wrongful conduct in question under another rule of law. Although they cannot be held liable for actions of hospitals or physicians, therapists can be held responsible and liable for their own negligent actions.[5]

Doctrine of Respondeat Superior

The doctrine of respondeat superior ("let the master answer") is a legal doctrine that states that an employer is liable for negligent acts of employees that occur while they are carrying out the orders or serving the interests of the employer. As early as 1698, courts declared that a master must respond to injuries and losses of persons caused by the master's servants. Nineteenth-century courts adopted the phrase respondeat superior, which is founded on the principle of social duty that all persons, whether by themselves or by their agents or servants, shall conduct their affairs in a manner not to injure others.[6] This principle is based on the concept that profit from the work of others, and the duty to select and supervise employees, are joined in liability.[7]

Doctrine of Res Ipsa Loquitur

In a malpractice action for negligence, the plaintiff has the burden of proving that a standard of care exists for the treatment of the medical problem, the healthcare provider failed to abide by the standard, this failure was the direct cause of the patient's injury, and damage was incurred. The legal community describes the aforementioned circumstances as the steps in a medical malpractice lawsuit, such as duty, breach of duty, and causation and damages. If the alleged negligence involves matters outside of general knowledge, an acceptable medical expert must establish these criteria. A long-accepted substitute for the medical expert has been the doctrine of res ipsa loquitur,[10] which means "the thing speaks for itself." Courts have decided to resolve the problem of expert unavailability in certain circumstances by applying res ipsa loquitur, which requires the defendant to explain the events and convince the court that no negligence was involved.[28] The Standards of Practice for Radiation Therapists may be used by either the defense or the prosecution to support or refute negligent behavior, as can expert witnesses. These standards are readily accessible to everyone via the ASRT website.

Doctrine of Foreseeability

The doctrine of foreseeability is a principle of law that holds an individual liable for all natural and proximate consequences of negligent acts to another individual to whom a duty is owed. The negligent acts could or should have been reasonably foreseen under the circumstances. A simpler definition is persons reasonably foreseeing that certain actions or inactions on their part could result in injury to others. In addition, the injury suffered must be related to the foreseeable injury. Routine radiation therapy equipment checks are important in overcoming this doctrine.[6]

RISK MANAGEMENT

Conceived little more than a decade ago, the concept of risk control, or risk management, was believed to be the key element in loss prevention from adverse medical incidents. Risk management links every quality improvement program with measurable outcomes necessary to determine overall effectiveness. Effectiveness here means success in reducing patient injury. An acute care hospital or medical center has the duty to exercise such reasonable care in looking after and protecting the patient. The legal responsibility of any healthcare practitioner is safe care. Risk management, which is a matter of patient safety, is the process of avoiding or controlling the risk of financial loss to staff members and the hospital or medical center. Poor-quality care creates a risk of injury to patients and leads to increased financial liability. Risk management protects financial assets by managing insurance for potential liability by reducing liability through surveillance. The job of risk management is to identify actual and potential causes of accidents or incidents involving patients and employees and to implement programs to eliminate or reduce such occurrences.[6] The number one reason for medical liability (malpractice) claims in medical imaging and radiation therapy is patient falls.

Hospital liability and malpractice insurance, also known as *patient liability insurance,* is intended to cover all claims against the hospital that arise from the alleged negligence of physician staff members and employees. Many have discussed whether radiation therapists should carry malpractice insurance. In making that decision, persons must determine the extent of provisions for malpractice coverage in their institutions. According to the doctrine of respondeat superior, the employer is liable for employees' negligent acts during work. The authority and responsibility of a physician supervising and controlling the activities of the employee supersede those of the employer, according to the doctrine of the borrowed servant. Regardless of how these legal doctrines may be applied, the fundamental rule of law that every therapist should clearly know and understand is the doctrine of personal liability. Persons are liable for their own negligent conduct, although most healthcare employees are covered under their employers' liability insurance. A wrongdoer may not be able to escape responsibility even though someone else may be sued and held legally responsible. In some situations, hospital insurers who have paid malpractice claims have successfully recovered damages from negligent employees by filing separate lawsuits against them.[6]

Hospital employees are instructed to report any patient injury to administration through the department manager. An incident report is routinely used to document unusual events in the hospital. An incident is defined as any happening that is not consistent with the routine operation of the hospital or the routine care of a particular patient. It may be an accident or a situation that could result in an accident.[23] Hospitals use incident reports in their accident-prevention programs to advise insurers of potential suits and prepare defenses against suits that might arise from documented incidents. Incident reports should be prepared according to the institution's published policies and procedures. An incident report is no place for opinion, accusation, or conjecture; it should contain only facts concerning the incident reported.[30] Incident reports should never be placed in the patient's written or electronic chart. There are usually written hospital and departmental procedures for completing and submitting incident reports. These reports ultimately end up in the office of risk management.

> Incident reports should not be placed in patients' written or electronic healthcare records.

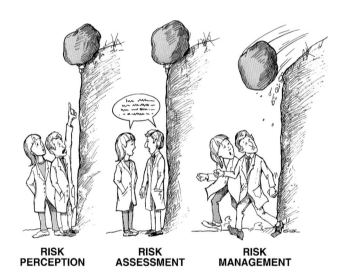

RISK PERCEPTION   **RISK ASSESSMENT**   **RISK MANAGEMENT**

MEDICAL RECORDS

The radiation oncology medical record is used to chronologically document the care and treatment rendered to the patient. All components of the patient's evaluation and cancer must be documented in the radiation oncology record. The format usually includes the following: a general information sheet listing the names of pertinent relatives, follow-up contacts, family physicians, and persons to notify in an emergency; an initial history and findings from the physical examination; reports of the pathology examinations, laboratory tests, diagnostic imaging procedures, and pertinent surgical procedures; photographs and anatomic drawings; medications currently used; correspondence with physicians and reimbursement organizations; treatment setup instructions; daily treatment logs; physics, treatment planning, and dosimetry data; progress notes during treatments;

summaries of treatment; and reports of follow-up examinations. Patients' radiation oncology records must be maintained and secured in the department separate from hospital and clinic records to ensure ready access at any time.[30] Radiation oncology medical records are commonly maintained in both paper and electronic formats. Medical record entries should be made in clear and concise language that can be understood by all professional staff members attending to the patient. Handwritten entries must be legible. An illegible record is worse than no record because it documents a failure by staff members to maintain a proper record and may severely weaken a hospital's or physician's defense in a negligence action. Entries into the paper record should be made in ink, and persons making entries should identify themselves clearly by placing their signatures after each entry. The hospital and physician should be able to determine who participates in each episode of patient care.[28] Entries should be made daily by the therapist operating the treatment machine. Any other therapist involved in the treatment of a patient that day should also check the daily entry for accuracy and initial the record.

Medical records are sometimes used by staff members to convey remarks inappropriate for a patient's chart. The following are examples of entries that should never be made:

- This is the third time therapist X has been negligent.
- Dr. A has mistreated this patient again.
- This patient is a chronic complainer and a nuisance.
- This patient smells; nursing staff should see that she gets a bath.

Such editorial comments are inevitably used against the physician and hospital in any negligence action filed by the patient. In addition, although the trend moves toward access by patients to their own medical records, patients are more likely to read and react with hostility to such comments.[28]

The general rule is to avoid the need for making corrections, but because humans are not perfect, corrections must be made from time to time. In the paper record, a staff member should simply draw a line through an incorrect entry because doing so allows others to identify what was initially written and corrected. The staff member should initial the correction, enter the time and date, and insert the correct information. Mistakes in the chart should not be erased, blacked out, or covered with a "white-out" product because doing so may create suspicion concerning the original entry.[30] Proper charting and documentation protocols should be taught in healthcare professional educational programs, as well as in the clinical setting. There are proper charting procedures.[7] The following lists contain information on charting information in the medical record in the "always" and "never" categories.

Always

1. Write so that others can read what is written (legibly, in paper records).
2. Make electronic entries so that others understand what is being communicated.
3. Use ink (in paper records).
4. Use correct spelling and approved standard medical abbreviations.
5. Enter accurate information: correct and precise.
6. Chart concisely.
7. Provide entries that are thorough.
8. Begin each new entry with the date and time (military notations) of the entry.
9. Chart information as it occurs.
10. Keep the information confidential.
11. Sign each entry with your name and title (electronic identification information or electronic signatures are acceptable).

Never

1. Chart with a pencil (in paper records).
2. Black-out, white-out, or erase entries.
3. Include unnecessary details.
4. Include critical comments about anyone (e.g., the patient, his or her family, or other healthcare professionals).
5. Leave blank spaces.
6. Use unapproved or improper abbreviations.
7. Record information for others.
8. Divulge patient information.
9. Use initials in place of your signature.
10. Chart for anyone else.
11. Leave a patient's electronic healthcare chart open.

Charting and other forms of documentation are written communication tools used to provide comprehensive healthcare data on an individual patient basis. Charting is the recording of patient information and observation regarding a specific patient in his or her long-term written or electronic record, such as the patient's chart. Documentation, on the other hand, is also the recording of any information relevant to patient care and treatment, but that information does not have to be entered into the patient chart.[7] There are forms used in a variety of healthcare departments that are specific to the services offered by that department. These documents are generally stored in the department only, for reference and use by that department only. What needs to be remembered most is that the patient's medical record is a legal document and as such is admissible in a court of law. It provides evidence concerning the care and treatment provided to the patient and the standards under which the care and treatment were administered.[27]

Radiation therapists under the direct supervision of the radiation oncologist and medical physicist carry out daily treatments. All treatment applications must be described in detail (orders) and signed by the responsible physician. Similarly, any changes in the planned treatment by the physician may require adjustment in immobilization, new calculations, and even a new treatment plan. Therefore, the therapist, physicist, and dosimetrist must all be notified of the changes.[27]

SUMMARY

- The ethical and legal considerations in cancer management are numerous and varied. The development of professional ethical characteristics begins with the discovery of an individual's personal values.
- Ethics are based on values, and knowing one's own values serves to enhance a person's concept of right versus wrong. Professional ethics is an extension of personal ethics. Healthcare professionals innately subscribe to the Principles of Biomedical Ethics.
- Professional standards guide the practice of medical imaging and radiation therapy. The Standards of Ethics, including the Code of Ethics and the Rules of Ethics, along with the Practice Standards for Medical Imaging and Radiation Therapy, are the prevailing structured professional guides and rules under which medical imaging technologists, radiologist assistants, radiation therapists, and aspiring students perform their healthcare duties.
- In healthcare, failure to perform according to ethical and other professional standards subjects practitioners to penalties under the law.
- In addition to the development of technical knowledge and skills, the foundation of radiation oncology includes standards of conduct and ideals essential to meeting the emotional and physical needs of patients.

- Radiation therapists must first view their profession as more than just a job. Student therapists should not pursue a simple goal to just pass a series of examinations and eventually the registry or earn a degree. Student therapists should set goals that establish them as professionals.
- An ideal professional has superior technical knowledge and works in harmony and cooperation with peers, physicians, and other healthcare personnel. With the appropriate educational background and determination to excel, a person can practice professionalism and achieve technical excellence.
- By delivering excellent patient care within professional standards, quality patient care can be provided by a healthcare team that is focused on the needs of the patients, both emotionally and physically, while recognizing and respecting patient rights.

Case I: Quality Care for All

As a student therapist, Susan observes many clinical situations. She is assigned to a treatment area that has an extremely high volume of patients. Susan observes that a staff member has treated a patient without an important treatment device in place. When she approaches the staff member about the situation, he mumbles something about the patient being palliative. Obviously, the treatment error must be corrected. How does Susan ethically and professionally handle this issue that her conscience dictates be addressed? Is this an ethical or a legal issue?

Case II: You Really Need This Treatment

Sam is a staff radiation therapist in a large center. He has a patient on his treatment schedule who is uncooperative and verbally abusive to the staff members. It is time for the patient's treatment, but once in the treatment room, he refuses to cooperate by not getting into the position required and holding still. Sam knows the patient is uncomfortable and needs the treatment to relieve symptomatic disease. Should Sam restrain the patient and force him to have the treatment? What legal and ethical considerations are involved in Sam's final decision?

Case III: To Tell or Not to Tell

Mrs. Smith is a 50-year-old woman with three adult children. She has been admitted to the hospital for tests to rule out cancer. While the tests are being processed, her husband and children meet with the doctor and ask him not to tell Mrs. Smith whether the results are malignant. They tell the doctor that she is afraid of cancer and that if she is given the diagnosis, she will become severely depressed and give up all desire to live. The physician is not comfortable with this request, but the family insists. The physician reluctantly agrees. What ethical and legal concepts are implicated in the family's request and physician's decision to comply with it?

Case IV: Maintaining a Standard of Care

Currently employed in a small radiation oncology center, Sandra has the task of orienting a new employee to the department and the treatment machine to which she is assigned. The new radiation therapist, Jane, although older than Sandra, is newly graduated from an educational program and has recently taken the American Registry of Radiologic Technologists Examination for Radiation Therapy. She has not yet received her credentials but is certainly qualified to begin her position in the department. In the course of working with Jane, Sandra begins to realize that there are some physical limitations for Jane. Jane has freely shared that she has a degenerative problem with her hands and has some loss of strength. When Sandra begins to make some suggestions to modify the handling of the custom blocks and other heavy treatment devices over the patient lying on the table, Jane becomes extremely defensive. Sandra is aware that the safety of her patients is at risk, and she must take some action. Discuss what that action might be and whether this might be an ethical or a legal situation.

Case V: Time Challenges in Treatment Delivery

A new patient is scheduled to start treatment on Jim's treatment machine on Monday. Everyone has warned him that the new patient is very angry and very difficult to schedule for procedures. Jim meets Mrs. Jones on Monday morning, greets her warmly, and does all that he can to put her at ease during the long process of starting her treatments. When the time comes for him to discuss her appointments, Mrs. Jones insists that she needs different appointment times daily. Jim carefully explains that they cannot accommodate quite that many changes in the schedule for the 7 weeks that she will be in treatment. Jim and Mrs. Jones reach an agreement that seems to satisfy them both. For the next several weeks, Mrs. Jones arrives at a different time every day. Sometimes she calls to reschedule; sometimes she just appears at the department with no notice. Jim and the other therapist he works with try very hard to accommodate their patient, but it begins to cause havoc with the rest of their schedule and inconvenience most of their other patients. Jim approaches Mrs. Jones with the question of whether another appointment time would be better for her. Mrs. Jones quickly becomes verbally abusive, screaming that she wishes she had gone elsewhere for treatment. She shouts that she doesn't want to talk about this anymore and she is tired of being chastised every time she is 5 minutes late. Because this is the first time Jim or his partner has mentioned her tardiness, they are surprised at her reaction. Discuss how they should handle the situation. Consider whether they will be able to discuss this with Mrs. Jones or should refer her to a supervisor, because she is so convinced that she has been harassed about her appointments since the beginning. What kind of legal or ethical issues does this case history contain?

Case VI: A Call to Intervene

Jim is a radiation therapist at Mercy Hospital. He learns that his widowed, childless, 89-year-old neighbor, Mrs. Dysart, has been admitted to the hospital where he works. She has some type of heart ailment and is on oxygen and a heart monitor. Every day Jim goes to visit her. She asks him to read scripture to her and he does. During a few days, Mrs. Dysart tells Jim that she knows that her time on earth may be nearing the end. He tries to convince her that she has plenty of life left and to not give up. She confides in Jim that she does not want to be resuscitated should her heart stop beating. He asks whether she has an advance directive, and she tells him no.

One evening after work, Jim goes to visit Mrs. Dysart, and she's not feeling well at all. She asks Jim to read to her again, and he does so. In the midst of his reading, Mrs. Dysart starts to cough and clutch her chest. Jim stands up and goes to her, asking if she's OK. Suddenly, the heart monitor beeps a warning, and Jim looks at the straight line it shows. He then looks back at Mrs. Dysart, and she has passed out. What should Jim do? What would you do if you were Jim?

Case VII: To Tell or Not to Tell: Is That a Question?

Lottie has just taken her American Registry of Radiologic Technologists (ARRT) Therapy Certification Examination, and was given a preliminary score of 97. She is extremely happy while she returns to work. Of course she has to tell everyone there and makes the announcement proudly. Everyone applauds and gives her congratulation accolades. Later, one of classmates and best friend, D.D., takes her aside and tells her that she is scheduled to take her exam the following morning. D.D. asks Lottie if she can tell her some of the questions on the exam. D.D. is not one of the intellectually brightest students in the class, and Lottie knows that any information she gives her will certainly help her score. What should Lottie do? What would you do?

Case VIII: Time: A Serious Matter

Trusty VanSmoot has had a very eventful year. He got married, had a child, moved several times, and his father was hospitalized numerous times for health problems. Given his wife, baby, father, and his job, Trusty has had little time for himself. Trusty receives his yearly registration renewal form from the American Registry of Radiologic Technologists (ARRT), and recognizes he may not have completed the requisite continuing education credits. He thinks about the situation and decides that there is little chance he will be audited. He signs the form, attesting that he has his continuing education, encloses a check, and mails the form. Two weeks later, Trusty receives an audit form from ARRT. What does Trusty do now? Is it ever feasible to lie to the ARRT? What are the possible repercussions for his actions? What would you have done and why?

Case IX: Pray for Me

Susan Sunshine is a radiation therapists a Saint Regis' Medical Center. Her best friends' mother, Mrs. Hart, is one of the patients receiving treatment at the facility. She sees Mrs. Hart on almost every visit and talks with her. On this particular, day Mrs. Hart seems troubled and confides in Susan that she is not feeling optimistic that her treatment is working or even if it will work. A very religious woman, Mrs. Hart asks Susan to pray for her. Susan agrees to do so. At church the next Sunday, when the pastor asks if there are any requests for special prayer, Susan stands and asks the pastor and congregation to pray for Mrs. Hart because she has cancer. Is there anything wrong with what Susan did? Did she violate any law or principle? What would you have done? Are there any possible legal or ethical ramifications?

REVIEW QUESTIONS

The answers to the Review Questions can be found by logging on to our website at: http://evolve.elsevier.com/Washington+Leaver/principles

1. Which of the following does not govern ethics?
   a. Professional codes
   b. Popular science
   c. Patient's Bill of Rights
   d. Technical practice

2. The foundation of law is:
   a. Autonomy
   b. Confidentiality
   c. Justice
   d. Ethics

3. Moral ethics are based on which of the following?
   a. Right and wrong
   b. Institutions
   c. Legal rights
   d. Codes

4. Which of the following is an ethical principle?
   a. Justice
   b. Individual freedom
   c. Egoism
   d. Confidentiality

5. Confidentiality, truth telling, and beneficence are which of the following?
   a. Ethical principles
   b. Legal rights
   c. Ethical characteristics
   d. Legal doctrines

6. A tort falls under which of the following?
   a. Criminal law
   b. Statutory law
   c. Civil law
   d. Common law

7. Res ipsa loquitur means which of the following?
   a. Things speak for themselves
   b. The thing speaks for itself
   c. Do no harm
   d. No negligence was involved

8. Which ethical theory group evaluates an activity by weighing good against bad?
   a. Deontology
   b. Teleology
   c. Virtue ethics
   d. Moral ethics

9. Which ethical model identifies the caregiver as a scientist dealing only with the facts and does not consider the human aspect of the patient?
   a. Collegial
   b. Covenant
   c. Engineering
   d. Priestly

10. Of the following, which model presents a more cooperative method of pursuing healthcare for patients and providers than the others?
    a. Analytical
    b. Engineering
    c. Covenant
    d. Collegial

11. Core beliefs concerning what is desirable and that help assess the worth of intangibles are called:
    a. Prospects
    b. Principles
    c. Theories
    d. Values

12. Informed consent must be secured:
    a. In writing
    b. Verbally
    c. Verbally and written
    d. Upon admission

13. Consent to release a patient's healthcare records:
    a. Must be secured from the patient orally
    b. Must be secured from the patient in writing
    c. Must be secured from the patient both orally and written
    d. Is not required

14. Copies of incident reports should be:
    a. Included in the patient's medical record
    b. Sent to the floor on which the patient is housed
    c. Given to the patient
    d. Sent to the office of risk management

15. The acronym HIPAA stands for:
    a. Health Improvement Policy and Accountability Act
    b. Health Information Policy and Action Act
    c. Health Insurance Portability and Accountability Act
    d. Health Improvement Privacy and Action Act

QUESTIONS TO PONDER

1. What does deontology emphasize?
2. Discuss the difference between law and ethics, and describe a situation in which the two may be in conflict.
3. Discuss and compare the analytical and covenant models of ethical decision-making. Discuss the way these models may be used in your profession and by whom.
4. What components are involved in ethical decision-making for the radiation therapist?
5. Discuss the required elements that make up an informed consent.
6. Explain the purpose of the scope of practice as it pertains to your performance as a radiation therapist.
7. Compare and discuss the different settings available in hospice care.
8. Discuss the differences in assault and battery. What kind of action can be taken in response to either of these?
9. Analyze the difference between negligence and carelessness. Can careful behavior still result in a charge of negligence? Describe such an instance.
10. Explain the purpose of a medical record, and note the components of a complete radiation oncology record.

REFERENCES

1. Kemp K. My battle scars can help others. *Birmingham News.* 2007.
2. Cancer facts and figures 2018. Estimated new cancer cases and deaths, US. American Cancer Society website. https://www.cancer.org/content/dam/cancer-org/research/cancer-facts-and-statistics/annual-cancer-facts-and-figures/2018/cancer-facts-and-figures-2018.pdf. Accessed November 2, 2018.
3. Kubler-Ross E. *On Death and Dying.* New York, NY: MacMillan. 1973.
4. American Registry of Radiologic Technologists. *The Standards of Ethics.* Revised. St. Paul, MN: The American Registry of Radiologic Technologists. 2019.
5. Beaucamp TL, Childers JF. *Principles of Biomedical Ethics.* 6th ed. New York, NY: Oxford University Press. 2001.
6. Warner S. Code of ethics: professional and legal implications. *Radiol Technol.* 1981;52:484–494.
7. Wilson B. *Ethics and Basic Law for Medical Imaging Professionals.* Philadelphia, PA: FA Davis. 1997.
8. *Merriam-Webster's New Collegiate Dictionary.* 11th ed. Springfield, MA: Webster, Inc. 2004.
9. Rath L, Harmin M, Simon S. *Values and teaching, 2nd ed. Columbus.* Charles Merrill. 1978.
10. Gurley LT, Calloway WJ. *Introduction to Radiologic Technology.* 7th ed. St. Louis, MO: Mosby.
11. Goleman D. Emotional Intelligence. New York, NY: Bantam Books. 2006.
12. Salovey P, Mayer J. Emotional intelligence, imagination, cognition and personality. *Imagin Cogn Pers.* 1990;9(3):185–211.
13. Edge RS, Groves JH. *Ethics of Health Care: A Guide for Clinical Practice.* 3rd ed. 2005. New York, NY: Delmar.
14. Kant I. *Groundwork of the Metaphysics of Morals.* Patton JJ, trans. New York, NY: Harper and Row. 2002.
15. Miller-Keane OTM, & O'Toole MT. *Miller-Keane encyclopedia and dictionary of medicine, nursing and allied health.* A Book. 7th ed. Philadelphia, Saunders. 2003.
16. Pozgar GD. *Legal and ethical issues for health professionals.* Jones & Bartlett Learning. 2019.
17. Parelli RJ, Weissman DK, Howles CM, & Shoham Z. *Medicolegal issues for diagnostic imaging professionals.* Auerbach Publications. 2008.
18. Towsley-Cook DM, Young TA. *Ethical and Legal Issues for Imaging Professionals.* 2nd ed. 2013. St. Louis, MO: Mosby.
19. HIPAA advisory. Phoenix Health Systems website. http://www.csun.edu/~lisagor/2006Fall/FCS494BEE/494BEE%20What%27s%20HIPAA_.pdf. Accessed November 2, 2018.
20. laby AE, & Glicksman AS. *Adapting to life-threatening illness.* Praeger Publishers. 1985.
21. Patient Protection and Affordable Care Act: HR-3590. 2019. https://congress.gov/bill/111th-congress/house-bill/3590. Accessed November 5, 2018.
22. Mill JS. *On Liberty: Collected Works of John Stuart Mill.* vol. 18. University of Toronto Press. Palgrave, London. 1966
23. Hall JK. *Law and Ethics for Clinicians.* Amarillo, TX: Jackhal Books. 2002.
24. Roy DJ. Ethical issues in the treatment of cancer patients. *Bull World Health Org.* 1989;67:341–346.
25. Sorajjakool S, Carr MF, Nam JM. *World Religions for Healthcare Professionals.* New York, NY: Routledge, Taylor & Francis Group. 2017.
26. Smith DH, McCarthy K. In the care of cancer patients. *Prim Care Cancer.* 1992;19:821–833.
27. Wright R. *Human Values in Health Care: The Practice of Ethics.* 1987. McGraw-Hill: New York.
28. A Sanbar SS. *Legal Medicine.* 7th ed. St. Louis, MO: Mosby. 2007.
29. Moffett P, Moore G. The standard of care: legal history and definitions: the bad and good news. *West J Emerg Med.* 2011;12(1):109–112.
30. Norris J. *Mastering Documentation.* PA: Springhouse Corporation.

3

Patient Assessment

Kristi L. Tonning, Maria Thompson

OBJECTIVES

- Describe the attributes and responsibilities of an effective healthcare provider in a cancer healthcare setting.
- Demonstrate effective verbal and nonverbal communication in a range of contexts.
- Identify the determinants that make up the interprofessional approaches to caring for the cancer patient.
- Discuss the importance of pain, psychosocial, nutritional, and cultural assessment with respect to the cancer patient and

identify how these are assessed and addressed in the healthcare setting.
- Discuss the importance of monitoring the patient while he or she is undergoing radiation therapy with respect to radiation dose and the expected timing of side effects.
- Discuss the significance of cultural competency of healthcare professionals and its relevance to the care of the patient and his/her relationship with the radiation therapist.

OUTLINE

KEY TERMS

Affective
Anemia
Assessment
Cachexia
Cancer rehabilitation
Cognitive
Coping strategies
Cultural competency
Depression
Empathy
End-of-life care

Interprofessional
Leukopenia
Myelosuppression
Palliative care
Pancytopenia
Patient navigator
Quality of life
Reflective listening
Therapeutic relationship
Thrombocytopenia

PATIENT ASSESSMENT DEFINED

The assessment (a clinical plan that identifies the unique needs of the patient and how those needs will be addressed by the healthcare team) of cancer patients and of systems in which they function provides the basis of effective cancer care. The diagnosis of cancer can precipitate significant changes in the lives of the patient and family. These changes can be physiologic, psychological, and spiritual. To understand the effect of the cancer diagnosis on a patient, significant other, or family, the diagnosis must be considered a process rather than an event. That process is dynamic and continuous and changes with time.

Information obtained through a continuous, systematic assessment allows the healthcare provider to (1) determine the nature of a problem, (2) select an intervention for that problem, and (3) evaluate the effectiveness of the intervention. Assessment can be accomplished most effectively through an interprofessional approach (a move toward patient care that may be defined as involving practitioners from different professions collaborating to deliver services and coordinating care programs), which requires the efforts of the entire oncology team, including surgical oncologists, medical oncologists, radiation oncologists, radiation therapists, oncology nurses, social workers, dietitians, spiritual counselors, and patient navigators. Patient navigators are designated individuals who provide personal guidance with medical, social, and financial services to patients while they move through the healthcare system.

Importance of Patient
Assessment in Radiation Oncology. In addition to obtaining a patient history, the assessment of cancer patients serves as the cornerstone for the structure of care. Patients arrive at the radiation oncology department in various states of emotional anxiety and physical pain. The patient and their loved ones often feel extremely vulnerable—in need of help, understanding, and guidance. They come expecting that healthcare providers are the experts and have the knowledge to help them. Most patients want not only physical and psychological support, but also a competent advocate to firmly stand alongside them with genuine empathy at this vulnerable time. Beginning with the point of initial contact through consultation, diagnosis, treatment delivery, and follow-up, the patient will inevitably experience an extreme range of emotions. Past coping skills may be challenged or modified while the patient may experience health changes, altered family dynamics, and varying degrees of ability to remain in control in an unknown environment.

Establishment of a Therapeutic Relationship

The radiation therapist must respect and support all patients by engaging in empathetic and therapeutic relationships. At the initial encounter with a patient, it is critical that the radiation therapist convey professionalism, competence, and empathy, the attributes that will serve as the foundation of the therapeutic relationship. A therapeutic relationship is defined as the relationship between a healthcare worker and a patient and the means by which a therapist and a patient hope to engage with each other and effect beneficial change in the patient. It is important to note that there is an inherent imbalance of power in the relationship between the patient and healthcare provider. The patient may feel at a distinct disadvantage and may not behave as he or she normally would. Health professionals must understand and recognize the hierarchy of patient needs, with the needs for food and fluids, safety, and comfort a priority. The patient's responses and behaviors are generally based on whether these needs are adequately met or not. For example, a patient who is in pain and distress may be unable to respond to a therapist's requests for the patient to remain still on the treatment couch. The use of verbal and nonverbal communication is instrumental in this relationship. To be effective in patient assessment, radiation therapists must use communication skills

---

BOX 3.1 Helpful Behaviors

Verbal
- Nonjudgmental.
- Avoid use of medical jargon.
- Reflect, clarify, and summarize patient's statements.
- Respond to patient messages expressed both verbally and nonverbally.
- Use verbal reinforcers such as "I see" and "Yes."
- Give information appropriately.
- Use humor at times to reduce tension.
- Have a moderately calm rate of speech.
- Have a moderate tone of voice.

Nonverbal
- Maintain appropriate eye contact.
- Use touch appropriately.
- Nod head occasionally.
- Display open body language.
- Exhibit animated facial expressions.
- Smile often and at appropriate times.

BOX 3.2 Nonhelpful Behaviors

Verbal
- Preaching.
- Blaming.
- Placating.
- Using words patient does not understand.
- Direct and demanding.
- Patronizing attitude.
- Straying from topic.
- Overinterprets.
- Questioning extensively.
- Talking about self too much.

Nonverbal
- Has poor eye contact.
- Inappropriate patient touch.
- Fidgety and impatient.
- Expressionless face.
- Rolling eyes or yawning.
- Shakes pointed finger at patient.

---

that involve hearing verbal messages, perceiving nonverbal messages, and responding verbally and nonverbally to both types of messages.

Box 3.1 lists helpful behaviors in effective communication with patients; Box 3.2 lists verbal and nonverbal behaviors that are not helpful in effective communication with patients.

> The radiation therapist must be an effective listener to successfully communicate with the patient and attempt to understand what the patient is really saying.

Some anthropologists believe that more than two-thirds of any communication is transmitted nonverbally. Therefore gestures, facial expressions, posture, personal appearance, and cultural characteristics must be interpreted to understand the patient. Nonverbal behavior provides clues to, but not conclusive proof of, underlying feelings. However, research has proved that nonverbal cues (Table 3.1) tend to be more reliable than verbal cues. Box 3.3 provides an exercise to help in recognizing nonverbal cues.

TABLE 3.1 Nonverbal Communication Cues

Cue	Examples
Eye contact[a]	Steady, shifty, or avoiding.
Eyes	Open, teary, closed, or excessively blinking.
Body position	Leaning toward or away.
Mouth	Loose, smiling, tight, or lip biting.
Facial expression	Animated, pained, blank, or distant.
Arms	Unfolded or folded.
Body posture	Relaxed, slouching, or rigid.
Voice	Slow, whispering, high-pitched, fast, or cracking.
General appearance	Clean, neat, well-groomed, or sloppy.

[a]Eye contact may vary in appropriateness based on cultural differences.

BOX 3.3 Exercise for Nonverbal Cues

What do the following gestures mean to you? When you have completed this exercise, compare your answers with those of your classmates. Do you have different perceptions?
1. A patient refuses to talk and avoids eye contact with you.
2. A patient looks directly into your eyes and stretches her hands out with the palms up.
3. The patient with whom you are talking holds one arm behind her back and clenches her hand tightly while using the other hand to clench her fist at her side.
4. A patient walks into the examination room for a radiation therapy consultation with the doctor, sits erect, and clasps his folded arms across his chest before saying a word.
5. A patient sits in the waiting room, slouches in his chair, says nothing, and has tears streaming down his cheeks.

BOX 3.4 Exercise for Cognitive and Affective Responses

1. Patient: "My skin is getting really red. I think you're burning me up."
   Cognitive response: "What are you putting on your skin?"
   Affective response: "It sounds like your skin is feeling uncomfortable. These are normal and temporary changes, and we're watching it every day."
2. Patient: "My throat is getting sore. How much more sore is it going to get? I don't want one of those feeding tubes."
   Cognitive response: "Are you drinking anything acidic, smoking, using your magic mouthwash?"
   Affective response: "It sounds like the idea of a feeding tube is really frightening. We'll continue to monitor your weight and side effects and give you a couple days break if necessary."
3. Patient: "It's only the second day of treatment and I have diarrhea!
   Cognitive response: "Well, what have you eaten?"
   Affective response: "It's pretty early for diarrhea, but I understand that it must be causing you discomfort. Do you have any other ideas of what might be causing it? Let's see the doctor and ask what she thinks."
4. Patient: "I'm still in so much pain! When does this radiation start to work?"
   Cognitive response: "Are you taking your pain medication?"
   Affective response: "I'm sorry you're hurting. Everybody is different, and sometimes it takes longer to get pain relief. Let's have you visit the doctor and review your pain medication."
5. Patient: "I sure am having trouble going to sleep. Is that normal?"
   Cognitive response: "Well, how long is it taking you to go to sleep? Are you napping during the daytime?"
   Affective response: "I imagine that must be making you feel tired. Tell me what kinds of things are going through your mind while you're going to sleep."
6. Patient: "I have a question and it's probably stupid, but I'm going to ask it anyway."
   Cognitive response: "No questions are stupid."
   Affective response: "I always appreciate patients who ask questions. It helps me know the things that are important to you."
7. Patient: "Is this going to cure me?"
   Cognitive response: "What did the doctor tell you?"
   Affective response: "I imagine this must be a big concern for you. Let's have you meet with the doctor and review what was discussed during your consultation."

Cognitive content is composed of the facts and words contained in the message. Affective content may be verbal or nonverbal and consists of feelings, attitudes, and behaviors. The ability to hear only the obvious cognitive content of a verbal message compared with the ability to hear both the cognitive and underlying affective messages distinguishes an ineffective from an effective listener. Affective messages express feelings and emotions. These messages are much more difficult to communicate, hear, and perceive than cognitive messages.

Although there is a wide spectrum of human feelings, they are often grouped into just four major categories: anger, sadness, fear, and happiness. It is not uncommon for one feeling to mask or cover up another. For example, anger may mask fear because fear is often at the root of anger. A cancer patient who appears to be extremely angry may be experiencing fear of death and loss of control and be unable to honestly show this feeling. Box 3.4 gives examples of cognitive and affective responses from a therapist interacting with a patient and demonstrates the difference between the two types of responses to patients.

Identifying underlying feelings in verbal messages is difficult at first and is related to a person's comfort level and proficiency in recognizing and expressing personal feelings. The healthcare professional must listen to patients' messages and identify his or her feelings rather than project personal feelings onto patients. This ability requires practice and awareness. Different people can interpret different underlying feelings for the same statement. Careful attention must be given to nonverbal and verbal cues when listening for the true feelings of patients.

> Affective communication involves feelings of anger, sadness, fear, and happiness. The radiation therapist needs to reflectively listen to the patient and to identify what the patient is feeling.

Reflective listening (reflecting the specific content or implied feelings of the patient's nonverbal observations or communication the patient feels has been omitted or emphasized) involves responding with empathy. Empathy is defined as identifying with the feelings, thoughts, or experiences of another person. To determine the way the other person feels, the healthcare provider may ask inwardly, "If I were in this person's position, how would I feel?" A critical part of empathy is sharing feelings about the person's verbal communication. For example, empathic responses include, "Yes, I understand that. I would feel angry, too," and "Yes, I'm glad that...It would make me feel good, too."

People rarely communicate in a direct manner concerning the thoughts and feelings that they are having. Reflective listening is a way for a person to listen and communicate effectively. The consequences of good reflective listening are as follows:
- The listener becomes aware of small problems and prevents them from developing into major problems.
- The listener is perceived by others as genuinely concerned, warm, understanding, and fair.
- The listener gains knowledge about others, which helps in relating to them in a genuine way.

Reflective listening is not the only form of verbal response that radiation therapists can use. Reflective listening is essential to developing verbal responses appropriate for the issues involved. The following are ten of the most commonly used and helpful verbal responses.

1. ***Minimal verbal response:*** Minimal responses are the verbal counterpart to occasional head nodding. These are verbal clues such as "Yes," "Uh huh," and "I see," and indicate that the healthcare provider is listening to and understanding the patient.
   Patient: "I have to go to the grocery store before picking up the children on the way home from treatment."
   Therapist: "Oh, I see."

2. ***Reflecting:*** Reflecting refers to healthcare providers who communicate their understanding of the patient's concerns and perspectives. Healthcare workers can reflect the specific content or implied feelings of their nonverbal observations or communication they feel has been omitted or emphasized. The following are examples of reflecting: "You're feeling uncomfortable about finishing your treatments," "Sounds as if you're really angry at this disease," and "You really resent being treated like you're sick."
   Patient: "I can't decide what to do. Nothing seems right."
   Therapist: "It sounds as if you're feeling frustrated with your choices, and you want me to help you figure it out?"

3. ***Paraphrasing:*** A paraphrase is a verbal statement that is interchangeable with a patient's statement. The words may be synonyms of words the patient has used. Paraphrasing acknowledges to patients that they are really being heard. The following is an example:
   Patient: "In our family, the children don't do any of the work around the house."
   Therapist: "The children in your family don't do any housework."

4. ***Probing:*** Probing is an open-ended statement used to obtain more information. It is most effective with statements such as "I'm wondering about…," "Tell me more about that," and "Could you be saying…?" are used in a smooth and flowing style. These statements facilitate much more open conversation than "how," "what," "when," "where," or "who" questions.
   Patient: "My wife made me late for treatment today."
   Therapist: "Could you tell me a little more about that?"

5. ***Clarifying:*** Clarifying is used to obtain more information about vague, ambiguous, or conflicting statements. Examples of clarifying include the following: "I'm confused about…," "I'm having trouble understanding…," "Is it true that…?," and "Sounds to me like you're saying…."
   Patient: "Anyway, I'm unable to do it because it's too expensive. Besides, they won't help me anyway."
   Therapist: "Sounds like you are saying that the tests will cost too much, and the results won't be worth the cost. Is that it?"

6. ***Interpreting:*** Interpreting occurs when the therapist adds something to the patient's statement or tries to help the patient understand underlying feelings. Healthcare providers may share their interpretation, the meaning, or the facts, thus providing the patient with an opportunity to confirm, deny, or offer an alternative interpretation. The patient may respond by saying, "Yes, that's it" or "No, it's not that, but..."
   Patient: "Nobody in this world cares about anyone else."
   Therapist: "It's scary to feel that nobody at all cares about you."

7. ***Checking out:*** Checking out occurs when therapists are genuinely confused about their perceptions of the patient's verbal or nonverbal behavior or have a hunch that should be examined. Examples are, "Does it seem as if…?" and "I have a hunch that this feeling is familiar to you; are you saying…?" Therapists ask the patient to confirm or correct their perception or understanding of the patient's words.
   Patient: "Everyone tells me how great I am doing. I guess I should be feeling less pain if my tumor is shrinking."
   Therapist: "Are you telling me that you are feeling more pain now? Is that right?"

BOX 3.5 **Exercise for Listening for Feelings**

For each of the following statements, write what you think the person is really feeling. Ask yourself, "What are the underlying feelings here?"

1. The doctor told me to come over here and have all these tests. I'll sit over here and wait until you're ready for me.
2. Have you heard anything about the new social worker? I'm supposed to see her at 3 PM.
3. Coming for treatment just doesn't seem to be helping me.
4. Are you going to see me again this week, Doctor?
5. Only 2 more weeks and I'm finished with my treatments.

Discuss your answers with a small group in your class. Then look at all the possible answers in the Answer Key on the Evolve website.

8. ***Informing:*** Informing occurs when the therapist shares objective and factual information. An example is, "Your white blood cell count is extremely low, so it would be safer for you to avoid large crowds where the chances are higher of being exposed to bacteria and viruses."
   Patient: "Do you think this is a good cancer center?"
   Therapist: "The XYZ Association has ranked this cancer center number one in the state."

9. ***Confronting:*** Confronting involves therapists making the patient aware that their observations are not consistent with the patient's words. This response must be done with respect for the patient and extreme tact so that a defensive response is not elicited. An example of confrontation would be the statement, "You say you're angry and depressed, yet you're smiling."
   Patient: "I don't want to talk about it."
   Therapist: "You've told me that being open and honest about your illness is important to you, but you aren't willing to do that just now."

10. ***Summarizing:*** By summarizing, the therapist condenses and puts in order the information communicated. This is extremely helpful when a patient rambles and has difficulty conveying the sequence of events. An example of summarizing is, "I hear you saying…"
    Patient: "I guess that about covers it."
    Therapist: "Let's see if we can review what we've talked about today. Does this seem right to you?"

Box 3.5 is designed to help the individual listen for feelings.

By using the 10 verbal responses, empathetic communication can be accomplished.

INTERPROFESSIONAL APPROACH TO THE ASSESSMENT OF CANCER PATIENTS

Interprofessional collaborative practice is an essential part of the radiation therapy treatment process for each patient, and the radiation oncology team works together with patients, families, and other healthcare workers in providing quality patient care. The World Health Organization defines interprofessional collaborative practice as "when multiple health workers from different professional backgrounds provide comprehensive services by working with patients, their families, caregivers, and communities to deliver the highest quality of care across multiple settings."[1] High-quality care includes the diagnosis and treatment of disease, communication between healthcare providers, and the education and social support for patients and their families. The radiation therapist plays an integral role in the assessment, care, and treatment of the oncology patient. The complexity of needs and the increasing diversity of patient populations have enhanced the demand for improved collaborative practice of healthcare professionals. Interprofessional practice can lead to improved communication between healthcare professionals, collaborative research endeavors, improved patient outcomes, and decreased medical errors or misadministration.[1]

General Health Assessment

A general health assessment is conducted by the oncology practitioner through the process of an interview. This interview is often done by the oncology nurse or radiation oncologist, but a radiation therapist may also conduct the interview in some instances. The history includes the collection of data about the past and present health of the patient. Although a history and physical evaluation is done and sent by a referring physician, a verification and current physical assessment and baseline laboratory information should also be completed.

One method of health assessment is the self-report survey. In such a survey, individuals disclose information about aspects of their lives that are important for the radiation oncology team in designing the patient's plan of care. A self-assessment tool generally collects comprehensive information including medical information (medical conditions, medications, allergies, dental health, and vision and hearing conditions), nutritional information (dietary patterns, elimination patterns, exercise), social information (family roles, support from friends and family, activities including sexual activity), lifestyle information (alcohol and tobacco use, sleep patterns, stress, values/beliefs), and, finally, the impact of cancer on the patient's life (e.g., pain, changes in roles and lifestyle).

Physical Assessment

The radiation therapist is often the first member of the oncology team who assesses critical changes in patient status, and it is within the scope of practice to make recommendations for interventions and referrals when warranted. Table 3.2 lists physical aspects that a therapist is responsible to assess daily and subsequent interventions. Some assessments of side effects are objective. They relate directly to the area receiving radiation therapy. These effects may be enhanced when the patient is undergoing adjuvant treatment. Fig. 3.1 displays a typical skin reaction that a patient may experience during treatment. Other effects of radiation are reported by the patient and are equally important to assess and to treat. Critical aspects of patient assessment include nutrition, pain, and biochemical balance (blood counts).

Nutritional Assessment

Nutritional assessments involve all members of the oncology team. Oncology nurses are in an ideal position to perform nutritional screenings and can provide referrals to the nutrition specialist or dietitian. In addition, therapists' awareness and knowledge in this area enable them to monitor patients under treatment, assess patients' current dietary habits or concerns, make diet and nutrition recommendations when appropriate, and make referrals when warranted.

Weight loss is often the first physical change that alerts individuals with cancer to seek medical treatment. It is an indicator of poor prognosis, and in some tumor sites, such as lung and upper gastrointestinal cancers, it is present in as many as 60% to 80% of patients at diagnosis, respectively.[2] Maintenance of a good nutritional status is one of the most difficult challenges in treating cancer patients. Nutritional assessment is the critical first step in developing a comprehensive approach to the nutritional management of individuals with cancer. Two screening/assessment tools, the PG-SGA (Scored-Patient Generated Subjective Global Assessment) and the MST (Malnutrition Screening Tool), have been identified as the best validated tools for use with cancer patients.[3] The MST is a pure screening tool, as seen in Box 3.6, and could be administered by any member of the team. The PG-SGA is a "gold standard" full-assessment tool that measures many factors that contribute to the complete nutritional picture. Patients fill in a simple checklist about their weight (or weight loss), dietary intake, symptoms that affect

their ability to eat, and their functional capacity, and the remainder of the tool is completed by a physician, nurse, or dietitian. Completion of the assessment includes a limited physical examination to determine physical indications of weight loss or edema; considerations of the cancer site, type, and stage; and an overall impression of the patient as healthy, partially malnourished, or severely malnourished.[4]

The percent of weight change is a good measure of nutritional status, and indicates the extent of tissue loss as a result of inadequate nutrition or metabolic factors. For this reason, weekly monitoring of weight change is imperative for patients who are undergoing radiation therapy. A sample of a relevant percent weight changes is found in Table 3.3.

Particular attention should be paid to patients with cancers that affect the head and neck area or gastrointestinal tract. For these patients, it is essential to address potential nutritional challenges at the initial stages of treatment and implement restorative measures early. Therapists who see these patients on a daily basis are in a good position to monitor changes and the effectiveness of interventions.

Nutritional Consequences of Cancer

A serious side effect of cancer can be the multidimensional problem known as cachexia. An international panel of experts developed this definition of cachexia: "Cachexia is a complex metabolic syndrome associated with underlying illness and characterized by loss of muscle with or without loss of fat mass. The prominent clinical feature of cachexia is weight loss in adults (corrected for fluid retention) or growth failure in children (excluding endocrine disorders). Anorexia, inflammation, insulin resistance and increased muscle protein breakdown are frequently associated with cachexia. Cachexia is distinct from starvation, age-related loss of muscle mass, primary depression, malabsorption and hyperthyroidism and is associated with increased morbidity."[5] Cachexia in cancer patients is associated with reduced physical function, reduced response to anticancer therapies, and reduced survival.[6] Some clinical indicators that may be introduced by patients might include comments about anorexia (loss of desire to eat), early satiation, taste changes, or physical barriers to eating caused by anatomic effects of the tumor or treatment. Nutritional intervention is often not effective in reversing cancer cachexia. Metabolic changes introduced by the presence of the tumor (e.g., inflammation) will also contribute to the condition of the patient. Current thinking has classified the stages of cancer cachexia into precachexia, cachexia, and refractory cachexia. In the earliest stages, monitoring and preventive nutritional support may be all that is needed. Patients in the refractory stage are beyond the ability to respond to nutritional or other interventions to reverse cachexia and will only benefit from palliation. In the midstage, patients will require more than nutritional supplements, including pharmacologic approaches to address the metabolic processes that are allowing cachexia to progress.[7] Treatment is most effective and easiest in the earliest stages, and close monitoring of patients with appropriate interventions may prevent progression of this life-threatening condition.[8]

Pain Assessment

Pain, one of the most feared consequences of cancer, is a complex process that has biologic, social, and spiritual dimensions. All pain is real, regardless of its cause, and most pain is a combination of physiologic and psychogenic factors. This phenomenon is connected to the essence of human existence and often precipitates questions about the meaning of life itself. Pain holds a great deal of power with the cancer patient experiencing it.

Pain assessment has several purposes. First, it establishes a baseline for treatment and interventions. Second, it helps the clinical team focus on which interventions are best for the patient. Third, it enables the evaluation of chosen interventions. Pain assessment should be systematic, organized, and ongoing. In general, certain principles should be followed in evaluating the cancer patient who experiences pain (Box 3.7).

TABLE 3.2 Components of Daily Physical Assessment—Specific and Nonspecific Effects

Side Effects	Dose[a]	Interventions
Specific Effects		
Skin reactions • Faint erythema • Erythema • Dry desquamation • Moist desquamation	1600 cGy 2000–3000 cGy 3000–4000 cGy 4000–6000 cGy	• Assess and monitor skin integrity and changes. • Use moisturizing lotion according to the physician's orders. • Avoid creams that contain alcohol. • Avoid exposing the treated area to heat, cold, wind, soaps, deodorant, and razor shaving. • Protect skin from further irritation, and wear loose cotton clothes. • If dry desquamation has occurred and the skin is tender, use cortisone cream as directed. • For moist desquamation, consult nurse and physician for prescriptions or moist healing techniques. • Try to aerate areas of skin breakdown, especially in skinfolds. • The physician may consider temporarily stopping further treatment with extreme skin reactions.
Epilation/alopecia (hair loss)	2000 cGy	• Protect the scalp from heat, cold, and wind. Suggest an appropriate head covering. • Avoid frequent shampooing. • Avoid using blow dryers, hairsprays, gels, or other hair preparations. • Apply moisturizing lotion to the scalp. • Explore issues related to body image (e.g., getting a wig or hairpiece at the start of treatment).
Mouth changes • Stomatitis • Xerostomia • Mucositis • Taste alterations	The following occur between 2000 and 3000 cGy	• Assess the presence of stomatitis, xerostomia, mucositis, and taste changes. • Instruct the patient about a soft, bland diet; avoid drying agents like alcohol; and practice gentle dental care. Use mouth rinses as directed by physician.
Pharyngitis Laryngitis Esophagitis	2000–3000 cGy 4000 cGy 2000–3000 cGy	• Assess pain during swallowing (odynophagia). • Optimize hydration. • Modify the diet to soft, nonspicy, and nonacidic foods. • Use topical anesthetics and analgesics as prescribed. • Assess cough.
Nausea and vomiting	1000–2000 cGy	• Anticipate nausea and vomiting in high-risk patients, and prevent nausea and vomiting by using antiemetics prophylactically before treatment and as needed continuously. • Provide fluids to prevent dehydration. • Refer or instruct the patient on a low-fat and low-sugar diet. • Eat small, frequent meals. • Use nonpharmacologic measures such as acupuncture, relaxation, and guided imagery.
Diarrhea/colic Cystitis	2000–5000 cGy 3000–4000 cGy	• Assess the bowel function. • Instruct the patient on a low-residue diet for use when diarrhea occurs. • Use antispasmodic medications as prescribed. • Instruct the patient on perianal care. • Assess the bladder function. • Monitor for urinary retention/urgency/frequency, dysuria, nocturia, or hematuria. • Use antispasmodic medications as prescribed. • Monitor for bladder infections. • Stress adequate hydration in both cases.
Pain		• Assess the location and intensity. • Instruct the patient on the importance of taking medications regularly.
Nonspecific Effects		
Skin pallor		Monitor low hemoglobin, white blood cell count, and platelet levels with weekly complete blood counts.
Weight loss		Monitor once per week, and chart the results. Determine eating problems.
Fatigue		Assess the energy level. Determine periods of increased fatigue. Assist patients to pace activities and listen to their bodies. Ensure adequate nutritional intake.
Sleep		Assess normal sleep patterns and changes. Evaluate the cause of problems.
Neurologic Changes		
Headaches Vision changes Gait and mobility changes Significant changes in temperament Changes in mental status		Should patients exhibit these changes, the radiation therapist should make an immediate referral to the radiation oncologist.

[a]All doses are based on a 180- to 200-cGy daily fractionation schedule, and side effects will occur earlier if the patient is having or has had chemotherapy. Side effects will also depend on the volume and critical components of the structure that is included in the field.

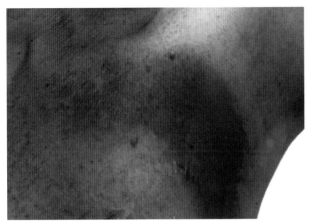

Fig. 3.1 Erythema and dry desquamation of the skin in response to external beam radiotherapy. (From Bland, KI, Copeland EM, Klimberg VS, Gradishar WJ. *The Breast: Comprehensive Management of Benign and Malignant Diseases.* 5th ed. Philadelphia, PA: Elsevier; 2018.)

BOX 3.6 Malnutrition Screening Tool

Appropriate measures are taken if they are at risk.
The Malnutrition Screening Tool is a simple screening test for malnutrition. Patients respond to the following questions; their answers are scored.
- Have you lost weight without trying?
- How much weight have you lost?
- Have you been eating poorly because of decreased appetite?
Scores are totaled to indicate the risk of malnutrition.

Modified from Leuenberger M, Kurmann S, Stanga Z. Nutritional screening tools in daily clinical practice: the focus on cancer. *Support Care Cancer.* 2010;18(Suppl 2):S17–S27.

TABLE 3.3 Evaluation of Weight Change

Time	Significant Weight Loss	Severe Weight Loss
1 mo	5%	>5%
3 mo	7.5%	>7.5%
6 mo	10%	>10%

Values charged are for percent weight change.
Modified from White JV, Guenter P, Jensen G, et al. Characteristics recommended for the identification and documentation of adult malnutrition (undernutrition). *J Acad Nutr Diet.* 2012;112:730–738.

A multidimensional conceptualization of cancer pain, as defined by Dalai and Bruera,[9] helps in understanding the scope of cancer pain. They propose six dimensions to consider in the assessment and management of the experience of cancer pain: (1) physiologic (organic cause of pain), (2) sensory (pain intensity, location, and quality), (3) affective (depression and anxiety), (4) sociocultural (cultural background and family dynamics), (5) behavioral (pain-related behaviors such as medication intake and activity level), and (6) cognitive (the meaning of pain, understanding, attitudes and beliefs, level of cognition).

Physiologic and Sensory Dimensions. Assessment of the physical dimensions of pain is a complex process. The components must include the severity of the pain, the location of the pain, the duration or temporal features, and the quality of the pain. The gold standard to assess patients' pain is always the self-report. Patients should be

BOX 3.7 Evaluation of the Cancer Patient's Pain

- Believe the patient's complaint of pain.
- Take a careful history of the patient's pain complaint.
- Evaluate the patient's psychological state.
- Perform a careful medical and neurologic examination.
- Order and review appropriate diagnostic studies.
- Treat the pain to facilitate the appropriate workup.
- Reassess the patient's response to therapy.
- Individualize the diagnostic and therapeutic approaches.

encouraged to feel that addressing pain issues is part of the overall treatment, not secondary to their anticancer treatments. Therapists can encourage discussions of daily pain with their patients. They can assist in the assessment of pain by identifying patients in need of urgent attention, including those who are not responding to pain medication; those whose daily activities (e.g., sleep, work, social interactions, and mood) are negatively affected by pain; and those whose pain remains constant. Referring these patients to the oncologist for immediate attention and taking a daily interest in other patients whose pain is not so acute can add a new dimension to the therapists' scope of practice and help the oncology team to address pain needs as soon as they are identified.[10]

Pain scales may be used during admission to the hospital and before or after surgery. In addition, pain scales are used in the radiation therapy department to assess pain daily (on treatment) and/or weekly during the physician's visit with the patient. Each facility will have a well-established policy for evaluating the fifth vital sign.

The pain severity is most often assessed with a one-dimensional tool. The numeric rating scale, the most commonly used scale, asks patients to choose a number from 0 to 10 that most closely describes their level of pain. On this scale, 0 = no pain, and 10 = the worst pain imaginable. Other similar tools include the verbal rating scale, the visual analog scale, and the "face scale," a pictorial scale that depicts faces expressing pain levels.[9] Fig. 3.2 illustrates examples of several pain scales.

The clinician can identify the location of pain by asking the patient to point to the spots or area that hurts or by presenting body diagrams so the patient can mark painful areas. The clinician should be conscious of the fact that pain may be present in many areas at once. The clinician can address the temporal nature of pain by asking the patient about the onset and duration of painful symptoms, the nature of the pain (constant, intermittent), and variations of pain throughout the day, with activity, and with treatments. A patient's description of the quality of the pain (the way that it feels) may help to identify the source of their pain. Use of adjectives such as sharp, stabbing, burning, and aching to describe the pain may help clinicians in their approach to treating the pain. Although a patient's own words are the best description, a list may be provided if they are unable to understand the concept of quality of pain or to find words for themselves.[9,11]

Acute and Chronic Pain

Acute pain is new, usually transient, and may come from diagnostic or surgical procedures. When the new pain is directly related to the growth or impact of the tumor (e.g., bowel obstruction or back pain with spinal cord compression symptoms), it should be treated as an emergency situation and addressed immediately. All new acute pain should be evaluated

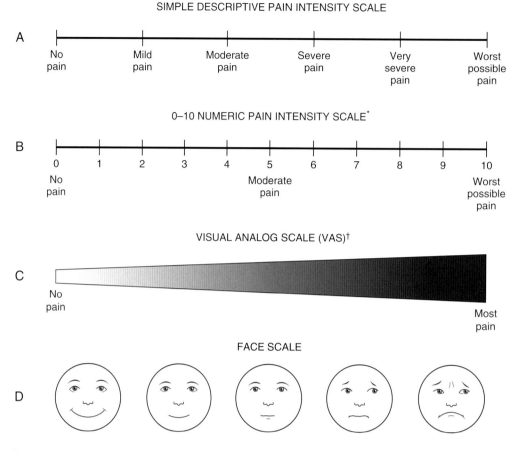

SIMPLE DESCRIPTIVE PAIN INTENSITY SCALE

A
No	Mild	Moderate	Severe	Very	Worst
pain	pain	pain	pain	severe	possible
				pain	pain

0–10 NUMERIC PAIN INTENSITY SCALE*

B
| 0 | 1 | 2 | 3 | 4 | 5 | 6 | 7 | 8 | 9 | 10 |

No pain　　　　　　Moderate pain　　　　　　Worst possible pain

VISUAL ANALOG SCALE (VAS)†

C

No pain　　　　　　　　　　　　　　Most pain

FACE SCALE

D

*If used as a graphic rating scale, a 10 cm baseline is recommended.
†A 10 cm baseline is recommended for VAS scales.

Fig. 3.2 Examples of pain scales. (From Swartz M. *Textbook of Physical Diagnosis: History and Examination.* 7th ed. Philadelphia, PA: Saunders; 2014.)

to find the source of the pain and to provide treatment as warranted. Pain that has been present for 3 months or longer is considered chronic pain. The majority of chronic pain is the result of tumor invading bone, soft tissue, viscera, blood, and nerves. Other sources of chronic pain may be the result of the surgeries, chemotherapy, and radiation that the patient has received (e.g., chronic radiation enteritis and proctitis).[9,12]

Affective Dimension

The emotional response to pain often results in depression, anxiety, and other psychological factors or personality traits that may increase patient suffering. Anxiety and depression are critical factors that affect a patient's response to pain and ability to tolerate and cope with pain, because anxiety often increases pain. Unfortunately, these symptoms are often not considered during a pain assessment. In patients with a past history of substance abuse, escalation of coping by use of drugs or alcohol may impair effective pain management and potentially complicate treatment of pain with opioids. A holistic assessment is especially important in pain assessment. Simple tools designed to measure distress (e.g., the visual analog scale, in which 0 = no distress and 10 = extreme distress) will give the team a chance to address the affective dimension of pain by supporting the patient or providing a referral to psychological or spiritual supportive services.[9]

Cognitive Dimension. Cognition impacts the way in which patients view their pain and express their needs to caregivers. In a cognitively intact individual, thoughts about pain may impact the effect of pain on their lives. If they feel that cancer pain is inevitable and that nothing can be done, they will be less likely to report increases in pain or to ask for help in managing pain. They may feel that the doctor is only concerned with treating the tumor and does not want to hear about pain. Some patients experience pain based on faulty logic. Past memories of relatives or friends with unresolved cancer pain may be unrealistic and cause them undue distress. A discussion with these patients about their feelings may alleviate distress and correct some of these faulty assumptions. If patients are cognitively impaired, talking about their fears should still be attempted. The assessment of their pain will require a combination of methods with strong dependence on their behaviors.

Behavioral Dimension. Cancer pain can cause changes in behavior that may contribute to increased pain or physical decline. Just the act of moving may cause the patient pain and avoidance of movement may increase adverse medical conditions such as respiratory complications. Therapists are in a good position to provide a daily observation of behaviors. How does a patient move when he or she is called from the waiting room? Is the patient dependent on chair arms or supportive devices to stand? Does the patient have difficulty getting on the treatment table and into position for treatment? And most importantly, do all these difficulties seem to be worsening, indicating potentially increased pain? The assessment of pain behavior should include verbal and nonverbal responses such as moans, grimaces, and complaints. Estimates of functionality (e.g., performing regular activities) are also

TABLE 3.4 Karnofsky Performance Status

Score (%)	Status
100	Normal: no complaints and no evidence of disease.
90	Ability to carry on normal activity: minor signs or symptoms of disease.
80	Normal activity with effort: some signs or symptoms of disease.
70	Self-care: inability to carry on normal activity or do active work.
60	Occasional assistance required, but ability to care for most needs.
50	Considerable assistance and frequent medical care required.
40	Disability: special care and assistance required.
30	Severe disability: hospitalization indicated, although death not imminent.
20	Extreme sickness: hospitalization and active supportive treatment necessary.
10	Moribund status: fatal processes progressing rapidly.
0	Death.

Modified from Yates JW, Chalmer B, McKegney FP. Evaluation of patients with advanced cancer using the Karnofsky Performance Status. *CA Cancer J Clin*. 1980;45:2220–2224.

TABLE 3.5 Eastern Cooperative Oncology Group Performance Status

Grade	Eastern Cooperative Oncology Group Status
0	Fully active, able to carry on all predisease activities without restriction.
1	Restricted in physically strenuous activity but ambulatory and able to carry out work of a light or sedentary nature (e.g., light housework and office work).
2	Ambulatory and capable of all self-care but unable to carry out any work activities. Up and about more than 50% of waking hours.
3	Capable of only limited self-care, confined to bed or chair more than 50% of waking hours.
4	Completely disabled. Cannot carry out any self-care. Totally confined to bed or chair.
5	Dead.

From Oken MM, Creech RH, Tormey DC, et al. Toxicity and response criteria of the Eastern Cooperative Oncology Group. *Am J Clin Oncol* 1982;5:649–655.

important aspects of pain behavior. Factors such as physical exercise, fatigue, and the ability to do chores have been used to measure pain. Two tools that are used to assess functional performance in cancer patients are the Eastern Collaborative Oncology Group (ECOG) performance status rating scale, with ratings from 0 to 5 (0 = unimpaired and 5 = dead) and the Karnofsky Performance Scale (with ratings from 100 to 0, in which 100 = normal functioning and 0 = dead).[11,13,14] Both the Karnofsky Performance Scale and the ECOG scales can be seen in Tables 3.4 and 3.5.

The use of analgesics and other treatments should also be considered in the assessment of pain behavior. The type and amount of medication and the way the dose is scheduled are important. Patients are often afraid of narcotic pain medications and take them only after they are in pain. Therapists should encourage regular dosing and explain the importance of a stable blood-serum level, which is needed to interrupt the pain cycle ("by the clock, not by the pain"). The duration of the effect of the drug and any mood change on administration should be noted.

When patients are seen with severely impaired cognitive abilities because of advanced cancer or other disease processes such as dementia or delirium, the oncology team may not be able to rely on patient self-reporting but should use alternative methods to assess pain. Although it may be possible to ask a few questions, pain assessment will rely on behavioral cues (e.g., crying, moaning, and grimacing), body movements (e.g., clenching fists, restlessness, and guarding), and social interactions (e.g., being withdrawn, silent, and irritable). The reports from caregivers will also contribute to the assessment of pain in this population.[9] An assessment tool such as the Pain Assessment in Advanced Dementia can provide a formally scored instrument and provide comparisons in pain levels during a period of time.[11,15]

Sociocultural Dimension. Everyone has feelings about the experience of pain. The sociocultural dimension of pain consists of a variety of ethnic, cultural, demographic, spiritual, and other related factors that influence a person's perception of and response to pain. Cultural and religious practices have a strong influence on the pain experience. Overt actions are accepted in some cultures, whereas other cultures consider such actions weak. A general value held by many Americans is that a good patient does not complain when in pain; a complainer has lost self-control. Unfortunately, healthcare professionals sometimes directly reinforce these beliefs.

Age, gender, and race may provide different pain experiences. Research shows that females and older individuals have increased verbal expressions of pain.

In considering the many dimensions of cancer pain, a holistic and multidisciplinary approach to assessment and management is essential. As stated, many factors contribute to the pain experience.

The multidimensional concept of cancer pain necessitates the involvement of various healthcare disciplines in assessment and management. Input is needed from many healthcare providers, including oncologists, primary physicians, nurses, radiation therapists, social workers, pharmacists, psychologists, anesthesiologists, and occupational therapists.

Tools to assess pain must be simple, short, and relevant for the patient. One-dimensional tools such as the numeric rating scale are used to measure one aspect of pain, such as the severity of pain. Multidimensional tools are likely to include the following: questions about pain intensity and mood, a body diagram to locate pain, verbal descriptors, and medication efficacy questions.[11] The McGill Pain Questionnaire is used to measure pain in complex pain situations such as chronic cancer pain.[16] It is widely used in both research and clinical situations and is reliable, valid, and available in many languages. The test has some limitations of difficulty in analysis for researchers/clinicians and test completion for patients. The Brief Pain Inventory was initially developed for oncology patients and has been shown to have reliability and validity.[17] It is easy to use, requiring only selections of values on a scale from 1 to 10 on most questions, and can be completed by the patient or by an interviewer from the oncology team. It includes measurements of pain intensity, a diagram for location of painful areas, a functional assessment, and questions on medication effectiveness.

Radiation therapists are vital in the ongoing assessment of a patient's pain. Awareness of personal beliefs and biases about pain, learning how to listen and communicate, being a keen observer, and asking key questions are imperative skills for holistic healthcare providers.

Accurate assessment of pain is the first step toward understanding the experience as the patient perceives it. Good assessment promotes an essential therapeutic relationship between patient and caregiver. Assessment is the foundation in the process of finding an effective intervention for the devastating experience of pain for the cancer patient.

Pain assessment has six dimensions, and all are important to consider when treating the whole patient. Radiation therapists are vital in the ongoing assessment of a patient's pain.

Blood Assessment

Hematologic changes in cancer patients are critical for ongoing assessments because hematopoietic tissue, such as bone marrow, exhibits a rapid rate of cellular proliferation. Hematopoietic tissue is especially vulnerable to cancer treatments (chemotherapy and radiation therapy). Myelosuppression, a reduction in bone marrow function, often results. The changes that occur can result in anemia, leukopenia, and thrombocytopenia.

Anemia is a decrease in the peripheral red blood cell count. Without sufficient red blood cells, the circulatory system's oxygen-carrying capacity is impaired. This results from a decrease in the hemoglobin level in the red blood cell, which serves as the carrier of oxygen from the lungs to tissues. Patients usually experience pale skin, muscle weakness, and fatigue (probably the most pervasive symptom). Normal blood values are found in Table 3.6.

Leukopenia is a decrease in the white blood cell count, thus increasing the risk of infection for the cancer patient. Because of chemotherapy, irradiation of a significant amount of bone marrow, or the disease process itself, patients may have compromised immune systems. Therefore, monitoring the white blood cell count during treatments is essential (refer to Table 3.6 for normal values). As a consequence of patients' inability to fight disease, they need to reduce their exposure risks. Patients should be told to have minimal contact with others, especially with sick individuals. If healthcare workers are sick and at work, they also need to keep a distance from patients.

Thrombocytopenia is a reduction in the number of circulating platelets. This decrease may be caused by a failure of the bone marrow to produce megakaryocyte cells, the precursors of platelets. This can be a result of various factors, such as chemotherapy, radiation therapy, the disease, or stress. The most significant factor that determines the risk of bone marrow depression related to radiation therapy is the volume of productive bone marrow in the radiation field. Therefore, with large fields, monitoring counts is extremely important. Normal values for platelets can be found in Table 3.6. Pancytopenia is the reduction in all circulating blood cells, including peripheral red blood cells, white blood cells and platelets.

Psychosocial Assessment

Quality of Life. A growing attention to the quality of life of cancer patients reflects the changing attitude of society and healthcare personnel. The value of cancer treatments is judged not only on survival but also on the quality of that survival. The term quality of life has emerged in recent years to summarize the broad-based assessment of the combined effect of disease and treatment and the trade-off between the two.

Cancer and its treatment, perhaps more than any other medical condition, are a major determinant of a patient's quality of life. The suggestion has been made that the emotional repercussions of cancer far exceed those of any other disease and that the emotional suffering cancer generates may actually exceed the physical suffering it causes. Therefore, good quality-of-life information can make a major contribution in improving the management of cancer patients.

A more general definition of quality of life is a person's subjective sense of well-being derived from personal experience of life as a whole. The areas of life, or domains, most important to individuals have the most influence on their quality of life. Fig. 3.3 diagrams the important domains and relationships that make life meaningful.

General agreement exists that the domains of quality of life for assessment should include physical, psychological, and social factors. In the physical domain, the quality of life is affected by loss of function, symptoms, and limited activity as a result of the disease process and physical effects of treatments. In the psychological domain, five major emotional themes have been identified: (1) fear and anxiety generated by the diagnosis and compounded by inadequate communication with caregivers, (2) loss of personal control associated with the need to be dependent on those administering treatment, (3) uncertainty about the outcome of treatments, (4) the physician's persistent enthusiasm for a cure, and (5) the debilitating effect of standard cancer treatments. In addition, loss of self-esteem and feelings of anxiety, depression, resentment, anger, discouragement, helplessness, hopelessness, isolation, and rejection are common.

Coping Strategies and Responses. During the past several decades, a great deal of interest has been focused on assessing the individual's psychosocial adjustment to illness. The areas that compose the realm of psychosocial issues are numerous.

TABLE 3.6 Normal Blood Values

Level		Percentage/Range
Hematocrit (Hct)		
Men		38.8–46.4
Women		35.4–44.4
Hemoglobin (Hgb)[a]		
Men		13.3–16.2 g/dL
Women		12.0–15.8 g/dL
Children[b]		11.5–14.5 g/dL
Blood Counts	**Per Cubic Millimeter**	**Percentage**
Erythrocytes (RBCs)		
Men	$4.30–5.60 \times 10^6$	100
Women	$4.00–5.20 \times 10^6$	100
Reticulocytes	0.8%–2.3% red cells	
Total leukocytes (WBCs)	3500–9050	100
Bands	0–450	0–5
Neutrophils	4530–6335	50–70%
Lymphocytes	710–4530	20–50
Eosinophils	0–540	0–6
Basophils	0–180	0–2
Monocytes	140–720	4–8
Platelets	165,000–415,000 (severely low <20,000)	

Values may vary slightly according to the laboratory methods used.
[a]Severely low <7.5 g/dL.
[b]Siparsky F, Accurso FJ. Chemistry & hematology reference values. In Hay WW, et al. *Current Diagnosis & Treatment: Pediatrics.* 21st ed. New York, NY: McGraw-Hill; 2012. From Kratz A, Pesce MA, Basner RC, et al. Appendix: laboratory values of clinical importance. In Longo DL, ed., et al: *Harrison's Principles of Internal Medicine.* 18th ed. New York, NY: McGraw-Hill; 2012.
RBCs, Red blood cells; *WBCs,* white blood cells.

The affective responses that occur most commonly among cancer patients are anxiety and depression. The discussion about tools for assessment focuses on these two major areas.

Anxiety. A working definition for anxiety is an individual's response to a perceived threat at an emotional level with an increased level of arousal associated with vague, unpleasant, and uneasy feelings. The instrument used most often to measure anxiety in cancer patients is the State-Trait Anxiety Inventory.[18] The State-Trait Anxiety Inventory is composed of two scales: the A-trait and A-state. The A-state consists of 20 items with a 4-point scale with the following possible responses: not at all, somewhat, moderately so, and very much. Responses are summed to measure the way the patient feels at a particular moment. Scores demonstrate the level of transitory anxiety characterized by feelings of apprehension, tension, and the autonomic nervous system–induced symptoms of worry, nervousness, and apprehension. The A-trait inventory is designed to measure a general level of arousal and predict anxiety proneness. Construct validity and reliability are established for this tool.

Another common tool used to measure anxiety is the Generalized Anxiety Disorder-7. It is used to screen and assess the severity of anxiety symptoms. The test asks patients to rate how often they experienced the seven states of anxiety (e.g., "Feeling afraid, as if something awful might happen") during the past 2 weeks. The ratings take values from 0 = not at all through 3 = nearly every day. Higher total scores represent greater severity of anxiety.[19]

Every patient brings a history of coping strategies to the cancer experience. Patients use whatever has worked for them in the past to manage their anxiety. Box 3.8 lists effective and noneffective coping strategies.

Depression. Depression is the second most common affective response in cancer patients. Depression is defined as the perceived loss of self-esteem that results in a cluster of affective behavioral (change in appetite, sleep disturbances, lack of energy, withdrawal, and dependency) and cognitive (decreased ability to concentrate, indecisiveness, and suicidal ideas) responses. Depression plays a major role in the quality of life for cancer patients and their families. However, empiric and clinical reports indicate that depression is an underdiagnosed and probably undertreated response among persons with cancer.

Knowing how to recognize depression is a critical skill for all oncology healthcare providers. Instances have been cited of patients with undiagnosed depression who returned home and committed suicide after receiving a radiation therapy treatment. The physicians, nurses, and therapists thought that the patient who was experiencing severe side effects for head and neck radiation treatments was just a "quiet person." The signs of depression were present, and no referral was made to a professional.

The criteria for a depressed condition are the following (usually five or more of these symptoms are present nearly every day for at least 2 weeks)[20]:

1. Depressed mood (feeling sad, empty, hopeless) reported by the patient or viewed by others (e.g., tears).
2. Diminished interest or pleasure in all or most activities most of the day.
3. Significant weight loss when not dieting or weight gain; decrease or increase in appetite or increased appetite or significant weight gain.
4. Insomnia or hypersomnia (e.g., difficulty falling asleep, awakening 30 to 90 minutes before time to arise, awakening in the middle of the night with difficulty going back to sleep, increased time of sleeping, frequent naps).
5. Psychomotor agitation or retardation (noticeable to others, not just subjective feelings).
6. Loss of energy or fatigue.
7. Feelings of worthlessness or excessive or inappropriate guilt.
8. Complaints or evidence of diminished ability to think or concentrate, such as slowed thinking or indecisiveness.
9. Recurrent thoughts of death, suicidal ideation, wishes to be dead, or suicide attempt.

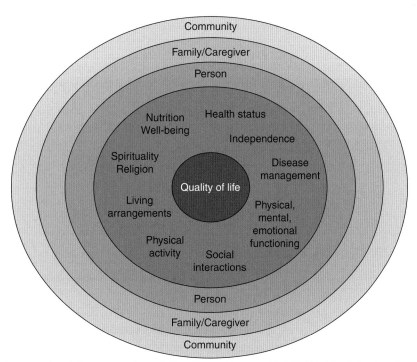

Fig. 3.3 Factors that influence quality of life. (From Kuczmarski MF, Weddle DO, American Dietetic Association. Position paper of the American Dietetic Association: nutrition across the spectrum of aging. *J Am Diet Assoc.* 2005;105:616–633.)

BOX 3.8 Effective and Noneffective Coping Strategies

Effective Strategies
- Information seeking.
- Participation in spiritual/religious activities.
- Practicing mindfulness, meditation, or prayer.
- Distraction.
- Expression of emotions and feelings.
- Positive thinking.
- Conservation of energy.
- Maintenance of independence.
- Maintenance of control.
- Goal setting.

Noneffective Strategies
- Denial of emotions.
- Minimization of symptoms.
- Social isolation.
- Passive acceptance.
- Sleeping.
- Substance abuse.
- Avoidance of decision-making.
- Blame of others.
- Excessive dependency.

(Modified from Miller JF. *Coping with Chronic Illness: Overcoming Powerlessness.* Philadelphia, PA: FA Davis; 2000.)

The radiation therapist who sees and talks to the patient daily is in an excellent position to recognize signs of depression. Questions about a patient's eating or sleeping habits or energy level are essential. Therapists must listen and discern carefully the answers to these questions. The danger of routine is when healthcare professionals ask how patients are doing but do not really hear what they are saying, whether through their words or nonverbal cues. Practicing and developing the skills discussed in the first part of this chapter are critical to take care of the whole patient.

Physiologic changes such as sleep disturbance, change in weight, appetite disturbance, and decreased energy are commonly experienced by cancer patients as a result of their disease or treatment. In addition, a level of depression is certainly appropriate because cancer represents a potential loss of not only life but also body parts, image, function, roles, and relationships. The oncology team must assess whether the level of the depression is a change from previous functioning and whether depression is persistent. The depression screening tools described below will help the team to decide whether referral to a specialist is indicated.

Focusing on systematic and continuous assessment for signs and symptoms of psychosocial problems can improve the quality and quantity of survival for patients who have cancer.

> Anxiety and depression are very important and common responses to a diagnosis of cancer and should be assessed for by specialists.

Rehabilitation. In cancer cases, the focus is most often on the disease rather than on its functional consequences. Cancer and its therapy can produce significant long-term and permanent functional losses, even in cases in which the goal is a cure. Each person with a disability needs opportunities to improve or at least maintain functional ability, regardless of the cause of the disability. Often, little

thought is given to aggressive rehabilitation of the cancer patient compared with patients with other conditions such as cardiac disease, a stroke, or a spinal cord injury. This omission occurs even though the overall 5-year survival rate for all patients with cancer is currently approximately 69.3%.[21] Rehabilitation in cancer is certainly relevant because the number of cancer survivors is growing. In the United States, cancer survivors totaled 15.5 million recently compared with 1.7 million newly diagnosed cases of cancer and 609,640 deaths from cancer.[22] The number of cancer survivors is expected to grow to 20.3 million by 2026.[23] Similar trends have been noted in the European Union.[24]

Cancer rehabilitation has been defined as the "the maximum restoration of physical, psychological, social, vocational, recreational, and economic functions within the limits imposed by the malignancy and its treatment."[25]

Following the passing of the National Cancer Act of 1971, the National Cancer Institute (NCI) was charged with conducting the national effort against cancer, including conducting research and setting up cancer centers and training programs.[26] The cancer rehabilitation initiative was defined through a 1972 conference sponsored by the NCI.

The National Cancer Rehabilitation Planning Conference identified four cancer rehabilitation objectives[27]:
1. Psychological support after the diagnosis of cancer.
2. Optimal physical functioning after the treatment of cancer.
3. Early vocational counseling when indicated.
4. Optimal social functioning as the ultimate goal of all cancer-control treatment.

Sadly, despite this national effort, cancer rehabilitation is still not available to many patients who could benefit, either from rehabilitation at initial diagnosis or as cancer survivors living with limitations that are the result of a tumor or of cancer treatment. Although inpatient cancer rehabilitation has been carried out in the past, a reduction of services has occurred, with reduced hospital stays and less acute side effects that traditionally were treated with rehabilitation because of improved cancer treatment techniques (e.g., less lymphedema following breast cancer surgery). The field of cancer rehabilitation is still struggling to be accepted as a necessary part of standard cancer care. Current barriers toward the adoption of widespread cancer rehabilitation in the United States are numerous. Stubblefield et al[28] state that of approximately 8300 board-certified physiatrists, very few practice in cancer rehabilitation centers. Financial barriers prevent many major medical institutions from adopting cancer rehabilitation centers. An innate prejudice also exists in the rehabilitation referral system. In cases of trauma, stroke, or cardiac event, the consideration of referral to rehabilitation is part of the primary treatment approach. Cancer rehabilitation referral my not be offered outside of major cancer treatment centers, and the trend in cancer care delivery is for patients to go to community-based centers where cancer rehabilitation may not be considered.[29] The focus has always been on curing the cancer and not on preventing future limitations through early rehabilitation efforts or on considering the quality of life in the surviving population.

As in other assessments, the evaluation for rehabilitative needs is a dynamic event. It should continue as new issues arise or past issues recur and is best accomplished by a multidisciplinary team meeting the specific needs of each patient.

Cultural Assessment

A culture embodies the wisdom, experience, convictions, values, and family and gender responsibilities assimilated by a fairly large aggregate of people over several generations.[30] Ethnocentrism is the belief that one way of doing things is the best way, in contrast to cultural

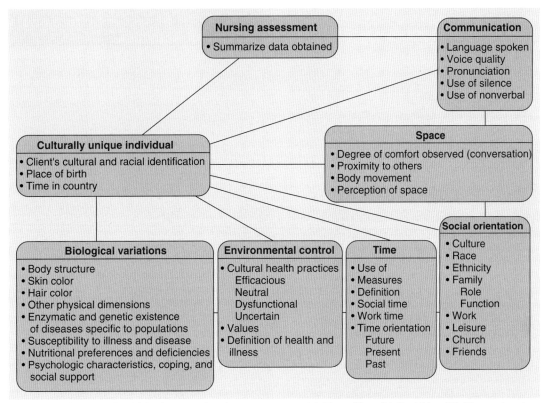

Fig. 3.4 Giger and Davidhizar's transcultural assessment model. (From Giger JN, Davidhizar RE. *Transcultural Nursing: Assessment and Intervention.* 7th ed. St. Louis, MO: Elsevier; 2017.)

relativism, which is the belief that other approaches and beliefs are as equally important. Stereotypes are the unjust convictions that all individuals or objects with a certain attribute are the same.

Cultural assessment refers to the systematic appraisal of the cultural beliefs, values, and practices of individuals and communities. Cultural beliefs and practices often influence health behaviors in families and cultural groups. Accepting and respecting the patient for their unique differences is an important attribute of the oncology caregivers. Fig. 3.4 illustrates a cultural assessment schema used in nursing. Cultural awareness and sensitivity is essential in appropriate assessment and holistic care of the patient. The U.S. Department of Health and Human Services has published standards for culturally and linguistically appropriate services. Standard 1 states that "Patients/consumers receive from all staff members effective, understandable, and respectful care that is provided in a manner compatible with their cultural health beliefs and practices and preferred language."[30]

A thorough patient assessment is a holistic process that involves evaluating and understanding the patient's values and beliefs. This is especially important when these values and beliefs are different from or in direct conflict with those of the healthcare provider and may impact the care of the patient. Customs that are the result of values and beliefs include dietary habits, religious practices, communication patterns, family structure, and health practices. Healthcare providers who practice cultural awareness and assessment skills are more likely to develop therapeutic relationships, better able to make effective interventions to the plan of care, and to alert the interprofessional team of the changing needs of the patient. Box 3.9 suggests ways to increase cultural sensitivity.

Cultural Competency. According to the U.S. Department of Health and Human Services Office of Minority Health, cultural and linguistic

---

BOX 3.9 Ways to Develop Cultural Sensitivity

- Recognize that cultural diversity exists.
- Demonstrate respect for persons as unique individuals with culture as one factor that contributes to their uniqueness.
- Respect the unfamiliar.
- Identify and examine your own cultural beliefs.
- Recognize that some cultural groups have definitions of health and illness and practices that attempt to promote health and cure illness. These definitions and practices may differ significantly from the healthcare giver's own definitions and practices.
- Be willing to modify healthcare delivery in keeping with the patient's cultural background.
- Do not expect all members of one cultural group to behave in exactly the same way.
- Appreciate that each person's cultural values may be ingrained and therefore extremely difficult to change.

Modified from Stulc P. The family as bearer of culture. In Cookfair JN, ed. *Nursing Process and Practice in the Community.* St. Louis, MO: Mosby; 1990.

competence is "a set of congruent behaviors, attitudes, and policies that come together in a system, agency, or among professionals that enables effective work in cross-cultural situations."[31] Organizations that promote cultural competency education for their employees can improve outcomes in healthcare quality and safety, and meet the needs of a wider range of patients. Radiation therapists are in a unique position of caring for people at one of the most vulnerable times in their lives. Developing culturally competent beliefs and practices will assist the patient in understanding the treatment delivery process, the goals of daily treatment field reproduction, supportive resources, and physical and psychosocial changes that they may experience.

Healthcare professionals cannot realistically possess knowledge and proficiency of each culture, but are expected to be culturally sensitive, inquisitive, and respectful of diverse patient populations while avoiding cultural stereotypes. The following generalization of cultures is an introductory overview of several predominant cultures in the United States and is not intended to promote cultural stereotypes. Generalizations are different from stereotypes in that they are a launching point for information, unlike stereotypes that act as the final point of view.[32] It is also important to note that cultural characteristics within groups may differ greatly and may change with varying levels of assimilation within the population.

Use of Interpreters. A radiation therapist would demonstrate cultural sensitivity by assessing the patient's level of understanding of the radiation therapy treatment delivery process and by evaluating the patient's emotional and physical response to treatment and interventions. It is important to assess the need for and to use patient translators when indicated. Although the practice of soliciting family members to act as translators between the therapist and the patient may be commonplace in some areas, care must be taken to avoid the use of family members for the interpretation and delivery of sensitive and/or private health information. Access to real-time translation in many languages is increasingly easier with emerging technologies and application software. Users of these technologies benefit from voice-to-voice or voice-to-text translations at point of care. The radiation therapist should investigate resources within the healthcare organization for language interpreters, as well as explore application software and use these resources whenever possible.

The radiation therapist may become aware of different cultural expectations related to the treatment delivery of their patients in a variety of ways and need to be sensitive to these differences. See Box 3.10 for some examples.

Spiritual Assessment

A holistic approach to patient care is one that addresses not only the physical, emotional, and familial dimensions experienced by a person, but one that includes the spiritual realm as well. A common misconception is that spirituality and religion are the same concept or that they are interchangeable. Spirituality encompasses a sense of fulfillment and connection with a power greater than oneself, whereas religion may entail distinctive principles and rituals practiced either alone or in established groups.

Traditionally, physicians are trained to focus on the physical aspects of the patient and consider the evaluation, diagnosis, and treatment of the human body to be their area of expertise. They often fail to address the spiritual dimension in assessment of the individual. Lack of clarity for the role of spiritual care has been shown to be based on a lack of education of both physicians and nurses as well as other oncology professionals.[33]

The spiritual dimension encompasses a person's need to find satisfactory answers to questions that revolve around the meaning of life, illness, and death. Spirituality is often a very important consideration in the quality of life of individuals and especially in those diagnosed with cancer. Healthcare professionals caring for oncology patients should make every effort to improve this area of their clinical practice.[33] Throughout the patient's course of radiation therapy treatment, he or she may begin to discuss religion or spirituality and reflect on its value in his or her life. The radiation therapist is often made aware of the spiritual needs and concerns that arise and has an opportunity to support the patient by actively listening, demonstrating empathy, and making appropriate referrals to chaplains or spiritual care

---

BOX 3.10   Impact of Culture on Daily Treatment Activities

- Involvement of family members (e.g., patients accompanied by large family groups); patients asking family members to translate.
- Gender restrictions (e.g., refusing care from therapists of the opposite sex).
- Differing attitudes toward appointment times and schedules.
- Modesty issues.
- Compliance and reluctance to ask questions or reveal symptoms.
- Dietary differences and their impact on nutritional interventions.
- Alternative medicine and practices.

---

providers within the healthcare organization or community. The spiritual, religious, and existential aspect of care is one of the identified clinical practice domains included in the National Consensus Project for Quality Palliative Care. It includes life review, evaluation of hopes and fears, meaning, purpose, feelings about afterlife, remorse, forgiveness, and achievement of life goals. A standardized spiritual assessment tool should be used to evaluate religious and/or spiritual history, inclinations, and associated principles and practices of the patient.[34]

The Joint Commission does not mandate that a particular spiritual assessment tool be used but does require healthcare organizations to survey the patient about any cultural, religious, or spiritual concerns that may affect care and their satisfaction with that care.[35]

Important considerations for those conducting spiritual assessments include how the questions are posed, with inquiries delivered without judgment, in a nonleading manner that allows for the individual to express his or her values and feelings.[36] The *Faith, Importance/Influence, Community and Address/Action in Care* spirituality history tool was created to provide physicians and healthcare professionals with an instrument to assess spiritual concerns of patients.[37]

Hope. Hope is the key concept and an essential ingredient in the religious and spiritual aspects of care and a major component in the healing process. Giving support with realistic hope is a powerful gift oncology caregivers can offer their patients. For some patients, hope is a major determinant between life and death.

A physician often becomes a symbol of hope. Through the physician's continued interest, the patient does not despair. The fear of being abandoned by this person of hope can clearly alter the patient's behavior. Patients may protect their relationships with their physicians by not questioning them, limiting their complaints to them, and treating them as they wish to perceive them—as miracle workers. When this occurs, the role of other members of the interprofessional team becomes paramount. Establishing a therapeutic relationship and applying effective communication skills are essential in caring for this patient.

Hope is a multidimensional construct that is more than goal attainment and has not been easily quantified. Hope is fundamental to meaning and transcendence for humans. For these reasons, including hope in holistic patient assessment and patient care is essential.

Awareness and respect for patient beliefs, values, and practices are essential in being an effective healthcare worker.

Family Assessment

The dynamics of a diagnosis of cancer reach beyond the patient and extend to the entire family. Responses will vary with respect to economic and psychosocial resources, across developmental stages of the family, and with differing demands of the illness.

Life for families of cancer patients becomes complex. Family members must often learn new roles, self-care skills, and ways of relating to and communicating with each other, friends, and the healthcare team. To support family members, an assessment of their functioning to reveal problem areas may be necessary.

In general, the focus of healthcare delivery is on the individual. Oncology care is unique in that it requires both an interprofessional and family systems approach to patient care. Viewing the family as the client promotes a holistic approach to the care of the patient.

Support resources and interventions can address both the physical needs and emotional adaptation to stressors related to illness for the entire family unit.

It is important for the healthcare provider to recognize that the patient's concept of family can include people who love and support each other, whether they are biologically related or not. Unmarried couples, same-sex couples, and blended families may play an important role in the care and support of the patient, and their value cannot be overlooked or diminished.

Most radiation therapists are aware of the integral role the family plays in the health of its members, and often meet the family and friends who accompany the patient to the radiation therapy treatment appointments. It is important to monitor the patient and family for signs of distress (emotionally, spiritually, and financially), as family dynamics can shift with changing roles and responsibilities of its members when one person is ill. The radiation therapist can demonstrate respect for the importance of family members by greeting them, teaching them aspects of the treatment delivery process, including them in changes in the plan of care or treatment schedules, and by making appropriate social service referrals when needed.

Special Cases in Assessment

Special attention must be given to meet the diverse needs of patients at different developmental stages in life and those with different sexual orientations because these aggregates may warrant additional support services and advocacy.

Children. To provide holistic care to a child with cancer, assessing the needs and concerns of the child's primary caregivers (usually the parents) is essential. Experiencing a life-threatening diagnosis for their child is an extremely stressful event for parents.

The assessment of children with cancer is a multidimensional task. Areas of functioning that should be considered are depression, withdrawal, anxiety, delinquency, achievement, family relations, and development.

The developmental level of children is directly related to the way they perceive, interpret, and respond to the diagnosis of cancer. A substantial amount of literature in nursing, medicine, psychiatry, psychology, and social work exists detailing the psychological effect of childhood cancer. The shock of diagnosis, discomfort and inconvenience of treatment, and the burden of living with a life-threatening disease are sources of distress and disruption for the child with cancer, parents, siblings, and extended family members.

Those who provide healthcare to children with cancer have a key role in helping the child and family cope with situations as they arise. The study by Wechsler and Sanchez-Iglesias[38] suggests that most children being treated for cancer are as psychologically adjusted as healthy children. This is due in part to the caregivers' concern and help with coping. However, adult survivors of childhood cancer are likely to have symptoms that are the result of their tumors or treatment and experience a decreased health-related quality of life.[39]

Adolescents. Developmental theory suggests that adolescence is a crucial stage in the process of building self-esteem, forming perceptions about body image, establishing autonomy, and developing social functions. The adolescent with cancer experiences a disruption of these vital processes. As a result, assessment for the adolescent must consider and address these unique areas. The adolescent with cancer may face a loss of self-esteem because of the unfamiliarity and vulnerability associated with the patient role. This role can cause the adolescent to feel inferior and dependent, thus inhibiting the developmental task of establishing independence.

Relationships with others and self-perception can change as the adolescent goes through treatment and is hospitalized. The unpredictability and uncertainty of cancer can limit the adolescent's sense of control and autonomy. Changes in body image, disruption of activities, and prescribed therapies can have a profound effect on the adolescent's self-image. Rapid changes in physical appearance as a result of treatments, disfigurement caused by the disease or amputation, or reduction in weight can confuse and impair the adolescent's self-perception.

These are complex processes that must be assessed and incorporated into the plan of care for the adolescent. The healthcare team must promote growth and developmental maturity while recognizing the burden that cancer places on the adolescent in meeting developmental tasks.

Elderly. When individuals enter the later stages of life, the risk of developing cancer increases. Specific attention to the sociologic issues for older persons is crucial for appropriate assessment and treatment of cancer.

An important problem to assess in older persons is the amount of sensory and cognitive impairment that may be present. Assessment of the ability of older patients to hear, see, or understand is paramount in their care and in their overall safety. Recognizing any change from normal behaviors, usual routines, and social interactions is extremely important. Loss of physical health, limited economic resources, changes in family structure, and losses of social status greatly affect the quality of life for older persons. Obtaining a complete medical history that includes medications, the family health experience and history, the functional status, and current concerns is crucial to sound healthcare. Box 3.11 lists some suggestions for therapeutic communication with an older patient.

Ongoing communication is the key to assessing and working effectively with the older patient. The best way to promote ongoing communication is to communicate well from the start and to take time to establish a therapeutic and healing relationship.

Lesbian, Gay, Bisexual, and Transgender. Every 10 years, the U.S. government creates and publishes Healthy People initiatives for health prevention and health promotion. The Healthy People 2030 national health initiative introduces the objectives for advancing the health, safety, and well-being of lesbian, gay, bisexual, and transgender people.[40] Lesbian, gay, bisexual, and transgender individuals have faced health disparities and hostile reactions to their sexual identity and preferences, which often contribute to barriers to healthcare and resistance to seeking medical attention.

1. Healthcare professionals are becoming more knowledgeable and aware of transsexualism and its related medical and surgical interventions.[41] Practicing culturally competent care with this population includes measures such as adding a selection option on intake surveys for transgender individuals, making nondiscriminatory

BOX 3.11　**Understanding Your Older Patient**

- Use proper form of address.
- Make older patients comfortable.
- Take a few moments to establish rapport.
- Try not to rush.
- Avoid interrupting.
- Use active listening skills.
- Write down takeaway points.
- Demonstrate empathy.
- Avoid jargon.
- Reduce barriers to communication.
- Be careful about language.
- Ensure understanding.
- Compensating for hearing deficits.
- Compensating for visual deficits.

Modified from National Institute on Aging, National Institutes of Health. *Talking With Your Older Patient: A Clinician's Handbook.* Bethesda, MD: National Institute on Aging, National Institutes of Health; 2008.

disclosures visible, having unisex bathrooms, and promoting education and sensitivity training to healthcare professionals.[42]

2. A radiation therapist caring for a transgendered patient should demonstrate care and consideration by discussing with the patient his or her sexual identity and preferred terms to use.[43]

3. As with other patient populations, the radiation therapist should respect the patient's dignity by properly draping the patient, maintaining confidentiality, recognizing significant others, and treating the patient holistically.

Palliative and End of Life. Cancer cure is believed to occur when the patient has undergone standard therapeutic interventions and the disease has not returned.[44] Some patients undergoing cancer treatment have diseases that are advanced and are deemed incurable by their healthcare providers. Palliative care is the delivery of interventions aimed at relieving symptoms and side effects of the disease and of the treatment and improving quality of life for the patient. Palliative care may include prescription and over-the-counter drugs, nutrition and hydration interventions, use of alternative medicines, and psychosocial supportive therapies combined with standard care. Many patients undergo radiation therapy treatments that are designed with a palliative intent. A common misconception is that palliative care is the same as end-of-life care. When oncology medical professionals have determined that the therapeutic interventions have ceased to work and cancer control is not sustainable, then end-of-life care may be initiated.[45] Radiation therapists are often one of the first of the interprofessional team to assess changes in the patient that may indicate not only advanced side effects of treatment, but of advanced disease as well. Not only should the radiation therapist refer the patient to the nurse and physician, but they should discuss with the team the reasons for this referral. An example of this assessment and referral would be when a patient that is being treated for their primary lung cancer demonstrates neurologic changes such as change in gait, personality, vision, or headaches. The physician may conduct a complete physical assessment and diagnostic workup in this patient to look for advancing disease such as brain metastasis. End-of-life care is delivery of physical and psychosocial interventions when the aim of treatment moves to one of comfort care only. Practitioners focused on treatment interventions and not on holistic care or quality of life for the patient and family can easily overlook this transition period. A referral to hospice services at this stage allows the patient and family to enjoy the time remaining and to prepare for end of life while not spending time on various invasive or painful medical interventions. The radiation therapist sees firsthand the physical and emotional toll on the patient receiving palliative radiation therapy, oftentimes to multiple areas of the body, and may play a role in having a conversation with the physician about the appropriateness of a hospice referral.

It is important for radiation therapists to be aware of the various needs of these aggregates, as they may warrant additional support services and advocacy.

SUMMARY

- Communication with the cancer patient can be achieved through verbal and nonverbal networks. The radiation therapist needs to be an effective listener to be able to successfully communicate with the patient via cognitive and affective means.
- Affective communication involves feelings of anger, sadness, fear, and happiness. The radiation therapist needs to reflectively listen to the patient and identify what the patient is feeling, and also be empathetic.
- Physical assessment of the patient on a daily basis by the radiation therapist is imperative to assess the onset of treatment-induced side effects. The therapist needs to be aware of all adjuvant treatments, such as chemotherapy, so that accurate patient assessment is made and the patient is referred to the doctor, dietitian, oncology nurse, or social worker for advice on caring for and treating any side effects.
- Pain assessment has many dimensions, and all are important to consider when treating the cancer patient as a whole being.
- Blood counts are affected by chemotherapy and radiation therapy and need to be monitored throughout a patient's treatment.
- Quality of life for the cancer patient needs careful assessment, and several tools can be used to determine the effect of cancer on the patient.

- Anxiety and depression are common affective responses and should be assessed by specialists.
- The family unit can also be disrupted by a cancer diagnosis, and some families need extra support to cope with the added dimension to family life. Assessment tools are available to help families determine whether they need help so that help can be established.
- When patients survive their cancer diagnoses, rehabilitation becomes a focus, and the aim is to encourage patients to function at their maximal level posttreatment.
- Awareness and respect for patient beliefs, values, and practices, even if they differ from the healthcare provider's values, are important aspects of being a culturally aware and culturally sensitive healthcare professional.
- Special attention must be given to meet the diverse needs of patients at different developmental stages in life and those with different sexual orientations.
- End-of-life care should be considered when the intent has shifted from curative intent to comfort care only.

Case I

A 61-year-old African-American man with a history of obesity, Crohn disease, and polyps presented with changes in stool caliber as well as blood in his stool. His staging workup included fecal occult blood test, sentinel node biopsy, and colonoscopy. His hematocrit was 30; hemoglobin, 10 g/dL. Pathology revealed stage IIIA (T3, N1, MO) adenocarcinoma of the ascending colon.

Family History

- Father, maternal uncle, and a 50-year-old brother had a history of colorectal cancer.

Social History

- Physically inactive.
- Married with three adult children.
- Practicing Muslim.

Physical Examination

Weight, 243 lb; pulse, 88 beats/min; blood pressure 132/92 mm Hg; temperature 98.6°F; Karnofsky status, 100; Eastern Collaborative Oncology Group (ECOG) performance of 1; bowel sounds hyperactive, X4 quadrants.

Treatment

- Surgery with postoperative radiation therapy and concurrent chemotherapy.

Discussion/Considerations

- Nutrition teaching.
- Medication side effects, doses, and interventions.
- Family and patient coping skills.
- Cultural and religious issues.

Case II

The patient is a 59-year-old Chinese female. While having her annual breast screening, a mass was revealed in her upper quadrant of the left breast. An excisional biopsy was taken, which revealed a 1-cm malignant mass. Further biopsies were taken of nodes, including the sentinel node. All biopsies were negative. Pathology revealed infiltrating ductal carcinoma stage T1N0M0.

Family History

- Patient is a mother of two children.
- Her mother was treated for postmenopausal breast cancer.

Social History

- Smokes 10 cigarettes per day.
- Has two healthy daughters.
- Speaks very limited English and often communicates through her children.

Physical Examination

Weight, 121 lb; pulse 74 beats/min; blood pressure, 112/78 mm Hg; temperature 98.4°F; Karnofsky status, 100; Eastern Collaborative Oncology Group (ECOG) status, 0. No lymphadenopathy was noted.

Treatment

- Lumpectomy followed by radiation therapy, tangential field approach, electron boost with bolus, and ongoing tamoxifen treatment.

Discussion/Considerations

- Medication side effects, doses, and interventions.
- Communication issues/need for interpreter.
- Cultural issues.
- Family/patient coping skills.

■ REVIEW QUESTIONS

The answers to the Review Questions can be found by logging on to our website at: http://evolve.elsevier.com/Washington/principles

1. Define patient assessment.
2. Explain what is included in the cognitive content of a message. Give an example.
3. Explain what is involved in an empathic response.
4. State the 10 most common verbal responses in effective communication.
5. Explain the assessment responsibility of radiation therapists for daily treatment in the following areas—relate this to daily dose and fractionation and when the side effects might happen.
   - Skin reactions
   - Diarrhea
   - Alopecia
   - Fatigue

   - Cystitis
   - Pain
   - Sleep
   - Nausea
   - Skin pallor
   - Oral changes and vomiting
   - Weight loss
   - Pharyngitis and esophagitis
   - Neurologic changes

6. State the frequent first sign of malnutrition.
7. State two important characteristics related to the cause of pain.
8. Define leukopenia and explain its signs and symptoms.
9. State the major symptoms of depression.
10. Define cultural competency and behaviors that demonstrate cultural awareness and sensitivity.

■ QUESTIONS TO PONDER

1. Why is doing an assessment in oncology important?
2. What is the basis of an effective therapeutic (communication) relationship?
3. Why is observing nonverbal communication so important?
4. What are the three purposes of pain assessment?
5. Why is rehabilitation of the cancer patient important?
6. What are some ways to support patients with spiritual needs?
7. What is the difference between ethnocentrism, cultural relativism, and stereotypes?

REFERENCES

1. Framework for action on interprofessional education and collaborative practice. World Health Organization website. http://whqlibdoc.who.int/hq/2010/WHO_HRH_HPN_10.3_eng.pdf?ua=1. Accessed October 12, 2018.
2. Nutrition in cancer care (PDQ). National Cancer Institute website. http://www.cancer.gov/cancertopics/pdq/supportivecare/nutrition/HealthProfessional. Accessed November 9, 2018.
3. Leuenberger M, Kurmann S, Stanga Z. Nutritional screening tools in daily clinical practice: the focus on cancer. *Support Care Cancer*. 2010;18(suppl 2):S17–S27.
4. Bauer J, Capra S, Ferguson M. Use of the scored Patient-Generated Subjective Global Assessment (PG-SGA) as a nutrition assessment tool in patients with cancer. *Eur J Clin Nutr*. 2002;56:779–785.
5. Evans WJ, Morley JE, Argiles J, et al. Cachexia: a new definition. *Clin Nutr*. 2008;27:793–799.
6. Fearon K, Strasser F, Anker SD, et al. Definition and classification of cancer cachexia: an international consensus. *Lancet Oncol*. 2011;12:489–495.
7. Bozzetti F. Nutritional support of the oncology patient. *Crit Rev Oncol Hematol*. 2013;87:172–200.
8. Argiles JM, Lopez-Soriano FJ, Busquets S. Mechanisms and treatment of cancer cachexia. *Nutr Metab Cardiovasc Dis*. 2014;23:s19–s24.
9. Dalal S, Bruera E. Assessing cancer pain. *Curr Pain Headache Rep*. 2012;16:314–324.
10. Kyie KA, Engel-Hills P. Pain assessment: the role of the radiation therapist. *South Afr Radiogr*. 2011;49(1):13–16.
11. D'Arcy Y. Assessing pain in patients with cancer. In: Davies P, D'Arcy Y, eds. *Compact Clinical Guide to Cancer Pain Management: An Evidence-Based Approach for Nurses*. New York, NY: Springer Publishing; 2013.
12. Portenoy RK. Treatment of cancer pain. *Lancet*. 2011;377:2236–2247.
13. Karnofsky DA, Burchenal JH. The clinical evaluation of chemotherapeutic agents in cancer. In: MacLeod CM, ed. *Evaluation of Chemotherapeutic Agents in Cancer*. New York, NY: Columbia University Press; 1949.
14. Oken MM, Creech RH, Tormey DC, et al. Toxicity and response criteria of the Eastern Cooperative Oncology Group. *Am J Clin Oncol*. 1982;5(6):649–655.
15. Warden V, Hurley AC, Volicer L. Development and psychometric evaluation of the Pain Assessment in Advanced Dementia (PAINAD) scale. *J Am Med Dir Assoc*. 2003;4(1). 19–15.
16. Melzack R. The McGill Pain Questionnaire: major properties and scoring methods. *Pain*. 1975;1:277–299.
17. Daut RW, Cleeland CS, Flannery RC. Development of the Wisconsin Brief Pain Questionnaire to assess pain in cancer and other disease. *Pain*. 1983;17:197–210.
18. Spielberger C, Gorusch R, Lushene R. *Manual for the State-Trait Anxiety Inventory*. Palo Alto, CA: Consulting Psychologists Press; 1970.
19. Spitzer RL, Kroenke K, Williams JBW, Lowe B. A brief measure for assessing generalized anxiety disorder. *Arch Intern Med*. 2006;166:1092–1097.
20. American Psychiatric Association. *Diagnostic and Statistical Manual of Mental Disorders: DSM-5*. 5th ed. Washington, DC: American Psychiatric Publishing; 2013.
21. Cancer trends progress report-February 2018. National Cancer Institute website. https://progressreport.cancer.gov/after/survival. Accessed November 9, 2018.
22. Cancer facts & figures 2018. American Cancer Society website: https://www.cancer.org/content/dam/cancer-org/research/annual-cancer-facts-and-statistics/annual-cancer-facts-and-figures/2018/cancer-facts-and-figures-2018.pdf. Accessed November 9, 2018.
23. Mariotto AB, Yabroff KR, Shao Y, et al. Projections of the cost of cancer care in the United States: 2010–2020. *J Natl Cancer Inst*. 2011;103:117–128.
24. Stubblefield MD, Hubbard G, Cheville A, et al. Current perspectives and emerging issues on cancer rehabilitation. *Cancer*. 2013;119(suppl 11):2170–2178.
25. Thomas DC, Ragnarsson KT. Principles of cancer rehabilitation medicine. In: Hong WK, Bast RC, Hait WN, et al., ed. *Holland-frei Cancer Medicine*. 8th ed. Shelton, CT: People's Medical Publishing House; 2010.
26. National Cancer Act of 1971. National Cancer Institute website. https://www.cancer.gov/about-nci/legislative/history/national-cancer-act-1971. Accessed November 9, 2018.
27. Cancer and rehabilitation. Medscape website. http://emedicine.medscape.com/article/320261-overview. Accessed November 9, 2018.
28. Stubblefield MD, Schmitz KH, Ness KK. Physical functioning and rehabilitation for the cancer survivor. *Sem Oncol*. 2013;40(6):784–795.
29. Alfano CM, Ganz PA, Rowland JH, et al. Cancer survivorship and cancer rehabilitation: revitalizing the link. *J Clin Oncol*. 2012;30(9):904–906.
30. Brusin JH. How cultural competency can help reduce health disparities. *Radiol Technol*. 2012;84(2):129–147.
31. What is cultural competency. USDHHS, Office of Minority Health website. https://minorityhealth.hhs.gov/omh/content.aspx?ID=2804. Accessed November 9, 2018.
32. Halbur K. *Essentials of Cultural Competency in Pharmacy Practice*. Washington, DC: American Pharmacists Association; 2019.
33. Ferrell B, Otis-Green S. Spirituality in cancer care at the end of life. *Cancer J*. 2013;19(5):431–437.
34. National Coalition for Hospice and Palliative Care website. https://www.nationalcoalitionhpc.org/. Accessed November 9, 2018.
35. Road map for hospitals. Joint Commission website. http://www.jointcommission.org/assets/1/6/ARoadmapforHospitalsfinalversion727.pdf. Accessed November 9, 2018.
36. Assessment of spirituality and religion. National Center for Cultural Competence website. https://nccc.georgetown.edu/body-mind-spirit/assessment.php. Accessed November 9, 2018.
37. FICA spiritual assessment tool. George Washington Institute for Spirituality and Health website. http://smhs.gwu.edu/gwish/clinical/fica. Accessed November 9, 2018.
38. Wechsler AM, Sanchez-Iglesias I. Psychological adjustment of children with cancer as compared with healthy children: a meta-analysis. *Eur J Cancer Care*. 2013;22:314–325.
39. Huang 1, Brinkman TM, Kenzik K, et al. Association between the prevalence of symptoms and health-related quality of life in adult survivors of childhood cancer: a report from the St. Jude Lifetime Cohort Study. *J Clin Oncol*. 2013;31(33):4242–4252.
40. Lesbian, gay, bisexual, transgender health. healthypeople.gov website. https://www.healthypeople.gov/2020/About-Healthy-People/Development-Healthy-People-2030/Framework. Accessed December 12, 2018.
41. Gooren L. Care of transsexual persons. *N Engl J Med*. 2011;354:1251–1257.
42. Health care for transgendered individuals. American College of Obstetricians and Gynecologists website. https://www.acog.org/Clinical-Guidance-and-Publications/Committee_Opinions/Committee_on_Health_Care_for_Underserved_Women/Health_Care_for_Transgender-Individuals. Accessed November 09, 2018.
43. Guidelines for the care of lesbian, gay, bisexual and transgender patients. GLMA (Gay and Lesbian Medical Association) website. http://www.glma.org/_data/n_0001/resources/live/GLMA%20guidelines%202006%-20FINAL.pdf. Accessed November 09, 2018.
44. Understanding statistics used to guide and evaluate treatment. cancer.net website. http://www.cancer.net/navigating-cancer-care/cancer-basics/understanding-statistics-used-guide-prognosis-and-evaluate-treatment. Accessed November 9, 2018.
45. ASCO recommends palliative care as a part of cancer treatment. cancer.net website. https://www.cancer.net/navigating-cancer-care/how-cancer-treated/palliative-care. Accessed November 9, 2018.

4

Overview of Radiobiology

Megan Trad

OBJECTIVES

- Define ionization and list the rules of reactions to ionizing radiation.
- Define the term radiobiology.
- Compare and contrast direct ionization and indirect ionization.
- Define LET.
- Define RBE.
- Compare and contrast high-LET and low-LET radiation.
- List the types of deoxyribonucleic acid (DNA) damage that may occur, including the consequences.
- List the gross structural changes to chromosomes.
- Diagram the cell cycle, labeling all phases.
- List the three categories of cellular response to radiation.
- Draw a cell survival curve for mammalian cells and label the different components.

- State the three external factors that influence cellular response to radiation and give examples of each.
- Explain the Law of Bergonié and Tribondeau.
- List each group of cell populations and give an example of each.
- Compare and contrast the two components of tissues and organs.
- State the two phases of response to radiation.
- Compare and contrast the processes of repair and regeneration.
- List the three syndromes of total body irradiation.
- Summarize the effects of radiation damage to the embryo and fetus.
- State the goal of radiation therapy.
- Define tissue tolerance dose and list several factors that alter the tolerance of tissue to radiation.

OUTLINE

KEY TERMS

Biologically effective dose (BED)

D_o

D_q

Extrapolation number (n)

Free radical

Functional subunits (FSUs)

Ionizing radiations

Law of Bergonié and Tribondeau

Linear energy transfer (LET)

Oxygen enhancement ratio (OER)

Radiolysis

Radioprotectors

Radiosensitizers

Relative biologic effectiveness (RBE)

Reproductive failure

Stereotactic ablative body radiotherapy (SABR or SBRT)

Stereotactic radiosurgery (SRS)

$TD_{5/5}$

$TD_{50/5}$

INTERACTION OF RADIATION AND MATTER

Since the discovery of x-rays by Roentgen in 1895, scientists and clinicians have investigated the interaction of ionizing[1] radiations and various target materials, including biologic tissue. When discussing the interaction of radiation with matter, two terms must be defined: *ionization* and *excitation*. In both ionization and excitation, the incoming radiation interacts with an atom. In ionization, the incoming radiation ejects an electron from the shell of the atom, thus causing the atom to be charged (ionized). In excitation, the electron in the outer shell of the atom is said to be excited (oscillating or vibrating) but is not ejected from the shell. *Radiation biology,* or *radiobiology,* has evolved since Roentgen's time and can be defined as the study of the sequence of events following the absorption of energy from ionizing radiations, the efforts of the organism to compensate, and the damage to the organism that may be produced.[2]

In evaluating the response of a living cell to ionizing radiation, the following must be considered[2]:

1. Radiation may or may not interact with a cell.
2. If an interaction occurs, damage may or may not be produced in the cell.
3. The initial energy deposition occurs extremely rapidly (much less than 1 second) and is nonselective or random in the cell. No specific areas of the cell are "chosen."
4. Visible tissue changes after irradiation are not usually distinguishable from those caused by other traumas. (The only exception to this may be cataracts, which are discussed later.)
5. Biologic changes that occur after irradiation do so after some time has elapsed. The duration of this latent period is inversely related to the dose administered and can range from minutes to years.

For convenience, it is typical to classify ionizing radiations as *electromagnetic* or *particulate*.

Types of Interactions

There are two types of interactions that occur when radiation initially interacts with a cell, direct or indirect ionization.[3] *Direct ionization* occurs when the incident particle itself interacts with the critical target of the beam (deoxyribonucleic acid [DNA]). This is most likely to occur when using alpha particles, protons, or electrons because of the relatively densely ionizing nature of these particulate radiations. The damage caused by alpha particles, protons, or electrons is termed direct effect because they produce damage directly to the critical target of the cell, which is the DNA.

The second type of interaction is called *indirect ionization* because of the effects of specific secondary particles on the target. This mechanism predominates when the incident beam is composed of x-rays, gamma rays, or neutrons. These indirectly ionizing radiations are not strong enough to directly cause damage to the DNA; instead, they give rise to fast (high-energy), charged secondary particles that can then directly or indirectly cause ionizations in the critical target. Indirect effect occurs predominantly when x-rays or gamma rays compose the primary beam, thus producing fast electrons as the secondary particles that interact with the most abundant cellular medium, water (H_2O). X-rays and gamma rays are considered sparsely ionizing radiations because their ionizing effects are not as densely packed as their particulate counterparts, such as alpha particles. Indirect effects involve a series of reactions known as radiolysis (splitting) of water. The initial event in radiolysis involves the ionization or ejection of an electron from a water molecule, thus producing a water ion (charged molecule):

$$H_2O \rightarrow H_2O + 1e^-$$

The ejected electron (e^-), known as a *fast electron* because of its high energy, may now be absorbed by a second water molecule forming another water ion (H_2O^-):

$$e^- + H_2O \rightarrow H_2O^-$$

The pair of water ions produced is chemically unstable and tends to rapidly break down or dissociate into another ion and a free radical (a highly reactive species with an unpaired valence [outer shell] electron):

$$H_2O \rightarrow H_2O + 1e^-$$

The free radical is symbolized by a dot (e.g., H· or OH·).

The ion pair (H^+ and OH^-) may recombine, thus forming a normal water molecule with no net damage to the cell. The probability of recombination is high if the two ions are formed close to each other. If these ions persist in the cell, they can react with and damage important macromolecules.

Free radicals may also recombine in the same manner as the previous ion pair, thus forming a normal water molecule:

$$H^\bullet + OH^\bullet \rightarrow H_2O$$

Free radicals may also combine with other nearby free radicals, thus forming a new molecule such as hydrogen peroxide that is toxic to the cell:

$$OH^\bullet + OH^\bullet \rightarrow H_2O_2 \text{ (hydrogen peroxide)}$$

Free radicals can participate in several other reactions involving normal cellular components, including DNA. Because the majority of the cell (80%) consists of water, the probability of damage by indirect effects is much greater than direct effects with the use of indirectly ionizing radiations. Of the several reactions just presented for indirect effects, the predominant pathway that accounts for approximately two-thirds of cellular damage involves the hydroxyl (OH·) radical. As discussed later, indirect effects predominate with sparsely ionizing or low linear energy transfer (LET) (average energy deposited per unit path length) radiations and can be modified by physical, chemical, or biologic factors. It is important to keep in mind that because the majority of the cell consists of water, the probability of damage occurring through indirect action is greater than the probability of damage through direct action.

Let's review:

Direct ionization:

- Occurs more often with densely ionizing radiations (protons and alpha particles).
- These are considered high LET radiations.
- The fast electron directly ionizes the DNA molecule, causing damage.

Indirect ionization:

- Predominant with sparsely ionizing radiations (x-rays and gamma rays).
- Causes damage to the DNA molecule mostly from splitting of H_2O (radiolysis).
- The free radicals created by the water splitting (H·, OH·), are highly reactive, and they in turn react with the DNA molecule.
- Two-thirds of the cellular damage caused by free radicals can be attributed to OH·.
- H_2O_2 (hydrogen peroxide) is toxic to the cell.

Linear Energy Transfer and Relative Biologic Effectiveness

Depending on the composition of the incident beam of radiation, various secondary particles are produced in the cell. These secondary particles may directly or indirectly ionize the critical target. The physical properties of these secondary particles (mass and charge) give rise to a characteristic path of damage in the cell. Radiations can therefore be categorized by the rate at which energy is deposited by charged particles (incident or secondary) while they travel through matter. This is the LET of the radiation.[4] The LET is an average value calculated by dividing the energy deposited in kiloelectron volts (keV) by the distance traveled in micrometers (μm or 10^{-6} m). *Sparsely ionizing* radiations such as x-rays and gamma rays are therefore classified as low LET because the secondary electrons produced are small particles that deposit their energy over great distances in tissue. Typical LET values for sparsely ionizing radiations may range from 0.3 to 3.0 keV/μm.[5] *Densely ionizing* radiations, which include charged particles such as protons and alpha particles, are classified as *high LET* because these particles are much bulkier in terms of mass than electrons, and therefore deposit their energy over much smaller distances in the cell (Fig. 4.1). LET is therefore directly proportional to the square of the charge (Q) and inversely proportional to the square of the velocity (v). The previously described relationship is expressed in the following equation:

$$LET = \frac{Q^2}{v^2}$$

Typical LET values may range from 30 to 100 keV/μm or greater, depending on the particle energy. Generally, a large charged particle such as a proton or alpha particle does not penetrate nearly as far as a smaller charged particle (electron) and not quite as far as an uncharged particle of equal mass (neutron). Neutrons usually have intermediate LET values (usually within the range of 5–20 keV/μm). While the neutron's energy increases, its penetration in tissue also increases; therefore, its LET decreases.

Knowledge of the LET of the radiation is important because it was discovered early in the study of radiation therapy that different LET radiations produce different degrees of the same biologic response. In other words, equal doses of different LET radiations do not produce the same biologic response. This fact is called the relative biologic effectiveness (RBE) of the radiation.[3] The RBE is related to the ability of radiations with different LETs delivered under the same conditions to produce the same biologic effect. The equation to determine the RBE of a test radiation is:

$$RBE \text{ of test radiation} = \frac{\text{Dose from 250-keV x-ray}}{\text{Dose from test radiation to produce the same biologic effect}}$$

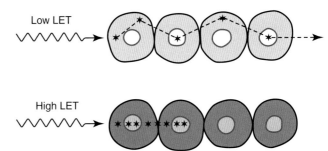

Fig. 4.1 Comparative effects of low– and high–linear energy transfer (LET) radiations on a population of cells. Low-LET radiation interacting with four cells emits an irregular path, whereas the straight path of high-LET radiation interacts with only two cells. High-LET radiation has produced two hits in the nuclei of two different cells, whereas low-LET radiation has produced only one hit in the same number of cells. (From Travis EL. *Primer of Medical Radiobiology.* 2nd ed. St. Louis, MO: Mosby; 1989.)

The test radiation referred to includes any type of radiation beam that is used. The effectiveness of the beam is determined by a historic comparison with a 250-keV x-ray beam that was the primary radiation beam available in the early days of radiation therapy. For example, if 400 cGy of 250-keV x-rays and 200 cGy of neutrons both result in 50% cell kill, the RBE of the neutrons equals 2. This result means that the neutrons are twice as effective as the x-rays. In general, while the LET of the radiation increases, so does its RBE. It is important to note that the biologic response, not the dose of radiation, is constant.

> While the LET of a radiation increases, the ionizations in the path become denser, creating more damage in the medium (tissue), and therefore more radiobiologic effect is observed. Therefore, while LET increases, RBE increases.

Radiation Effects on Deoxyribonucleic Acid

As mentioned earlier, the critical target in the nucleus of the cell for radiation damage is thought to be DNA. Damage to this key molecule may be lethal to a cell and has led to the development of a target theory for radiation damage. This theory states that when ionizing radiation interacts with or near a key molecule, the sensitive area is termed a *target*. An ionization event that occurs in the target is termed a *hit*. These terms are applied only under conditions in which radiation interacts with the target by direct effects. This theory does not account for damage to DNA that is the result of free radical–mediated pathways (indirect ionization).

Regardless of whether DNA is damaged by direct or indirect effects caused by radiation, several types of damage can occur.[6] DNA is a large molecule with a well-known double-helix structure. The double helix consists of two strands, held together by hydrogen bonds between the bases. The "backbone" of each strand consists of alternating sugar and phosphate groups. Attached to this backbone are four bases, the sequence of which specifies the genetic code. Two of the bases are termed *pyrimidines*: thymine and cytosine. The remaining two bases are termed *purines*: adenine and guanine.[3] One form of damage involves the change in or loss of one or more of the four nitrogenous (nitrogen-containing) bases: adenine (A), thymine (T), cytosine (C), and guanine (G). A second form of damage may involve breakage of hydrogen bonds between the A-T and C-G base pairs, which function to keep the two DNA strands together. Bonds may also be broken between the components of the backbone of each DNA strand (i.e., between the deoxyribose sugar and phosphate groups connected to each base and known collectively as a *nucleotide*). This may lead to intrastrand or interstrand cross-linking of DNA.

The consequences of these types of DNA damage vary. Loss or change of a base results in a new base sequence, which can cause minor or major effects on protein synthesis. A change in base sequence not rectified by the cell is an example of a mutation (change in the genetic

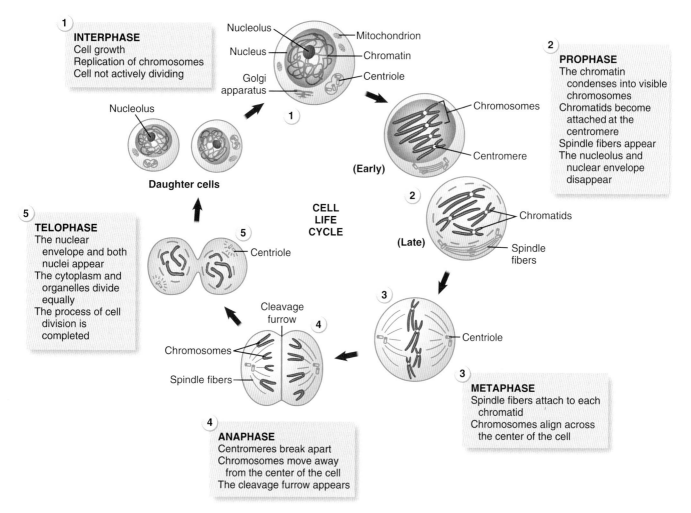

Fig. 4.2 The major events of mitosis. (From Patton KT, Thibodeau GA. *The Human Body in Health & Disease.* 7th ed. St. Louis, MO: Elsevier; 2018.)

material). Agents such as ionizing radiation that cause mutations are mutagenic. Single-strand breaks in the DNA backbone (common after irradiation with low-LET radiations) may or may not be repaired. If they are not repaired, damage may occur. Single-strand breaks, more commonly caused by low-LET radiations, are more readily repaired than double-strand breaks, which are more apparent after exposure to high-LET radiations. The production of multiple-strand breaks compared with single-strand breaks correlates much more strongly with cell lethality and therefore supports the theory that high LET produces more biologic effects (RBE). Radiation interaction with DNA does not always result in damage, and most of the damage can be and probably is repaired. Consequences of DNA damage in somatic (body) cells involve the irradiated organism or individual, whereas DNA damage in germ (reproductive) cells may also affect future generations.

Radiation Effects on Chromosomes

A review of the four phases of mitosis, which is a continuous process of organizing and arranging nuclear DNA during cell division, is helpful in understanding radiation effects on chromosomes. Fig. 4.2 shows the major events of mitosis. Because DNA molecules form genes and thousands of genes compose a chromosome, studying genetic damage from ionizing radiation in terms of gross structural damage to chromosomes is often easiest.[7]

Early studies in this area often involved plant chromosomes because their small diploid number (number of chromosomes in each somatic cell) and large relative size facilitated study under the light microscope.

The fact that radiation is an efficient breaker of chromosomes by indirect or direct pathways is now well documented. Gross structural changes in chromosomes are referred to as *aberrations, lesions,* or *anomalies.* A distinction also exists between chromosome and chromatid aberrations. A chromosome aberration occurs when radiation is administered to cells in the G1 phase or before the cell replicates its DNA in the S phase (cell duplication). A chromosome aberration may involve both daughter cells after mitosis, because if the break is not repaired, the cell replicates it during the S phase. A chromatid aberration results when radiation is administered to cells in the G2 phase or after they have completed DNA synthesis (cell duplication). This term applies to the arms (chromatids) of a replicated (duplicated) chromosome. In this situation, only one of the two daughter cells formed after cell division is affected if the damage is not repaired.

Structural changes induced in chromosomes by radiation include single breaks, multiple breaks, and a phenomenon known as *chromosome stickiness,* or *clumping.* Consequences of these structural changes may include healing with no damage and loss or rearrangement of genetic material.

A single radiation-induced break in any part of a chromosome results in two chromosome fragments. One fragment contains the centromere (the place the mitotic spindle attaches during mitosis), and the other (known as the *acentric fragment*) does not.[2] The rejoining of these fragments, termed *restitution,* has a high probability of occurring because of their proximity.[7] Approximately 95% of all single breaks heal by restitution with no resulting damage to the cell.

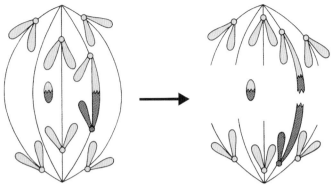

Fig. 4.3 The fate of the dicentric and acentric fragments during anaphase, thus leading to anaphase bridge formation. The dicentric fragment attaches to the mitotic spindle at each centromere and is pulled toward both poles of the cell *(left)* and ultimately breaks again *(right)*. The acentric fragment does not attach to the spindle, thus resulting in loss of genetic material to the new daughter cells. (From Travis EL. *Primer of Medical Radiobiology*. 2nd ed. St. Louis, MO: Mosby; 1989.)

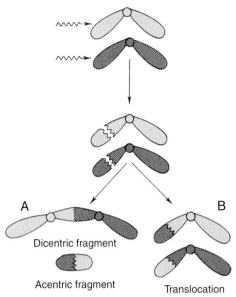

Fig. 4.4 Two different chromosomes *(top)* may sustain a single break in one arm *(center)* and result in formation of dicentric and acentric fragments (A) or translocation of genetic material between the two (B). In the latter process, two complete chromosomes are formed. However, the exchange of chromosome parts and therefore genetic information should be noted. (From Travis EL. *Primer of Medical Radiobiology*. 2nd ed. St. Louis, MO: Mosby; 1989.)

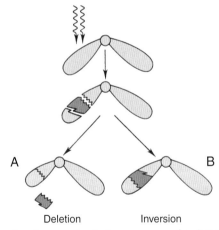

Fig. 4.5 Two breaks occurring in the same arm of a chromosome *(top* and *middle)* may result in deletion of the fragment between the breaks (A) or inversion of the fragment, which is illustrated by the change in positions of the break lines (B). (From Travis EL. *Primer of Medical Radiobiology*. 2nd ed. St. Louis, MO: Mosby; 1989.)

If irradiation occurs in G1 cells and restitution does not occur, both fragments are replicated during the S phase, thus resulting in four fragments (each with a broken end).[2] Two of these chromatids contain a centromere, whereas the other two do not. The two centromere-containing chromatids may now join, thus forming a *dicentric* fragment. The other two fragments may also join, thus forming an acentric fragment.

These structural aberrations become evident during the metaphase and anaphase stages of mitosis. Because the acentric fragment does not contain a centromere, the spindle fibers do not attach to it during the metaphase stage. Therefore the genetic material it contains probably will not be transmitted to either daughter cell. The dicentric fragment, however, has two centromeres and will therefore be attached to the mitotic spindle at two sites instead of one. Therefore, this fragment is pulled simultaneously toward both poles of the cell. The fragment between the two centromeres then becomes stretched, thus giving rise to a characteristic *anaphase bridge*, which eventually tears by the end of the anaphase stage, resulting in an unequal transmission of genetic information to each daughter cell (Fig. 4.3).

A single break in one chromatid in two different chromosomes also produces four fragments. Two fragments contain a centromere, and two do not.[2] Again, dicentric and acentric chromosomes may result by the joining of the broken fragments (Fig. 4.4A). In addition, the acentric fragment from one broken chromosome may join to a centromere-containing fragment of the other broken chromosome, thus forming a new normal-appearing chromosome. This rearrangement is known as *translocation* (Fig. 4.4B). Although translocation does not necessarily result in a loss of genetic information, the sequence of genes in the new translocated chromosome is different from the original sequence before radiation damage. The consequences of radiation-induced translocations can vary from no effects in somatic cells to malformed or nonviable offspring if these translocations occur in germ cells.

A double break in one arm (chromatid) of a chromosome results in three fragments, each with a broken end.[2] Of these three, one fragment contains the centromere, and the other two are acentric. The major consequences of a double break are known as *deletions* and *inversions* (see Fig. 4.3). A deletion of genetic material results when the fragment between the breaks is lost and the remaining two fragments join (Fig. 4.5A). The effect of a deletion varies depending on the amount and significance of the genetic information that was in the lost fragment. An inversion of genetic material results when the middle fragment with two broken ends turns around or inverts before rejoining the other two fragments (Fig. 4.5B). Although no loss of genetic material occurs after an inversion, the DNA base sequences, and therefore the gene sequence, are altered. This

alteration affects the types and amounts of critical proteins synthesized by the cell and can certainly affect the long-term viability of the cell.

Because of the random absorption of ionizing radiation in the cell, a single break can be induced in each chromatid of the same chromosome, thus again producing three fragments. The fragment with two broken ends contains the centromere, and the other two fragments are acentric. This may result in the formation of a ring chromosome and an acentric chromosome (Fig. 4.6).[2] The ring chromosome is replicated and transmitted to the daughter cells, whereas the acentric fragment and its genetic information are not passed on. If a replicated ring chromosome becomes tangled before the metaphase stage, unequal separation of each ring during the anaphase stage may result; therefore, the daughter cells do not inherit equal amounts of genetic information.

Several factors influence the type and extent of chromosome damage induced by ionizing radiations. The number of single breaks

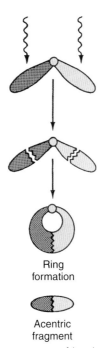

Ring
formation

Acentric
fragment

Fig. 4.6 One possible consequence of breaks in both arms of a chromosome by radiation is that the broken arms join to form a ring. The remaining fragments join but are left without a centromere (acentric fragment). (From Travis EL. *Primer of Medical Radiobiology.* 2nd ed. St. Louis, MO: Mosby; 1989.)

produced is directly proportional to the total dose of radiation administered. The frequency of single breaks, or simple aberrations, also increases as the LET of the radiation decreases. Therefore, low-LET radiations, such as x-rays and gamma rays, produce a higher amount of simple versus complex (multiple-break) aberrations.

Aberrations can be divided into two groups: *stable or unstable. Stable* aberrations may result in genetic mix-up, leading to mutations, but the cell's viability generally remains. Examples would be translocations, or inversion aberrations. Aberrations that usually kill the cell or result in its inability to indefinitely reproduce are called *unstable* aberrations. Rings, dicentrics, and anaphase bridges fall into this category.

Radiation Effects on Other Cell Components

Although nuclear DNA is the critical target for radiation-induced cell damage, other structures in the cell are also damaged by ionizing radiations and contribute to cell damage and death.[8] Among these cellular components is the plasma or cell membrane. Absorption of energy by the structural components of the plasma membrane (i.e., the phospholipid bilayer and proteins) can result in membrane damage and therefore changes in the permeability of the membrane with regard to the transport of substances in and out of the cell. Damage to the mitochondrial and lysosomal membranes in the cytoplasm can also result in drastic consequences to the cell. All cellular components (including vital proteins, enzymes, carbohydrates, and lipids) can undergo structural and functional changes after irradiation that can be deadly to the cell. Because the deposition of energy from secondary particles (electrons, protons, or alpha particles) is random in matter, any site in the cell can be at risk for damage from radiation exposure.

CELLULAR RESPONSE TO RADIATION

Since the mid-1950s, when Puck and Marcus[9] first irradiated human cervical carcinoma cells in a Petri dish, the response of human, animal, and plant cells to radiation has been intensely studied. The response of cells after irradiation can now be placed into one of three categories: division delay, interphase death, or reproductive failure.

The line of cervical carcinoma cells that have been used since the 1950s are termed *HeLa cells.* The New York Times bestseller *The Immortal Life of Henrietta Lacks* by Rebecca Skloot describes how HeLa cells have become one of the most important tools in medicine and examines the life of Henrietta Lacks, whose cervical cancer provided the first diagnosis of HeLa cells. Reading *The Immortal Life of Henrietta Lacks* as a class might create a beneficial discussion on how HeLa cells have impacted the field of radiation therapy.

Division Delay

Disruption in the mitotic index (MI), the ratio of the number of mitotic cells to the total number of cells in the irradiated population, a disruption that is caused by irradiated cells, is known as *division delay.* This process results in cells in interphase at the time of irradiation to be delayed in the G2 phase. This is also known as *mitotic delay.*

The consequence of mitotic delay is a decrease in the MI for the cell population, which means that fewer cells than normal will enter mitosis and divide. Therefore, fewer new daughter cells will be produced. The magnitude of this response to radiation is dose dependent; the higher the radiation dose, the longer the mitotic delay and therefore the greater the decrease in MI. If the dose is less than 1000 cGy, most cell lines recover and eventually proceed through mitosis. This results in a higher-than-normal number of cells dividing and is termed *mitotic overshoot.*

Canti and Spear[10] first observed division delay in 1929 when they exposed chick fibroblasts in vitro to various doses of radiation. The mechanism behind division delay is thought to involve the inhibition or delay of DNA and/or protein synthesis after irradiation. Apparently, cells attempt to repair radiation damage before mitosis by stopping in the G2 phase to confirm that the DNA and proteins are intact. Any damage found is repaired during this phase of the cell cycle so that it does not disrupt cell division or possibly lead to cell death. Division delay occurs in both lethally and nonlethally damaged cells.

Interphase Death

If irradiation of the cell during the G1, S, or G2 phase results in death, this mode of response is termed an *interphase death.*[11] Interphase death is defined as the death of irradiated cells before these cells reach mitosis, also known as *nonmitotic* or *nondivision death.*[2] This form of cell response can occur in nondividing cells (such as adult nerve cells) and rapidly dividing cells. In general, radiosensitive cells (vegetative intermitotic [VIM] and differentiating intermitotic [DIM]) succumb to an interphase death at lower radiation doses than radioresistant cells (reverting postmitotic [RPM] and fixed postmitotic [FPM]). The exception to this is the mature lymphocyte, which is sensitive to interphase death at a dose as low as 50 cGy. The mechanism of interphase death is not clear but may involve damage to one or more biochemical pathways involved in cell metabolism. In most cell types, interphase death is not the primary mode of response to irradiation.

Reproductive Failure

The third and most common end point for response of cells to radiation is reproductive failure (also known as *mitotic death*), which is defined as a decrease in the reproductive integrity or cells' ability to undergo an unlimited number of divisions after irradiation.[9] This effect on the reproductive capacity of cells can be traced to the extent of chromosome damage induced by the radiation dose.

Apoptosis

Although unrelated to mitosis, because it is not an unsuccessful attempt by the cell to divide, another form of cell death that has been associated with the cellular response to radiation is apoptosis (programmed cell death). Cellular apoptosis appears to have gene (*p53* and *bcl-2*)

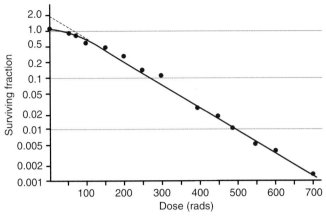

Fig. 4.7 The first survival curve with HeLa cells by Puck and Marcus. Below 150 cGy, the curve exhibits a shoulder region and becomes exponential (straight) at higher doses. (From Puck TT, Marcus TI. Action of x-rays on mammalian cells. *J Exp Med.* 1956;103:653.)

TABLE 4.1	**The Exponential Relationship Between a Radiation Dose and Surviving Fraction**		
Original Cell Number	**Dose Delivered (Gy)**	**Fraction of Cells Killed**	**Number of Cells Killed**
100,000	5	50	50,000
50,000	5	50	25,000
25,000	5	50	12,500
12,500	5	50	6,250
6,250	5	50	3,125

From Travis EL. *Primer of Medical Radiobiology.* 2nd ed. St. Louis, MO: Mosby; 1989.

involvement following exposure to radiation.[3] A characteristic apoptotic cell death involves nuclear fragmentation, cell lysis, and phagocytosis of the chromatin bodies by neighboring cells.[2]

CELL SURVIVAL CURVES

The most common way of evaluating the cellular response to radiation was first introduced by Puck and Marcus[9] in 1956, when they irradiated human cervical cancer cells (known as *HeLa cells*) in vitro and plotted the results (number of colonies formed) on a semilogarithmic graph. Their results, termed a *survival curve*, was a plot of the radiation dose administered on the x-axis versus the surviving fraction (SF) of cells on the y-axis (Fig. 4.7).

This survival curve is characteristic of the survival of cells exposed to low-LET radiations such as x-rays or gamma rays. A shoulder region or flattening of the curve occurs at doses below 150 cGy and indicates that cells must accumulate damage in multiple targets to be killed. Because this survival curve is graphed on a semilog plot, the linear portion of the curve (doses of >150 cGy) indicates that equal increases in dose cause equal decreases in the SF of cells but the absolute number of cells killed varies (Table 4.1).[2]

This exponential response of cells to radiation is caused by the random probability of radiation interacting with critical targets in the cell. Upon irradiation of a cell population with n targets/cell (with n > 1), several results are observed:

1. Some cells are lethally damaged (all targets are hit).
2. Some cells are sublethally damaged (a few targets are hit).
3. Some cells are not damaged (no targets are hit).

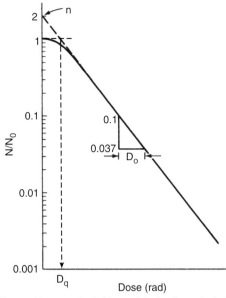

Fig. 4.8 The multitarget, single-hit model of cell survival characteristic low–linear energy transfer (LET) radiations (x-rays and gamma rays). The parameters n, D_o, and D_q should be noted. (From Bushong SC. Radiologic Science for Technologists: Physics, Biology, and Protection. 10th ed. St. Louis, MO: Mosby; 2013.)

While the radiation dose increases, the probability of cellular targets being hit also increases.

Three important parameters that allow interpretation of survival curves are the extrapolation number (n), quasithreshold dose (D_q), and D_o dose. A characteristic survival curv for cells exposed to x-rays is shown in Fig. 4.8.[12]

The n, originally known as the *target number*, is determined by extrapolating the linear portion of the curve back until it intersects the y-axis. In Fig. 4.8, the n equals 2, which theoretically means two critical targets are in the cell and must be inactivated. For mammalian cells exposed to x-rays, the n ranges from 2 to 10.

Another measure of cell response at low doses is the D_q. This parameter represents the dose at which survival becomes exponential, meaning that below this threshold dose, there appears to be no effect on cell death. The D_q is a measure of the width of the shoulder region of the survival curve and is determined by drawing a horizontal line from an SF of 1 on the y-axis to the place it intersects the line extrapolated back from the linear portion of the curve for determination of *n*. The D_q is also a measure of the cell's ability to accumulate and repair sublethal damage.[13,14]

If a cell population has a high D_q value, one could assume that it is good at repairing sublethal damage; therefore, radioresistant D_q is a measurement of radiosensitivity.

The third parameter, known as the D_o (or D37) dose, reduces the SF of cells by 63%. In other words, 37% of the cells survive. The D_o equals the reciprocal of the slope of the curve's linear portion and is a measure of the cells' radiosensitivity. Radiosensitive cells have a low D_o, whereas radioresistant cells have a high D_o. For mammalian cells, the D_o usually is between 100 and 220 cGy.[3]

Several equations describe the dose-response relationships expressed by survival curves.[12] The three survival curve parameters are described by the equation $\log_e n = D_q/D_o$. The SF can be calculated as $SF = 1 - (1 - e^{-D/D_o})^n$. In this equation, n is the extrapolation number, and D is the total dose.[12] This equation accurately predicts the response of complex cell types, including most mammalian cells, in which the

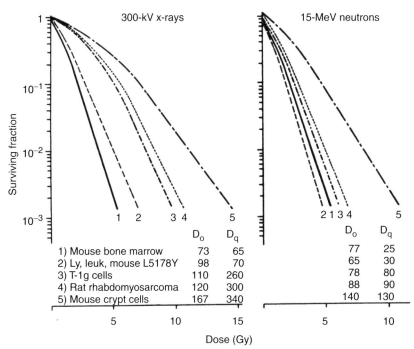

Fig. 4.9 Survival curves for various types of mammalian cells irradiated with 300-kV x-rays or 15-MeV neutrons. The wide variability in the shoulder (D_q) and slope (D_o) seen in the x-ray survival curves is reduced after neutron irradiation. The D_o and D_q values shown are expressed in Gy. (From Broerse JJ, Barendsen GW. Current topics. *Radiat Res Q.* 1973;8:305–350.)

number of targets is presumed to be greater than one. (This is known as the *multitarget, single-hit model*.)

Factors That Influence Response

As proposed by Ancel and Vitemberger[15] in 1925, various external factors influence cellular response to radiation. This change in response is termed *conditional sensitivity*. Three groups of factors can affect cellular radioresponse and therefore change the overall appearance of a cell line's survival curve and magnitude of the parameters n, D_q, and D_o. These factors are:

1. Physical: LET and dose rate.
2. Chemical: radiosensitizers and radioprotectors.
3. Biologic.

Physical Factors. The response of cells to high-LET radiation differs from that seen after exposure to low-LET radiation.[16] The response of five mammalian cell lines to 300-kV x-rays and 15-MeV neutrons is shown in Fig. 4.9. The shoulder region (D_q) is usually decreased or even absent after irradiation with high-LET radiations such as alpha particles and neutrons. In addition, survival curves tend to be steeper (the D_o is lower) after high-LET treatment. The effects of LET on biologic response result from differences in the density of energy deposition in the cell. Because DNA is thought to be the critical target in cells, the most efficient radiation with the highest RBE induces two strand breaks in the DNA molecule, thus leading to a high probability of cell death. This optimal LET is thought to be approximately 100 keV/μm. Therefore, all radiations with LETs above or below the optimal level are less efficient (have a lower RBE) in terms of cell killing (Fig. 4.10). At this density of ionizations, the average separation between ionizations coincides with the diameter of the DNA double helix (2 nm), thereby increasing the probability of double-stranded breaks with a single particle.[3]

A second physical factor that influences cellular radioresponse is dose rate.[17] A dose rate effect has been observed for reproductive

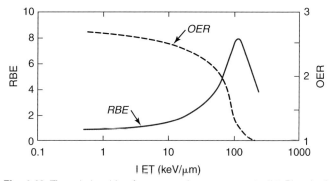

Fig. 4.10 The relationship of oxygen enhancement ratio *(OER)* and relative biologic effectiveness *(RBE)* as a function of linear energy transfer *(LET)*. The data were obtained by using T1 kidney cells of human origin, irradiated with various naturally occurring alpha particles. (From Barendsen GW. *Proceedings of the Conference on Particle Accelerators in Radiation Therapy*; LA-5180-C. Washington, DC: U.S. Atomic Energy Commission, Technical Information Center; 1972.)

failure, division delay, chromosome aberrations, and survival time after whole-body irradiation. Low dose rates are less efficient in producing damage than high dose rates. Survival curves generally shift to the right, thus becoming shallower (D_o increases), and the shoulder becomes indistinguishable at low dose rates (Fig. 4.11). This change in the appearance of the survival curve is explained by the cells' ability to repair sublethal damage from radiation treatment during and after exposure when given at sufficiently low dose rates. This dose rate effect is significant with low-LET radiations such as x-rays and gamma rays but is not observed with high-LET radiations.

Chemical Factors. Two major chemical factors influence the cellular response to radiation. Certain chemicals that enhance response to radiation are known as radiosensitizers. Other chemicals, termed

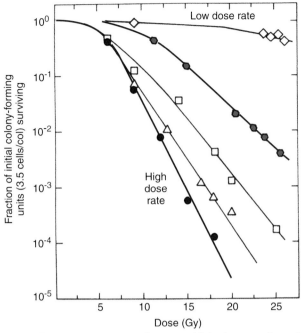

Fig. 4.11 Dose-response curves for an established mammalian cell line irradiated with a wide range of dose rates from a high of 1.07 Gy/min to a low of 0.0036 Gy/min. Reduction of the dose rate makes the survival curve more shallow and causes the shoulder to eventually disappear. (From Bedford JS, Mitchell JB. Dose-rate effects in synchronous mammalian cells in culture. *Radiat Res.* 1973;54:316–327.)

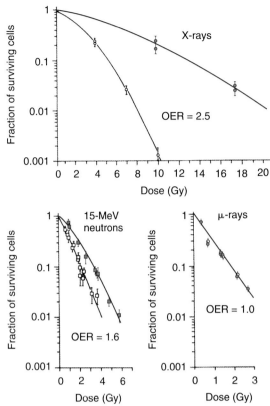

Fig. 4.12 A comparison of the oxygen effect after x-ray, neutron, or alpha particle irradiation. The oxygen enhancement ratio *(OER)* is highest after sparsely ionizing radiation (OER = 2.5), compared with densely ionizing radiations such as alpha particles (OER = 1.0). In the x-ray and neutron curves shown, the curve to the left represents the response of oxic cells, and the curve to the right represents the hypoxic cell response. The oxic and hypoxic curves overlap when alpha particles are used. (From Broerse JJ, Barendsen GW, van Kersen GR. Survival of cultured human cells after irradiation with fast neutrons at different energies in hypoxic and oxygenated conditions. *Int J Radiat Biol.* 1967;13:559–572.)

radioprotectors, have the opposite effect (i.e., they decrease the cellular response to radiation).

The most potent radiosensitizer to date is molecular oxygen. The oxygen effect has been observed in all organisms exposed to ionizing radiation.[18] Although the exact mechanism of the oxygen effect is unknown, the presence of oxygen is thought to enhance the formation of free radicals and "fix" or make radiation damage permanent that would otherwise be reversible. This is also known as the *oxygen fixation hypothesis.* Oxygen must be present during the radiation exposure for sensitization to occur. The sensitizing effects of oxygen are most significant with low-LET radiations in which indirect effects caused by free radical formation predominate over direct effects.

Cell survival curves differ for oxic (normal oxygen level) versus hypoxic (reduced oxygen level) cell populations.[19] While the availability of oxygen decreases, cell response also decreases such that the survival curve shifts to the right because D_q and D_o increase. This effect is most pronounced with x-rays and gamma rays. The effects are less while the LET of the radiation increases (Fig. 4.12). The magnitude of the oxygen effect is termed the oxygen enhancement ratio (OER).[3] The OER compares the response of cells with radiation in the presence and absence of oxygen. The equation to determine the OER for ionizing radiations is:

$$OER = \frac{\text{Radiation dose under hypoxic / anoxic conditions}}{\text{Radiation dose under oxic conditions to produce the same biologic effect}}$$

One common end point used to determine the OER is the D_o. For example, if the $D_o = 300$ cGy under hypoxic conditions but is reduced to 100 cGy under oxic conditions, the OER for the radiation in the experiment is 300/100 = 3.0. For mammalian cells, the OER for x-rays and

gamma rays is generally 2.5 to 3.0. This means that hypoxic cells are 2.5 to 3.0 times more resistant than oxic cells to a dose of low-LET radiation. Fig. 4.10 illustrates a strong correlation between the OER and RBE as a function of LET. This figure illustrates that the maximum RBE and the rapid decrease in OER occur at an LET of approximately 100 keV/μm.

Whereas oxygenation conditions are easily modifiable with cells in vitro, measurements of oxygen levels (known as *oxygen tension* or P_{O_2}) are more difficult to determine and modify in vivo. In vivo oxygen tensions of 20 to 30 μm Hg appear to render cells fully sensitive to low-LET radiations. The radiosensitivity of cells decreases while the P_{O_2} decreases, thus limiting the response of hypoxic cells in tumors treated with radiation.

Other compounds have also been tested as radiosensitizers. Most notable among these are halogenated pyrimidines and nitroimidazoles. Halogenated pyrimidines such as 5-bromo-deoxyuridine and 5-iodo-deoxyuridine are analogs of the DNA base thymidine.[20] These agents act as nonhypoxic cell sensitizers and are taken up by cycling cells during DNA synthesis (S phase). If enough of these compounds are substituted for thymidine, the DNA of the cell becomes more susceptible to radiation by a factor approaching 2. The rationale for the clinical use of these compounds is based on the shorter cycle times observed for tumor cells versus their normal cell counterparts. This should result in preferential uptake by tumors.

Nitroimidazoles such as misonidazole are oxygen-mimicking agents (i.e., they behave chemically like oxygen in terms of indirect effects involving free radicals).[1] In addition, nitroimidazoles may diffuse farther than oxygen from blood vessels, thereby reaching radioresistant hypoxic cells in a tumor. These agents are classified as *hypoxic cell sensitizers*. The idea behind their use is to selectively increase the radiosensitivity of hypoxic tumor cells. This desired selective sensitization of tumors has not been achieved in the clinic. Two major reasons for this are that (1) neither of these sensitizing agents exclusively localizes in malignant tissue, and (2) both of these agents cause side effects at therapeutic doses. New and improved sensitizing agents that localize in malignant tissues without toxic side effects are under development in the United States and England.

In some clinical situations, attempts have been made to protect normal tissues instead of sensitizing tumors to a dose of radiation. The agents used are known as *radiation protectors,* or *dose-modifying compounds.*[21] The most important group of protectors are sulfhydryls, agents that contain a free or potentially free sulfur (S) atom in their structure. Examples of sulfhydryls include cysteine, cysteamine, and WR-2721(Amifostine). Sulfhydryls act as free radical scavengers that compete with oxygen for free radicals formed after the radiolysis of water. If the sulfhydryl binds to the free radical before the oxygen does, the free radical can decay back to a harmless chemical species instead of causing damage to vital structures in the cell. The ability of a radioprotector to diminish the effects of a dose of radiation is called the *dose reduction factor (DRF).* The equation for determining the DRF is as follows[3]:

$$DRF = \frac{\text{Radiation dose with the radioprotector}}{\begin{array}{c}\text{Radiation dose without the radioprotector}\\\text{to produce an equal biologic effect}\end{array}}$$

Similar to the oxygen effect, radioprotectors must be present during the irradiation. In practice, radioprotectors are administered at short time intervals (within 30 minutes) before radiation therapy. In general, this allows uptake by normal tissues so that they are protected without allowing enough time for significant tumor uptake. This therefore precludes protection of the tumor. If the radioprotector is effective, a DRF of 2.0 to 2.7 may be achieved, depending on the normal tissue that is involved. Similar to the oxygen effect, protection by sulfhydryls is much more significant against low-LET radiations that depend on free radical mechanisms, whereas little or no protection against high-LET radiations can be achieved. As with radiosensitizers, therapeutic doses of radioprotectors often cause side effects in patients. This fact has limited the widespread clinical use of radioprotectors.

> Sulfhydryls act as "free radical scavengers" that compete with oxygen for free radicals formed after the radiolysis of water.

Biologic Factors. Cellular response is also affected by two important biologic factors: position in the cell cycle and ability to repair sublethal damage. Cellular radiosensitivity is dependent on the specific phase of the cell cycle containing the cells at the time of irradiation (this fact is also referred to as *age response*). In general, cells are most sensitive in the G2 and M phases, of intermediate sensitivity in the G1 phase, and most resistant in the S phase, especially during late S (Fig. 4.13).[22] This variation in response of cells should not be discounted because the D_o for late S-phase cells may be as much as 2.5 times higher than for the same cells in the G2 and M phases. During irradiation of asynchronous cells with low doses, the majority of survivors are expected to be S-phase cells.

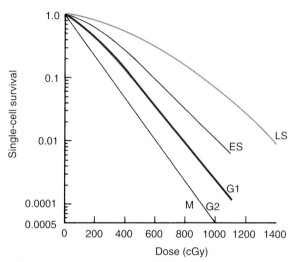

Fig. 4.13 The effect of cell-cycle position on survival of a synchronous population of cells. The M and G2 phases are the most radiosensitive, whereas the early S period *(ES)* and late S period *(LS)* are the most resistant. (From Sinclair WK. Cyclic responses in mammalian cells in vitro. *Radiat Res.* 1968;33:620.)

In addition to the variation in sensitivity caused by position in the cell cycle, Elkind and Sutton-Gilbert[14] showed in 1960 that cell survival increases if a dose of radiation is administered in fractions as a split dose instead of as a single dose (with the total dose remaining the same). Elkind and Sutton-Gilbert also showed that, depending on the time interval between each fraction, the survival curve parameters *n*, D_q, and D_o can remain the same as expected after a single-dose treatment. With low-LET radiations, Elkind and Sutton-Gilbert showed that the shoulder on the survival curve repeated after each fraction. This result indicated that cells were repairing sublethal damage from the first fraction before exposure to the second fraction.[14] This repair of sublethal damage after low-LET irradiation appears to be completed in most cell lines tested within several hours of each exposure, depending on the dose/fraction. This repair of sublethal damage in normal tissues during fractionated radiation therapy in the clinic may account for the sparing of normal tissues relative to tumors. In addition, hypoxia reduces a cell's capacity to repair sublethal damage. This may partially account for the favorable tumor responses after fractionation compared with single-dose radiation therapy.

RADIOSENSITIVITY

Law of Bergonié and Tribondeau

In 1906, two scientists, Bergonié and Tribondeau,[23] performed experiments by using rodent testes to investigate reported clinical effects of radiation known at the time. Testes were chosen as the model for the experiments because they contain cells differing in function and mitotic activity. These cell types ranged from immature, mitotically active spermatogonia to mature, nondividing spermatozoa (sperm).

The results of the animal experiments indicated that immature, rapidly dividing cells were damaged at lower radiation doses than mature, nondividing cells. This result led to the formation of the Law of Bergonié and Tribondeau, which states that ionizing radiation is more effective against cells that (1) are actively mitotic, (2) are undifferentiated, and (3) have a long mitotic future. Bergonié and Tribondeau therefore defined radiosensitivity in terms of the mitotic activity and the level of differentiation. These two characteristics determined a normal cell's sensitivity to radiation. Therefore, cells that divide more often are more radiosensitive than cells that divide less often or not at all.

TABLE 4.2 Classification of Mammalian Cells According to Their Characteristics and Radiosensitivities

Cell type	Characteristics	Examples	Radiosensitivity
VIM	Divide regularly and rapidly, are undifferentiated, and do not differentiate between divisions	Type A spermatogonia, erythroblasts, crypt cells, and basal cells	Extremely high
DIM	Actively divide, are more differentiated than VIMs, and differentiate between divisions	Intermediate spermatogonia and myelocytes	High
Vessels/connective tissue	Irregularly divide and are more differentiated than VIMs or DIMs	Endothelial cells and fibroblasts	Intermediate
RPM	Do not normally divide but retain capability of division and are variably differentiated	Parenchymal cells of liver and lymphocytes[a]	Low
FPM	Do not divide and are highly differentiated	Nerve cells, muscle cells, erythrocytes, and spermatozoa	Extremely low

[a]Lymphocytes, although classified as relatively radioresistant by their characteristics, are extremely radiosensitive.
DIM, Differentiating intermitotic; *FPM*, fixed postmitotic; *RPM*, reverting postmitotic; *VIM*, vegetative intermitotic.
From Travis EL. *Primer of Medical Radiobiology.* 2nd ed. St. Louis, MO: Mosby; 1989.

The level of maturity or differentiation of a cell refers to its level of functional and/or structural specialization. According to Bergonié and Tribondeau, cells that are undifferentiated (i.e., immature cells, the primary function of which is to divide and replace more mature cells lost from the population) are extremely radiosensitive. These cells are also known as *stem* or *precursor cells*. In the testes, a spermatogonia is an example of a stem cell. A fully differentiated cell, known as an *end cell*, has a specialized structure or function, does not divide, and is radioresistant. Two examples of end cells are spermatozoa in the testes and erythrocytes in the circulating blood. In 1925, Ancel and Vitemberger[15] added to the findings of Bergonié and Tribondeau. Ancel and Vitemberger proposed that the environmental conditions of a cell before, during, or after radiation treatment could influence the extent and appearance of radiation damage. Current knowledge indicates that the expression of radiation damage generally occurs when the cell is stressed, usually during reproduction. The sensitivity of a cell to radiation can also be modified. This change in sensitivity is known as *conditional sensitivity*.

Cell Populations

In 1968, Rubin and Casarett[24] grouped mammalian cell populations into five basic categories based on radiation sensitivity (Table 4.2). The end point chosen was radiation-induced cell death. The most radiosensitive of these groups is known as *VIM cells*. VIM cells are rapidly dividing, undifferentiated cells with short life spans. Examples include basal cells, crypt cells, erythroblasts, and type A spermatogonia.

The second most radiosensitive group is known as *DIM cells*. These cells are also actively mitotic but a little more differentiated than VIM cells. In fact, VIM cells such as type A spermatogonia divide and mature into DIM cells such as type B spermatogonia.

The third group of cells, known as *multipotential connective tissue cells*, is intermediate in radiosensitivity. These cells (such as endothelial cells of blood vessels and fibroblasts of connective tissue) divide irregularly and are more differentiated than VIM and DIM cells.

The fourth group, *RPM cells*, normally do not divide but are capable of doing so. RPM cells typically live longer and are more differentiated than the three previously discussed groups. These cells, including liver cells, are relatively radioresistant. Another example of an RPM cell is the mature lymphocyte. This cell, however, is very radiosensitive despite its characteristics and is therefore an exception to the Law of Bergonié and Tribondeau.

The most radioresistant group of cells in the body is known as *FPM cells*. FPM cells are highly differentiated, do not divide, and may or may not be replaced when they die. Examples include certain nerve cells, muscle cells, erythrocytes, and spermatozoa.

Tissue and Organ Sensitivity

Because radiosensitivities of specific cells in the body are now known, that information can be used to determine radiosensitivities of organized tissues and organs. Structurally, tissues and organs are composed of two compartments: the parenchyma and stroma. The parenchymal compartment contains characteristic cells of that tissue or organ. VIM, DIM, RPM, and FPM cells are examples of parenchymal cells. The parenchyma is considered the functional unit of the cell. Regardless of the types of parenchymal cells in a tissue or organ, they also have a supporting stromal compartment.[25] The stroma consists of connective tissue and the vasculature and is generally considered intermediate in radiosensitivity, according to Rubin and Casarett.[24]

The radiosensitivity of a tissue or an organ is a function of the most sensitive cell it contains.[24] For example, the testes and bone marrow are considered radiosensitive because of the presence of VIM stem cells in their parenchymal compartments. In these two organs, parenchymal cells are damaged at lower radiation doses than stromal cells (fibroblasts and endothelial cells). Radiation-induced sterility in males can occur after high doses because of destruction of immature spermatogonia cells that were destined to become mature spermatozoa.[26] A decrease in circulating erythrocytes in the blood after irradiation is caused by destruction of the more sensitive stem cell (erythroblast) in the bone marrow.[11]

Tissues and organs that contain only RPM or FPM parenchymal cells are therefore more radioresistant. Examples include the liver, muscle, brain, and spinal cord. In this situation, stromal cells are damaged at lower doses than parenchymal cells. Blood vessels in these organs become damaged, thus decreasing blood flow and therefore the supply of oxygen and nutrients to the parenchymal cells. Therefore, radiation-induced death of parenchymal cells in these organs is predominantly caused by stromal damage. This form of indirect cell death is a significant mechanism of radiation damage in radioresistant tissues and organs.

SYSTEMIC RESPONSE TO RADIATION

Response and Healing

Response to ionizing radiation treatment refers to visible (detectable) structural and functional changes that a dose produces in a certain period. Response at all levels (whether in a cell, a tissue, an organ, a system, or the entire organism) is a function of the dose administered, the volume irradiated, and the time of observation after exposure. With the exception of cataracts of the ocular lens, radiation-induced changes are neither unique nor distinguishable from biologic effects caused by other forms of trauma.

Structural or morphologic response after irradiation is usually grouped into two phases: early or acute changes observed within 6 months of treatment and late or chronic changes occurring more than 6 months later.[2] The appearance of late changes is a consequence of early changes that were irreversible and progressive. The probability of late changes occurring depends on the dose administered, the volume irradiated, and the healing ability of the irradiated structure (organ).

Organ healing can occur after radiation exposure by the process of regeneration or repair.[2] *Regeneration* refers to the replacement of damaged cells by the same cell type. Regeneration results in partial or total reversal of early radiation changes and is likely to occur in organs containing actively dividing VIM and DIM parenchymal cells. Examples include the skin, small intestine, and bone marrow. Regeneration is the desired healing process and can restore an organ to its preirradiated state.

Irreversible early changes, however, heal by the process of repair. *Repair* refers to the replacement of damaged cells by a different cell type, thus resulting in scar formation or fibrosis. Healing by repair does not restore an organ to its preirradiated state. Repair can occur in any organ and is more likely after high doses ($\geq$1000 cGy) that destroy parenchymal cells, thus making regeneration impossible. Repair is the predominant healing process in radioresistant organs containing RPM and FPM parenchymal cells that do not divide or have lost the ability to do so.

Under conditions that produce massive and extensive damage to the organ, neither healing process may occur, and tissue death or necrosis results. Therefore, the type of healing, if any, that occurs is a function of the dose received and the volume of the organ receiving it.

The total dose that is tolerated depends on the volume of the tissue irradiated and the architecture of their functional subunits (FSUs).[3] Enough FSUs must remain clonogenic for the tissue repair to occur. If the tissue has *structurally defined* FSUs, then it can only repair a predetermined area or functional space of the organ (e.g., kidney glomerulus and spinal cord). *Structurally undefined* FSUs, such as those located in the skin, allow cells to migrate throughout the organ and repair the necessary damage.

The other important factor that must be considered is the time after the treatment. In general, radiosensitive organs (e.g., the skin) respond faster and more severely than radioresistant organs.[2] The reverse situation may hold true at a later time. For example, irradiation of skin and lung tissue with a dose of 2000 cGy induces severe early skin changes but minimal early lung changes (within 6 months). However, if the same tissues are examined 6 to 12 months after irradiation, minimal late changes are found in the skin, but severe late changes are observed in the lung. This rate of response depends mostly on the cell cycle or generation times of the parenchymal cells in each organ. Because most cells die when attempting to divide after irradiation, cells with short cycle times show radiation damage sooner than cells with long cycle times. In comparing skin and lung parenchymal cells, cycle times are considerably shorter for parenchymal cells of the skin.

General Organ Changes

The most common early or acute changes after irradiation include inflammation, edema, and possible hemorrhaging in the exposed area. If doses are high enough, these early changes may progress to characteristic late or chronic changes, including fibrosis, atrophy, and ulceration. These late changes are not reversible and therefore are

permanent. The most severe late response is tissue necrosis or death. The sensitivity of the most radiosensitive organ of a system determines the general response of that system in the body. The Radiation Therapy Oncology Group[27] has summarized the acute and chronic effects of radiation into various categories or grades based on the severity of the clinical response[28] (Tables 4.3 and 4.4).

These are categorized as *deterministic effects* because they have a dose threshold associated with a clinical response.

> Deterministic effects occur when the number of cells lost is sufficiently large and affects the function of the organ. The probability of the effect is zero below a threshold dose, and the severity of harm also increases above this threshold dose.[3]

TOTAL-BODY RESPONSE TO RADIATION

This section involves specific signs and symptoms induced by exposure of the entire body at one time to ionizing radiation. The total-body response to radiation is presented in terms of three radiation syndromes.[3] Characteristics of each syndrome are dependent on the dose received and exposure conditions. Three specific exposure conditions apply in dealing with radiation syndromes: (1) exposure must be acute (minutes), (2) total-body or nearly total-body exposure must occur, and (3) exposure must be from an external penetrating source rather than ingested, inhaled, or implanted radioactive sources.[2]

Radiation Syndromes in Humans

Although an abundance of animal data regarding the effects of total-body exposure to radiation exists, considerably less human data under the same conditions are available. However, human data are available from (1) industrial and laboratory accidents, (2) fallout from atomic bomb test sites, (3) therapeutic medical exposures, (4) individuals exposed at Hiroshima and Nagasaki, and (5) the nuclear reactor accident at Chernobyl in the Soviet Union. As with lower animals, humans suffer the three radiation syndromes if the same exposure conditions are met.[3] Table 4.5 contains a summary of the acute radiation syndromes in humans after whole-body irradiation.

Each syndrome occurs in three phases:
1. Prodromal phase:
   a. Symptoms correlate to dose and can be gastrointestinal, neurologic, or both in nature.
2. Latent phase:
   a. Period in which victim appears to have no symptoms of exposure.
3. Manifest illness phase
   a. The effects of the exposure become evident and correlate with dose.

Hematopoietic Syndrome. The hematopoietic syndrome in humans is induced by total-body doses of 100 to 1000 cGy.[3] The median lethal dose, $LD_{50/60}$, for humans is estimated to be between 350 and 450 cGy but varies with age, health, and gender. Typically, females are more resistant than males, and the extremely young and old tend to be a little more sensitive than middle-aged persons. The prodromal stage or syndrome is observed within hours after exposure and is characterized by nausea and vomiting. The latent stage then occurs and lasts from a few days to as long as 3 weeks. Although the affected individual feels well at this time, bone marrow stem cells are dying. Peripheral blood cell counts decrease during the subsequent manifest illness stage at 3 to 5 weeks after exposure. Depression of all blood cell counts, termed *pancytopenia*, results in anemia (from a decreased number of

TABLE 4.3 Radiation Therapy Oncology Group Acute Radiation Morbidity Scoring Criteria

Organ/Tissue	Grade 0	Grade 1	Grade 2	Grade 3	Grade 4
Skin	No change from baseline	Follicular, faint, or dull erythema; epilation; dry desquamation; decreased sweating	Tender or bright erythema; patchy, moist desquamation; moderate edema	Confluent, moist desquamation other than skin folds; pitting edema	Ulceration, hemorrhage, necrosis
Mucous membrane	No change from baseline	Injection/patient may experience mild pain not requiring analgesic	Patchy mucositis that may produce an inflammatory serosanguineous discharge, patient may experience moderate pain requiring analgesic	Confluent fibrinous mucositis, patient may experience severe pain requiring narcotic	Ulceration, hemorrhage, necrosis
Eye	No change	Mild conjunctivitis with or without scleral injection, increased tearing	Moderate conjunctivitis with or without keratitis requiring steroids and/or antibiotics, dry eye requiring artificial tears, iritis with photophobia	Severe keratitis with corneal ulceration, objective decrease in visual acuity or in visual fields, acute glaucoma, panophthalmitis	Loss of vision (unilateral or bilateral)
Ear	No change from baseline	Mild external otitis with erythema, pruritus secondary to dry desquamation not requiring medication, audiogram unchanged from baseline	Moderate external otitis requiring topical medication, serious otitis media, hypoacusis on testing only	Severe external otitis with discharge or moist desquamation, symptomatic hypoacusis, tinnitus, not drug related	Deafness
Salivary gland	No change from baseline	Mild mouth dryness, slightly thickened saliva, may have slightly altered taste such as metallic taste; these changes not reflected in alteration in baseline feeding behavior, such as increased use of liquids with meals	Moderate to complete dryness; thick, sticky saliva, markedly altered taste	—	Acute salivary gland necrosis
Pharynx and esophagus	No change from baseline	Mild dysphagia or odynophagia, patient may require topical anesthetic or nonnarcotic analgesics, patient may require soft diet	Moderate dysphagia or odynophagia, patient may require narcotic analgesics, patient may require pureed or liquid diet	Severe dysphagia or odynophagia with dehydration or weight loss (>15% from pretreatment baseline) requiring NG feeding tube, IV fluids, or hyperalimentation	Complete obstruction, ulceration, perforation, fistula
Larynx	No change from baseline	Mild or intermittent hoarseness, cough not requiring antitussive, erythema of mucosa	Persistent hoarseness but able to vocalize; referred ear pain, sore throat, patchy fibrinous exudate, or mild arytenoid edema not requiring narcotic; cough requiring antitussive	Whispered speech, throat pain or referred ear pain requiring narcotic, confluent fibrinous exudate, marked arytenoid edema	Marked dyspnea, stridor, or hemoptysis with tracheostomy or intubation necessary
Upper GI tract	No change from baseline	Anorexia with ≤5% weight loss from pretreatment baseline, nausea not requiring antiemetics, abdominal discomfort not requiring parasympatholytic drugs or analgesics	Anorexia with ≤15% weight loss from pretreatment baseline, nausea and/or vomiting requiring antiemetics, abdominal pain requiring analgesics	Anorexia with >15% weight loss from pretreatment baseline or requiring NG tube or parenteral support; nausea and/or vomiting requiring tube or parenteral support; abdominal pain, severe despite medication; hematemesis or melena; abdominal distention (flat plate radiograph demonstrates distended bowel loops)	Ileus, subacute or acute obstruction, perforation, GI bleeding requiring transfusion; abdominal pain requiring tube decompression or bowel diversion
Lower GI tract including pelvis	No change from baseline	Increased frequency or change in quality of bowel habits not requiring medication, rectal discomfort not requiring analgesics	Diarrhea requiring parasympatholytic drugs (e.g., diphenoxylate/atropine [Lomotil]), mucous discharge not necessitating sanitary pads, rectal or abdominal pain requiring analgesics	Diarrhea requiring parenteral support, severe mucous or blood discharge necessitating sanitary pads, abdominal distention (flat plate radiograph demonstrates distended bowel loops)	Acute or subacute obstruction, fistula, or perforation; GI bleeding requiring transfusion; abdominal pain or tenesmus requiring tube decompression or bowel diversion

Continued

TABLE 4.3   Radiation Therapy Oncology Group Acute Radiation Morbidity Scoring Criteria—cont'd

Organ/Tissue	Grade 0	Grade 1	Grade 2	Grade 3	Grade 4
Lung	No change from baseline	Mild symptoms of dry cough or dyspnea on exertion	Persistent cough requiring narcotic, antitussive agents; dyspnea with minimal effort but not at rest	Severe cough unresponsive to narcotic antitussive agent or dyspnea at rest, clinical or radiologic evidence of acute pneumonitis, intermittent oxygen or steroids may be required	Severe respiratory insufficiency, continuous oxygen or assisted ventilation
Genitourinary	No change from baseline	Frequency of urination or nocturia twice pretreatment habit; dysuria, urgency not requiring medication	Frequency of urination or nocturia, which is less frequent than every hour; dysuria, urgency, bladder spasm requiring local anesthetic (e.g., phenazopyridine [Pyridium])	Frequency with urgency and nocturia hourly or more frequently; dysuria, pelvic pain, or bladder spasm requiring regular, frequent narcotic; gross hematuria with or without clot passage	Hematuria requiring transfusion; acute bladder obstruction not secondary to clot passage, ulceration, or necrosis
Heart	No change from baseline	Asymptomatic but objective evidence of ECG changes or pericardial abnormalities without evidence of other heart disease	Symptomatic with ECG changes and radiologic findings of congestive heart failure or pericardial disease, no specific treatment required	Congestive heart failure, angina pectoris, pericardial disease responding to therapy	Congestive heart failure, angina pectoris, pericardial disease, arrhythmias not responsive to nonsurgical measures
CNS	No change from baseline	Fully functional status (i.e., able to work) with minor neurologic findings, no medication needed	Neurologic findings present sufficient to require home care; nursing assistance may be required; medications including steroids, antiseizure agents may be required	Neurologic findings requiring hospitalization for initial management	Serious neurologic impairment that includes paralysis, coma, or seizures >3 per week despite medication; hospitalization required
Hematologic WBC (×1000)	≥4.0	3.0–4.0	2.0–3.0	1.0–2.0	<1.0
Platelets (×1000)	>100	75–100	50–75	25–50	<25 or spontaneous bleeding
Neutrophils	≥1.9	1.5–1.9	1.0–1.5	0.5–1.0	≤0.5 or sepsis
Hemoglobin (g %)	>11	11–9.5	9.5–7.5	7.5–5.0	—
Hematocrit (%)	≥32	28-32	≤28	Packed cell transfusion required	—

Guidelines: The acute morbidity criteria are used to score and grade toxicity from radiation therapy. The criteria are relevant from day 1, the commencement of therapy, through day 90. Thereafter, the European Organization for Research and Treatment of Cancer/Radiation Therapy Oncology Group criteria of late effects are to be used. The evaluator must attempt to discriminate between disease- and treatment-related signs and symptoms. An accurate baseline evaluation before commencement of therapy is necessary. All toxicities grade 3, 4, or 5+ must be verified by the principal investigator.

CNS, Central nervous system; *ECG,* electrocardiogram; *GI,* gastrointestinal; *IV,* intravenous; *NG,* nasogastric; *WBC,* white blood cell.

From Trotti A, Byhardt R, Stetz J, et al. Common toxicity criteria: version 2.0. An improved reference for grading the acute effects of cancer treatment: impact on radiotherapy. *Int J Radiat Oncol Biol Phys.* 2000;47:13–47.

erythrocytes), hemorrhaging (from a decreased number of platelets), and serious infection (from a decreased number of leukocytes).

The probability of survival decreases with an increasing dose. Most individuals receiving doses less than 300 cGy survive and eventually recover during the next 3 to 6 months. Survival time decreases with an increasing dose. After a dose of 300 to 500 cGy is reached, death may occur in 4 to 6 weeks. With a dose of 500 to 1000 cGy, death is likely within 2 weeks.[2] No record exists of human survival when the total body dose exceeds 1000 cGy.[3] The primary causes of death from the hematopoietic syndrome are infection and hemorrhaging after destruction of the bone marrow.

Gastrointestinal Syndrome. If the total body dose is between 1000 and 10,000 cGy, the gastrointestinal syndrome is induced.[3] This syndrome may also be induced by a dose as low as 600 cGy and overlaps with the cerebrovascular syndrome at doses of 5000 cGy or more.

The mean survival time for this syndrome is 3 to 10 days or as long as 2 weeks with medical support and is largely independent of the actual dose received. The prodromal stage occurs within hours after exposure and is characterized by nausea, vomiting, diarrhea, and cramps. The latent stage then occurs 2 to 5 days after exposure. At 5 to 10 days after exposure, nausea, vomiting, diarrhea, and fever mark the manifest illness stage. Death occurs during the second week after exposure.

The gastrointestinal syndrome occurs as a result of damage to the gastrointestinal tract and bone marrow. As discussed previously, the small intestine is the most radiosensitive portion of the digestive system.[29] After exposure to doses in excess of 1000 cGy, severe depopulation of crypt cells leads to partial or complete denudation of the villi lining the lumen of the small intestine. Consequences of this damage include decreased absorption of materials across the intestinal wall, leakage of fluids into the lumen (resulting in dehydration),

TABLE 4.4 Radiation Therapy Oncology Group/European Organization for Research and Treatment of Cancer Late Radiation Morbidity Scoring Schema

Organ/Tissue	Grade 0	Grade 1	Grade 2	Grade 3	Grade 4	Grade 5[a]
Skin	None	Slight atrophy, pigmentation change, some hair loss	Patchy atrophy, moderate telangiectasia, total hair loss	Marked atrophy, gross telangiectasia	Ulceration	Death directly related to radiation is a late effect for all tissue types
Subcutaneous tissue	None	Slight induration (fibrosis) and loss of subcutaneous fat	Moderate fibrosis but asymptomatic; slight field contracture (<10% linear reduction)	Severe induration and loss of subcutaneous tissue, field contracture (>10% linear measurement)	Necrosis	
Mucous membrane	None	Slight atrophy and dryness	Moderate atrophy and telangiectasia; little mucus	Marked atrophy with complete dryness, severe telangiectasia	Ulceration	
Salivary glands	None	Slight dryness of mouth, good response on stimulation	Moderate dryness of mouth, poor response on stimulation	Complete dryness of mouth, no response on stimulation	Fibrosis	
Spinal cord	None	Mild Lhermitte syndrome	Severe Lhermitte syndrome	Objective neurologic findings at or below cord level treated	Mono-paraquadriplegia	
Brain	None	Mild headache, slight lethargy	Moderate headache, great lethargy	Severe headaches, severe CNS dysfunction (partial loss of power or dyskinesia)	Seizures or paralysis, coma	
Eye	None	Asymptomatic cataract, minor corneal ulceration or keratitis	Symptomatic cataract, moderate corneal ulceration, minor retinopathy or glaucoma	Severe keratitis, severe retinopathy or detachment, severe glaucoma	Panophthalmitis; blindness	
Larynx	None	Hoarseness, slight arytenoid edema	Moderate arytenoid edema, chondritis	Severe edema; severe chondritis	Necrosis	
Lung	None	Asymptomatic or mild symptoms (dry cough), slight radiographic appearances	Moderate symptomatic fibrosis or pneumonitis (severe cough), low-grade fever, patchy radiographic appearances	Severe symptomatic fibrosis or pneumonitis; dense radiographic changes	Severe respiratory insufficiency, continuous O_2, assisted ventilation	
Heart	None	Asymptomatic or mild symptoms, transient T-wave inversion and ST changes, sinus tachycardia >110 beats/min (at rest)	Moderate angina on effort, mild pericarditis, normal heart size; persistent abnormal T wave and ST changes, low QRS	Severe angina; pericardial effusion, constrictive pericarditis, moderate heart failure, cardiac enlargement, ECG abnormalities	Tamponade; severe heart failure, severe constrictive pericarditis	
Esophagus	None	Mild fibrosis, slight difficulty in swallowing solids, no pain on swallowing	Unable to take solid food normally, swallowing only semisolid food, dilation may be indicated	Severe fibrosis, able to swallow only liquids, may have pain on swallowing, dilation required	Necrosis, perforation, fistula	
Small and large intestine	None	Mild diarrhea, mild cramping; bowel movement 5 times daily, slight rectal discharge or bleeding	Moderate diarrhea and colic, bowel movement >5 times daily, excessive rectal mucus or intermittent bleeding	Obstruction or bleeding requiring surgery	Necrosis, perforation, fistula	
Liver	None	Mild lassitude; nausea, dyspepsia, slightly abnormal liver function	Moderate symptoms, some abnormal liver function tests, serum albumin normal	Disabling hepatic insufficiency, liver function tests grossly abnormal, low albumin, edema, or ascites	Necrosis, hepatic coma or encephalopathy	
Kidney	None	Transient albuminuria; no hypertension; mild impairment of renal function, urea 25–35 mg/dL, creatinine 1.5–2.0 mg/dL, creatinine clearance >75%	Persistent moderate albuminuria (2+), mild hypertension; no related anemia; moderate impairment of renal function; urea >36–60 mg/dL, creatinine clearance 50%–74%	Severe albuminuria, severe hypertension, persistent anemia <10%, severe renal failure, urea >60 mg/dL, creatinine >4.0 mg/dL, creatinine clearance <50%	Malignant hypertension, uremic coma, urea >100%	

Continued

TABLE 4.4   Radiation Therapy Oncology Group/European Organization for Research and Treatment of Cancer Late Radiation Morbidity Scoring Schema—cont'd

Organ/Tissue	Grade 0	Grade 1	Grade 2	Grade 3	Grade 4	Grade 5[a]
Bladder	None	Slight epithelial atrophy, minor telangiectasia (microscopic hematuria)	Moderate frequency, generalized telangiectasia, intermittent macroscopic hematuria	Severe frequency and dysuria, severe generalized telangiectasia (often with petechiae), frequent hematuria; reduction in bladder capacity (<150 mL)	Necrosis; contracted bladder (capacity <100 mL), severe hemorrhagic cystitis	
Bone	None	Asymptomatic; no growth retardation, reduced bone density	Moderate pain or tenderness, growth retardation, irregular bone sclerosis	Severe pain or tenderness, complete arrest of bone growth, dense bone sclerosis	Necrosis, spontaneous fracture	
Joint	None	Mild joint stiffness, slight limitation of movement	Moderate stiffness, intermittent or moderate joint pain, moderate limitation of movement	Severe joint stiffness, pain with severe limitation of movement	Necrosis, complete fixation	

[a]Any toxicity that caused death is graded 5.
CNS, Central nervous system; ECG, electrocardiogram.
From Trotti A, Byhardt R, Stetz J, et al. Common toxicity criteria: version 2.0. An improved reference for grading the acute effects of cancer treatment: impact on radiotherapy, *Int J Radiat Oncol Biol Phys.* 2000;47:13–47; Cox JD, Stetz J, Pajak TF. Toxicity criteria of the Radiation Therapy Oncology Group (RTOG) and the European Organization for Research and Treatment of Cancer (EORTC). *Int J Radiat Oncol Biol Phys.* 1995;31:1341–1346.

TABLE 4.5   Summary of Acute Radiation Syndromes in Humans After Whole-Body Irradiation

Syndrome	Dose Range	Time of Death	Organ and System Damaged	Signs and Symptoms	Recovery Time
Hematopoietic	100–1000 cGy[a]	3 weeks–2 months	Bone marrow	Decreased number of stem cells in bone marrow, increased amount of fat in bone marrow, pancytopenia, anemia, hemorrhage, and infection	Dose dependent, 3 weeks to 6 months; some individuals do not survive
Gastrointestinal	1000–5000 cGy[b]	3–10 days	Small intestine	Denudation of villi in small intestine, neutropenia, infection, bone marrow depression, electrolyte imbalance, and watery diarrhea	None
Cerebrovascular	>5000 cGy	<3 days	Brain	Vasculitis, edema, and meningitis	None

[a]Median lethal dose, $LD_{50/60}$, for humans in this dose range (450 cGy).
[b]Median lethal dose, LD_{100}, for humans in this dose range (1000 cGy).
From Travis EL. *Primer of Medical Radiobiology.* 2nd ed. St. Louis, MO: Mosby; 1989.

and overwhelming infection as bacteria gain access to the circulating blood. Significant changes in bone marrow also occur, highlighted by a severe decrease in circulating leukocytes. However, death occurs before the other peripheral blood cell counts significantly decrease. Despite attempts at regeneration of crypt cells in the small intestine, bone marrow damage likely leads to death as a result of the overwhelming infection, dehydration, and electrolyte imbalance.

Cerebrovascular Syndrome. The third and final radiation syndrome is the cerebrovascular syndrome. This syndrome, which was formerly known as the *central nervous system syndrome*, occurs exclusively after doses of 10,000 cGy or more but can overlap with the gastrointestinal syndrome because it can be induced by a dose as low as 5000 cGy.[3] Death after such high total-body doses occurs in several days or less. The prodromal stage lasts only minutes to several hours (depending on the dose) and is characterized by nervousness, confusion, severe nausea and vomiting, loss of consciousness, and a burning sensation in the skin. The latent period (if distinguishable) lasts only several hours or less. Within 5 to 6 hours after exposure, the manifest illness stage begins and is characterized by watery diarrhea, convulsions, coma, and death.

The cause of death from cerebrovascular syndrome is not completely known at this time. At autopsy, brain parenchymal cells appear almost completely normal despite the high dose. These parenchymal cells are extremely radioresistant FPM cells, according to Rubin and Casarett.[24] Autopsy findings show extensive blood vessel (stromal) damage in the brain, thus resulting in vasculitis, meningitis, and edema in the cranial vault. The resulting increase in intracranial pressure is probably the major cause of death. In addition, peripheral blood counts and the villi of the small intestine do not exhibit significant changes in these individuals when examined at autopsy. This is the result of the exposed person not living long enough for these effects to become evident.

Response of the Embryo and Fetus

Radiation exposure can also damage the developing embryo and fetus in utero. Generally, in utero radiation damage manifests as lethal effects, congenital abnormalities present at birth, or late effects observed years later. These effects can be produced by (1) irradiation of the sperm or ovum before fertilization, thus resulting in inherited effects; or (2) exposure of the fetus to radiation, thus resulting in congenital defects. This section deals only with congenital abnormalities resulting from radiation exposure.

Stages of Fetal Development. Extensive mouse studies have established that the effect induced by radiation depends not only on the radiation dose, but also on the time of the exposure's occurrence during gestation.

The husband-and-wife research team of Russell and Russell[30] divided fetal development into three stages:

1. Preimplantation: In humans, the preimplantation stage occurs from conception (day 0) to 10 days after conception. During this time, the fertilized ovum is actively dividing, thus forming a ball of highly undifferentiated cells.[31]
2. Organogenesis: The newly formed ball of cells, known as the *embryo*, then implants in the uterine wall and begins the major organogenesis stage (from day 10 to week 6). During this time, on specific gestational days, embryonic cells differentiate into the stem cells that eventually form each organ in the body.
3. Fetal growth stage: At the end of the sixth week, the embryo is known as a *fetus* and enters the fetal growth stage, and continues to grow until birth. The central nervous system in the fetus differs from that in the adult because the neuroblasts (stem cells) of the fetus are still mitotically active and not fully differentiated. Therefore, unlike that of the adult, the fetal central nervous system is responsive to radiation and can be damaged at relatively low doses.

Radiation Effects on Humans in Utero. Radiation effects on human embryos have been investigated with data sources that were described previously (atomic bomb survivors in Japan after World War II, fallout exposures, occupational exposures, and diagnostic or therapeutic exposures of pregnant women).[32,33] A definitive cause-and-effect relationship between radiation and a specific abnormality is difficult to prove in human beings. The two primary reasons for this are (1) the background incidence of spontaneous congenital abnormalities is approximately 6%, and (2) radiation does not induce unique congenital abnormalities (excluding cataracts). Therefore, implicating a certain radiation exposure as the sole cause of a specific congenital abnormality is difficult. The results of animal studies have been extrapolated to humans to allow predictions with regard to effects that might occur in irradiated human embryos and fetuses (Fig. 4.14).

Unfortunately, human data exist for radiation effects from in utero exposure. A report in 1930 by Murphy and Goldstein[34] described congenital defects (microcephaly) attributed to radiation exposure in utero. In one study of children born to 11 women who were pregnant and received high doses from the bomb dropped in Hiroshima, 7 of the 11 children (64%) had microcephaly and were mentally retarded.[35] In another study of 30 children who were irradiated in utero at Nagasaki, 17 (57%) were affected (7 fetal deaths, 6 neonatal deaths, and 4 surviving children who were mentally retarded).[36] Table 4.6 illustrates the correlation between gestational stage and the probability of developing congenital malformations.

Dekaban[37] in 1968 studied children born to women irradiated with a therapeutic dose of 250 cGy during various stages of gestation. The results of this study indicated that exposure to the dose during the first 2 to 3 weeks of gestation produced a high frequency of prenatal death but few severe abnormalities in surviving children who were brought to term (similar to the mouse studies). This was later coined the "all or nothing" response. This theory supported that irradiation during

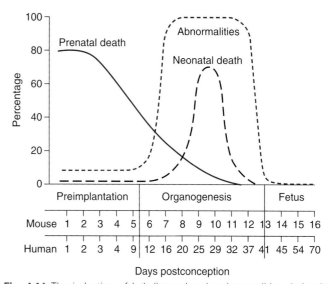

Fig. 4.14 The induction of lethality and major abnormalities during in utero exposure on different gestational days in the mouse embryo by using 2.0 Gy. Lower scale indicated Rugh's time estimates for the three stages in the human embryo. (From Travis EL. *Primer of Medical Radiobiology*. 2nd ed. St. Louis, MO: Mosby; 1989.)

TABLE 4.6 Summary of Radiation Effects on the Embryo and Fetus			
Stage of Gestation	Growth Retardation	Death	Microcephaly and Mental Retardation
Preimplantation	None	Embryonic death and resorption	None
Organogenesis	Temporary	Neonatal death	Very high risk
Fetal	Permanent	Approximately equal to the LD$_{50}$ in adults	High risk

LD$_{50}$, Median lethal dose, 50%.
From Hall EJ, Giaccia AJ. *Radiobiology for the Radiobiologist*. Philadelphia: Lippincott Williams & Wilkins; 2005.

this phase would either cause the fetus to spontaneously abort and be reabsorbed, or the fetus would continue to develop without any malformations or obvious effects of the exposure.[3] Irradiation between 4 and 11 weeks correlated with severe central nervous system and skeletal abnormalities, and corresponded to the organs in development during the exposure. The same dose (250 cGy) administered between the 11th and 16th week frequently resulted in mental retardation and microcephaly, whereas irradiation after the 20th week resulted in functional defects such as sterility.

> The maximum permissible dose to the fetus during the entire gestational period from occupational exposure of the mother should not exceed 0.5 rem (5 mSv), with monthly exposure not exceeding 0.05 rem (0.5 mSv).

In summary, although difficult to prove conclusively, the embryo and fetus are considered to be the most radiosensitive forms of animals and humans. Radiation, if it must be administered during a known pregnancy, should be delayed as much as possible because the fetus is more radioresistant than the embryo. In 1993, the International Commission on Radiological Protection recommended the 28-day rule, which states that the safe period for exposure of the possibly pregnant uterus is 28 days after menstruation.[6] As mentioned previously, the most radiosensitive period for induction of abnormalities in humans is between days 23 and 37. These effects usually involve the central nervous system and most commonly include microcephaly, mental retardation, sensory organ damage, and stunted growth. Skeletal changes appear to be most prevalent when radiation is administered between weeks 3 and 20.

> In regard to the fetal effects of radiation, the principal factors of importance are the dose and the stage of gestation at which it is delivered.

LATE EFFECTS OF RADIATION

The previous section dealt with the total-body response to high doses of radiation, which usually results in lethality. Of equal and possibly even more concern is the biologic response resulting from exposure to much lower doses of radiation. Because the latent period for an effect is inversely proportional to radiation dose, the biologic response to low doses is not observable for extended periods, ranging from years to generations.[3] These effects are therefore known as *late effects* and are termed *somatic effects* if body cells are involved or *genetic effects* if reproductive (germ) cells are involved.

> Latent period: The time interval between irradiation and the appearance of a malignancy is known as the latent period.

Somatic Effects (Carcinogenesis): Stochastic and Deterministic

Historic Background. The most important late somatic effect induced by radiation is carcinogenesis.[38–40] Radiation is therefore classified as a *carcinogen*, or *cancer-causing agent*. In 1902 (only 7 years after Roentgen's discovery of the x-ray), the first reported case of radiation-induced carcinoma appeared in the literature. By 1910, at least 100 cases of skin cancer were reported in radiologists and radiation oncologists who were unaware of the potential hazards of this new modality.

Carcinogenesis is considered to be an "all-or-nothing" event. This means that any dose, no matter how low, has some potential of inducing cancer. Cancer induction is therefore a nonthreshold event with the probability of an effect increasing as the dose increases. Carcinogenesis is therefore an example of a *stochastic effect*, in which every dose carries some magnitude of risk.[3]

Sufficient human data exist to implicate radiation as a cancer-causing agent. Most of the early data involve occupational exposures by radiation scientists, clinicians, and therapists who were chronically exposed to various radiation sources before the risks of such exposures were known. Ionizing radiation has been implicated as a cause of skin cancer, leukemia, osteosarcoma, lung cancer, breast cancer, and thyroid cancer.

> Stochastic effects occur when somatic cells are exposed to radiation. The probability of cancer increases with dose, with no threshold dose, but the severity of the cancer is not dose related.[3]

Leukemia. Radiation was first implicated as a cause of leukemia in 1911. That study involved 11 cases of leukemia in occupationally

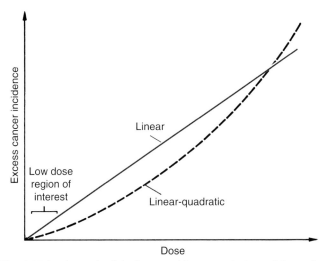

Fig. 4.15 A schematic of the linear and linear-quadratic models used to extrapolate the incidence of cancer from high-dose data down to low doses. Both models fit high-dose data as well, but at low doses, the estimated incidence depends on the model. (From Travis EL. *Primer of Medical Radiobiology*. 2nd ed. St. Louis, MO: Mosby; 1989.)

exposed individuals.[2] Atomic bomb survivors in Hiroshima and Nagasaki had higher incidences of leukemia than the nonexposed population.[3] Early radiologists in the United States who died between 1948 and 1961 had a much higher frequency of leukemia (300%) than the general population.[41,42] However, a similar study involving British radiologists showed no increased leukemia incidence in an early group (before 1921) compared with later groups who used some level of radiation safety.[43]

The latent period for leukemia induction by radiation is usually 4 to 7 years, with peak incidence approximately 7 to 10 years after exposure. This period is much shorter than that observed for radiation-induced solid tumors, which have latent periods ranging from 20 to 30 years or longer.[3]

Radiation induction of leukemia is somewhat specific in that only certain types of leukemia show an increased incidence in irradiated individuals. For example, only acute and chronic myeloid leukemia types are more prevalent in irradiated adults, whereas acute lymphocytic leukemia is more common in irradiated children.[44] Radiation exposure does not seem to affect the incidence of chronic lymphocytic leukemia. The available evidence suggests that leukemia induction is a nonthreshold (stochastic), linear response to radiation[11] (Fig. 4.15). However, other cancers induced by radiation may follow a linear-quadratic rather than a linear relationship to radiation dose.[3]

Skin Carcinoma. The first reported case of radiation-induced skin cancer (which occurred on the hand of a radiologist) was in 1902.[45] Because early x-ray machines were crude, radiologists placed their hands in the beam path to check its efficiency. This led to early skin changes (erythema) that were used to gauge the output of the beam, but skin tumors were observed years later in many of these individuals. Patients treated with radiation for several benign conditions such as acne and ringworm of the scalp also showed an increased incidence of skin cancer years later.[46] As a result of modern radiation safety procedures, skin cancers in radiation workers are no longer observed.

> Squamous cell and basal cell carcinomas have been the most frequently observed skin cancers in patients who have had radiation exposure.

Osteosarcoma. The most striking example of radiation-induced osteosarcoma, or bone cancer, is a group of radium watch-dial painters. These workers regularly licked their brushes (which contained radium paint) to make the brush tip come to a point before painting the watch dials. The radium, once ingested, was absorbed into the workers' bones. Of the several hundred workers exposed this way, approximately 40 cases of osteosarcoma were observed years later. The dose-response for bone cancer in this group followed a linear-quadratic relationship that was dependent on the activities of the two radium isotopes (^{226}Ra and ^{228}Ra) contained in the paint.[47]

Lung Carcinoma. More than 500 years ago, German pitchblende miners suffered from a condition known as *mountain sickness*, which was later determined to be lung cancer.[3] Inhaling chronic amounts of radon gas in the air of the mines, these miners' lungs were exposed to high-LET alpha particles that were emitted while the radon decayed. Uranium miners in the United States who were studied from 1950 to 1967 also had an increased incidence of lung cancer, most likely for the same reasons.[48] Radon gas and its decay products are now known to be significant contributors (200 mrem/year) to annual background radiation levels and are the major risk factors for lung cancer in nonsmokers.

> The naturally occurring deposits of radioactive materials in the rocks of the earth decay through a long series of steps until they reach a stable isotope of lead. One of these steps involves radon gas.

Thyroid Carcinoma. Irradiation of enlarged thymuses in children before the 1930s over the dose range from 1200 to 6000 cGy was a popular treatment.[5,49] Unfortunately, a 100-fold increase in thyroid cancer was observed in these children. An increased incidence of thyroid cancer also occurred in individuals who were exposed as children to fallout from the bombings in Hiroshima and Nagasaki. Some of these individuals who developed thyroid cancer may have received doses as low as 100 cGy. Extensive follow-up is required to track the occurrence of these tumors because of the typical latent period of 10 to 20 years (which varies inversely with the dose that is received).

Breast Carcinoma. Three major groups of irradiated women with increased incidences of breast cancer seem to implicate radiation as the causative agent[3]: (1) irradiated female survivors in Hiroshima and Nagasaki, Japan; (2) Canadian women in a Nova Scotia sanitorium who had tuberculosis and were subjected to numerous fluoroscopic procedures; and (3) women treated for benign breast diseases such as postpartum mastitis. The best data that are available (with the Canadian study as the largest source) indicate that radiation induction of breast cancer most closely follows a linear dose-response relationship.[50]

Nonspecific Life-Shortening Effects

Research studies have shown that animals chronically exposed to low doses of radiation die younger than nonexposed animals.[51] Autopsy examinations (known as *necropsies* in animals) revealed a decreased number of parenchymal cells and blood vessels and an increased amount of connective tissue in organs. These changes resembled those seen in older animals and have been referred to as *radiation-induced aging*.[52] The effect on life span in these animals indicated a nonthreshold, linear relationship with radiation dose. However, more recent studies indicate that the life-shortening effect in these animals was probably the result of cancer induction at moderate doses and

organ atrophy, cell killing, and cell loss at high doses. Therefore the life-shortening result can be explained by the occurrence of specific rather than nonspecific effects. Most of the human data available support the statement that specific causes of radiation-induced life shortening are identifiable, although some exceptions to this probably exist.

Genetic Effects

Somatic late effects can occur in an irradiated individual, and exposure of reproductive (germ) cells in that individual may affect future generations. As mentioned previously, ionizing radiation is a known mutagen (i.e., it can induce mutations in the genetic material [DNA/genes] found in the cell nucleus). Mutations (which are permanent, heritable [transmittable to subsequent generations], and generally detrimental) occur spontaneously in genes and DNA. The number of spontaneous mutations that occur in each generation of an organism is described as the *mutation frequency,* which can be increased by any mutagenic agent, including radiation.[53] If the mutation frequency in a generation is doubled by exposure to radiation, the radiation dose is then known as the *doubling dose.*[54] In humans, the doubling dose is estimated to range from 50 to 250 rem (0.5–2.5 Sv), with an average figure given as 100 rem (1.0 Sv).[3]

The classic study that demonstrated the mutagenic potential of radiation was performed by H. J. Müller[55] in 1927 and involved the use of the *Drosophila melanogaster,* or fruit fly. Müller irradiated male and female fruit flies under a number of conditions and observed the mutation frequencies in the next several generations. The fruit fly was used as the model for these experiments because it has a number of easily identifiable mutations such as those involving its wing shape and eye and body color. In addition, large populations of fruit flies can be maintained and bred relatively quickly and easily.

The results of Müller's fruit fly experiments (which have not been contradicted by subsequent studies with mice) include the following[55]:

1. Radiation does not produce new or unique mutations but increases the frequency of spontaneous mutations in each generation.
2. Mutation frequency is linearly related to radiation dose.
3. Radiation induction of mutations has no clear threshold; it is a stochastic effect similar to carcinogenesis.

In addition to Müller's experiments, subsequent animal studies have indicated that high dose rates can cause more genetic damage than low dose rates, males are more sensitive than females at low doses and low dose rates to genetic effects, and that not all mutations show the same susceptibility to induction by radiation.[3] The estimated doubling dose for humans is based on extrapolations from the numerous animal experiments.

RADIATION THERAPY
Goal of Radiation Therapy

The goal of radiation therapy in the treatment of cancer is to eradicate the tumor while not destroying normal tissues in the treatment field. This is easier said than done because radiation interaction in matter is a nonspecific, random process that does not distinguish between malignant and normal tissues. Biologic damage can be induced in tumor and normal tissues. Therefore, the tolerance of the normal tissue in the treatment field limits the dose that can be administered to the tumor. Several methods have been attempted to deal with this limiting factor during treatment so that more effective tumor treatments can be given. Several of these methods are discussed in this section.

General Tumor Characteristics

Parenchymal and Stromal Compartments. Similar to normal tissue, malignant tumors are composed of parenchymal and stromal compartments. A tumor parenchyma may contain as many as four sub-populations or groups of cells.[2]

Cells belonging to group 1 are viable, actively mitotic (cycling) cells that are responsible for tumor growth. The percentage of group 1 cells in a tumor type usually varies from 30% to 50% and is termed the *growth fraction* (GF).[56] The GF typically decreases while the size (volume) of the tumor increases.

Group 2 cells are typically viable but nondividing (not cycling). These cells, also known as *G0 cells,* have retained the ability to reenter the cell cycle and divide if properly stimulated.

Groups 3 and 4 are composed of nonviable cells. Group 3 cells appear structurally intact, whereas group 4 cells do not. Groups 3 and 4 cells therefore do not contribute to tumor growth.

The exact percentage of cells in each group varies with the size and type of tumor. In addition, each tumor contains a stromal compartment of blood vessels and connective tissue. In small, newly formed tumors, the stroma may be entirely composed of normal host vessels, whereas large, older tumors contain a mix of normal and tumor vessels, or the supporting vasculature may be the result of angiogenesis factors released by the tumor cells themselves. As discussed later, the tumor vasculature plays an important role in tumor growth and the oxygen effect.

Factors That Affect Tumor Growth. The rate at which tumors grow depends on three major factors: (1) the division rate of proliferating parenchymal cells, (2) the percentage of these cells in the tumor (GF), and (3) the degree of cell loss from the tumor.[57] The division rate of factor 1 cells in a tumor tends to be faster than the division rate for normal parenchymal cells from the same tissue.[58] For example, malignant skin cells cycle faster than normal skin cells. This might seem to imply that tumors have short doubling times (the time it takes to double in volume), but tumor doubling times in vivo are actually much longer than expected. The two major reasons for this are GF and cell loss. Although factor 1 cells have short cycle times versus normal cells of the same origin, only an average of 30% to 50% of all cells in the tumor are included in this category.[56] In addition, of the new cells produced by mitosis at the end of each cycle, as many as 90% may be lost from the primary tumor itself. This cell-loss factor (f), which is manifested by metastases, cell death, and exfoliation (shedding of cells as in gastrointestinal tumors), is thought to be the most significant in vivo factor with regard to tumor growth.[57] A high cell-loss factor slows the growth of the primary tumor, but if cells are lost by metastasis, new tumors form in other sites in the body and limit the curative potential of any treatment, including radiation therapy.

Oxygen Effect. Tumor growth is characteristically unorganized compared with that of normal cells. During their early growth stages, tumors begin to outgrow their vascular supply. This results in differing levels of oxygen availability (known as *oxygen tension,* or Po_2) for the tumor cells, depending on their proximity to functioning blood vessels. This was first observed clinically in 1955 by Thomlinson and Gray,[25] who examined human bronchial carcinoma specimens. Thomlinson and Gray observed that the amount of necrotic (dead) tissue in the tumor was related to the size of the tumor itself. A tumor with a radius of less than 100 μm did not contain necrotic areas. A tumor with a radius of greater than 160 μm showed a necrotic area surrounded by a viable rim of cells approximately 100 to 180 μm thick.

Thomlinson and Gray concluded that tumor cells located more than 200 μm from the nearest blood vessels (capillaries) are anoxic (no oxygen available) and unable to proliferate. These cells then die, thus forming the necrotic area. Tumor cells closest to blood vessels, however, are well oxygenated (known as *oxic* cells), are actively dividing, and compose the GF of the tumor. Between the oxic and anoxic cells are cells exposed to gradually decreasing oxygen tensions. These are known as *hypoxic cells.* Although hypoxic cells do not have normal levels of oxygen available to them, they are viable and capable of dividing. Data from animal tumors estimate that approximately 15% or more of the tumor-cell population may be hypoxic. This is known as the *hypoxic fraction* of the tumor.[59] Thomlinson and Gray's study estimated that the oxic, hypoxic, and anoxic populations in tumors were a result of the limited ability of oxygen to diffuse large distances in tissue. They estimated this diffusion distance of oxygen to be approximately 160 to 200 μm.[25] More recent studies indicate that a diffusion distance closer to 70 μm for oxygen may be more accurate.[3]

The vasculature network that forms in each growing tumor with factors such as division rate, GF, and cell loss ultimately gives rise to oxic, hypoxic, and anoxic cell populations in that tumor. The radioresponse of a tumor depends (among other factors) on these cell populations. Anoxic cells do not contribute to the GF and therefore do not affect clinical outcome. Cells that are fully oxygenated (oxic) are highly radiosensitive to low-LET radiations (see the previous discussion on OER). The third group (viable hypoxic cells) is resistant to low-LET radiations by a factor of as high as 2.5 to 3.0. The hypoxic fraction in each tumor is presumed to be responsible, at least in part, for tumor regrowth after radiation therapy. One of the reasons for the fractionation of a radiation dose is an attempt to increase the radioresponse of these hypoxic cells (see the discussion on reoxygenation).

Theory of Dose-Fractionation Techniques

Modern radiation therapy treatments are given in daily fractions during an extended period (as long as 6 or 8 weeks) so that a high total dose is given to the tumor while ideally sparing normal tissues.[60] This technique, known as fractionation, originated in 1927 and replaced a single high-dose radiation treatment. The type of tumor and tolerance of the normal tissue in the treatment field determine the total dose, size, and number of fractions, and treatment duration.

A fractionated dose of radiation is less efficient biologically than a single dose. Therefore, higher total doses are necessary during fractionation to produce the same damage compared with a single dose. For example, a single dose of 1000 cGy causes more damage than two fractions of 500 cGy separated by 24 hours, although the total delivered dose remains the same.

A typical fractionation scheme may involve a daily fraction size of 180 to 200 cGy given 5 times a week for 6 weeks for a total of 30 fractions. This results in a total treatment dose ranging from 5400 to 6000 cGy (54 to 60 Gy). Depending on the tumor to be treated, the actual total dose may be higher or lower than this. *Hyperfractionated* schedules for radiation include treatments BID (twice a day) and TID (three times a day). *Hypofractionation* involves the use of dose fractions substantially larger than the conventional level of around 2 Gy.[3]

The biologic effects on tissue from fractionated radiation therapy depend on the "four Rs" of radiation biology:

1. Repopulation
2. Redistribution
3. Repair
4. Reoxygenation

Repopulation. During protracted radiation therapy, surviving cells in the tumor and adjacent normal tissues may divide, thus repopulating these tissues partially or completely. Normal tissue repopulation is highly desirable and decreases the risk of late effects. Fractionated doses take advantage of normal tissue repopulation that occurs between fractions. This can result in the sparing of normal tissues in the treatment field.[61] In contrast, tumor repopulation is highly undesirable and contributes to tumor regrowth during or after treatment.

Redistribution.
Irradiation of an asynchronous cell population (in which cells are distributed in all phases of the cell cycle) typically results in death to cells in the most sensitive phases (G2 and M), whereas more resistant cells (especially in the late S phase) survive. This process, known as *partial synchronization*, results in a redistribution or reassortment of surviving cells after irradiation.[62] The ideal clinical situation for radiation treatment exists when tumor cells have moved into a sensitive phase and normal cells have moved into a resistant phase. Theoretically, the timing of each radiation fraction can be based on the progression of cells into a sensitive or resistant phase. However, because this cannot be determined clinically, the partial synchronization of cell populations by radiation and other modalities (e.g., hydroxyurea) that may occur has not yet been successfully exploited.

Repair of Sublethal Damage.
Repair of sublethal damage has occurred within hours of radiation exposure in normal and tumor cells in vitro.[37] Fractionated radiation treatment takes advantage of repair processes in normal tissues that are active between radiation fractions. This partially accounts for the sparing effect on normal tissues that fractionation can achieve. Repair of sublethal damage is oxygen dependent (i.e., cells require a certain amount of oxygen to efficiently carry out repair mechanisms). Because a proportion of tumor cells are thought to be hypoxic, tumors in general are presumed to be incapable of repairing sublethal radiation damage as efficiently as normal tissues.[17] Although demonstrated in animal models, this differential repair between tumors and normal tissues may not be clinically significant in human tumors.

Reoxygenation.
The fourth R of radiobiology, unlike the other three, is presumed to apply only to tumors. This phenomenon, termed *reoxy-genation*, is the process by which hypoxic cells gain access to oxygen and become radiosensitive between radiation fractions.

As discussed previously, the OER for x-rays and gamma rays is 2.5 to 3.0 when delivered as a single dose. However, the OER decreases during fractionation of x-rays and gamma rays. This decrease implies that a proportion of hypoxic cells reoxygenate and therefore become more sensitive to the next fraction. Although the exact mechanisms of reoxygenation are not clear, clinical trials of fractionated radiation therapy seem to indicate that tumor response is improved compared with that from single-dose treatment. During fractionation, the initial dose fraction should kill a significant proportion of well-oxygenated (oxic), radiosensitive cells near blood vessels in the tumor. The effects on hypoxic, radioresistant cells are considerably less from the same dose fraction. Therefore, immediately after exposure, the percentage of hypoxic tumor cells increases significantly and may even reach 100% for a short time. Within 24 hours, hypoxic cells somehow gain access to oxygen. Because cells nearest the blood vessels are likely killed by the radiation fraction, oxygen may diffuse beyond these dead cells and reach a percentage of the hypoxic cells. Studies on animal tumors have demonstrated that the hypoxic fraction reestablishes itself in the tumor, usually within 24 hours of treatment.[63] In other words, if a tumor had a hypoxic fraction of 15% before treatment, it eventually reestablishes this percentage after reoxygenation is complete. The standard time interval of 24 hours between radiation fractions in human

tumors was extrapolated from animal experiments. This time interval coincides with the range of reoxygenation rates in animal tumors and presumably occurs in human tumors. Because healthy normal tissues do not usually have hypoxic cells, the process of reoxygenation does not apply to these tissues.

Methods to Improve Tumor Radioresponse.
Reoxygenation does not rid the tumor of all hypoxic cells. If it did, fractionated treatments with low-LET radiations would be highly curative. Unfortunately, some tumors remain resistant to fractionated radiation therapy. This fact has given rise to a number of methods to overcome this persistent oxygen effect.

One early method involved the use of a chamber of hyperbaric (high-pressure) oxygen.[2] Patients were placed in sealed chambers containing pure oxygen at a pressure of 3 atmospheres. The rationale behind this was that the diffusion distance of oxygen would increase as a result of the high pressure used in the chamber so that it might reach the hypoxic areas in the tumor. However, this technique did not produce improved clinical results and only complicated the treatment delivery because of increased length of time for treatments and patients' claustrophobia.

A related method involved the administration of perfluorochemicals (drugs that can carry oxygen) with 100% oxygen or carbogen (95% O_2/5% CO_2) breathing before and during radiation treatment.[2] The clinical results seemed to indicate improved response for several tumor types (most notably head and neck tumors), but the overall results were disappointing.

Radiosensitizers, radioprotectors, high-LET radiations, chemotherapy agents, and hyperthermia (heat) have all been used with varying degrees of success in terms of improved tumor response. However, each method is limited by biologic or technical constraints.[3]

Concept of Tolerance
Strandquist Isoeffect Curves.
Although the preference of fractionated radiation treatments versus high single doses is now established, the exact protocol for administration of fractionated doses continues to evolve. In 1944, Strandquist[64] made the first attempt to establish a relationship between radiation dose and treatment time. He developed plots of total dose (on a logarithmic scale) versus treatment duration (time in days on a linear scale) and called them isoeffect curves (Fig. 4.16). These *isoeffect curves* related the treatment schedule in terms of total dose and time with the clinical outcome, including early effects, late effects, and tumor cure. The use of isoeffect curves led to treatment schedules for fractionated radiation therapy that gave a high probability of tumor control without exceeding the tolerance of normal tissue. Also during this time, the discovery was made that the tolerance of normal tissue is more dependent on the number and size of fractions than on the overall duration between the first and last fractions.

Tolerance and Tolerance Dose.
Because the radiation dose applied to the tumor mass is limited by the tolerance of the normal tissue in the treatment field, identifying doses that can be used on normal tissues and factors that affect these doses is important. Historically, tolerance doses were established for normal tissues in terms of the total dose delivered by a standard fractionation schedule that caused a minimal (5%) or maximal (50%) complication rate within 5 years ($TD_{5/5}$ or $TD_{50/5}$, respectively). These doses were commonly known as *normal tissue tolerance doses*. The $TD_{5/5}$ and $TD_{50/5}$ tolerance doses for various organs were classified as mild to moderate or severe to fatal morbidity.[65] According to Rubin and Casarett,[24] for example, the $TD_{50/5}$ for

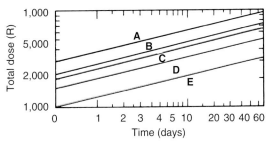

Fig. 4.16 Isoeffect curves from Strandquist's data that relate various treatment schedules to the following clinical results: *A*, Skin necrosis; *B*, cure of skin cancer; *C*, moist desquamation; *D*, dry desquamation; *E*, skin erythema. (From Strandquist M. Studien über die cumulative Wirkung der Röntgenstrahlen bei Fraktionierung, *Acta Radiol.* 1944;55[suppl]:1–300.)

the heart was 55 Gy if 60% of the heart was irradiated. If only 25% of the heart was irradiated, the $TD_{50/5}$ increased to approximately 80 Gy. The two dose levels ($TD_{5/5}$ or $TD_{50/5}$) expressed by Rubin and Casarett are still important concepts in radiation therapy treatment planning.

In 1991, Emami et al published a paper that addressed the need for more accurate knowledge of the time-dose-volume relationships for normal tissues, especially as it concerned three-dimensional (3D) treatment planning. His group of researchers divided the total volume of each of the 28 critical sites of normal tissue (organs) into "thirds": one-third, two-thirds, and whole organ (Table 4.7). Only conventional fractionations of 180 to 200 cGy/day for 5 days/week were considered.[66]

Nominal Standard Dose. In an attempt to design treatment schedules that result in optimal tumor response with acceptable normal tissue damage, Ellis[67] in 1968 proposed the concept of nominal standard dose (NSD). Ellis derived the following equation from the isoeffect curves of Strandquist that took into account several parameters of fractionated radiation therapy:

$$D = NSD \times T^{0.11} \times N^{0.24}$$

In the equation, D is the total dose, NSD is the nominal standard dose, T is the overall treatment time in days between the first and last fractions, and N is the number of fractions.[67] Ellis[68] proposed the unit of rets (rad equivalent therapy) for NSD, and in many situations, NSD1800 rets was considered the standard for comparison. The NSD equation allowed radiation oncologists to enter their treatment data, calculate the NSD for their centers, and compare this with the findings of other centers. The limitations of this concept, however, include the following: (1) the equation is based on connective tissue response and therefore is not useful for late-responding normal tissues, and (2) the equation does not take into account the volume irradiated, which is critical to determining the tolerance of normal tissues. Although the NSD concept was popular in the 1970s, it is now useful for only an extremely limited number of clinical situations in radiation therapy.

Biologically Effective Dose. The concept of the biologically effective dose (BED) is an important tool to understand tumor and normal tissue control by using different treatment times and dose fractionation schedules. This approach may be more common with treatment modalities that use a high dose per fraction during a shorter time for the delivery of the total radiation dose. For example, conventional fractionation is delivered at a dose of 180 to 200 cGy per fraction during a period of 4 to 7 weeks. Stereotactic radiosurgery (SRS) and stereotactic ablative body radiotherapy (SABR) doses tend to be much larger per fraction and are delivered over a shorter period of time. When a BED is calculated for a combination of dose per fraction, total dose, and overall treatment time,

it allows the physician's prescription to be converted into a dose that describes the biologic effect of the radiation on tumor and normal tissue.

Historically, isoeffect curves have been used for fractionation schedules and continue to be used today. With time, methods of dose escalation for treatment planning have evolved integrating known dose limits on normal tissues and organs. These new methods are necessary to estimate how much dose is acceptable when given in nonstandard fractionation schedules, as is common with SRS and SABR. The benefits of these techniques not only offer shorter treatment schedules, but also boast better local tumor control.

According to Fowler,[69] two important improvements occurred in the BED formula. First, in 1999, high-LET radiation was included, second, in 2003 overall times could be "triangulated" to optimize tumor BED and cell kill. With this "triangulated" approach, the goal of these newest techniques (SRS and SABR) in radiation therapy were aimed at delivering radiation with surgical precision, reducing the dose to normal tissues, and gaining important ground on local control of tumors that historically have been resistant to standard fractionation.

PRESENT STATUS OF RADIATION THERAPY

The use of intensity-modulated radiation therapy and image-guided radiation therapy (IGRT) in recent years has revolutionized the field of radiation oncology. IGRT uses ultrasound, cone beam computed tomography (CT), kilovoltage imaging, and MV beam portal imaging to improve tumor targeting. Four-dimensional CT is a simulation technique that tracks tumor motion during the respiratory cycle. Improved immobilization devices increase patient comfort and reproducibility.[70] These devices allow physicians to reduce target expansions and decrease the amount of surrounding normal tissues receiving significant radiation dose. Reduction of the dose to normal tissues provides an opportunity to increase the dose to the tumor and offer better local control for some of the most difficult cancers.

Stereotactic treatment, delivering ablative doses in a few fractions, has been used in radiation therapy for decades, principally for the treatment of intracranial lesions. The ability to target tumors with stereotactic doses outside of the cranium has only been realized with the mainstream use of image guidance, motion management, and better immobilization. Stereotactic body radiation therapy has shown very promising results for the treatment of lung cancer. Lung cancer treatment with stereotactic body radiation therapy offers significantly higher fractional doses than the conventional 3D treatments with a low incidence of serious toxicity and improved local control. Image guidance continues to evolve with the use of fiducial markers and beam transponders that allow radiation therapists and physicians the ability to track the tumor with real time movement.

A number of treatment techniques combine the use of radiation therapy with other modalities. This is now the method of choice for many human malignancies. Because of the limited effect of low-LET radiations on hypoxic and S-phase tumor cells, the use of hyperthermia[71] and chemotherapeutic agents[3] in conjunction with radiation has increased with improved clinical results for a number of tumor types. In addition, the use of high-LET forms of radiation, such as protons, has certain benefits versus conventional x-ray therapy.[72] The energy deposition of protons increases slowly with depth and reaches a sharp maximum near the end of the particles' range in a region called the *Bragg peak*. Clinical applications have attempted to use this Bragg peak region to maximize the delivery dose to the target organ while sparing the surrounding normal tissues. With the knowledge gained from clinical trials and preclinical experimentation, improvements in tumor responses and survival rates after radiation therapy continue to be realized.

TABLE 4.7 Tolerance Doses of Emami et al.[66] Predicted Tolerance Doses

Organ	Injury	One-Third	Two-Thirds	Whole Organ
Bladder	Contracture	—	8,000	6,500
Brain	Necrosis/infarction	6,000	5,000	4,500
Brainstem	Necrosis/infarction	6,000	5,300	5,000
Colon	Obstruction/perforation	5,500	—	4,500
Ear mid/external	Acute serous otitis	3,000	3,000	3,000[a]
Ear mid/external	Chronic serous otitis	5,500	5,500	5,500[a]
Esophagus	Perforation, stricture	6,000	58,000	5,500
Femoral head	Necrosis	—	—	5,200
Heart	Pericarditis	6,000	4,500	4,000
Kidney	Nephritis	5,000	3,000	2,300
Larynx	Necrosis	7,900[a]	7,000[a]	7,000[a]
T-M joints mandible	Marked limitation of joint function	6,500	6,000	6,000
Liver	Liver failure	5,000	3,500	3,000
Lung	Pneumonitis	4,500	3,000	1,750
Brachial plexus	Nerve damage	6,200	6,100	6,000
Optic chiasma	Blindness	—	—	5,000
Eye lens	Cataract	—	—	1,000
Optic nerve	Blindness	—	—	5,000
Retina	Blindness	—	—	4,500
Rectum	Proctitis/necrosis/fistula/stenosis	—	—	6,000
Parotid gland	Xerostomia	—	3,200[a]	3,200[a]
Skin	Necrosis/ulceration	7,000	6,000	5,500 100 cm^2
Small intestine	Obstruction/perforation	5,000	--	4,000[a]
Spinal cord	Myelitis/necrosis	5,000 5 cm^2	5,000 10 cm^2	4,700 20 cm^2
Stomach	Ulceration/perforation	6,000	5,500	5,000

[a]<50% of volume does not make a significant change.
TD$_{5/5}$, Tissue dose associated with a 5% injury rate within 5 years.
Modified from Emami B, Lyman J, Brown A, et al. Tolerance of normal tissue to therapeutic radiation. *Int J Radiat Oncol Biol Phys*. 1991;21:109–122.

■ SUMMARY

- In both ionization and excitation, the incoming radiation interacts with an atom. In ionization, the incoming radiation ejects an electron from the shell of the atom, thus causing the atom to be charged (ionized). In excitation, the electron in the outer shell of the atom is said to be excited (oscillating or vibrating) but is not ejected from the shell.
- Radiation effects on tissue can be direct or indirect. When a beam of charged particles is incident on tissue, direct ionization of DNA is highly probable because of the relatively densely ionizing nature of most particulate radiations. Indirect effect occurs predominantly when x-rays or gamma rays compose the primary beam, thus producing fast electrons as the secondary particles that interact with water (H_2O). Indirect effects involve a series of reactions known as radiolysis (splitting) of water.
- A cell survival curve is a plot of the radiation dose administered on the x-axis versus the SF of cells on the y-axis. This survival curve is characteristic of the survival of cells exposed to low-LET radiations such as x-rays or gamma rays.
- The Law of Bergonié and Tribondeau states that ionizing radiation is more effective against cells that (1) are actively mitotic, (2) are undifferentiated, and (3) have a long mitotic future.

- The Radiation Therapy Oncology Group has summarized the acute and chronic effects of radiation into various categories or grades based on the severity of the clinical response (see Tables 4.3 and 4.4).
- There are three syndromes described in humans as a result of total-body irradiation. (1) The hematopoietic syndrome in humans is induced by total-body doses of 100 to 1000 cGy. (2) The gastrointestinal syndrome results if the total-body dose is between 1000 and 10,000 cGy. (3) The cerebrovascular syndrome occurs exclusively above 10,000 cGy but can overlap with the gastrointestinal syndrome because it can be induced by a dose as low as 5000 cGy.
- Biologic response resulting from exposure to lower doses of radiation may not be observable for extended periods, ranging from years to generations. These effects are therefore known as late effects and are termed somatic effects if body cells are involved or genetic effects if reproductive cells are involved.
- The biologic effects on tissue from fractionated radiation therapy depend on the four Rs of radiation biology, which are repopulation, redistribution, repair, and reoxygenation.

REVIEW QUESTIONS

The answers to the Review Questions can be found by logging on to our website at: http://evolve.elsevier.com/Washington+Leaver/principles

1. The term that relates biologic response to the quality of radiation is:
   a. Linear energy transfer.
   b. Oxygen enhancement ratio .
   c. Relative biologic effectiveness.
   d. Therapeutic ration (TR).
2. Generally, which is the most radiosensitive phase of the cell cycle?
   a. G1.
   b. G2.
   c. M.
   d. S.
3. Which of the following tissues is the most radiosensitive?
   a. Muscle.
   b. Ocular lens.
   c. Liver.
   d. Bone and cartilage.
4. Which of the following is *not* one of the four Rs of radiation therapy?
   a. Reconfirmation.
   b. Reoxygenation.
   c. Redistribution.
   d. Repopulation.
5. Strandquist's isoeffect curves are related to which of the following?
   a. Oxygen enhancement.
   b. Translocation of DNA.
   c. Fractionation.
   d. Radiation syndromes.
6. According to the Law of Bergonié and Tribondeau, ionizing radiation is more effective against cells that are:
   a. Actively mitotic and differentiated and have a long mitotic future.
   b. Actively mitotic and differentiated and have a short mitotic future.
   c. Not actively mitotic and undifferentiated and have a long mitotic future.
   d. Actively mitotic and undifferentiated and have a long mitotic future.
7. Which of the following particles do not contribute to the direct effect of radiation?
   a. Protons.
   b. Positrons.
   c. Alpha particles.
   d. Heavy nuclear fragments.
8. Gross structural changes in chromosomes resulting from radiation damage are referred to as:
   a. Chromosome stickiness or clumping.
   b. Aberrations, lesions, or anomalies.
   c. Deletions and inversions.
   d. Interphase death or replication failure.
9. What is another term for the cellular response that results in the delay of division of cells in the cell cycle?
   a. Mitotic delay.
   b. Interphase death.
   c. Reproductive failure.
   d. Apoptosis.
10. Carcinogenesis as a result of radiation exposure:
    a. Is higher if individuals are exposed in their youth as compared with adulthood.
    b. Has a decreased latency period for all cancers.
    c. Is described as deterministic.
    d. Is all of the above.

QUESTIONS TO PONDER

1. Discuss the interactions of radiation and matter (specifically, the indirect and direct effects on the cellular level).
2. Describe the relationship between LET, RBE, and OER. Be able to graphically support your answer.
3. How does radiation sensitivity relate to the goals of radiation oncology in terms of tumor control and the sparing of normal tissue structures?
4. Relate the three graphic components of the cell survival curve (n, D_o, and D_q) to the administration of radiation treatments.
5. Describe the five classifications of mammalian cells according to their radiosensitivities and characteristics, listing examples for each classification.
6. Briefly describe the three total-body responses to radiation. Remember to include the dose ranges at which each of these responses occur.
7. Discuss the three main stages of fetal development and the common effects of radiation exposure on the fetus during each stage.

REFERENCES

1. Adams GE, Flockhart IR, Smithen CE, et al. Electron-affinic sensitization. VII. A correlation between structures, one-electron reduction potentials, and the efficiencies of nitroimidazoles as hypoxic cell radiosensitizers. *Radiat Res.* 1976;67:9–20.
2. Travis EL. *Primer of Medical Radiobiology.* 2nd ed. St. Louis: Mosby. 1989.
3. Hall EJ, Giaccia AJ. *Radiobiology for the Radiologist.* 7th ed. Philadelphia, PA: Lippincott Williams & Wilkins. 2012.
4. Zirkle RE. Partial cell irradiation. *Adv Biol Med Phys.* 1957;5:103.
5. Pifer JW, Toyooka ET, Murray RW, et al. Neoplasms in children treated with x-rays for thymic enlargement. II. Tumor incidence as a function of radiation factors. *J Natl Cancer Inst.* 1963;31:1357.
6. Selman J. *The Fundamentals of Imaging Physics and Radiobiology.* 9th ed. Springfield, IL: Charles C Thomas. 2000.
7. Dewey WC, Humphrey RM. Restitution of radiation-induced chromosomal damage in Chinese hamster cells related to the cell's life cycle. *Exp Cell Res.* 1964;35:262.
8. Simic MG, Grossman L, Upton AC. *Mechanisms of DNA Damage and Repair.* New York, NY: Plenum Press. 1986.
9. Puck TT, Marcus TI. Action of x-rays on mammalian cells. *J Exp Med.* 1956;10:653.
10. Canti RG, Spear FG. The effect of gamma irradiation on cell division in tissue culture in vitro, part II. *Proc R Soc Lond B Biol Sci.* 1929;105:93.
11. Till JE, McCulloch EA. A direct measurement of the radiation sensitivity of normal mouse bone marrow cells. *Radiat Res.* 1961;14:213–222.
12. Bushong SC. *Radiologic Science for Technologists: Physics, Biology and Protection.* 10th ed. St. Louis: Mosby. 2012.

13. Belli JA, Dicus GJ, Bonte FJ, et al. Radiation response of mammalian tumor cells. I. Repair of sublethal damage in vivo. *J Natl Cancer Inst.* 1967;38:673–682.
14. Elkind MM, Sutton-Gilbert H. Radiation response of mammalian cells grown in culture. I. Repair of x-ray damage in surviving Chinese hamster cells. *Radiat Res.* 1960;13:556.
15. Ancel P, Vitemberger P. Sur la radiosensibilitie cellulaire. *C R Soc Biol.* 1925;92:517.
16. Broerse JJ, Barendsen GW. Current topics. *Radiat Res Q.* 1973;8:305–350.
17. Bedford JS, Mitchell JB. Dose-rate effects in synchronous mammalian cells in culture. *Radiat Res.* 1973;54:316–327.
18. Wright EA, Howard-Flanders P. The influence of oxygen on the radiosensitivity of mammalian tissues. *Acta Radiol (Stockholm).* 1957;48:26.
19. Broerse JJ, Barendsen GW, van Kersen GR. Survival of cultured human cells after irradiation with fast neutrons at different energies in hypoxic and oxygenated conditions. *Int J Radiat Biol.* 1967;13:559–572.
20. Kinsella T, Mitchell JB, Russo A, et al. The use of halogenated thymidine analog as clinical radiosensitizers: rationale, current status, and future prospects: non-hypoxic cell sensitizers. *Int J Radiat Oncol Biol Phys.* 1984;10:1399–1406.
21. Patt HM, Tyree EB, Straube RL, et al. Cysteine protection against x-irradiation. *Science.* 1949;110:213.
22. Sinclair WK. Cyclic x-ray responses in mammalian cells in vitro. *Radiat Res.* 1968;33:620–643.
23. Bergonié J, Tribondeau L. De quelques resultats de la radiotherapie et essai de fixation d'une technique rationelle. *C R Acad Sci.* 1906;143:983.
24. Rubin P, Casarett GW. *Clinical Radiation Pathology.* vols. 1 and 2. Philadelphia, PA: W.B. Saunders. 1986.
25. Thomlinson RH, Gray LH. The histological structure of some human lung cancers and the possible implications for radiotherapy. *Br J Cancer.* 1955;9:539.
26. Withers HR, Elknid MM. Radiation survival and regeneration characteristics of spermatogenic stem cells of mouse testis. *Radiat Res.* 1974;57:88–103.
27. Cox JD, Stetz J, Pajak TF. Toxicity criteria of the radiation therapy oncology group (RTOG) and the European organization for research and treatment of cancer (EORTC). *Int J Radiat Oncol Biol Phys.* 1995;31:1341–1346.
28. Trotti A, Byhardt R, Stetz J, et al. Common toxicity criteria: version 2.0. An improved reference for grading the acute effects of cancer treatment: impact on radiotherapy. *Int J Radiat Oncol Biol Phys.* 2000;47:13–47.
29. Withers HR, Elkind MM. Microcolony survival assay for cells of mouse intestinal mucosa exposed to radiation. *Int J Radiat Biol.* 1970;17:261–267.
30. Russell LB, Russell WL. An analysis of the changing radiation response of the developing mouse embryo. *J Cell Physiol.* 1954;43(suppl 1):103–149.
31. Rugh R. X-ray-induced teratogenesis in the mouse and its possible significance to man. *Radiology.* 1971;99:433–443.
32. Griem ML, Meier P, Dobben GD, et al. Analysis of the morbidity and mortality of children irradiated in fetal life. *Radiology.* 1967;88:347–349.
33. MacMahon B. Pre-natal x-ray exposure and childhood cancer. *J Natl Cancer Inst.* 1962;28:231.
34. Murphy DP, Goldstein L. Micromelia in a child irradiated in utero. *Surg Gynecol Obstet.* 1930;50:79.
35. Plummer C. Anomalies occurring in children exposed in utero to the atomic bomb at Hiroshima. *Pediatrics.* 1952;10:687.
36. Otake M, Schull WJ. In utero exposure to A-bomb radiation and mental retardation: a reassessment. *Br J Radiol.* 1984;57:409–414.
37. Dekaban AS. Abnormalities in children exposed to x-irradiation during various stages of gestation: tentative timetable of radiation injury to the human fetus. *J Nucl Med.* 1968;9:471.
38. Court-Brown WM, Doll R. Mortality from cancer and other causes after radiotherapy from ankylosing spondylitis. *Br Med J.* 1965;2:1327.
39. Upton AC. Radiation carcinogenesis. In: Busch H, ed. *Methods in Cancer Research.* Vol. 4. New York, NY: Academic Press. 1968.
40. Warren S. Radiation carcinogenesis. *Bull N Y Acad Med.* 1970;46:131–147.
41. Dublin LI, Spiegelman M. Mortality of medical specialists, 1938-1942. *J Am Med Assoc.* 1948;137:1519.
42. March HC. Leukemia in radiologists in a 20-year period. *Am J Med Sci.* 1950;220:282.
43. Court-Brown WM, Doll R. Expectation of life and mortality from cancer among British radiologists. *Br Med J.* 1958;2:181.
44. Court-Brown WM, Doll R, Bradford Hill A, et al. The incidence of leukemia after the exposure to diagnostic radiation in utero. *Br Med J.* 1960;2:1599.
45. Pack GT, Davis J. Radiation cancer of the skin. *Radiology.* 1965;84:436.
46. Albert RE, Omran AR. Follow-up studies of patients treated by x-ray epilation for tinea capitis. I. Population characteristics, postttreatment illnesses, and mortality experience. *Arch Environ Health.* 1968;17:899–918.
47. Rowland RE, Stehney AF, Lucas HF. Dose response relationships for radium-induced bone sarcomas. *Health Phys.* 1983;44:15–31.
48. Saccomanno G, Archer VE, Saunders RP, et al. Lung cancer of uranium miners on the Colorado plateau. *Health Phys.* 1964;10:1195.
49. Simpson CL, Hempelmann LH. The association of tumors and roentgen-ray treatment of the thorax in infancy. *Cancer.* 1957;10:42.
50. McKenzie I. Breast cancer following multiple fluoroscopes. *Br J Cancer.* 1965;19:1.
51. Rotblat J, Lindop P. Long-term effects of a single whole body exposure of mice to ionizing radiation. II. Causes of death. *Proc R Soc Lond B Biol Sci.* 1961;154:350.
52. Curtis HJ. *Radiation-Induced Aging in Mice.* London, UK: Butterworth. 1961.
53. Krall JF. Estimation of spontaneous and radiation-induced mutation rates in man. *Eugenics Q.* 1956;3:201.
54. Schull WL, Otake M, Neal JV. Genetic effects of the atomic bomb: a reappraisal. *Science.* 1981;213:1220–1227.
55. Müller HJ. On the relation between chromosome changes and gene mutations. *Brookhaven Symp Biol.* 1956;8:126.
56. Mendelsohn ML. The growth fraction: a new concept applied to tumors. *Science.* 1960;132:1496.
57. Steel GG. Cell loss as a factor in the growth rate of human tumors. *Eur J Cancer.* 1967;3:381–387.
58. Lyskin AB, Mendelsohn ML. Comparison of cell cycle in induced carcinomas and their normal counterparts. *Cancer Res.* 1964;24:1131.
59. Van Putten LM, Kahlman LF. Oxygenation status of transplantable tumor during fractionated radiotherapy. *J Natl Cancer Inst.* 1968;40:441–451.
60. Peters LJ, Withers HR, Thames HD. Radiobiological considerations for multiple daily fractionation. In: Kaercher KH, Kogelnik HD, Reinartz G, eds. *Progress in Radio-Oncology.* vol. 2. New York, NY: Raven Press. 1982.
61. Withers H. The 4 R's of radiotherapy. In: Lett JT, Adler H, eds. *Advances in Radiation Biology.* vol. 5. San Francisco, CA: Academic Press.
62. Withers HR. Cell cycle redistribution as a factor in multi-fraction irradiation. *Radiology.* 1975;114:199–202.
63. Thomlinson RH. Effect of fractionated irradiation on the proportion of anoxic cells in an intact experimental tumor. *Br J Radiol.* 1966;39:158.
64. Strandquist M. Studien über die kumulative Wirkung der Roentgenstrahlen bei Fraktionierung. *Acta Radiol.* 1944;55(suppl):1–300.
65. Kramer S. Principles of radiation oncology and cancer radiotherapy. In: Rubin P, Small W, eds. Clinical oncology: a multidisciplinary approach for physicians and students. Philadelphia, PA: W.B. Saunders.
66. Emami B, Lyman J, Brown A, et al. Tolerance of normal tissue to therapeutic radiation. *Int J Radiat Oncol Biol Phys.* 1991;21:109–122.
67. Ellis F. Dose. time, and fractionation in radiotherapy. In: Ebert M, Howard A, eds. *Current Topics in Radiation Research.* Amsterdam, Netherlands: North Holland Publishing.
68. Ellis F. Nominal standard dose and the ret. *Br J Radiol.* 1971;44:101–108.
69. Fowler JF. 21 years of biologically effective dose. *Br J Radiol.* 2010;83(991):554–568.
70. Khan F. *The Physics of Radiation Therapy.* 4th ed. Philadelphia, PA: Lippincott Williams & Wilkins. 2010.
71. Arcangeli G, Cividalli A, Nervi C, et al. Tumor control and therapeutic gain with different schedules of combined radiotherapy and local external hyperthermia in human cancer. *Int J Radiat Oncol Biol Phys.* 1983;9:1125–1134.
72. Barendsen GW. Proceedings of the Conference on Particle Accelerators in Radiation Therapy, (pp 120-125), LA-5180-C, Oak Ridge, TN, 1972, US Atomic Energy Commission, Technical Information Center.

5

Detection and Diagnosis

Dennis Leaver

OBJECTIVES

- Discuss the three fundamental questions a physician would ask if someone were sick.
- Explain the value of the interview as a diagnostic tool.
- Describe the importance of the medical record.
- Compare and contrast the four aspects of the physical examination: inspection, palpation, percussion, and auscultation.
- Discuss the benefits of cancer screening.
- Explain the significance of sentinel node biopsy in the detection of breast cancer.
- Define prevalence, incidence, sensitivity, and specificity.
- Discuss the benefits of digital mammography.
- Evaluate the various methods of screening for colorectal cancer.
- Discuss DNA testing for human papillomavirus and how it relates to cervical cancer.
- Compare PET, MRI, and CT as diagnostic tools.
- Describe the TNM system used for staging cancer, specifically the three components used to describe the extent of the disease.

OUTLINE

KEY TERMS

Auscultation
Baseline
Diagnosis
Excisional biopsy
Edema
Incisional biopsy
Incidence
Inspection
Lymphadenopathy
Metastases
Mutation
Palpation
Paraneoplastic syndrome
Percussion

Premalignant
Prevalence
Prevention
Respiratory rate
Rhythm
Screening
Sentinel lymph node
Sensitivity
Sign
Specificity
Staging
Symptom
Syndrome

INTRODUCTION TO DETECTION AND DIAGNOSIS

The improvement in cancer survival reflects several factors, including the increased emphasis on detection and diagnosis of particular cancers at an earlier stage, the use of new treatment methods, and a better understanding of how some cancers behave. Survival rates vary significantly by cancer type and stage at diagnosis, so careful observation of signs and symptoms may help diagnose disease at an earlier stage.

The 5-year relative survival rate for all cancers is 69.7%.[1] Over the past three decades, the 5-year relative survival rate for all cancers combined increased 20% among whites and 24% among blacks, yet it remains lower for blacks (70% vs. 63%, respectfully). Improvements in survival, which varies greatly by cancer type and stage at the time of diagnosis, reflect improvements in treatment as well as earlier diagnosis for some cancers.[2]

Relative survival rates for cancer compares survival among cancer patients with that of people not diagnosed with cancer. It represents the percentage of cancer patients who are alive after a designated time period (usually 5 years) relative to persons without cancer. It includes patients who have been cured and those who have relapsed or are still in treatment.[2] The National Cancer Institute compiles cancer statistics for doctors, therapists, researchers and cancer registries through a program called SEER (Surveillance, Epidemiology, and End Results). Data for major cancer sites can be accessed by age, sex, race/ethnicity. Check out an interactive tool on their website called "Fast Stats" at http://seer.cancer.gov/faststats.[3]

In this chapter, we will explore the process and many of the tools and procedures used to detect and diagnose disease, especially cancer. This will include a discussion on the interview as a diagnostic tool, the importance of the medical record and medical history, details involved in the physical examination, screening tools, the recommendations of the American Cancer Society (ACS) for detecting cancer, and laboratory/medical imaging studies useful in detecting cancer.

The detection and diagnosis of disease, especially cancer, have come to rely increasingly on two specialties: imaging and pathology. With continued advances in computer technology, diagnostic imaging and its application to the detection of disease provide increased effectiveness in managing diseases such as cancer. Medical imaging modalities include nuclear medicine studies, positron emission tomography (PET), mammography, computed tomography (CT), magnetic resonance imaging (MRI), ultrasound, x-ray, and newer molecular imaging technologies. Some medical imaging modalities are able to show both anatomic detail and physiologic/functional detail. The physician is still needed to understand the application of these new imaging modalities and to establish a relationship with the patient.

The physician who wishes to establish a relationship with the patient and help someone who is sick should try to answer these three fundamental questions for the patient, posed originally by Reinertsen and LeBlond:[4]

"What's happening to me and why?"
"What does this mean for my future?"
"What can be done about it, how will that change my future?"

The routine physical examination is an important tool in maintaining good health and detecting conditions or diseases early so that intervention is possible before the patient demonstrates signs or experiences more advanced symptoms. Failure to pursue a diagnosis may permit a disease to progress from curable to incurable.[4] Early detection

has proved important in cancer management. According to the ACS,[5] prevention (strategies and measures that stop cancer from developing) and early detection are two of the most important and effective strategies of saving lives from cancer, diminishing suffering from cancer, and eliminating cancer as a major health problem. Prevention includes measures that stop cancer from developing. Early detection includes examinations and tests intended to find the disease as early as possible, before it has spread. The earlier a cancer can be found, the more effectively it can be treated. This may result in fewer side effects. In fact, the relative survival rate for people with cancers for which the ACS has specific early detection recommendations (breast, colon, rectum, cervix, prostate, testes, and skin) is approximately 81%.[5] Early detection and effective screening (selecting appropriate tests and studies to check for disease) programs translate into increased survival.

Anatomical sites that are easier to access, such as the breast, cervix, larynx and colon, generally have better 5-year cancer survival rates as compared with anatomical sites that are more difficult to access, such as pancreas and ovaries. Early detection is important. Cancers of the pancreas and ovary are rarely detected early. Not only does the ACS have limited early detection recommendations for cancer sites like these, but the anatomic position of the pancreas (deep in the upper abdomen) and ovary (deep in the lower abdomen) are difficult, if not impossible to palpate on physical examination. Usually sites like these do not present with symptoms until the cancer has advanced.

Broad cancer education may lead to less cancer incidence in our society. For example, limiting our exposure to harmful ultraviolet rays from the sun will reduce our risk of skin cancer. Smoking is the most preventable cause of death in our society. Certainly, our diet may play a role in preventing colon cancer. Find out more information by visiting the American Cancer Society at www.cancer.org.

The actual physical examination (whether routine or a result of the patient experiencing signs or symptoms) is a methodical process of detection that covers all the anatomic systems. A sign is "an objective finding as perceived by an examiner." For example, the examining physician may notice signs such as a rash, feel a mass, or note the color of the patient's skin. A symptom is a "subjective indication of a disease or a change in condition as perceived by the patient." For example, the patient may complain of pain, numbness, dysphagia, dyspnea, difficulty in sleeping, or lack of appetite. These are symptoms.

If a patient is experiencing symptoms, it is usually an indication that the condition or disease process is more advanced. If a set of signs or symptoms arises from a common cause, it is referred to as a syndrome. Many diseases share the same signs and symptoms. Grouping signs and symptoms into a syndrome with results of tests and medical procedures helps the physician to eliminate some diseases and narrow the choices for a correct diagnosis.

A diagnosis is defined as the identification of a disease or condition. A diagnosis can be subjective or objective. A subjective diagnosis is based on several factors. The patient's complaints and medical history are considered subjective. The physician's preliminary diagnosis with no hard evidence for support is also considered subjective. An objective diagnosis is based on results of current medical procedures and tests (such as a tissue biopsy or laboratory data) and observations by the physician and other medical personnel.

The process for obtaining an objective diagnosis begins with the interview and physical examination to help assess the patient's current status and determine the necessary steps (if any) to take. During a physical examination, the physician follows a step-by-step process that includes the acquisition of data or clues through the interview process, a review of past medical records, a physical examination, and a list of the patient's chief complaints.[4] Each disease process has distinguishing features that may serve as "clues." The physician must search for clues that may correspond to a list of problems. The list is then used to generate hypotheses, which in turn may lead to a diagnosis. Clues are sought by taking a history, performing a physical examination, and ordering laboratory and medical imaging tests. The physician must then consider several hypotheses, which might explain the problems the patient is having in terms of diseases in another list called *differential diagnoses.* The clues or facts obtained during the interview, physical examination, and diagnostic testing are then used to support or refute each hypothetical disease in the differential diagnosis list in the hope of finally arriving at "the diagnosis."[4]

PATIENT INTERVIEWS AS A DIAGNOSTIC TOOL

The most powerful diagnostic tool of the physician is the initial interview. By this means, one learns the chronologic events and symptoms of the patient's illness. Diagnostic hypotheses are generated and tested as the patient's history unfolds, resulting in the formulation of the most likely diagnoses at the completion of the interview and testing.[4] The physician must interview the patient to acquire accurate information. If the patient is too ill or handicapped to provide the information, the physician uses other sources such as family, friends, prior medical records, and other healthcare providers.

In the interview process, the physician asks questions, and the patient provides answers. The physician determines the patient's chief complaints and current status and obtains the patient's medical and psychosocial history. The interview is also used to establish the physician-patient relationship and demonstrate to the patient a caring, empathetic attitude. In a study of 103 cancer patients by Sapir et al,[6] patients overwhelmingly expected their oncologists to be patient and skilled in diagnostic procedures (98%); tactful, considerate, and therapeutically skilled (90% to 95%); and skilled in the management of pain and the psychosocial consequences of cancer (75% to 85%). When there is bad news to be communicated, patients want the truth. Breaking bad news to the cancer patient can be stressful, especially when the physician is inexperienced, the patient is young, or where there are few options for a successful outcome.[7,8] In addition, over the past 40 years, there has been a shift from patients accepting a paternalistic role from their physician to patients desiring a more active role for themselves.[9]

Allowing enough time for an interview is important. If the interview is rushed, the patient may feel that the physician is not empathetic. Bram et al provide guidelines for a successful interview of the cancer patient. The recommendations include arranging for privacy, involving significant others, sitting down to help relax the patient, making connections with the patient through eye contact, and managing interruptions.[9]

The initial interview may be a long process in the radiation oncology setting because the physician must not only assess the patient, but also provide information regarding the goals, benefits, and risks involved in a course of treatment. Radiation therapists, nurses, and midlevel practitioners, such as physician assistants or advanced practice nurses, may also interview the patient during the treatment process to obtain information about the patient's concerns, questions, and treatment-related side effects. During the treatment process, the therapist must select words that are clear and convey the correct meaning to the patient. The meaning of words is relative. A radiation therapist may ask, "What medications are you taking?" The response may be "None," although the patient is taking aspirin for pain and an

TABLE 5.1	Examples of Facilitating Verbal Responses
Type of Response	**Examples**
Minimal	"I see."
	"I understand."
Reflecting feelings	"I see you are very angry."
	"It is very scary."
Clarifications	"How bad did it hurt?"
	"This only bothers you at night?"

antacid for indigestion. In the patient's mind, these are not medications because they were not prescribed. Verbal and nonverbal communication are important.

Verbal communication involves the manner, quality, and intonation of speech. Forms of nonverbal communication include facial expressions, posture, personal appearance, and manner of movement. The radiation therapist may be at a distinct advantage in assessing verbal and nonverbal communication from the patient because of their daily interaction with the patient. Patients young and old will see their radiation therapist on average five to six times more often than their physician, assuming that the physician sees the patient during the initial consultation and weekly thereafter. This increased exposure to the therapist allows a sense of mutual confidence and trust to develop. In many situations, the patient may divulge more specific information to the therapist, especially concerning treatment-related side effects, pain management, and other issues important to the patient.

Observing nonverbal communication while the patient is talking can help determine the real meaning of the patient's words. Listening is an essential component of effective communication used by many healthcare disciplines and has always been considered a crucial component to any meaningful conversation involving the patient (see Chapter 3, Patient Assessment). Certain characteristics that are essential to effective listening have been identified and include empathy, silence, attention to both verbal and nonverbal communication, and the ability to be nonjudgmental and accepting.[4]

The patient may say one thing but really mean another. For example, the radiation therapist asks the patient, "Are you having any pain?" The patient says, "No." However, the patient's appearance, posture, and facial expressions may contradict the verbal response. The patient sits slouched over, grimaces during movement, and moves slowly with great deliberation. These are all nonverbal signs of pain. These signs may be related to a medical problem other than pain or a psychological problem, or they may simply have no significance. A slouched posture may indicate pain, low self-esteem, depression, or some other unexplained phenomenon. A grimace may be a psychological response to the question or physician, a sign of indigestion, or a facial tic. Slow, deliberate movement may mean unfamiliarity with the surroundings, discomfort, or distraction. Observing this type of nonverbal communication requires probing further to rule out pain.

Some of the verbal responses that can facilitate the interview are minimal responses, reflecting feelings, and seeking clarification (Table 5.1). Responses that may hinder the interview are the use of social clichés, imposition of the interviewer's own values, and devaluing or minimizing the patient's feelings or responses (Table 5.2). In addition, the interviewer should present themselves as unhurried, interested, and sympathetic in an effort to obtain the patient's confidence and rapport.[4]

TABLE 5.2 Examples of Hindering Verbal Responses	
Type of Response	**Examples**
Social clichés	"You will feel better soon." "Don't worry; everything will be alright."
Imposing values	"You should not be having sex outside of marriage." "Someone your age should be more responsible."
Devaluing the patient's feelings or responses	"I wish I had a nickel for every time I heard this." "This is just part of the aging process."

TABLE 5.3 Information Gathered During the Medical History Interview	
Type of Data	**Information Obtained**
Demographic data	Age, race, gender, marital status, and current occupation
Chief complaints	Symptoms, current illness, and current condition
Medical history	Childhood illnesses, allergies, immunizations, injuries, prior hospitalizations, psychological problems, and medications
Family history	Illnesses, causes of death, genetic disorders, and mental disorders
Personal history	Occupation, lifestyle, and sexual activity and preferences

MEDICAL RECORD AND MEDICAL HISTORY

The medical record documents the patient's past medical experience. The format of the medical record may differ from institution to institution and according to whether the person was an inpatient or outpatient seen in the clinic or emergency department. It may be a paper or electronic chart or a combination of both forms. The use of electronic health records and telemedicine (the remote diagnosis and treatment of patients) is expected to grow at a compounded annual rate by more than 14% in the next several years. This is expected to improve access to healthcare while reducing costs.[10]

The hospital medical record is a legal public document that is available to the medical staff; medical departments of the hospital, clinic, and insurance companies; or by subpoena to a court of law. Patients do not own their medical records, but they may review them on request and have copies released. The medical record contains the medical history, results of laboratory tests and medical procedures, progress notes, copies of consent forms, correspondence, and even images produced in the radiation therapy department.

The format for taking a medical history may vary from physician to physician but should be done in a logical manner. Table 5.3 contains a summary of the type of information obtained that is important. This information may also become part of a separate radiation therapy paper or electronic chart.

Need for Demographic Data

Demographic data provide an overview of the patient, including information on the patient's age, gender, race, and, possibly, national origin. The reason for obtaining demographic data is that certain disease conditions are found to be more prevalent for groups according to age, gender, race, and national origin.

For example, although cancer occurs at any age, the incidence (the number of new cases of a disease during a period of time) is higher among older persons, especially those older than age 65 years. However, certain types of cancer occur more frequently in other age groups. The classic presentation of Wilms tumor (a cancer of the kidney) is that of a healthy child in whom abdominal swelling is discovered by the child's mother, pediatrician, or family practitioner during a routine physical examination.[11]

Some types of cancer occur more frequently by gender. For example, men are affected more often than women by lung cancer, whereas the incidence of thyroid cancer is higher in women.

The incidence of cancer among races and nationalities varies. For example, the incidence of esophageal cancer is extremely high in the Bantu of Africa, China, Russia, Japan, Scotland, and the Caspian region of Iran.[11] In the United States, the rate of prostate cancer is significantly higher in African-American men than in Caucasian men.[5]

Importance of the Medical History

The medical history provides a snapshot of the patient's prior medical problems and treatments. The determination of prior medical problems may establish risk factors for acquiring diseases in the future. For example, a patient who has a long history of indigestion and gastric reflux caused by a hiatal hernia may be at risk for ulcers or carcinoma of the esophagus.[11] Gastric reflux is the backward flow of contents of the stomach into the esophagus. A hiatal hernia is a congenital or acquired condition that is the result of movement of the stomach through the esophageal opening of the diaphragm into the thorax. Certain symptoms, illnesses, or conditions may indicate the possibility of a predisposing factor, premalignant condition (physiologic characteristics or predisposing factors that may lead to malignancy), paraneoplastic syndrome (a collections of symptoms that result from substances or hormones produced by the tumor, and they occur remotely from the tumor), or other risk factors. Paraneoplastic syndrome is a rare condition that sometimes occurs with the diagnosis of lung cancer.

Certain types of cancer appear to repeat in families. Leukemia may develop in more than one sibling. If the mother has breast cancer, the daughter may be at greater risk for the disease because of inherited genetic mutations, which are changes to the base pair sequence of either DNA or RNA and are passed down to descendants (BRCA1 and BRCA2).[5,11] The risk of colon cancer increases with age and may be associated with certain inherited genetic mutations or a family history of colon cancer. In some cases, health insurance plans will cover the cost of genetic testing, especially when it is recommended by a physician.

Genetic testing looks for specific mutations in a person's genes, chromosomes, or special proteins. Overall, inherited changes are thought to play a role in about 5% to 10% of all cancers.[12] More than 50 hereditary cancer syndromes have been identified. Box 5.1 includes some of the more common inherited cancers for which genetic testing is available.

The personal history encompasses the patient's lifestyle (past and present). Questions should be asked about close relatives that have the same type of cancer. The physician asks questions regarding dietary, exercise, alcohol, cigarette, and drug habits. The physician must also determine the patient's sexual activity, frequency, and preferences. Determining the patient's past occupations is important. For example, the patient may have been employed in an occupation that carried the risk of exposure to asbestos, disease, certain chemicals, or other carcinogens.

BOX 5.1   Common Inherited Cancers With Genetic Testing Available

Listed below are common inherited cancer syndromes for which genetic testing is available, the gene(s) that are mutated in each syndrome, and the cancer types most often associated with these syndromes are listed for each inherited cancer syndromes.[12]

Hereditary Breast Cancer and Ovarian Cancer Syndrome
- Genes: *BRCA1, BRCA2*
- Related cancer types: Female breast, ovarian, and other cancers, including prostate, pancreatic, and male breast cancer

Li-Fraumeni Syndrome
- Gene: *TP53*
- Related cancer types: Breast cancer, soft tissue sarcoma, osteosarcoma (bone cancer), leukemia, brain tumors, adrenocortical carcinoma (cancer of the adrenal glands), and other cancers

Cowden Syndrome (*PTEN* Hamartoma Tumor Syndrome)
- Gene: *PTEN*
- Related cancer types: Breast, thyroid, endometrial (uterine lining), and other cancers

Lynch Syndrome (Hereditary Nonpolyposis Colorectal Cancer)
- Genes: *MSH2, MLH1, MSH6, PMS2, EPCAM*
- Related cancer types: Colorectal, endometrial, ovarian, renal pelvis, pancreatic, small intestine, liver and biliary tract, stomach, brain, and breast cancers

Familial Adenomatous Polyposis
- Gene: *APC*
- Related cancer types: Colorectal cancer, multiple nonmalignant colon polyps, and both noncancerous (benign) and cancerous tumors in the small intestine, brain, stomach, bone, skin, and other tissues

Retinoblastoma
- Gene: *RB1*
- Related cancer types: Eye cancer (cancer of the retina), pinealoma (cancer of the pineal gland), osteosarcoma, melanoma, and soft tissue sarcoma

Multiple Endocrine Neoplasia Type 1 (Wermer Syndrome)
- Gene: *MEN1*
- Related cancer types: Pancreatic endocrine tumors and (usually benign) parathyroid and pituitary gland tumors

Multiple Endocrine Neoplasia Type 2
- Gene: *RET*
- Related cancer types: Medullary thyroid cancer and pheochromocytoma (benign adrenal gland tumor)

Von Hippel-Lindau Syndrome
- Gene: *VHL*
- Related cancer types: Kidney cancer and multiple noncancerous tumors, including pheochromocytoma

---

PHYSICAL EXAMINATION

The physical examination, medical history, and test results help the physician detect variations in the normal state of the patient. The physical examination is an extremely organized, detailed exploration of the patient's anatomic regions. Performing a physical examination requires all of the clinician's senses and skills.

The following paragraphs list some examples of aspects in the physical examination and information the clinicians may be seeking. The information in this section is extremely general and far from comprehensive regarding all aspects of the physical examination. Inspection, palpation, percussion (the act of striking or tapping the patient gently), and auscultation are the four classic techniques of the physical examination.

Inspection

Inspection is the use of sight to observe. A distinction must be made between seeing and observing. Something may be seen but not observed. For example, a person may see a group of people, but on further observation of the group, the person begins to make distinctions. The person may be able to say that 10 people were in the group and may then observe differences in gender, race, age, appearance, and behavior.

The physician observes the color of the patient's skin, which may indicate signs of a disease condition. Many diseases and conditions affect skin coloration. The skin may be dark, pale, gray, flushed, jaundiced, or cyanotic. Dark skin may be natural or caused by irritation of another medical condition. Pale skin may be natural or caused by anemia. Flushed or reddened skin may be caused by hormones, a reaction to external beam radiation therapy, infection, or burns. Jaundice, a yellow coloration of the skin, may be caused by obstruction of the bile ducts. Cyanosis, a blue coloration of the skin, may be caused by a lack of oxygen in the blood.

The physician looks for scarring or lesions such as warts, moles, ulcerations, tumors, and asymmetry on the surface of the skin. Scarring is an indication of prior medical procedures or injury. The presence of lesions or changes in warts and moles may be benign, a sign of malignant transformation, or cancer. Asymmetry may be an indication of edema, thrombosis, hematoma, injury, or an underlying tumor. Edema is a swelling of the tissue caused by the accumulation of excessive amounts of fluid. Thrombosis is the abnormal accumulation of blood factors in a blood vessel that causes a clot. A hematoma is the abnormal accumulation of blood in tissue from a blood vessel that has ruptured. An inspection may also use the sense of smell to help in making a diagnosis. For example, the smell of the patient's breath, vomitus, wound, urine, or sputum may indicate infection, ketoacidosis, or some other condition.

Olfactory (smell) inspection can be a valuable tool in the assessment process. Each time a patient is assessed, it provides an opportunity to train the four senses: sight, touch, hearing, and smell. Consider the following examples[4]:

Breath: Odors on the breath from acetone, alcohol, and other substances may lead to further questions and diagnosis.

Sputum: Foul-smelling sputum suggests bronchiectasis (an abnormal stretching and enlarging of the respiratory passages caused by mucus blocking the airway, which may lead to infection and inflammation) or lung abscess.

Vomitus: The gastric contents may emit odors of alcohol, phenol, or other poisons, or the foul smell of fermenting food. A fecal smell from the vomitus may indicate an intestinal blockage.

Feces: Particularly foul-smelling stools are common in pancreatic insufficiency.

Urine: An ammonia odor in the urine may result from fermentation within the bladder. A sweet smell may indicate diabetes.

Pus: A nauseating sweet odor, like the smell of rotting apples, is evidence that pus is coming from a region of gas gangrene.

Palpation

Palpation is the use of touch to acquire information about the patient. The physician palpates the patient by using the tips of the fingers. Light palpation is used for a superficial examination. Heavy pressure may be necessary for deep-seated structures. Through palpation, the physician tries to distinguish between hard and soft, rough and smooth, and warm and dry. Vibrations in the chest or abdomen can be felt through palpation. Palpation of an artery can help determine the pulse. Palpation is also used to determine whether pain is present. For example, the patient may not experience pain from an inflammatory process until pressure is applied or applied and released quickly. Areas where superficial lymph node groups exist, such as the neck, axilla, and groin, are important to palpate to determine whether there is any lymphadenopathy (swelling of any lymph nodes). The use of touch in these areas can help determine how many lymph nodes, if there are any, are palpable and whether they are mobile or fixed to underlying structures. Palpation is commonly used in a pelvic examination to examine the vaginal tissues in female patients and the smoothness or nodularity of the prostate gland through the rectal wall in male patients.

Percussion

Percussion is different from palpation in that percussion is the act of striking or tapping the patient gently. The purpose of percussion is to determine pain in underlying tissue or cause vibrations. Making a fist and pounding it gently over the kidney area does not normally produce pain. However, if the patient has an underlying kidney infection, percussion may produce pain.

Placement of the examiner's third finger of one hand flat on the surface of the patient over the lung or abdomen produces another form of percussion. With the third finger of the other hand, the examiner gently raps the dorsal surface of the third finger that is resting on the patient. Depending on the location of the percussion, different sounds are produced. For example, if percussion is done over the lung (which is an air-filled cavity), the vibrations have a different sound than that of the abdominal cavity. Percussion over a normal lung produces a resonant sound, whereas percussion over the abdomen produces a distinctively duller sound. For the radiation therapist, percussion is helpful in determining the place the abdomen ends and the lung begins.

Auscultation

Auscultation is the act of listening to sounds within the body. With a stethoscope, the physician or respiratory therapist performs auscultation by listening to the lungs, heart, arteries, stomach, and bowel sounds. Sounds in the lungs vary depending on the presence or absence of air, fluid, and disease, producing distinct sounds to the trained ear. A pumping heart produces sounds that can be altered by changes or abnormalities of its structure and function.

Vital Signs

Vital signs are almost always taken during the physical examination. Vital signs include temperature, pulse, respirations, blood pressure, and a pain assessment of the patient and will be discussed one by one to help the student understand their importance. These measurements of basic body functions can vary from patient to patient depending on the time of day and physical activity, condition, and age of the patient. Taking baseline, or initial, values at various times to establish the patient's norm is important.

Temperatures are taken orally, rectally, in the ear, on the skin, or in the axilla. Oral temperatures should not be taken on unreliable patients. This includes patients who are irrational, comatose, prone to convulsions, and young children. Patients in these categories should have temperatures taken rectally or in the ear. The rectal temperature

TABLE 5.4 Normal Adult Values for Vital Signs	
Vital Signs	**Values**
Temperature	
Oral	96.8°F–98.6°F (36°C–37°C)
Rectal	99.6°F
Axillary	97.6°F
Pulse	60–100 beats per minute
Respirations	12–18 breaths per minute
Blood pressure	90–140 mm Hg
	60–80 mm Hg
Pain	Subjective scales may be used indicating the intensity of pain

is considered the most accurate. Devices most commonly used for taking temperatures are electronic thermometers. The electronic ear thermometer can be used on adults and children. Temperatures are measured in Fahrenheit (F) or Celsius (C), and some values are given in ranges. Textbooks may list slightly different values for normal and abnormal temperatures (Table 5.4).

Factors observed during the taking of a pulse are rate, rhythm, size, and tension. Rate indicates the number of beats per second. Rhythm is the pattern of beats. Size has to do with the size of the pulse wave and volume of blood felt during the ventricular contraction of the heart. Tension refers to the compressibility of the artery (e.g., soft or hard) (see Table 5.4).

Respiratory rate is the number of breaths that are taken in a minute. Factors that are observed during the evaluation of respiration are rate, depth, rhythm, and character. Depth refers to shallow or deep breathing. The deeper the breath, the greater is the amount of air that is inhaled. Rhythm refers to the regularity of breathing (slow, normal, or rapid). Character refers to the type of breathing, from normal to labored (see Table 5.4).

When blood pressure is taken, the systolic and diastolic pressures are noted. Systolic blood pressure represents the pressure in the blood vessels during the contraction of the heart and is the first sound heard through the stethoscope when blood pressure is taken. Diastolic pressure represents the pressure in the blood vessels during the relaxation phase of the heart after the contraction. The diastolic pressure is the last sound heard through the stethoscope when blood pressure is taken (see Table 5.4).

Blood Pressure Procedure. The most common site for taking blood pressure is the upper arm near where the brachial artery crosses the elbow joint (antecubital fossa). Fig. 5.1 illustrates a radiation therapist assessing blood pressure. The patient may be sitting or lying supine and should be resting in that position for a few minutes before the blood pressure is taken. The cuff, which contains an inflatable rubber bag, should be wrapped snugly around the arm, not too snug, but snug enough to place a finger between the cuff and the patient's arm. The arm should be kept at the level of the heart. The cuff should be centered over the brachial artery with the distal end of the cuff at least 3 cm above the antecubital fossa.[4,13,14]

After the brachial artery is located (it is usually medial to the insertion of the biceps brachii tendon but can be located lateral to the tendon's insertion in some patients), the flat portion of the stethoscope, called the diaphragm, should be gently placed over the artery. The cuff should be inflated to 180 to 200 mm Hg or approximately 30 mm Hg above the point at which the palpable

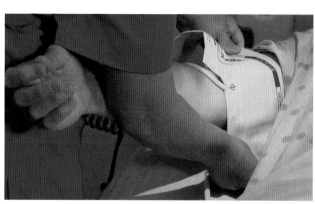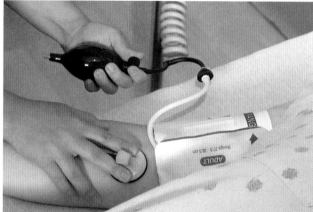

Fig. 5.1 Assessing blood pressure with a blood pressure cuff, sphygmomanometer, and stethoscope. (Copyright © Mosby's Clinical Skills: Essentials Collection.)

pulse disappears. The therapist should then open the valve slowly (no more than 2–3 mm Hg/s), listening for the sounds of the first heartbeat, noting the reading on the sphygmomanometer as the systolic pressure. While deflation continues, the sounds will become louder and maintain a consistency for a considerable range before becoming muffled or the sound stops. The therapist should note the reading on the sphygmomanometer as the diastolic pressure.[4,14] (See Box 5.2 for a more detailed description of taking a blood pressure.)

Pain. Recognizing pain as a major, yet largely avoidable, public health problem, The Joint Commission (TJC) developed standards that have created expectations for the assessment and management of pain in accredited hospitals and other healthcare settings. According to TJC, pain is considered the "fifth" vital sign. Pain intensity ratings should be recorded along with temperature, pulse, respiration, and blood pressure. Fig. 5.2 illustrates a Brief Pain Inventory (BPI) instrument commonly used to evaluate pain.

Despite the increased attention to pain management in the last decade, there is continuing evidence that pain is undertreated. Undertreated pain was first documented in a study by Marks and Sachar, in which they found that 73% of hospitalized patients had moderate to severe pain.[15] Recent studies suggested that when patients had moderate to severe pain, they had only approximately a 50% chance of obtaining adequate pain relief.[16]

In a more recent study by Basch et al of 461 prostate cancer patients, pain was undertreated in patients with metastatic castration-resistant prostate cancer. Even patients in the study with severe pain reported underuse of analgesics. Researchers used the BPI instrument, which measures pain by using a 0 to 10 numeric rating scale in which 0 indicates "no pain," and 10 indicates "pain as bad as you can imagine" to evaluate pain in the prostate cancer patients. Results showed that 40% of patients with a pain intensity of 4 or higher reported no current narcotic analgesic use. Among patients with BPI scores of 7 or higher ("severe" pain), only 27% reported use of a long-acting narcotic, and 18% reported no analgesic at all.[17]

Cancer pain includes pain caused by the disease itself, such as direct tumor invasion of tissue, compression on or infiltration of nerves or blood vessels, organ obstruction, infection, inflammation, and toxicities from chemotherapy or radiation treatment.[16] The International Association of Pain defines **pain** as an unpleasant sensory and emotional experience associated with actual or potential tissue damage.

BOX 5.2   Blood Pressure Procedure

Step 1: Prepare the patient: Introduce yourself. Make sure the patient is sitting or in the supine position, allowing 5 minutes to relax before taking the blood pressure (BP). The patient's arm should be positioned so it is level with his or her heart. Remove any excess clothing that might interfere with the BP cuff or constrict blood flow in the arm.

Step 2: Choose the proper BP cuff size: The arm cuff should be at least 10 cm wide. Wrap the cuff around the patient's arm and use the INDEX line to determine whether the patient's arm circumference falls within the RANGE area. Otherwise, choose the appropriate smaller or larger cuff.

Step 3: Place the cuff on the patient's arm: Palpate/locate the brachial artery and position the cuff so that the ARTERY marker on the cuff points to the brachial artery. Wrap the cuff snugly around the arm, positioned so the inferior portion of the cuff is at least 3 cm above the antecubital fossa.

Step 4: Position the stethoscope: Palpate the arm at the antecubital fossa with the middle and index finger to locate the strongest pulse sounds and place the diaphragm (flat portion) of the stethoscope over the brachial artery.

Step 5: Prepare the cuff: Holding the rubber bulb in the palm of one hand, close the valve on the bulb with thumb and finger, then begin pumping the cuff bulb.

Step 6: Inflate the cuff. By pumping the bulb rapidly, inflate the cuff to approximately 20 to 30 mm Hg above the expected systolic reading. If this value is unknown, inflate the cuff to 160 to 180 mm Hg. (If pulse sounds are heard right away, inflate to a higher pressure.) Inflation of the cuff should take 7 seconds or less.

Step 7: Slowly deflate the BP cuff: Begin deflation by opening the valve slowly. The American Heart Association recommends that the pressure fall at 2 to 3 mm Hg/s. A faster rate is likely to result in an inaccurate measurement.

Step 8: Listen for the systolic reading: The first occurrence of rhythmic sounds heard as blood begins to flow through the artery is the patient's systolic pressure. This may resemble a tapping noise at first. After the first sound, the pulsing will get louder as the pressure is slowly released.

Step 9: Listen for the diastolic reading. Continue to listen while the cuff pressure drops and the sounds fade. Note the gauge reading when the rhythmic sounds stop. This will be the diastolic reading.

Step 10: Complete the procedure. Remove the cuff and record the values as systolic/diastolic (e.g., 120/80). Wipe the eartips and diaphragm of the stethoscope with alcohol before storing the equipment.

Some radiation therapy facilities require the radiation therapist to record the BPI score in the electronic medical record along with daily treatment doses and other important information. This provides much needed up-to-date information on the patient's "fifth vital sign."

Pain Scales Combined: NRS + FACES

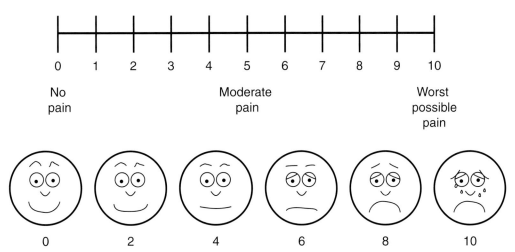

Fig. 5.2 The Brief Pain Inventory instrument, which measures pain by using a 0 to 10 numeric rating scale, in which 0 indicates "no pain" and 10 indicates "pain as bad as you can imagine," is used to evaluate pain in prostate cancer patients. Example of how the Numerical Rating Scale *(NRS)* can be combined with the Wong-Baker FACES Pain Rating *(FACES)* in a horizontal format. If the NRS is not easily understood, the FACES scale is an alternative. (From Hockenberry MJ, Wilson D, Rodgers CC. *Wong's Essentials of Pediatric Nursing.* 10th ed. St. Louis, MO: Elsevier; 2017:116; and Pasero C, McCaffery M. *Pain: Assessment and Pharmacologic Management.* St. Louis, MO: Mosby; 2011:56.)

Clinical Application of Vital Signs

As a therapist who interacts with the patient daily, there is a greater opportunity to assess, observe, and/or interact with the patient than the nurse or radiation oncologist (who might see the patient as needed or at least weekly). If, in the course of interacting with the patient, the therapist recognizes some abnormality, further evaluation of the patient may be indicated. Vital signs may provide additional information quickly before other laboratory test or scans. Vital signs are sensitive indicators of the presence of disease and are strongly correlated with severity of illness.[4] Table 5.5 provides some clinical correlations with increased or decreased values of temperature, pulse, respiration, and blood pressure. Well-trained therapists will use their clinical skills to probe the patient, seeking information on how the patient is tolerating the treatment and look for signs of risk to the patient's health and well-being.

SCREENING

Screening refers to testing in individuals who are asymptomatic for a particular disease. In addition to detecting cancer early, screening for certain cancers can identify abnormalities that may become precancerous and prevent potential progression to cancer. An estimated 20% of all cancers diagnosed in the United States are caused by a combination of excess body weight, physical inactivity, excess alcohol consumption, and poor nutrition and thus could also be prevented. A great deal of suffering and death from cancer could be avoided by more systematic efforts to reduce tobacco use, control obesity, improve diet, increase exercise, and the routine use of established screening tests.[18] Early detection of cancer through screening has been determined to reduce mortality from cancers of the colon and rectum, breast, uterine cervix, and lung.[19]

Screening is the cornerstone of the diagnosis and management of the patient. It is done for large, asymptomatic populations at risk to detect deviations from the norm or signs of disease. Specific screening is performed for patients who are symptomatic, undergoing treatment, or being followed up. The determination to do mass screening is

based on the results obtained, the cost-effectiveness, and the risk to the patient. Areas of screening performed today are aimed at identifying cancer at its earliest stage, which translates into increased cure rates for most cancers. Until the early 1960s, there were a small number of tests that were available for asymptomatic patients such as a chest x-ray, a complete blood count, a blood chemistry test, a urinalysis, and a stool test for occult blood. With the development of multichannel automated analyzers, many laboratory tests could now be obtained for the same cost as that of the few tests that had been performed previously. Most screening studies can be grouped into two major categories: laboratory studies and medical imaging. Hundreds of laboratory tests and medical imaging procedures exist today. Discretion must be exercised in selecting appropriate tests to be done, and studies are not performed unless logical reasons exist for doing so. Cost can be a factor.

The ACS believes that early detection examinations and tests can save lives and reduce suffering from cancers of the breast, colorectal, prostate, cervix, endometrial, testes, oral cavity, and skin. Some of these cancers can be found by self-examination, physical examination, and laboratory tests (such as mammography, the Papanicolaou [Pap] test, and the prostate-specific antigen [PSA] blood test).[5] Cancer screening can be effective if a disease has a high incidence or prevalence in a population and the test has the ability to produce results with the appropriate sensitivity (defined as the ability of a test to give a true-positive result) and specificity (defined as the ability of a test to obtain a true-negative result).

There are four measures used to assess the impact of cancer in the general population. The incidence rate is the number of new cases per year per 100,000 persons. The death (or mortality) rate is the number of deaths per 100,000 persons. The survival estimate is the proportion of patients alive at some point subsequent to the diagnosis of their cancer. The prevalence count is the number of people alive that have ever been diagnosed with a cancer.[20]

In the United States, the leading cause of cancer in women is breast cancer, and the leading cause of cancer in men is prostate cancer. Therefore, a significant portion of the population benefits from mass

TABLE 5.5   Clinical Application of Vital Signs

Vital Sign	Increased/Decreased	Possible Causes	Related Information
Temperature	Increased	Decreased white blood cell (WBC) count	A drop in WBC can be caused by irradiation of a significant amount of bone marrow and/or certain chemotherapy drugs.
	Increased	Infection caused by bacteria, virus, fungus, or parasite (occult abscess is common)	It should be noted that some patients, especially the elderly, those with renal failure, or those receiving high doses of corticosteroids, are not always able to mount a response to infection
	Increased	Inflammatory	Lupus, rheumatic fever, radiation therapy, and other diseases
	Increased	Tissue necrosis	Myocardial infarction, pulmonary infarction, stroke, and tumor
	Increased	Neoplastic	Leukemia, lymphoma, and solid tumors; some lymphomas produce night sweats, which mark the end of the fever at night
	Decreased	Hypothermia	Heat stroke, poverty, homelessness, and psychosis
Pulse	Increased	Infection	Tachycardia (>100 beats/minute) usually accompanies fever; the pulse rate is proportionate to the temperature elevation
	Increased	Anxiety, hyperthyroidism, anemia, exercise, and beta-adrenergic medications	Radiation treatments and a diagnosis of cancer can contribute to anxiety
	Decreased	Some healthy persons, especially well-conditioned athletes, and occasionally in severe infections	Rare
Respirations	Increased	Hypoxia, caused by superior vena cava (SVC) syndrome, a type of advanced lung cancer	Some primary or metastatic lung tumors can wrap around the SVC, restricting blood flow back to the heart
	Increased	Fear, anemia, some lung cancers, and pain	More likely to be seen among some cancer patients
	Increased	Exertion, obesity, cardiac insufficiency, pulmonary embolism, infections, emphysema, pneumothorax, hyperthyroidism	Breathing is faster when restricted by weakness of or restriction of respiratory muscles
	Decreased	A result of central nervous system–depressant drugs such as opiates, benzodiazepines, barbiturates, and alcohol	Drugs used to reduce pain are commonly seen with palliative care in radiation oncology
	Decreased	Intracranial tumors, especially those that cause an increase in intracranial pressure (ICP)	An increase in intracranial pressure is often seen with tumors blocking the flow of cerebral spinal fluid, such as that seen in pediatric medulloblastoma
Blood pressure	Increased	Causes for hypertension are numerous, including stroke, heart failure, and chronic kidney failure	Each patient's blood pressure should be checked weekly, both to detect hypertension and establish a baseline for comparison
	Increased	Neurologic causes of hypertension include adrenal adenoma, pituitary adenoma, and some primary brain tumors	Rare
	Decreased	Dehydration	A 20-mm drop in blood pressure may indicate dehydration, especially for radiation therapy patients treated in the head and neck area, abdomen, and pelvic area, because of nausea, vomiting, and/or diarrhea
	Decreased	Hypotension may be the result of bleeding, ascites, burns, diabetes, shock, high fever, or other causes	Each patient's blood pressure should be checked weekly, both to detect hypotension and establish a baseline for comparison
	Decreased	Anaphylactic shock	Can occur with the administration of iodine-based contrast agents used during the computed tomography simulation process

Data from LeBlond, RF, Brown DD, Sunja M, et al. *DeGowin's Diagnostic Examination.* 11th ed. 2019. New York, NY: McGraw-Hill.

medical screening. If the disease is caught early enough, morbidity and mortality rates may be reduced. Mass screening for breast cancer in China is not effective because the at-risk population is low. However, the reverse is true for cancer of the esophagus; the number of persons at risk for cancer of the esophagus is extremely high in certain regions of China. Because the population at risk for cancer of the esophagus is much lower in the United States, mass screening for esophageal cancer would not be beneficial in terms of outcome and cost effectiveness.

Diseases for which mass screening tools have received more attention in recent years include cancers of the breast, lung, prostate, colon,

TABLE 5.6 Screening Guidelines for the Early Detection of Cancer in Average-Risk Asymptomatic People

Cancer Site	Population	Test or Procedure	Recommendation
Breast	Women, age 40–54 years	Mammography	Women should undergo regular screening mammography starting at the age 45 years.
			Women ages 45 to 54 years should be screened annually.
			Women should have the opportunity to begin annual screening between the ages of 40 and 44 years.
	Women, age ≥55 years		Transition to biennial screening or have the opportunity to continue annual screening. Continue screening as long as overall health is good and life expectancy is ≥10 years.
Cervix	Women, age 21–29 years	Pap test	Screening should be done every 3 years with conventional or liquid-based Pap tests.
	Women, age 30–65 years	Pap test and human papillomavirus (HPV) DNA test	Screening should be done every 5 years with both the HPV test and the Pap test (preferred), or every 3 years with the Pap test alone (acceptable).
Women, age ≥66 years	Pap test and HPV DNA test		Women age ≥66 years who had ≥3 consecutive negative Pap tests or ≥2 consecutive negative HPV and Pap tests with in the past 10 years, with the most recent test occurring in the past 54 years should stop cervical cancer screening.
	Women who have had a total hysterectomy		Stop cervical cancer screening
Colorectal†	Men and women, age ≥50 years	Guaiac-based fecal occult blood test (gFOBT) with at least 50% sensitivity or fecal immunochemical test (FIT) with at least 50% sensitivity, OR	Annual testing of spontaneously passed stool specimens. Single stool testing during a clinician office visit is not recommended, nor are "throw in the toilet bowl" tests. In comparison with guaiac-based tests for the detection of occult blood, immunochemical tests are more patient friendly and are likely to be equal or better in sensitivity and specificity. There is no justification for reporting FOBT in response to an initial positive finding.
		Stool DNA test, OR	Every 3 years
		Flexible sigmoidoscopy (FSIG), OR	Every 5 years alone, or consideration can be given to combining FSIG performed every 5 years with a highly sensitive gFOBT or FIT performed annually.
		Double-contrast barium enema, OR	Every 5 years
		Colonoscopy, OR	Every 10 years
		CT colonoscopy	Every 5 years
Endometrial	Women at menopause		Women should be informed about risks and symptoms of endometrial cancer and encouraged to report unexpected bleeding to their physician.
Lung	Current or former smokers age 55–74 years in good health with 30+ pack-year history	Low-dose helical CT (LDCT)	Clinicians with access to high-volume, high-quality lung cancer screening and treatment centers should initiate a discussion about annual lung cancer screening with apparently healthy patients aged 55–74 years who have at least 30 pack-year smoking history and who currently smoke or have quit within the past 15 years. A process of informed and shared decision-making with a clinician related to the potential benefits, limitations, and harms associated with screening for lung cancer with LDCT should occur before any decision is made to initiate lung cancer screening. Smoking cessation counseling remains a high priority for clinical attention discussions with current smokers, who should be informed of their continuing risk of lung cancer. Screening should not be viewed as an alternative to smoke cessation.
Prostate	Men, age ≥50 years	Prostate-specific antigen test with or without digital rectal examination	Men who have at least a 10-year life expectancy should have an opportunity to make an informed decision with their healthcare provider about whether to be screened for prostate cancer after receiving information about the potential benefits, risks, and uncertainties associated with prostate cancer screening. Prostate cancer screening should not occur without an informed decision-making process.

From Cancer prevention and early detection: facts and figures. American Cancer Society website. www.cancer.org, Accessed July 2018; Cancer facts and figures 2018 supplemental data. American Cancer Society website. http://www.cancer.org, Accessed on July 15, 2018.

cervix, and endometrium. These screening guidelines have evolved with the implementation of new scientific data. As new screening technologies become available, the standards for creating guidelines evolve and are adapted to the changing population.

The ACS strongly recommends mass screenings for breast, colorectal, prostate, lung, cervical, and endometrial cancers. Table 5.6 provides an excellent overview of recommendations for screening and detection by site and symptoms.

Breast

For women between the ages of 40 and 44 years, the ACS recommends that they should have the opportunity to begin annual screening for

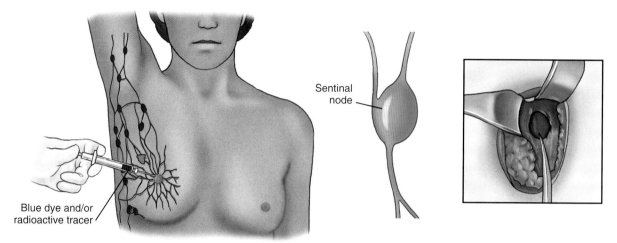

Fig. 5.3 The sentinel lymph node procedure focuses on finding lymph nodes that are the first to receive draining fluid from breast tumors. A blue dye or radioactive tracer is injected near the tumor site and is then absorbed locally, traveling to the sentinel node(s).

breast cancer. For women 45 years of age and older, the ACS recommends an annual mammogram, which can demonstrate small lesions before they can be palpated. More detailed recommendations include the following:

- The ACS recommends that women with an average risk of breast cancer should undergo regular screening mammography starting at age 45 years (strong recommendation).
- Women aged 45 to 54 years should be screened annually (qualified recommendation).
- Women 55 years and older should transition to biennial screening or have the opportunity to continue screening annually (qualified recommendation).
- Women should have the opportunity to begin annual screening between the ages of 40 and 44 years (qualified recommendation).
- Women should continue screening mammography as long as their overall health is good and they have a life expectancy of 10 years or longer (qualified recommendation).
- The ACS does not recommend clinical breast examination for breast cancer screening among average-risk women at any age (qualified recommendation).

Note that a strong recommendation conveys that the benefits of adherence to that intervention outweigh the undesirable side effects that may result from screening. Qualified recommendations indicate there is clear evidence of benefit of screening but less certainty about the balance of benefits and harms, or about patients' values and preferences, which could lead to different decisions about screening.[21]

Mammography screening has been shown to reduce breast cancer mortality across a range of studies, including randomized controlled trials and several observational studies.[22,24,28,29] Screening mammography in women aged 40 to 69 years is associated with a reduction in breast cancer deaths and inferential evidence supports breast cancer screening for women 70 years and older who are in good health.[19]

What is average risk? The ACS recommendations for women at average risk of breast cancer include women without a personal history of breast cancer, women without a history of suspected or confirmed genetic mutation known to increase risk of breast cancer, and/or women without a history of previous radiation therapy to the chest at a young age.

In addition, the ACS provides recommendations for breast MRI screening as an adjunct to mammography and/or ultrasound for women at high risk, based on a genetic mutation known to increase the risk of breast cancer, a history of radiation to the chest at ages 10 to 30 years, or an estimated lifetime risk of approximately 20% to 25% or greater.[21]

The sentinel lymph node biopsy procedure focuses on finding lymph nodes that are the first to receive draining fluid from breast tumors and, therefore, the first to collect cancer cells. A blue dye, radioactive substance (technetium-99m sulfur colloid), or both, is injected near the tumor site and is then absorbed locally through the lymph system, traveling to the sentinel node(s). The node is then more easily identified by the surgeon so it can be removed and examined for cancer cells (Fig. 5.3). If there are no cancer cells present, an axillary lymph node dissection may not be necessary.

The understanding of cancer biology associated with breast cancer is demanding more and more attention to the detection and treatment of breast cancer. Biologic factors help guide treatment strategies. Increasing evidence suggests that breast cancers defined by expression of the estrogen receptor, progesterone receptor, and human epidermal growth factor represent unique biologic expressions. Breast cancers that are estrogen receptor positive, progesterone receptor positive, or both, are associated with a more favorable prognosis because they generally respond to hormonal therapy. For women whose cancer tests positive for human epidermal growth factor 2/neu, approved targeted therapies are available.[5]

Lung

Improvements in the biologic understanding of lung tumors, the advent of spiral CT scanning, and advances in the treatment of lung cancer have led many investigators to evaluate the use of CT in screening for lung cancer. Several studies have shown a benefit with the use of CT for screening in lung cancer. Low-dose spiral CT scans and molecular markers in sputum have produced promising results in detection of lung cancers at earlier, more operable stages in high-risk patients.[23] One study, the National Lung Screening Trial (NLST), has shown promising results.

The NLST compared low-dose helical CT with chest radiography in the screening of heavy smokers for early detection of lung cancer.[25] The NLST examined 53,454 smokers, aged 55 to 74 years, who had a smoking history of at least 30 pack-years (calculated by multiplying the average number of packs of cigarettes smoked per day by the number of years a person smoked. For example, 30 pack-years could be calculated as a smoker of one pack per day for 30 years or two packs a day for 15 years) and had no signs or symptoms of lung cancer. The study showed that those who were screened with low-dose CT scans had a 15% to 20% lower chance of dying from lung cancer as compared with those screened with a standard chest x-ray. Within the three rounds of screening over a 7-year period, data revealed a positive result in 24.2% for those screened with a CT scan compared with 6.9% of those with a chest x-ray. In both arms of the trial, the majority of positive screens led to further testing.[25]

Lung cancer is the leading cause of cancer-related death in the United States. Five-year survival rates approach 70% with surgical resection of early stage disease; however, the overall 5-year survival rate for lung cancer is low: 17% for men and 24% for women, due in part to the large number of cases diagnosed with advanced stage disease.[5] Early-stage lung cancer is now treated in some cancer centers with a complex treatment-planning process that incorporates respiratory motion of the mass into the treatment planning process. Early detection is essential for patients to benefit from this highly specialized type of external beam radiation therapy treatment. The ACS estimates that there are about 6.8 million current and former smokers eligible for screening; in one study, only 262,700 received it.[5,25]

Prostate

Screening for prostate cancer, which is one of the leading causes of death in American men older than 50 years, remains controversial. Two European studies found a lower risk of death from prostate cancer among men who received PSA screening, whereas a study in the United States found no reduction.[19] Current research is exploring new biologic markers for prostate cancer, as well as alternative patient ages for screening initiation and timing of testing, with the goal of identifying and treating men at highest risk for aggressive disease while minimizing unnecessary testing and overtreatment of men at low risk for prostate cancer death.[5] The two most common methods used to screen for prostate cancer are digital rectal examination and PSA blood test. Consensus is lacking on whom to screen, when to screen, and what to do if cancer is discovered.

In its 2016 recommendations for prostate cancer, the ACS encourages men to have a discussion with their healthcare provider regarding the risks and benefits of prostate screening.[5] The discussion about screening men depends on their risk level and should include the following:

- At age 50 years for men who are at average risk for prostate cancer and are expected to live at least 10 years.
- At age 45 years for men at high risk for developing prostate cancer. This includes African Americans and men who have a first-degree relative (father, brother, son) diagnosed with prostate cancer at an age younger than 65 years.
- At age 40 years for men at even higher risk, which includes those with more than one first-degree relative diagnosed with prostate cancer before the age of 65 years.

If cancer is discovered during the screening process, the time between future screenings will vary depending on the PSA level detected. Men who choose to be tested who have a PSA of less than 2.5 ng/mL may only need to be tested every 2 years. Screening is recommended every year for those with a PSA level of 2.5 ng/mL or higher. Because prostate cancer tends to grow slowly, men who are asymptomatic and who do not have a 10-year life expectancy should not be tested.[2,5,19]

Interestingly, a sharp increase in prostate cancer incidence rates began in 1988 after the introduction of screening for PSA. This increase was not the result of prostate cancer developing in more men, but rather the ability of the new test to find more cases at an earlier stage. The incidence leveled off after a few years and has recently started to decline. This is a pattern typically observed after the introduction of a new early detection test. Most importantly, death rates have begun to decline in recent years, likely resulting from earlier detection.[5]

TABLE 5.7   Actions That May Alter Test Results

Person Responsible	Actions
Caregiver	Incomplete or inaccurately filled-out requisitions
	Incomplete or inaccurate coordination of activities
	Incomplete or inaccurate patient instruction
	Incorrectly performed procedure
	Incorrect labeling of specimens
Patient	Incorrect interpretation of instructions
	Lack of cooperation
	Inability to follow instructions or noncompliance

Sensitivity, Specificity, and Predictive Values

Other measures for determining the value of a study are the sensitivity, specificity, and predictive values. *Sensitivity* is defined as the ability of a test to give a true positive result when the disease is present. In other words, a person who tests positive for cancer from a high-sensitivity test probably has cancer. *Specificity* is defined as the ability of the test to obtain a true-negative result. When the results of a high-specificity test are negative, that person probably does not have cancer.[4]

The ideal situation is for a test to yield a high sensitivity and high specificity. However, that is almost impossible. Because of the morbidity and mortality rates of cancer, the ability to detect cancer early in all individuals tested is important. High sensitivity is selected when the disease prevalence is low. A positive finding of cancer from a high-sensitivity test can be confirmed by subjecting the patient to a second test of high specificity. High specificity is selected when the disease prevalence is high. Determining the sensitivity and specificity of the test can affect its *predictive value*. The predictive value of a positive test increases with an increase in the sensitivity and specificity of the test. Sensitivity and specificity are the most widely used statistics used to describe a diagnostic test. Unfortunately, they are not always helpful to clinicians trying to determine the probability of disease. Reviewing the definitions of prevalence, sensitivity, and specificity may be helpful:

Prevalence: Probability of disease in the entire population at any point in time.
Incidence: Probability that a disease will develop in a disease-free patient during an interval.
Sensitivity: Probability of a positive test among patients with disease.
Specificity: Probability of a negative test among patients without disease.

Common Sources of Errors

The sources of errors in medical studies are many. Any medical examination always has a margin of error in the results. The possibility of errors exists in the ordering of a study. Request must be entered into the computer completely and correctly, and may include the patient's demographic data, symptoms, or diagnosis, if available, and the purpose of the test.

Coordination of the patient's activities is important. Special consideration must be given to patients who are handicapped, disabled, diabetic, or infirm. Extra time may be necessary to accommodate these patients in scheduling a battery of activities before the study, preparing the patient, and performing the procedure. Care must be taken in the ordering of the study and test, coordination of activities, and preparation of the patient (Table 5.7). For example, if a patient on the treatment schedule is receiving both radiation therapy and chemotherapy every fifth day, it may be helpful to the patient to attempt to schedule both appointments as close as possible on the days chemotherapy is scheduled, unless there are expected adverse side effects from combining both treatments too closely together. Some tests require coordination so that they do not interfere with each other. For example, a glucose tolerance test takes place during a period of 2 hours, at which time blood must be drawn. If the patient is not available when the blood is to be drawn, the results of the test are invalid. Some tests must be done before others because they may interfere with the next test. Improper coordination may result in the patient having to go through an uncomfortable preparation for the test again. In addition, many of the tests are invasive, can be uncomfortable, and carry certain risks. Repeated radiographic procedures result in unnecessary exposure of the patient to ionizing radiation.

LABORATORY STUDIES

Hundreds of laboratory studies are available today. Some studies are used to analyze the composition of the blood and bone marrow and rule out blood disorders. Blood studies are concerned with blood cells, whereas blood chemistry tests examine chemicals in the blood, such as glucose, electrolytes, and proteins. Microbiologic studies are helpful in detecting specific organisms that may cause infection. Urine studies are done to analyze the composition and concentration of the urine. These studies are helpful to detect diseases and disorders of the kidney and urinary system and endocrine or metabolic disorders. Fecal studies are done to examine the waste products of digestion and metabolic disorders. These studies are useful to detect gastrointestinal diseases and disorders such as bleeding, obstruction, obstructive jaundice, and parasitic disease. Studies are also done to investigate the immune system. Immunologic studies examine the antigen-antibody reactions. Serologic tests are done to diagnose problems such as neoplastic disease, infectious disease, and allergic reactions. Baseline values should always be obtained to observe any deviation. Table 5.8 contains normal ranges for a complete blood cell count. The values may vary from institution to institution, depending on the methods used.

MEDICAL IMAGING

The physiology and anatomy of the body can be imaged in many ways, and the procedures used can be extremely simple or complex. Every procedure provides some element of risk to the patient. For example, noninvasive procedures provide very little risk to the patient. Whereas an invasive procedure such as a biopsy provides some risk, the exact amount of acceptable risk depends on many factors. The physician and patient should discuss the risks and benefits of any diagnostic imaging procedure.

Electrical Impulses

Some medical imaging techniques use electrical impulses of the body to determine the ability of the heart, brain, and muscles to function. The electrocardiogram demonstrates the electrical conductivity of the heart muscle. This aids in the detection and diagnosis of heart disease. During the examination, wave patterns representing the electrical pulse are recorded. The physician studies the wave patterns to check for any deviations. The electroencephalogram records brain-wave activity; this study helps to detect and diagnose seizure disorders, brainstem disorders, brain lesions, and states of consciousness. An electromyogram measures the electrical conductivity of the muscle, thus aiding in the detection and diagnosis of neuromuscular problems.

TABLE 5.8   Normal Ranges for Complete Blood Count

Blood Component	Range
White blood cells	5,000–10,000/mm³
Red blood cells	3.90–5.40 million/mm³
Platelets	150,000–425,000/mm³
Hemoglobin	12–16 g/dL
Hematocrit	37%–47%
Differential White Blood Cells (WBC)	
Neutrophils	42%–72%
Lymphocytes	17%–45%
Monocytes	3%–10%
Eosinophils	0%–4%
Basophils	0%–2%

Nuclear Medicine Imaging

Nuclear medicine imaging introduces a special radionuclide (radioactive substance) into the patient. A radionuclide, or radiopharmaceutical, is an isotope that undergoes radioactive decay. In doing so, it gives off radiation, often in the form of gamma rays. It is an unstable element that attempts to reach stability by emitting several types of ionizing radiation. The radionuclide may be injected, swallowed, or inhaled, depending on the diagnostic procedure. After the introduction of the radionuclide into the patient, it follows a specific metabolic pathway in the body. Several minutes to several hours later, an imaging device is placed outside the patient's body, and the resultant radiation from the radionuclide is measured and imaged.

The three most common imaging devices are the gamma camera, rectilinear scanner, and the PET scanner. The large circular gamma camera does not move and views the whole area of interest at one time. The rectilinear scanner starts at the top or bottom of the area of interest and scans from side to side until the entire area of interest has been imaged. This method may be used to detect metastatic cancer in the bone. PET imaging has proved especially useful in oncology in recent years and is used more commonly as a diagnostic tool. This modality makes possible the viewing of an organ's function and blood flow in addition to the image of its anatomy.[14] The PET scanner works by creating computerized images of chemical changes that take place in tissue. The patient is given an injection of a combination of a sugar (glucose) and a small amount of radioactive material. The radioactive sugar can help locate a tumor, because cancer cells take up or absorb sugar faster than other tissues in the body and glucose is the essential building block for cell metabolism.[14]

Routine Radiographic Studies

Routine radiographic studies consist of contrast and noncontrast types. The use of contrast media such as barium and iodine helps to visualize anatomy that is radiolucent. If the anatomic structure is radiolucent, the x-rays are not completely absorbed by the structure and therefore cannot be demonstrated on an image. For example, gas and fecal material in the colon may be visualized without contrast. However, to visualize the structure, position, filling, and movement of the colon, a barium-based contrast agent is necessary. For the esophagus to be visible, the patient must drink barium. Bone has a relatively high density and can be demonstrated without the aid of contrast media.

Routine noncontrast studies consist of chest x-ray studies; mammograms; images of the abdomen that include the kidneys, ureters, and bladder; and radiographs of the skull, spine, and other bones. Contrast studies include but are not limited to the kidneys, upper and lower gastrointestinal tract, and blood vessels. Contrast examinations are also used in CT and MRI studies.

Computed Tomography

CT, which was first introduced in Great Britain in the early 1970s, was initially developed to study the brain in cross section. Since then, other applications have become useful, and today, CT scans of the head, chest, abdomen, and pelvis are routine. The CT scanner digitizes a complex x-ray image and stores it in a computer. Scanners that can produce a three-dimensional image are available and are used for reconstructive surgery and radiation therapy treatment planning.

CT imaging has several advantages versus routine radiography procedures. By rotating an x-ray tube 360 degrees around the patient, data are gathered that can be reconstructed digitally in more than one plane, allowing the healthcare provider to see structures in a three-dimensional display. This eliminates the problem of overlying structures commonly seen on radiographs and gives significantly more data to evaluate for diagnostic purposes. In addition, density data are more easily distinguished between air, soft tissue, and bone. In other words, one can see a greater degree of contrast of gray shades between various structures. CT scanning is also less expensive than MRI scanning.

Magnetic Resonance Imaging

MRI is a method of creating diagnostic images of the body by using a combination of radiofrequency waves and a strong magnetic field. Unlike nuclear medicine and radiology, MRI does not use ionizing radiation to produce an image. MRI units have the ability to demonstrate soft tissue to a much greater degree than CT units. However, CT units can demonstrate bone better than MRI units.

MRI has become increasingly popular clinically because it is a noninvasive procedure that has, to date, shown no harmful late side effects. In addition, the image quality is better in specific anatomic areas, such as the brain and spinal cord. The diagnostic scanning tool has several disadvantages compared with CT scanning: it is expensive to use; it cannot be used in patients with metallic devices, such as pacemakers; and it cannot be used with patients who are claustrophobic (however, new MRI systems with a more open design are available). MRI technology offers image reconstruction in multiple planes, including transverse, sagittal, and coronal.

Diagnostic Ultrasound

Diagnostic ultrasound is one of the least expensive imaging techniques. It is also quick and simple and usually causes only minimal patient discomfort. Ultrasound also differs from radiography in that its images are produced with high-frequency sound waves instead of ionizing radiation. Ultrasound, also called sonography, is an imaging technique in which high-frequency sound waves are bounced off of tissues and internal organs, producing an image called a *sonogram*. During an ultrasound examination, the clinician spreads a thin coating of lubricating jelly over the area to be imaged. This jelly improves the conduction of the sound waves. A handheld device called a *transducer* directs the sound waves through the skin toward specific tissues or organ. While the sound waves are reflected back from the tissues, the patterns formed by the waves create a two-dimensional image on a computer.[10] Ultrasound has been used for breast cancer screening and prostate localization and volume calculations.

In breast cancer screening, ultrasound may be used as part of other diagnostic procedures, such as mammography or fine-needle biopsy.

Ultrasound is not used for routine breast cancer screening because it does not consistently detect certain early signs of cancer such as microcalcifications of calcium in the breast that cannot be felt but can be seen on a conventional mammogram. Sometimes, a cluster of microcalcifications may indicate that cancer is present.

Ultrasound has been used extensively in gynecologic and prenatal imaging. Fetal weight, growth, and anatomy can be studied without exposure to ionizing radiation. The ability of ultrasound to demonstrate soft tissue structures is helpful in demonstrating gallstones, kidney stones, and tumors.

CANCER DIAGNOSIS (BIOPSY)

Histologic evidence is vital in making a diagnosis of cancer. Tissue for diagnosis is obtained through scraping, needle aspiration, needle biopsy, incisional biopsy, and excisional biopsy.

Exfoliative cells can be found in all parts of the body. These are cells that have been scraped off deliberately or sloughed off naturally. They are found in the urine, sputum, feces, and mucus.

Exfoliative cytologic studies are extremely helpful in identifying neoplastic disease, especially in the management of cervix and lung cancer. The only problem with cytologic studies is that individual cells are viewed and the determination of cells as invasive or noninvasive is not possible.

Other methods of obtaining tissue are needle, incisional, and excisional biopsies. Needle biopsies and incisional biopsies can be done on an outpatient basis by using local anesthesia. Only small amounts of tissue can be obtained by needle and incisional biopsies. An incisional biopsy (see Figure 1.6) involves the removal of only a portion of the tumor for diagnosis. With all biopsy specimens, the sample is then viewed under a microscope by a pathologist. The tissue sample may be stained with chemicals to highlight specific parts of the cell's cytoplasm and nucleus or to amplify specific regions of DNA.

An excisional biopsy involves the removal of the entire tumor for diagnosis. This procedure provides for a more definitive diagnosis because the margins of the tumor are examined by the pathologist to see whether the cancer has spread beyond the area that is biopsied. If the margins are "clear" or "negative," that means that no disease was found at the edges of the biopsy specimen. A "positive margin" means that disease was found at the edge of the specimen and that the tumor has directly invaded beyond the area biopsied. Additional investigation or treatment may be necessary.[26]

When cancer is detected, determining the presence of metastatic disease is necessary. The use of a tumor marker may help detect widespread disease. A tumor marker is a substance produced and released by the tumor. Tumor markers refer to a molecule that can be detected in serum, plasma, or other body fluid. Tumor markers are useful in detecting the presence of specific types of tissue, such as prostatic tissue in the case of PSA, metastatic disease, and determining the effect of the treatment.

STAGING SYSTEMS

After a histologic diagnosis of cancer has been made, the cancer must be staged. Staging helps to determine the anatomic extent of the disease. Treatment decisions are based on the histologic diagnosis and extent of the disease. The natural growth for most cancers if untreated is that they extend beyond their original site by direct extension or move into the lymphatic and circulatory systems. They ultimately metastasize to distant sites. Staging systems are based on this concept.[27]

Recommendations regarding staging of cancer by individual researchers, specialties, committees, and other groups have not been uniform. The major groups that have been involved in staging and are working together to establish common terminology are the International Union Against Cancer, the International Federation of Gynecology and Obstetrics, and the American Joint Commission on Cancer.[27]

Specific definitions of the tumor, node, metastasis (TNM) staging system are shown in Table 5.9 (subdivisions are not included). Another aspect of the staging system is the histologic type and histologic grade. *Histologic type* refers to cell type, and *histologic grade* refers to the differentiation of the cell. For example, the histologic type may be squamous cell carcinoma, and the histologic grade indicates the closeness of the cells' resemblance to a normal squamous cell. Table 5.10 lists the histopathologic grades.

Another aspect of the staging system is the use of the numbered stages 0 through IV to indicate the stages of the tumor. Stage 0 usually indicates carcinoma in situ. Stages I and II indicate the smallness of the tumor, involvement of early local and regional nodes with no distant metastases (defined as the spread of cancer beyond the primary site), or both. Stage III indicates that the tumor is more extensive locally and may have regional node involvement. Stage IV indicates locally advanced tumors with invasion beyond the regional nodes to other areas. The categorizations of stage 0 through IV are often grouped with the TNM system of staging. For example, stage 0, TisN0M0, indicates an extremely localized early disease, whereas stage II, T2N0M0, indicates a more advanced disease. Stage IV, any NM1, indicates an extremely late advanced disease.

There are several reasons for the precise clinical description and accurate classification (staging) of cancers, specifically:

- To aid the physician and radiation therapy team in the planning of the treatment
- To provide some indication of prognosis. It may be one of many factors in determining prognosis
- To assist in the evaluation of the results of treatment. It helps in comparing groups of cases, especially as it relates to various therapeutic procedures
- To assist in the exchange of information from one treatment center to another

TABLE 5.9 TNM Clinical Classification*

TNM Classification	Description
Primary Tumor (T)	
TX	Primary tumor not assessable
T0	No evidence of primary tumor
Tis	Carcinoma in situ
T1, T2, T3, T4	Increasing size and/or local extent of the primary tumor
Regional Lymph Nodes (N)	
NX	Regional lymph nodes not assessable
N0	No regional lymph node metastasis
N1, N2, N3	Increasing involvement of regional lymph nodes
Distant Metastasis (M)	
MX	Presence of distant metastasis not assessable
M0	No distant metastasis
M1	Distant metastasis

*The American Joint Committee on Cancer (AJCC) and the International Union Against Cancer (UICC) maintain the TNM classification as a tool for healthcare providers to stage different cancers.
(Data from American Cancer Society. https://www.cancer.org/treatment/understanding-your-diagnosis/staging.html. Accessed November 20, 2019

TABLE 5.10 Histopathologic Grade (G)

GX	Grade not assessable
G1	Well differentiated
G2	Moderately differentiated
G3	Poorly differentiated
G4	Undifferentiated

SUMMARY

- As stated earlier in this chapter, medicine is the accumulation of knowledge that has been developed through discovery, systematic scientific study, and research. These processes help to detect, diagnose, treat, and manage disease.
- According to the ACS, prevention and early detection are effective strategies of saving lives, diminishing suffering, and eliminating cancer as a major health problem.
- Vital signs are almost always taken during the physical examination and at intervals throughout the radiation therapy treatment process. They include temperature, pulse, respirations, blood pressure, and a pain assessment of the patient.
- Prevention includes measures that stop cancer from developing.

- Early detection includes examinations and tests intended to find the disease as early as possible. Screening examinations include mammography, Pap test, colonoscopy, and PSA blood test.
- The sentinel lymph node procedure focuses on finding lymph nodes that are the first to receive draining fluid from breast tumors and other tumors, therefore, the first to collect cancer cells.
- After a diagnosis of cancer is made and the extent of the disease has been determined, appropriate treatment can be initiated. The TNM staging system is applied to the disease process in an effort to direct treatment options that may use molecular biomarkers and predict outcomes from treatment, which may include guided precision therapy.

REVIEW QUESTIONS

The answers to the Review Questions can be found by logging on to our website at: http://evolve.elsevier.com/Washington/principles

1. Cancer screening can be effective if a disease has a high incidence or prevalence in a population and the test has the ability to produce results having the appropriate _____ and specificity.
   a. incidence
   b. sensitivity

   c. range
   d. cost factor

2. What are essential factors that must be observed when taking the pulse?
   I. Rate
   II. Rhythm
   III. Character

   a. I and II.
   b. I and III.
   c. II and III.
   d. I, II, and III.

3. Which of the following is not a screening procedure recommended by the American Cancer Society for the early detection of cancer?
   a. Mammography for breast cancer.
   b. Pap test.
   c. Prostate-specific antigen blood test.
   d. CT scanning for brain cancer.

4. Which of the following statements is false?
   a. Ultrasonography uses high-frequency sound waves.
   b. CT scans have a higher resolution than radiographs.
   c. MRI scans use ionizing radiation.
   d. Most invasive procedures provide some risk to the patient.

5. A drop in the white blood cells (WBCs) can be caused by irradiation of a significant amount of bone marrow, certain chemotherapy drugs, or both. What test would most likely detect a problem in the patient as a result in a drop in WBCs?
   a. Complete blood count.
   b. Pulse.
   c. Blood pressure.
   d. Respirations.

6. Exfoliative cytology is a means of collecting tissue through:
   a. Needle biopsy.
   b. Scraping cells.
   c. Incisional biopsy.
   d. Blood test.

7. Factors that help to facilitate the patient interview include all of the following *except:*
   a. Interviewer's ability to put the patient at ease.
   b. Asking clear and concise questions.
   c. Use of technical jargon.
   d. Use of terminology having the same meaning to the patient and interviewer.

8. Sensitivity, as it relates to screening examinations, is defined as:
   a. The ability of a test to give a true-positive result.
   b. The ability of the test to obtain a true-negative result.
   c. The number of new cases of a disease during a period of time.
   d. The effectiveness of the therapist in assisting the patient toward understanding the test results.

9. Mass screening is based on all of the following *except:*
   a. Specific results obtained.
   b. Cost effectiveness.
   c. Risk to the patient.
   d. Geographic location.

10. Using the TNM staging system, _____ describes the size and local extent of the primary tumor.
   a. T
   b. N
   c. M
   d. G

QUESTIONS TO PONDER

1. Why do you think that the detection and diagnosis of disease, especially cancer, have come to rely more and more on two specialties: radiology and pathology?
2. Discuss three clinical applications of obtaining vital signs specific to radiation therapy treatments.
3. What is a sentinel node biopsy procedure, and why is it performed?
4. Predict the benefits of mass screening for at least three specific types of cancer.
5. Describe, step by step, the process of obtaining a blood pressure by using the brachial artery.
6. Apply the general aspects of the TNM staging system in assisting with the treatment decision.
7. Compare the screening recommendations for the following cancer sites: breast, prostate, cervix, and colon.
8. Discuss at least three diagnostic imaging procedures used in the workup of a typical patient with breast cancer. Do the same for prostate cancer and for colon cancer.

REFERENCES

1. Noone AM, Howlader N, Krapcho M, et al, eds. SEER Cancer Statistics Review, 1975–2015. National Cancer Institute website. https://seer.cancer.gov/csr/1975_2015/, based on November 2017 SEER data submission, posted to the SEER website, April 12, 2018.
2. Cancer facts and figures 2018 supplemental data. American Cancer Society website. https://www.cancer.org/content/dam/cancer-org/research/cancer-facts-and-statistics/annual-cancer-facts-and-figures/2018/cancer-facts-and-figures-2018.pdf. Accessed July 16, 2018.
3. Fast Stats: an interactive tool for access to SEER cancer statistics. Surveillance research program. National Cancer Institute website. https://seer.cancer.gov/faststats/index.html. Accessed April 20, 2018.
4. LeBlond RF, Brown DD, Suneja M, Szot JF. *DeGowin's Diagnostic Examination.* 10th ed. New York, NY: McGraw-Hill, 2019.
5. American Cancer Society. *Cancer Facts and Figures.* Atlanta, GA: American Cancer Society, 2018.
6. Sapir R, Catane R, Kaufman B, et al. Cancer patient expectations of and communication with oncologist and oncology nurses: the experience of an integrated oncology and palliative care service. *Support Care Cancer.* 2000;8:458–463.
7. Baile WF, Buchman R, Lenzi R, et al. SPIKES—a six step protocol for delivering bad news: application to the patient with cancer. *Oncologist.* 2000;5:302–311.
8. Fujimori M, Uchitomi Y. Preferences of cancer patients regarding communication of bad news: a systematic literature review. *Jpn J Clin Oncol.* 2009;39(4):201–216.
9. Brom L, Pasman HRW, Widdershoven GAM, et al. Patient preferences for participation in treatment decision-making at the end-of-life: qualitative interviews with advanced cancer patients. *PLoS One.* 2014;9(6):1–15.
10. Slow repeal of the ACA and its effect on technology. HuschBlackwell Website. https://www.healthcarelawinsights.com/2017/02/slow-repeal-of-the-aca-and-its-effect-on-healthcare-technology/.
11. Halperin E, Wazer DE. *Perez and Brady's Principles and Practice of Radiation Oncology.* 7th ed. Philadelphia, PA: Wolters Kluwer.
12. Genetic testing for hereditary cancer syndrome. National Cancer Institute website. https://www.cancer.gov/about-cancer/causes-prevention/genetics/genetic-testing-fact-sheet. Accessed April 16, 2018.
13. Anderson K. 10 steps to accurate manual blood pressure measurement. Suntech medical website. http://blog.suntechmed.com/blog/32-bp-measurement/220-10-steps-to-accurate-manual-blood-pressure-measurement. Accessed July 12, 2018.
14. Waterstram-Rich KM. *Nuclear Medicine and PET/CT: Technology and Technique.* St. Louis, MO: Elsevier, 2016.
15. Marks RM, Sachar EJ. Undertreatment of medical inpatients with narcotic analgesics. *Ann Intern Med.* 1973;78:173–181.

16. Pain: current understanding of assessment, management and treatments. National Pharmaceutical Council website. www.npcnow.org/publication/pain-current-understanding-assessment-management-and-treatments. Accessed June 1, 2018.

17. Bahl A, Oudard S, Tombal B, et al. Impact of cabazitaxel on 2-year survival and palliation of tumour-related pain in men with metastatic castration-resistant prostate cancer treated in the TROPIC trial. *Ann Oncol.* 2013;24(9):2402–2408.

18. Smith RA, Andrews K, Brooks D, et al. Cancer Screening in the United States, 2017: a review of current American Cancer Society guidelines and current issues in cancer screening. *CA Cancer J Clin.* 2017;67(2):100–121.

19. American Cancer Society. *Cancer Prevention and Early Detection Facts and Figures.* Atlanta, GA: American Cancer Society.

20. Cancer survival statistics-surveillance research program. National Cancer Institute website. https://surveillance.cancer.gov/statistics/typs/survival.html. Accessed April 20, 2018.

21. Oeffinger KC, Fontham ETH, Etzioni RE, et al. Breast cancer screening for women at average Risk, 2015 guideline update from the American Cancer Society. *J Am Med Assoc.* 2015;314(15):1599–1614.

22. Berry DA, Cronin KA, Plevritis SK, et al. Cancer intervention and surveillance modeling network (CISNET) collaborators. Effect of screening and adjunct therapy on mortality from breast cancer. *N Engl J Med.* 2005;353(17):1784–1792.

23. Boiselle PM. Computed tomography screening for lung cancer. *J Am Med Assoc.* 2013;309(11):1163–1170.

24. Gøtzsche PC, Jørgensen KJ. Screening for breast cancer with mammography. *Cochrane Database Syst Rev.* 2013;6:CD001877.

25. National Lung Screening Trial Research Team. The National Lung Screening Trial: overview and study design. National Cancer Institute website. https://www.cancer.gov/types/lung/research/nlst. Accessed July 3, 2018.

26. Lewis SM, Dirksen SR, Heitkemper MM, et al. *Medical-Surgical Nursing: Assessment and Management of Clinical Problems.* 8th ed. St. Louis, MO: Mosby.

27. American Joint Commission on Cancer. *AJCC Cancer Staging Manual.* 9th ed. New York, NY: American Joint Commission on Cancer, 2014.

28. Broeders M, Moss S, Nyström L, et al. EUROSCREEN working group. The impact of mammographic screening on breast cancer mortality in Europe: a review of observational studies. *J Med Screen.* 2012;19(suppl 1):14–25.

29. Smith RA, Cokkinides V, Brawley OW. Cancer screening in the United States, 2012: view of current American cancer society guidelines and current issues in cancer screening. *CA Cancer J Clin.* 2012;62(2):129–142.

6

Medical Imaging

Ronnie G. Lozano

OBJECTIVES

- List and describe the components and the operation of a radiographic imaging system and computed tomography imaging system.
- Describe the components of a typical x-ray tube and how x-rays are produced.
- Compare and contrast x-ray interactions in the diagnostic range with matter.
- Describe factors that impact image details and image distortion.
- Solve problems associated with magnification.
- Compare various imaging techniques, including conventional films, photostimulable plates, and flat-panel detectors.
- Compare and contrast the use of megavoltage and kilovoltage onboard imaging applications.

- Explain the basic principles of image formation for each of the following modalities: computed tomography, cone-beam computed tomography, magnetic resonance imaging, ultrasound, and nuclear medicine.
- Describe the concept of image-guided radiation therapy and its application.
- Discuss the impact of spiral pitch ratio upon the ALARA principle.
- Describe the evolution of slip ring technology and its impact upon computed tomography technology.
- Discuss the emerging trends and innovations in imaging technology for radiation therapy

OUTLINE

KEY TERMS

ALARA
Anode
Aperture size
Artifact
Attenuation
Backscatter
Bremsstrahlung
Cathode
Classical scatter
Characteristic radiation
Coherent scatter
Compton scattering
Cone-beam computed tomography
Contrast
Computed radiography
Density
Detectors
Detector array
Differential absorption
Filament
Film/image density
Flat-panel detectors
Fluorine-18 fluorodeoxyglucose (FDG)
Functional and molecular magnetic resonance imaging

Gadolinium
Image contrast
Image fusion
Interfraction uncertainties
Inverse square law
Ionization
Onboard imaging
Magnetic resonance imaging
Magnetic resonance imaging safety zones
Noise
Nuclear medicine imaging
Photoelectric effect
Pixels
Positron emission tomography
Positron emission tomography-computed tomography
Resolution
Scatter
Slip ring technology
Spatial resolution
Spiral pitch ratio
Ultrasound
Voxels
Window level

INTRODUCTION

Medical imaging plays a critical role in the diagnosis and treatment of cancer patients. X-rays used in this process penetrate the body to create a useful image. This information helps members of the cancer management team achieve an important goal in radiation oncology: to maximize the radiation dose to cancer cells and minimize the dose to the surrounding normal tissue.

Medical imaging has improved as a result of advances in digital imaging technology and computerization. Advances in microprocessor speeds and computer memory that handle large amounts of data have had a great impact on diagnostic medical procedures and radiation therapy imaging.

Medical imaging modalities such as computed tomography (CT), magnetic resonance imaging (MRI), positron emission tomography (PET), and ultrasound use a variety of digital imaging concepts. Radiation therapy imaging has also become more robust to produce higher-quality images that integrate or fuse the different modalities. Advancements in medical imaging have revolutionized how we simulate and plan radiation therapy treatments. The imaging technologies have provided valuable information that is often incorporated into the simulation planning process by a complex process of image fusion. This multidisciplinary approach has allowed for more accurate treatment simulation, treatment planning, and treatment delivery. Please refer to the CT Simulation chapter for detailed information on CT simulation (Chapter 21).

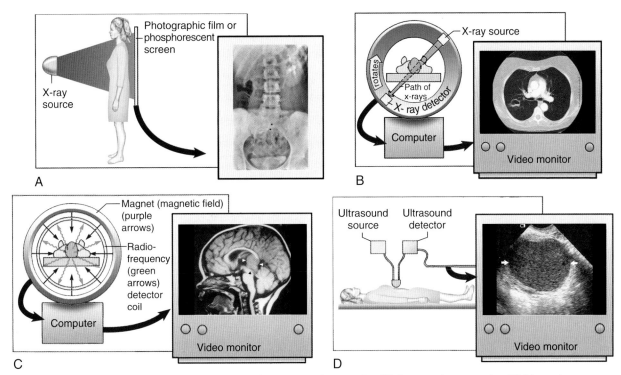

Types of medical imaging. (A) Radiography, or x-ray photography. (B) Computed tomography. (C) Magnetic resonance imaging. (D) Ultrasonography. (From Patton KT, Thibodeau GA. *The Human Body in Health and Disease.* 7th ed. St. Louis, MO: Elsevier; 2018,. Imaging scans from Eisenberg RL, Johnson NM. *Comprehensive Radiographic Anatomy.* 4th ed. St. Louis, MO: Mosby; 2007.)

CT technology continues to evolve with other new imaging technologies that combine modalities, such as CT/PET for enhanced imaging. In this chapter, several concepts are introduced, including the history of x-rays, their production, the design of the tube from which they are produced, their interaction with matter, the art of creating high-quality medical images (both conventional and digital), and the basic principles of image formation for CT, MRI, ultrasound, and nuclear medicine.

HISTORIC OVERVIEW

The roentgen (R) is the conventional unit of measurement for x-ray and gamma rays, replaced today by the standard international unit air kerma (Gy_a). The conventional unit reflects the name of the German mechanical engineer and physicist, Wilhelm Conrad Rontgen, who discovered x-rays in 1895. Medical imaging conventional units for ionizing radiation were initially designated as the Roentgen for exposure in air, the Rad for absorbed dose in tissue, and the Rem for occupational dose. All historical conventional units have standard international unit equivalents that now correspond to the international metric system. These are the air kerma, the grey, and the sievert. Additional detailed information may be found in the chapters on Photon Dose Distribution (Chapter 23) and Photon Dosimetry Concepts and Calculations (Chapter 22).

The essential elements of x-ray production have not changed; however, x-rays have changed regarding their application in medicine. Modern x-ray tubes (Fig. 6.1) still require a source of electrons (the cathode), a current capable of liberating them from their tungsten filament home, a target toward which they can be directed (the anode), and the extremely high voltage necessary to persuade this reluctant electron cloud to flow at the velocity required to produce x-rays.

Digital imaging has nearly replaced conventional methods of obtaining a medical image. X-rays have a variety of diagnostic and therapeutic purposes, and because of that, many modalities such as diagnostic radiology, nuclear medicine, mammography, cardiovascular imaging, and CT scanning exist to aid the physician in the precise diagnosis of disease and treatment planning. In addition, MRI and ultrasound, which produce images without x-rays, contribute greatly as well.

MEDICAL IMAGING TECHNOLOGY OVERVIEW

The X-Ray Tube

The production of x-rays requires a source of accelerated electrons, an appropriate target material, a high voltage, and a vacuum in a closed system. The production of x-rays occurs inside the tube because of high-speed electrons colliding with a metal object called the *anode*. The components of the tube, the cathode and anode, are enclosed in a glass envelope and protective housing (Fig 6.1 and 6.2). These are described as follows.[1-6]

The Cathode

The cathode is one of the electrodes found in the x-ray tube and represents the negative side of the tube. It consists of two parts: the filament and focusing cup. As a first step in x-ray production, the primary function of the cathode is to produce electrons and focus the electron stream toward the metal anode.

The Filament

The filament is a small coil of wire made of tungsten, which has an extremely high melting point (3380°C). The coil of wire is a smaller version of that found inside of a light bulb or toaster. A current, which heats the filament, is passed through the small coil of wire where electrons boil off and are emitted from the filament.

Most modern x-ray tubes have dual filaments, thus permitting the selection of a large or small source of electrons. The length and width of the filament control the ability of the x-ray tube to produce fine imaging detail. Most modern x-ray machines are equipped with a rotating

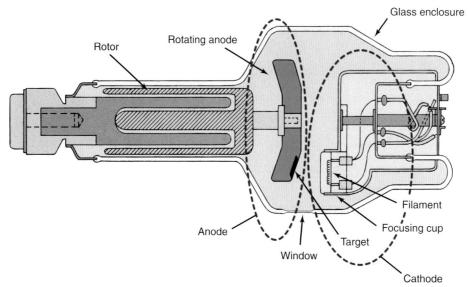

Fig. 6.1 Diagram of a rotating-anode x-ray tube illustrating the fundamental parts. (From Bushong S. *Radiologic Science for Technologists: Physics, Biology, and Protection.* 10th ed. St. Louis, MO: Mosby; 2013.)

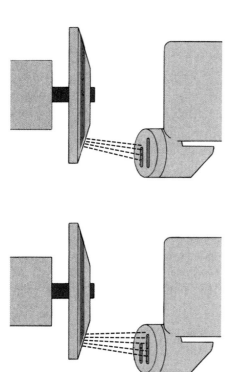

Fig. 6.2 In a dual-focus x-ray tube, focal spot size is controlled by heating one of the two filaments. (From Bushong S. *Radiologic Science for Technologists: Physics, Biology, and Protection.* 11th ed. St. Louis, MO: Mosby; 2017.)

anode tube having 0.6-mm (small) and 1.0-mm (large) focal spots. Other x-ray machines with focal spots as small as 0.1 mm and as large as 2.0 mm are also commercially available.

The Focusing Cup. The selection of a small or large focal spot is associated with the small and large filaments, which are embedded in a small oval depression in the cathode assembly called a focusing cup. The negative charge of the focusing cup helps direct electrons toward the anode in a straighter, less divergent path.

The Anode

The anode is the positive side of the x-ray tube. It receives electrons from the cathode as a target, dissipates the great amount of heat as a result of x-ray production, and serves as the path for the flow of high voltage. Aspects of anode assembly include the composition of the anode, the target, and the line focus principle. The anode is a circular disk composed of many different metals, each designed to contribute to the effectiveness of x-ray production (Fig. 6.3). The rotating tungsten disk serves as the target and can range as large as 13 cm in diameter. Rhenium-alloyed tungsten serves as the target focal track material because of its ability as a thermal conductor and the source of x-ray photons. The rotor, which allows most anodes to reach 3400 rpm, is an excellent device to help dispel the great amounts of heat created.

The Target. Electrons from the cathode strike the portion of the anode called the *target*. Within the target is the actual area where interaction occurs to produce x-rays, the focal spot. This is the point at which x-ray photons are produced and begin to fan out in a divergent path. There are small and large focal spots that may be programmed to correspond with low kVp/mAs and high kVP/mAs applications. The small focal spot provides more detail; however, more heat is created by bombarding a smaller area of the target. To overcome the disadvantage of creating more heat and still maintain image detail, the target is angled as shown in Fig. 6.4. In this way, a larger geometric area can be heated while a small focal spot is maintained. Fig. 6.4 displays the line focus principle. The actual focal spot size of the target is larger than the effective focal spot size. Most x-ray tubes have a target angle from 7 to 20 degrees.[1–6]

The Glass Envelope

The cathode and anode are in a vacuum in the x-ray tube. The removal of air from the glass envelope or x-ray tube permits the uninterrupted flow of electrons from the cathode to the anode. The efficiency of the tube is increased because no air molecules are floating around inside the x-ray tube to collide with the accelerated electrons. The tube may measure from 20 to 30 cm in length and be as large as 15 cm in diameter at the central portion. Some x-ray tubes today are made of metal, reducing the buildup of tungsten deposits on the glass envelope, which is a result of numerous target interactions during the life of the x-ray

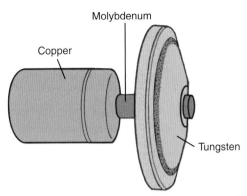

Fig. 6.3 The tungsten anode of a dual focus x-ray tube. The actual source of x-ray is the surface area hit by the accelerated electrons shown in blue. (From Bushong S. *Radiologic Science for Technologists: Physics, Biology, and Protection*. 11th ed. St. Louis, MO: Mosby; 2017.)

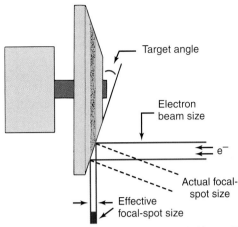

Fig. 6.4 By angling the target of the rotating anode (thus taking advantage of the line focus principle), a larger geometric area can be heated while a small focal spot is maintained. (From Bushong S. *Radiologic Science for Technologists: Physics, Biology, and Protection*. 11th ed. St. Louis, MO: Mosby; 2017.)

tube. Tungsten deposits on the inside of the glass envelope can reduce tube life and cause arcing.

The Protective Housing

To control unwanted radiation leakage and electrical shock, the x-ray tube is mounted inside the protective housing. Lead lining in the protective housing helps prevent radiation leakage during an exposure. A special oil fills the space between the protective housing and glass envelope to insulate the high-voltage potential and provide additional cooling capacity.

X-RAY PRODUCTION

X-rays are one of the many forms of electromagnetic energy organized according to wavelength on the electromagnetic spectrum (Fig. 6.5). X-rays share wave characteristics with radio waves and microwaves, visible light, cosmic radiation, and a host of other energy forms. However, all these radiant energies share certain properties. They all travel at the speed of light (3×10^{10} cm per second); they all take the form of a wave expressed as wavelength (the distance between the crests in the wave) and frequency (the number of complete wave cycles per second).

X-ray radiations and gamma radiations are located at the high end of the spectrum and possess extremely short wavelengths (see Fig. 6.5). The relationship between wavelength and frequency is an inverse proportion (i.e., as wavelength decreases, frequency increases). In 1900, the German physicist Max Planck showed through his quantum theory that frequency and energy are directly proportional. Despite their constant velocities, different forms of electromagnetic radiation may have widely varying energies from the low end of the spectrum, where radio waves exist, to the high end, where x-ray radiations, gamma radiations, and cosmic radiations are found. While the wavelength decreases and frequency increases, so does the associated quantum energy.

Thermionic Emission

X-ray production is a result of a stream of electrons liberated from the cathode and accelerated across the tube at high speeds to collide with the anode. These cathode electrons are emitted from the tungsten filament atoms in a process called *thermionic emission,* which refers to heat and the release of ions.

Thermionic emission begins when the filament circuit is energized causing it to heat up. The process of liberating electrons from the filament wire is a result of heat. An electrical current (mA) is applied to the filament, which begins to glow, much like a toaster or an electric oven. While the current or the flow of electrons increases, the filament

reaches the hot state necessary for outer-shell electrons to leave their orbits, resulting in electrons called *thermions*.

Potential Difference

The electron cloud produced from thermionic emission hovers by the cathode (filament side of tube) indefinitely, unless something is done to encourage it to move. Applied voltage creates a potential difference between the negative cathode (filament) and positive anode (target). This causes the negatively charged electrons to be strongly repelled from the negatively charged cathode side of the tube and drawn at extreme speeds by the attracting force of the positively charged anode side. In modern three-phase radiographic equipment, the velocity of this electron stream can approach the speed of light.

Target Interactions: Characteristic and Bremsstrahlung Radiation

The interactions described here occur within an x-ray tube. Care should be taken not to confuse these with the interactions occurring outside the x-ray tube within the body, referred to as interactions with matter. The principal interaction in x-ray production results in the output of bremsstrahlung (German for "braking") radiation (Fig. 6.6). Bremsstrahlung accounts for approximately 75% to 80% of the tube's output and is produced by the sudden deceleration of the high-speed electron while it is deflected around the nucleus of the tungsten atom. Within the target atoms of the anode, the kinetic energy of the decelerating electron is given off as a bundle of pure energy, or an x-ray photon.

A second, lesser interaction also contributes to the production of x-rays. Characteristic radiation is created by the direct interaction of cathode electrons with inner-shell electrons of the target material. Although bremsstrahlung interaction is dependent on "braking" electrons, characteristic x-ray is dependent on "breaking" the bonds holding the electrons within the inner orbital shell. The photon produced is a direct conversion from binding energy to a photon of energy when the bonds are "broken."

Some electrons may collide with tungsten orbital electrons that have sufficient energy to overcome their binding energy and eject them from orbit. This process is called *ionization* (Fig. 6.7). When an inner-shell electron is ejected from orbit, leaving a void, an outer shell electron moves in to fill the orbital void. The energy of x-rays produced in this manner is dependent on the binding energy of the target atom's electrons.

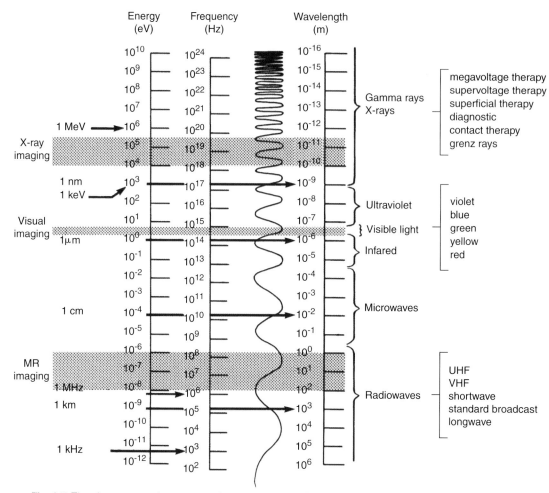

Fig. 6.5 The electromagnetic spectrum demonstrates specific values of energy, frequency, and wavelength for some regions of the spectrum. *keV,* Kiloelectron volt; *kHz,* kilohertz; *MeV,* million electron volts; *MHz,* megahertz; *MR,* magnetic resonance; *nm,* nanometer; *UHF,* ultrahigh frequency; *VHF,* very high frequency.

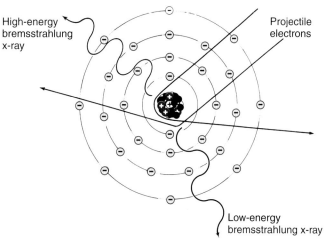

Fig. 6.6 The bremsstrahlung interaction. (From Bushong S. *Radiologic Science for Technologists: Physics, Biology, and Protection.* 10th ed. St. Louis, MO: Mosby; 2013.)

While the atomic number of an element increases, so does the energy level of each shell. This is the rationale for the use of materials of high atomic number (such as tungsten) in the targets of x-ray tubes. Binding energy drops with each successive electron orbit away from the nucleus. Outer-shell, or valence, electrons have an extremely low binding energy

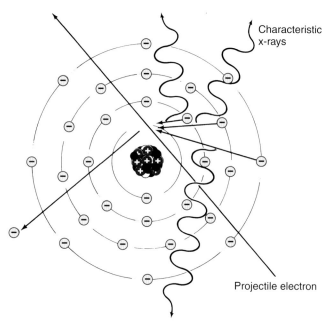

Fig. 6.7 The characteristic interaction. (From Bushong S. *Radiologic Science for Technologists: Physics, Biology, and Protection.* 10th ed. St. Louis, MO: Mosby; 2013.)

and are easily ejected from orbit. Therefore ionization events in the O or P shell of the tungsten atom do not produce characteristic x-ray photons of sufficient energy to be useful. Tungsten K-shell electrons, however, have a binding energy of 69.5 kiloelectron volts (keV). When a K-shell electron is ejected from orbit and replaced with a tungsten L-shell electron, a surplus energy of 57.4 keV is released in the form of a characteristic x-ray photon. Energies of this magnitude are well within the useful range for diagnostic x-rays.[1-6]

Fundamental Physics of X-Ray Production

Albert Einstein's principle of conservation involved the theoretical relationship between the kinetic energy of moving matter and the production of light quanta (photons). In his historic theory of relativity, Einstein demonstrated that matter accelerated to a sufficient velocity can become pure energy.

This principle applies to the production of the x-ray. The velocity (and kinetic energy) of the cathode electron racing towards the target is determined by the potential difference created by the energy applied to the tube in volts. Increasing voltage (kVp control) across the tube increases the net positive and net negative polarity of the tube; the increased potential difference across the tube results in higher photon energy. As the applied tube voltage increases, so does the kinetic energy of the racing electron available for conversion into x-ray photons. High-energy photons pass through matter more readily than low-energy photons. The ability of the photon to pass through matter such as human body tissues is called *penetration*. A radiation beam of high-energy photons penetrates structures with greater ease than a low-energy photon beam.

This resulting photon beam energy may be described in terms of beam quality. A beam of radiation produced using high kVp may be described as a high-quality beam (i.e., it contains a large percentage of highly penetrating, extremely energetic photons). However, quality addresses only a portion of the x-ray beam characteristics. The number of photons in the beam may describe the photon beam characteristics in terms of beam quantity.

Thermionic emission is defined as the "boiling off" of electrons from the filament as the filament is heated, and when an electrical current (milliampere, or mA) is applied to the filament, which begins to glow hot, much like a toaster or a hair dryer. It is reasonable that as the current to the filament increases, the number of electrons boiling off increases. Disregarding target attenuation factors, in the most general terms, each electron racing towards the target with higher kinetic energy may produce one photon. The relationship between the number of cathode electrons released during thermionic emission and the production of x-ray photons is proportional. As the electrical current applied specifically to the filament (mAs control) is increased, a predictable increase in the number of electrons released occurs. The relationship between filament current (expressed in milliampere second, or mAs) and the quantity of electrons liberated is a direct proportion. The relationship has no bearing on beam energy or penetrating ability but describes the beam's characteristics in terms of beam quantity.[1-6]

X-RAY INTERACTIONS WITH (BODY) MATTER

Overview

The language used to describe x-ray interactions within the body and within the x-ray tube may be confusing to the student. For example, the term "target atom" is used frequently to describe interactions in the body. It does not refer to the target of the x-ray tube. It refers to the intended destination of the x-ray delivered to the body part—outside the x-ray tube. Characteristic and bremsstrahlung radiation refer to

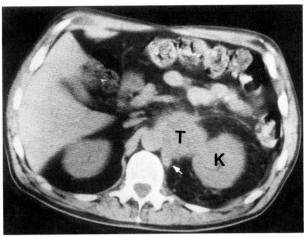

Fig. 6.8 A transverse computed tomography image demonstrates an adrenal carcinoma. Large soft tissue tumor *(T and arrow)* invades the medial aspect of the left kidney *(K)*. (From Eisenberg RL, Johnson NM. *Comprehensive Radiographic Anatomy*. 4th ed. St. Louis, MO: Mosby; 2007.)

interactions occurring inside an x-ray tube. These involve an accelerated electron racing towards the target inside the x-ray tube to produce x-rays.

While an x-ray beam passes through matter, the beam undergoes a gradual reduction in the number of photons or exposure rate. This process is termed *absorption* or, more correctly, attenuation. Photons in the original or primary beam may also be scattered (i.e., they may change direction as they collide with atoms in their path). In the human body, the rate of beam attenuation and degree of scattering is determined by tissue thickness, density, and atomic number. The net effect is a wide variation in the quantity of photons reaching the film, image receptor, or CT detector.

The human body consists of varying quantities of air, fat, water, muscle, and bone, each with its own absorption properties or absorption coefficient. A CT scan of the abdomen (Fig. 6.8) provides an ideal demonstration of these differential absorption characteristics. Denser structures and those of higher-than-average atomic numbers appear as lighter areas on the image because of their higher rates of attenuation. Air, as a result of its extremely low density and fat and of its relatively low atomic number, appears as dark areas, whereas bone, which is dense and has a high atomic number (Z), appears as a light shadow. These differential absorption characteristics of anatomy is the basis of radiographic imaging.[7]

As we discuss the interactions with matter in this section, it will be helpful to remember that as energy increases, penetration increases. At lower energies, the emitted x-ray will interact with the whole atom—classical scatter, unmodified scatter, also known as coherent scatter, Rayleigh, and Thompson scattering. Moderate energy x-ray tends to interact with the orbital electrons within the atom—Compton scatter or Compton effect and photoelectric effect; and high-energy x-rays penetrate through the electron orbital shells interact deep in the nucleus—pair production and photodisintegration. As energy increases, the interaction with the atom goes from superficial to deep within the nucleus. It is also helpful to remember that three interactions exist within what is referred to as the "diagnostic range," that is, the energy level from 40-kVp to 150-kVp machine settings. These are the low to moderate energy level interactions, classical scatter, Compton effect, and photoelectric effect. Two interactions exist in the high-energy levels, (MeV energy level). These are pair production and photodisintegration.[1-6]

Interaction at Low Energies (<10 keV): Classical Scatter

General Description: Also known as unmodified scatter, Coherent scatter, Rayleigh, and Thompson scattering, this interaction primarily involves low-energy x-ray less than 10 keV. The interaction is described as follows. See Fig. 6.9.

Interaction Process: The incident x-ray interacts with the atom, causing excitation. That means that the electrons are "excited" and vibrate at the photon frequency, but there are no electrons ejected, and there is no ionization. There is no "net" transfer of energy. The result is simply the change in the direction of the x-ray trajectory with no change in its energy level. The interaction is at such a low energy level that the x-ray that penetrates the human body typically does not exit the body.[1–6]

Interaction at Moderate Energy Levels (80 to120 keV): Compton Scatter and Photoelectric Effect

Compton Scatter. General Description: Compton scatter occurs within moderate energy levels; however, it exists throughout the diagnostic energy range machine settings (40 to 150 kVp). It is the predominant interaction within the moderate energy levels. At these energy levels, the incident x-ray penetrates the atom and interacts with an outer-shell electron. The net result is ionization of the atom with a change in the exiting photon's direction, with less energy than the incident photon. Most of the energy is divided between the electron hit by the incident photon and the resulting scattered photon. However, the scattered x-ray photon usually retains most of its energy after the first interaction and may undergo additional ionization interactions with other atoms. This scattered photon emits its energy with every ionization eventually being absorbed, or at higher initial energy settings, it may retain its energy and exit the body. The electron is ejected and referred to as the "Compton electron" or "recoil electron." This ejected electron has sufficient energy to attach itself to another atom. See Fig. 6.10.

Although specific steps are taken by staff to reduce exposure in radiology, the following generalizations should be considered regarding Compton scatter. In the radiology department, Compton scatter poses the most serious exposure hazard during fluoroscopy procedures. Especially with procedures such as cardiac catherization, large amounts of radiation scatter are emitted from the patient to the radiology staff

standing near. In terms of image quality, it is responsible for the deterioration of image resolution, producing "fog" on the image. As a general rule, a scattered photon may be referred to as a "contaminated" photon in terms of imaging because it is a result of striking not one but several anatomical structures before it reaches the image detector. This means that the information it transfers is not that of a pure image and does not represent any one anatomical structure clearly. If the scattered photon reaches the CT detectors or image receptor, it strikes it at random. It produces unwanted "optical" density as a result of the multiple collisions within the body during the photon's trajectory.

Interaction Process: The incident x-ray photon approaches the atom with considerable energy. The photon penetrates the atom colliding with an outer shell. The outer-shell electrons exist farthest from the nucleus and therefore has the least binding energy as compared with the inner-shell electrons. They are referred to as "loosely bound" electrons. The collision results in a transfer of energy from the photon to the electron. The result is the breaking of the bonds holding the electron to the orbital shell. Because outer-shell bonds are weak bonds, the binding energy has a negligible role. The electron now has sufficient energy to be ejected from the atom, causing ionization. The photon is simply deflected from its original path and exits the atom with less energy. The principle focus is a scatter photon.[1–6]

Photoelectric Effect

General Description: The best way to remember the results of the photoelectric effect is "total absorption." It is said that differential absorption, or "differences in absorption," is the basis of radiographic imaging. Image receptors or detectors react to exposure by producing a darker shade that represents the anatomy as levels of exposure to the receptor or detector increase. It should be noted that the photoelectric effect is very dependent on the atomic number (Z) of an atom. The more protons in the nucleus of an atom, the more probable an incident photon will be absorbed through the photoelectric effect. See Fig. 6.11.

Although less dense tissue like lung tissue tends to allow x-rays to penetrate and be transmitted, dense tissue like bone tends to reduce the amount of x-ray transmitted through absorption (high Z number). The resulting image for lung is a dark shade, whereas the image for bone is a much lighter shade.

Interaction Process: The incident x-ray photon approaches the atom with considerable energy. The photon penetrates the atom, colliding with an inner-shell or K-shell electron. The electron is ejected from the atom. The electron is referred to as a "photoelectron." The incident photon disappears and is considered to be absorbed. The

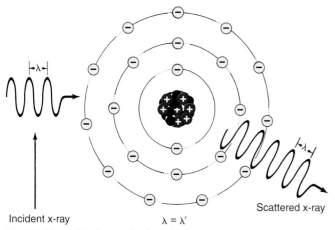

Fig. 6.9 Unmodified scattering is an interaction between extremely low energy (generally <10 kiloelectron volts) and is of little importance in radiation therapy. (From Bushong S. *Radiologic Science for Technologists: Physics, Biology, and Protection.* 10th ed. St. Louis, MO: Mosby; 2013.)

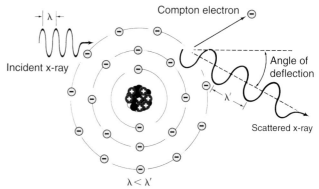

Fig. 6.10 The Compton effect is produced when an x-ray photon interacts with an outer-shell orbital electron. The photon must possess sufficient energy to eject it from orbit and alter its own path. (From Bushong S. *Radiologic Science for Technologists: Physics, Biology, and Protection.* 10th ed. St. Louis, MO: Mosby; 2013.)

principle focus of the photoelectric effect is the absorption of the incident x-ray. The human body is composed primarily of carbon, hydrogen, and oxygen atoms, and none of these materials has sufficiently high k-shell energies to produce secondary photons of any magnitude. For this reason, most photoelectric interactions in tissue result simply in absorption with no appreciable secondary effect. This is desirable because to clearly define anatomic structures of differing densities and atomic number on an image, their relative variation in absorption rates, however slight, must be used to the fullest imaging advantage.

Normal human anatomy provides a predictable variation in tissue densities. For example, kidneys can be seen in a radiograph of the abdomen, not because of their density difference compared with the greater surrounding tissue, but because they are outlined by a thin band of fat called the *adipose capsule*. Fat has a higher density than soft tissue, so it absorbs more x-ray photons creating a variation in tissue density (a lighter shade on the image). Contrast materials, such as iodine, barium, and other agents of high atomic number, may be used to enhance the visibility of structures with similar composition that would otherwise remain unseen.

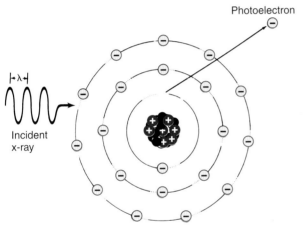

Fig. 6.11 The photoelectric effect, sometimes described as true absorption, occurs when the incident photon penetrates deep into the atom and ejects an inner-shell electron from orbit. (From Bushong S. *Radiologic Science for Technologists: Physics, Biology, and Protection.* 10th ed. St. Louis, MO: Mosby; 2013.)

> Attenuation of the radiation beam is the reduction of the number of photons remaining in the beam after passing through a given thickness of material. The amount of attenuation is the result of the thickness of the absorber (for example, the patient's body) and type of material irradiated (fat, bone, soft tissue, or air).

TECHNICAL FACTORS AND IMAGE CHARACTERISTICS

The function of kVp and mAs machine settings in medical imaging involves factors that impact the quality and quantity of the x-ray produced. This then relates to characteristics and accuracy of the radiographic image representing the anatomy in terms of image contrast and image density.

Image Density

Image density is defined as the degree of darkening on the image. This is not to be confused with tissue density, which refers to the compactness of molecules in the atomic structure of different body parts. Image density is a relatively simple concept to grasp because it is easy to visualize. An image of high density is dark, and an image of low density is light. The rules governing density are equally straightforward. When more photons reach the image receptor, density increases; when fewer photons reach the image receptor, density decreases (Figs. 6.12 and 6.13).

There is a clear and predictable role that mAs have in image density. When all other factors remain the same, the relationship between mAs and density is a direct proportion (i.e., as mAs are doubled, so is the resulting density on the image). In addition, kVp may be used to change image density. A far smaller increase in kVp is needed to significantly affect the image receptor than is required by using mAs. When all other factors remain the same, a kVp increase of only 15% doubles the image density. This may be referred to the 15% rule for kVp.[1-6]

Distance

Another major extrinsic factor influencing density is distance, which refers to the gap between the focal spot (target) of the x-ray tube and the recording medium. The terminology used to describe this gap varies with the equipment in use and its application. Target-to-image receptor distance (TID), focal film distance, and source-to-image receptor distance refer to the same idea.

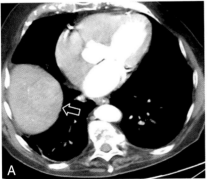
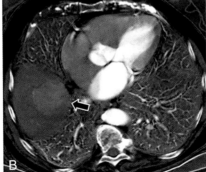
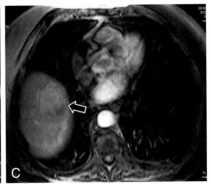

Fig. 6.12 An 87-year-old male patient with a liver lesion in the dome of the liver. (A) Mono-energetic computed tomography (CT) image (scaled at 65 keV). (B) Quantitative material density image. (C) Corresponding magnetic resonance (MR) image. In this case, the lesion was large, but still very difficult to detect in the mono-energetic image (A), mainly because of the localization next to the dome of the liver and the very small HU difference to the surrounding liver tissue, respectively. It is more clearly differentiated in the material density iodine image (C). (From Muenzel D, Lo GC, Parakh A, et al. *Eur J Radiol.* 2017;95:300–306.)

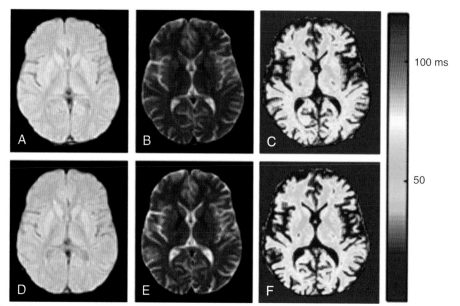

Fig. 6.13 Magnetic resonance imaging. Images (A) and (D) illustrate significantly lighter density than images (B) and (E). Images (C) and (F) illustrate T2 weighting from proton density images with a T2 intensity contrast scale. (From Uddin N, McPhee KC, Blevins G, et al. Recovery of accurate T_2 from historical 1.5 tesla proton density and T_2-weighted images: Application to 7-year T_2 changes in multiple sclerosis brain. *Magnetic Resonance Imaging.* 2017;37:21–26.)

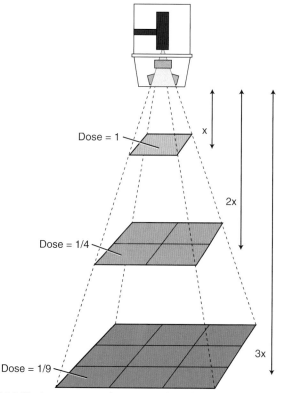

Fig. 6.14 The inverse square law means that while distance is doubled, a quantity of radiation is spread over an area four times as great, thereby reducing the intensity of the beam in any area to one-fourth its original value.

Distance can have a profound effect on image density (Fig. 6.14). The relationship between distance and density follows the inverse square law, which states that the intensity of the beam of radiation is inversely proportional to the square of the distance. Put more simply, when distance is doubled, the quantity of radiation reaching the

image receptor (or occupationally exposed personnel) is reduced to one-fourth. The inverse square law works because of the property of x-rays stating that they travel in straight lines and diverge from a point of origin. As distance is doubled, a quantity of radiation is spread over an area four times as great, thereby reducing the intensity of the beam in an area to one-fourth of its original value.

Image Contrast

Image contrast is the element of imaging that provides visual evidence of differential absorption rates of various body tissues. Image contrast has been described as the tonal range of densities from black to white or the number of shades of gray in the image. Fig. 6.15 illustrates the difference between high and low contrast. Image contrast may also be referred to as the "scale of contrast." One may describe an image with high contrast as having a short scale of contrast. The short scale quickly goes from white to black with very few number of shades or tonal ranges in between, simply white to black offering very little image information. One may describe an image with low contrast has having a long scale of contrast; see Fig. 6.16. The long scale quickly has a longer number of shades or tonal ranges between white and total blackness. A long scale of contrast or an image with lower contrast may offer more detailed information such as fine hairline cracks, surface texture within the subject, or perhaps a small lung nodule that is represented by a medium shade of gray.

Optimal contrast results when technical factors (primarily kVp) are selected that maximize the rate of differential absorption between body parts of varying tissue density and effective atomic number. Optimal kVp ranges exist for all body parts. The most important factor in determining optimal kVp is subject thickness, but numerous other factors, such as scatter radiation and field size, may also influence the selection.

Physical Factors of Imaging. Many components should be considered, such as geometric factors, control of unwanted scatter radiation, and problems associated with contrast and density of the image. An understanding of the many factors affecting the production of good-quality simulation and portal images is essential.

Asym. SE, B_{SL}= 0   Asym. SE, B_{SL}= 7.1 µT

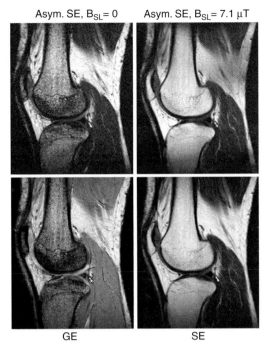

GE   SE

Fig. 6.15 Magnetic resonance imaging (MRI). An MRI of the knee and related anatomy structures demonstrates different image contrast. Image contrast is described as the tonal range of densities from black to white or the number of shades of gray in an image. (From Martirosian P, Rommel E, Schick F, Deimling M. Control of susceptibility-related image contrast by spin-lock techniques. *Magnetic Resonance Imaging*. 2008;26(10): 1381–1387.)

Geometric Factors

This principle of divergence, in which photons move in straight but different directions from a common point (focal spot), contributes greatly to the magnification and distortion seen on CT simulation images and portal images. Two geometric factors are important in radiation oncology: magnification and distortion.

Magnification. All images on a CT simulation image, portal image, or liquid-crystal display monitor appear larger or smaller than they are in reality. When the image appears larger, this condition is known as *magnification*. The images represent objects in the path of the beam. These objects can be located closer to the common point source (e.g., objects near the multileaf collimator) or nearer to the image receptor (anatomy in the patient). The degree of magnification depends on several factors, all of which have to do with the geometric arrangement of the x-ray target, the patient (object), and the medium on which the image is displayed.

Magnification can be measured and expressed as a factor. Magnification is directly proportional to the distance of the object from the target or source and is dependent on the distance of the object from the image receptor. The magnification factor is defined as follows:

Magnification factor = image size / object size

Example: If an object in the patient, such as the maximum width of a vertebral body, measures 5.3 cm, and its image on the image receptor measures 7.5 cm, what is the magnification factor?
Answer:

Magnification factor = 7.5 cm/5.3 cm = 1.4

Another method of determining the magnification factor is to use the geometric relationship between similar triangles. Two triangles are similar if the corresponding angles are equal and corresponding sides are proportional. In many radiation therapy imaging procedures, determining the size of an object (especially in a patient) is not possible. In these situations, the magnification factor can be calculated by using the ratio of TID and target-to-object distance (TOD):

Magnification factor = TID/TOD

Example: An image taken at 140 cm TID during a treatment verification procedure produces a portal image measuring 6.5 cm on the image receptor. The distance from the target (source) to the object is 100 cm. What is the magnification factor?
Answer:

Magnification factor = 140 cm/100 cm = 1.4

Magnification, expressed as a factor or ratio, is inherent in the production of most portal images. This is the result, in part, of limitations of the treatment equipment used in radiation oncology. A greater degree of magnification is tolerated in radiation oncology than in diagnostic radiology, in which loss of radiographic detail from magnification is more critical to image quality. The radiation therapist should possess an understanding of the practical applications of magnification and demonstrate the ability to measure its effects in the clinical setting.[1–6]

Distortion. Distortion is a change in the size, shape, or appearance of the structures that are examined. Magnification is a good example of size distortion. More magnification occurs with large TODs. Conversely, the greater the TID, the less is the magnification of the object on the image. For minimal distortion, the distance and angulation of the x-ray beam in relationship to the anatomic part (object) and image receptor must be given special attention, especially with portal imaging.

Shape distortion is the misrepresentation of the actual shape of the structure that is examined. This occurs when the object plane or part examined is not parallel with the image plane (Fig. 6.17). If these two planes are parallel, only size distortion occurs, and that distortion is directly proportional to the TOD and TID.[1–6]

Scatter Radiation

During an exposure, some x-rays are absorbed photoelectrically, and others pass through the patient to reach the image receptor. This is partially a result of the kilovoltage (kVp) of the x-ray. If more photons pass through the patient, then the radiographic image has a greater density. The opposite is true if fewer photons reach the image receptor and more photons are absorbed in the body: radiographic density decreases. A considerable amount of the radiographic density results from scatter radiation, in which photons arrive at the image receptor after bouncing off matter haphazardly. However, the density on the image receptor from scatter photons does not directly correlate to the anatomic structures of interest. Instead, the unwanted scatter radiation decreases contrast and reduces image quality.

Less scatter radiation is produced by restricting the beam through careful collimation of the x-ray beam. If fewer primary photons are emitted from the x-ray tube, fewer scatter photons are created. Collimating the primary x-ray beam is the first line of defense in controlling unwanted secondary radiation.

Patient Factors of Imaging: Tissue Thickness, Field Size, Subject Density, and Pathology. Large patients absorb and scatter more radiation than smaller patients. Not only does the amount of tissue irradiated influence the production of scatter, but the density of

- In general , low kVp gives high subject contrast (short scale contrast)
- High kVp gives low subject contrast (longscale contrast)

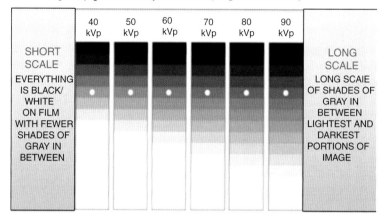

Fig. 6.16 Short and long scales of image contrast. (Modified from Alipour A, Soran-Erdem Z, Utkur M. A new class of cubic SPIONs as a dual-mode T1 and T2 contrast agent for MRI. *Magnetic Resonance Imaging.* 2018;49:16–24.)

the tissue irradiated also affects the quantity of scatter. While the volume of tissue irradiated and atomic number of the material irradiated increases, the amount of scatter increases. The atomic number of the material irradiated affects the amount of scatter radiation produced because the x-ray photons have a greater chance of interacting with an electron in a material with a higher density. For example, more scatter occurs in the pelvis, which has more bone (higher atomic number), than in the thorax, which has more air (lower atomic number). The patient's thickness and the field size greatly influence the volume of tissue irradiated. Larger patients and larger field sizes produce more scatter.

Any diseased state in the body can dramatically alter the body's absorption characteristics. In many situations, the changes that accompany pathology can actually improve the image. This phenomenon is of obvious value in diagnostic radiography and can also prove useful in radiation therapy treatment planning. After all, localizing disease that is not visible with the use of x-rays is difficult.

Tissue changes that occur in pathology are often characterized as additive or destructive (Fig. 6.18) Additive pathologies are those with increased tissue density and therefore appear as light regions on the radiographic image or CT image. Most nonmalignant disease entities are additive. They include edema, Paget disease, atelectasis, abscesses, pleural effusions, and several other common illnesses. Hilar masses commonly associated with lung tumors are universally additive, and any large, fluid-filled mass also appears as an additive pathology. Necrotic areas in a tumor are generally destructive in appearance (typical of a high-grade brain tumor called an *astrocytoma*), but the band of actively mitotic, highly vascularized malignant tissue that surrounds this dead mass is often seen as additive in density.

Most patients with multiple myeloma or any osteolytic metastatic disease have a destructive pathologic disease. Metastases from breast and prostate cancer can sometimes be seen as pathologically additive or destructive on the CT or radiographic image when they are present in bone.

The individual nature of healthy and diseased body tissues makes generalizations on levels of absorption difficult. Far more important is the radiation therapist's understanding that dense structures absorb

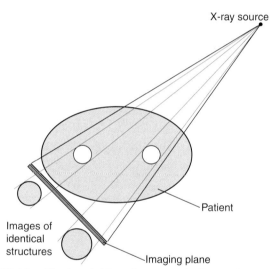

Fig. 6.17 Magnification of objects from an angled beam, demonstrating unequal magnification and distortion.

more photons photoelectrically and produce more Compton scattering. Conversely, tissues that are thin, less dense, and aged result in dramatically decreased attenuation and thus produce a disproportionately darker image.

AN OVERVIEW OF EARLY ADVANCES IN IMAGING MODALITIES

Imaging Media Technology

A medium is a source or channel that may convey data or information. Media is the collective and plural noun of many different types of mediums. In addition to the older conventional recording media (processing film), medical imaging technology has developed many other radiographic image receptors such as fluoroscopic screens, image intensifiers, electronic portable imaging devices (EPID), photostimulable phosphor plates, scintillation and piezoelectric crystals,

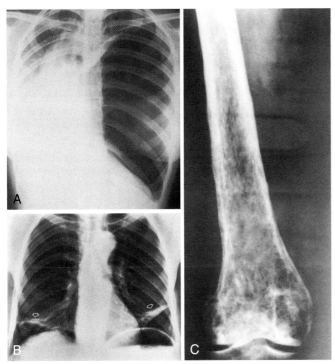

Fig. 6.18 (A) This pleural effusion in the left hemithorax is an example of an additive pathology. (B) This figure demonstrates atelectasis in the lower portion of both lungs (another example of an additive pathology [an opacity on the radiograph]). (C) An Ewing sarcoma has destroyed part of the distal femur. (From Eisenberg RL, Johnson NM. *Comprehensive Radiographic Anatomy*. 4th ed. St. Louis, MO: Mosby; 2007.)

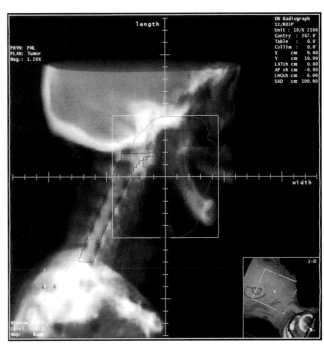

Fig. 6.19 An example of a digital reconstructed radiograph demonstrating the treatment area on a lateral neck field of a radiation therapy patient with a tumor in the tonsillar fossa.

and flat-panel detectors (FPDs). Digitally reconstructed radiographs (DRRs) are used with CT simulation, a type of computer image similar in appearance to a conventional radiograph but displayed on a video monitor or stored on x-ray film. In digital imaging, radiation detectors for which electrical output is proportional to the radiation intensity are used to convert an output signal to a digital form that the computer can display as an image (Fig. 6.19).[1-6]

Screen Film and Cassettes

Contemporary practice in radiation therapy has moved toward digital imaging technology replacing the use of screen film and the radiographic film cassette. However, the use of technology varies greatly from region to region across our country and across international practice. The best candidate for any radiation therapy staff is the one with the broadest skill set and knowledgeable practice that may be incorporated when needed or called upon. A brief description of film and cassette follows with this in mind.

The cassette provides the light-tight conditions necessary for a photostimulable phosphor plate or x-ray film to work properly. The cassette, which opens similar to a book, is made of material with a low atomic number such as cardboard, plastic, and carbon fiber. The back of the cassette is designed differently from the front of the cassette. Lead, copper, or other metal backing prevents unwanted scatter radiation from returning to the film or other image receptor after it has exited the cassette. This type of backscatter radiation can cause unnecessary fog and reduce image quality.[1-5] A digital radiation therapy portal image taken on the treatment machine is of similar or slightly better quality than analog images acquired by using traditional methods of film and cassettes. A computerized digital image of a patient in his or her radiation therapy treatment position can be captured in a matter of moments, uploaded to a computer to check or enhance the image quality, and then sent to a physician in another part of the hospital for viewing. This process is faster and more efficient than conventional methods of obtaining and viewing medical images. The ability to archive the digital image and transmit these images from one workstation to another is vastly better than the traditional methods of sharing and storing conventional simulation and portal images.[1-6]

From Analog to Digital Imaging

What does analog-to-digital conversion mean? Traditional direct reading devices are "analog"; that is, they provide information in a nonnumeric format and are usually mechanical, electromechanical, or photographic. To provide a digital image, the analog image must undergo computerized conversion to a series of minute bits of information initially recorded as a series of binary numbers. The numbers must be collected through some method of analog scan, stored, and then reconstructed to form pixels (picture elements). This provides the basic information necessary to make a two-dimensional image, the cornerstone of CT scanning technology. An even more complex system can create a three-dimensional image by using voxels (volume elements) and is the basis for some CT imaging and most MRIs. This permits the manipulation of images so that they may be viewed from all aspects. Fig. 6.20A and B illustrates that each cell in a CT scan is a two-dimensional representation (pixel) and a three-dimensional representation (voxel).[1-6]

The relationship between the number of pixels or voxels is crucial to image quality. This is described as "resolution." The greater the number of pixels in the matrix, the higher is the resolution of the image. A matrix of 1024 × 1024 is the minimum required, and adequate for cardiac catheterization, CT, and other forms of digital imaging. Fig. 6.21 demonstrates high and low resolution depicting various levels of matrices and elements of "noise" shown on imaging data.[1-6]

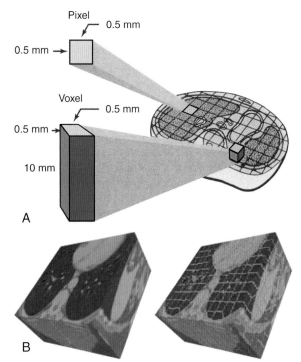

Fig. 6.20 (A) Each cell in a computed tomography scan is a two-dimensional representation (pixel) and a three-dimensional representation (voxel). (B) Each cell in a computed tomography scan is a two-dimensional representation (pixel) with reference to the X and Y axis of the image and a three-dimensional representation (voxel) with reference to the Z axis of the image—head to toe direction. (A, From Bushong S. *Radiologic Science for Technologists: Physics, Biology, and Protection.* 10th ed. St. Louis, MO: Mosby; 2013. B, Reproduced From Buyssens P, Gardin I, Ruan S. Eikonal based region growing for superpixels generation: application to semi-supervised real time organ segmentation in CT images. *IRBM* 2014;35(1):20–26. Copyright © 2013 Elsevier Masson SAS. All rights reserved.)

The Digital Cassette and Computed Radiography

Computed radiography (CR) comprises several types of image receptors. It has served as a transition between film-based image receptors and digital imaging. It is another form of imaging in which a latent image of the subject is obtained that is not visible until the image is processed. However, unlike radiographic film in which the latent image exists as an unseen change in the silver halide crystal's atomic structure, CR uses photostimulable plates, which convert x-rays into the digital image. The flat plate contains a 0.3-mm layer of phosphor powder mixed with binder protected by a surface coating. This layer, when exposed to x-rays, stores the latent image as a distribution of electron charges. The number of trapped electrons is proportional to the number of x-rays absorbed locally, constituting the latent image. Because of normal thermal motion, the electrons will slowly be liberated from the traps. The latent image should be readable for as long as 8 hours after the initial exposure, depending on the room temperature. The image plate is then inserted into a machine in which a small helium-neon laser converts the stored electron energy to light energy. The emitted light energy is collected by a special photomultiplier tube and converted to an electrical signal, which is then digitized and stored on a computer.

The photostimulable phosphor plate is also known as an *imaging plate*, *storage phosphor plate*, or *digital cassette*. The plate is reusable and very portable. To prepare the plate for an x-ray exposure, the plate is exposed to high-intensity light to erase any previous image. The image plate is then placed in a cassette and may be used in the same manner as a film-screen exposure. A cassette similar to a regular film cassette is

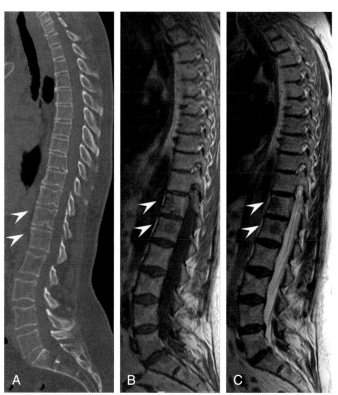

Fig. 6.21 The image illustrates extremely high resolution using a multidetector (MD) computed tomography (CT)/magnetic resonance imaging (MRI) system to assess bone lesions and metastases. The blending of the image data results in the highest resolution. The image is that of a 67-year-old female suffering from breast cancer. In MDCT, (A) no osteolytic or osteoblastic lesion was detected. In contrast, on MRI in the 12th thoracic and 1st lumbar vertebral body hypointense lesions *(arrows)* were detected. In T2-w SE images, these lesions also appeared with hypointense signal (C), thus suspective of osteoblastic lesions. Despite this critical detection with the systems, the lesions proved to be false positives. Histology identified hematopoietic islands as the underlying cause; metastases were ruled out. (From Buhmann S, Becher C, Duerr HR, et al. Detection of osseous metastases of the spine: Comparison of high resolution multi-detector-CT with MRI. *Eur J Radiol.* 2009;69(3):567–573, Copyright © 2007 Elsevier Ireland Ltd.)

used to house the digital imaging plate. Conventional x-ray equipment can therefore easily accept the CR cassettes, making a smooth adaptation of the digital technology. Some radiation therapy departments may use CR when EPID or kV imaging is not available, or if treatment is at an extended distance where field size and treatment distance are not conducive for EPID or kV imaging.

Several advantages are seen with the phosphor imaging plate versus the film screen method of producing an image. With most exposures, a uniform density will be present on the plate despite overexposure and underexposure. This is one of the benefits of the system compared with the older film screen combination. If there is an underexposure, the digital system allows the addition of contrast, density, and brightness to modify the original image within a certain exposure latitude. Even if the original image was overexposed and too "dark," the digital image can be "lightened" by varying contrast and brightness by using simple computer controls.[1-6]

The Electronic Network: Picture Archiving and Communication Systems

Today, almost all patient medical records are electronic. Computers store and share all kinds of information. For example, in an imaging department within the hospital setting, a picture archiving and communication system (PACS) is used to store images, which can be conveniently accessed from the radiation therapy department as well as other areas of the hospital. To ensure that images are communicated properly, standards have been established that use specific protocols, such as HL-7 (Health Level-7) and digital imaging and communication in medicine (DICOM). HL-7 is the most common protocol used in health information systems. DICOM, developed by the American College of Radiology (ACR), is used for PACS (see chapter 24 for additional information).[1-6]

IMAGING MODALITIES IN RADIATION THERAPY

Onboard Imaging

In the past, to verify the isocenter and treatment fields, MV portal images were the only method available. MV portal image quality is poor because of increased amounts of scatter radiation common at higher energy levels, at which Compton interaction predominates. MV imaging usually results in poor subject contrast, making it difficult to distinguish between soft tissues, bony anatomy, and other important structures on the image. Onboard imaging (OBI) systems, with the use of kV x-rays and FPDs, provide better contrast and improved detail, and generate high-resolution soft tissue images.[8,9] Currently, many vendors equip their linear accelerator with two imaging systems (MV and kV). Fig. 6.22 illustrates the kV x-ray source (tube) and the kV imager (FPD) at right angles to the MV source (same as treatment) and the MV imager (EPID). The kV imaging system (OBI) can provide the therapist with three imaging options:

1. Two-dimensional image acquisition, useful in obtaining orthogonal images.
2. Fluoroscopy, so that the body part and its potential motion can be seen in detail.
3. Three-dimensional image acquisition, or cone-beam CT (CBCT), to be compared with the CT simulation images.[8,9]

Megavoltage Imaging

MV imaging can be of two types: a traditional flat-panel megavoltage system or a megavoltage CT imaging (MVCT) system. Flat-panel MV is arguably the most versatile imaging tool in the radiation therapy department. FPDs, a type of amorphous silicon imaging device, attached to the linear accelerator via a retractable carriage or robotic arm system, allow on-demand image acquisition. The imaging system consists of the FPD hardware as well as the associated workstation and imaging software. MV image acquisition obtains real-time electronic images of the patient that can, in turn, be compared with the patient's DRRs that were created during the planning process to validate the setup position before treatment.[8,9]

In MVCT imaging used, for example, with a tomotherapy treatment unit, data are collected with a set of 640-xenon image detectors located on the opposite side of the gantry ring, making it possible to verify the patient's position on the treatment table by comparing MVCT images with CT simulation images obtained earlier for treatment planning purposes. The nominal voltage of the linear accelerator in the imaging mode is lowered to 3.5 MV, providing better image quality and improving the soft tissue contrast.[8,9]

Kilovoltage Imaging

A similar imaging modality to MV imaging is kV imaging. With energies in the keV range, kV imaging uses a separate x-ray source and amorphous silicon detectors for imaging. The kV imaging hardware is mounted to the linear accelerator via a retractable carriage or robotic arm system, which allows on-demand image acquisition.[8,9] In addition,

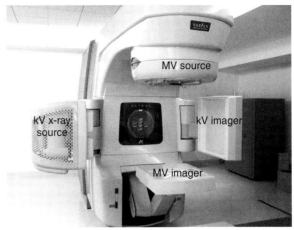

Fig. 6.22 A typical linear accelerator equipped with an onboard imaging (OBI) system and traditional megavoltage *(MV)* imaging system. The kilovolt *(kV)* imaging system (OBI) can provide the therapist with three imaging options: (1) two-dimensional image acquisition, useful in obtaining orthogonal images; (2) fluoroscopy, so that the body part and its motion can be seen in detail; and (3) three-dimensional image acquisition or cone-beam computed tomography.

the imaging system consists of the hardware as well as the associated workstation and imaging software. kV imaging systems can obtain not only real-time electronic images of the patient, which can be compared with DRR images, but also many systems offer fluoroscopic image acquisition and CBCT acquisition (a form of CT that uses wider x-ray beam angles for scanning, thus yielding the ability to scan a much larger volume within one rotation). The benefits of kV imaging rest in the nature of the predominant photon interaction at the kilovoltage energy range, namely the photoelectric interaction. The differential absorption of kV x-rays within bone (higher density), soft tissue, and air (lower density) improves contrast. The tonal range between blacks and whites on the image provides the therapists viewing the image with more information related to bony anatomy and surrounding structures. In the MV range, Compton scattering predominates, decreasing soft tissue contrast and making it more difficult for the therapist to distinguish between soft tissue structures and bony landmarks. In addition, kV imaging uses a substantially lower dose to image the patient as compared with MV imaging. The kV dose is approximately 100 times smaller than that for MV imaging, maintaining exposures as low as reasonably achievable (ALARA). When comparing kV and MV imaging, there are several important concepts to remember, such as dose to the patient, image quality, and the ability of the therapist to evaluate setup uncertainties.[8,9]

Computed Tomography

Godfrey Hounsfield was a British physicist/engineer who shared the 1979 Nobel Peace Prize in physics with Alan Cormack, a Tufts University medical physicist, who earlier developed the mathematics now used to reconstruct CT images. The 1972 invention continues to be a leading imaging modality in radiation oncology, offering "high spatial resolution at the submillimeter level."[1-6,10] A CT scanner consists of an x-ray tube that rotates around the patient. Reconstruction yields a single image that corresponds to an object's x-ray absorption along a straight but diverging line. While the x-ray tube rotates around the patient, a panel of detectors measures the amount of radiation exiting the patient. To acquire a complete volume, several acquisitions must be performed with a short table movement in between.

Other more sophisticated and useful methods of CT scanning, such as spiral CT (See Fig. 6.23) CBCT, and cardiac CT imaging, are

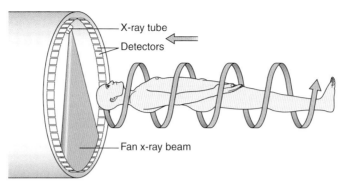

Fig. 6.23 The principle of spiral (helical) computed tomography. The patient moves into the scanner with the x-ray tube continuously rotating and the detectors acquiring information. In the case of lung cancer, the rapidity of data acquisition allows a complete examination of the thorax to be performed. (From Spiro SG, Silvestri GA, Agusti A. *Clinical Respiratory Medicine.* 4th ed. Philadelphia, PA: Saunders; 2012.)

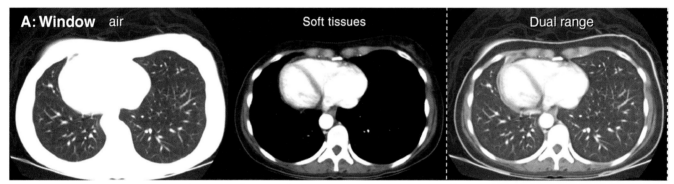

Fig. 6.24 A computed tomography scan of the thorax demonstrating three different windows for viewing. The data collected from the detectors, in terms of bone, soft tissue, and air, are the same in each image. The display of information has been manipulated by the computer to change the contrast of the image. (From Bidaut LM, Humm JL, Mageras GS, et al. Imaging in radiation oncology. In: Leibel SA, Phillip TL, eds. *Textbook of Radiation Oncology.* 3rd ed. Philadelphia, PA: Saunders; 2010.)

available. While the CT scanner rotates around the patient, the transmission of x-rays through the patient are measured and recorded. The x-rays travel through different types of tissue, such as bone, soft tissue, and air-filled cavities, all with varying densities. Multiple measurements of x-ray transmission obtained from different angles of the x-ray source and detectors allow for the computation and representation of various tissue densities within the patient. Varying thicknesses detected by the transmission of the x-rays are also computed and represented as a cross-sectional image through the body.[1-6]

A CT scan of the thorax (Fig. 6.24) demonstrates three different windows for viewing. The data collected from the detectors, in terms of bone, soft tissue, and air, are the same in each image. The display of that information has been manipulated by the computer to change the contrast of the image. By changing the contrast of the image through a process of electronic manipulation of the CT data, digital images can be processed to modify, enhance, or suppress some of their characteristics. This is especially useful in the thorax area, where it may be difficult to see lung detail and, at the same time, examine the anatomy around the heart and mediastinum. Additional information on CT follows later in this chapter.

Cone-Beam Computed Tomography. CBCT is an imaging technique that can be used throughout the course of treatment and has rapidly become the standard daily imaging modality for rigid-body registration.[8,9,11] A CBCT provides imaging data that can recognize

and assess any positioning errors. These errors may be corrected with shifts applied to the treatment table. Researchers report that using CBCT it offers good contrast between structures of large density differences.[8,9,11] CBCT also allows the ability to monitor tumor response throughout the course of treatment, although it is not diagnostic.

All CT scanners are technically CBCT systems. The application of wider cone beam angles has its associated benefits and trade-offs. The benefits of the use of wider cone angles for scanning are the ability to scan a much larger volume (whole organs) within one rotation. Conversely, some challenges are associated with the use of the wider cone beam angle. These include an increase in the amount of scatter radiation reaching the detector and, consequently, the associated reduction in image quality. Included in the trade-off of wider cone beam angles are the creation of imaging artifacts, which are the result of the nature of the system's design. Some benefits have been exploited in image-guided radiation therapy (IGRT) through the integration of CBCT used with linear accelerator technologies. A CBCT-equipped linear accelerator features an imaging source perpendicular to the treatment source, which is coupled to a detector panel. Several projection images are obtained of the patient at multiple intervals through a 180- or 360-degree rotation. These images provide information to reconstruct patient anatomy in three dimensions and are displayed for the therapist to view in all three anatomic planes.[8,9]

Commercial CBCT scanners are available in both kV and MV energies, with benefits and drawbacks to each. In kV-CBCT, a kV tube operating in the energy range of 40 to 130kV is required. The x-ray tube is typically mounted perpendicular to the linear accelerator treatment head and coupled with an FPD for imaging. For the case of MV-CBCT, the imaging MV x-rays are the same used for treatment. The beam coming from the treatment head is directed at the FPD of the unit and used for routine portal imaging.

Because volumetric images are obtained throughout the scan, image reconstruction does not require interpolation (the recreation of information not captured between slices), and true image reconstructions are available in all three anatomic planes. CBCT image quality has not yet matched that of diagnostic CT. Although the CBCT systems currently available provide bony and soft tissue visualization acceptable for the applications of CBCT in radiation therapy, there are some contributing factors that result in a reduction of the image quality.[8,9] CBCT is a volume image obtained during a period of time while the gantry rotates around the patient. Therefore it is particularly susceptible to motion artifacts during scanning. The resulting image is an average of motion within the patient during the scanning window. Similarly, the use of FPDs and the larger cone angle for scanning contributes to several issues, including more scatter, geometric imaging problems, and motion considerations. KV imaging has been shown to reduce the overall dose to the patient while providing improved soft tissue visualization.

Magnetic Resonance Imaging

In 2003, Paul C. Lauterbur and Sir Peter Mansfield were awarded the Nobel Peace Prize in Medicine for their work with MRI with the first image created in the 1970s.[12] Medical imaging applications of MRI is a result of earlier work and research on nuclear magnetic resonance (NMR). NMR was used for analyzing the chemical structure of compounds in the chemistry lab for decades. Lauterbur, a chemist, and Manfield, a physicist, worked with corporations, such as Dow Corning and Stanford University and other research institutes and universities, to develop what we know today as MRI.

The MRI system can be identified as having three key components integral to its operation: the magnet and associated coils, the couch, and the computer processing system. In appearance, an MRI machine resembles a CT scanner; however, it differs greatly in function. The typical MRI bore is deeper and smaller than that of a CT scanner and is surrounded by the radiofrequency (RF) coils, imaging coils, and the electromagnetic coils. Because of the nature of the magnetic coils, they must be supercooled by liquid nitrogen and liquid helium to near-absolute zero temperatures to function. Units designed for radiation therapy scanning and MRI simulation have become commercially available. These systems have wider bores and indexed flat therapy tabletops that can be used with a variety of MRI-compatible accessories for immobilization and positioning to match departmental needs. Adjustable coil bridges are available to keep the coil close to the patient for optimal imaging. Gradient distortion functionality is available for these oncology MRI units. MRI-compatible patient marking lasers are also available for patient alignment.

Strict policies and procedures must be followed because of the potential risks for patients and healthcare workers who enter the magnetic field. The ACR has published a special manuscript referred to as the ACR Guidance Document on MR Safe Practices: 2013. The safety guide outlines various potential risks not only to the patient, but to family members, the medical staff, and others such as first responders for emergencies and housekeeping personnel. In addition to risks related to the magnetic environment, the guide outlines warnings and recommended actions in cases of exposure to the supercooling gases, claustrophobia and anxiety, contrast agents, pregnancy precautions, and screening various metal used for past medical treatments such as surgical clips and cardiac pacemakers or implantable cardioverter defibrillators.[13]

The radiation therapist must be familiar with these policies and procedures. Before the exam, patients must be screened for implanted devices such as a pacemaker, hearing aid, defibrillators, or prosthetic devices. These devices may prohibit the patient from receiving the MRI. It is important to have the patients completely disrobe and remove all metal. The loud and lengthy procedure should be explained to the patient before the exam. Proper signs need to be posted alerting patients and staff regarding the magnet in use.

The ACR describes four zones to limit access to the MRI.

a. Zone 1: Area accessible to the general public.
b. Zone 2: More strictly supervised area. This is usually the area where patients are screened.
c. Zone 3: Area restricted to MR personnel; located outside the treatment room.
d. Zone 4: MR scanner room.[13]

Patient positioning and stability are extremely important during an MRI scan. It is best that the treatment planning MRI be performed with the patient in the treatment position. This facilitates image registration with the CT data set. Unlike CT scanning, in which motion during a slice impacts local artifact effects to the slice in question, motion in MRI has the potential to affect the entire image. Therefore positional accuracy and the maintenance of patient position throughout the duration of the examination are key for successful imaging. MRI has better soft tissue contrast and resolution than CT. Therefore it is useful in defining the tumor volume, especially in the brain, head and neck, liver, pelvis, prostate, and in sarcomas. MRI has the ability to display detailed anatomic information (in the sagittal, coronal, and transverse planes), such as the presence and extent of tumors, the shape of normal structures adjacent to the tumor volume, and the distinction between recurrent tumor and necrosis. Its application has grown rapidly in recent years, especially with the ability to capture the MRI information and apply it to the radiation therapy treatment planning process either alone or fused with other imaging modalities such as CT or PET.

MRI does not use ionizing radiation, but rather uses the body's natural magnetic properties. The human body is made up of specific elements, such as carbon, hydrogen, oxygen, and others—all with specific and unique characteristics. In many cases, electrons orbit around a central nucleus of protons and neutrons. Because of this, both protons and neutrons behave like tiny magnets as they spin about their own axis within the nucleus. Hence these nuclei have what physicists call a "residual magnetic moment." Only those nuclei with an odd number of protons and neutrons behave as a small atomic magnet. Ordinary hydrogen with only one proton, and hence a net positive charge, has the strongest magnetic moment. Other nuclei with an odd number of nucleons (protons + neutrons) exhibit a smaller magnetic moment. Because the human body is composed mostly of H_2O (between 60% and 80%), there is an abundant number of hydrogen atoms that express a magnetic moment. When the nuclei of hydrogen atoms or other atoms with weaker magnetic moments are placed in an intense magnetic field, they tend to align themselves either with or against the applied magnetic field, as is the case with the large and powerful magnets used in MRI.[1-6] MRI is a noninvasive procedure that uses strong magnetic fields and radio waves to produce images in any plane through the patient. Researchers report that magnetic fields that are used with MRI clinically are "between 1.5 and 3 Tesla, whereas human research scanners go up to 7 Tesla."[1-6,10]

Pulses of RF energy are applied to the patient within the MRI scanner, and then the return signal from the patient is collected by a signal coil, measured, and reconstructed into an image. Because the signal produced is fairly small, it is best if the receiving coils are close to the

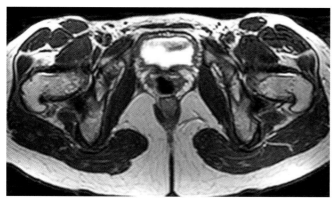

Fig. 6.25 A transverse (axial) T2-weighted magnetic resonance imaging scan of the female pelvis taken at a level just inferior to the symphysis pubis. Note the normal anatomy of the bladder, vagina, and rectum. (From Kelley LL, Petersen CM. *Sectional Anatomy for Imaging Professionals.* St. Louis, MO: Mosby; 2007.)

area being imaged. There are head coils for brain imaging, spine coils, and surface coils for various extremities. This can pose challenges in the use of diagnostic MRI units for radiation therapy imaging because of positioning and immobilization devices for radiation therapy treatment.[10]

The RF energy returning from the patient is based on three characteristics: (1) the intensity of the signal (representative of the spin density related to the concentration of rotating nuclei within the patient); (2) the time constant T1, known as the *longitudinal relaxation time*; and (3) the time constant T2, known as the *transverse relaxation time*. These three characteristics form the basic parameters used to produce a magnetic resonance image. A variety of methods, known as *pulse sequences*, have been developed to apply the RF energy to a patient and to collect and measure the RF signal radiated from the patient. The MRI computer processing system allows the technologist to select the appropriate pulse sequences required for the organ of interest. Pulse sequences yield images with valuable spatial and contrast information about atomic structure and function in the patient. Fig. 6.25 demonstrates a T2-weighted transverse MRI scan of the female pelvis.[1-6,10]

NUCLEAR MEDICINE IMAGING

Although CT revolutionized the field of radiation therapy, it continues to have some limitations; CT imaging provides a low tissue contrast, resulting in the construction of differing tumor volumes from physician to physician. In contrast, CT imaging does provide better imaging of bony structures and organs like the lungs that move too much for MRI.[12]

Nuclear medicine can provide additional information about the tumor, which includes metabolic activity and function. Nuclear medicine uses radioactive isotopes (radionuclides) that are injected into the patient. The specific radionuclides can localize to specific organs, which allows the ability to image the extent of a disease. The radioactive decay is recorded by a gamma camera, which detects and records radiation output. One form of nuclear medicine imaging is PET.

Positron Emission Tomography

PET was developed in the 1970s and can be used to diagnose, stage, and follow up cancers because of the physiologic functional information it provides. PET is a form of imaging in which the physiology, metabolism, and biochemistry, rather than the anatomic structure, are displayed in the image.[1-6,10,12,14] Physiology describes how a tissue,

an organ, or a system may function. Anatomy is related to the structure of a specific tissue, system, or organ. CT imaging is an excellent example that displays anatomic structure. PET alone can be difficult to interpret in the absence of anatomic imaging. PET can be performed along with a CT scan (known as a PET-CT), which provides anatomic detail. Images can be "registered," which allows the CT and PET to be fused and viewed together. This aids in identifying the tumor volume and surrounding patient anatomy. A PET-CT can also be fused with the CT acquired during the simulation process and used for treatment planning. This is very desirable and assists the radiation oncologist and medical dosimetrist with target volume definition and treatment planning.[8,9,10,12] PET images may be displayed in the transverse, sagittal, or coronal planes. Functional differences seen on the image may represent normal or abnormal pathology as areas of increased density.[1-6]

PET takes advantage of the body's natural process of metabolism and exploits some of the molecular building blocks of life, for example, the amount and rate of amino acids, molecular oxygen, or glucose used by the tissue or organ. This is done by labeling a radioactive nuclide, usually tagged to a specific gamma-emitting radioactive pharmaceutical selected for its tendency to concentrate in a specific tissue of interest in the patient. An analog of glucose, fluorine-18 fluorodeoxyglucose (FDG) is currently the most common agent used in PET imaging. FDG is a positron emitter.[1-6,10,12,14]

A positron is an antiparticle that, when released from the nucleus, pairs up with an electron. This pairing is known as an annihilation event and results in the conversion of matter into energy according to Einstein's equation $E = mc^2$. The result of the annihilation event is a pair of annihilation photons of equal energy traveling in opposite directions. The photons emitted by FDG escape from the body and are measured by an external detector positioned very close and on opposite sides of the patient. Malignant cells utilize more glucose to meet their energy needs. The measurement process yields a "physiologic map" of the accumulation, distribution, and excretion of the radioactive material in the organ or tissue of interest. Several types of radioactive tracers have been developed for imaging with PET, but most clinical oncology PET studies use FDG. The use of FDG to image glucose metabolism takes advantage of the observation that malignant cells have higher rates of aerobic glycolysis than does normal tissue. Malignant cells divide more rapidly and need more glucose to meet their energy needs.

A thorough knowledge of normal anatomy and normal FDG distribution in the body is necessary before any evaluation of pathologic accumulations can be attempted. Fig. 6.26 demonstrates normal distribution of FDG in a total-body PET/CT scan. Its application has grown rapidly in recent years, especially with the ability to capture the PET information and apply it to the radiation therapy treatment planning process either alone or fused with other imaging modalities such as CT or MRI. Other agents, such as the isotope gallium-68, are also useful with the fused imaging modalities (Fig. 6.27).[8,9,10,12]

Positron Emission Tomography/Computed Tomography Hybrid Imaging. Researchers report that PET/CT is "important for the delivery of modern conformal therapy and essential for implementing involved-node radiation therapy in lymphoma." Because of its ability to provide more defined and accurate data, PET/CT imaging can play a key role in the planning of treatments, showing more accurate tumor volumes.[6]

Use of a dedicated CT/PET scanner that performs both imaging sequences during one examination provides both detailed structural information from the CT scan and functional information from the PET scan. Because of all its advantages, the use of PET imaging had been combined with CT imaging to create a PET/CT

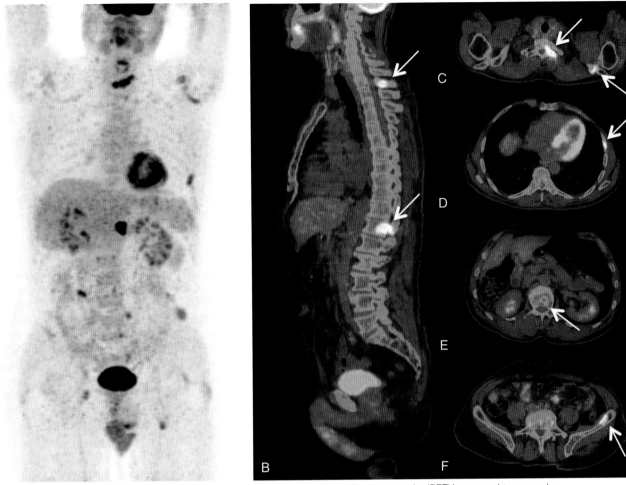

Fig. 6.26 Fluorine-18 fluorodeoxyglucose (FDG)-positron emission tomography (PET)/computed tomography (CT) of a 59-year-old female with a clinical suspicion of multiple myeloma and "salt-and-pepper" aspect of the whole bone marrow compartment on the magnetic resonance (MR) examination of the spine. Maximum intensity projection PET (A), sagittal PET/CT fused (B), axial PET/CT fused (C), axial CT related (D) of the left arm, axial PET/CT fused of the pelvis (E), and CT-related (F) images. A diffuse bone marrow involvement was observed in the whole bone compartment, both axial and appendicular (vertebrae, costal arch, sternum, pelvis, humeri, and femora) (A and B), with focal lesions at the left humerus (C and D) and left sacrum (E and F). These lesions do not correspond to osteolytic areas on CT exam, indicating early bone marrow involvement. (From Rubini G, Niccoli-Asabella A, Ferrari C, et al. Myeloma bone and extra-medullary disease: role of PET/CT and other whole-body imaging techniques. *Crit Rev Oncol Hematol.* 2016;101:169–183, Copyright © 2016 Elsevier Ireland Ltd.)

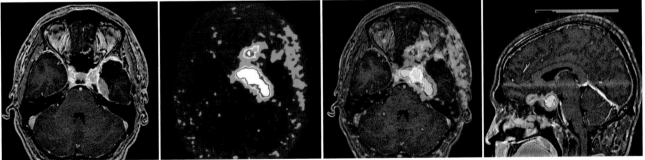

Fig. 6.27 The images illustrate gross tumor volume (GTV) with magnetic resonance imaging (MRI)/computed tomography (CT) with positron emission tomography (PET) and a gallium-68 isotope, and with PET/computed tomography (CT)/MRI fusion that illustrates functional imaging showing areas with high 68 Ga uptake, enabling GTV delineation. Without PET data, the GTV MRI/CT included a volume that would have been irradiated that was not tumorous. (From Graf R, Nyuyki F, Steffen I, et al. Contribution of 68 Ga-DOTATOC PET/CT to target volume delineation of skull base meningiomas treated with stereotactic radiation therapy. *Int J Radiat Oncol Biol Phys.* 2013;85(1):68–73. Copyright © 2013 Elsevier Inc.)

hybrid imaging, which is being implemented more often in planning and treatment.[15] PET/CT provides better detailed images, aiding in more accurate staging and response assessment of lymphomas. A study reported that PET/CT "identified more than 97% of disease sites of Hodgkin lymphoma (HL) and aggressive non-HL," leaving just around 3% unaccounted for.[15] Currently, PET/CT is mainly used to help with staging and response assessment of HL and diffuse large B-cell lymphoma (DLBCL), although it is lately being used more often in other domains. As the tumor changes throughout the course of treatment of lymphomas, PET/CT can be used to follow these changes and potentially modify the chemotherapy treatment in response to the changes seen on the images taken during the treatment course.[15] When contrast is used during PET/CT imaging, the "sensitivity in detecting involved lymph nodes" is also increased in comparison to CT imaging alone.[16]

The development of a dedicated CT/PET scanner has overcome many previous problems involved in fusing CT and PET images. Diagnostic PET-CT scanners have curved tabletops, which cause difficulty in fusing the images to the treatment planning CT acquired with a flat tabletop. It is preferable to have the patient in the treatment position in the appropriate immobilization devices for both procedures to ensure accurate fusion. Flat tabletops are available for most diagnostic PET-CT scanners. PET-CT simulators designed for radiation therapy use have large bores and a flat couch very similar to CT simulators. Some radiation oncology centers have purchased PET-CT scanners to use for simulation and/or treatment planning purposes. If the PET-CT resides in the radiation therapy department, the facility must staff nuclear medicine technologists or share staff with the nuclear medicine department. The radiation therapists are able to perform the CT scans but are not able to perform the PET portion because of the use of the radioactive isotope. If the scanner is located in the nuclear medicine department, the radiation therapists must be present to assist with patient positioning, immobilization, the simulation procedure (if applicable), and any patient marking.[8,9,10,12]

Positron Emission Tomography/Magnetic Resonance Imaging.

According to researchers, combining PET and MRI "represents a unique hardware approach to visualization and quantification of functional processes with high sensitivity and to providing high-resolution, high-contrast anatomical images, respectively within a single imaging system."[17] PET/MRI obtains better data when used together rather than when each is used on its own, because it utilizes the advantages of both (Fig. 6.28).

With the use of PET/MRI imaging, a photomultiplier tube (PMT) cannot be used like it is with standard, single-modality PET. The PMT is combined with "standard PET detectors" containing a scintillating material; an electrical signal is eventually converted out by the PMT. Based on the acceleration of electrons, PMT technology cannot be used in a combined PET/MRI imaging system because of the magnetic field from MRI.[18] New concepts have been introduced to try to find a way around the challenge of PMTs being used when PET is combined with MRI; PMTs have been replaced with semiconductor detectors, which are not sensitive to magnetic fields. Because of the use of a semiconductor rather than a PMT, "the design of fully-integrated PET/MRI systems that permit simultaneous acquisition of PET and MRI data of the same axial field of view" is possible.[18]

Information gained from the combined modalities includes "MRI-based motion estimation and correction, PET reconstructions incorporating MRI information, MRI-based partial volume correction for PET and the enhanced definition of regions-of-interest for the extraction of quantitative values." Researchers report that when PET/MRI fusion is "in the hands of trained, motivated

and collaborative teams," it can turn into a "multi-facetted imaging modality that bears many potentials for improved diagnostic work-up of patients."[18]

Ultrasound

Ultrasound, also known as *sonography,* is a useful medical imaging tool for delineating surface contours and localizing internal structures such as the prostate gland.[8,9,10,12]

Ultrasound may include color-Doppler flow imaging to enhance imaging of vascular flow direction. Ultrasound may be further enhanced with MRI/ultrasound fusion.

In this imaging technique, a transducer is used to generate a mechanical disturbance (pressure wave) that moves through the tissue. While the sound wave moves through the body, it encounters a variety of interfaces between tissue that reflect and refract (change the direction of) the ultrasound energy. The amount of energy reflected back to the transducer depends on the physical density of the tissue and the speed of the ultrasound through the tissue. A piezoelectrical crystal within the transducer is used to create the ultrasound waves. The wave is initiated by applying a momentary electrical shock to the piezoelectrical crystal, which sets the crystal into a vibration mode. Ultrasound energy reflected from an interface between tissues returns as a pressure wave of reduced amplitude to the transducer, where a small electrical signal is generated, captured, and processed.[1-6]

The application of ultrasound is particularly useful in delineating tissues that differ only slightly. For example, ultrasonography may be used to localize the prostate gland or prostate bed in the lower pelvis before external beam radiation treatment is administered.[8,9,10,12] It is also used to distinguish between solid and cystic lesions in the breast following mammography. This works well because the sound waves travel well through fluid-filled cavities and cysts.

Because the prostate gland moves relative to bony anatomy between the time of initial image acquisition for treatment planning and treatment delivery, real-time imaging, such as ultrasound, is sometimes used to accurately localize the target at the time of treatment delivery.[9,10,12] Freehand ultrasound imaging is used to acquire data at any anatomic orientation by either sliding or arcing the probe across the region of interest. One acquires many arbitrary two-dimensional images until enough images have been collected to fill a three-dimensional matrix covering the volume of interest. This information is then used through an in-room coordinate system each day to determine the absolute position of the prostate volume within the patient. Daily adjustments may be made relative to the linear accelerator isocenter.

Pressure variations applied in the suprapubic area during prostate localization procedures and the interuser (from one therapist to another) variation of the contour alignment process may affect the accuracy of prostate localization.[8,9,10,12]

Principles of Image-Guided Radiation Therapy.

IGRT allows for the correction of positional setup errors. These corrections can be of two types: interfraction and intrafraction uncertainties, which can increase the confidence in the target treated, allowing for dose escalation and reduction of margins around the tumor. Interfraction uncertainties refer to variations in setup that exist between each setup, that is, inaccuracies in positioning, variations in machine characteristics, and changes in patient anatomy and target shape over time. Intrafraction uncertainties refer to the variations that occur within a fraction (i.e., organ or patient motion). IGRT, or online correction, is the process of correcting uncertainties that result during treatment. This is accomplished by imaging before and, in some cases, throughout treatment, using an imaging system such as CBCT, which allows for online image

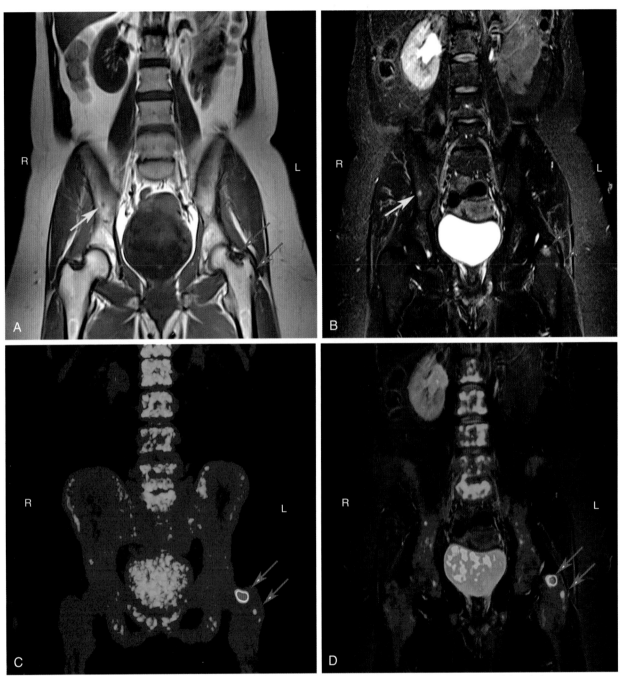

Fig. 6.28 [18F]-NaF positron emission tomography (PET)/magnetic resonance (MR) imaging of the abdominal and pelvic region in a patient with known prostate cancer referred for staging assessment. (A) Coronal T1-weighted spin-echo MR image, and (B) coronal short-TI inversion recovery (STIR) MR image show three osseous metastases *(arrows)* involving the proximal left femur and right iliac bone. (C) Coronal [18F]-NaF PET maximum intensity projection image, and (D) fused coronal [18F]-NaF PET/STIR MR image show concordance between both imaging modalities for the presence of the two proximal left femoral bone lesions *(red arrows)*, but discordance for the presence of the right iliac bone lesion, which is detected on MR imaging but not on [18F]-NaF PET *(yellow arrow)* given its small size. This case illustrates the added value of combined PET and MR imaging modalities. *L,* Left; *R,* right. (From Anderson KΓ, Jensen KΕ, Loft A. PET/MR imaging in musculoskeletal disorders. *PET Clinics* 2016;11(4):453–463. Copyright © 2016 Elsevier Inc.)

review and subsequent positional corrections. With the increased use of three-dimensional treatment planning, including intensity-modulated radiation therapy (IMRT), volumetric modulated arc therapy, stereotactic radiosurgery (SRS), and stereotactic body radiation therapy, it has become more useful to consider interfraction and intrafraction uncertainties that affect treatment planning and treatment delivery methods. With multiple fraction treatment, all of the following effects should be considered[8,9]:

- Daily setup variations.
- Geometric uncertainties.

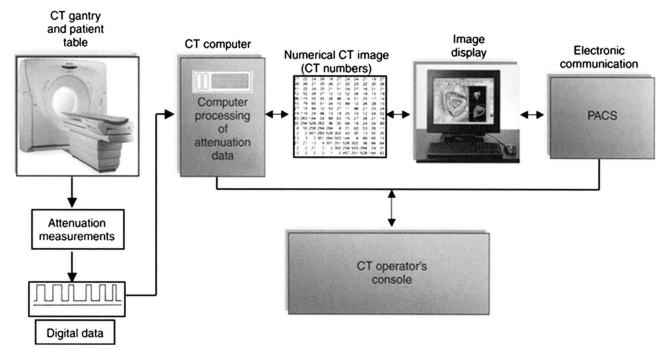

Fig. 6.29 General schematic of the computed tomography *(CT)* system and related subsystems and communication assemblies. The CT scanner gantry sends all data signals to the computer for image reconstruction. The results of computer processing are images that are displayed on a television monitor for viewing by an observer. *PACS,* Picture archiving and communication systems. (From Seeram E. *Computed Tomography: Physical Principles, Clinical Applications, and Quality Control.* St. Louis, MO: Saunders Elsevier; 2009.)

- Changes in patient anatomy and target shape with time.
- Patient movement and internal organ movement during treatment.
- Education and experience of the radiation therapists.

Daily imaging, compared with weekly portal imaging of the patient's skeletal and/or soft tissue anatomy, and/or implanted fiducial markers with a combination of EPID, IGRT, and CBCT (kV or MV) has reduced random and systematic variations.

Regardless of the imaging modality used, IGRT follows the same basic principles. Images obtained at the time of treatment are compared with a reference image. This reference image is typically obtained at the point of planning and represents the optimal patient position included in the treatment planning process. The treatment image is then registered or matched to the reference image. Once matched, variations in the patient's position can be identified and corrections calculated and applied, either through manual adjustments or automatic robotic couch correction.[8,9]

Computed Tomography Design and Technology. The essential mechanical and electrical components of a CT scanner include the CT gantry, patient table, intercom, CT computer with array processor, and a high-voltage generator. Located in the external part of the gantry are the controls for couch movements, emergency off buttons, and CT localizer lasers. Located in the internal aspect of the gantry are the detector array, x-ray tube, and generator. A second set of very stable and accurate external lasers (in addition to the CT localizer lasers) are also necessary. Fig. 6.29 provides a general schematic of the CT system and related subsystems, including communication assemblies.

The Gantry. The gantry of a CT scanner, which contains the rotating x-ray tube, is essentially the circular "doughnut" into which the patient is inserted during the scan. Aperture size (the diameter of the hole into which the patient is positioned), also commonly called *bore size*, is an important factor in radiation oncology. Ideally, the aperture should be 80 to 90 cm to accommodate a variety of patient setups, especially for breast simulations and wider body sections such as the pelvis. The exact treatment position may not always be possible on a scanner with the small aperture that is found on some units.

The gantry includes the x-ray tube, the detector array, the high-voltage generator, the slip ring (S-R), and the mechanical support devices. These subsystems receive electronic commands from the operating console and transmit data to the computer, where image production takes place.[1-6]

The X-Ray Tube. An x-ray tube used for CT imaging is similar in design to those used in the conventional simulator, diagnostic x-ray equipment, and angiography, with a few special features. Because a great deal of stress is placed on the CT x-ray tube, the tube must be able to withstand large amounts of heat from multiple exposures during a short period of time on numerous patients scheduled each day. Heat may be dissipated by using a large-diameter, thick anode disk, rotating at fast as 10,000 rpm. Cooling oil, circulated around the x-ray tube, small fans, and, in some cases, a heat exchanger, may be used to reduce the amount of heat buildup around the x-ray tube. Manufacturers will usually list the anode heat capacity in MHU (million heat units) and the maximum anode heat dissipation (how quickly the heat is removed from the tube assembly) rate in KHU (thousand heat units). With spiral CT, greater thermal demands are placed on the x-ray tube because the tube may be energized continuously for as long as 120 seconds. High heat capacity and high cooling rates are trademarks of x-ray tubes designed for spiral CT.[1-6]

The Detectors. Solid-state detectors are designed to convert radiation to light. Then photodiode assemblies convert light to an electronic signal that receives and measures the attenuated beam from a rotating x-ray tube. Spacing of the detectors varies, depending on the design; however, generally, one to eight detectors per centimeter or one to five detectors per degree are available. Some 90% of the incident x-ray is absorbed and contributes to the output. Because of the spacing of the detectors, the net output is nearly 90%. Positioned between the detector array and the computer, the data acquisition system serves several functions, such as measurement of the transmitted radiation beam, binary coding of the measurements, and transmission of the binary data to the computer.[1-6]

The Couch. The CT couch tabletop for radiation therapy is similar to that of a conventional simulator in that it is made of low-Z material such as carbon fiber. Diagnostic CT scanners use a curved couch top; thus an insert should be purchased to provide a flat surface to scan patients in the treatment position. Most CT scanners allow for the installation of a flat radiation therapy couch tabletop that mimics the table of the linear accelerator. Some come with predrilled holes or notches along the lateral edge of the couch to provide a suitable locking location to register (index) immobilization devices such as head holders, prone pelvis immobilization devices, and breast boards. This feature is important with the increased use of three-dimensional conformal therapy and IMRT. The CT couch for radiation therapy use must be very accurate in terms of mechanical positioning. Precise patient positioning is essential, especially when indexing the patient to a specific position within the gantry opening. A carbon fiber tabletop provides little attenuation of the x-ray beam and, at the same time, provides good longitudinal support of the patient. These features are critical while the couch travels through the gantry. The couch and tabletop should not deflect or sag while it extends and travels through the CT bore. Regular quality assurance testing is important to ensure that the treatment couch position and movement are accurate for treatment planning purposes.[1-6]

The Computer Console. While computer technology increases with faster processors and larger memory, procedure time and image reconstruction time are reduced. Depending on the image format, numerous equations (hundreds of thousands) must be solved simultaneously, requiring a large-capacity computer to process the images. Images are typically processed by an image reconstruction server that resides at the computer console or in close proximity. Reconstruction time, the time it takes the image reconstruction system to analyze and process the information received from the detectors and display it on the computer monitor, is an important variable in the application of CT simulation. With the use of special array processors, multiple images are reconstructed per second. The array processor takes the raw data from the detector measurements and reconstructs the data by performing simultaneous calculations. The images are rapidly displayed at the CT control console on one or more computer monitors and become available to load into various applications for manipulation and viewing. Images are typically exported to a PACS system for radiation oncologist review and storage. With radiation therapy CT simulation, they can be loaded into CT simulation software, exported to a CT simulation workstation, or exported to a treatment planning system. The reconstructed images can be reformatted into various planes by using the image data.[1-6]

Generations of Computed Tomography

The first generation of data acquisition geometry consisted of a pencil beam and single detector. An x-ray tube and detector assembly moving axially across the patient in a straight line completes a translation. After the first translation, the tube and detector rotate one degree and complete another translation. This continues until at least 180 degrees of data have been collected. This process is known as *translate-rotate scanning motion*. The second-generation scanners, which produced faster scans, were based on translate-rotate motion, but the detectors (solid-state devices designed to convert radiation to light), consisted of a fan beam of 5 to 30 detectors. The third-generation scanners were based on a curved array of detectors in which the x-ray tube and the detectors rotated continually around the patient, which is the current technology used in the scanners today. The fourth generation of scanners, no longer used, consisted of stationary detectors, and only the tube rotated around the gantry.

Other variations of scanner geometries have been developed and marketed and may be referred to by some as *later-generation scanners* (i.e., fifth-, sixth-, and seventh-generation scanners).[1-6]

Slip Ring Technology

The first CT scanners, known as *conventional or axial scanners*, required the patient to be positioned at a fixed point and the x-ray tube to be rotated 360 degrees around the patient. The tube stopped rotating, and then the table moved a fixed distance into the scanner. The tube had to return to its original position, then repeat the rotation around the patient, stopping again to return to its starting point. This was necessary to keep the cables inside the machine from twisting by unwinding cables attached to the tube and other components by reversing the rotation. Continuous revolutions are made possible today through S-R technology. S-R technology allows rotation without cables or electrical wiring connected to the moving gantry parts. S-Rs are electromechanical devices that conduct electricity and send electric signals using rings and brushes. One surface is a smooth ring; one is a ring with brushes that sweeps the smooth ring to transmit power or electric signals without wiring or cables. This same technology is used in computers that utilize a mechanical hard drive disk, and CD, or DVD drives. The hard drive disk rotates continuously within the computer. Brushes glide in contact with the smooth surface of the disk to transmit signals. Conductive brushes made of conductive material serve as the sliding contact. S-R technology has made fast scanners incorporating helical or spiral CT possible. Helical scanning provides the acquisition of continuous data sets without having to stop the gantry rotation. Data sets can be stacked to form a three-dimensional image reconstruction based on the continuity of the anatomic data acquired. Spiral or helical scanning is referring to the motion of x-ray tube during the scan. The tube rotates continuously around the patient from head to toe, resembling a coiled spring pattern. Fig. 6.30 illustrates S-Rs, x-ray detector, and PET detectors in a PET/CT scanner. See also Fig. 6.23 illustrating the coiled helical scanning pattern.

The data points are recorded as the tube travels from head to toe. The large data set can be used to reconstruct any part of the patient being imaged. The images are converted reconstructions of the data set and may be viewed as sagittal and coronal planes in addition to the conventional transverse/axial plane.[1-6] The advantages of helical scanners include the following:

- A fast scan with the capability of acquiring a large data set of the patient in a single breath hold.
- Capturing critical anatomical data points with a continuous scan that may have been missed using slice-to-slice technology.
- Useful in CT angiography and radiation therapy treatment planning and imaging of uncooperative or critically ill patients.

Multislice Spiral Computed Tomography. CT scanners are designed with a finely collimated x-ray fan beam and a detector array (group of detectors) that rotate around the patient in a

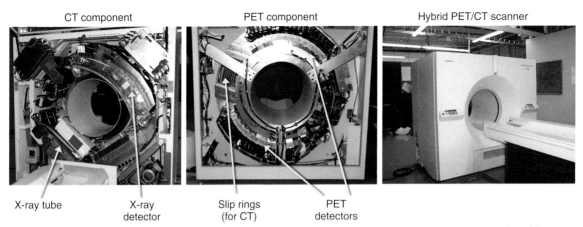

CT component   PET component   Hybrid PET/CT scanner

X-ray tube   X-ray detector   Slip rings (for CT)   PET detectors

Fig. 6.30 The first hybrid positron emission tomography *(PET)*/computed tomography *(CT)* scanner. The CT component (left) consists of an x-ray tube and single row of x-ray detectors mounted on a rotating gantry. The PET detector system (center) is mounted on the rear of the same rotating gantry and consists of a partial ring of block detectors made from the scintillator bismuth germanate. The photograph on the right shows the completed prototype system. Note the slip rings and detector assemblies. (From Townsend DW. Combined positron emission tomography–computed tomography: The historical perspective. *Seminars in Ultrasound, CT, and MRI* 2008;29(4):232-235.)

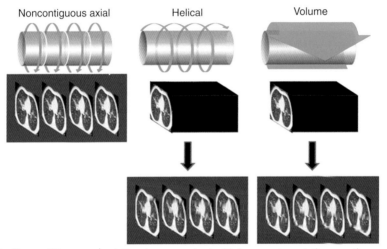

Noncontiguous axial   Helical   Volume

Fig. 6.31 Significant differences in data volume acquired with less gantry rotations as the scanning technology improves from the single detector row and single "nonhelical" rotation to the helical scanner using multiple channels ranging as high as 64- to 320-detector row technology. One great benefit of acquiring more data is less exposure to the patient. During noncontiguous axial acquisition, the x-ray tube is collimated to a narrow beam width and rotates around the patient for one rotation. The tube is then turned off while the patient table is translated 10 mm, at which point the tube is turned back on and undergoes another rotation. This process repeats until the desired scan length is covered. During helical acquisition, a wider nominal beam width is used, and the tube rotates continuously while the patient table simultaneously translates. During volume mode, a single rotation covers the entire anatomy, and there is no table translation during the acquisition. (From Podberesky D, Angel E, Yoshizimi T. Comparison of radiation dose estimates and scan performance in pediatric high-resolution thoracic CT for volumetric 320-detector row, helical 64-detector row, and noncontiguous axial scan acquisitions. *Acad Radiol.* 2013;20(9):1152–1161, Copyright © 2013 AUR.)

continuous fashion (see Figs. 6.23 and 6.31). The finely collimated beam is created by the prepatient and postpatient (predetector) collimator via metal plates attached to the x-ray tube. Collimation absorbs photons that would enter the patient's body at several angles, producing unwanted scatter radiation. This prepatient collimation in a conventional (single-slice) CT scanner determines the slice thickness. While the x-ray tube and opposing detector make one complete rotation (360 degrees) around the patient, thousands of x-ray transmission measurements are recorded by the detectors. CT information is generally recorded by a group of solid-state image detectors.

The advantages of multislice detector imaging technology include shorter imaging times per scan or the ability to image more anatomy in the same or less time, ultimately sparing the patient unnecessary radiation exposure. One essential difference between single-slice CT scanners and multislice CT scanners is how slice thickness is determined. For single-slice CT, slice width is determined by a combination of the physical prepatient and postpatient (predetector) collimators. Multislice systems utilize multiple detector rows to use the x-ray beam more efficiently and acquire greater amounts of data per sweep. Fig. 6.31 illustrates significant differences in data volume acquired with less gantry rotations as the scanning technology improves from the single detector row and single "nonhelical" rotation to the helical scanner using multiple channels ranging as high as 64- to 320-detector row technology. One great benefit of acquiring more data is less exposure to the patient. For these CT scanners, the x-ray beam must be wide enough to irradiate all active detector rows required for a particular scan. In multislice scanning, the combination of beam collimation and detector array size is controlled by the protocol parameter collimation. The selected collimation can affect the x-ray beam geometry both before the patient (similar to a traditional collimation) and after exiting the patient (usually called *postpatient collimation*). Collimation can be used to mask parts of the detectors and decrease the effective size of the remaining exposed detectors. The collimation mode also determines the detector rows that are active and used for data collection. The detector array affects how the raw data are collected, which will determine slice width selections available for reconstruction (the process in which the CT computer analyzes and processes the information received from the detectors and displays it on a TV monitor). Slice thickness is a CT reconstruction parameter that determines the thickness of reconstructed images. Slice increment is a CT reconstruction parameter that determines the distance between the center of CT slices.[1-6] With smaller effective detector sizes, thinner slices are available for reconstruction. Wider slice thicknesses (3 mm, 5 mm, and 10 mm) can be reconstructed by combining or fusing the signal from multiple rows (see Fig. 6.31). Because the detector array is wider for 16-, 32-, or 64-channel CT, it takes a lower number of rotations to cover the region of interest. Acquisition time and patient exposure are dramatically reduced. This also results in much greater image detail of internal structures. Fig. 6.32 illustrates the improved image detail of a 4-channel detector row, a 16-channel detector row, and a 32-channel detector row multislice CT.

Data Acquisition

Data acquisition, information collected from the patient to produce the CT image, occurs with conventional CT or helical CT, as described previously. The patient is positioned in the center of the bore so that the patient's contour is not cut off laterally. Otherwise, it is possible that the patient's anatomy will not be visible in the diameter of the scanning window or scanning field of view (SFOV). The SFOV is smaller than the aperture of the gantry. CT scanners typically have a set or defined SFOV. The operator defines the display field of view (DFOV) to include the anatomy to be viewed. The DFOV, also called the reconstruction field of view, can be less than or equal to the SFOV in the area reconstructed seen on the image monitor. A smaller or narrow DFOV results in a larger image size, an increase in spatial resolution (the clarity or the measure of detail in a CT image), and an increase in noise.[1-6]

The x-ray tube rotates around the patient. The detectors measure the amount of radiation transmitted through the patient. The intensity of radiation detected varies based on the density and effective atomic number of structures in the beam (bone, air, and soft tissue). The numerous intensity profiles or projections are converted by an analog-to-digital converter and stored in digital form in the computer as raw data.

Spiral Pitch Ratio

Spiral pitch ratio, or simply "pitch," describes the relationship between the patient couch movement through the CT scanner and the x-ray beam width. It is a ratio between couch movement and beam width. The equation for pitch ratio is as follows:

$$\text{Spiral Pitch Ratio} = \text{Couch Movement Each 360 Degrees/Beam Width}$$

The effect of changing the pitch in a scan may result in either overlap of beam width or gaps between beam width as the table moves in toward the gantry during a scan. In other words, the pitch is the relationship of beam width and gantry rotation speed to rate of table movement. This pertains to multislice spiral CT imaging, where, instead of one beam and only one slice per revolution, you may acquire several wide slices per revolution with potential of overlapping if the table movement is not appropriately coordinated with the speed of the CT gantry rotation producing the beam. In practice, the pitch for multislice CT is usually 1.0.

The following is an example of a typical spiral pitch ratio word problem.

Problem: During a 360-degree x-ray tube rotation, the patient couch moves 8 mm. The beam width is 5 mm. What is the pitch?

Solution: 8 mm/5 mm = 1.6:1

Spiral Beam Ratio and Radiation Protection

So, what does spiral pitch ratio mean regarding patient exposure as it relates to the ALARA principle?

The implications of pitch and radiation protection are critical to know. The standard pitch in practice is 1.0 and may be expressed as 1.0:1. However, pitch ratios may be:

- 0.5:1
- 1.0:1 (standard pitch)
- 1.5:1
- 2.0:1

Studying the figures will help the student understand the following critical concepts regarding pitch and exposure to the patient. Increasing the pitch to above 1:1 increases the tissue volume that can be imaged at a given time. This is an advantage of multislice CT, because a large volume may be scanned in a single breath hold. This means that a pitch of 2:1 results in extended tissue volume imaged per revolution. The benefit is that the patient dose is reduced with higher pitch settings. It is easy to visualize the beam width as a larger "bandwidth" of beams together. A pitch less than 1.0:1, a pitch of 0.5, for example, results in overlapping images and higher patient dose. A pitch of less than 1.0 actually images part of the tissue volume of the previous band width, exposing the patient anatomy more than once. If you think of the width of the beam as "bandwidth," a larger bandwidth covers more tissue; therefore less gantry revolutions are required. The entire scan is faster because more tissue is covered with less actual "beam-on" time exposing the patient.

Spiral Pitch Ratio and Data Acquisition. An increase in pitch increases the volume that can be imaged in a given time, but at the cost of data sampling. A too-high pitch may result in image artifacts, especially in moving targets. In CT, the term artifact is applied to any systematic discrepancy between the CT numbers in the reconstructed image and is an undesired alteration of data. Lower pitches may be beneficial in increasing resolution. On a multislice scanner, if mA remains constant, dose is inversely proportional to pitch. However, on some systems, mA is automatically adjusted so that dose remains

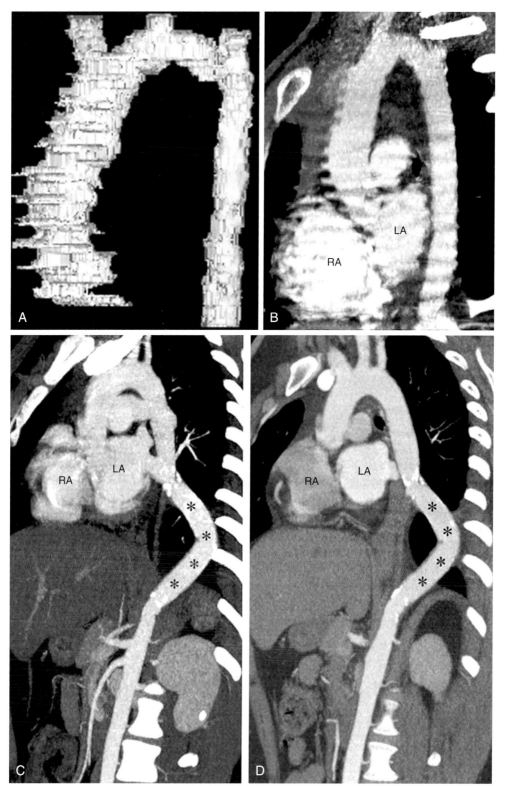

Fig. 6.32 The figure illustrates the improved image detail from a 4-channel detector row to a 16-channel detector row, and 32-channel detector row multislice computed tomography *(CT)*. (A) Three-dimensional image of the aorta obtained with single-detector row CT scan shows severe cardiac pulsation artifacts and a short coverage that includes only the upper half of the thoracic aorta. (B) Oblique sagittal image obtained with 4-detector row multidetector (MD) CT reveals slight decrease in cardiac pulsation artifacts and a slight increase in longitudinal coverage, including the entire thoracic aorta. (C) Oblique sagittal image obtained with 16-detector row MDCT shows a considerable decrease in cardiac pulsation artifacts and a substantial increase in longitudinal coverage. An aortic bypass graft *(asterisks)* is noted. (D) Oblique sagittal image obtained with 32-detector row MDCT. right atrium *(RA)*, left atrium *(LA)*. (From Goo HW. Cardiac MDCT in children: CT technology overview and interpretation. *Radiol Clin North Am.* 2011;49(5):997–1010, Copyright © 2011 Elsevier Inc.)

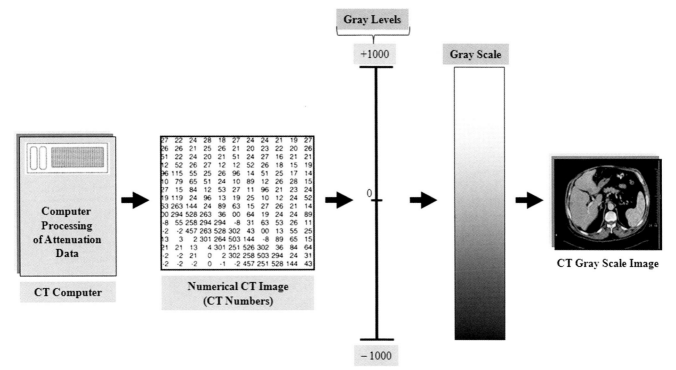

Fig. 6.33 The conversion of computed tomography *(CT)* numbers into a gray scale image. (From Seeram E. Computed tomography: physical principles and recent technical advances. *J Med Imaging Radiat Sci.* 2010;41(2):87–109, Copyright © 2010 Elsevier Inc.)

constant. Because helical scanners collect data in a spiral fashion, the data must be interpolated to construct the data to create a transverse (axial) plane. This mathematic process called interpolation estimates attenuation between two known points. Interpolation is completed before reconstruction of an image.[1-6]

Image Reconstruction

Enough transmission data must be collected to produce an acceptable image. Therefore the CT scanner must rotate around the patient for at least 180 degrees. Numerous algorithms, a specific set of instructions to get a specific output, have been developed to reconstruct the raw data into reconstructed data. One common algorithm applicable to CT is filtered back projection (FBP), a commonly used method of reconstructing CT data, called the *convolution method*. The term *filter* here refers to a mathematic function, not a metal filter.

Filtered-back projection has been the industry standard for CT image reconstruction for decades. Although it is a very fast and fairly robust method, FBP is a suboptimal algorithm choice for poorly sampled data or for cases in which noise overwhelms the image signal. Such situations may occur in low-dose or tube power-limited acquisitions (e.g., scans of morbidly obese individuals). While the dose is lowered, the signal to the detectors decreases, and noise is increased. When these very high levels of noise are calculated through the reconstruction algorithm, the result is an image with significant artifacts and high noise levels.

Newer iterative reconstruction (IR) techniques attempt to find the image that is the "best fit" to the acquired data. The measurements that are the noisiest contribute very little to the final image in the iterative process. Hence IR techniques reduce the noise and artifacts present in the resulting reconstructed image. More recent innovations in computer hardware design and algorithm optimizations have allowed widespread clinical use of IR techniques in CT.[1-6]

Computed Tomography Numbers. Structures represented on the scan may range from black to white, depending on the density of the structure and the amount of information received by the detectors. This is one of the advantages of CT simulation compared with fluoroscopy-based simulation. CT can differentiate between soft tissue structures, such as the pancreas and stomach, much better than radiographic images. While the beam is attenuated by the patient, varying degrees of absorption of the x-ray beam occur, depending on how much tissue (patient thickness) the beam travels through and the tissue type. The detectors will register more of the x-ray beam while it passes through lung tissue in the thorax versus when the x-ray beam passes through the soft tissue of the abdomen. Attenuation coefficients of body tissue are directly related to its atomic number, or how many protons and neutrons are packed in the nucleus of an atom. The more protons and neutrons in the nucleus, the higher the atomic number and the greater chance for the x-ray beam to be absorbed or attenuated through the photoelectric effect and Compton scattering. Bone and metal, such as surgical clips, fiducial markers, or dental fillings, have the greatest chance of absorbing or attenuating the x-ray beam and appear as whiter areas on the scan. The same principle applies to the use of contrast agents such as barium sulfate or iodine-based contrast. Black areas on the CT scan represent low-density areas such as gas in the stomach or air in the lungs. As mentioned previously, Hounsfield units are named after Sir Godfrey Hounsfield, an English engineer who invented CT. After his initial scans were performed first on a preserved human brain, then on a fresh cow brain, he allowed a scan of his own brain to further document one of the greatest medical breakthroughs in imaging. He assigned values from +1000 for dense bone to −1000 for air, and represented water as "0." Structures with a beam attenuation of less than 0 are represented by a negative number, and structures with an attenuation number greater than 0 have a positive HU. Fig. 6.33 illustrates the system conversion of HU of various tissues and linear attenuation coefficients to an image. HUs, which correspond to the electron density of a specific tissue such as lung, soft tissue, and bone, are set at less than1000 for air (zero density), 0 for water (unit density), 15 for cerebrospinal fluid, 20 for blood, 40 for gray matter, 50 for muscle, and 1000 for dense bone. Originally, the scale had the value of greater than 1000; however, with patients having metal replacements (e.g., hip replacements), which have a high atomic number, CT scanners now report HUs much higher than 1000.[1–6]

Image Display

The digital image structure can be described with respect to several characteristics, including matrix pixels, voxels, and bit depth. The signal is analyzed by the computer and reconstructed on a monitor, giving a transverse cross section of the body. Images seen on the screen are a display of cells in rows and columns, called the image matrix. Matrix size can be selected; however, 512 × 512 is commonly used in CT. In a 512 × 512 matrix, there are a total of 262,144 pixels of information. Each cell on the image matrix is called a pixel (picture element), which is a two-dimensional representation of a corresponding tissue. Each pixel and the slice thickness or volume is called a voxel (volume element). Fig. 6.20A illustrates how pixels and voxels are used in viewing an image for CT scanning application. *Bit depth* refers to the number of bits per pixel. A single bit would show the image as black or white. A bit depth of 2 implies that each pixel will have 22 or 4 gray levels per pixel. Each pixel contains a numeric value (discrete value) that represents a brightness level. For a typical bit depth of 16 bits (2 bytes), there can be more than 10,000 different brightness levels, and the image size would be on the order of 512 kB. Pixel size, the physical length and width of each pixel, can be determined by dividing the field of view by the matrix size. The pixel size can be determined by using the follow formula:

$$\text{pixel size} = \text{FOV (mm)/matrix size}$$

The smaller the pixel size, the greater the potential for better spatial resolution, but the greater the noise. While the pixel size decreases, the matrix size increases for the same FOV. Three factors determine the voxel size: slice thickness, matrix size, and field of view. Voxel size can be described as an isotropic or anisotropic display. Isotropic display means that the length, width, and height (x, y, and z) dimensions are equal, or the voxel is a perfect cube. Isotropic imaging increases spatial resolution and enhances 3-D reconstructions.

The radiation therapist is able to manipulate the appearance of the image after it has been acquired by the CT scanner by a technique called *windowing*. Two characteristics of windowing are window level (WL) (this represents the central Hounsfield unit of all the CT numbers within the window width [WW]) and WW (the range of numbers displayed or the contrast on a CT image). These options allow the image to be manipulated to view a specific type of tissue by adding or subtracting contrast, density, or both.[1–6, 8,9,10,12]

A computer monitor can display only 256 gray levels, of which only approximately 80 are visually discernible to the human eye. The display can be optimized by changing how the HUs are displayed on the screen. This can be related to the brightness and contrast of a television screen. If WW is narrowed, greater contrast or sharper changes in the shades of gray result. This is useful in visualizing tissues with similar densities. A clinically useful gray scale is achieved by setting the WL and WW on the computer console to a suitable range of HUs, depending on the tissue examined. The term WL represents the midpoint HU of all the CT numbers within the

WW. The WW covers the HU of all the tissues of interest, and these are displayed as various shades of gray. Tissues with CT numbers outside this range are displayed as either black or white. Both the WL and WW can be set independently on the computer console by the radiation therapist. Their respective settings affect the final displayed image. The effect of a wide window will decrease contrast, and a narrow WW will increase contrast, as seen in Fig. 6.24. The WW/WL equation is used to determine the WL and gray scale range. The first step is to take the WW number and divide it in half. Then add it and subtract that number from the WL. This will provide a gray scale range.

Example:

$$WW = +600$$

$$WL = +100$$

$$Range = -200 \text{ to } +400$$

It is recommended that wide WW should be used for tissues with attenuation that is greatly different. Narrow WWs should be used for soft tissues. WLs should be near the tissues of interest attenuations average. Scanners often have preset windows available to optimize windowing.

IMAGE QUALITY

Key components of CT image quality include spatial resolution, image noise, low contrast, temporal resolution, and dose. Spatial resolution refers to the degree of blurring in a CT image or the ability to discriminate between two adjacent high-contrast objects. Low-contrast resolution refers to the ability to see differences in objects that are similar shades of gray in tissue. Image **noise** is the grainy appearance of an image. Parameters such as mAs, kVp, slice thickness, table increment, pitch reconstruction interval, FOV, matrix size, and reconstruction filter affect the desired quality of the image.[1–6]

Spatial Resolution

Spatial resolution, also known as *high contrast*, is specified in terms of line pairs that are equal-sized black and white bars. Factors that affect spatial resolution that are inherent to the equipment are focal spot size, detector cell size, scanner geometry, and sampling frequency. The smaller the focal spot size and the smaller the detector size, the better the resolution. Factors that the therapist has control over are pixel size, slice thickness, and the reconstruction filter used. A small pixel size creates better spatial resolution; however, the image is noisy. The FOV and the matrix size affect the pixel size and, in turn, the spatial resolution.

If the matrix size in CT is 512 × 512, and if there is a 40 × 40 FOV, the pixel size is 0.8 × 0.8 mm. If there is a 20 × 20 FOV, the pixel size is 0.4 × 0.4 mm. Using the same FOV, resolution will be improved with a larger image matrix. Fig. 6.21 illustrates images with different matrix sizes.

Reconstruction filters are applied to the raw data. Two basic options are a smooth filter or a sharp filter. A smooth filter is used to reduce noise and improve the contrast between soft tissues (low-contrast resolution). Smooth filters may also decrease the finer structural details (high contrast resolution) and edge definition. A sharp filter used for musculoskeletal examinations may improve the spatial resolution, but it will increase noise.[1–6]

Noise

If a homogeneous medium such as water is scanned, each pixel should have a value of zero. This naturally occurring variability is known as scan noise. The following factors affect image noise:

- kV(p)
- mA
- Exposure time
- Collimation/reconstructed slice thickness
- Reconstruction algorithm or filter
- Helical pitch/table speed
- Helical interpolation algorithm
- Others (e.g., focal spot to isocenter distance and detector efficiency)

An increase in kVp and mAs decreases noise. The more photons detected by the image receptor, the less noisy the image. A sharper reconstruction filter increases noise. An increase in image matrix increases noise because the smaller the pixel size, the fewer photons per image receptor. Increased FOV and slice thickness decrease noise.[1-6]

Low-Contrast Resolution

Image contrast is inherent in the various tissue densities such as soft tissue, air in the lungs, and bony anatomy. CT is superior in displaying better image contrast compared with a conventional radiographic image. CT can distinguish tissue density differences of less than 0.5%, compared with conventional radiography that can only differentiate densities as low 10%. For example, the liver on a CT scan can be differentiated from other soft tissue structures in the abdomen much better than a conventional radiographic image of the abdomen. Low-contrast resolution is influenced by a large number of factors that include a similar list to that described for image noise. An increase in noise can decrease low-contrast resolution.[1-6]

Temporal Resolution

Temporal resolution is the ability to freeze or decrease motion of the scanned object. An increase in gantry rotation speed will increase temporal resolution. Temporal resolution is a key component on four-dimensional CT and is further discussed in the CT Simulation chapter.

Dose of Exposure

Dose delivered to a patient in a single CT slice at the skin surface is in the range of 2 to 10 mSv, which is considerably greater than other imaging modalities. It is approximately equivalent to 100 to 500 chest x-rays. Factors that affect dose include patient size, patient centering, mAs, and kVp selection, gantry rotation, pitch, collimation, and scan length. Dose to the patient increases with an increase in mAs. Wider beam coverage and a greater pitch may decrease the dose to the patient. In scanning a smaller region of anatomy, the dose to the patient will decrease. Last, minimizing repeat scans by reducing motion artifacts will help reduce the dose. Recent advances in image reconstruction allow images to be created at lower dose levels. Scanners may use an automatic current selection tool to suggest mAs, based on patient size and shape. Other tools such as tube current modulation, automatic exposure control, or IR, which maintains noise levels at lower mAs values, may also vary the intensity of the beam throughout the scan, yielding varying mAs levels per slice. This may allow the user to, in turn, lower patient exposure and still achieve acceptable image quality. A balance must be achieved between spatial resolution, noise, and patient dose.[1-6]

In CT, there are several ways that dose or exposure is represented. CT dose index (CTDI) is a normalized value that is computed from measurements on a standard phantom. CTDI is usually displayed in milligrays and is useful for measuring scanner output, but it does not

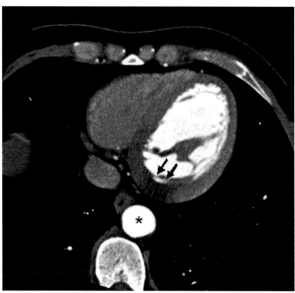

Fig. 6.34 Axial image from a multidetector computed tomography coronary angiogram with significant beam hardening artifact. Note the area of transmural attenuation density *(arrows)* in the basal inferior wall emanating from the descending aorta *(asterisk)* and vertebral spine. (From George RT, Lima J, Lardo A. CT detection of myocardial perfusion, infarction, and viability. In: *Atlas of Cardiovascular Computed Tomography: Imaging Companion to Braunwald's Heart Disease*. Philadelphia, PA: Saunders; 2010.)

equate to patient absorbed dose or differences in total exposure resulting from scan length. Another tool to measure dose is dose length product, which is CTDI multiplied by the length of the scan, and represents the total absorbed dose in a phantom during the length of a scan and is also measured in milligray-centimeter. Both of these metrics, although helpful, do not measure patient dose because they do not include specifics such as patient size. They can be useful in comparing the amount of radiation exposure between different scan protocols or scanners. A measurement termed *effective dose* is used to estimate biologic risk. It can be calculated by multiplying DLP by a dose conversion coefficient that is specific to the anatomic area or organ of interest.[1-6]

It is important to have the patient in the center of the bore. Off-centering may decrease image quality and may increase patient dose. The average positioning error is 2 cm too low. A 4 cm off-centering can result in a 30% increase in noise and a 68% increase in mA. Altering kVp changes the reported CT number, which can alter the treatment planning dose calculations. If a lower technique is desired, lower the mAs. Only modify kVp after consulting with the physicist before the scan. Gantry rotation speed is the time that it takes for the gantry to rotate 360 degrees. It is directly proportional to dose. If all other factors remain constant, and the rotation time is reduced by half, the dose is reduced by half.[1-6]

Artifacts

CT artifacts are unwanted image abnormalities that can be caused by patient motion, anatomy, design of the scanner, or system failure. Common CT artifacts that can greatly degrade the quality of the images, sometimes to the point of making them diagnostically unusable, are beam hardening, partial volume effect, star artifact, ring artifact, and motion and helical artifacts.

Some CT imaging artifacts can be avoided with careful planning and the use of critical thinking skills by the radiation therapist. Beam-hardening artifacts (Fig. 6.34) can be seen as dark bands. To

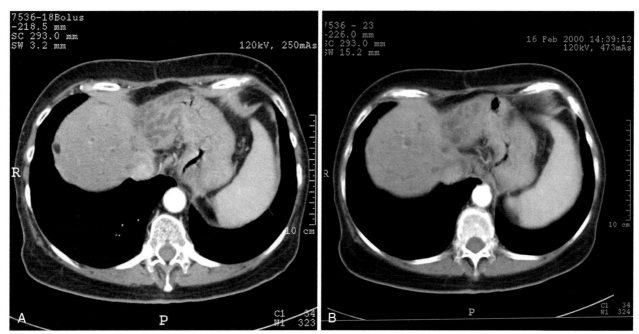

Fig. 6.35 Liver scan showing partial-volume artifact. (A) A 2.5-mm slice thickness shows good visibility of small liver lesions. (B) A 10-mm slice thickness shows reduced lesion detectability with partial-volume averaging. (From Jordan DW, Haaga JR. *CT and MRI of the Whole Body*. 6th ed. Philadelphia, PA: Elsevier; 2017. Images courtesy Dr. John Hagga.)

minimize these artifacts, thin slices should be used, and extremely dense contrast media should be avoided. Partial-volume artifacts are a result of a large scanning tissue thickness. These occurs when tissues of widely varying absorption properties occupy the same voxel; the beam attenuation is proportional to the average value of the attenuation coefficient of the voxel. A volume average is computed for such voxels, leading to the partial-volume error. A partial-volume artifact can be subtle and gradual, requiring care in interpretation. Partial-volume artifacts can obscure the appearance of small lesions that are averaged together (Fig. 6.35). Star artifacts (Fig. 6.36) can occur from surgical clips or other metallic objects within the patient. The presence of metal objects such as pacemakers, electrodes, stents, and surgical clips, or simply very dense contrast media in the scan field can generate severe streak artifacts (Fig. 6.37). They occur because the metal object absorbs the radiation, resulting in incomplete projection profiles. Avoiding the metal object within the FOV, if possible, would be the only way to eliminate this type of artifact. Reconstruction algorithms that reduce metal artifacts have been developed. These IR algorithms can select optimal data projections, thus reducing the effect of the metal in the resulting images. A ring artifact (Fig. 6.38) can occur if a detector is not working properly, and may be more common in third-generation CT scanners. Artifacts similar to the ring artifact occurring in a spiral or helical scanner appear as an arc. Motion artifacts (Fig. 6.39) appear as streaks or less resolution, and are commonly seen in and around the diaphragm when the abdomen and thorax are scanned. Faster scanners help reduce motion artifacts, especially when patients can hold their breath during a scan. Stair-step artifact occurs when the reconstruction interval on a spiral CT scan is too large and a stepped appearance in the vessels is created. Stair-step artifacts appear as horizontal lines through the image, visible especially around the edges of structures in multiplanar and three-dimensional reformatted images, when wide collimations and

nonoverlapping reconstruction intervals are used. Patient positioning before scanning and proper selection of scanning parameters are the most important factors in avoiding CT artifacts.[1-6]

INTRAVENOUS CONTRAST AGENTS USED IN MEDICAL IMAGING

Iodine-Based Contrast Agents

Iodine based contrast is commonly used in radiological diagnostic imaging. According to the US National Library of Medicine medical journal, there are four types of iodine contrast agents (ICAs); these contrast agents are categorized as polymers such as ionic monomer, ionic dimer, nonionic monomer, and nonionic dimer.[19] One ICA may have more attenuation, whereas the other ICA has lower attenuation but has a higher osmolarity rate; this can be dangerous for the patients' blood if not administered adequately. Some ICAs attenuate more than others; therefore some ICAs need to have higher intravenous dose administration to produce an excellent-quality image. All of the ICAs may be traced back to the early 1950s. According to several studies, iodine has been known to be the most common contrast used in the radiologic imaging (owing to its high Z number), mainly for use with CT scans.

Allergic reactions can be caused by ICA, and the professional staff must be aware of the typical signs of reactions. Studies describe patients with only minor reactions such as pruritus, erythema, nausea, and vomiting within the first hour. These minor reactions require only observation for the patient. The literature also describes patients with severe reactions within seconds that, if not treated in a timely manner, could have severe consequences. Most of the time, patients with severe anaphylactic shock can be medicated with methylprednisolone that will prevent severe reactions. Several of these situations can be avoided if the staff have the appropriate patient medical history.[19]

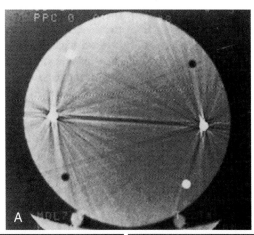

Fig. 6.36 Streak artifacts. (A) Uniform medium with metallic pin; note the large amount of streak artifact. (B) A hip prosthesis. (C) Streaks from metal clips in the heart. (From Jordan DW, Haaga JR. *CT and MRI of the Whole Body.* 6th ed. Philadelphia, PA: Elsevier; 2017.)

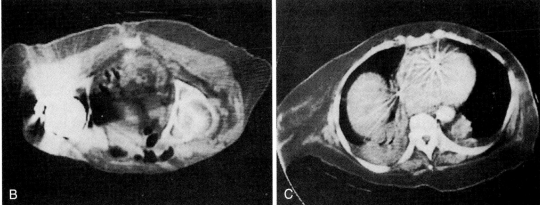

Fig. 6.37 Metal objects, such as surgical wires (A), pacemaker electrodes (B), and dense contrast material (C), can generate severe streak artifacts. (From Gaspar T. Interpretation and reporting in obstructive coronary disease. In: Ho VB, Reddy GP, eds. *Cardiovascular Imaging.* St. Louis, MO: Saunders; 2011.)

Gadolinium-Based Contrast Agents

Gadolinium agents are used as contrast agents with MRI. These are most commonly used to enhance vessels in MR angiography. Another use involves brain tumors that have affected the blood-brain barrier. These agents are useful in localizing tumors where the blood-brain barrier has been comprised. Gadolinium based agents are not as safe as iodine-based agents and are known to be nephrotoxic and neurotoxic. Because these agents cross over the blood-brain barrier and are associated with a higher incidence of anaphylactoid reactions, extra precautionary measures are taken to avoid overdose or repeated scans.[20,21]

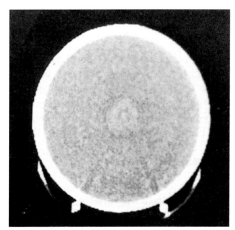

Fig. 6.38 Ring artifact demonstrated in the center of a uniform water phantom. Note that streak artifacts are also pictured, caused by metal pins or feet supporting the bottom of the phantom. (From Jordan DW, Haaga JR. *CT and MRI of the Whole Body.* 6th ed. Philadelphia, PA: Elsevier; 2017.)

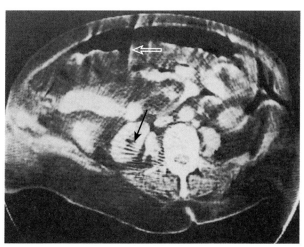

Fig. 6.39 Streak artifact *(open arrow)* caused by motion of bowel gas in a slow abdominal scan on a conventional single-slice computed tomography (CT) scanner. Machine-caused streaks are also seen. Streak artifact *(solid arrow)* is caused by an unstable rotor in the x-ray tube, producing unstable focal spot motion during the scan. (From Jordan DW, Haaga JR. *CT and MRI of the Whole Body.* 6th ed. Philadelphia, PA: Elsevier; 2017.)

However, the US Food and Drug Administration (FDA) published a report in 2017 addressing the concern of "gadolinium remaining in patients' bodies, including the brain, for months to years after receiving these drugs. Gadolinium retention has not been directly linked to adverse health effects in patients with normal kidney function, and we have concluded that the benefit of all approved gadolinium-based contrast agents (GBCAs) continues to outweigh any potential risks." In 2018, a follow-up report by the FDA stated the following, "This is an update to the FDA Drug Safety Communication: FDA identifies no harmful effects to date with brain retention of GBCAs for MRIs; review to continue issued on May 22, 2017." The only effect that is absolutely identified is that of nephrotoxicity. The FDA has stated the following regarding kidney damage: "To date, the only known adverse health effect related to gadolinium retention is a rare condition called nephrogenic systemic fibrosis (NSF) that occurs in a small subgroup of patients with preexisting kidney failure. We have also received reports of adverse events involving multiple organ systems in patients with normal kidney function. A causal association between these adverse events and gadolinium retention could not be established."[22]

Emerging Imaging Innovations in Radiation Therapy and Cancer Management

The current body of literature includes multiple publications with positive outcomes relating innovation in some type of imaging modality and cancer management. What follows are only a few selected applications where medical imaging technology has improved cancer management.

Advances in Positron Emission Tomography-Computed Tomography

The treatment of certain head and neck cancers has been traditionally challenged by poor survival rates. For some, the quality of life has been compromised solely because of surgeries that impact cosmetic appearance and oral function. One study points out that residual nodal disease attributed to necrosis and radiation resistance has improved as a result of combining chemotherapy with radiation. With chemoradiation becoming standard practice, a study by the GETTEC-French Head and Neck Intergroup revealed that PET-CT may be used to monitor the treatment response of nodal groups at risk. It is reported that with PET-CT showing a complete response to chemoradiation treatment,

eliminating a neck dissection is becoming the most common strategy for advanced nodal disease among centers for that group.[23]

Advances in Positron Emission Tomography Hypoxia-Tracing Radioisotopes

Tumor hypoxia remains one of the leading causes of treatment failure. It is responsible for increased radioresistance, distance metastasis, and increased tumor growth because of angiogenesis. We have expressed previously that FDG is currently the most commonly used agent in PET imaging. PET has become an effective tool for assessing hypoxia with the use of certain hypoxia-specific radioisotopes. However, FDG has been found to have properties that are not effective as a radiotracer for hypoxic cells. The most studied hypoxia-specific radiotracer is ^{18}F-fluoromisonidazole (F-MISO). Although research is ongoing, this is referred to as "dynamic" F-MISO PET imaging of hypoxia. Recent reports confirm that it is effective in detecting hypoxic tumor volumes in several types of cancers; however, results have not been consistent. PET scans of head and neck cancer patients using F-MISO detected tumors exhibiting high tracer uptake with implications of high risk for treatment failure.[24]

Another study refers to the use of several types of hypoxia-specific radioisotopes as PET radiotracers, used for head and neck and lung cancers. The study relates using "adaptive" radiotherapy in response to image-guided alterations in normal tissue or characteristics of hypoxia. Scanning the patient between treatments may guide the treatment strategy in terms of changing the treatment field, escalating dose without overdosing critical structures such as the parotid and spinal cord, and guiding modulation of dose delivery based on tumor growth. Additionally, hypoxic tissue may be targeted with radiosensitizers or hypoxia cytotoxins.[25]

Dual- or Twin-Beam Dual-Energy Computed Tomography

The CT system with two x-ray tubes provides a beam with two different energies that are simultaneously captured or blended for multiple benefits, one being to improve quality, such as patient motion artifacts.[26] Dual-energy or spectral CT have the two independent tubes and detector systems at 90 degrees from each other on the same gantry (Fig. 6.40). Some dual-energy CT systems are single-source systems that

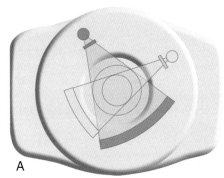 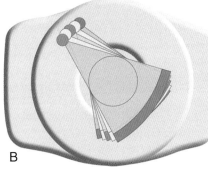 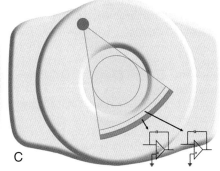

A B C

Fig. 6.40 Schematic illustration of the main dual-energy computed tomography CT (DECT) systems. (A) Dual-source DECT consists of two source-detector combinations in a nearly orthogonal configuration, allowing the same section to be scanned simultaneously at the two energies (Siemens AG, Forchheim, Germany). (B) Single-source DECT with rapid tube potential switching (Gemstone spectral imaging; GE Healthcare, Waukesha, WI, USA). This system consists of a single source-detector combination. DECT projection data are acquired by very fast switching between low- and high-energy spectra combined with fast sampling capabilities of a proprietary detector for spectral separation at each successive axial or spiral view. (C) Layered or sandwich detector DECT (Philips Healthcare, Andover, MA, USA). This scanner also consists of a single source-detector combination, but spectral separation is achieved at the level of the detector. The system takes advantage of the polychromatic nature of the c-ray beam and highly specialized detectors consisting of two layers with maximal sensitivity for different energies for separation of different energy spectra. For all images, yellow is used to illustrate the low-energy spectrum and blue the high-energy spectrum. (From Forghani R, Mukherji SK. Advanced dual-energy CT applications for the evaluation of the soft tissues of the neck. *Clin Radiol.* 2018;73(1):70–80. Copyright © 2017 The Royal College of Radiologists.)

use a spectral filter that splits the x-ray beam into a low-energy and a high-energy beam. The beam energy is switched from low to high after each rotation. The fusion image of high- and low-kVp images uses a weighting of 60% from 80 kVP and 40% from 140 kVp for the best images of head and neck squamous cell carcinomas. However, the different types of systems include the dual-source CT (DECT) by Siemens Healthcare, the single-source CT (DECT) with rapid kVp switching by GE Healthcare and Cannon Medical Systems, and layered or sandwich detector DECT by Philips Healthcare. DECT can differentiate structures with high atomic numbers, including iodine-53 and calcium-20. The types of images that are produced by DECT are referred to as virtual monochromatic (VMI) images, weighted average (WA) images, and material decomposition maps, also referred to as an iodine map. VMI images are reconstructed images at prescribed energy levels. The image represents what the image would look like if the study was acquired with a monochromatic beam at a given energy. WA images are reconstructed by blending data from low- and high-energy acquisitions using the dual-source scanners. Material decomposition maps display the estimated distribution and quantity of a material of interest based on its elemental composition and unique spectral characteristics, also referred to as the iodine map. In treatment of head and neck cancers, DECT is useful in the evaluation of tumor extension for laryngeal cartilage invasion and characterization of cervical lymph nodes, among other general observations, such as the reduction of dental metal artifacts. In addition, the detection of heavy metals in the body can also be utilized in the evaluation of diffused calcium deposits in the brain, silicone in lymph nodes, and iron deposits in the liver.[27,28]

A special challenge involves bone marrow imaging. Calcium and soft tissue have similar dual-energy attenuation coefficients more than the similarity between calcium and iodine contrast. What does this mean if the imaging of the spine is complicated because of the marrow composition of calcium in the vertebrae? Despite using the iodine-based contrast media, distinguishing marrow from other tissue is difficult. This is especially true for young patients with small anatomy who are subject to motion artifacts.

Emerging Trends in Magnetic Resonance Imaging for Radiation Therapy. What follows is a short preview and brief description of advances in the MRI discipline of medical imaging. Much work with great detail on functional and molecular MRI techniques that assess physiological and functional parameters relevant to tumor biology such as diffusion, perfusion, and oxygenation has been published. These advances offer new ways and improved methods of tumor delineation, confirming dosimetry or guiding patient-specific adaptive radiation therapy treatment planning, thereby offering safe dose escalation and/or reducing toxicity to normal tissue as compared with standard ultrasound or CT- or MRI-based imaging techniques.

One limitation identified with standard MRI occurs when the morphologic appearance of residual or recurrent disease overlaps with normal anatomy, or with treated tissue that has changed its morphology. Functional and molecular MR imaging has new capabilities of identifying these different tissue types.

Previous work includes advances with dynamic contrast-enhanced MRI and diffusion-weighted MRI that identify and demonstrate changes in tissue perfusion and the "Brownian motion" of water molecules leading to enhanced radiation therapy response assessment.[29] To clarify, perfusion is the transport or passage of fluid through the circulatory system or lymphatic system to an organ or a tissue, usually referring to the delivery of blood to a capillary bed in tissue. Adequate perfusion is a part of a patient's assessment process. Brownian motion or pedesis is the random motion of particles suspended in a fluid or gas resulting from their collision with the quick atoms or molecules in the gas or liquid. This relates to the Wiener process, which is a mathematical model used to describe such Brownian motion, which is often called a particle theory.[30,31]

The most recent advances include intravoxel incoherent motion MRI. Much technical detail is not included in this description; however, the process results in new information on both tissue perfusion and cell density without the use of contrast agents, as is required with conventional methods of perfusion assessment.

Another recent innovation consists of blood oxygenation level–dependent (BOLD) and tissue oxygenation level–dependent

(TOLD) MRI. BOLD measures hypoxia through signal loss in tissue because of "paramagnetic deoxygenated" red blood cells, which generate local magnetic field gradients. TOLD MRI distinguishes oxygenated tissue from hypoxic tissue through a signal increase in oxygenated tissue because of the absence of "paramagnetic deoxyhemoglobin." Differentiating normal from hypoxic tissue guides adaptive radiation therapy planning, since normal tissue may be spared the higher dose required of malignant tissue.[29]

Magnetic resonance spectroscopy has been used to measure metabolism in vivo, but sensitivity is poor, and only hydrogen molecules may be identified. Hyperpolarization increases the MR signal intensity of MR visible nuclei by a factor of 10,000. This greatly improves detection sensitivity, which allows molecules other than hydrogen to be imaged. Hyperpolarization involves enhancing or increasing the polarization levels of the nuclear spin of small molecules. Publications on hyperpolarized MRI for cancer management uses ^{13}C-pyruvate. ^{13}C-pyruvate has been studied to detect treatment response to glioma tumors. The studies involve the level of tumor lactate fraction measurements immediately following a radiation therapy treatment as compared with normal tissue. Studies also involve lactate level measurements before treatment with implanted tumors of squamous cell carcinoma and colon tumors in mice. The studies suggest that hyperpolarized ^{13}C-pyruvate MRI may serve as a useful biomarker to evaluate radiation therapy treatment effects at the early stages of treatment or at various other time points.[29]

The limitations of using these new MRI techniques for treatment planning are being explored. The major factors involve CT as the primary imaging modality in radiation therapy with CT-based calculations of the mass attenuation coefficient as the primary factor for dose calculations. Although advances have been made, MRI is unable to calculate mass attenuation coefficients as accurately as CT. Although research has shown positive implications for radiation therapy treatments, adaptive studies in radiation therapy have not been investigated with the emerging MRI techniques. However, the literature suggests that these methods have unique advantages compared with conventional modalities of medical imaging currently in use.[29]

The Magnetic Resonance Linear Accelerator. The MR-linear accelerator offers real-time MRI of tumor locations during treatment delivery. It is expected to facilitate adaptive treatment planning with real-time assessment to improve the identification of radiosensitive tissue. This is expected to improve conformal beam sculpting, beam modulation, and to improve dose escalation without overdosing normal tissue. In essence, this is expected to improve the therapeutic ratio of aggressive tumors while sparing normal tissue. Technical challenges include the lack of electron density data obtained, which limits the measurement accuracy of dose calculation and the production of secondary electrons caused by the magnetic field within the MR-Linac interferes with the radiation dose distribution. Research continues to improve these challenges with strategies that also include a real-time Monte Carlo approach to account for the influence of the magnetic field on dose calculations.[29]

SUMMARY

- X-rays have a variety of diagnostic and therapeutic purposes, and, because of that, many modalities such as diagnostic radiology, nuclear medicine, mammography, cardiovascular imaging, and CT scanning exist to aid the physician in the precise diagnosis of disease.
- X-rays are capable of causing certain substances to fluoresce, ionizing materials through which they pass, and causing chemical and biologic changes in tissue. These properties are the basis of x-ray interactions with matter.
- In the production of x-rays, electrons are accelerated in a vacuum toward the target and, as the electrons are stopped suddenly, 75% to 80% of the target interaction is bremsstrahlung radiation, released in the form of x-rays.
- Target interactions include bremsstrahlung interactions, which occur with the nucleus, and characteristic radiation, which occurs mostly with inner-shell electrons of the target material.
- In the diagnostic energy range, three interactions occur. Photons may be absorbed photoelectrically or undergo coherent (unmodified) or Compton scattering during an interaction.
- Density is the overall blackening of the film or image receptor. Contrast is the tonal differences (scale of grays) between the blacks and whites on an image.
- Magnification can be measured and expressed as a factor. Magnification on an image receptor is directly proportional to the distance of the object from the target or source and is dependent on the distance of the object from the image receptor.
- CT and MRI scans provide the most useful information for treatment planning purposes in radiation therapy.
- Converting a series of numbers to a viewable image is the basis of digital imaging. The numbers are collected through some method of analog scan, stored, and then reconstructed to form pixels (picture elements). An even more complex system can create a three-dimensional image by using voxels (volume elements) and is the basis for some CT imaging and most MRI imaging. This permits the manipulation of images so that they may be viewed from all aspects.
- Flat panel detectors, with the use of amorphous silicon, are based on solid-state integrated circuit technology and thin-film transistor technology to produce useful digital images.
- MV and kV energy can be used to obtain images; however, kV energy has the advantage of improved image quality and reduced dose to the patient.
- Cone-beam CT uses a larger cone angle than a CT scanner to scan an entire volume of the patient rather than a single slice per rotation.
- Unlike x-rays and CT scans, which use radiation, MRI uses a large magnet and radiofrequency waves to produce an image.
- PET is a form of imaging in which the physiology, metabolism, and biochemistry, rather than the anatomic structure, are displayed in the image. Physiology describes how a tissue, organ, or system may function.
- Ultrasound, also known as *sonography,* is a useful medical imaging tool for delineating surface contours and localizing internal structures such as the prostate gland. In this imaging technique, a transducer is used to generate a mechanical disturbance (pressure wave) that moves through the tissue.

■ REVIEW QUESTIONS

The answers to the Review Questions can be found by logging on to our website at: http://evolve.elsevier.com/Washington+Leaver/principles

1. Which of the following are considered x-ray interactions occurring with (body) matter?

    I. Bremsstrahlung x-rays.

  II. Compton scattering.

 III. Photoelectrical absorption.

 IV. Rectification.

    a. I and II.
    b. II and III.
    c. II, III, and IV.
    d. I, III, and IV.
2. Which of the following best refers to the digital imaging process?
    a. Analog image intensifier.
    b. Flat panel detector.
    c. Bremsstrahlung radiation effect.
    d. Characteristic radiation effect.
3. If a radiograph taken at 120-cm TID produces an image measuring 3.5 cm through the use of a 90-cm TOD, what is the magnification factor?
    a. 0.75.
    b. 1.33.
    c. 2.63.
    d. 4.66.
4. Amorphous silicon is commonly found in:
    a. Intensifying screens.
    b. MRI image receptor.
    c. Flat panel detectors.
    d. X-ray target material.
5. Kilovolt cone-beam CT has certain advantages versus megavoltage cone-beam CT, including:
    a. A Lower dose delivered to the patient.
    b. Ability to use the linear accelerator's MV source to generate x-ray images.
    c. Better contrast of soft tissue and bone.
    d. Both a and c.
6. Image guided radiation therapy can use a number of different imaging modalities to correct for:
    I. Interfraction uncertainty.
    II. Intrafraction uncertainty.
    III. Random error.
    IV. Beam flatness.
       a. I.
       b. I and II.
       c. II and III.
       d. I and IV.
7. In multislice CT, the protocol parameter collimation is:
    a. Detector array size only.
    b. Beam collimation only.
    c. A combination of beam collimation and detector array size.
    d. Neither detector array size nor beam collimation.
8. Black areas on a CT scan represent_____.
    a. Low density.
    b. Medium density (average).
    c. High density
    d. Greater pixel size.
9. A/an _____is an unwanted pattern on an image that does not represent anatomy.
    a. Algorithm.
    b. Filter.
    c. Artifact.
    d. Diode.
10. Spatial resolution is improved by:
    1. Smaller pixel size.
    2. Thicker slices.
    3. Sharp algorithm filter.
       a. 1 and 2.
       b. 2 and 3.
       c. 1 and 3.
       d. 1, 2, and 3.

QUESTIONS TO PONDER

1. What does a spiral beam ratio of 2 to 1 mean in terms of ALARA and exposure to the patient? Explain.
2. What does a spiral beam ratio of 0.5 to 1 mean in terms of ALARA and exposure to the patient? Explain.
3. Compare and contrast bremsstrahlung and characteristic target interactions.
4. Describe the two interactions in (body) matter (keV energy level) that have the most effect in the diagnostic imaging range.
5. Define the terms *pixel* and *voxel* and explain how they relate to digital imaging.
6. Describe how S-R technology works and how it impacted the evolution of CT imaging technology.
7. Describe the basis for PET.
8. Explain to a patient how the CT scanner obtains an images. What do you say to a patient who is concerned about receiving too much dose during their scan?
9. When imaging a pediatric patient, how would you alter the CT scan? What parameters would be altered?

REFERENCES

1. Bushong SC. *Radiologic Science for Technologists: Physics, Biology, and Protection.* 11th ed. St. Louis, MO: Mosby; 2017.
2. Adler AM, Carlton RR. *Introduction to Radiologic and Imaging Sciences and Patient Care.* 7th ed. St. Louis, MO: Elsevier; 2019.
3. Adler AM, Carlton RR. *Introduction to Radiologic and Imaging Sciences and Patient Care.* 6th ed. 6. St. Louis, MO: Elsevier Saunders; 2015.
4. Fauber TL. *Radiographic Imaging and Exposure.* 5th ed. St. Louis, MO: Mosby; 2016.
5. Johnston J, Fauber TL. *Essentials of Radiographic Physics and Imaging.* 2nd ed. St. Louis, MO: Mosby; 2015.
6. Carlton RR, Adler EM. *Principles of Radiographic Imaging: An Art and a Science.* 5th ed. New York, NY: Delmar Cengage Learning; 2012.
7. ICRP. ICRP. Publication 135: diagnostic reference levels in medical imaging. *Ann ICRP.* 2017;46(1):1–44.
8. Pawlicki T, Scanderbeg DJ, Starkschall G. *Hendees' Radiation Therapy Physics.* 4th ed. Hoboken, New Jersey, NJ: Wiley and Sons, Inc.; 2016.
9. Khan FM, Gibbons JP, Sperduto PW. *Khan's Treatment Planning in Radiation Oncology.* 4th ed. Philadelphia, PA: Wolters Kluwer; 2016.
10. Rist C, Belka C, Cyran CC, et al. Visualization, imaging and new preclinical diagnostics in radiation oncology. *US National Library of Medicine.* 2014;9(3):1–15.
11. Kim A, Sahgal A, Keller BM, Al-Ward S, Lim-Reinders S. Online adaptive radiation therapy. *Int J Radiat Oncol Biol Phys.* 2017;99(4):994–1003.
12. Pereira GC, Traughber M, Muzic RF Jr. The role of imaging in radiation therapy planning: past, present, and future. *BioMed Res Int.* 2014;2014:231090.

13. Kanal E, Barkovich AJ, Bell C, et al. ACR guidance document on MR safe practices: 2013. *J Magn Reson Imaging.* 2013;37:501–530.

14. Glaudemans AWJM, de Vries EFJ, Galli F, Dierckx RAJO, Slart RHJA, Signore A. The use of ¹⁸F-FDG-PET/CT for diagnosis and treatment monitoring of inflammatory and infectious diseases. *Clin Dev Immunol.* 2013;2013:623036.

15. Mikhaeel NG, Yeoh K. Are we ready for positron emission tomography/computed tomography-based target volume definition in lymphoma radiation therapy? *Int J Radiat Oncol Biol Phys.* 2012;85(1):14–20.

16. Celebic A, Auperin A, Ruelle C, et al. Role of FDG-PET in the implementation of involved-node radiation therapy for Hodgkin lymphoma patients. *Int J Radiat Oncol Biol Phys.* 2014;89(5):1047–1052.

17. Sattler B, Cal-Gonzales J, Rausch I, Quick HH, Boellaard R, Beyer T. Technical and instrumentational foundations of PET/MRI. *Int J Radiat Oncol Biol Phys.* 2017;94(1):A3–A13.

18. Mohamed ASR, Fuller CD, Hansen C, et al. Prospective analysis of in vivo landmark point-based MRI geometric distortion in head and neck cancer patients scanned in immobilized radiation treatment position: results of a prospective quality assurance protocol. *Clin Transl Radiat Oncol.* 2017;7:13–19.

19. Pasternak JJ, Williamson EE. Clinical pharmacology, uses, and adverse reactions of iodinated contrast agents: a primer for the non-radiologist. *Mayo Clin Proc.* 2012;87(4):390–402.

20. Ranga A, Agarwal Y, Garg KJ. Gadolinium based contrast agents in current practice: risks of accumulation and toxicity in patients with normal renal function. *Indian J Radiol Imaging.* 2017;27(2):141–147.

21. Murphy KJ, Brunberg JA, Cohan RH. Adverse reactions to gadolinium contrast media: Aa 1996 review of 36 cases. *Am J Roentgenol.* 1996;167(4):847–849.

22. US Food and Drug Administration. FDA drug safety communication: FDA warns that gadolinium-based contrast agents (GBCAs) are retained in the body; requires new class warnings. https://www.fda.gov/Drugs/DrugSafety/ucm589213.htm; 2018. Accessed January 15, 2019.

23. Mehanna H, McConkey CC, Rahman JK, et al. PET-CT surveillance versus neck dissection in advanced hand and neck cancer. *N Engl J Med.* 2016;374(15):1444–1454.

24. Marcu LG, Moghaddasi L, Bezak E. Imaging of tumor characteristics and molecular pathways with PET: developments over the last decade toward personalized cancer therapy. *Int J Radiat Oncol Biol Phys.* 2018;102(4):1165–1182.

25. McKay MJ, Taubman KL, Foroudi F, et al. Molecular imaging using PET/CT for radiotherapy planning of adult cancers: current status and expanding applications. *Int J Radiat Oncol Biol Phys.* 2018;102(4):783–791.

26. Yang X, Wang T, Ghavidel B, et al. Optimal virtual monochromatic image in "twin beam" imaging of dual-energy CT for head and neck cancer radiation therapy. *Int J Radiat Oncol Biol Phys.* 2018;102(3S):S104–S105.

27. Krauss B. Dual-energy computed tomography technology and challenges. *Radiol Clin N Am.* 2018;56:497–506.

28. Yabuuchi H, Kamitani T, Sagiyama K, et al. Clinical application of radiation dose reduction for head and neck CT. *Eur J Radiol.* 2018;107:209–215.

29. Jones KM, Michel KA, Bankson JA, et al. Emerging magnetic resonance imaging technologies for radiation therapy planning and response assessment. *Int J Radiat Oncol Biol Phys.* 2018;101(5):1046–1056.

30. Dictionary.com Unabridged (v 1.1). from Dictionary.com website: http://dictionary.reference.com/browse/perfusion. Assessed January 15, 2019

31. Thomas DL, Lythgoe MF, Pell GS, et al. The measurement of diffusion and perfusion in biological systems using magnetic resonance imaging. *Phys Med Biol.* 2000;45(8):R97–R138.

7

Treatment Delivery Equipment

Amy Heath

OBJECTIVES

- Discuss the historic development of radiation therapy treatment delivery equipment.
- Compare and contrast the clinical applications of kilovoltage equipment, including superficial treatments and orthovoltage therapy.
- Describe the four major components of the linear accelerator stand: the klystron, waveguide, circulator, and cooling system.
- Explain how x-rays are produced in the linear accelerator.
- Describe the major components located in the gantry of the linear accelerator, including the electron gun, accelerator structure (guide), and treatment head.
- Explain the concept of indexing as it applies to patient immobilization and positioning.
- Identify where multileaf collimators are located in the treatment head, and explain how they operate.
- Describe the importance of the robotic couch in the implementation of intensity-modulated radiation therapy and image-guided radiation therapy.
- Discuss the characteristics of a cobalt-60 treatment unit.
- Describe several modern trends in radiation therapy treatment delivery equipment.
- Discuss medical accelerator safety considerations.

OUTLINE

KEY TERMS

Accelerator structure
Beam-flattening filter
Bending magnet
Circulator
Dose maximum (D_{max})
Dynamic wedge
Electron gun
Electronic portal imaging device

Gantry
Interlocks
Isodose line
Klystron
Linear accelerator
Magnetron
Microwaves
Multileaf collimator

OVERVIEW OF TREATMENT DELIVERY EQUIPMENT

While there are many different types of radiation oncology treatment devices, the linear accelerator is by far the most popular treatment machine used in radiation oncology. These machines have evolved to deliver both photon and electron beams in a variety of methods external beam radiation therapy (EBRT). X-ray beam energy used in linear accelerators ranges from as low as 60 kilovoltage (kV) (to check patient positioning) to as high as 25 megavoltage (MV) (for treatment). Photon beams consist of x-rays or gamma rays. The majority of cancer treatment today, that uses electrons, protons, and x-rays, is delivered with the use of MV treatment beams in the range of 6 to 25 MV.

The linear accelerator has evolved in the past 10 years and continues to do so, mostly because of advances in computer technology. Computer technology advances included a faster central processing unit (CPU), allowing the computer to run more efficiently, reconstruct digital images with greater speed, and provide more stability and safety features to the overall treatment delivery process. This speed has doubled approximately every 18 months since the 1970s. According to Moore's law, the number of transistors incorporated in a computer chip will approximately double every 24 months.[34] For example, the first computer processor, released in 1971, was the Intel 4004. This was only a 740-kHz processor and was only capable of processing 92,000 instructions per second. Current processors are multicore GHz processors that can process more than 100 billion instructions per second.[12] This advance in speed has also allowed linear accelerators to increase the focus of radiation with greater accuracy to a moving target, a changing target, or both, and at the same time, reduce the dose to surrounding healthy tissue. Today, linear accelerators use sophisticated treatment planning programs and multileaf collimators (MLCs) to focus the dose to the tumor volume with intensity-modulated radiation therapy (IMRT), volumetric-modulated arc therapy (VMAT), stereotactic radiosurgery (SRS), and stereotactic body radiation therapy (SBRT) beams. High-dose, flattening filter-free (FFF) beams have allowed increased dose rates in the several thousand monitor units (MU)/minute (Varian TrueBeam and Halcyon, Accuray's TomoTherapy, Radixact, and CyberKnife).[1,14,50] Image-guided radiation therapy (IGRT) has taken advantage of advances in kV imaging (an imaging device that consists of a flat panel detector and a simple x-ray tube that has become very useful in improving the application of radiation therapy dose delivery) equipment and image reconstruction technology (faster CPUs, multicore processors, and more computer storage) to more efficiently evaluate the accuracy of treatment delivery. With the increase in computer technology, Van Dyke[49] mentions several modern trends in radiation therapy treatment delivery that have evolved and continue to do so, including:

- Increased concern about uncertainties and errors in radiation oncology.
- Increased doses per fraction (hypofractionation).
- Increased imaging for radiation therapy planning, guidance, and monitoring.
- More emphasis on dose volume end points (normal tissue complications) for treatment planning (inverse planning).
- Increased educational and regulatory requirements.
- Financial resource considerations and cost-benefit analysis.
- Future technology developments that include more sophisticated treatment planning algorithms, more compact machines, and more patient-focused three-dimensional (3D)/four-dimensional quality assurance.

This chapter introduces the student to a variety of radiation therapy equipment, including low-energy machines such as superficial equipment, and orthovoltage machines. Characteristics of cobalt-60 (^{60}Co) are also discussed. A large portion of the chapter provides a detailed overview of the operation of the linear accelerator, including several modern trends in radiation therapy treatment delivery equipment.

EQUIPMENT DEVELOPMENT

Conventional low-energy equipment, which typically uses x-rays generated at voltages as high as 300-kV(p) (kV peak), have been used in radiation therapy since the turn of the twentieth century. These kV units (low x-ray voltage radiation therapy treatment machines) include Grenz, contact, superficial, and orthovoltage machines. The use of this equipment dramatically decreased after 1950. This decrease was in part the result of the increased popularity of ^{60}Co units and the subsequent development of the linear accelerator (a radiation therapy treatment machine that uses high-frequency electromagnetic waves to accelerate charged particles, such as electrons, to high energies via a linear tube). However, kV equipment is still used in many departments today, in part because of the low cost and simplicity of design compared with MV units. The primary application of kV equipment is in the treatment of skin and superficial lesions.

The introduction of MV therapy equipment, which generates x-ray beams of 1 MV or higher, was a natural progression from low-energy units. Although kV units were and are beneficial, they still have two principal limitations that are clinically essential: they cannot reach deep-seated malignancies with an adequate dosage of radiation, and they do not spare skin and normal tissue. In addition, because the photoelectric effect is the dominant interaction in this energy range, the dose is heavily deposited in high Z (atomic number) materials, such as bone. Treating tumors behind or near bones with these machines is difficult and can lead to long-term complications. As a result of these shortcomings, manufacturers began concentrating their efforts on addressing these and other shortcomings of low-energy equipment.

The early to middle part of the twentieth century marked a period of tremendous development of the equipment used to treat tumors (Fig. 7.1). The medical physics community began experimenting with the acceleration of electrons, protons, neutrons, and heavy ions. An attempt was made in medicine to find a better way to deliver a curative dose of radiation therapy. In North America, the Van de Graaff (1937), betatron (1941), ^{60}Co (1951), and linear accelerator (1952) were introduced.[24]

Until the early to mid-1950s, most cancer patients undergoing radiation therapy were treated with low-energy equipment. Physicians did their best with the equipment available to them, but it was difficult to deliver a high-enough dose of radiation needed for tumor control without causing significant toxicities. As a result, surgery was still the treatment of choice for most cancers.

CHARACTERISTICS OF KILOVOLTAGE X-RAY EQUIPMENT

Central axis depth dose and physical penumbra are related to beam quality. In treatment planning, the central-axis-depth dose distribution for a specific beam depends on the beam's energy. The depth of an

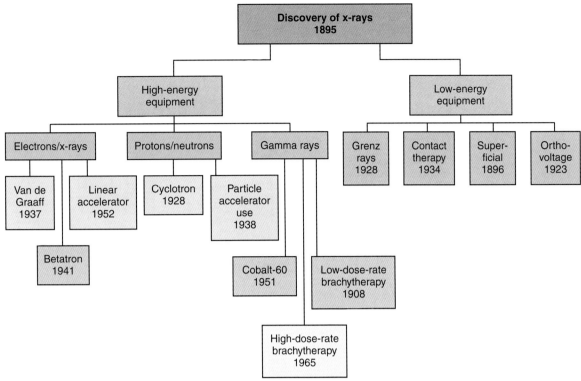

Fig. 7.1 A timetable chart illustrates the development of high- and low-energy treatment equipment since the discovery of x-rays in 1895. Every effort has been made in researching the accuracy of the information in this chart. However, several sources and experts in the field sometimes disagree about the exact dates that equipment was introduced clinically. (For more information, refer to Bentel C. *Radiation Therapy Planning*, New York, NY: McGraw-Hill;1993; and Grigg EM. *The Trail of the Invisible Light.* Springfield, IL: Charles C Thomas; 1965.)

isodose curve increases with beam quality. For example, a 50% isodose line (a line representing various points of similar value in a beam along the central axis and elsewhere) for a 200-kVp beam reaches a deeper tumor than a 50% isodose curve of a 100-kVp orthovoltage beam. Orthovoltage beams demonstrate an increased scatter dose to the tissue outside the treatment region, thus exhibiting a marked disadvantage compared with MV beams.[32] In other words, the absorbed dose in the medium outside the primary beam is greater for low-energy beams than for those of a higher energy.[26] Limited scatter outside the field for MV beams occurs because of predominantly forward scattering of the beam. Superficial treatment and orthovoltage units are extremely reliable and free of electromechanical problems. This contributes to a lack of downtime, which is a problem more often with MV treatment machines.

CLINICAL APPLICATIONS OF KILOVOLTAGE EQUIPMENT

Superficial Treatments

Superficial therapy relates to treatments with x-rays produced at potentials ranging from 40 to 150 kV.[26,31] Usually, 1- to 6-mm-thick aluminum filters are inserted in a slot in the treatment head to harden the beam by filtering out very low photons. The degree of hardening is measured in half-value layers (HVLs). Typical HVLs used in superficial treatments range from 1 to 8 mm of Al.[26,27] Skin cancer and tumors no deeper than 0.5 cm can be treated with superficial treatments because of the rapid falloff of the radiation dose (Fig. 7.2).

Superficial treatment administration uses a cone or applicator, which is attached to the diaphragm of the treatment head by the radiation therapist. Cone sizes are generally 2 to 5 cm in diameter, and

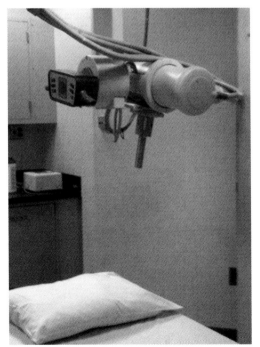

Fig. 7.2 Superficial treatment unit. (Courtesy Linda Alfred.)

lead cutouts are tailored to fit the treatment area if needed. The lead cutout will be placed on the skin. The cone then lies directly on the skin (or lead cutout) with a source skin distance (SSD) of 15 to 20 cm.[26] Because no standard treatment table comes with the system, the patient can lie on a stretcher or sit in a chair for treatment. Three parameters are set at the console area for treatment delivery: kV, mA (x-ray current

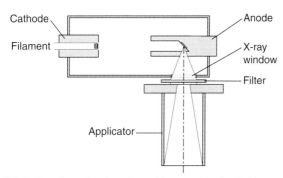

Fig. 7.3 Orthovoltage treatment machine used to treat skin cancers. (From Mills JA, Porter H, Gill D. Radiotherapy beam production. In: Symonds P, Deehan C, Mills JA, et al. *Walter and Miller's Textbook of Radiotherapy: Radiation Physics, Therapy and Oncology.* 7th ed. London, UK: Churchill Livingstone; 2012.)

measured in milliamperes), and treatment time. Patients are monitored through a lead glass window and with as audio contact.

Orthovoltage Therapy

Orthovoltage therapy describes treatment with x-rays produced at potentials ranging from 100 to 500 kV.[26] Most orthovoltage equipment operates at 200 to 300 kV and 10 to 20 mA. Much like the superficial units, orthovoltage units use filters designed to achieve HVLs from 1 to 4 mm of copper.[6,26,27] Aluminum and Thoraeus filters may also be used. Thoraeus filters are made of tin, copper, and aluminum. The filter is placed so that tin is closest to the x-ray tube, absorbing the lowest-energy photons. Copper and aluminum then absorb characteristic x-rays caused by the transmission through the filter, as well as other low-energy photons that are missed.[45] Orthovoltage units use cones to collimate the beam or a movable diaphragm consisting of lead plates can be used to adjust the field size. Lead cutouts placed on the skin may further shape the field. Conventionally, the SSD is 50 cm (Fig. 7.3).[26]

The types of tumors treated with orthovoltage units include skin, mouth, and rectal carcinoma (with the use of cones inserted into the patient). As with superficial treatments, the average treatment time can range from seconds to several minutes, depending on the filtered kV, prescribed dose, collimator, or cone size. The penetrating depth depends on the kV and filter. Usually, orthovoltage units experience limitation in the treatment of lesions deeper than 2 to 3 cm.

Orthovoltage units are still present in some clinics and hospitals. They are reliable alternatives to the use of electrons in the treatment of many superficial skin lesions. Most skin lesions treated with orthovoltage units are squamous cell and basal cell cancers, as well as benign keloids. Some clinicians prefer the orthovoltage unit for treating skin tumors because of beam characteristics, especially treatments requiring small fields.

> The 100- to 300-kV x-ray beam is usually more effective to treat superficial tumors such as skin cancer because it limits the dose to normal tissue underneath. However, orthovoltage therapy is not as easy to find today in many radiation therapy centers because of the increased emphasis on new methods of treating patients such as 3D-conformal radiation therapy (3D-CRT), intensity-modulated radiation therapy, and volumetric-modulated arc therapy.

MEGAVOLTAGE EQUIPMENT

Treatment delivery machines producing x- X-ray beams of 1 MV or greater can be classified as MV equipment. Examples of clinical MV machines are accelerators such as the linear accelerator. Cobalt-60 units, popular in developing countries, are also classified as *MV treatment units.*

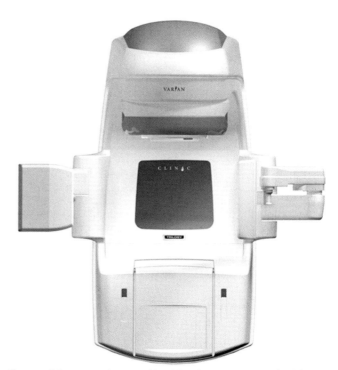

Fig. 7.4 A linear accelerator with a kilovoltage source on the left and a flat panel detector on the right. (Courtesy Varian Medical Systems, Palo Alto, CA.)

Linear Accelerator

The term *linear accelerator* means that charged particles travel in straight lines while they gain energy from an alternating electromagnetic field. The linear accelerator (Fig. 7.4) is distinguished from other types of particle accelerators, such as the cyclotron, in which the particles travel in a spiral pattern, and the older outdated betatron, in which the particles travel in a circular pattern.[32]

In the linear accelerator, x-rays and electrons are generated and used to treat a variety of tumors. The accelerator structure (guide), which resembles a length of pipe, is the basic element of the linear accelerator. The accelerating structure (guide) allows electrons produced from a hot cathode (electron gun) to gain energy until they exit the far end of the hollow structure.[28] Understanding of the proper use of this equipment is significant to the radiation therapist because it is one of the essential tools that enables the radiation therapist to deliver a prescribed dose of radiation.

Aspects of the linear accelerator that are discussed in this section include a history of the linear accelerator, its design features, and a description of the major components. An explanation of the key components in a linear accelerator provides a basic overview of its operation and will aid in the student's understanding of this complex piece of equipment. These components include the klystron, waveguide, circulator, water-cooling system, electron gun, accelerating structure (guide), bending magnet (used in high-energy linear accelerators to bend the electron stream at a variety of angles so that it is pointed at the target), flattening filter, scattering foil, and other accessories.

History. The first 100-cm source-axis distance (SAD) "fully isocentric" linear accelerator was manufactured in the United States and installed in 1961 (Fig. 7.5). Compared with kV machines or other MV machines, the linear accelerator can generate higher-energy beams with greater skin sparing; sharper, more defined field edges with less penumbra; treatment beams shaped with computer technology, and they can decrease the exposure to personnel from radiation leakage.

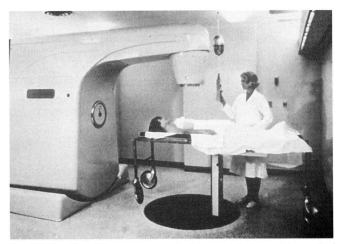

Fig. 7.5 The first 100-cm source-axis-distance fully isocentric medical linear accelerator manufactured in the United States in 1961 by Varian Associates. (Courtesy Varian Medical Systems, Palo Alto, CA.)

Development. The development of the linear accelerator has its roots in England and the United States. In these countries, many men and women have contributed significantly to the research and development of the linear accelerator. The magnetron and klystron proved an invaluable and important component in today's high-energy linear accelerator. The klystron is a form of radiowave amplifier that greatly multiplies the amount of introduced radiowaves. The magnetron and klystron are two special types of electron tubes that are used to provide microwave power to accelerate electrons. Microwaves are similar to ordinary radiowaves but have frequencies thousands of times higher. The microwave frequencies needed for linear accelerator operation are approximately 3 million cycles per second (3000 MHz).[28] A major difference between the klystron and magnetron is that a klystron is a linear-beam microwave amplifier requiring an external oscillator or radiofrequency (RF) source (driver), whereas the magnetron is an oscillator and amplifier. The introduction of the magnetron and klystron assisted in the transfer of energy needed to accelerate electrons, which in turn were converted to high-energy x-rays used in the medical application of the linear accelerator in the treatment of malignant disease.

Medical Application. In the late 1940s, the chief radiologist of Stanford's x-ray department, Dr. Henry Kaplan, became interested in the medical application of the linear accelerator. Work on a linear accelerator had also begun in England, but the Stanford University project proved most practical, in part because of the support of President Eisenhower in 1959 and subsequent funding by the U.S. Congress in 1961.

In 1948, the British Ministry of Health brought together the three main groups who were working on the linear accelerator project in England—the Medical Research Council, headed by Dr. L.H. Gray; the Atomic Energy Research Establishment, headed by D.W. Fry; and the Metropolitan Vickers Electric Company (later to become Associate Electrical Industries), led by C.W. Miller. The resulting linear accelerator was installed at Hammersmith Hospital in London in June 1952. The first treatment was delivered on August 19, 1953, with an 8-MV photon beam. Another 4-MV linear accelerator was installed at Newcastle General Hospital in August 1953, and another was installed at Christie Hospital in Manchester, England in October 1954. The first single gantry unit (Fig. 7.6) could be rotated over an arc of 120 degrees by lowering part of the treatment room floor.[29]

The linear accelerator was introduced in England and the United States in the 1950s. In England, a 2-MV magnetron and 3-m stationary accelerator were used to produce an output of 100 cGy/min with the 8-MV machine.[29] This was a major achievement, even by today's standards. In the United

States, a linear accelerator was first clinically used at Stanford University Hospital in January 1956 to treat a child suffering from retinoblastoma.[22]

A joint venture between the British industrial team and the Stanford University group under the direction of C.S. Nunan produced the first ergonomic linear accelerator (a 6-MV, isocentric linear accelerator with the ability to rotate 360 degrees around a patient lying supine on the treatment couch).

The evolution of the linear accelerator is discussed in this section with reference to three types of linear accelerators: the early linear accelerators (produced in 1953–1961); second-generation, 360-degree rotational units (produced 1962–1982); and new computer-driven, third-generation treatment machines.

Early Accelerators. The early linear accelerators were extremely large and bulky compared with today's design features. In 1952, the first linear accelerator was installed at Hammersmith Hospital in London and had an 8-MV x-ray beam and limited gantry motion. Several other linear accelerators with improved design features were also installed in England in the early to mid-1950s. As mentioned previously, the Stanford University linear accelerator in the United States treated its first patient in 1956. Since then, several manufacturers have designed and built linear accelerators for clinical purposes.

Second-Generation Accelerators. Second-generation linear accelerators can be referred to as the older, 360-degree rotational units, which are less sophisticated than their modern offspring. These isocentric units, some of which are still operational today, allow treatment to a patient from any gantry angle. They offered an improvement in accuracy and dose delivery versus the extremely early models, primarily because of their 360-degree rotational ability around an isocenter.

Second-generation linear accelerators are similar to some older cars on the road today. They may have more bumps, dents, and high mileage. They may work well at times but usually require a considerable amount of maintenance. An older car has the same basic components as a newer one, such as an engine, transmission, and operator's panel (with fewer knobs and buttons), to accomplish the task. A third-generation linear accelerator is similar to the newer car of today. The newer car is equipped with many of the basic components of the older, less-sophisticated automobile but has added features, such as an aerodynamic design, antilock brakes, and computer-integrated components.

Third-Generation Accelerators. In general, third-generation accelerators have improved accelerator structures (guides), magnet systems, and beam-modifying systems to provide wide ranges of beam energy, dose rate, field size, and operating modes with improved beam characteristics. These accelerators are highly reliable and have compact design features. Today, linear accelerators account for more than 80% of all operational MV treatment units in the world.[30]

Third-generation computer-driven linear accelerators are available with a wide variety of options, which may include dual-photon energies, dynamic wedging, multileaf collimation, a choice of several electron energies, electronic portal verification systems, and image-guided apparatus (kV x-ray generator and imaging flat panel detector).[28,32,51] Because of the advances in 3D treatment planning, some new linear accelerators provide additional features. Before some of these newer features are discussed, a basic understanding of components and design features of a linear accelerator are necessary.

Linear Accelerator Components

A typical linear accelerator consists of a drive stand, gantry, treatment couch, and console electronic cabinet. Some linear accelerators may also have a modulator cabinet, which contains components that distribute and monitor primary electrical power and high-voltage pulses to the magnetron or klystron. Each of the components is critical to

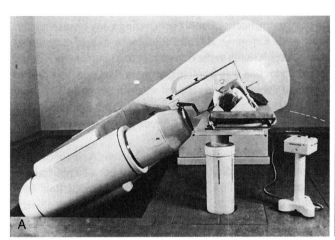
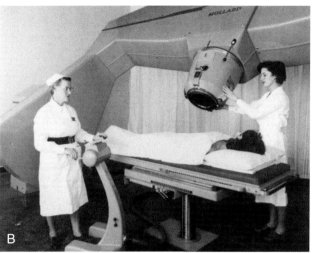

Fig. 7.6 (A) The first single gantry unit installed at Christie Hospital in Manchester, England, in October 1954. It could rotate over an arc of 120 degrees by lowering part of the treatment floor. (B) The first clinical linear accelerator manufactured by Mullard (later purchased by Phillips Medical Systems) in the United Kingdom, circa 1953. (A, Courtesy Christie Hospital, Manchester. B, Courtesy Phillips Medical Systems, Shelton, CT.)

TABLE 7.1 Major Components of the Linear Accelerator

Component	Purpose
Electron gun	Source of electrons to be accelerated, injects electrons into accelerating structure
Magnetron	Source of microwave power in machines ≤10 MV
Klystron	Amplifies microwaves (supplied by radiofrequency [RF] driver) in machines >10 MV
Waveguide	Carries microwave power from its source to the accelerating waveguide
Circulator	Prevents backflow of microwaves into klystron
Accelerating structure	Accelerates electrons through multiple coupled cavities in a linear fashion
Bending magnet	Magnet system that focuses and directs the electron beam from the accelerating structure toward the treatment head
Target	Placed in electron beam to create an x-ray beam
Primary collimator	Shapes the beam; sets maximum field size of the beam at isocenter
Carrousel	Houses scattering foils and flattening filter, moves specific component into beam as needed
Scattering foils	Scatter electrons to create a uniform beam of electrons for treatment
Flattening filter	Flattens the x-ray beam exiting the target
Monitor chambers	Ionization chambers in the treatment head that measure dose, beam flatness and symmetry
Secondary collimators	Jaws of the machine, sets field size of the beam; often asymmetric

From Bourland JD. Radiation oncology physics. In: Gunderson S, Tepper J, eds. *Clinical Radiation Oncology.* 4th ed. Philadelphia, PA: Elsevier.

the total function and operation of the linear accelerator. Table 7.1 describes each major component of the linear accelerator and its function.[7]

Design Features

In the treatment room, the major components of a linear accelerator can be divided into three specific areas: drive stand, gantry, and

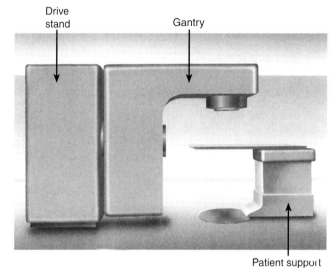

Fig. 7.7 The major components of a linear accelerator include a drive stand, gantry, patient support assembly (treatment couch), control console (not shown), and modulator cabinet (also not shown). (Courtesy Robert Morton and Medical Physics Publishing, Madison, WI.)

treatment couch (Fig. 7.7). A typical treatment room is designed with thick concrete walls for shielding purposes. In this space, the gantry is mounted to the drive stand, which is secured to the floor. Most radiation therapy machines have three rotating parts: gantry, collimator, and couch. The treatment unit is positioned in a way that permits 360-degree rotation of the gantry. A treatment couch is mounted on a rotational axis around the isocenter. This permits the positioning of a patient lying supine or prone on the treatment couch. One ceiling and two side lasers project small dots or lines onto predetermined marks (established during the simulation process) on the patient. Sometimes a fourth midsagittal laser is mounted opposite the drive stand, high on the wall in a way that directs a continuous line along the sagittal axis of the patient. This laser may be used to position the patient's midsagittal plane along the long axis of the treatment couch. One or more closed-circuit television cameras may be mounted on the wall of the treatment room to enable the radiation therapist to monitor the patient

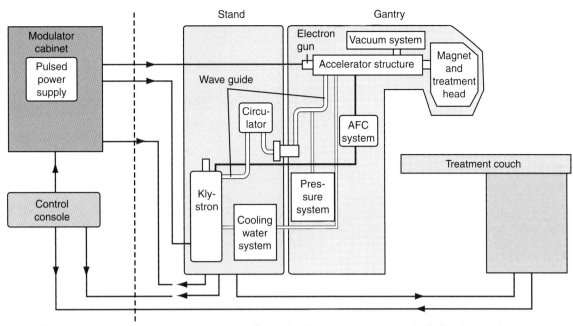

Fig. 7.8 Block diagram of a linear accelerator illustrating the major components, including the stand, gantry, treatment couch, modulator cabinet, and control console. *AFC,* Automatic frequency control. (Courtesy Robert Morton and Medical Physics Publishing, Madison, WI.)

during treatment. Computer monitors are also mounted in the room to view patient setup instructions and treatment machine parameters.

Drive Stand. The gantry rotates on a horizontal axis on bearings within the drive stand, which is firmly secured to the floor in the treatment room. The drive stand appears as a large, rectangular cabinet, at least as large as the gantry. As its name indicates, the drive stand is a stand containing the apparatus that drives the linear accelerator. The drive stand can open on both sides with swinging doors for easy access to gauges, valves, tanks, and buttons. Some facilities house the stand behind a false wall in the treatment vault to improve the aesthetics of the room, shield noise, and to make the room less intimidating to patients. Four major components are housed in the stand: the klystron or magnetron, waveguide, circulator, and cooling system (Fig. 7.8).

Treatment machines are either equipped with a magnetron or klystron, both serving as the source of microwave power used to accelerate electrons.[28] Magnetrons are capable of producing microwaves and are used in low-energy treatment machines. Klystrons, on the other hand, amplify microwaves and require a separate RF driver. Klystrons are used in high-energy linear accelerators (>10 MeV).[7] Although magnetrons are less expensive than klystrons, klystrons last longer. Once created and amplified, the microwave power is directed toward the waveguide, much like a copper wire delivers electricity to an outlet in a home. However, the waveguide is a hollow, tubelike structure that may be rectangular or cylindrical in shape. A circulator is placed between the klystron and the waveguide. It directs the RF energy into the waveguide and prevents any reflected microwaves from returning to the klystron, which could lead to damage and breakdown. The circulator acts much like the valves found in human veins and the lymphatic system, which are designed to prevent the backflow of blood and lymphatic fluid.[26,28,32]

The water-cooling system, which is actually a thermal stability system, allows many components in the gantry and drive stand to operate at a constant temperature. The cold water carries excess heat away from these components, as well as keeps them at a constant temperature. Components cooled by circulating water include the accelerator structure, klystron, circulator, target, and other important assemblies and components. Often the water-cooling system is part of

the hospital or medical center's water supply that may first be filtered through a "chiller," which cools the water before it reaches the treatment machine.[32] Ultimately, the microwaves from the magnetron or klystron are directed to the accelerator structure by the hollow-tubed waveguide where the microwaves work to speed up electrons.

> If the engineering department within the hospital needed to shut down the water supply to the radiation therapy department temporarily to repair a valve in another part of the hospital, what would happen? Discuss with other students in your class what impact a lack of water would have on the safe operation of a linear accelerator.

Gantry. The gantry is responsible primarily for directing the photon (x-ray) or electron beam at a patient's tumor. It can accomplish this goal through rotational fields or fixed fields positioned at the isocenter. For isocentric-type treatment, this point is usually positioned in the patient's tumor or clinical target volume. With newer treatment couches, as much as six degrees of translations of the treatment couch (left/right, up/down, and in/out, pitch, roll, and rotational movement) move the patient in relationship to the isocenter, thus allowing for precise patient positioning (Fig. 7.9). The standard couch is equipped with four degrees of translation (left/right, up/down, in/out, and rotational movement).[42]

The controls to the gantry motions are located on a control pendant(s) or the dedicated keyboard outside the room at the console area. Digital readings are also displayed at various locations on the machine, pendant, computer monitors, or console. Gantry angle, collimator rotation, field size (defined by the X_1, X_2, Y_1, and Y_2 collimators or jaws), and additional information are commonly displayed for easy reference at the base of the gantry or on a separate monitor located in the treatment room.

> The major components in the gantry are the electron gun, accelerator structure (guide), and treatment head (Fig. 7.10).

Electron Gun. The electron gun is responsible for producing electrons and injecting them into the accelerator structure. Electron

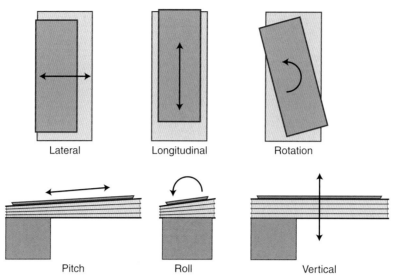

Lateral   Longitudinal   Rotation

Pitch   Roll   Vertical

Fig. 7.9 Six degrees of freedom equipped on a modern robotic treatment couch include: vertical, lateral, and longitudinal movement; pitch; roll; and rotation.

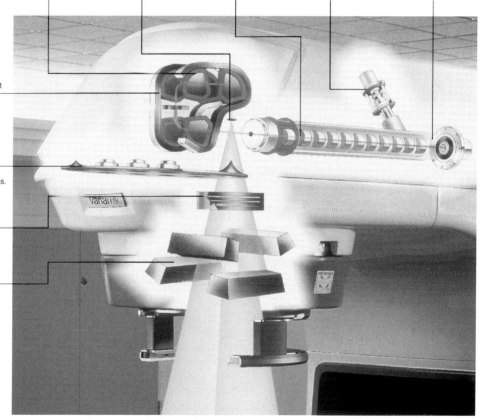

Steering System
Radial and transverse steering coils and a real-time feedback system ensure beam symmetry to within ±2% at all gantry angles.

Focal Spot Size
Even at maximum dose rate, the circular focal remains less than 3.0 mm, held constant by the achromatic bending magnet. Ensures optimal image quality for portal imaging.

Standing Wave Accelerator Guide
Maintains optimal bunching for different acceleration conditions, providing high dose rates, stable dosimetry, and low-stray radiation. Transport system minimizes power and electron source demands.

Energy Switch
Patented switch provides energies within the full therapeutic range, at consistently high, stable dose rates, even with low energy X-ray beams. Ensures optimal performance and spectral purity at both energies.

Gridded Electron Gun
Controls dose rate rapidly and accurately. Permits precise beam control for dynamic treatments because gun can be gated. Demountable, for cost-efffective replacement.

Achromatic Dual-Plane Bending Magnet
Unique design with ±3% energy slits ensures exact replication of the input beam for every treatment. Clinac 2300C/D design enhancements allow wider range of beam energies.

10-Port Carousel with Scattering Foils/Flattening Filters
Extra ports allow future specialized beams to be developed. New electron scattering foils provide homogeneous electron beams at therapeutic depths.

Ion Chamber
Two independently sealed chambers, impervious to temperature and pressure changes, monitor beam dosimetry to within 2% for long-term consistency and stability.

Asymmetric Jaws
Four independent collimators provide flexible beam definition of symmetric or asymmetric fields.

Fig. 7.10 The major components of the gantry include the electron gun, accelerator guide, and treatment head, which includes components such as the bending magnet, beam-flattening filter, ion chamber, and upper-lower collimator jaws. (Courtesy Varian Medical Systems, Palo Alto, CA.)

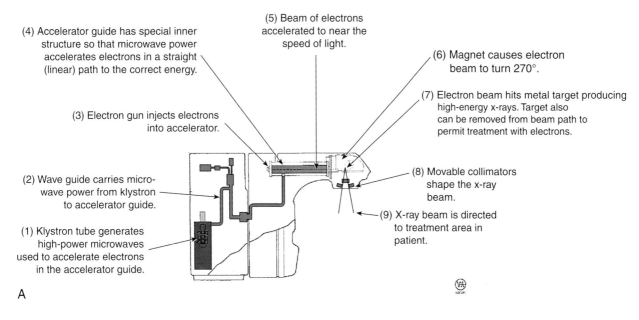

(4) Accelerator guide has special inner structure so that microwave power accelerates electrons in a straight (linear) path to the correct energy.

(5) Beam of electrons accelerated to near the speed of light.

(6) Magnet causes electron beam to turn 270°.

(3) Electron gun injects electrons into accelerator.

(7) Electron beam hits metal target producing high-energy x-rays. Target also can be removed from beam path to permit treatment with electrons.

(2) Wave guide carries micro-wave power from klystron to accelerator guide.

(8) Movable collimators shape the x-ray beam.

(1) Klystron tube generates high-power microwaves used to accelerate electrons in the accelerator guide.

(9) X-ray beam is directed to treatment area in patient.

A

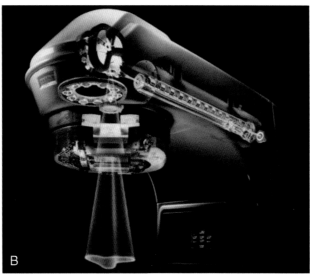

B

Fig. 7.11 (A) This high-energy radiation therapy treatment machine illustrates the horizontally mounted accelerator structure and 270-degree bending magnet. (B) The horizontally mounted accelerator structure and treatment head depict the path of the electron and x-ray beam. (Courtesy Varian Medical Systems, Palo Alto, CA.)

production in a linear accelerator is similar to that in a diagnostic x-ray tube. In the linear accelerator, the cathode is a spherically shaped structure made of a material with a high atomic number, such as tungsten. Tungsten is the element of choice because of the high temperatures required (between 800°C and 1100°C). As the cathode is heated, electrons are boiled off (thermionic emission) and enter the accelerator structure.[28]

Accelerator Structure. The accelerator structure, sometimes called the *accelerating waveguide or guide,* can be mounted in the gantry horizontally, as illustrated in Fig. 7.11 (high-energy machines), or vertically, as illustrated in Fig. 7.12 (low-energy machines). The accelerator structure accelerates and bunches the electrons after they are created by the electron gun. Microwave power (produced in the klystron or magnetron) is transported to the accelerating structure, by the hollow-tubed waveguide, and in the accelerator structure corrugations are used to slow the waves (sometimes analogous to small jetties at a beach used to break up ocean waves). As a result, the crests

of the microwave electrical field are made approximately synchronous with the flowing bunches of electrons.[29,33] After the flowing electrons leave the accelerator structure, they are directed toward the gantry. In the gantry, x-rays are produced or a treatment beam of electrons is shaped.

> A vertically mounted accelerator structure provides a short distance to accelerate the electrons in a low-energy treatment machine, and a horizontally mounted accelerator structure provides a longer distance to accelerate electrons and equates to a higher-energy linear accelerator treatment machine.

From basic radiologic physics, microwave means "extremely small wavelengths." Because the length of waves is inversely proportional to its energy, energy is high. The microwave frequency needed for the linear accelerator is in the range of 3 million cycles per second (3000 MHz). Amplification that occurs in the accelerating structure is in the closed-ended, precision-crafted copper cavities. Here the electrical power provides momentum to the low-level electron stream mixed with the microwaves. An alternating positive and negative electrical charge accelerates the electrons toward the treatment head.

Medical linear accelerators accelerate by traveling or standing electromagnetic waves (Fig. 7.13A and C) Each design feature accelerates the electrons by using a source of microwave power. In the traveling wave design, the microwaves enter the accelerator structure at one end (near the electron gun) and travel in one direction to the other end. In this design, the electrons are moved on the accelerating wave (very similar to the way a surfer is moved powerfully forward by the ocean wave). In the standing wave design microwaves move forward and are reflected backwards within the accelerator structure. This forward and backward flow of microwaves creates a standing wave and a condition where every other cavity has no electric field, meaning half of the cavities do not contribute to the acceleration of electrons. The cavities that do not contribute to acceleration are repositioned to the sides of the accelerator structure (since electrons do not need to move through them) yielding a structure that is about one-half as long as the traveling wave design.[7,33,49]

The length of the accelerator structure varies depending on the beam energy of the linear accelerator. The length may vary from 30 cm for a 4-MV unit to 1 m or more for high-energy units, regardless if x-rays or electrons are used for treatment.[28,29] For modern, high-energy linear accelerators, as many as five cavities are sometimes used to accelerate the electron bunch enough to generate the desired energy. The radiation therapist should remember that as more cavities are used, higher energy is derived. After electrons leave the accelerating structure (guide), they are directed toward the treatment head. The treatment head may contain various beam-shaping devices, radiation monitors, and possibly a bending magnet if a horizontal accelerator structure is used.

Treatment Head. Several components designed to shape and monitor the treatment beam are located in the treatment head (Fig. 7.14). These components may consist of a bending magnet, x-ray target, primary collimator, beam-flattening filter or scattering foil, ion chamber, secondary collimators, and one or more slots for hard wedges and other accessories. Horizontal accelerator structures requiring high-energy beams need a bending magnet to direct the electrons toward the patient (otherwise, the electrons would continue straight out horizontally through the treatment head of the gantry). A magnet system may bend the electron group through a net angle of approximately 90 to 270 degrees.[28,33] When a 90-degree bending magnet is used, the electrons

would be spread out and be of varying energies. In linear accelerators with a 270-degree bending magnet, or an achromatic bending magnet, the electron beams converge after being deflected, resulting in a smaller focal spot. This will translate to sharper field edges and smaller penumbra.[28,32] After being deflected by the bending magnet, the electrons will either strike the x-ray target if photons are needed for treatment or continue on for electron treatment.

When photons are used for treatment, the x-rays are next shaped by a primary collimator, which is designed to limit the maximum field size. In modern linear accelerators, this is typically a 40 × 40 cm field projection at the isocenter. Next, the beam passes through a beam-flattening filter, which is located on the carousel with the scattering

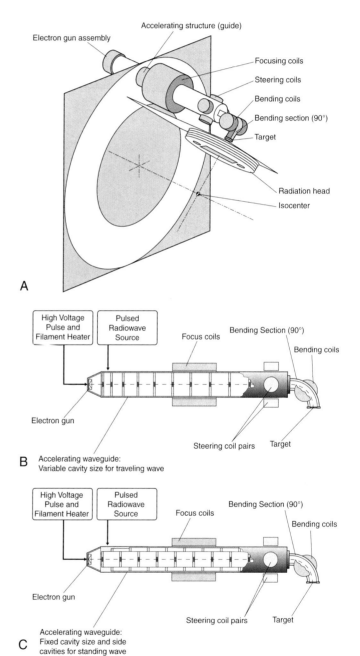

Fig. 7.13 A view of a horizontally mounted accelerating waveguide (A) and crossectional view of (B) traveling waveguide and (C) standing waveguide. (From Symonds P, Deehan C, Mills JA, et al. *Walter and Miller's Textbook of Radiotherapy: Radiation Physics, Therapy and Oncology.* 7th ed. London, UK: Churchill Livingstone; 2012.)

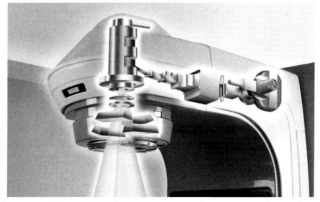

Fig. 7.12 A low-energy linear accelerator demonstrates the vertically mounted, straight-through beam design, which eliminates the need for complex beam-bending magnet systems. (Courtesy Varian Medical Systems, Palo Alto, CA.)

foil (Fig. 7.15). Beam-flattening filters are used for x-ray treatment, whereas scattering foils are used for electron treatment. When photons are used for treatment, the beam is forward peaked after hitting the x-ray target. The beam-flattening filter is a conical metal absorber that absorbs more photons from the center of the beam and fewer from the edges, resulting in a uniform beam across the field.[28] If the linear accelerator offers duel-energy photons, then two beam-flattening

filters, one for each energy, are used to provide more uniform treatment fields. Flattening filters have been constructed of tungsten, steel, lead, uranium, aluminum, or some combination of these metals depending on the x-ray energy.[25] Modern treatment machines also have a flattening filter–free option (FFF), which is used when the dose rate needs to be increased.[28] The scattering foil, also positioned on the carousel, is used in the electron mode. When electrons are used for treatment instead of x-rays, the target is retracted, and a scattering foil that matches the electron energy selected for treatment is moved into place to spread out the pencil-like electron beam and produce a flat field across the treatment field. A different scattering foil is used for each electron energy. The scattering foil system usually consists of dual lead foils, where the first foil scatters most of the electrons with a minimum of bremsstrahlung x-rays. The second foil may be thicker in the central region to flatten the field. The small amount of bremsstrahlung contamination produced with an electron beam is usually less than 5% of the beam.[25]

Once the beam passes through the flattening filter or scattering foil, it travels through a series of ion chambers. In most cases, the monitoring system consists of several transmission-type parallel plate ionization chambers. These ion chambers monitor the beam for its symmetry in the right-left and inferior-superior directions for both photon and electron treatments. They also monitor field symmetry and dose rate.[25] In addition to monitoring characteristics of the beam, the ion chambers are responsible for terminating the beam when the desired MU have been delivered. The system is designed so that if one ion chamber fails to terminate the beam, the other will serve as a backup to decrease the likelihood that a patient receives a higher dose than prescribed.[28]

Next, the beam passes through the secondary collimators, also known as the jaws. The upper and lower collimator jaws, usually made of lead or tungsten, are controlled be a remote hand pendant or the treatment machine console with the use of software to preset the patient's field size. Modern linear accelerators are equipped with independent or asymmetric jaws so that each axis (X1, X2, Y1, Y2) can

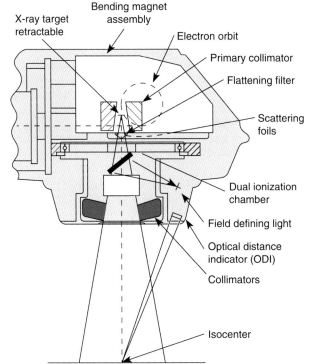

Fig. 7.14 Cross section of the treatment head of a high-energy linear accelerator. (Courtesy C.J. Karzmark and Varian Associates, Palo Alto, CA.)

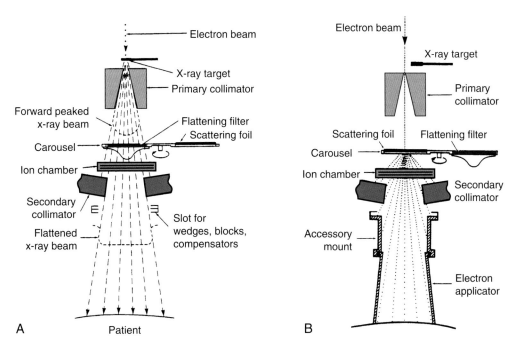

Fig. 7.15 The subsystem components with the treatment head of a high-energy linear accelerator. (A) Note the beam subsystem is in the x-ray mode, indicated by the position of the flattening filter. (B) The subsystem in the electron mode is indicated by the position of the scattering foil. (Courtesy Robert Morton and Medical Physics Publishing, Madison, WI.)

move independently. The secondary collimator allows the beam to be shaped in rectangles on varying field sizes from 0 × 0 cm to 40 × 40 cm at the isocenter.[28,32] In addition to setting the field size, the jaws can rotate around the isocenter if needed. Additional beam-shaping and modifying devices in addition to MLCs, such as a wedge, electron cone, compensator, or custom shielding blocks, can be placed in accessory slots just below the secondary collimators.

The light localizing system, or field light, is also located in the treatment head. Light from a quartz-iodine bulb outlines the dimensions of the radiation field as it appears on the patient. This alignment of the radiation and light fields allows accurate positioning of the radiation field in relationship to reference points on the patient. MLCs may further define the light field to correspond to the desired treatment field shape. Linear accelerators are also equipped with an optical distance indicator, or rangefinder, which projects the target-skin distance onto the patient's skin.[26,28,32]

Control Console.

Monitoring and controlling of the linear accelerator occur at the control console. Located outside the treatment room, the control console may take the form of a digital display, push-button panel, and/or video display terminal (VDT) in which the machine status and patient treatment information are incorporated into the computerized treatment unit. The ready state of the equipment allows the therapist to confirm the treatment parameters. All interlocks (safety switches blocking or terminating radiation production) must be satisfied for the machine to allow the beam to be started. A lighted message on the VDT usually indicates that the machine is in the ready state. An indicator for the beam-on state remains on throughout the patient's treatment until the prescribed dose is delivered.

Monitoring the patient visually with a remote video monitor(s) and a sound system during treatment is essential. Both the visual and aural monitors must be functional to safely deliver a prescribed dose of radiation therapy. This is especially important for lengthy treatment sessions. Visual monitoring should be designed so that the radiation therapist can watch the patient for movement and overall condition, as well as to avoid collision with the gantry and table during imaging or rotational treatment.

Interlock displays can occur before or during a treatment. The interlock system is designed to protect the patient, staff members, and equipment from hazards. Patient protection interlocks, including beam energy, beam symmetry, dose, and dose-rate monitoring, prevent radiation and mechanical hazards to the patient. For example, interlocks protect the patient against extremely high dose rates, especially if the treatment unit provides x-ray and electron beams. Interlocks can also ensure the correct beam modifying device is used. Because of the high electron beam currents used for x-ray production, extremely high dose rates can result if the target or flattening filter does not intercept the beam. Machine interlocks protect the equipment from damage, which may include problems detected in the machine's high-voltage power supply, water-cooling system, or vacuum system. Other interlocks designed to protect the staff, patient, and machine include door interlocks and collision avoidance systems.[32]

Emergency "off" buttons, which can terminate irradiation and machine functions, are located on the control panel and at several other locations in the treatment room. These switches terminate all electrical power to the equipment and require a complete start-up procedure before the treatment machine can produce an electron or photon beam.

As a radiation therapist, you witness the table begin to rise after the correct dose has been delivered for the first treatment field. You press the emergency "off" button located on the wall near the gantry, but nothing happens. What would you do next?

Besides displaying the operational mode of the treatment unit, the control console serves several other functions. It may provide a digital display for prescribed dose (monitor units), mechanical beam parameters, such as collimator setting, MLC settings (on a separate monitor) or gantry angle, and possibly as many as 50 other status messages.[29] The radiation therapist will also use the control console for IGRT. All aspects of imaging (scheduling, acquiring, and evaluation) takes place at the control console. Overall, the treatment control console provides a central location for controlling and operating the linear accelerator.

Treatment Couch.

The treatment couch is the area on which patients are positioned to receive their radiation treatment. Several unique features of the carbon fiber treatment couch provide the tabletop with mobility. The carbon fiber couch top facilitates higher image quality and improved dose distribution by reducing scatter radiation. The tabletop moves mechanically vertically, horizontally, and laterally, as well as rotates through the isocenter via the hand pendant or switches on the control console. The movement of the table must be smooth and accurate with the patient in the treatment position, thus allowing for precise and exact positioning of the isocenter during treatment positioning. Some tabletops support as much as 250 kg (550 lb) and range in width from 45 to 50 cm. If the couch width on the computed tomography (CT) simulator is not similar to that of the treatment unit, reproducibility may become a problem, especially with large patients. Treatment couches are designed to be lightweight, rigid, and flat. Some couches had been equipped with a mylar insert or mesh insert, which allowed for maximum radiation transmission.[32]

Some newer treatment couches are now referred to by many as *robotic correction tables,* or *robotic couches.* They are made of carbon fiber, similar to the previous generation of couches, but they feature six degrees of movement, which allow the table to move around the patient's isocenter.[42] Along with the standard vertical, lateral, longitudinal, and rotation movements, pitch (moving the head of the table up or down) and roll (rotation on the side to side axis) corrections are possible. Because of this, the robotic couch may also be referred to as a 6-degree-of-freedom couch. After the therapist positions the patient on the table, the treatment position is verified by using online imaging. The patient's position is corrected, if necessary, with couch corrections, rather than by moving the patient. This is typically automatically completed from the control console without the radiation therapist having to enter the room, and then the treatment is delivered. With the increased use of cone beam CT (CBCT) imaging before treatment, many facilities are using robotic couch corrections for all treatment sites.[42]

Most treatment machine manufacturers offer the same indexed carbon fiber couch top for the CT simulator and treatment units. Indexing allows for increased accuracy in treatment setup reproducibility from simulation to treatment delivery and through multiple treatments during the course of daily radiation therapy delivery. The transfer of information, such as the exact location of immobilization devices, from CT simulation to the treatment machine is improved when devices are referenced or indexed to the treatment table. The patient and immobilization device are then "locked" into place on the treatment table using a system of numbered or lettered holes, or notches, along the lateral edge of the carbon fiber tabletop (Fig. 7.16). Indexing is essential for accurate treatment, especially when IMRT is used. The robotic couch is beneficial for IMRT. The robotic couch acts as a mechanism to efficiently and accurately reposition the target with respect to the reference image before each treatment.

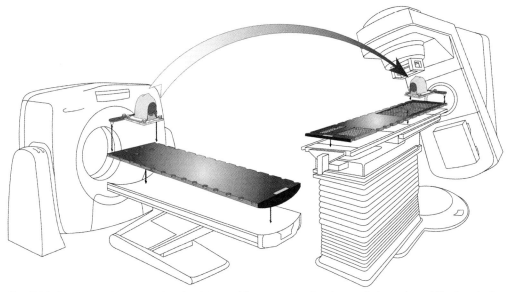

Fig. 7.16 A computed tomography simulator and linear accelerator demonstrate an immobilization device indexed in the same location on the carbon fiber tabletop. Note the small notches along the lateral edge of the tabletop used to index the immobilization devices. (Courtesy MEDTEC, Orange City, IA.)

Modulator Cabinet. This important component of the linear accelerator is usually located in the treatment room or adjacent closet and is the noisiest part. The modulator cabinet stores the pulsed power supply, which supplies the electrical power to the klystron and electron gun. In some systems, the modulator cabinet contains three major components: the fan control, auxiliary power distribution system, and primary power distribution system. The fan control switch automatically turns the fans off and on as the need arises for cooling the power distribution (auxiliary and primary) in the modulator cabinet. The auxiliary power distribution panel contains the emergency "off" button that shuts off the power to the treatment unit. Circuit breakers used to disconnect power to different components of the linear accelerator, often used by physics and service personnel, may also be located in the modulator cabinet.[28]

Applied Technology

Computer-controlled accelerators include multimodality treatment units. Because of their increased flexibility in design and dose delivery, these accelerators are used by more radiation treatment centers. Dual-photon energies (ranging from a 6-MV low-energy x-ray beam to high-energy x-ray beams of 15 to 25 MV) provide the radiation oncologist with more options in treating a wide range of diseases. In addition, several electron energies ranging from 4 to 22 MeV are available to treat more superficial tumors. Multimodality treatment units offer several advantages. Because of their dual photon energies, they can provide backup for other treatment units that may experience downtime as a result of electrical, mechanical, or software problems. In addition, patients can be treated with multiple beam energies on the same treatment unit. In some centers with multiple treatment units, identical calibrations for each treatment machine are completed to allow for additional flexibility in managing treatment delays.

Modern Treatment Technologies. Numerous technologies have become standard in the past 10 years, allowing radiation oncologists and radiation therapists to increase radiation doses to various tumor sites. These include 3D-CRT, MLCs, micro-MLCs, kV imaging, and IGRT.

Three-dimensional CRT, in which the field shape and beam angle change while the gantry moves around the patient, requires sophisticated computer-controlled equipment. Conformal therapy has certain advantages over traditional forms of therapy. IMRT, which is a type of 3D-CRT, has provided a significant technologic advance in radiation therapy treatment planning. This method of delivering the prescribed dose of radiation therapy has proven beneficial in escalating the dose to the tumor volume and reducing the dose to normal tissue.[15,26,52] VMAT is another type of CRT where a modulated beam is delivered through a rotational field.

Traditionally, with the process of 3D-CRT, images from CT, magnetic resonance imaging (MRI), and positron emission tomography are transferred to treatment planning computers where normal tissues and tumor volumes are defined. Treatment plans developed by using 3D-CRT are done so with a "forward planning" process, where beam arrangements are tested by trial and error until a satisfactory dose distribution is produced. This can be very time-consuming for complex cases. IMRT develops treatment plans using "inverse treatment planning." With inverse treatment planning, the radiation oncologist selects dose parameters for normal tissues and the target volume, and the computer calculates the desired dose distribution and beam arrangements.[17,51] The IMRT targeting computer also adjusts the intensity of radiation beam across the field with the aid of MLC moving in and out of the beam portal under precise computer guidance.[32,38]

A dynamic wedge, also called a virtual wedge, is used for computerized shaping of the treatment field (Fig. 7.17). It has the ability, under computer control, to modify and shape the desired isodose distribution using the large field-defining collimator or jaw. In the Elekta linear accelerator, the virtual wedge is positioned just below the ion chamber and above the MLC and is used instead of one of the field-defining collimators to create a dynamic wedge effect.[51] The computer-controlled dynamic wedge can be used in place of a 15-, 30-, 45-, or 60-degree "hard" wedge. Dynamic wedges are designed in such a way that wedge dose distributions using varying field sizes yield acceptable wedged isodose distributions compared with physical wedges. This design relies strongly on computer software to vary the dose rate and mechanical motion of the collimator during treatment.[16,51]

As previously mentioned, linear accelerators are equipped with x and y jaws, with one setting field length and the other setting field width. Modern treatment machines are equipped with dual asymmetric jaws, which provide a variety of options for treatment purposes. For some treatments that require abutting fields, independent motion of one or both sets of jaws may be desirable. A sharp, nondivergent field edge is obtained by closing one of the jaws to the beam's central axis, thereby shielding half the radiation field. Use of the independent jaw motion necessitates accurate and precise treatment positioning to avoid treatment field overlap.

Shaping the Beam

Shaping the radiation beam to conform to the target volume is extremely important, especially with 3D-CRT. Beam shaping involves the use of wedges, primary and secondary collimators, Cerrobend blocks, compensators, and, more importantly, MLCs. Improvements in MLC design by linear accelerator manufacturers in recent years have allowed for improved treatment precision and conformality. With the widespread use of 3D-CRT, IMRT, and VMAT, there has been a demand for more focused beams and faster treatment delivery time. Improvement in MLC design helped meet these goals.

Several aspects of MLC systems exist that shape the radiation therapy volume by using approximately 52 to 160 leaves, whose movements are computer controlled. Usually made of tungsten, these metal collimator leaves slide into place to form the desired field shape by projecting 0.25-cm to 1-cm beam widths at the isocenter.[28,32,38] The most common leaf width is 1 cm. MLCs used for SBRT or SRS may be even smaller (micro-MLCs or mini-MLCs), which are used to conform the dose to very small treatment volumes receiving larger or single-fraction doses than those used in conventional fractionation of 180 to 200 cGy per fraction. Fig. 7.18 demonstrates MLC position in the treatment head for the Elekta linear accelerator. This example of beam shaping with the use of MLCs is especially critical for full-field beam shaping with the use of IMRT, VMAT, SRS, and SBRT. Table 7.2 compares three major vendors: Elekta, Siemens, and Varian as they are applied to the MLC construction, position within the treatment head, leaf configuration, leakage, leaf speed, positioning accuracy, and penumbra.

A type of binary MLC is used in TomoTherapy units. Sixty-four MLC collimator leaves either block or let in radiation in individual

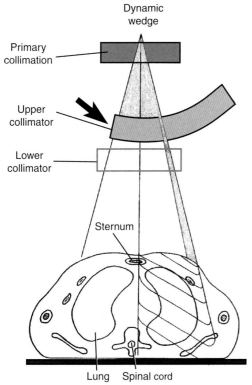

Fig. 7.17 The upper collimator moves during treatment to create a dynamic wedge effect. (Courtesy Varian Medical Systems, Palo Alto, CA.)

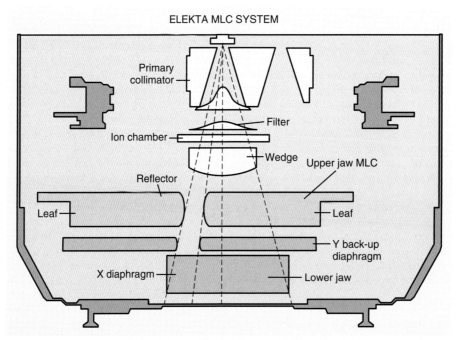

Fig. 7.18 A schematic drawing of the Elekta multileaf collimator *(MLC)* position in the treatment head. In this design, the MLC unit replaces the upper collimator used to shape the radiation beam. (From Xia P, Xing L, Amols HI, et al. Three dimensional conformal radiation therapy and intensity modulated radiation therapy. In: Hoppe RT, Phillips TL, Roach M. *Leibel and Phillips Textbook of Radiation Oncology.* 3rd ed. Philadelphia, PA: Saunders; 2010.)

parts of the fan beam. Each leaf produces a beamlet by moving from a closed to open position and back to a closed position. The collimator works in a binary fashion, either "on" or "off." In other words, an individual leaf can be fully open or fully closed. The open/close cycle lasts only 20 ms while the beam rotates around the patient delivering IMRT treatment.[36]

Fig. 7.19 illustrates a schematic of MLC beam shaping. There are many characteristics of MLC construction that affect the shape of the radiation beam, such as the position of the MLCs within the gantry head (distance from the target), total thickness of each leaf, and several other factors (see Table 7.2). We will examine three important characteristics of MLC construction related to leakage and how they affect the dose delivered:

1. Transmission through the thickness of the MLC.
2. Leakage between the MLC leaves.
3. Penumbra at the end or tip of the leaf.

The thickness of each leaf is important in reducing the amount of radiation transmitted through the tungsten alloy MLC leaf. As with Cerrobend blocking, transmission through the entire thickness is as low as 2% to 5%. Collimator thickness is strongly dependent on how far the MLCs are located from the target. Fig. 7.20 illustrates the MLC configuration within the head of the gantry for three major vendors: Elekta, Siemens, and Varian. If one were to measure through-the-leaf distance, the tungsten alloy would measure 7.5 cm for Elekta, 6.5 cm for Siemens, and 5.5 cm for the Varian MLC leaf.[8,18]

> What effect does the weight of multileaf collimators within the treatment head of the gantry have on treatment?

For MLCs to operate efficiently, the leaves need to slide smoothly between each other with thin gaps between leaves to reduce radiation transmission and leakage. The more leaves, the greater the challenge in design. A tongue-and-groove design for each MLC helps to reduce radiation leakage. Carpenters are familiar with the design of tongue-and-groove construction used to fit similar objects together edge to edge, as is common in expensive cabinet work and other woodwork designs. A groove is cut into one piece of the wood along its edge where a corresponding tongue fits in neatly from a second piece of wood, joining the two pieces together. This construction provides strength and support to the cabinet. With MLC construction, strength and support are important, but more important is a reduction in radiation transmission and leakage.

Fig. 7.21 illustrates a schematic "end-on" view of an MLC, showing the tongue-and-groove design and the resulting beam transmission. Treatment planning calculations are affected by which portions of the MLC the beam passes through. Does the beam pass through the proximal portion (closest to the target), central tongue-and-groove portion, or the distal portion of the MLC?[52] Tongue-and-groove designs may differ slightly from one vendor to the next, but all designs attempt to reduce radiation transmission and leakage, which is especially important in IMRT treatment in which the beam time needed to deliver the necessary dose to the tumor volume is increased.

A third design consideration is the penumbra at the tip of the leaf. It is important to match as closely as possible the radiation field beam divergence with the position of the end or tip of the MLC leaf. This

TABLE 7.2 Multileaf Collimator Characteristics of Three Major Radiation Therapy Vendors

MLC Feature	Elekta	Siemens	Varian
Maximum field size (cm)	40 × 40	40 × 40	40 × 40
Number of leaves	160	160	120
Leaf width (mm)	2.5, 5.0	5.0	2.5, 5.0, 10.0
Leaf speed	6.5 cm/s	4.3 cm/s	2.5 cm/s
MLC position	Replaces upper "X" collimator	Replaces lower "Y" collimator	Mounted below both "X" and "Y" collimators as a tertiary collimator
Leaf positional accuracy (leaf tip)	1.0 mm	1.0 mm	2.0 mm
MLC distance from target (cm)	37.3 cm	46.0 cm	51.4 cm
Penumbra (leaf tip)	5.0–6.0 mm	4.0–8.5 mm	2.4–5.1 mm
Transmission leakage (intertip gap)	0.45%	0.63%	1.34%

MLC, Multileaf collimators.
From Kim S, Palta JR. Advances in radiation therapy techniques on linear accelerators. In: Van Dyk J, ed. *Modern Technology of Radiation Oncology*. Vol. 3. Madison, WI: Medical Physics Publishing; 2013; Xia P, Xing L, Amols HI, et al. Three-dimensional conformal radiotherapy and intensity-modulated radiotherapy. In: Hoppe RT, Phillips TL, Roach M. *Leibel and Phillips Textbook of Radiation Oncology*. 3rd ed. Philadelphia, PA: Saunders; 2010; and Multileaf collimators. ElektaAB website. www.elekta.com. Accessed September 25, 2019

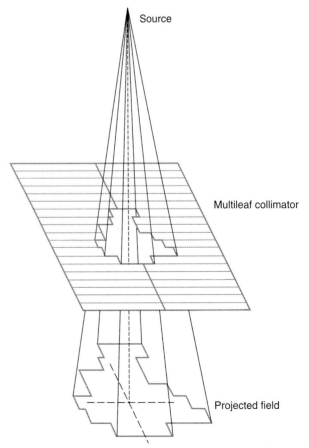

Fig. 7.19 A schematic of multileaf collimator beam shaping. Each leaf is moved independently, controlled by a separate small motor within the head of the collimator, to create the desired beam shape. (From Bourland JD. Radiation oncology physics. In: Gunderson S, Tepper J, eds. *Clinical Radiation Oncology*. Philadelphia, PA: Churchill Livingston; 2012.)

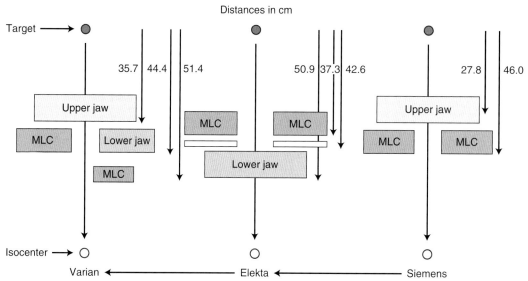

Fig. 7.20 Schematic drawing demonstrating the multileaf collimator position in the gantry head for three major vendors: Elekta, Seimans, and Varian. Note the position of the multileaf collimator *(MLC)* and its distance from the source of radiation. Multileaf collimators are located a specific distance from the target: Varian, 51.4 cm; Elekta, 37.3 cm; and Siemens, 46 cm.

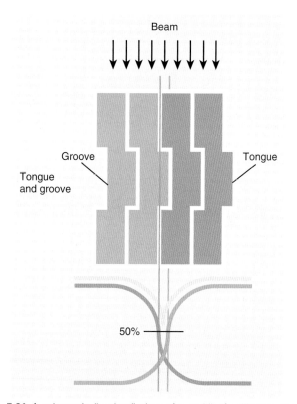

Fig. 7.21 A schematic "end-on" view of a multileaf collimator showing the tongue-and-groove design and the resulting beam transmission. (From Xia P, Xing L, Amols HI, et al. Three dimensional conformal radiotherapy and intensity modulated radiotherapy. In: Hoppe RT, Phillips TL, Roach M. *Leibel and Phillips Textbook of Radiation Oncology.* 3rd ed. Philadelphia, PA: Saunders; 2010.)

depends a great deal on where the leaf is in relation to the central axis of the beam. The further away the leaf tip, the more divergences it must accommodate. Fig. 7.22 illustrates a typical rounded-leaf-end design of an MLC. Generally, the leaf edge maintains a reasonable penumbra over all field sizes and, because of its curved design at

the tip of the leaf transmission, can be as high as 20% or more when apposing leaves abut each other.[52]

Several concerns should be evaluated in the use of MLC beam shaping. Penumbra at the end of individual leaves may be increased depending on the angle of the leaf and its position within the treatment field (along the field edge or near the central portion of the treatment beam). Penumbra adds to a small amount of dose uncertainty along the edge of the shaped field. With multiple fields, as is common with 3D-CRT, the problem is minimized because the dose is spread out over multiple fields.[26] Another physics consideration is the interleaf transmission leakage. This leakage may average 2.5% and reach as high as 4% in some MLC configurations. This leakage should be considered when treating a large number of fields (especially when using IMRT) that require a higher number of monitor units to deliver the prescribed dose.[17,52]

> **Multileaf collimators** have a variety of characteristics that play an important role in achieving optimal dose distribution for patients. Geometric and physical characteristics, such as transmission, leaf width, penumbra, and leaf speed interact to optimally shape the beam.

Radiation Therapy Imaging

An electronic portal imaging device (EPID) is another method to improve treatment field accuracy and verification. Most electronic portal imaging systems are lightweight and come with a retracted arm along the gantry's axis. The arm is equipped with amorphous silicon imaging technology, which provides a quick and accurate comparison of its images with reference images without loss of patient data or duplicate entry. Images can be reviewed immediately online in the control room or later with traditional offline review tools. Despite the poor image quality common with regular port films (as a result of Compton and pair-production interactions), comparable quality images are possible with EPID.

The position of the image detector in relationship to the patient can affect image quality through magnification and scatter radiation. Bissonnette et al[5] have shown that a magnification factor of 1.6 is optimal for television-based camera portal imaging systems. Swindell et al[48]

CALCULATION OF LEAF END TRANSMISSION

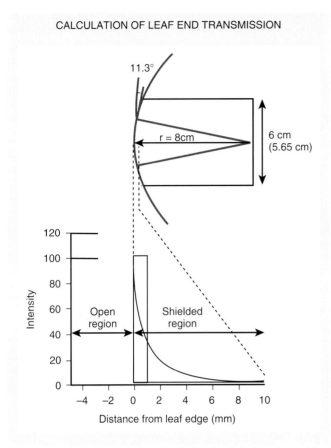

Fig. 7.22 Illustration of a typical rounded-leaf-end design of a multileaf collimator. (From Xia P, Xing L, Amols HI, et al. Three dimensional conformal radiotherapy and intensity modulated radiotherapy. In: Hoppe RT, Phillips TL, Roach M. *Leibel and Phillips Textbook of Radiation Oncology*. 3rd ed. Philadelphia, PA: Saunders; 2010.)

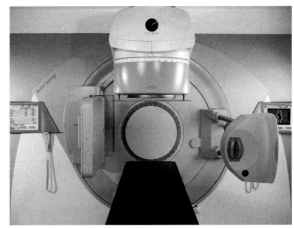

Fig. 7.23 An Elekta linear accelerator with kV imaging system perpendicular to the megavoltage treatment beam/imaging system.

found that an object-image-receptor distance of 40 cm is sufficient to reduce the effects of scatter radiation on image quality. Attention to details such as scatter radiation and magnification is an important factor in improving an already somewhat poor image quality with traditional portal imaging.

Image-Guided Radiation Therapy. IGRT has the potential to improve the application of radiation therapy dose delivery. It may be used in a variety of forms, including EPID, an in-room CT scanner, kV cone beam, MV CBCT, ultrasound, and others. The rationale for IGRT is to image the patient just before treatment and compare the position of external setup marks and internal anatomy with the treatment plan. Shifts in patient position are made for each fraction just before treatment delivery. Studies have indicated that there are substantial interfractional and intrafractional variations in the shape, volume, and position of treatment targets and the normal surrounding tissue.[17] The cause of such variations may include respiratory motion, movement of the body or internal structures, weight loss, and radiation-induced changes such as tumor shrinkage. IGRT can track changes in patient positioning resulting from some of these variations.

Traditional EPID utilizing MV x-ray beams are used to check patient position before or at the end of treatment. Disadvantages of the pretreatment MV imaging include high imaging dose (1–5 cGy) and poor image quality because of the high energy x-ray beams. All three major manufacturers—Elekta, Varian, and Siemens—offer a type of kV x-ray imaging system that is installed at right angles to the treatment beam and may provide radiographic and CBCT modes to visualize patient anatomy.[26,51]

The use of kV imaging systems, which use a source of kV x-rays and a flat panel image detector, represents a major breakthrough in radiation therapy portal imaging (Fig. 7.23). The traditional MV x-ray beams that were used for EPIDs demonstrated poor image quality (poor contrast) and made bony anatomy difficult to see. The better-detailed kV image resembles conventional simulation images and diagnostic-quality x-ray images and provides more information about soft tissue and bony anatomy comparison. Some centers use embedded fiducial markers to track patient setup inaccuracies. The use of onboard imaging enables the tracking of these fiducial markers after the daily setup of the patient and before the delivery of treatment. With or without fiducial markers, this type of IGRT will allow daily checks of patient positioning before and/or during treatment for every patient scheduled on the treatment unit.[32]

Verification and Recording Devices. Computers are used to assist the radiation therapist in the verification of treatment parameters. If the average number of patients treated on a linear accelerator is assumed to be between 25 and 30 patients per day and each patient may have an average of 20 separate parameters (e.g., gantry angle, treatment distance, field size), this equals 500 to 600 parameters that must be matched each day. Verification systems not only allow incorrect setup parameters to be corrected before the machine is turned on, but may also provide data in other areas, such as computer-assisted setup, recording of patient data, allowing for data transfer from the simulator or treatment planning computer, and assisting with quality control. See Chapter 25 on e-charting and image management for a more detailed discussion.

Specialized Treatment Machines

Smaller, more compact, medical linear accelerators were introduced in the 1990s as an alternative to the conventional linear accelerators. The field of radiation therapy continues to evolve, bringing new treatment technology. In addition to proton beam radiation therapy (which will be covered in Chapter 16), there are numerous specialized radiation therapy treatment machines available. These include helical delivery machines, such as TomoTherapy and Radixact (both by Accuray) and Varian Halcyon; stereotactic treatment machines, such as CyberKnife and Gamma Knife; portable intraoperative radiation therapy (IORT) devices; and MRI-guided radiation therapy machines, such as MRIdian

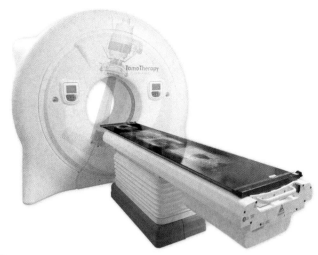

Fig. 7.24 TomoTherapy Hi-Art linear accelerator, which uses a megavoltage source for treatment and imaging.

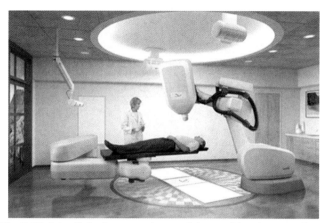

Fig. 7.25 CyberKnife linear accelerator. It is considered a type of stereotactic radiosurgery, a noninvasive treatment in which high doses of focused radiation beams are delivered from several locations.

by ViewRay and Elekta Unity. Each of these will be briefly discussed (see Chapter 15 for more information).

Helical Delivery Machines. Helical delivery treatment machines have been available since 2003. The TomoTherapy system, also known as "slice therapy," was the next evolution of IMRT and advanced imaging capability.[4] The TomoTherapy concept combined conventional linear accelerator technology with CT technology, enabling rotational or direct method IMRT treatment and daily IGRT. Daily IGRT is accomplished with a vertically mounted 6-MV accelerator powered by a magnetron. For treatment delivery, the linear accelerator rotates continuously while the treatment couch moves through the gantry bore (Fig. 7.24), producing a spiral treatment beam. The machine is also capable of treating with static beams.[40] The 6-MV linear accelerator x-ray beam resembles the shape of a fan, 40 cm wide and 1 cm, 2.5 cm, or 5 cm thick, as measured at the isocenter.[32,39,46] Sixty-four collimator leaves either block or let in radiation in individual parts of the fan. Each leaf produces a beamlet, by moving from a closed to open position and back to a closed position. As mentioned, the collimator works in a binary fashion. The open/close cycle lasts only 20 ms while the beam rotates around the patient.[36]

The set of xenon image detectors located on the opposite side of the ring makes it possible to verify the patient's position on the treatment table by comparing MV CT images with CT simulation images gathered earlier for treatment planning purposes. The nominal voltage of the linear accelerator in the imaging mode is lowered to 3.5 MV, providing better image quality.[36,43] Unlike a conventional linear accelerator, there is no light field for patient setup. The isocenter is 85 cm from the source (SAD), which is also the bore diameter. A shorter SAD also helps to increase the dose rate to approximately 850 cGy/min.[43]

The Radixact Treatment System is Accuray's latest development in helical treatment delivery. This technology builds on the traditional TomoTherapy delivery system but has changed components within the gantry to improve treatment delivery. Faster image acquisition and processing, as well as faster treatment delivery (dose rate of 1000 cGy/min) is possible on the Radixact system. Motion management techniques have been developed. Additional changes to the traditional TomoTherapy treatment planning and treatment delivery software were made to improve and enhance workflow and integration with other software systems.[40,41,44]

In 2017, the Halcyon treatment system (Varian Medical Systems) was introduced into radiation therapy clinical practice. The Halcyon treatment machine is a ring-based helical treatment delivery system with several unique features. The linear accelerator produces a 6-MV FFF beam with a dose rate of 800 MU/min. The linear accelerator is capable of rotating up to four rotations per minute. The treatment bore is 100 cm wide. The treatment machine lacks jaws, and the field is shaped by dual layer MLC, with a nominal field size of 28 × 28 cm². Imaging can be acquired through kV-CBCT and MV-CBCT, as well as produce 2D or 3D image sets.[13,50]

Stereotactic Radiosurgery Machines. One treatment machine used for stereotactic radiosurgery (SRS) is the CyberKnife system (Accuray, Inc.) This radiation therapy treatment machine is a versatile, small, and compact 6-MV linear accelerator. It is considered a type of stereotactic radiosurgery, a noninvasive treatment in which high doses of focused radiation beams are delivered from several locations outside the body (Fig. 7.25). The objective is to minimize dose to the surrounding normal tissue. Although it is used for precise treatment to small tumors, it is possible to perform full-body radiation therapy by using image-guided robotics. The parts of the CyberKnife system include an image-guided camera, which is used to localize the tumor, and a linear accelerator, which is attached to the robotic arm. The CyberKnife can treat vascular lesions, tumors throughout the body, and functional disorders of the body with submillimeter accuracy. The system continually tracks and monitors patient position during the treatment. The image information stored in the computer's operating system is used by the machine to adapt to variance in the patient's position by repositioning the treatment unit.

With the use of x-rays to locate the position of the lesion during treatment, the CyberKnife dynamically aligns the radiation beam with the observed position of the treatment target. Unlike most conventional external beam radiation therapy (EBRT) treatments, each beam is aimed independently with no fixed isocenter. The system literally tracks in real time the movement of the target volume. The CyberKnife, similar to the historic ⁶⁰Co, defines the field size at 80-cm SAD, but with a reference depth of 1.5 cm.[1,35]

The Leksell Gamma Knife was the first treatment machine designed exclusively for SRS. Gamma Knife machines use 192 to 201 ⁶⁰Co sources (depending on the model) directed at a single point to deliver a high dose of radiation at the target while minimizing dose to surrounding tissue. Recent updates to the Gamma Knife system include the addition of CBCT option to treat patients with a frameless system, as well as continuous motion monitoring. Chapter 15 provides further details about this technology.[11,47]

Portable Intraoperative Radiation Therapy. The application of radiation directly to the tumor or tumor bed while still exposed during surgery is termed IORT. It is not a new concept. Beck[2] used it as a cancer treatment modality as early as 1909 when he attempted to treat patients with gastric and colon cancer by using kV x-rays. The practice of IORT was started in the United States in the late 1970s by Goldson at Howard University.[20,23] It is the ultimate tissue-sparing procedure because the surrounding tissue and organs at risk (OAR) are displaced or retracted out of the radiation beam. An OAR may be defined as normal tissues (critical structures) that may influence treatment planning, the delivery of a prescribed dose of radiation, or both because of their sensitivity to radiation damage. The effective dose of radiation to the tumor cells is substantially increased. In theory, IORT can also improve the therapeutic ratio.

IORT can be used as a "boost dose," literally replacing several weeks of a conventional fractionated course of treatment while avoiding the unnecessary radiation to normal tissues that occurs when EBRT is used. It also practically eliminates the possibility of a geographic miss that could occur with EBRT because the target is visualized. From a radiobiologic standpoint, the application of direct radiation to microscopic residual tumor cells during surgery when they are most vulnerable can assist the effectiveness of subsequent adjuvant therapy.

However, there were historic challenges to the implementation of IORT. The existence of operating rooms that are shielded for radiation was rare. This required a patient under anesthesia to be transported from the operating suite to the radiation therapy department, adding significant time to the process and thus increasing patient risk. The process also demanded very complex logistics and a significant commitment of specialized personnel. There were also the economic realities of the linear accelerator setup for IORT, which could not be used for conventional patient treatment easily. Even when facilities constructed operating suites that were fully shielded using modified conventional linear accelerators, the cost was still a barrier.

Mobile units can be used in unshielded rooms, are a magnitude lighter in weight and more compact compared with traditional linear accelerators, and can easily be moved from one operating suite to another or shared between facilities. Mobile IORT technology has opened the doors for an expansion of this application. It is also patient friendly in that the patients receive a dose in one treatment with fewer side effects than would have been possible with EBRT.

IORT either alone or as an adjuvant treatment to EBRT is now used for early-stage breast cancer, stage II nonsmall cell lung cancer along with chemotherapy, and stage II/III rectal cancer. Some studies have shown that because OAR can be literally removed from the radiation path, the ability to intensify the dose exists without the risk of significant side effects.[19] If the dose is limited to less than 15 Gy, complications from the IORT are also significantly diminished. The combination of low complication rates and high local control is formidable. In practice, the dose intensification can be applied to any anatomic site that is surgically accessible and is at risk for undesirable complications with EBRT. IMRT is also thought to lower side effects, but it can be more time-consuming in treatment delivery and overall course duration than conventional EBRT. Given these characteristics, it is not feasible to deliver IMRT to every patient. IORT as a partner to IMRT shortens the overall time of delivery while providing adequate tumor dose control and decreased complications.[19]

Magnetic Resonance Imaging-Guided Radiation Therapy Treatment Machines. Although traditionally used for diagnosis, MRI is now being used in the radiation therapy treatment process. Two MR-IGRT treatment machines are clinically available: MRIdian by ViewRay and Elekta MR-Linac (Unity). These helical treatment devices are equipped with both MRI and linear accelerators, allowing the patients to be imaged while the treatment is delivered. MR-IGRT has the capability of tracking tumor motion during treatment, as well as the soft tissue imaging superiority of MR scans. Tumors of the abdomen and pelvis, as well as those that move during treatment, are ideal targets for MR-IGRT. In addition to radiation safety, MRI safety guidelines must be followed.[3,9,10,21]

Medical Accelerator Safety Considerations

With the increased use of multimodality treatment units, potential hazards exist that usually were not present in single-modality treatment units.[37,49] Monitoring and controlling safe operating conditions for a computer-driven linear accelerator are more difficult than for the more conventional, electromechanical type.

Emergency Procedures. Emergency procedures, if implemented properly, can prevent serious accidents and possibly save a patient's life. Written emergency procedures should be located at or near the treatment control console (some state regulatory agencies require this). Radiation therapists should be familiar with written procedures in the event of a patient emergency. Knowledge of the location of emergency stop buttons (inside and outside the treatment room), couch evacuation mechanism, and other emergency tools is critical in the event of a machine malfunction. Other emergencies involving the patient's medical condition may also require the radiation therapist's attention.

Safety Considerations. Electrical, mechanical, and radiation safety considerations must be more elaborate with multimodality treatment units because of the accelerator's increased flexibility. Errors with the treatment machine, or the related software, can cause significant consequences or harm. For example, if a large electron beam current intended for x-ray production is used for an electron treatment, an extremely large dose rate can result. If the scattering foil is in place or the beam scanning is operational, an estimated dose comparable with a typical 2-Gy dose fraction can be delivered to a patient in 0.03 seconds at 4000 Gy/min. This dose rate can create hazards for the patient. To address this type of problem, digital logic and microprocessors have been incorporated into the linear accelerator control and monitor functions.[37]

Potentially dangerous problems can result from a harmful incident of a prescribed radiation dose, which can be minor or major and may cause death or serious injury to the patient, depending on the extent of the dose. The World Health Organization (WHO) has developed a system for the international classification for patient safety terms in an effort to standardize definitions. Runciman et al[39] provide a description of WHO definitions related to patient safety.

- An *error* is the failure to carry out a planned action as intended or the application of an incorrect plan. Errors may manifest by doing the wrong thing (commission) or by failing to do the right thing (omission), at either the planning or execution phase.
- An *event* is something that happens to or involves a patient.
- A *harmful incident* (adverse event) is an incident that results in harm to a patient.
- *Healthcare-associated harm* is harm arising from or associated with plans or actions taken during the provision of healthcare, rather than from an underlying disease or injury.
- A *patient safety incident* is an event or circumstance that could have resulted, or did result, in unnecessary harm to a patient.
- A *near miss* is an incident that did not reach the patient.
- A *no harm incident* is one in which an event reached a patient, but no discernable harm resulted.

- A *reportable circumstance* is a situation in which there was significant potential for harm, but no incident occurred.
- A *violation* is a deliberate deviation from an operating procedure, standard, or rule. Both errors and violations increase risk, even if an incident does not actually occur.

In 1993, the American Association of Physicists in Medicine Radiation Therapy Committee Task Group Number 35 published a list containing most of the causes of potentially life-threatening problems associated with electrical, mechanical, human, and software errors involving medical linear accelerators (Table 7.3).[37] Although technology has advanced and evolved since this report was published, the potential for errors within the radiation therapy process still remains. In 2012, as part of *Safety is No Accident: A Framework for Quality Radiation Oncology and Care*, suggestions for tools that would facilitate safety in a radiation oncology department were shared.[2] These are summarized in Box 7.1.[2]

A comprehensive understanding of and familiarization with the design, characteristics, performance parameters, and control of the linear accelerator are essential for many of the members of the cancer management team.

> This "Safety is No Accident" report was updated in 2019 and provides even more detail about safety incorporating key concepts like systems thinking, human factors engineering, and incident learning. More information is available at: https://www.astro.org/Patient-Care-and-Research/Patient-Safety/Safety-is-no-Accident

Cobalt-60 Characteristics

Today, increasingly fewer ^{60}Co units are used to treat cancer in the United States, but they still may be used in developing countries. Although the gamma knife, which uses ^{60}Co sources, is still used in many institutions as an effective form of SRS treatment, in the 1980s, ^{60}Co units were the mainstay of most radiation oncology departments. The decrease of ^{60}Co units began in the 1960s with the introduction of the linear accelerator because linear accelerators provided better isodose distribution (a larger dose to the tumor and a smaller dose to normal tissue), faster dose rate, smaller penumbra, and more manageable radiation protection concerns. Despite the decline in popularity of ^{60}Co units in the United States, they are the backbone of many radiation therapy departments in low- and middle-income countries. For

example, according to the International Atomic Energy Association's Directory of Radiotherapy Centers, only 26 of the 53 African countries have radiation therapy equipment, and of those that do, many rely on the dependability of the ^{60}Co unit. This popularity is probably the result of the unit's cost, simpler design, and reliability.[45]

In the early 1950s, ^{60}Co units became popular because they could deliver a significant dose of radiation below the skin surface. Compared with earlier teletherapy (treatment at some distance) units, such as radium and cesium treatment machines, ^{60}Co units were faster at delivering the dose and more cost effective at producing and using the isotope. At the time, mining the ore necessary to produce a small amount of radium was extremely expensive. The ^{60}Co units were the first practical radiation therapy treatment units to provide a significant dose below the skin surface and simultaneously spare the skin the harsh effects of earlier methods. These elements allowed the radiation oncologist and radiation therapist to deliver larger doses of radiation to greater depths in tissue. When a greater percentage of dose occurs below the skin surface, the term dose maximum (D_{max}) is used to describe the process. D_{max} is the depth of maximum buildup, in which 100% of the dose is deposited. Table 7.4 describes the depth of D_{max} for a variety of beams. For ^{60}Co, D_{max} occurs at 0.5 cm below the skin surface. This was a tremendous advantage versus the other types of equipment (especially orthovoltage) used to treat cancer at the time.

There are several methods to turn the beam "on": rotating wheel, sliding drawer, and use of a shutter or jaws. To protect personnel, the ^{60}Co source must be shielded when the source is in the "off" position. Radiation therapists working with ^{60}Co machines must be aware of what to do if the source fails to retract after the machine is turned off. Compared with linear accelerators and other electrically operated therapy equipment, these machines constantly emit radiation. A great deal of high-density material, such as lead or depleted uranium, surrounds the source in the head of the machine (Fig. 7.26). To help the machine rotate smoothly and provide additional shielding, it must have a counterweight. In part, this is to balance the lead shielding in the head of the machine housing the radioactive ^{60}Co source. This counterweight, extending from the opposite end of the gantry in which the source is housed, is called a *beam stopper*.

Production

Cobalt-60 is an artificially produced isotope. Similar to many other isotopes used in the diagnosis and treatment of disease, ^{60}Co becomes radioactive when its atomic number is altered. This may happen in a particle accelerator called a *cyclotron*, or *nuclear reactor*. The

TABLE 7.3   Medical Accelerator Hazards

Type	Cause	Consequences
Incorrect dose delivered	Electrical, software, and therapist	Serious injury, increased complications, genetic effects, second primary, and compromised tumor control
Dose delivered to the wrong area	Mechanical, software, patient motion, and therapist	Serious injury, increased complications, genetic effects, second primary, and compromised tumor control
Machine collision	Mechanical, software, patient motion, and therapist	Significant injury and death
Incorrect beam	Electrical, software, and therapist	Serious injury, increased complications, genetic effects, second primary, and compromised tumor control
General hazards	Electrical and mechanical	Significant injury and death

BOX 7.1   Tools to Improve Safety in Radiation Oncology Departments

- Well-defined procedures
- Standardization of procedures and tasks
- Increased utilization of human factors engineering
- Incorporation of quality assurance tasks into radiation oncology software
- Peer review
- Daily morning meetings
- Safety rounds
- Regular safety announcements and updates
- Adequate staffing levels
- Realistic process and treatment times

From Safety is no accident: a framework for quality radiation oncology and care. American Society for Radiation Oncology website. https://www.astro.org/Patient-Care-and-Research/Patient-Safety/Safety-is-no-Accident. Accessed September 24, 2019.

production of ^{60}Co begins with the stable form of cobalt, which has an atomic mass number of 59. The atomic mass number is the sum of the number of protons and neutrons in the nucleus. After ^{59}Co is bombarded or irradiated in a nuclear reactor with slow neutrons, the nucleus of ^{59}Co absorbs one neutron and becomes radioactive ^{60}Co. This can be expressed in the following formula:

$$^{59}\text{Co} + {}^{1}\text{n} \cong {}^{60}\text{Co}$$

As in any radioactive substance, ^{60}Co emits γ radiation in an effort to return to its more stable state.

Cobalt-60 activity may be expressed in curies (Ci), the historical unit of radioactivity, which equals 3.7×10^{10} becquerel (Bq). Bq, the standard international unit of radioactivity, equals 1 disintegration per second. Most sources have an activity of 750 to 9000 Ci and may be referred to as *kilocurie sources*.[27] In addition, the activity may be defined in rhm units (1 rhm unit represents 1 roentgen per hour at 1 m). The quality of the radiation produced by the source does not depend on the number of curies. With a 3000-Ci source, the equipment can be operated at an 80-cm distance and have a 10-cm depth dose of 56%.[26] Sources used in radiation therapy typically range from 3000 to 9000 Ci and have a specific activity of 75 to 200 Ci/g.

Specific activity is the number of transformations per second for each gram of radionuclide decaying at a fixed rate. Specific activity is the number of curies per gram. The specific activity for a ^{60}Co source can be as high as 400 Ci/g, but for radiation therapy treatment, it is usually 200 Ci/g. A smaller source at the standard 80 SSD produces a beam of lower intensity requiring longer treatment time.

The radioactive ^{60}Co source and its shielding (in the form of a protective casing) are referred to as the *cobalt capsule*. The diameter of the capsule can range from 1 to 3 cm for radiation therapy purposes; 1.0 to 2.0 cm is the preferred diameter. The radioactive cobalt source contains disks, slugs, or pellets grouped in a cluster or solid cylinder, encased in a stainless steel capsule, and sealed by welding. The capsule is placed inside a second steel capsule that is also welded. The multiple layers of metal prevent leakage of the radioactive material and absorb the beta particles produced during the decay process.[27]

Characteristics. The radioactive ^{60}Co nucleus emits ionizing radiation in the form of high-energy gamma rays. ^{60}Co decays by first emitting a beta particle with an energy of 0.31 MeV that is absorbed in the source's steel capsule. After emitting the beta particle, the nucleus enters an excited state of nickel-60. The nickel-60 decays to a ground state by emitting two gamma rays per disintegration. Of the two gamma rays emitted, one has an energy of 1.17 MeV, and the

TABLE 7.4 Depth of Maximum Dose for Various Photon Energies

Beam Energy	D_{max} (cm Below SKIN Surface)
Superficial	0.0
Orthovoltage	0.0
Cobalt-60	0.5
4 MV	1.0
6 MV	1.5
10 MV	2.5
15 MV	3.0
20 MV	3.5
25 MV	5.0

MV, Megavoltage.
From Stanton R, Stinson D. *Applied Physics for Radiation Oncology*. Madison, WI: Medical Physics Publishing; 1996.

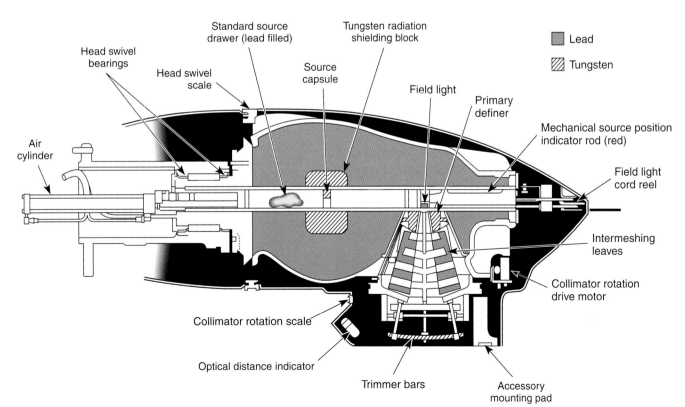

Fig. 7.26 A cross section of typical cobalt-60 components. (Courtesy Atomic Energy of Canada Limited, Medical Products, Kanata, Ontario, Canada.)

other is 1.33 MeV.[27] The beam can be considered polyenergetic or heterogeneous because more than one energy is decaying from the isotope. For practical purposes, the two energies are averaged to give an effective energy of 1.25 MeV. The large source size of the ^{60}Co created large penumbra at field edges. Because of this, trimmer bars were often added below the treatment head to 'trim" penumbra off the edges of the field.

Because ^{60}Co is a radioactive isotope, it has a half-life ($t_{1/2}$), the time necessary for a radioactive material to decay to half or 50% of its original activity. Cobalt-60 decays to 50% of its activity after a $t_{1/2}$ of 5.26 years. To compensate for the reduction in beam output each month, a correction factor of approximately 1% per month must be applied to the output. The correction factor increases the treatment time necessary to deliver the appropriate dose. To maintain adequate output for patient treatment and thus eliminate longer treatment times, the ^{60}Co source should be replaced at least every 5.3 years.

Shielding blocks were either made of lead, or more commonly Lipowitz metal, similar to the ones used for electron treatment on a linear accelerator. Cerrobend is a form of Lipowitz metal used for designing custom shielding blocks for photons and electrons and consists of 50.0% bismuth, 26.7 lead, 13.3% tin, and 10.0% cadmium. Cerrobend melts (70°C) at a much lower point than lead (327°C). Therefore, Cerrobend is easier and safer to use. However, cadmium (a toxic metal) can get into the bloodstream of individuals who work with Lipowitz metal. Some manufacturers have a type of Lipowitz alloy without cadmium available for a slight increase in cost.[27]

SUMMARY

- Historically, radiation therapy treatment delivery equipment has evolved from low-energy, low-skin-sparing, unsophisticated systems (such as orthovoltage units) to today's computerized, MV linear accelerators that can treat a variety of deep-seated tumors.
- In the treatment room, the major components of a linear accelerator can be divided into three specific areas: drive stand, gantry, and treatment couch.
- Four major components are housed in the stand: the klystron, waveguide, circulator, and cooling system.
- The major components in the gantry are the electron gun, accelerator structure (guide), and treatment head.
- The transfer of information, such as the exact location of immobilization devices, from simulation to the treatment machine is improved when devices are referenced or indexed to the treatment tabletop.

- MLC systems are used to shield areas by using approximately 52 to 160 leaves. These heavy metal collimator leaves slide into place to form the desired field shape by projecting 0.25- to 1-cm beam widths per leaf.
- Specialized treatment machines are becoming increasingly popular in radiation therapy departments, used to increase the dose to the target while minimizing dose to the surrounding normal tissue.
- The radioactive ^{60}Co nucleus emits ionizing radiation in the form of high-energy gamma rays, with a D_{max} of 0.5 cm. Of the two gamma rays emitted, one has an energy of 1.17 MeV and the other an energy of 1.33 MeV. For practical purposes, the two energies are averaged to give an effective energy of 1.25 MeV.

REVIEW QUESTIONS

The answers to the Review Questions can be found by logging on to our website at: http://evolve.elsevier.com/Washington+Leaver/principles/ Megan Trad's

1. Which of the following does not relate to MLC leakage or transmission?
   a. The shape of the curved end or tip of MLC.
   b. The thickness of MLC.
   c. Cerrobend used to increase the speed of MLC.
   d. The tongue-and-groove effect of MLC.
2. Which of the following kV x-ray machines would be used to treat a skin cancer that was estimated to be nearly 2 cm in thickness?
   a. Contact therapy.
   b. Superficial treatments.
   c. Orthovoltage therapy.
   d. Linear accelerator.
3. If an electron beam does not demonstrate consistency in dose across the treatment field, what might be at fault?
   a. Scattering foil.
   b. Flattening filter.
   c. Wedge.
   d. Multileaf collimator.
4. What is the average energy with which ^{60}Co emits gamma rays used for radiation therapy treatments?
   a. 1.17.
   b. 1.25.
   c. 1.33.
   d. 2.50.
5. A TomoTherapy unit is best described as:
   a. A 6-MV linear accelerator x-ray beam resembling the shape of a fan, 40 cm wide and 1 cm, 2.5 cm, or 5 cm thick as measured at the isocenter.

   b. Primary and secondary collimators made of tungsten and these metal collimator rods slide into place to form the desired field shape.
   c. The beam can be considered polyenergetic or heterogeneous because more than one energy is decaying from the isotope.
   d. For practical purposes, the two energies are averaged to give an effective energy.
6. Which of the following would not be used for IGRT?
   a. EPID.
   b. kV cone beam CT.
   c. kV image.
   d. Orthovoltage x-ray unit.
7. When were linear accelerators first commercially available for clinical use?
   a. 1895.
   b. 1930s.
   c. 1950s.
   d. 1980s.
8. A beam-flattening filter is placed in the path of the beam when _____ are used for treatment purposes.
   a. Protons.
   b. Electrons.
   c. X-rays.
   d. Gamma rays.
9. What does a klystron or magnetron produce?
   a. Microwave power.
   b. Alternating current.
   c. Accelerated electrons and photons.
   d. Magnetic fields used to bend the beam.

10. Trace the path of an electron in a linear accelerator by selecting the best route from the following.
    I. Electron gun.
    II. Collimator.
    III. Accelerator guide.

IV. Bending magnet.
    a. I, II, III, IV.
    b. I, III, IV, II.
    c. II, I, IV, II.
    d. III, I, II, IV.

■ QUESTIONS TO PONDER

1. Why do you think IGRT may be a better way to check the delivery of radiation therapy?
2. Discuss the application and use of superficial and orthovoltage treatment in radiation therapy.
3. Why must a monthly calculation correction be made for the ^{60}Co treatment?
4. Discuss the integration of computerization and the linear accelerator operation. What are the benefits and drawbacks?
5. Compare MLC characteristics of the three major vendors: Elekta, Siemens, and Varian.

6. Discuss the major components of the linear accelerator, including the klystron, waveguide, circulator, electron gun, accelerator guide, and bending magnet.
7. Describe the difference between a beam-flattening filter and a scattering foil.
8. Describe the advantages of a treatment couch with 6 degrees of freedom.
9. What type of specialized treatment machine does your facility have? How does it compare to a standard linear accelerator?

REFERENCES

1. Products. Accuray, inc. website. www.accuray.com. Accessed December 4, 2018.
2. Safety is no accident: a framework for quality radiation oncology and care. American Society for Radiation Oncology website. https://www.astro.org/Patient-Care-and-Research/Patient-Safety/Safety-is-no-Accident. Accessed December 4, 2018.
3. Avivarasan I, Anuradha C, Subramanian S, et al. Magnetic resonance image guidance in external beam radiation therapy planning and delivery. *Jpn J Radiol.* 2017;35:417–426.
4. Beavis AW. Is tomotherapy the future of IMRT? *Br J Radiol.* 2004;77:285–294.
5. Bissonnette JP, Jaffray DA, Fenster A, et al. Optimal radiographic magnification for portal imaging. *Med Phys.* 1994;21:1435–1445.
6. Bushong SC. *Radiologic Science for Technologists: Physics, Biology, and Protection.* 11th ed. St. Louis, MO: Elsevier; 2017.
7. Bourland JD. Radiation oncology physics. In: Gunderson S, Tepper J, eds. *Clinical Radiation Oncology.* 4th ed. Philadelphia, PA: Elsevier; 2015.
8. Boyer A, Biggs P, Galvin J, et al. *Basic Applications of Multileaf Collimators.* AAPM Report No. 72. Madison, WI: Medical Physics Publishing; 2001.
9. Cao Y, Tseng CL, Balter JM, et al. MR guided radiation therapy: transformative technology and its role in the central nervous system. *Neuro Oncol.* 2017;19:16–29.
10. Chen AM, Cao M, Hsu S, et al. Magnetic resonance imaging guided reirradiation of recurrent and second primary head and neck cancer. *Adv Radiat Oncol.* 2017;2:167–175.
11. Chung HT, Park WY, Kim TH, et al. Assessment of the accuracy and stability of frameless Gamma Knife radiosurgery. *J Appl Clin Med Phys.* 2018;19(4):148–154.
12. Computer Hope Website. www.computerhope.com. Accessed December 7, 2018.
13. Cozzi L, Fogliata A, Thompson S, et al. Critical appraisal of the treatment planning performance of volumetric modulated arc therapy by means of a dual layer stacked multileaf collimator for head and neck, breast and prostate. *Technol Cancer Res Treat.* 2018;17:1–11.
14. Dieterich S, Famimian B. Stereotactic and robotic radiation therapies. In: Van Dyk J, ed. *Modern Technology of Radiation Oncology.* Vol. 3. Madison, WI: Medical Physics Publishing; 2013.
15. Elshaikh M, Ljungman M, Ten Haken R, et al. Advances in radiation oncology. *Annu Rev Med.* 2006;57:19–31.
16. Faddegon BA, Garde E. A pulse-rate dependence of dose per monitor unit and its significant effect on wedged-shaped fields delivered with variable dose rate and a moving jaw. *Med Phys.* 2006;33(8):3063–3065.
17. Fraass BA, Eisbruch A, Feng M. Intensity-modulated and image-guided radiation therapy. In: Gunderson LL, Tepper JE, eds. *Clinical Radiation Oncology.* 4th ed. Philadelphia, PA: Elsevier; 2015.

18. Galvin JM. The multileaf collimator—a complete guide. American Association of Physicists in Medicine website. www.aapm.org/meetings/99AM/pdf/2787-9625.pdf. Accessed December 7, 2018.
19. Goer DA, Musslewhite CW, Jablonw DM. Potential of mobile intraoperative radiotherapy technology. *Surg Oncol Clin N Am.* 2003;12:943–953.
20. Goldson AL. Preliminary clinical experience with intraoperative radiotherapy. *J Natl Med Assoc.* 1978;70:493–495.
21. Green O, Henke LE, Parikh P, et al. Practical implication of ferromagnetic artifacts in low-field MRI-guided radiotherapy. *Cureus.* 2018;10(3):e2359.
22. Grigg FRN. *The Trail of the Invisible Light: From X-Olyahlen to Radio (Bio) logy.* Springfield, IL: Charles C Thomas; 1965.
23. Gunderson LL, Shipley WU, Suit HD, et al. Intraoperative irradiation: a pilot study combining external beam photons with 'boost' dose intraoperative electrons. *Cancer.* 1982;49:2259–2266.
24. Hansen WF. The changing role of the accelerator in radiation therapy. *IEEE Trans Nucl Sci.* 1983;30:1781–1783.
25. Halperin EC, Wazer DE, Brady LW, Perez CA. *Perez and Brady's Principles and Practice of Radiation Oncology.* 7th ed. Philadelphia, PA: Walters Klower; 2018.
26. Kahn FM, Gerbi BJ, Sperduto PW. *Treatment Planning in Radiation Oncology.* 4th ed. Philadelphia, PA: Lippincott Williams & Wilkins; 2016.
27. Khan FM, Gibbons JP. *Khan's The Physics of Radiation Therapy.* 5th ed. Philadelphia, PA: Lippincott Williams & Wilkins; 2014.
28. Karzmark CJ, Morton RJ, Lamb J. *A Primer on Theory and Operation of Linear Accelerators in Radiation Therapy.* 3rd ed. Madison, WI: Medical Physics Publishing; 2018.
29. Karzmark .J, Nunan CS, Tanabe E. *Medical Electron Accelerators.* New York, NY: McGraw-Hill; 1992.
30. Kim S, Palta JR. Advances in radiation therapy techniques on linear accelerators. In: Van Dyk J, ed. *Modern Technology of Radiation Oncology.* Vol. 3. Madison, WI: Medical Physics Publishing; 2013.
31. Ma CM, Coffey CW, DeWerd LA, et al. AAPM protocol for 40-300 kV x-ray beam dosimetry in radiotherapy and radiobiology. *Med Phys.* 2001;28(8):868–893.
32. McDermott PM, Orton CG. *The Physics and Technology of Radiation Therapy.* 2nd ed. Madison, WI: Medical Physics Publishing; 2018.
33. Mills JA, Porter H, Gill D. Radiotherapy beam production. In: Symonds P, Deehan C, Mills JA, et al, eds. *Walter and Miller's Textbook of Radiotherapy: Radiation Physics, Therapy and Oncology.* 7th ed. London, UK: Elsevier Churchill Livingstone; 2012.
34. Moore's Law and the Intel Innovation. Intel Website. http://www.intel.com/content/www/us/en/history/museum-gordon-moore-law.html. Accessed December 5, 2018.
35. Podder TK, Fredman ET, Ellis RJ. Advances in radiotherapy for prostate cancer treatment. *Adv Exp Med Biol.* 2018;1096:31–47.
36. Piotrowski T, Skórska M, Jodda A, et al. Tomotherapy—a different way of dose delivery in radiotherapy. *Contemp Oncol.* 2012;16(1):16.

37. Purdy JA, Biggs PJ, Bowers C, et al. Medical accelerator safety considerations: report of AAPM radiation therapy committee task group No. 35. *Med Phys.* 1993;20:1261–1275.

38. Purdy JA, Mutic S. Principles of radiologic physics and dosimetry. In: Halperin EC, Wazer DE, Brady LW, Perez CA, eds. *Perez and Brady's Principles and Practice of Radiation Oncology.* 7th ed. Philadelphia, PA: Walters Klower.

39. Runciman W, Hibbert P, Thomson R, et al. Toward an international classification for patient safety: key concepts and terms. *Int J Qual Health Care.* 2009;21(1):18–26.

40. Saw CB, Katz L, Gillette C, Koutcher L. 3D treatment planning on helical tomotherapy delivery system. *Med Dos.* 2018;43:159–167.

41. Scharr E, Beneke M, Casey D, et al. Feasibility of real-time motion management with helical tomotherapy. *Med Phys.* 2018;45(4):1329–1337.

42. Schmidhalte D, Fix MK, Wyss M, et al. Evaluation of a new six degrees of freedom couch for radiation therapy. *Med Phys.* 2013;40(11):111710-111711-11710-11.

43. Sen A, West MK. Commissioning experience and quality assurance of helical tomotherapy machines. *J Med Phys.* 2009;34(4):194–199.

44. Smilowitz JB, Dunkerley D, Hill PM, et al. Long term dosimetric stability of multiple TomoTherapy delivery systems. *J Appl Clin Med Phys.* 2017;18(3):137–143.

45. Stanton R, Stinson D. *Applied Physics for Radiation Oncology.* Madison, WI: Medical Physics Publishing, WI

46. Sterzing F, Uhl M, Hauswald H, et al. Dynamic jaws and dynamic couch in helical tomotherapy. *Int J Radiat Oncol Biol Phys.* 2010;76:1266–1273.

47. Steiler F, Wenz F, Schweizer B, et al. Validation of frame-based positioning accuracy with cone beam computed tomography in Gamma Knife Icon radiosurgery. *Phys Med.* 2018;52:93–97.

48. Swindell W, Morton EJ, Evans PM, et al. The design of megavoltage projection imaging systems: some theoretical aspects. *Med Phys.* 1991;18:651–658.

49. Van Dyk J, Battista JJ. Technology evolution in the twenty-first century. In: Van Dyk J, ed. *Modern Technology of Radiation Oncology.* Vol. 3. Madison, WI: Medical Physics Publishing.

50. Halcyon. Varian Medical System Website. https://www.varian.com/oncology/products/treatment-delivery/halcyon. Accessed December 4, 2018.

51. Verhey LJ, Petti PL. Principles of radiation physics. In: Hoppe RT, Phillips TL, Roach M, eds. *Leibel and Phillips Textbook of Radiation Oncology.* 3rd ed. Philadelphia, PA: Elsevier Saunders; 2010.

52. Xia P, Xing L, Amols HI, et al. Three dimensional conformal radiotherapy and intensity modulated radiotherapy. In: Hoppe RT, Phillips TL, Roach M, eds. Leibel and Phillips *Textbook of Radiation Oncology.* 3rd ed. Philadelphia, PA: Elsevier Saunders; 2010.

8

Treatment Procedures

Annette M. Coleman

OBJECTIVES

- Construct an action plan for patient treatment setup and delivery.
- Describe the radiation therapist's role in the quality assurance program.
- Review the radiation treatment chart for information to decide to treat and prepare the room for treatment.
- Given a specific situation, select and describe the safest transfer method for the patient and the radiation therapist.
- Describe a step-by-step process to align the patient and treatment volume with the machine isocenter and coordinate system.

- Discriminate between setup and field imaging goals.
- List and define beam-shaping and beam-modification devices.
- Compare treatment setup implications between photon and electron beams: (1) collimation, (2) bolus, and (3) adjacent fields.
- Describe multileaf collimators and their application as both beam-shaping and beam-modification devices in treatment delivery.
- Categorize common external beam treatment techniques
- List appropriate responses to treatment interruptions.

OUTLINE

KEY TERMS

Beam modifiers
Beam's eye view
Collimation
Compensators
Elapsed days
Feathering
Fiducial
Field

Fraction
Fractionation
Hinge angle
Immobilization devices
Interlocks
Interfraction
Intrafraction
Isocenter

Radiation treatment is essential to quality oncologic care and its delivery under a radiation oncologist's direction, which constitutes the radiation therapist's core professional practice. Conscientious attention to precision in simulation and treatment delivery and to patients' physiologic and psychologic needs highlights the radiation therapist's contribution to the cancer management team. Radiation therapists deliver radiation therapy treatments, monitor and operate sophisticated radiation-producing equipment, and maintain detailed, accurate treatment history records.

Consistent treatment depends on abilities and limitations imposed by equipment, treatment beam geometry, and the patient. Quality radiation patient care depends on the radiation therapist's specialized knowledge and skills in radiation treatment techniques, equipment operation, spatial proficiency between patient anatomy and equipment capabilities, radiation exposure response, communication, and empathy for patients' personal needs. Knowledge in anatomy, oncology, treatment planning, physics, radiation biology, and legal considerations are a prerequisite to clinical judgment formation necessary to execute responsibilities safely and responsibly.

Well-developed organization and communication skills are called on to execute each patient's unique treatment plan while directing a full and varied patient load. The action plan for each patient is unique and complex but effectively achieves a core task set. A baseline task analysis can provide a framework for organizing an action plan (Box 8.1). Details and alternative pathways build on this foundation, addressing individual treatment technique complexities, specialized equipment, and procedures. Acronyms can be powerful memory devices, assuring critical tasks are consistently executed (Box 8.2).

RADIATION ONCOLOGY RECORD

The patient chart is the communication nucleus for the radiation care team. As a legal record, its completeness, organization, and accuracy are critical. Traditionally dependent on treatment team members' handwritten accounts, electronic medical records (EMR) are now the routine charting medium, integrating text and image information with radiation oncology workflow. Information centrally stored can be presented uniquely to each treatment team member by task, and access is limited only by the facility's information technology network.

With electronic charting, the medium for medical charting evolves, not the requirements. Record integrity and security remains each care team member's responsibility. Information access and entry is associated with a log-in identification and is managed much more securely than with paper. In addition to accuracy, the radiation therapist is ethically and legally accountable to patient privacy and confidentiality of medical records.

Medical Record: Treatment: Rational and Response

A radiation treatment chart captures relevant patient medical history, including diagnostic and staging results along with general medical conditions that might impact treatment outcomes. Before receiving treatment, patients must provide their informed consent to any procedures. Informed consent requires the patient or their legal guardian receives an explanation and understands his or her disease status, treatment alternatives, and consequences associated with and without treatment. As patient advocate, the radiation therapist verifies patient understanding and ensures informed consent is documented in the chart.

Patient response to treatment is monitored and recorded throughout and following treatment completion. Radiation treatment responses often require medication, nutrition, or psychosocial intervention; all care activities are recorded in the chart. The entire treatment team monitors radiation reactions through direct observation, blood counts or other lab test reviews, and questioning regarding nutritional intake, skin reactions, and other treatment related symptoms. Weekly radiation oncologist on-treatment visits document weight changes, symptom emergence and care, and other treatment response indicators. Ancillary care team members, such as nutritionists and social workers, may also include their assessments and instructions in the radiation therapy chart.

BOX 8.1 Treatment Procedure Task Analysis

1. Review the chart.
2. Prepare the room. Position immobilization devices on the treatment table, and place treatment accessories within reach.
3. Greet and identify the patient.
4. Assist the patient onto the treatment table and into the prescribed position.
5. Identify treatment site and procedure; document the Time Out.
6. Raise the couch, bringing the area to be treated to the beam area.
7. Locate surface landmarks.
8. Refine the patient position relative to the isocenter using lasers, light field, and surface landmarks.
9. Perform setup verification procedures, imaging, etc.
10. Rotate gantry and collimator to prescribed positions.
11. Position beam-shaping accessories and visually verify using the light field.
12. Perform portal verification procedures.
13. Position beam modifiers (wedge, compensator, and bolus).
14. Inform the patient that you are leaving, and treatment will begin.
15. Monitor the patient.
16. Set appropriate machine controls, and review correspondence with prescribed values in the record and verification system.
17. Initiate beam-on. Monitor patient and equipment function. When multiple fields are to be treated, do the following:
18. Validate parameters downloaded to accelerator and enable accelerator motion, or enter the room and check the patient, field position, and beam modifiers.
19. Repeat steps 7 through 15 for all fields until the treatment completion.
20. Assist the patient from the couch and room.
21. Complete the treatment record.

Image Record

As with the text chart, electronic imaging practices now predominate. Integrated text and images present a far more robust patient story than independently managed paper and film records. Treatment planning and delivery communications and workflow are dramatically improved with diagnostic and planning data readily transferable between systems.

Verification imaging completes the treatment record, and verification image communication between the radiation therapist and radiation oncologist is critical to treatment accuracy. Verification imaging documents treatment localization reproduction (hidden anatomy identification relative to observable or palpable surface landmarks). Images are acquired with the patient in the treatment position, compared with reference images from the treatment plan. This provides critical confirmation and documentation that the planned treatment was accurately reproduced.

Radiation Treatment Record

The radiation treatment record is truly unique to the radiation oncology EMR. The radiation prescription, treatment plan, and treatment record are highly specialized information not applied by other medical specialties.

BOX 8.2 Treatment Procedure Mnemonics

For PATIENT IDENTIFICATION: "**CONFIRM**"
- **C**heck name, **O**n screen, **F**ind data, **R**eview data with patient, **M**ove to sim/treatment room.
- Ask the patient for two forms of identification. Once assured this is the correct patient, verify the patient picture on the screen and ask the patient where they are having treatment. The patient and treatment are reviewed; ask the patient to move to the treatment room.

For SIMULATION and TREATMENT UNIT: "**SAME**"
- **S**traighten, **A**lign, **M**ove couch, and **E**nsure immobilization.
- Use the "**SAME**" standard for every patient. Straighten the patient on the simulation or treatment couch. Align the patient to the table for both longitudinal and lateral directions. Once straight and aligned, move the couch/patient support assembly (PSA) vertically, longitudinally, and laterally as needed. Then ensure immobilization is enough to begin simulation or treatment.

For CT SIMULATION: "**SIMMED**"
- **S**et BBs/wires, **I**mage, **M**ark, **M**easure, **E**ducate, and **D**ocument.
- Once the "**SAME**" standard and proper immobilization is demonstrated, execute the "**SIMMED**" routine. Set the BBs/wires to prepare for scout/images. Once imaged, mark the patient and make any necessary measurements. After marking, educate the patient on marks care and future appointments. Once the patient leaves, document required information.

For TREATMENT UNIT: "**LASER**"
- **L**evel, **A**lign, **S**creen check, **E**xit, and **R**eview chart.
- Once the "**SAME**" standard and proper immobilization is demonstrated, perform the "**LASER**" routine. Level the patient to the lateral lasers. Once level, align the patient to isocenter. After the patient is positioned correctly, check the in-room screen/monitor for any notes or changes that must be made before exiting the room. Once at the console, review the chart again. "**STEPS**"
- **S**tudy plan, **T**hink about the console, **E**yes on patient, **P**ort film verification, and **S**afe to treat.
- After reviewing the chart, study the treatment plan and know what fields are to be treated. Watch the console and the patient. Image if necessary, check and verify, move couch accordingly. Affirm it is safe to treat and beam on.

From RL Wegener, MS, RT(R)(T). Delgado Community College, Radiation Therapy Technology Program. With permission.

Radiation dose and equipment settings under which it was delivered is recorded at each treatment session. The treatment history identifies the treatment date(s) and increments the delivered treatment number and elapsed days (total time over which treatment is protracted) and fractional and total dose delivered to the prescribed volume and critical structures near or in the treatment volume. Notations are made regarding procedures completed during a treatment session, such as verification imaging (radiographic or electronic treatment documentation) and addition or deletion of bolus or other beam modifiers. All treatment record entries must identify the treating radiation therapists. When multiple fractions are delivered on a single day, delivery time is also required.

As accelerator capabilities and treatment plans increased in complexity, equipment settings became too numerous to manually set, confirm, and chart in the treatment history. Modern treatment delivery requires verification and record (V&R) systems integration with the radiation chart.

V&R systems send prevalidated treatment plan parameters to the treatment machine for setup and delivery. Actual machine settings are compared against those most recently prescribed and prevent treatment beam initiation if settings vary outside a specified tolerance range. On beam delivery conclusion, the machine returns data documenting what settings were in place and meterset (monitor units [MU]) delivered.

V&R systems can extend verification and documentation beyond the treatment machine, from patient identification to secondary equipment not integrated with the treatment machine itself. Field sequences may be defined, automating selection and machine movement to settings and beam delivery.

As with the EMR, V&R functions change the method, not the responsibilities. Appropriate decision making for the entire care team is dependent on accurate and complete records, and treatment history integrity is the radiation therapist's responsibility, not the equipment. Data accuracy must be confirmed by the treatment team before inclusion; observed deviations from what actually took place must be reported and investigated.

Quality Assurance: Chart Review

The treatment chart is both a tool and a focus for the facility's quality assurance (QA) program. The activities and documentation performed to reduce errors and optimize patient care comprise the QA program. The treatment chart must include information identifying and supporting the treatment rationale, a detailed treatment plan description, informed consent documentation, and detailed treatment delivery records. Treatment must not proceed if any information is unavailable or in question.

The radiation therapist's primary role in the QA program is ensuring accurate radiation delivery as prescribed by a radiation oncologist. This requires reviewing patient records, monitoring radiation-producing equipment functioning, maintaining accuracy in treatment reproduction, monitoring changes in patient status, and maintaining complete and accurate treatment records.

Examples of weekly chart reviews may include monitoring treatment verification checks, such as source-skin distance (SSD) records, diode measurements, verification imaging frequency and radiation oncologist review status, fractional and cumulative tracked dose accuracy, physics chart check completion, and charge verification.

Chart reviews include previous entry verification. With traditional paper records, the most common charting errors were numeric: addition or transpositions often in the dose record. As the chart is the primary document referenced in litigation processes, corrections require the original entry to be apparent. Legible corrections and reasonable

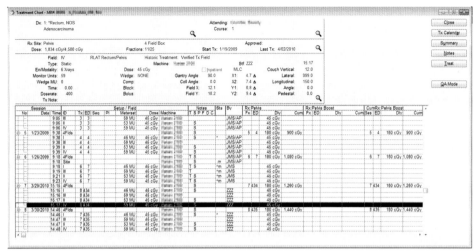

Fig. 8.1 Treatment chart.

explanations are required. With paper, one line is drawn through the entry, followed by the correct value, the correcting individual initials, and the date. Correction fluid or other methods hiding original entries are viewed with suspicion and must be avoided.

Changes to treatment orders or corrections to entries must be apparent in electronic records as with paper records. The EMR assists chart QA with time-stamped data entries and access to detailed change histories. The ability to selectively filter and display information relevant to tasks or timelines can greatly streamline chart review. Prospectively, required information and processes can be reinforced by blocking actions when information or authorization is not available.

TREATMENT SESSION PREPARATION

Before initiating treatment, review the chart's treatment section for completeness and accuracy. Information necessary for treatment reproduction includes an identification image and patient confirmable data, such as birth date, street address, or phone number. Confirm that the radiation prescription is signed; detailed patient- and equipment-positioning information, dosimetric plans, calculations, and the treatment history record are complete with fractional and cumulative doses, machine settings, verification imaging, and prescribed changes (Fig. 8.1).

Radiation Prescription

Radiation may be delivered only under a radiation oncologist's direct order. As with drug and other therapies, radiation orders are written as prescriptions that must be signed by the radiation oncologist before radiation treatment initiation. No exceptions are allowed. The prescription must provide specific information supporting consistent interpretation by qualified professionals, including the radiation therapist. Recommendations have been published by the American Society of Therapeutic Radiation Oncology, identifying key external beam prescription elements and sequencing. Anatomic treatment site is identified first, followed by method of delivery (minimally, photons, electrons, or identifying an isotope). Prescription definition begins with (1) dose per fraction (individual dose intended for a treatment session), followed by (2) number of fractions, and (3) total radiation dose to be delivered. Additional prescription components, including protraction (time over which the treatment will be given) schedule, planning instructions, information specifying beam energy, portal sizes and entry angles, and beam modifiers (devices that change treatment field shape or radiation distribution at depth) may be included in the prescription and with patient-positioning information.[1] Some

guidance on treatment sites naming may be found in reports by the American Association of Physicists in Medicine and the American College of Surgeons.[2,3]

Great responsibility is accepted by the radiation therapist when dispensing the prescription. In preparation, review the prescription before starting the treatment course, applying knowledge on radiation effects, tumor-lethal doses, and radiation tolerance limits for normal tissue. Prescriptions appearing to exceed tissue limits or deviate from standard practice must be reviewed with the physician before delivery. Great care is taken by every team member to eliminate errors and ensure the safest treatment delivery.

The prescription is again reviewed immediately before each treatment fraction. Changes may be ordered at any time, and the radiation therapist provides the "last line of defense" that changes are implemented as ordered. The physician's signature and date must accompany any changes in the prescription. Common prescription changes include fraction and total dose or changes to bolus or beam apertures. Changes affecting dose calculation require plan review to ensure corrections have been made before treatment delivery.

Treatment Plan and Reference Images

Treatment plan review ensures critical information is available for treatment plan reproduction before treatment initiation. Setup instructions, diagrams, and/or photographs illustrate patient positioning, immobilization, and surface landmark locations indicating the treatment isocenter position (the intersection point for the linac's three axes rotation [gantry, collimator, and couch base]). Any adjustments to the original information must be clearly identified.

One or more **treatment fields** compose a treatment plan. A treatment field is the tissue volume exposed to radiation from a single radiation beam. Treatment fields expose target volumes, maximizing the dose delivered to the tumor while minimizing the dose to normal structures. Each treatment field, or portal, is assigned an identifier and name indicating the prescription site and beam direction (Fig. 8.2). Field identifiers follow department-established protocols. In general, some incremental format is applied to distinguish fields from distinct projections. Subscript letters, numbers, or prime marks (', ") denoting changes in the field size, shape, or isocenter from the original field are used when the prescription volume and beam direction have not changed. Field names further clarify beam orientation and targeted anatomy. The complete field definition includes detailed console and beam-shaping parameters necessary to deliver dose objectives.

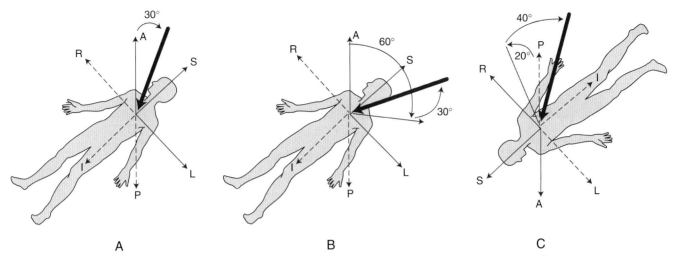

Fig. 8.2 Three-dimensional beam nomenclature. Beams are named referencing the patient coordinate system. (A) The A30S beam is 30 degrees superior from the anterior axis. (B) The A60L30S beam is 60 degrees left from the anterior axis and 30 degrees superior. (C) The P20R40I beam is 20 degrees right from the posterior axis and 40 degrees inferior. (From Bourland D. Radiation oncology physics. In: Gunderson LL, Tepper JE, eds. *Clinical Radiation Oncology.* 2nd ed. Philadelphia, PA: Churchill Livingstone; 2007.)

> Treatment field dimensions are stated width by length in centimeters.
> International Commission on Radiation Units and Measurements Reports 50 and 62 define treatment volumes to be used for prescribing and reporting radiation doses.

Dose distributions and meterset calculations, typically prepared by the medical dosimetrist,[4] are reviewed and signed by at least two treatment-planning team members before being made available for treatment. Before treatment, radiation therapists independently review the treatment plan for calculation factor faithfulness against treatment parameters. Field sizes, beam modifiers, and treatment depths used in calculations must be consistent with those identified in the treatment setup instructions. Results may be further verified by direct dose measurements at treatment course start using electronic diodes or other dosimeters placed on the patient in the treatment field during treatment. The value of these checks cannot be overstated; therapists are the last defensive line in the collective review series performed to eliminate errors. Radiation therapists are consistently reported as discovering the most errors or near-miss incidents to a US national incident learning system.[5]

Medical images further illustrate treatment plans. Planning images are the standard images which on-treatment images are compared in order to verify treatment position and to document treated volumes. Planar radiographs from simulation procedures or digital reconstructed radiographs from computed tomography (CT) data by treatment planning or virtual simulation systems may serve as treatment field or isocenter reference images. Treatment field reference images show the beam's eye view (BEV) area to be irradiated and the beam shape and direction as it passes through the patient and surrounding radiopaque references, such as bones or implantable fiducials (placed object used as a point reference). Isocenter reference images may additionally be required if field image projections are insufficient, or the planning CT itself may be used with advanced in-room imaging systems.

Treatment History

At treatment record review, therapists evaluate completeness and accuracy to date and determine actions to be taken at the treatment session about to commence. Questions may include the following:
- "When was the patient's last treatment?"

- "Have any changes to the prescription or treatment plan been ordered? Is current information sufficient to execute those changes?"
- "How far along is the patient in his or her treatment course?"
- "What treatment site and fields are intended for today's treatment session?"
- "Has the weekly on-treatment visit schedule been met? Are any changes to the patient's physical or emotional state identified?"

Attention to the dose delivered informs expectations for the patient's physical reactions to the treatment. As the treatment team member seeing patients at each treatment session, the radiation therapist is key to treatment response monitoring. Understanding radiation reactions and management methods informs the decision to proceed or withhold treatment pending radiation oncologist consultation.

Verification Image History

Before treatment, review the historic images, implement and document any related treatment modification orders, or call unreviewed images to the radiation oncologist's attention.
- "Have previous images been reviewed?"
- "Are setup changes ordered?"
- "Which setup verification method is required today?"
- "Are treatment field images needed today?"

THE TREATMENT ROOM

The organization and maintenance of the treatment room is the radiation therapist's responsibility. Ergonomic movement, lighting, orderliness, and infection precautions are emphasized, enhancing safety for patients and therapists. In addition to monitoring treatment unit performance, inspect treatment accessories regularly for wear or damage, and assure proper lighting levels are maintained. Enough shelf and cabinet space must be available to securely store equipment off the floor. Treatment accessories and positioning or immobilization devices touching patients must be cleaned and disinfected after each use. Isolate custom devices, avoiding cross contamination between patients. Sustain nonreusable or disposable items, such as tape, laundry, and bolus materials. Report and correct any unsafe conditions.

Treatment room design may be viewed as radiating outward from the isocenter. The isocenter is the intersection point for three machine rotation axes (gantry, collimator, and couch base), allowing beam redirection without repositioning the patient. A well-planned treatment room encourages efficient movement around this focal point. Shelves and storage cabinets form the perimeter, leaving the area around the treatment unit clear. Treatment accessory and device storage is generally concealed and organized at heights not requiring stepstools or ladders for retrieval.

> Universal precautions are infection control methods in which any human blood or body fluid is treated as if it were known to be infectious.

Maintain vigilance in infection control. Remember that undiagnosed infections may be present in any individual, and handle all blood and body fluids as if they were infectious. Remember the often immunodeficient oncology patient state, and take responsibility for preventing disease transmission. Clean treatment table and positioning accessories with disinfectant cleaners after each use. Replace linens after each patient, covering the treatment table and keeping the treatment window clear. Apply universal precautions with all patients. Remember, the most important practice toward preventing infection transmission is thorough handwashing after patient contact.

Isocentric linear accelerator mounting facilitates complex treatment plan reproducibility. These versatile units accommodate exquisitely complex field arrangements. Treatment setup seeks coincidence between the treatment unit isocenter and treatment plan isocenter. Yet, because both are effectively hidden from view, alignment requires spatial awareness and visual assistance.

Laser systems installed at the treatment room perimeter generate points or lines intersecting at the treatment machine isocenter. Three or four sources project from the walls and from the ceiling (or opposite the gantry), providing visual references to the machine isocenter location. Using vertical and horizontal planes, the light effectively references a location obscured within a patient (Fig. 8.3). Thus, laser alignment with external patient landmarks directs positioning the accelerator's isocenter to its planned position within the patient. A second laser set may be available at a position lower and outside the gantry's rotation arc. This set allows patient leveling at an ergonomic table height for the therapists. Lasers are highly focused light. Red or green helium neon lasers are generally used. Green lasers project more sharply than red, with their shorter wavelength scattering less at the skin surface. In-room lasers are not harmful to skin but do have the

ability to damage vision. The laser source must not be looked directly into—this precaution applies to everyone entering the treatment room and must be communicated to patients.

Treatment rooms require both standard and dim lighting. Full, standard lighting provides safety for patients and therapists entering and exiting the room and assists when locating accessory equipment. Reducing the light in the treatment room adds clarity to lasers and field light, thus assisting the patient positioning and treatment setup process. While treatment is in progress, full lights are on, aiding patient observation.

Treatment Room Preparation

Room preparation begins before the patient arrives. Treatment setup dimensions, field size, gantry, collimator, and table positions are reviewed. A beam aperture is set and the gantry positioned so that lasers are visible at the isocenter and the field light crosshairs project in a vertical or horizontal direction. The treatment table (couch) is raised or lowered appropriate to the patient's transportation method. Position the table window where treatment fields will reach the patient without intercepting the couch. Mylar covers the table windows, supporting the patient without attenuating the treatment beam. Support may be enhanced by carbon fiber supports beneath the Mylar. The primary window is open across the table and supported by side bars, meeting most field arrangement needs. For oblique or rotational field arrangements that might pass through the side rails, an alternative configuration supports the table center with windows on either side.

Comfort affects the patient's ability to maintain a treatment position; therefore, care is taken at simulation to define a reproducible and sustainable position. Improvements in treatment planning and image evaluation methods are supporting increasingly narrow margins on normal tissue, demanding increased immobilization for all treatment sites. Complexity varies depending on anatomic site mobility. Considerations at the time of simulation include general patient condition (e.g., age, disability, pain), normal structure location, treatment area skin folds, ability to treat all fields in one position, and minimizing normal tissue exposure. Positioning and immobilization devices, such as sponges, casts, masks, and/or bite blocks, support the elected position. Matching devices are oriented on the treatment table relative to the expected patient orientation and location. Interfraction setup variation may be further minimized using indexing systems where immobilization devices are aligned or fitted to incremented positions on the treatment table.

Treatment accessories, such as electron cone, wedges, and bolus, are placed in a readily accessible location away from initial setup activity.

THE PATIENT

Patient Preparation and Communication

From first introductions, initiate and take responsibility for the rapport characterizing the radiation therapist-patient relationship. Seek to establish a relationship that encourages confidence and cooperation. Patients entrust the radiation therapist with their care, and your relationship will typically extend over a period ranging from 2 to 8 weeks. Over this period, the radiation therapist is a patient resource, and this relationship's caliber directly affects the patient's care quality perception. Anticipate questions and concerns associated with radiation treatment, and create an environment sensitive to patient needs. With daily contact, the radiation therapist acts as a liaison, directing the patient to resources designed to meet his or her physical and psychosocial needs. Developing a constructive patient-professional relationship may provide insight into the individual's experience and coping mechanisms, and observations may reveal social service needs or changes in disease state. Notify the physician when changes are observed.

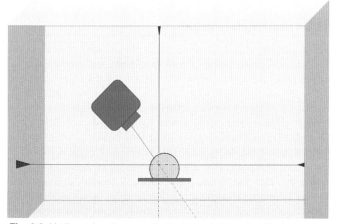

Fig. 8.3 Horizontal and perpendicular lasers intersect at the isocenter.

Understanding expectations during treatment empowers patients and fosters cooperation through mutual respect. Provide clear directions at a level the patient understands. Prioritize cultural sensitivity and linguistic competency. Consider age, mental status, and native language. Use questioning techniques to discover acute radiation reaction onset and severity. Use open-ended questioning, starting with who, what, when, and why questions not answerable with a simple yes or no to encourage dialogue. Avoid closed questioning: "are, do, is, will, can, should," and so on. Brief answers may be followed with gently probing questions to ensure the patient's treatment reactions are understood.

When starting treatment, extend every effort to help patients feel safe. Explain reasons for requiring inconvenient or uncomfortable procedures, such as removing restrictive clothing that may alter skin marks and inhibit treatment position reproduction. Where department practice requires undressing before entering the treatment room, guide them through the gown and robing location and any secure places provided for belongings. Demonstrate audio and visual monitoring systems. Prepare them for gantry proximity, machine motion, and treatment sounds. Offer assurance that their privacy and contact will be maintained always, even as the radiation therapists observe from outside the treatment room.

Through the treatment course, provide counseling in proper skin mark maintenance, general skin care, and nutritional guidelines. Recognize scope of practice boundaries, and demonstrate appropriate decision-making when referrals become necessary. Assess verbal and observable responses (e.g., skin reactions, weight change, changes in demeanor), evaluating whether treatment should continue or be withheld until the patient may be seen by the physician.

Patient Identification, Time Out

When room preparations are complete, greet and confirm patient identification, leading him or her to the treatment room.

Confirm patient identity using at least two methods. Many factors contribute to potential misidentification, and consequences range from discontent in the waiting room to treatment misadministration. Patients may have the same or similar names, illness or anxiety may hinder their ability to respond to their own name, and some will be anxious enough to answer to whichever name you call. As a result, be cautious when identifying patients, and do not become reliant on your own recognition.

The treatment chart includes an identification image for visual confirmation. The most important identification tool for inpatients is their wrist bracelet, which is read before moving a patient into the treatment room. Outpatients typically carry identification cards and may be asked to state their own name, address, or phone number, distinguishing them from those with the same name. Electronic charting and patient management systems offer further security with bar coding and biometric identity confirmation matching chart to patient.

Globally, there is increased awareness regarding wrong site, wrong procedure, and wrong person treatment incidents. Protocols mandated in most countries bring attention to the 3 Rs (right) or 3Cs (correct), patient, site, and procedure. In the United States, The Joint Commission requires accredited organizations to comply with the following Universal Protocol and Time Out.[6]

1. Preprocedure verification (chart and room preparation): verify procedure, patient site, identify items which must be available for procedure, and match items to patient.
2. Mark procedure site.
3. Time out:
   - standardized process within organization
   - initiated by a designated team member at every instance

- immediate team members performing the procedure actively communicating
- correct patient confirmed using at least two methods
- correct site, markings verified
- correct procedure to be undertaken
- document, organization determines form and amount

PATIENT TRANSFERS

Patients require varying assistance onto the treatment table and thus a plan for assuring their comfort and safety. Include the patient whenever possible in your transfer planning. He or she may be able to move themselves or have pain they wish considered, and they have experience informing suggestions for their safe transfer. Have the table prepared with the correct window, and align the patient so their treatment area will be over the window when the transfer is executed. When planning a patient transfer, do not forget to assess your own assistance needs.

> Underestimating the need for assistance can result in injury to the patient and the caregiver.

Many ambulatory patients require minimal assistance. However, even ambulatory patients can find traditional treatment table height a challenge. Extended-range treatment tables can be a great assistance; in their absence, stepstools are routinely employed. Unstable patients, such as those experiencing weakness or injury, may require only a supportive arm or guidance; instruct them to lead with their strong foot, whether stepping up or down from the stool. Still others will arrive in a wheelchair or on a stretcher.

Evaluate transfer requirements, mindful of auxiliary medical equipment in use. Although most extensively in place with inpatients, outpatients also arrive with oxygen or nutritional support or even portable medication pumps. Tubes and catheters must be recognized and carefully handled so as not to disrupt placement or introduce infection.

Understand and apply proper body mechanics when assisting or transferring patients. General rules require a wide support base with the feet apart and one foot placed slightly forward. Keep weight to be moved close, bending at knees and hips, not waist, maintaining a flat to normal curve in the lower back. Never twist or bend sideways while supporting weight.

Wheelchair Transfers

For patients unable to stand unassisted, consider patient size and general stability relative to your own abilities. A second caregiver moving equipment and supporting the primary lifter can significantly improve safety for everyone involved. Prepare by positioning the wheelchair parallel to the table. If the patient has weakness or impairment on one side, position the stronger side in the direction of movement. Lock chair wheels. Raise footrests and stand facing the patient. With the patient's feet together, the assister positions their feet on either side of the patients' and leans forward, bending at the knees and hips while maintaining a flat to natural lower spine curve. The patient reaches around the lift assister's shoulders while the lift assister reaches under the patient's arms, locking arms around the patient's back. The patient is raised to his or her feet and pivoted 90 degrees so his or her back faces the table. Next, ease the patient into a sitting position. Once steadied, with an arm behind the patient's shoulders and the other behind the knees, ease the patient into the supine position in one smooth motion.

Reverse these actions when getting the patient off the table. Give the patient a moment to adjust after sitting up and continue supporting them; dizziness is not unusual on such positional changes. Do not leave the patient unaided until he or she is securely back into the wheelchair.

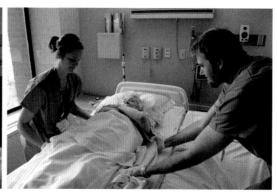

Fig. 8.4 Patient transfer using a slide board. (From Ehrlich RA, Coakes C. *Patient Care in Radiography*. 9th ed. St Louis, MO: Elsevier; 2017.)

If, for any reason (e.g., paralysis, pain), the patient requires more assistance onto the table, stretcher transport should be arranged. This is a safety consideration for the patient and caregivers.

Stretcher Transfers

Stretcher transfers should be completed with no fewer than two caregivers. The stretcher is placed alongside the treatment table with the side rails lowered and wheels locked. The table is positioned at the same level as the stretcher. If the patient can slide over, one lift assistant may secure the stretcher while another stands opposite the treatment table, providing guidance and ensuring the patient does not fall.

Immobile patient transfer across both treatment table and stretcher will force breaches in good body mechanics. At some point, weight will be held away from the assisters' own center of gravity, and someone will push rather than pull. Extra care and concentration must be used for these reaches. A draw sheet and slide board can assist these transfers, reducing injury risk to the people performing the transfer. Slide boards are relatively thin plastic sheets, large enough to support the patient but generally used only to bridge the space between the stretcher and treatment table so the patient may be pulled rather than lifted from one to the other. Patients bring their hands to their chest. The slide board is positioned by rolling the patient and placing the board under the draw sheet. After the patient is eased back onto the slide board, the board may be pulled to the treatment table or the patient slid across the bridge created over the gap between the stretcher and treatment table. The slide board must be removed if it is in the treatment beam path or will affect the treatment position (Fig. 8.4).

Slide boards should not be used when rolling puts the patient at risk for injury. In this situation, several individuals are needed. The appropriate number depends on factors such as patient size or special considerations such as pain. Lifters position themselves to support the patient's head, shoulders, hips, and feet during the entire lift. Ideally, a draw sheet is in place from the move from bed to stretcher, or the stretcher sheet may be sufficient to avoid rolling the patient. Pull sheets taut, rolling edges and gripping firmly. The team leader specifies a count, so everyone lifts at the same time. The patient is lifted just high enough to clear the treatment table and stretcher surfaces, moved over, and eased down (Fig. 8.5). Ensure the patient is secure and any accessory equipment, intravenous lines, catheters, oxygen, and other tubing are cleared from treatment machine motion from before moving the stretcher away.

PATIENT POSITION, ISOCENTER, AND FIELD PLACEMENT

Advances in imaging and treatment planning encourages continuous precision as radiation medicine evolves. With increasing confidence, the physician, dosimetrist, and radiation therapist focus beams to the target while minimizing the radiation delivered to surrounding normal tissues. V&R systems communicate detailed machine settings to set, verify, and document treatment plan reproduction at the treatment unit. Clinical value, however, is achieved only with beam coincidence with the patient and his or her tumor. Surface landmark instability and laxity in treatment position reproduction or immobilization contribute greatly to treatment variation and thus represent the greatest obstacle to applying advances in treatment planning. Minimizing these factors is a primary technical challenge for the radiation therapist.

Patient Positioning

The treatment session positioning goal is planned position reproduction. Landmark alignment with internal targets relies on vertical and horizontal planes; even slight body position variation can mean large discrepancies with the internal location a surface landmark represents (Fig. 8.6).

On arrival to the treatment room, the patient will remove artificial devices (e.g., dentures, temporary prostheses) consistent with simulation and planning. Prescribed shielding, such as wax/tin mouth guard reducing scatter from fillings to the buccal mucosa, may be positioned before settling the patient into the treatment position.

With the area to be treated over the appropriate treatment table window, the patient is coarsely aligned straight and level. Orienting the patient's treatment plan isocenter as close as possible to the table center provides maximum clearance for techniques requiring 360-degree gantry rotation. Alternatively, treatment beams with small gantry angles off the vertical axis, such as lung boost fields, may be accommodated by biasing the patient toward the side that the anterior field enters. Larger angles off the vertical axis (such as those used in breast tangents) may be accommodated by moving the patient closer to the treatment side.

> Many opposing oblique or tangential fields may be accommodated without treatment table rotation by making lateral patient shifts (consequently isocenter) relative to the table surface.

Using setup instructions from the chart, the treatment position refinement begins. Setup instructions include illustrations, photographs, and descriptive statements, such as supine versus prone, arm placement, and names and locations of other positioning devices. Measurements indicating the relative anatomy position (e.g., chin to suprasternal notch or sternal slope) may be used. The patient's treatment area is positioned relative to the machine isocenter where final fine-tuning is completed.

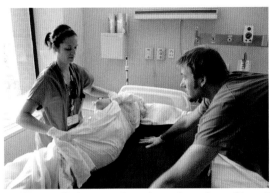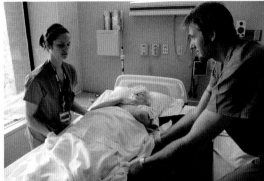

Fig. 8.5 Patient transfer using a draw sheet. (From Ehrlich RA, Coakes C. *Patient Care in Radiography*. 9th ed. St Louis, MO: Elsevier; 2017.)

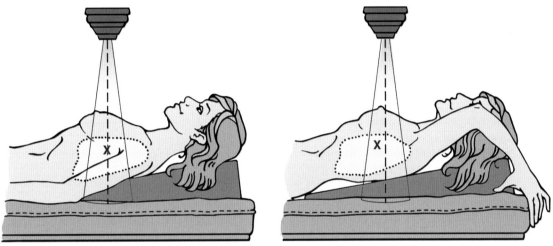

Fig. 8.6 Change in patient position changes landmark location relative to interest point.

Localization Landmarks

The treatment isocenter moves with, and is hidden within, the patient. Because neither the machine isocenter nor its planned position in the patient can be seen directly, treatment setup is dependent on aligning observable references distant to the actual interest point. In combination with topographic anatomy knowledge, localization landmarks are reference points used to direct patient positioning relative to the treatment machine. Landmarks include natural anatomy or artificial fiducials (fixed reference points against which other objects can be measured) positioned at a fixed relationship to unseen anatomy. Fiducials may be permanent or semipermanent, at the skin surface, internal, or fixed external to the patient.

Surface landmarks (references) include visible and palpable anatomy (bones or other identifiable points that can be seen or felt), tiny permanent marks created in the skin (aka tattoos), or semipermanent ink. Permanent marks are made by a sterile dye speck to the dermis layer, just under the skin surface, with a sterile hypodermic needle. Permanent marks allow for normal bathing during treatment. Very tiny, they are not obvious in public and do not damage clothing. For treatment, tiny permanent marks offer precision and stability without spreading or migrating. Traditionally, permanent marks were depended on for follow-up care and as references to avoid previous treatment area overlap. These purposes have waned as precision and previous treatment records improve. Drawbacks include a psychological perspective, and the term *tattoo* has societal connotations to manage when communicating with the patient. Permanent marks may

be an unnecessary cancer reminder long after they are needed. An alternative to dark ink, ultraviolet ink offers similar effectiveness that may lessen factors contributing to posttreatment body image.[7,8] Surface-guided radiation therapy (SGRT), systems using stereo camera, and computer systems match and monitor the patient's treatment area surface offering opportunities to eliminate skin marks.

Semipermanent marks, alone or in combination with minimal permanent marks, may enhance triangulation coordinates and identify field corners or edges. Permanent ink markers and paint pens easily mark skin and are difficult to remove; the varying colors can be useful for clarity across multiple plans and against different skin tones. Cross contamination between patients is a concern. Although studies have shown permanent markers to have effective bactericidal action, this lessens as the pen dries, and the immunocompromised cancer patient is more susceptible to transmissions.[9] Patient education and cooperation is necessary as potential removal or drift exists when refreshing over the treatment course. Clear patient-sensitive tape or markers with adhesives designed to resist removal while remaining gentle to sensitive skin may cover marks to aid in retention during bathing.

Implanted fiducial markers can be used, including radiopaque gold seeds or radiofrequency beacons, that provide internal references for mobile soft tissue, such as the prostate. These, however, require an invasive procedure to implant and added cost and risks to a treatment course. The use of these should be evaluated for each patient's situation, and risk should be low relative to the precision gained when used.

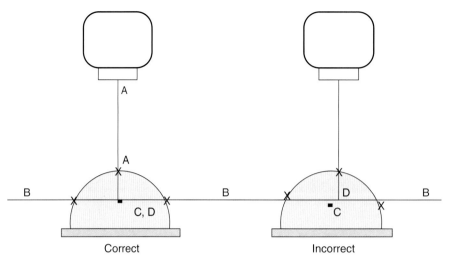

Fig. 8.7 Three-point positioning: tattoos (x). (A) Crosshairs. (B) Lasers. (C) Planned location isocenter. (D) Actual isocenter location.

Thermoplastic masks or stereotactic frames provide temporary, external fiducial references. Thermoplastic molds may be formed with enough immobilization that marks applied to the mask remain coincident with a treatment volume. Stereotactic frames use rigid and a highly reproducible means to orient precise incremental references beyond the skin surface. Head frames may be screwed directly into the skull, rendering the head immobile for the use of treating intracranial structures. Other variations using palate or other custom molds enable repeated frame use for fractionated treatment while increasing immobility over thermoplastic masks alone.

Isocenter Alignment

The treatment unit isocenter position is static. It can be located by following the room lasers and field crosshairs to their intersection point. Begin treatment volume alignment to the machine using triangulation references, which are three points forming intersecting horizontal, vertical, and transverse planes. In order to align the patient to the isocenter, the patient will be raised on the treatment couch until the lateral side lasers coincide with the patients marks on the right and left side. The patient can then be moved superiorly/inferiorly to alight the transverse position. Finally the treatment couch is moved left to right in order to align the sagittal laser or the field crosshair.

With the patient in the approximate treatment position and the observable landmarks identified, the treatment table is positioned to bring the patient close to the location for treatment. While maintaining patient dignity with drapes, locate external landmarks referenced in the setup instructions. Dim the room lights, and refine patient position relative to machine coordinates using lasers and the treatment field light. Using lateral marks, straighten and level the patient. The Z plane position may be determined from the table surface or the SSD. Several methods may be used to determine SSD. Table height has an advantage when the patient is lying directly on the table. There will be less interfraction or therapist variability. When a supporting device, such as an angle board, is in use, an optical distance indicator (ODI) or range finder may be necessary. The ODI or range finder light projects onto the patient's skin and is matched at the intersecting crosshairs that coincide with the beam's central ray. Mechanical distance indicators include incrementally marked rods or a measuring tape mounted to the collimator assembly extended to touch the patient's surface at the central axis. Treatment position is refined, aligning three observable landmarks on the patient with isocenter references, lasers, and beam crosshairs; treatment position is refined.

With the patient in treatment position, the isocenter is positioned relative to the localization landmarks. The planar intersection identified

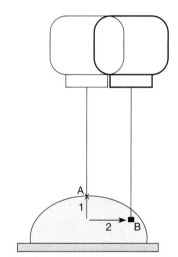

Fig. 8.8 Landmark and coordinate method. (A) Surface landmark (tattoo). (B) Planned isocenter location. 1, Shift to depth; 2, lateral shift.

by the three positioning points may coincide with the treatment isocenter (Fig. 8.7); however, this is not always practical. Anatomic references are seldom conveniently located, and many treatment sites do not lend themselves to stable localization mark placement. Mobile skin surfaces, such as the breast or axilla; older or obese persons; sloping surfaces, such as those treated with tangential fields; and irregular surfaces, and areas covered by dressings are imprecise or inaccessible. For these situations, apply a landmark and coordinate system (Fig. 8.8). Align stable surface landmarks with lasers followed by table motion in the X, Y, and Z planes. Indexed couches with digital linear position readouts contribute valuable precision in making these adjustments.

VERIFICATION IMAGING (ISOCENTER)

Traditional isocenter position accuracy is accomplished comparing planar images with corresponding reference images. The exposure projections may be a treatment portal subset or defined specifically for setup verification.

A single planar (two-dimensional) image or opposing image pair with coincident central ray projections, however, is insufficient to verify point position in three-dimensional space (Fig. 8.9A,B). The isocenter position on a planar image is distorted as all information is when compressed into two dimensions; distance to a point from the

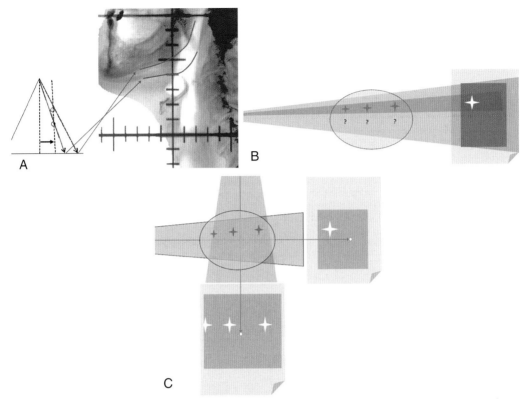

Fig. 8.9 Geometric distortion. (A) Parallel structures offset from central axis (B) Overlying structures along beam divergence. (C) Orthogonal projections.

radiation source cannot be determined. Stereoscopic images are two images from different angles focused on the same point.

Adding a second image, rotated on the isocenter from the first, approximates the third dimension.

The isocenter position is at the central axis's intersection. Accuracy for stereoscopic image review increases as beam coincidence decreases. This occurs because the increasing angle between incident beams reduces geometric distortion. The greatest possible noncoincidence is two beams at 90-degree angles. Orthogonal images are two beams perpendicular to one another with a 90-degree angle between them (Fig. 8.9C). Accuracy for stereoscopic image review is at its greatest with perpendicular orthogonal beam sets. Adding image projections also improves results; cone beam CT (CBCT) perhaps being the best illustration where accumulating multiple planar exposures produces precise spatial results.

Classic film imaging requires skill and attention to limitations, including beam geometry, image quality, evaluator subjectivity, and time. Image magnification varies, and distortion is introduced by poor cassette placement. Image quality is fixed and inferior contrast unavoidable because of megavoltage (MV) Compton scatter obscuring radiographic landmarks. Beam position interpretation has shown measurable assessment variability between individuals. Also, images evaluated after treatment (offline), even on subsequent days, offer no opportunity to correct treatments already delivered. Even when films are taken immediately before treatment delivery (online), patient movement is possible while patients wait for processing and evaluation.

The graticule (bb tray or dot tray) is a calibrated device fitting into the collimator and projecting field information to radiographic images, central ray, aperture size, rotation, and magnification.

Electronic imaging introduces enhanced image quality and registration tools. The phosphor plates of the computed radiography (CR) are exposed in a similar manner as film. Electronic portal imaging devices (EPIDs) eliminate geometric distortion from misaligned cassettes. EPIDs capture near real-time planar images or multiple exposures while the gantry rotates to produce a CBCT. CBCT visualizes soft tissue with or without implanted markers and produces three-dimensional images for the most accurate position evaluation. Images available in moments at the treatment console minimize time for patient movement between imaging and correction. Enhancement algorithms produce visualization clarity, automated image registration, and fusion, and display produce rapid, consistent results reducing subjectivity. Electronic MV portal and kilovoltage (kV) imaging accelerate isocenter and treatment field alignment verification.

Image-Guided Radiation Therapy, Online Setup Correction

Electronic imaging's efficiency and quality make routine pretreatment online correction viable. Online, image-guided radiation therapy (IGRT) techniques correct interfraction setup variation or changes occurring between treatment sessions. Image- and nonimage-based systems are used. Precise online corrections support reduced normal tissue in treatment volumes.

Motion observation and correction may be applied pretreatment, or during treatment (intrafraction), ensuring moving target inclusion. Options include radiographic systems, planar (cine) or four-dimensional CBCT, and nonradiographic means, such as ultrasound, SGRT, and radiofrequency tracking systems monitoring implanted beacons. Intrafraction motion monitoring may be combined with motion-reducing equipment and/or beam interruption (gating) mechanisms should the target move outside the treatment beam path.

Offline Systematic Setup Correction

Online image review most effectively minimizes daily setup variation; however, time and exposure factors may not outweigh this benefit for all treatment protocols. Setup variation includes systematic (e.g., changes in equipment between simulation and treatment room) and random components (e.g., bladder or bowel filling, organ motion), with systematic variation the more significant source.

Systematic variation is the consistent component in daily setup variation, primarily resulting from planned treatment setup transfer from the simulator to the treatment unit. Systematic isocenter setup variation may be approximated offline by determining the average setup correction from the first few treatment sessions. This correction may be added to setup instructions for subsequent treatment sessions. Remaining random variation includes inherent setup and organ motion variation that cannot be prospectively eliminated. Anticipated random error range varies with anatomic site and must be accommodated for in treatment planning. Random error is minimized by immobilization and online imaging techniques.

> Offline protocols determining systematic setup variation can identify setup adjustments, producing more accurate results preimaging or pretreatment. Judicious online and offline protocols, in combination with trend analysis, can produce improved results for all patients.

BEAM POSITION AND SHAPE

Once isocenter coincidence is accepted, rotate the gantry to the projection angle for treatment initiation. Basic linac collimation (arrangement of shielding material designed to define the x an y dimensions of the field) limits beam shape to rectangles. Large blocking systems with movable, opposing "jaws" are positioned in the treatment machine head. Field (jaw) settings define the overall radiation field dimensions at the isocenter. Electron therapy and stereotactic techniques add tertiary collimation systems and cones, improving dose distribution by reducing penumbra (Fig. 8.10).

Because neither people nor tumors present in squares and rectangles, treatment plans generally require further treatment aperture shaping. Standard lead or spent uranium blocks were a common, useful accessory in the treatment room. Modern radiation therapy beam shaping requires custom shielding using low melting point lead alloys, such as Cerrobend, or multileaf collimation (MLC).

> Cerrobend's bismuth (50%), lead (26.7%), tin (13.3%), and cadmium (10%) composition has a 165°F (74°C) melting point. Alternative alloys with similar characteristics and lower toxic metal concentrations are available to further protect workers.

Beam Shaping and Multileaf Collimators

Linear accelerators equipped with MLC (Fig. 8.11) systems customize field shapes using jaws sliced into leaf banks where opposing leaf banks form leaf pairs. Independently positioned, leaf pairs quickly and flexibly produce complex treatment field shapes. For additional information on MLC configuration, see Chapter 7, Figure 7.21.

The number of leaf pairs, available leaf widths, leaf design, and control systems vary between manufacturers, with some manufacturers offering several models. Design considerations include minimizing leakage between leaves with an interlocking leaf design or by positioning the primary jaws outside the field as backup jaws during treatment delivery. Leaf end shape optimizes a divergent field edge and will be rounded on systems that move leaves on a single plane. Leaf width is measured at the isocenter and impacts field edge smoothness. Micro-MLC units with leaf widths less than 5 mm provide greater refinement. Micro-MLC units

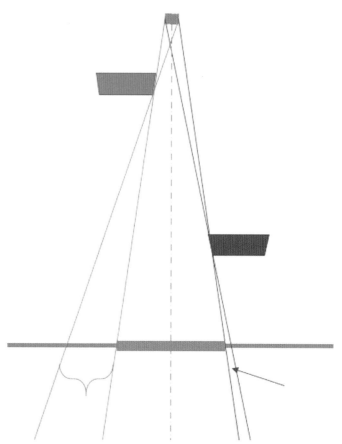

Fig. 8.10 Penumbra decreases as source to collimation distance increases.

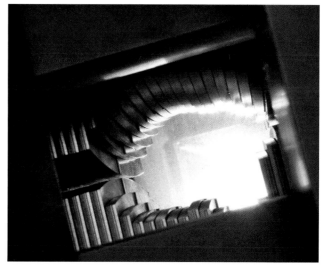

Fig. 8.11 Multileaf collimator. (Courtesy of Elekta Systems.)

may be removable, offering treatment unit flexibility. Control systems may be integrated with the accelerator console or may be separate, which has implications for field parameter selection and MLC files as well as backup options should network access be interrupted.

In addition to treatment volume customization, MLCs improve safety and satisfaction. Without heavy blocks, strain injuries or injuries caused by dropping heavy equipment is reduced for patients and radiation therapists. MLCs repositioned from the console reduces overall treatment session time, improving patient comfort and department efficiency.

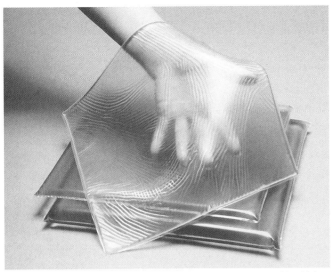

Fig. 8.12 Superflab bolus. (Courtesy Civco, Inc., Orange City, IA.)

PORTAL VERIFICATION IMAGING

Portal images verify the BEV path, the beam shape, and projection using the MV treatment beam. Exit dose exposes an EPID, CR plate, or classic radiographic film. As verification portal images are taken before the first treatment, systematic errors may be corrected before treatment is delivered.

Portal images use single- or double-exposure techniques. Single-exposure images are enough when radiographic landmarks are located within the treatment area. Classic, slow exposure rate verification film (v-film) is an option where film is in place during the entire treatment exposure. Double exposures include a short exposure to the treatment area and a second exposure following field-shaping retraction, which exposes a larger area surrounding the treatment area. Double exposures include treatment field and surrounding anatomy information, increasing interpretation landmarks while also increasing normal tissue dose.

Department policy defines portal imaging frequency. Partially based on historic studies showing a reduction in treatment errors associated with increased portal imaging, portals at treatment course initiation and weekly thereafter for most cases are an accepted standard. Unstable landmarks or treatment volume proximity to critical structures may prompt increased frequency. IGRT protocols where daily isocenter position is verified may support reducing individual treatment portal imaging frequency.

BEAM-MODIFYING DEVICES

The primary treatment planning goal is treating a target to an even (homogeneous) dose while minimizing the dose delivered to normal tissue. With assurance, the radiation is directed *toward* the prescribed volume; static devices or dynamic collimation systems may further modify radiation dose distribution *across* the treatment field.

Bolus

In radiation therapy, *bolus* refers to materials whose interactions with the radiation beam mimic tissue. Bolus comes in many forms and has many applications. Bolus must conform to the treatment surface without air gaps and build up or attenuate dose equivalently to tissue to be effective. Commercially available gel sheets developed specifically for use in radiation therapy are available in standard-thickness sheets (Fig. 8.12). Other commercial sheet materials for surfaces include brass mesh. Materials for custom bolus shapes include paraffin wax, Vaseline gauze, wet gauze or towels, water bags, and even three-dimensional printed materials. These materials can be variable in tissue equivalence; measurements may be appropriate to assure treatment intentions are met.

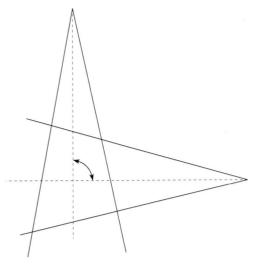

Fig. 8.13 A 90-degree orthogonal hinge angle.

Bolus thickness equivalent to maximum dose depth for the treatment energy eliminates the beam's skin-sparing effect, bringing maximum dose deposition to the patient's surface. Bolus may be applied with this goal over entire treatment areas or simply over scars, superficial nodes, or other areas of concern.

Bolus may be used to compensate for surface contour variations or to eliminate cavity air gaps. For example, surgical procedures leaving anatomic defects, such as sinus or eye removal, produce significant irregularities. Filling the cavity with bolus material such as Vaseline gauze or a water-filled balloon significantly improves dose distribution in the target volume. This application is useful only in situations where skin-sparing loss is acceptable or desired. When skin sparing is to be maintained, individualized compensators should be evaluated.

Compensators

MV treatment unit design produces a beam delivering a relatively even dose across the perpendicular plane. Patients, however, rarely provide a flat surface perpendicular with the incident treatment beam. As just discussed, dose distribution skewing caused by irregular surfaces can be addressed with bolus material, yet it eliminates skin sparing. Compensators (beam modifier changing radiation output across the beam profile) are positioned in the treatment machine head; skin sparing is retained. As with bolus, materials vary; copper, brass, lead, or Lucite may be used.

Tissue deficits are generally most significant over one dimension (width or length), and a standardized two-dimensional compensator addresses this treatment situation. With modern treatment techniques, two-dimensional compensators are infrequently encountered. Complex contours may necessitate custom three-dimensional compensators.

Wedges

Combining multiple treatment fields may produce inhomogeneous dose distributions over the target volume. Dose distribution for a single treatment field meeting a flat surface is relatively parallel to the surface. When a second beam is positioned directly opposite this beam, the dose distribution combines relatively consistently across the exposed volume. However, as the hinge angle (angle between two intersecting treatment beams' central rays) (Fig. 8.13) decreases, the dose delivered to overlapping areas varies significantly; high- and low-dose regions appear in the desired target volume.

Although physical wedges appear like two-dimensional compensators, their application differs significantly. Wedges are designed to change the isodose angle relative to the beam axis at a specified depth within the patient. Wedges reduce the dose overlap between fields with hinge angles less than 180 degrees. The thick wedge end, the heel, attenuates the greatest radiation, thus drawing isodose lines closer to the surface. Attenuation decreases along the wedge to the thin end, or toe, where the dose delivered to the patient will be greater than the dose at the opposite side. When wedges are used, heels are typically positioned together, reducing high-dose regions inside the hinge angle.

External wedges must be lifted and slid into position. The manufacturer usually provides wedges that are customized for specific treatment units. Standard wedge sizes are 15, 30, 45, and 60 degrees. Field sizes are limited with standard compensators and wedges. Care must be taken to ensure that treatment fields do not extend beyond the beam modification device's heel or sides (flash or extension beyond the toe is acceptable).

Internal wedge units allow wedge angle optimization. The machine positions a physical 60-degree "universal" wedge in the beam path for a specified number of MU. The beam is interrupted, the wedge removed, and the remaining MU are delivered; the wedged-to-unwedged beam ratio results in a custom wedge angle.

Nonphysical wedges slope dose distribution using jaw motion. Jaws are positioned together at one field edge. As the moving jaw sweeps away, the wedge toe forms as more dose is delivered to the field edge. This lessens the dose across the field when the last exposure is made and the wedge is in full position.

> The photon beam interaction with attenuating materials produces scatter electrons contaminating the photon beam and producing increased skin dose for patients. Air attenuates low-energy electrons absorbed in about 15 cm; therefore, all beam-shaping and modification devices for photon beams must be secured at least 20 cm from the patient surface.

ASSESS AND ACCEPT TREATMENT PARAMETERS

Before leaving the room, perform a final treatment setup review, verifying patient positioning, beam direction, and beam modifier placement. If arc therapy is being applied or if subsequent treatment fields will be positioned from outside the treatment room, ensure free clearance for gantry motion throughout the treatment rotation. Check that the patient, accessory medical equipment, treatment table, and all stretchers, chairs, and stools are all free from the gantry path. Once satisfied that set parameters meet those prescribed by the treatment plan, notify the patient that you are exiting the treatment room to administer the radiation. Communicate the approximate time that the beam will be on, and reassure the patient that he or she is always being monitored. Exit confirming the patient is the only person in the treatment room.

Patient Monitoring Systems

To protect radiation therapists from radiation exposure, the patient must be left alone in the treatment vault during radiation delivery. In some situations (orthovoltage or other low-energy treatments), treatment may be monitored directly through leaded glass windows. This is impractical with MV units, however, and indirect monitoring systems are used. To maintain patient safety and treatment accuracy, audio and visual contact must be maintained at all times. At least two cameras maintain visual contact with the patient. Generally, at least one long-view camera visualizes the whole patient, allowing observation for general distress or movement, whereas another provides a closer view of the treatment area for subtle patient movement observation. Visual monitors must be positioned so that the patient and gantry motion is always visible; a changing gantry angle must not obstruct patient monitoring at any time.

Two-way audio communication between the treatment room and console remains continuously audible in the console area. A switch allows communication into the treatment room. A stop at the console area before the first treatment allows monitoring system demonstration to new patients, reassuring them they are heard and seen during treatment delivery and that their privacy is protected.

Console

Radiation delivery is controlled at the treatment console area located outside the treatment room. Console configuration varies widely and may include multiple computer-controlled screens operating the treatment unit and ancillary systems.

The console provides information regarding treatment unit status and operation. Beam modifier use may require placement confirmation to release safety interlocks. Interlocks prevent beam initiation and include alerts prompting treatment setup and safety procedure completion. Interlocks include closing doors, beam modifier placement (wedges, compensators, electron cones), and machine operation requirements (water, vacuum, etc.). Disagreement with interlock requirements triggers a fault indicator on the console. Fault-light panels provide diagnostic information regarding proper functioning and equipment problem sources.

Although equipment maintenance is ultimately the radiation physicist's responsibility, monitoring equipment function and reporting problems to the physics or engineering department is a critical radiation therapist responsibility. Any equipment malfunctions or setup errors affecting treatment delivery must be reported to the radiation oncologist and corrective actions documented in writing. Malfunctions or errors resulting in misadministration must be reported following Nuclear Regulatory Commission or state reporting requirements. Reportable events and misadministration definitions may change over time, so reportable event determination is made by the radiation safety officer. Equipment malfunctions causing serious injury or death are reported through the US Food and Drug Administration's Medical Device Reporting Act.

TREATMENT DELIVERY

Beam On and Beam Off

Set the parameters for treatment delivery, or confirm settings downloaded from the V&R system, including the calculated primary and backup monitor unit (or timer) settings.

Initiate the treatment beam. Red "radiation on" lights in and outside the treatment room indicate radiation activity in the treatment room. Monitor the patient and console meterset (e.g., MU, time) administered.

At beam on, ion chambers within the beam measure radiation output. The relative dose delivered is displayed in MU on the linear accelerator console. Primary, secondary, and backup systems function to interrupt the treatment beam after the prescribed dose has been delivered. Backup systems may be manually or automatically set depending on treatment unit sophistication and function as safety interlocks, terminating the beam if the primary counter malfunctions. The accelerator is designed to deliver the dose at specified rates; decreases in that rate may indicate malfunctions. Backup systems include secondary ion chambers calibrated a percentage lower than the primary ion chamber and timers that interrupt the beam after a set period.

After radiation delivery to the first treatment port, assess patient and treatment unit position for each subsequent field. Set new field size, table, gantry, collimator angles, and position-changing treatment accessories. With computer-controlled field shaping through MLCs and beam modification through dynamic wedges, V&R systems provide parameters for sequential treatment field setup, and multiple treatment fields may be delivered from the console without treatment room reentry. Motion may be initiated using functions at the accelerator console or on the pendant in the treatment room. Such auto-setup procedures, reducing treatment time and incorrect treatment parameters, must be accompanied by diligence observing patient movement and proximity to moving equipment.

Treatment Interruptions

Machine conditions might cause a machine to turn off before a beam is completely delivered. Patient movement, improper machine motion, or treatment beam failure to stop may also require the radiation therapist to interrupt the treatment beam. Options for beam interruption by the radiation therapist include pressing a beam-off button, turning the operation key to the "off" position, or opening the treatment unit door. If these actions fail to stop the beam, an emergency off switch must be available, completely turning off the treatment unit. An emergency off switch is a final choice, as a machine warm-up period before reuse is generally necessary.

Depending on the interruption circumstances, the beam may be resumed or treatment terminated. The treating radiation therapist determines the actions following beam interruption. Whenever possible, treatment will be resumed and completed; however, when equipment operation or beam quality are in question, the physician must be involved in the assessment.

When treatment termination is necessary, accurately record the partial treatment. Subsequent treatments may require revision to achieve the intended treatment plan. Validate and write down machine settings, including MU, at interruption. Check electronic and physical backup counters, recording readouts in a manual system. Compare machine readouts with those sent to the V&R system. Record and report any discrepancy for investigation.

TREATMENT TECHNIQUES

Field arrangement decisions depend on tumor location and nearby critical structures. At simulation, the radiation therapist works with the radiation oncologist and dosimetrist to plan field arrangements within treatment machine capabilities to include target volumes, minimize traversing normal tissues, and avoid critical structures.

Multiple Fields

Most treatment plans require radiation delivery through multiple portals to achieve optimal dose homogeneity through the target volumes. As fields overlap, an increased dose is deposited relative to tissues receiving radiation from only one portal. Accuracy in multiple field irradiation is greatly enhanced with isocentric treatment techniques. With the treatment unit isocenter precisely positioned in the target volumes, the machine may be moved to direct radiation beams at the target from many directions without repositioning the patient, thus preserving accuracy.

The most basic multiple-field technique is the parallel opposed portal (POP). The hinge angle for POP fields equals 180 degrees. POP fields may enter the patient from any two directions relative to the patient and are often identified by those directions, for example, right-and-left lateral (laterals), anteroposterior and posteroanterior, and anterior oblique and posterior oblique (obliques). Parallel opposed fields are not used frequently and usually require few treatment accessories beyond beam shaping. Opposing fields for superficial volumes on curved surfaces, such as the breast or ribs, which flash off the patient's surface, are referred to as *tangential fields or tangents*. The hinge angle between tangential fields may vary slightly from 180 degrees, accommodating beams divergence so the deep field edge is coincident rather than the beam axes (Fig. 8.14).

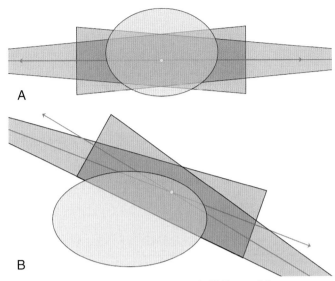

Fig. 8.14 (A) Parallel opposed. (B) Tangentials.

The wedge pair technique changes the volume receiving radiation by decreasing the hinge angle between two treatment fields. The relative dose in the area formed between the narrowing hinge angle increases as the angle between the field pairs decreases. Overlapping isodose lines are parallel to the treatment surface, not parallel to one another, and combining them produces high dose deposition in the shallow target portion relative to dose deposited more deeply. By reducing the radiation delivered to the shallow region, wedges distribute the dose more homogeneously throughout the target (Fig. 8.15). Three-field techniques often require wedges to achieve the same dose homogeneity goal, as the dose increases on the side where the third field enters.

Adding fields increases dose where beams intersect while decreasing dose to surrounding tissues. Deep-seated tumors rely on increasing beams to reduce normal tissue dose while increasing dose where beams overlap. The four-field technique, sometimes referred to as a *four-field box,* was commonly used in pelvis or abdomen treatment. These fields are arranged 90 degrees from one another and generally require no more than beam shaping for optimal dose distribution.

Conformal therapy applies three-dimensional tumor volume localization to treatment field definition. Adding couch rotations may position the beam in directions that acquisition devices cannot be positioned. With CT simulation, treatment planning systems can define beam directions that cannot be viewed with two-dimensional imaging. Fields are defined through a derived BEV and shaped to include the target with minimal normal tissue margins. Six or more fields, often in arrangements noncoplanar with the gantry rotation, may be used to increase the dose to the target while producing sharp dose falloff to surrounding tissue. Immobilization devices are carefully designed, and treatment is delivered in the same manner as in other multiple-field techniques. With high-energy beams, dose distributions are comparable with arc therapy.

Arc therapy demonstrates the ultimate multiple-field technique, and arcs may be defined in co-planar and noncoplanar arrangements. In standard arc therapy, radiation is delivered through a static field as the gantry moves through its rotation arc. In doing this, arc therapy effectively delivers radiation through a continuous, overlapping treatment portal sequence. Conformal arcs add a jaw and MLC movement conforming exposure to the outermost target width as it changes through the rotation (Fig. 8.16).

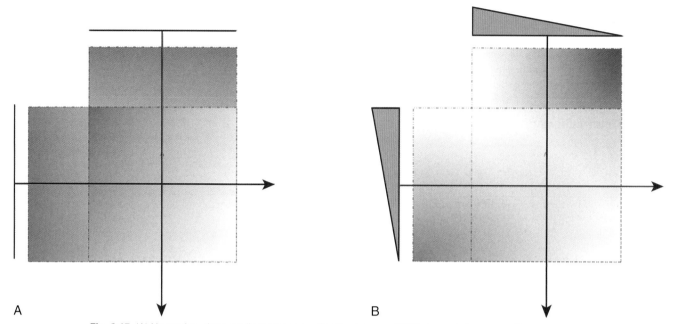

Fig. 8.15 (A) No wedge, dose gradient across overlapping beams. (B) Wedge pair, homogeneity across overlapping region reduced.

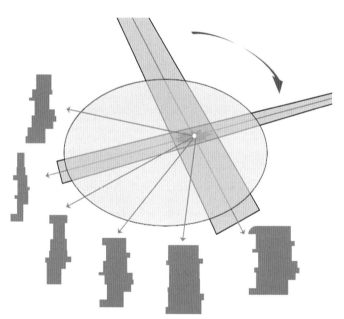

Fig. 8.16 Conformal arc, beam aperture conforms to changing target dimensions.

Adjacent Fields

Photon beam divergence and electron dose distribution bulging at depth poses challenges for adjacent treatment field alignment. Over and under dose areas are concerning. Methods include abutting fields at the skin surface or at some depth with or without coplanar treatment beam edge alignment. Abutting field edges produce "hot" matches where beams overlap immediately below the surface. The overlap area must be carefully evaluated for total dose tolerance. When a low-dose area is acceptable at or near the surface, adjacent fields may be separated by a calculated gap. Positioning the field edge correctly, planes coplanar to one another may be accomplished through using blocks or independent jaws eliminating divergence (Fig. 8.17A) or using gantry, collimator, and table rotations to align treatment field edges (Fig.

8.17B,C). Although abutting geometrically matched fields theoretically provides a match without inhomogeneity, setup variation must be a recognized risk. Abutting or gapped, feathering (junction migration through the treatment course) may be used to blur dose inhomogeneities at a junction.

Intensity-Modulated Radiation Therapy

Conventional and conformal treatment plans distribute a relatively uniform dose across each field. Normal tissue is protected by controlling field direction and shape, areas in which treatment fields overlap, and receive an increased radiation dose relative to areas that receive radiation from only one field. Intensity-modulated radiation therapy (IMRT) alters this model, delivering nonuniform, *modulated* exposure across the BEV. As radiation intensity varies across the exposed field, critical structures in its path are given less dose. Target areas receiving a low dose from one direction are compensated by larger doses delivered through another gantry angle not intersecting the protected structure. By overlapping multiple intensity-modulated fields, high radiation doses are delivered to targets that are irregularly shaped or close to critical structures. These nonuniform exposures create even dose distribution to target volumes with steep dose gradients to adjacent normal tissue. IMRT treatment planning requires "inverse" planning algorithms where the clinical objectives are specified first, and the planning system works in reverse to determine optimal beam parameters.

Beam modulation may be accomplished using three-dimensional compensators with material thickness increasing over protected structures in each beam path. MLC motion, however, revolutionized radiation treatment delivery. In addition to field shaping, MLCs moving through beam delivery modulate radiation intensity across the BEV. Planning and QA is accomplished in-house; treatment delivery is efficient without the need to change physical compensators between each treatment field.

MLC-modulated beams apply to one of two modes of delivery. *Step and shoot,* or segmental MLC, positions MLC leaves and then initiates beam. The therapist initiates the treatment field once; the MLC controller manages beamlet off/on and leaf motion sequence. Once the

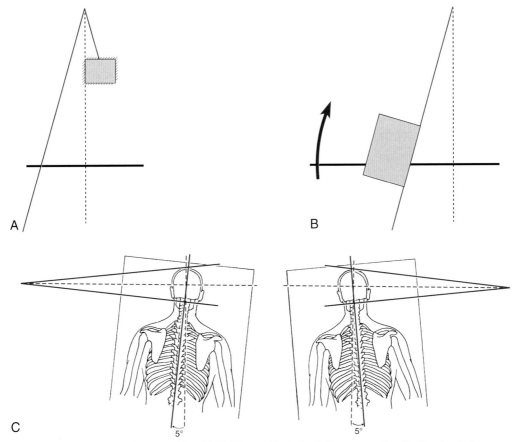

Fig. 8.17 Geometric field matching. (A) Half-beam block. (B) Collimator rotation. (C) Couch rotation.

first beamlet (an IMRT field subdivision) is complete, the beam turns off, leaves move to the next position, beam turns on/off, and so forth, proceeding through each beamlet until treatment is delivered. Sliding window, or dynamic MLC, moves leaves throughout a single beam on/off sequence. Modulated arc therapy delivers IMRT through rotational arcs, with moving MLCs and variable dose rate, further conforming dose delivery.

Highly physics intensive, IMRT requires specially equipped accelerators, inverse treatment planning, sophisticated dose measurement, QA tools, and V&R systems to manage large and complex treatment plans. At treatment delivery, immobilization and IGRT setup verification is emphasized, as volumes with highly defined treatment margins are particularly sensitive to positioning and isocenter alignment.

Stereotactic Radiation Therapy

Stereotactic techniques treat small targets with many intersecting beams creating concentrated dose areas with very sharp dose falloff. By distributing the dose delivered to normal tissue over greater areas, the high dose area is increasingly focused on the target. Linear accelerator–based stereotactic radiosurgery (SRS) or stereotactic radiation therapy (SRT) reduce penumbra with cones sharpening dose gradients and multiple noncoplanar arcs directed at the tumor. The Gamma Knife uses fixed cobalt-60 sources to produce similar dose distributions. CyberKnife's robotics direct a highly focused beam through complex patterns not constrained by mounted systems.

SRS delivers a single large treatment fraction without overdosing nearby normal tissue. SRT adds the fractionation radiobiological benefits to the treatment. Stereotactic body radiation therapy combines conformal or modulated radiation therapy elements with stereotactic coordinate techniques and motion management for areas outside the cranium, including spine, lung, and liver.[10] Treatment is hypofractionated with a single or few high-dose treatment sessions. Targets are precisely defined while motion is minimized and monitored. Setup verification procedures are applied at each treatment session, seeking submillimeter accuracy. Sophisticated immobilization and localization include integrated external fiducial and immobilization devices, such as head or body frames, identifying the isocenter and treatment field localization.

Total-Body Irradiation

Total-body irradiation (TBI) positions patients at an extended distance to produce a sufficiently large field size. On treatment units not specifically designed for this purpose, this usually means lying on the floor or standing or sitting against a treatment room wall with the gantry rotated 90 degrees. To achieve dose homogeneity, patients must be treated with POP fields, requiring repositioning halfway through the treatment. Several dedicated TBI treatment machines have been developed in centers with a high demand for this treatment. These machines simplify treatment by using fixed, extended distance, or double-headed treatment units to deliver radiation through both anterior and posterior surfaces with the patient in a comfortable, constant position.

Adaptive Radiation Therapy

Adaptive radiation therapy (ART) accommodates anatomic changes occurring over a treatment course. Tumors and normal structures change shape and size from one day to the next and as tumors respond to treatment. Structure movement in or out of beam paths disrupts intended dose distribution. Repositioning via IGRT accommodates for some interfraction variation; ART adapts dose distribution with changing beam apertures and modulation. Strategies include on- and

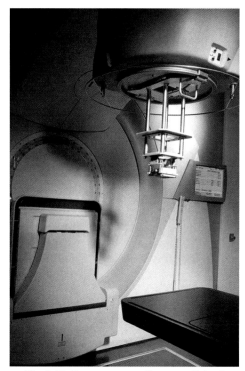

Fig. 8.18 Electron cones. (Courtesy Elekta.)

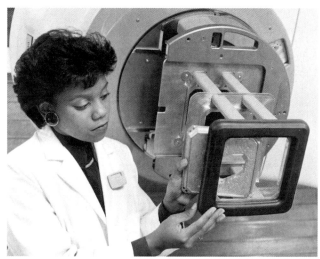

Fig. 8.19 Electron cutouts. (Courtesy Varian Medical Systems.)

offline plan adaptation. Offline adaptation may entail resimulation and planning after several completed treatment sessions or establishing a treatment plan "library" across a predictable organ position range, such as bladder filling. Plan selection from the library is informed at each session using pretreatment imaging. Online ART takes place during the treatment session, requiring advanced imaging and fast planning tools. A treatment planning system modifies a reference plan using contours generated from pretreatment imaging. System integration is prized, saving time and reducing opportunities for error. As plan conformality increases, normal tissue dose decreases, and tumor dose escalation may be supported.

ELECTRON BEAM

Superficial treatment volumes may be addressed using electron beams. Electrons provide rapid dose buildup and a uniform dose region, followed by rapid dose falloff. Setup procedures are less reliant on the isocenter, with distance, collimation, and SSD having greater significance to dose distribution. Optimal gantry rotation brings the beam cross plane parallel with the treatment surface. The orientation may be referred to as *en-face*, meaning directly facing. Special considerations for electron beam treatments include beam collimation, shielding, and bolus requirements.

Electron Collimation and Beam Shaping

Electron mass and charge give rise to increased interactions in air than occur with photon beams. Electron beam scattering causes lateral dose bowing at depth. Tertiary collimation, extensions close to the treatment surface, sharpens dose gradient at the beam edges. Collimation systems for electron therapy include static field size cones attached to the gantry accessory tray or trimmer bars adjustable to varying field sizes. Trimmer bars attached to the collimator provide greater flexibility in field size, but increased distance from the patient increases penumbra and

lateral dose scattering. Cones or trimmer bars are usually secured on the treatment unit before the patient is positioned, as the patient will be positioned close to collimation (Fig. 8.18).

Electron field shaping may be positioned on the patient or within the electron cone. Attenuated much more efficiently than photon beams, surface field shaping require lead equivalent thicknesses measured in millimeters (general rule: half energy in lead millimeters). Surface shaping may be cut and formed to the patient except where the weight is uncomfortable. Electron interaction with surface-positioned metals produce low-energy scatter radiation, increasing dose and reactions to surfaces. Covering with a low Z-number material, such as aluminum, tin, or paraffin wax, absorbs these low-energy photons. Alternatively, field-defining apertures, or "cutouts," fit directly inside the electron cone end (Fig. 8.19). Planning field-shaping cutouts may be accomplished through a simulation or manual procedure where the required field shape is drawn on a template positioned on the patient's surface. The template is then used to form a mold and Cerrobend cutout.

Electron Therapy Shielding: Underlying Structures

Thin structures, such as the nares, auricle, eyelids, and lips, are often treated with electron therapy. Use additional shielding to protect underlying normal tissue such as medial nasal membranes, skin behind the ear, optic lens, lacrimal ducts and glands, and gingiva from unnecessary radiation exposure. Because of the proximity of the beam collimation and the constraints of superficial beam alignment, these shields will typically be positioned before the treatment field is positioned.

Electron Therapy and Bolus

Bolus materials in electron therapy are the same as those used with photons; however, applications differ. Three applications for bolus exist in electron therapy. First, electron beam dose distribution is exquisitely sensitive to irregular surfaces and air cavities, and so cavity filling is often necessary. Bolus over an even contour will generally be positioned following beam alignment, whereas bolus to fill a cavity or irregular surface may require placement in advance. Second, as with photons, bolus may be used to eliminate skin sparing. In contrast with photons, bolus only applies for low-energy electron beams, as skin sparing decreases with increasing electron energy. Third, overall treatment depth can be customized by combining electron energy choice and bolus to decrease penetration.

SUMMARY

- The radiation therapist is an active participant in the treatment planning and delivery processes with a primary responsibility to care quality. To meet treatment goals, whether palliative or curative, the radiation therapist remains vigilant in accurate treatment reproduction and delivery as prescribed by the physician.
- As the expert in treatment delivery, the radiation therapist is highly skilled in MV treatment units' operation and accessories used to customize each patient's treatment. Through treatment delivery and documentation, treatment unit function monitoring, and inclusion on the departmental QA committee, radiation therapists actively engage in continuous patient care improvement.
- Patient safety and care are the radiation therapist's responsibility. As the treatment team member interacting with the patient most frequently, the radiation therapist routinely assesses patient mobility, pain, and social or other factors affecting well-being. Physical and emotional reactions to radiation treatment are addressed within the scope of practice guidelines. Patients are directed to the physician or other professionals as needs are discerned.
- Treatment room maintenance is critical to safe and efficient patient care and treatment delivery. The radiation therapist ensures access and proper treatment accessory handling, both standard and customized for an individual patient.
- Before each patient's arrival, the radiation therapist team carefully reviews the treatment record to determine current treatment status and the imminent session's prescribed plan. An action plan is prepared for, including positioning, beam-shaping and beam-modification devices collection and placement, and team agreement on verification procedures and treatment field delivery sequence.
- Responses to treatment interruptions are understood and appropriately applied with resumption protocols ranging from immediate to delayed to deferring completion from the session.
- Technical advances in diagnostic imaging, treatment planning computers, and MV treatment units have created great flexibility in treatment plans. Tumor volumes are identified and localized with greater confidence, and treatment beams are focused more narrowly. Normal tissue is increasingly spared from radiation exposure and damage. Reduction in setup error through improvements in positioning, immobilization, and localization landmarks, then performing precise pretreatment setup verification, is attained through radiation therapist diligence, knowledge, and commitment to their patients.

REVIEW QUESTIONS

The answers to the Review Questions can be found by logging on to our website at: http://evolve.elsevier.com/Washington+Leaver/principles

1. The patient arrives in the radiation oncology department and is only able to stand and walk several steps at a time. What is the most appropriate transportation and transfer method?
   a. Walk with assistance.
   b. Wheelchair.
   c. Stretcher without slide board.
   d. Stretcher with slide board.
2. Recommended setup landmarks include:
   I. Tattoos.
   II. Palpable bony points.
   III. Semipermanent ink marks.
      a. I and II.
      b. I and III.
      c. II and III.
      d. I, II, and III.
3. Which is added daily to the treatment record?
   I. Treatment number.
   II. Cumulative dose.
   III. Elapsed days.
      a. I and II.
      b. I and III.
      c. II and III.
      d. I, II, and III.
4. The period over which radiation is delivered is:
   a. Fractionation.
   b. Exposure time.
   c. Protraction.
   d. Treatment plan.
5. Treatment beam shape and projection is verified through:
   a. BEV evaluation.
   b. Stereoscopic imaging.
   c. CBCT.
   d. Portal imaging.

6. Wedge systems include all the following *except:*
   a. Global.
   b. Universal.
   c. Standard tray mounted.
   d. Virtual.
7. Multileaf collimators may be used to:
   I. Shape a beam.
   II. Reduce dose to normal tissue.
   III. Vary dose delivered across the beam.
      a. I and II.
      b. I and III.
      c. II and III.
      d. I, II, and III.
8. The feathering technique may be used to:
   a. Eliminate overlap.
   b. Increase dose to a gapped region.
   c. Decrease dose to a gapped region.
   d. Decrease dose between abutted fields.
9. The angle between two treatment beams' central axes is the:
   a. Central angle.
   b. Gantry angle.
   c. Wedge angle.
   d. Hinge angle.
10. Which is not a bolus use with electron treatments?
    a. Eliminate high-energy electron skin sparing.
    b. Eliminate low-energy electron skin sparing.
    c. Decrease dose penetration depth.
    d. Compensate for tissue deficits.

QUESTIONS TO PONDER

1. Differentiate between an immobilization device and a positioning aid.
2. Analyze information to be included in the radiation therapy treatment chart.
3. Describe the treatment setup process.
4. Discuss factors contributing to decisions regarding portal imaging frequency.
5. Discuss the radiation therapist's role in continual patient care quality improvement.
6. Practice converting closed- to open-ended questions.

REFERENCES

1. Evans SB, Fraass BA, Berner P, et al. Standardizing dose prescriptions: an ASTRO white paper. *Pract Radiat Oncol.* 2016;6(6):e369–e381.
2. Mayo CS, Moran JM, Bosch W, et al. American association of physicists in medicine task Group 263: standardizing nomenclatures in radiation oncology. *Int J Radiat Oncol Biol Phys.* 2018;100(4): 1057–1066.
3. American College of Surgeons. *Standards for Oncology Registry Entry.* Effective January 1, 2018.
4. American Society of Radiologic Technologists. *The Practice Standards for Medical Imaging and Radiation Therapy: Radiation Therapy Practice Standards.* Effective June 23, 2019. Available at https://www.asrt.org/docs/default-source/practice-standards/ps_radiationtherapy.pdf?sfvrsn=18e076d0_22. Accessed September 25, 2019.
5. RO-ILS, ASTRO, AAPM. *Radiation Oncology Incident Learning System RO-ILS Year in Review 2015.* Available at https://www.astro.org/uploadedFiles/_MAIN_SITE/Patient_Care/Patient_Safety/RO-ILS/2015YIR.pdf. Accessed September 25, 2019.
6. The Joint Commission website. www.jointcommission.org. Accessed January 2019.
7. David JE, Castle SKB, Mossi KM. Localization tattoos: an alternative method using flourescent inks. *Radiat Ther.* 2006;15:11–15.
8. Landig SJ, Kirby AM, Lee SF, et al. A randomized control trial evaluating fluorescent ink vs dark ink tattoos for breast radiotherapy. *Br J Radiol.* 2016;89(1068):20160288.
9. Tadiparthi S, Shokrollahi K, Juma A, Croall J. Using marker pens on patients: a potential source of cross infections with MRSA. *Ann R Coll Surg Engl.* 2007;89(7):661–664.
10. Timmerman RD. (PI): RTOG 0618, A phase II trial of stereotactic body radiation therapy (SBRT) in the treatment of patients with operable stage I/II, non-small cell lung cancer. *Therapy Oncology Group.* 2012. Available at https://clinicaltrials.gov/ct2/show/NCT00591838. Accessed September 25, 2019.

9

Infection Control in the Radiation Oncology Facilities

Zachary D. Smith, Charles M. Washington, Megan Trad

OBJECTIVES

- Interpret and apply the processes of isolation techniques used in healthcare facilities.
- Discuss the evolution and necessity of standard precautions.
- Select protective equipment to be worn that is appropriate for a given medical procedure or situation.

- Use actions that will protect the patient, public, and yourself in regard to the transmission of infectious disease.
- Identify processes used in the sterilization and disinfection of medical equipment and the medical environment.
- Describe laws and regulations that are in place to ensure a safe work environment for healthcare workers.

OUTLINE

KEY TERMS

Autoclave
Critical items
Droplet nuclei
Fomite

Incubation
Isolation
Standard precautions
Sterility

INFECTION CONTROL IN RADIATION ONCOLOGY FACILITIES

Evolution of Isolation Practices

Healthcare-associated infections (HAIs) have been a serious problem ever since sick patients were placed together in a common setting. Even in biblical times, the need to isolate or quarantine persons with leprosy was recognized. In the early part of the twentieth century, healthcare workers (HCWs) wore special gowns, washed their hands with disinfecting agents, disinfected contaminated equipment, and practiced a wide variety of isolation or quarantine measures to contain contagious diseases such as tuberculosis (TB). In 1970, the US Centers for Disease Control and Prevention (CDC) published its first guidelines for HAIs and isolation techniques.[1] These guidelines recommend the use of seven isolation categories based on the routes of disease transmission.

Because not all diseases in a given category required the same degree of precautions, this approach, although simple to understand and apply, resulted in overisolation for many patients. Over the next decade, it became evident that although this approach helped prevent the spread of classic contagious diseases, it neither addressed new drug-resistant pathogens or new syndromes, nor focused on HAIs in special care departments. Thus, in 1983, the CDC published new guidelines.[2] Contact isolation, acid-fast bacilli (AFB, another name for TB), and blood and body fluids were added, and the protective isolation category was deleted. These significant changes encouraged the hospital's infection control committee to choose between category-specific and patient-specific isolation categories.

The Health Infection Control Practices Advisory Committee issued a *Special Report: Guideline for Isolation Precautions in Hospitals* in January 1996.[3] This guideline consisted of two tiers of precautions, which are still endorsed in the 2007 guideline and still in use as of 2019.[4] In the first and most important tier were precautions designed for the care of all hospital patients regardless of their diagnosis or presumed infection status; these were known as standard precautions.[3] The second tier, known as *transmission-based precautions,* consisted of precautions designed only for the care of specific patients.[3]

Standard Precautions

Standard precautions apply to (1) blood; (2) all body fluids, secretions, and excretions except sweat; (3) nonintact skin; and (4) mucous membranes. *Standard precautions* are designed to be the primary strategy to control HAIs by reducing transmission risk from both known and unknown sources of infection. Major components of standard precautions are shown in Box 9.1.

> Always practice standard precautions. Imagine that all patients have undiagnosed infections.

Transmission-Based Precautions

Transmission-based precautions are aimed at patients with a confirmed diagnosis or a suspected diagnosis of an epidemiologically important pathogen that warrants additional precautions beyond standard precautions. Table 9.1 lists some of the diseases that require transmission-based precautions. Airborne, droplet, and contact precautions are the three designated types of transmission-based precautions. Each

---

BOX 9.1   Synopsis of Standard Precautions

Hand Hygiene
- Wash hands with soap and water (40–60 seconds (s)) if visibly soiled (blood, body fluid) and after caring for patient with known or suspected diarrhea.
- Alcohol-based hand rub preferred with exceptions noted above because of superior microbial activity, reduced skin drying, and convenience. Apply enough to cover all hand areas and rub till dry (20–30 s).
- Before touching a patient or performing an aseptic task, even if gloves will be worn disinfect hands.
- Immediately after glove removal; after final contact with patient disinfect hands.
- If hands will be moving from contaminated body site to clean body site during patient's care disinfect hands.
- Disinfect hands after contact with inanimate objects in the immediate vicinity of where the patient was (i.e., treatment table).

Gloves
- Clean, nonsterile gloves are adequate for most procedures.
- Wear gloves when touching blood, body fluids, secretions, excretions, and any contaminated items, mucous membranes, or nonintact skin.
- Change gloves between tasks and procedures on the same patient after contact with potentially infectious material.
- Remove gloves promptly and before touching noncontaminated items, equipment, and environmental surfaces and immediately perform hand hygiene.

Mask, Eye Protection, and Face Shield
- Wear these devices to protect mucous membranes of your eyes, nose, and mouth during procedures likely to generate splashes or sprays of blood, body fluids, secretions, or excretions. Use care in removing mask; don't touch the front with your hands.
- Wear a mask when performing an aseptic task.
- Do not confuse a mask and a particulate respirator.

Gown
- A clean, nonsterile gown is adequate for most purposes.
- Wear a gown to protect your skin and to prevent soiling your clothing where splashes or sprays are likely. Select one that is appropriate for the amount of fluid likely to be encountered (cloth vs. plastic).
- Remove a soiled gown promptly.

Needlestick Safety
- Wearing gloves when tattooing is optional (no consensus at this time by professional groups). Do wear gloves if blood anticipated or broken skin in area where hand will be placed to perform tattoo.
- Clean area with alcohol wipe and allow area to dry.
- Never administer a tattoo with the same ink syringe even if the needle is changed.
- Dispose of needle at point of use in sharps container.

Patient Care Equipment
- Handle used items/equipment in a careful manner to prevent transfer of pathogens.
- Clean, disinfect, or reprocess reusable items before use with another patient.

Environmental Control
- This pertains to routine care, cleaning, and disinfection of environmental surfaces such as treatment couches, treatment equipment, and other frequently touched surfaces.

Linen
- Handle, transport, and process all used linen soiled with blood, body fluids, secretions, or excretions in a careful manner so as not to spread pathogens.

Occupational Health and Bloodborne Pathogens
- Take care to prevent injuries when using anything sharp and when lifting heavy blocks, wedges, or other radiation therapy devices.
- Do not recap a used needle; do not manipulate a used needle using both hands or use any technique that involves directing the point of a needle toward any part of your body.
- Use mouthpieces, resuscitation bags, or other ventilation devices as an alternative to mouth-to-mouth resuscitation methods.

Respiratory Hygiene/Cough Etiquette
- Implement measures to isolate patients/accompanying persons who have signs/symptoms of a respiratory infection beginning at entry to facility and continuing throughout visit. Offer masks to coughing patients upon entry.
- Post signs to cover mouth and nose when sneezing or coughing. Provide tissues and no-touch trash receptacles for disposal.
- Provide alcohol rub stations throughout the facility for staff and visitor use.
- Place a patient who contaminates the environment or who does not (or cannot be expected to) assist in maintaining appropriate hygiene or environmental control in a private room or area.

Modified from Centers for Disease Control and Prevention. Guide to infection prevention in outpatient settings: minimum expectations for care. 2016 (website). https://www.cdc.gov/infectioncontrol/pdf/outpatient/guide.pdf. Accessed October 2, 2019.

TABLE 9.1 Type of Precautions Recommended for Selected Infections

Infection/Condition	Precaution Type[a]
Anthrax	S
Clostridium difficile	S, C
Diphtheria	S, D
Ebola[a]	S, C, D
Flu (influenza) (if at pandemic/epidemic level)	S, D
Hanta virus	S
Hepatitis A, if diapered/incontinent	S S, C
Hepatitis B, C, D, E, G	S
Leprosy	S
Measles (rubeola)	S, A (for up to 2 hours in a room)
Monkeypox	S, C [a]A, until smallpox ruled out
Multidrug-resistant organisms (MRSA, VRE, VISA/VRSA, ESBLs, resistant pneumonia)	S,C
Mumps	S, D
Noroviruses (cruise ships, schools, etc.)	S [a]D if diapers, incontinent, vomit
Pertussis (whooping cough)	S,D
Pneumococcal pneumonia	S
SARS	S, A, C, D
Smallpox	S, A, C
Staphylococcus aureus (not MRSA), if major skin, wound, burn	S S, C
Streptococcus, group A -if major skin, wound, burn -if pneumonia	S,D S, C, D S, D
Rubella (German measles)	S, D
Tuberculosis -Extrapulmonary (draining lesions) -Pulmonary or pharyngeal	S, A, C S, A
Varicella (chickenpox, shingles)	S, A, C
Viral (other common)	S

[a]Based on research to date.

ESBL, Extended-spectrum beta-lactamase; *MRSA*, methicillin-resistant *Staphylococcus aureus*; *SARS*, severe acute respiratory virus; *VRE*, vancomycin-resistant enterococci; *VISA*, vancomycin-intermediate *S. aureus*; *VRSA*, vancomycin-resistant *S. aureus*. Types of precautions: S, Standard precautions; A, airborne; C, contact, D, droplet. Where A, C, D occur, one should also use S level of precaution, which does not correlate with death rate. S means use of hand hygiene, gloves, mask, eye protection, or face shield depending on anticipated exposure and nature of the healthcare worker (HCW)-patient interaction.

Modified from Siegal JD, Rhinehart E, Jackson M, et al. 2007 Guideline for isolation precautions: preventing transmission of infectious agents in health-care settings. CDC website. http://www.cdc.gov/hicpac/2007ip/2007isola-tionprecautions.html. Accessed November 14, 2018.

of the three can be used alone or in combination for a disease that has more than one transmission route. An empiric approach to admission and diagnosis can be important because often a patient's definitive diagnosis cannot be made until a multitude of tests and procedures have been completed and may take several hours to several days. In the meantime, precautions can be taken to prevent the transmission of the disease if the suspected diagnosis ends up being the definitive diagnosis.

ISOLATION FUNDAMENTALS

Behind any effective isolation program are the basic practices and procedures used around the clock by all HCWs. Radiation therapists are at the forefront of patient care within the radiation oncology department. As such, it is imperative to be aware of steps that can be taken to protect the patients for whom we care. If the following fundamental infection control measures are routinely observed, the risk of transmitting disease can be greatly diminished.

Hand Hygiene

Hand hygiene remains the single most crucial way to prevent the spread of HAIs. Hand hygiene consists of actions taken to reduce the transient flora that colonize the superficial layers of normal skin. The transient flora is acquired by a HCW during direct contact with patients or contact with contaminated environmental surfaces, which in turn are transferred to other HCWs, patients, or even the same patient through cross contamination if hand hygiene is inadequate or omitted.[4] Hand hygiene has been cited frequently as the single most important practice to reduce the transmission of infectious agents in healthcare settings and is clearly an essential element of standard precautions.

Most HCWs worldwide know that hand hygiene is mandatory in surgical settings, when blood is obviously present, or in other similar "dirty" activities. However, transient pathogenic flora can be picked up by a HCW through lifting a patient, taking a pulse or blood pressure, touching an intravenous pole or stretcher rail, touching linear accelerator hand controls and keyboards, touching a patient's hand or any skin surface, and touching a patient's gown or bed linen.[5,6,7] These so-called "clean" activities also contribute to the overall HAI rate and warrant hand hygiene measures after each episode.

Although soap and water still plays an important and active role, we now have medicated (antimicrobial) soap, alcohols, chlorhexidine, chloroxylenol, iodine and iodophors, quaternary ammonium compounds, and other agents.[7,8] Skin irritation from hand hygiene products, especially soap and other detergents, can be addressed with the addition of emollients and humectants.[9]

In Box 9.2 and Table 9.2, emphasis is placed on work habits that are most likely to be encountered by a radiation therapist.[10] Surgical hand hygiene procedures have also changed substantially. Box 9.3 shows the highlights of current surgical hand antisepsis. As more studies and agents are analyzed, changes to these guidelines can be expected and are warranted.

> Hand hygiene is the single most crucial and effective weapon for reducing healthcare-associated infections. Use hand agents routinely and frequently; wash when appropriate.

Fingernails are the primary reservoir of microflora on the hands, even after intense washing.[4] The underside of the nail, the subungual region, harbors the highest number of microorganisms.[11] Today, most healthcare facilities with well-informed epidemiologic personnel have policies stating that nails must be neat and trimmed to a length typically around one-quarter inch and that the wearing of artificial nails of any type is prohibited.

> Fingernails should be natural, unpolished, short, and neat.

BOX 9.2 Nonsurgical Hand Hygienic Technique and Characteristics

Alcohol-Based Hand Rubs	Soap (Detergent) and Water Washing
• Current gold standard based on cost, effectiveness, and efficiency except for clinical situations calling for hand wash. • Apply to palm; rub together to cover all surfaces of hands and fingers. • Rub until completely dry. • Use volume specified by manufacturer. • Takes less time to apply; comes in pocket-size containers. • Causes less skin irritation and dryness than water and soap.	• Wet hands with water that is not hot (hot water is irritating to the skin). • Apply product covering all hand and finger surfaces. • Rub hands together vigorously for at least 40–60 seconds (friction promotes removal of microorganisms). • Rinse well (more water usage removes more microorganisms). • Pat until completely dry with single-use, disposable towel (friction when drying irritates the skin). • Use paper towel to turn faucet off. • Soap may be in bar, liquid, powdered, or leaflet form (if bar soap is used, a drainage rack should be in place). • Should be performed for every 10 to 15 alcohol-based hand-rub applications. • Should be followed with lotion/cream to decrease skin irritation.

Modified from Centers for Disease Control and Prevention. Guideline for hand hygiene in health-care settings: recommendations of the Healthcare Infection Control Practices Advisory Committee and the HICPAC/SHEA/APIC/IDSA Hand Hygiene Task Force. *MMWR* 2002;51:1–44.

TABLE 9.2 Actions and Indications for Hand Hygiene

Action Needed	Indication
• Use alcohol-based hand rub, less skin irritation and more effective for most routine patient care.	• Not visibly soiled • Simple routine touching of patient or patient environment • Before having direct contact with patient • Before inserting a urinary catheter or other invasive nonsurgical procedure • After contact with patient's intact skin (e.g., lifting or shaking hand) • When moving from contaminated body site to "clean" body site during same patient care • After contact with inanimate objects (including medical equipment) in the immediate vicinity of patient (e.g., bed rails, wheelchairs, treatment couch) • After removing gloves
• Wash hands with water and soap (plain or antimicrobial).	• Visibly dirty or contaminated by blood or other body fluid/excretion, mucous membrane contact, nonintact skin, wound dressing • Before eating • After using restroom • After caring for patient known to have *Clostridium difficile* or diarrhea
• Nonalcohol-based hand rubs that smell good and are available in the stores/malls are not FDA approved unless so stated. • Alcohol-based hand rubs are flammable and should be stored only in approved areas.	

FDA, US Food and Drug Administration.
Modified from WHO guidelines on hand hygiene in health care: first global patient safety challenge, clean care is safer care 2009. WHO website. http://whqlibdoc.who.int/publications/2009/9789241597906_eng.pdf. Accessed November 14, 2018; Centers for Disease Control and Prevention. Guideline for hand hygiene in health-care settings: recommendations of the Healthcare Infection Control Practices Advisory Committee and the HICPAC/SHEA/APIC/IDSA Hand Hygiene Task Force. *MMWR* 2002;51:1–44.

Also worth noting is that rings worn by HCWs have been studied to determine whether bacterial counts are higher in ring wearers than in those who do not wear rings. Several studies have shown that the area underneath the ring is more heavily populated by bacteria than on ringless fingers.[12,13,14] However, at this time, it has not been firmly established whether the wearing of rings results in greater transmission of pathogens, and thus, no recommendation has been made.[13] Until further studies are performed, it would be prudent to wear no ring or fewer rings while performing radiation therapy duties and to take special care to make sure that hand hygiene products reach the skin area under the ring.

With the development of blood-transmitted diseases, spore-driven *Clostridium difficile*–associated diarrhea, multidrug resistant organisms (e.g., vancomycin-resistant enterococci [VRE] and methicillin-resistant *Staphylococcus aureus* [MRSA]), legal actions by patients, and the cost of healthcare-associated infections, hand hygiene is in the healthcare and public spotlight. Patients and the public are very aware that HCWs are not always practicing hand hygiene as they should. Infection rates at specific healthcare facilities are becoming publicly available by law in more than half of the states; thus, it is worthwhile at the institutional level to mount and maintain an active hand-hygiene educational campaign.[15,16] Institutions worldwide are revamping their HCW educational and safety strategies to promote adherence to implemented hand-hygiene protocols. Some facilities are actually monitoring employee compliance and counseling them for individual improvement in techniques; others are rewarding employees when goals are achieved, placing reminders and posters in the workplace, changing hygiene agents, and making cleansing agents more readily

BOX 9.3 Surgical Hand Antisepsis

• Remove rings, watches, and bracelets before starting scrub.
• Use either an antimicrobial soap or an alcohol-based surgical hand rub with "persistent activity" (e.g., continues to work for a prolonged time period).
• Scrub all surfaces of hands, under nails, fingers, and forearms for time recommended by manufacturer (typically 2–3 minutes). Longer times (e.g., 10 minutes) are not necessary.
• If alcohol *surgical* hand rub is preferred, hands and forearms should be prewashed with a nonantimicrobial soap to remove spores and dried completely before application of the alcohol agent.
• Hands, fingers, and forearms should be thoroughly dry before putting on sterile gloves.
• A brush to scrub with is not recommended. Brushes and sponges may be used but are no longer required because they contribute to skin irritation.

Data from Centers for Disease Control and Prevention. Guideline for hand hygiene in health-care settings: recommendations of the Healthcare Infection Control Practices Advisory Committee and the HICPAC/SHEA/APIC/IDSA Hand Hygiene Task Force. *MMWR* 2002;51:1–44; WHO Guidelines on Hand Hygiene In Health Care: First Global Patient Safety Challenge, Clean Care Is Safer Care 2009. WHO website. http://whqlibdoc.who.int/publications/2009/9789241597906_eng.pdf. Accessed November 14, 2018.

assessable.[17] Facilities also provide hand lotions and creams to minimize hand irritation.[17]

Radiation therapists should perform hand hygiene in front of the patient so they have a visual confirmation. Patients should be told to feel free to remind them if they don't see them cleanse their hands before procedures. Finally, the therapist should always thank the patient if they receive a reminder and perform hand hygiene immediately, even if it had already been done out of sight of the patient. Radiation therapists should never act irritated at the patient for requesting to visually see the washing of hands.

Gloving

There are several important reasons for the wearing of gloves. One is to provide the HCW a protective barrier and to keep his or her hands from becoming grossly contaminated. A second reason is to keep the patient safe from any microorganisms that may be present on the HCW's hands. A third reason is that when gloves are removed immediately after a patient contact and disposed of immediately, they cannot serve as a fomite and infect other patients. A massive increase in glove cost and glove use occurred when the Occupational Safety and Health Administration (OSHA) mandated that gloves be made available and worn if blood or body fluids were present.[18]

Gloves manufactured for healthcare purposes are subject to US Food and Drug Administration (FDA) evaluation and approval.[19]

The wearing of gloves does not guarantee safety, however, because they can have manufacturing defects too small to be seen, and they can be easily torn or punctured by equipment. Hands can also be easily and unknowingly contaminated upon glove removal. Because of these reasons, CDC guidelines state that hands should always be cleaned promptly after removing gloves.

Gloves are made of different polymers, including latex, a natural rubber, or synthetic materials (e.g., vinyl, nitrile, or neoprene). With the increase of glove use, it was quickly realized that a significant and increasing number of HCWs were sensitive or even highly allergic to latex. Gloves must be available as powdered latex, powder-free latex, or synthetic to accommodate latex-sensitive HCWs.[20] Although a single pair usually is sufficient, note that vinyl gloves have higher failure rates.[20] The use of petroleum-based hand lotions or creams has been negatively associated with latex barrier protection, and thus, their use should be avoided. Sharp or ragged nails should be avoided because they easily produce punctures or tears that are not visually detectable.

Radiation therapists should always remove gloves before handling the hand pendant and couch controls, operating the accelerator console, answering the telephone, pushing the door close button, or touching any other treatment accessory. Two to three therapists typically make up the treatment team, so one can remove his or her gloves after a patient assist or lift and act as the "clean" therapist who will be responsible for handling equipment. Alternately, therapists can remove gloves as needed and put on another pair when indicated.

> Wear gloves when patient care dictates but not when handling accelerator controls or other objects. Apply hand hygiene after removing gloves.

Masks, Respiratory Protection, Eye Protection, and Face Shields

The use of masks is intended for three purposes in healthcare. They are (1) worn by the HCW to protect them from contact with infectious materials (sprays of blood or body fluids and respiratory secretions), even if droplet precautions are not in place; (2) placed on the coughing patient to protect the HCW; and (3) worn by the HCW performing a procedure requiring a sterile technique to protect the patient. Mucous membranes of the mouth, nose, eyes, and compromised facial skin (acne) all serve as entry portals for infection. Two mask types are available: (1) surgical masks that must be fluid resistant and FDA approved, and (2) procedure/isolation masks that are not fluid resistant or approved by the FDA.[4] If a procedure will generate splashes or sprays of blood, body fluids, secretions, or excretions (suctioning, bronchoscopy), a face mask or goggles and mask are required; personal eyeglasses are not adequate. A cloth or paper mask gradually becomes damp with exhalation of respiratory moisture. Because transmission risk increases with the degree of wetness, damp masks should be replaced with dry ones as needed. Radiation therapists are usually trained on proper removal of a face shield, goggles, and a mask. The OSHA bloodborne pathogens final rule mandates the wearing of masks, eye protection, and face shields during activities likely to generate splashes or sprays.[21,22] A mask should not be confused with a particulate respirator.

Particulate Respirators

A special kind of device called a particulate respirator is needed to protect against pathogens that consist of small droplet nuclei and are transmitted via the airborne route. Respiratory protection per OSHA and the CDC calls for a fit-tested National Institute for Occupational Safety and Health–certified N95 or higher particulate filtering respirator, educational training, and periodic reevaluation.[21,23] Particulate respirators come in a variety of types, such as tight or loose fitting and atmosphere supply respirators (provide clean air from an uncontaminated source), and are assigned a protection factor (the higher the number, the greater the protection). A user-seal check should be done each time a HCW puts one on.[23] A person with facial hair cannot wear one.[24] They were first recommended for TB in 1989; they continue to be recommended for TB, bioterrorism anthrax, smallpox, avian influenza (bird flu), SARS (severe acute respiratory virus, which emerged in and was imported from China), and other emerging hemorrhagic fevers in which transmission data is still limited.[24-26]

Gowns and Protective Apparel

Gowns are to be worn as a protective barrier over an HCW's uniform or street clothes. To protect clothing and underlying skin, one should anticipate the amount of fluid contamination and choose between ordinary cloth gowns and gowns that are impermeable to liquids. Leg coverings, boots, or shoe coverings are also needed when splashes or large quantities of liquids are present or anticipated.[22]

Patient Placement

A vital component of any infection control plan is designating whether it is crucial for a patient to have a private room or not. When direct contact or indirect contact transmission pathogens are involved, a private room is needed when the source patient has poor hygiene practices, contaminates the environment, or cannot be expected to participate in infection control measures. If a private room is not available, then patients infected with the same pathogen can be housed together. A private room with special air handling and negative ventilation is important in airborne transmission diseases and referred to as an AIIR (airborne infection isolation room).[4]

Transport of Infectious Patients

Patients with epidemiologically significant microorganisms should leave their rooms only for essential procedures to decrease the risk of transmission. For essential procedures, the patient should wear a mask, dressings, or whatever barrier is deemed necessary for the specific pathogen that he or she carries. The personnel who will be performing the essential procedure should be notified in advance so that they can be prepared to receive the patient, and the patient should receive instruction on how he or she can help prevent the spread of the pathogen to others.

Patient Care Equipment and Articles

Equipment and articles used for patient care require proper handling once contaminated. Many items are disposable, whereas others may be reused after reprocessing. The method of disposal or reprocessing is determined by the severity of the associated disease, the environmental stability of the pertinent pathogen, the physical characteristics of the item, and the facility's infection control plan. If a disposable item is sharp and could cause injury, it must be placed in a puncture-resistant container immediately after use to meet OSHA standards.[22] Other items may simply be bagged. Only one bag is needed if the bag is sturdy and remains uncontaminated on the outside; if not, then two bags are used. Items that can be reprocessed are divided into three categories: critical, semicritical, and noncritical and are covered in a later section of this chapter.

Laundry

A clean pillowcase or sheet should always be used for each patient. Contaminated laundry presents a very low risk of disease transmission provided it is handled, transported, and laundered in a manner that prevents transfer of pathogens. Federal standards state that used laundry is to be handled as little as possible with a minimum of agitation and bagged or placed in a container at the location where it is used.[22] For a radiation therapy department, this translates to a container in every treatment room, dressing room, and examination room. If laundry is contaminated and wet, gloves should be worn, and the laundry must be placed in a bag, which prevents soak-through or leakage. Contaminated laundry also has to be placed in labeled or red bags unless the medical facility treats all laundry as if it was contaminated and all employees are aware of the practice.[27] Commercial laundries often use water at a temperature of 160°F and 50 to 150 ppm (parts per million) and chlorine bleach for grossly contaminated linen.[28] For home laundry, use water as hot as possible, and make smart shopping choices in regard to fabrics that can withstand heat. Some hospitals provide uniforms as part of employment. Many centers suggest that HCWs remove work shoes and bag them in the parking lot and then switch to a clean pair before entering their car to avoid tracking infectious pathogens into their home environment. Once home, promptly changing out of work clothes and using a separate laundry basket is also a smart practice.

Routine Cleaning of Environment

Equipment used on patients who have been placed on one or more of the transmission-based precautions should be cleaned in the same manner as patients on standard precautions unless the pathogen or the amount of environmental contamination is such that special procedures are necessary. In addition to routine cleaning, disinfectants may be required for specific pathogens that are capable of surviving in the inanimate environment for prolonged periods of time. Treatment tables and supporting equipment, stepstool handles, prone pillows, breast boards, head and neck supports, and any other positioning device used on more than one specific patient should be cleaned after each patient contact.

The method of cleaning and choice of cleaning and/or disinfecting products should be based on recommendations of the manufacturer of the equipment and infection care consultation and be part of the exposure control plan.

> Clean treatment room after treating each and every patient. Wipe down anything the patient makes contact with.

Blood or Body Fluid Spills

Blood or body fluid spills should be cleaned up immediately. OSHA does not specify a specific procedure or a single specific disinfectant. Either a disinfectant approved by the Environmental Protection Agency (EPA) for hospital use or a 1:10 fresh solution of household bleach (sodium hypochlorite) should be used, with 1 part bleach and 10 parts water.[22] Household bleach has a broad spectrum of antimicrobial activity and is inexpensive and fast acting; however, it is corrosive and relatively unstable and therefore must be fresh to be effective. It is also inactivated by organic matter, which means that it becomes useless as it kills microorganisms; thus, it does not provide a prolonged effect and must be available in an appropriate quantity for the size of the spill. Choice of product(s) should be in the exposure control plan.

Student Education

Students should receive blood and body fluid instruction at the earliest stage of their professional education. Orientation to OSHA rules and regulations and medical facilities' overall infection control programs and hazardous materials programs should take place before active participation in the clinical component of education. In some educational programs, students rotate through multiple healthcare facilities. These programs must ensure that a student is thoroughly familiar with each facility's bloodborne pathogens program before any active participation occurs. Students are required to *immediately* report any known or possible bloodborne exposure to clinical supervisors, followed by prompt contact of educational program officials.

RIGHTS OF THE HEALTHCARE WORKER

Today's HCW should never have to wonder what to do if an employer does not provide proper protection equipment, but if this occurs, HCWs have legal rights. OSHA helps provide job safety and health protection for employees by promoting safe and healthful working conditions throughout the nation. State laws are also in place. HCWs can lawfully refuse to work in truly unsafe conditions and have the right to insist on wearing protective equipment, but they cannot "walk out" on their job if they want their rights protected.[29] HCWs must inform their employer of the unsafe conditions. If an employer does not respond, the employee should contact OSHA to file a complaint and request an inspection be conducted.[29] OSHA will withhold, on request, the name of the employee filing the complaint.[29] Before filing a complaint, a HCW should be sure that the unsafe condition is indeed serious (i.e., the situation could have caused death or serious harm). Retaliation against the employee for reporting such working conditions is against the law.

The opposite situation can also occur. On occasion, HCWs may have unreasonable fears and be overly cautious. Examples include the HCW who refuses to go anywhere near a human immunodeficiency virus/acquired immunodeficiency syndrome (HIV/AIDS) patient or the worker who insists on wearing full-body protective gear when unnecessary. This type of reaction is usually caused by lack of proper education about the risk of transmission and proper protective actions that the HCW should take. The employer should let the HCW explain fears and perceptions and should then educate the HCW with the necessary information in understandable language. The HCW cannot be discharged or discriminated against in any way just because of a misperception or because of a complaint or call to OSHA. HCWs who believe they have been discriminated against should file a complaint with their nearest OSHA office within 30 days of the alleged discriminatory act.[29] However, if after counseling and if the situation is deemed to be reasonably safe and proper equipment was provided, and the HCW still refuses to provide care, as in the AIDS patient example, the employer may have the right to dismiss the worker.

HCWs also have legal rights if they develop an occupationally acquired infection. Workers' compensation laws, determined by each state, are in place to protect the employee who is injured, disabled, or killed while on the job. For compensation to be awarded, the injury must have occurred while practicing within his or her scope of practice. Bungee jumping off the 17th floor of the hospital during lunch hour, for example, would not be covered because it is outside the scope of practice of a radiation therapist. In most cases, HCWs do not have the right to file a negligence or criminal suit in addition to a workers' compensation claim unless they can prove that their employer intentionally disregarded an infection risk. The HCW must also be able to establish that the infection was acquired on the job, not in the community.

Another extremely important right HCWs have is complete confidentiality. To protect privacy, most healthcare facilities take special steps to avoid placing the HCW's "patient" chart where other employees have access to it. In addition, such a diagnosis might not be placed on computerized charting systems. It is not appropriate to view a patient chart that is not in the direct line of your care. For example, if a coworker is diagnosed with cancer and being treated at the same facility but on another machine, you are not permitted to view his or her chart at any time.

ROLE OF THE CENTRAL SERVICES DEPARTMENT

With the concerns of bloodborne pathogens and emerging diseases, many healthcare centers have chosen to leave the reprocessing of medical supplies and equipment in the hands of experts. Some radiation therapy centers are now choosing to send items needing sterilization out for processing and hiring expert consultants to do onsite inspections, recommend appropriate products, write infection control performance protocols, and conduct staff in-service training. In large healthcare facilities, this area of expertise typically is found in a department known as *central services*, or *central supply.* The central service department (CSD) is accountable for preparing, processing, sorting, and distributing the medical supplies and equipment required in patient care. This central location is economical and subjected to stringent levels of quality control according to The Joint Commission (TJC) standards.[30,31] Accreditation by TJC is available for traditional hospitals as well as ambulatory healthcare facilities. Several major cancer centers are accredited and listed online.[30]

A student or employee tour through a major center's CSD can be an extremely enlightening and educational experience. Contaminated equipment is first precleaned and decontaminated by trained, specially clothed workers. This clothing includes items such as waterproof aprons and face shields. Reprocessing may include disassembly and sending equipment through devices that remind a person of a commercial car wash, complete with a presoak cycle, wash cycle, and dry cycle. Instruments are then prepared for sterilization by the most appropriate method. Ideally, each package sterilized is labeled with a control number in case any item needs recalling. The labeling process may also identify the sterilizing unit used, its load, the time and date an item was sterilized, the item's expiration date, and sometimes even the individual who packaged the item (Fig. 9.1)

After a package has been disinfected or sterilized, it should be handled as little as possible and stored in a low-traffic, clean, dry, closed area. If an item comes into contact with something and becomes soiled, is dropped on the floor, is exposed to moisture, or is physically

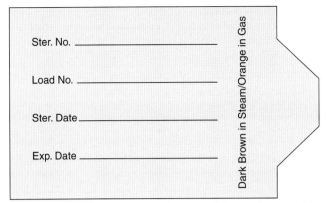

Fig. 9.1 Sterilization labels are used as part of the quality control program in a central services department. If an item must be recalled, it can be tracked by its control number.

penetrated, it is deemed contaminated and should not be used. Sterile items should be stored away from the floor, ceiling, outside walls, vents, pipes, doors, and windows. The temperature should be approximately 75°F (24°C) degrees with a relative humidity not to exceed 70% with four air exchanges per hour.[32] Closed shelves are preferred over drawers because the risk of damaging a sterilized package is greater in opening and closing a drawer than opening the door to a cabinet. If a closed cabinet is not an option, open shelves are a feasible solution. Placing a plastic designated sterility maintenance dust cover over the sterilized packages can decrease the chance of damage and contamination.[32]

Each healthcare facility determines the amount of time that a sterilized item can be stored and is event related.[32] Important factors in determining shelf-life include packaging material and an open or closed shelf design, both of which combined are more important than time alone. It is further assumed that after the opening of a sterilized package, a sterile technique will be used, and the date of expiration will be checked. Package dating assists in the rotation process, and the older items that have not yet expired should be used first. Commercially prepared items should be discarded upon reaching the expiration date provided by the manufacturer.

STERILIZATION AND DISINFECTION TECHNIQUES

In general, medical supplies and equipment can be divided into risk categories based on each item's use.[33,34] Critical items are products or instruments inserted into normally sterile areas of the body or into the bloodstream and must be sterile for use. Items in this category include needles, surgical instruments, urinary catheters, and implants. *Semicritical items* are those that contact mucosal surfaces but do not ordinarily penetrate body mucosal surfaces. Nonintact skin is also included in this group. Items included in this group are endoscopes, thermometers, laryngoscopes, and anesthesia equipment. It is preferable to sterilize items in this category, but high-level disinfection may be used.[33,34] *Noncritical items* do not ordinarily touch the patient or touch only the patient's intact skin; therefore, they do not need to be sterile. This category includes items such as tabletops, bedpans, crutches, and blood pressure cuffs.[33,34] Radiation therapists have the potential to come into contact with all three risk categories within their practice. Therefore, having a solid understanding of sterilization and disinfection techniques is critical.

The FDA requires that medical devices be sold with explicit instructions stating whether the devices are single use or reusable and the way they must be processed if reusable.[34,35] Reuse of items labeled single use has been a very controversial topic regarding regulatory, ethical, medical, legal, and economical issues. In 2000, the FDA mandated that hospitals or other third-party reprocessors who choose to reprocess a single-use item would be subjected to the same stringent processes as the original manufacturers and assume their risk.[34] Reuse rules continue to evolve; for the latest guidance, refer to the FDA.

> Critical items, semicritical items, and noncritical items are labels used to classify risk of contamination for medical equipment utilization.

Sterilization is a process that destroys all microbial life forms, including resistant spores. Sterilization can be achieved through physical or chemical processes. There are no degrees of sterilization; an item is either sterile or it is not sterile. Processes used for sterilization include steam under pressure, dry heat, low-temperature sterilization (ethylene oxide gas, hydrogen peroxide gas plasma, ozone), and specific liquid chemicals (peracetic acid immersion).[34]

Disinfection is a process that reduces microbial life forms and can range from *high-level disinfection* to *intermediate-level disinfection* and even *low-level disinfection*.[34,36] Low-level disinfection is synonymous with sanitization. High-level disinfection eliminates all microbial life forms except situations in which there are high numbers of bacterial spores or prions.[34] Intermediate-level disinfection kills the TB bacterium, most viruses, and most fungi but not most bacterial spores.[34] Low-level disinfection inactivates most bacteria, some viruses, and some fungi but is mostly ineffective against TB bacterium and bacterial spores.[34] The major point to remember is that some microbial life forms cannot be eliminated by disinfection processes. In the healthcare setting, disinfection is typically achieved through the use of liquid chemicals or wet pasteurization (very hot water).

Antiseptics are different from disinfectants. The term *antiseptic* is reserved for antimicrobial substances applied to skin surfaces. Methods of sterilization and disinfection are addressed in the following text and differ with regard to the biocidal agent, biocidal action, contact between the biocidal agent and the microorganism, and severity of treatment.[37] Regardless of whether sterilization or disinfection is appropriate for a given situation, neither process is likely to be successful if meticulous cleaning does not precede the process. A basic premise is that the fewer organisms remaining after simple cleaning, the fewer there are left to kill, which in turn increases the safety margin. Simple sorting, disassembly, soaking, scrubbing and brushing, rinsing and draining, or drying is used before sterilization or disinfection processes. Foreign matter that remains after inadequate cleaning and processing generally renders an item unusable.

Heat

The use of heat, moist or dry, is the most reliable, available, and economical method of destroying microorganisms. Boiling water (100°C, 212°F) is probably the oldest method used. Although boiling greatly decreases the number of microorganisms, it does not destroy all microorganisms, such as spores; thus, boiling fits into the category of disinfectants rather than sterilants. In fact, temperatures lower than boiling (50°C–70°C, 122°F–158°F) are sufficient to kill most viruses, bacteria, and fungi.[36] HIV is destroyed by moist heat at 60°C (140°F) in 30 minutes, a temperature well below the requirement for boiling water.[38,44]

Hot water pasteurization is a process using water at a temperature of 145°F (63°C) for 30 minutes, but again, it must be stressed that this is not considered a sterilization process.[33,38] Steam under pressure, however, is capable of destroying all life forms, provided that a proper combination of temperature and time is achieved. Older references typically quoted a specific time, temperature, and pressure combination, and the student accepted this combination as an absolute. In reality, steam sterilization works as an inverse relationship, and many

combinations are equally effective; thus, steam sterilization is analogous to the various time-dose relationships used in treating cancer. Simply put, the time required for steam sterilization decreases as the temperature increases, but temperatures above 134°C (273.2°F) should not be used.[39]

Steam sterilizers are commonly referred to as *steam autoclaves* and can be described as closed metal chambers. Autoclaves can be grouped into two general categories: gravity displacement and high-speed prevacuum devices.[34] The gravity displacement type uses a lower temperature of 121°C (250°F) but requires a longer exposure time of 30 minutes.[34] The prevacuum type uses 132°C (270°F) for 4 minutes.[34] These time/temperature combinations are standard recommendations for wrapped articles and represent time minimums. Steam sterilization is the most commonly used method of sterilization for healthcare facilities because of its low cost, its absence of toxic residue, and the fact that it can sterilize an extremely wide assortment of materials. A drying cycle follows exposure to the steam and is often the longest portion of the autoclave cycle.

With a special exception of an infectious life form known as a *prion* (proteinaceous infectious particle), which causes diseases such as Creutzfeldt-Jakob disease (CJD), no life forms survive if exposed to steam under pressure at 30 pounds per square inch at 121°C (250°F).[36] An exposure that lasts 15 to 20 minutes at this temperature and pressure is adequate for killing most life forms; however, the heat-resistant Creutzfeldt-Jakob agent requires 1 hour of exposure at a temperature of 132°C (270°F) in a gravity displacement unit.[39,41]

The term *prion* (pronounced *pree-on*), introduced in 1982 by SB Prusiner (for which he won a 1997 Nobel Prize), is used to describe unique, infectious central nervous system (CNS) agents composed of protein but lacking identifiable nucleic acid.[40] Prions, whose functions are still not fully understood, consist of long strands of protein that are normal components of the brain and other tissues.[39] They cause disease only when they deteriorate and start folding themselves into three-dimensional structures different from their normal structure.[39,40] Prion diseases do not initiate an immune response, include in a noninflammatory pathologic process confined to the CNS, have an incubation period of years, and usually are fatal in less than 1 year after diagnosis.[39] Symptoms of CJD present as rapidly progressing dementia, changing to coma and then death, and there is no cure.[42,43] A better-known prion variant of CJD-related disease is bovine spongiform encephalopathy, commonly referred to as mad cow disease, which is passed to humans through contaminated beef products.[42] CJD has been associated with corneal transplants, dura mater graphs, pituitary growth hormone injections, and other neurosurgical procedures.[37] Extreme caution should be taken with brain tissue and CNS fluids because HCWs have died from an occupational exposure.[37]

Another device known as a terminal sterilizer (formerly known as a flash sterilizer) can be used in an emergency situation (but not with CJD reprocessing).[32] This device is operated at a temperature of 132°C (270°F), exposure time of 4 minutes at 27 to 28 lbs of pressure (if gravity design), or specific manufacturer requirements for the unit or the instrument to be flashed.[34] Flash autoclaving should not routinely be substituted for standard autoclaving procedures to save time or as an alternative to purchasing additional instrument sets.

Cotton fabric and special steam-permeable plastics or paper can be used as packaging materials. Other criteria essential to the selection of appropriate packaging materials for any sterilization method include the resistance to puncture and tears, penetration by microorganisms, and absence of toxic or biologically harmful particles. Care must be exercised in packing items for steam sterilization to ensure that the steam can reach all surfaces and cavities of a specific item. For example, lids must be taken off containers, and many items may require disassembly. Items in a package must be arranged loosely because over-packing may lead to problems with sterilization.

Steam sterilization also has its limitations. Instruments such as needles and scalpels may be dulled. Oxidation and corrosion may also occur with certain metals. Powder and oil products should not be auto-claved because the steam has difficulty in penetrating such substances. Many products such as rubber and synthetic polymers are heat sensitive and could melt or deteriorate. Other products such as injectable solutions may lose their biologic usefulness when subjected to high heat levels.

Because of packing precautions, packaging material differences, product sensitivity to heat, and TJC quality control standards, comprehensive knowledge is required of anyone in charge of steam sterilization or any method of sterilization. For these reasons, sterilization is best done by experts, the employees of the CSD.

To summarize, steam sterilization techniques and combinations of pressure, temperature, and time are influenced by the type of microorganism to be destroyed, the instruments, and the unit used.

Dry heat is also used for sterilization. Although its use declined since the introduction of single-use syringes and needles sterilized by other methods, dry heat is still useful for reusable needles, glass syringes, sharp cutting instruments and drills, powders and oily products, and metals that oxidize or corrode with exposure to moisture. The advantage of dry heat is its ability to penetrate solids, nonaqueous powders or oils, and closed containers. The dry heat units are easily installed and have relatively low operational costs.[34] Its primary disadvantage when compared with steam is that higher temperatures and longer exposure times are required to achieve sterilization. Commonly referenced temperatures are 150°C (300°F) for 150 minutes, 160°C (320°F) for 120 minutes, and 170°C (350°F) for 60 minutes.[34] Similar to cooking in a home oven, aluminum foil or aluminum containers are commonly used for packaging. Items that are heat sensitive should be sterilized by other available techniques.

Incineration, another form of heat, is frequently applied to biohazardous waste materials generated in healthcare settings. Some incinerators are located on hospital grounds, but most are commonly located away from hospitals, residential areas, and high-occupancy buildings. Because incinerators are typically located some distance away, designated vehicles are required to transport biohazardous waste to the incinerator site. As a final note, all use of glass bead "sterilizers" should be discontinued because they are not FDA approved.[34]

Gas

Gas sterilizers are available for medical products that cannot withstand high temperatures, such as endoscopes and plastic items. When they were first introduced, the use of gas sterilizers became increasingly important because of the use of a greater number of instruments and products that could not tolerate high heat exposure. More recently, however, even though gas is still widely used, new methods are being introduced because of environmental concerns, the impact of the Clean Air Act, and EPA and OSHA oversight.[34] Gas is a more complex and expensive method than dry or wet heat. Ethylene oxide (usually written as ETO) is the gas used in most gas sterilizers.[34,43]

In the past, ETO was mixed with Freon, but carbon dioxide (CO_2) is now the additive of choice because of Freon's harmful effect on the ozone layer.[34] The operation of a gas sterilizer should be attempted only by qualified experts because the gases present fire and explosion hazards. Gas sterilizers are equipped with special detectors to alert personnel in the event of a gas leak.

To recap, gas is slower and more expensive and has the possibility of toxic residue. Very few hospitals have an ethylene oxide sterilizer. Large medical institutions frequently cooperate and provide gas sterilization access to medium and small medical institutions to assist with cost. Gas sterilization is not applied to liquids or products packaged in gas impervious wrappers. Products can be wrapped in the same packaging materials used for steam sterilization.

Hydrogen peroxide gas plasma units, marketed since 1993, consist of gas in a highly charged vacuum state.[34] The free radicals created interact with the microorganisms to destroy them. The entire process takes anywhere from 28 to 75 minutes, depending on the model. There is no toxic emission, so no aeration is necessary. More of these exist now, but there are still some associated technical problems.[45] They cannot be used with cellulose-based products, such as paper and linen, and may not be able to penetrate small lumens, so their use is restricted for many items.

Ozone

Ozone was FDA cleared for sterilization in 2003.[34] Ozone units use US Pharmacopeia–grade oxygen, steam-quality water, and electricity to sterilize, with a cycle duration of about 4 hours, 15 minutes at 30°C to 35°C (86°F–95°F).[34] The process can be used on stainless steel, titanium ceramic, glass, polyvinyl chloride, silicon, and other materials.[34] Low temperature, no toxic emission, and no residue to aerate make it an attractive alternative for many items.

Radiation

Although not routinely used in the healthcare setting, ionizing radiation is widely applied at industrial sites for medical products and equipment that cannot withstand heat. Gamma radiation from cobalt-60 sources or linear accelerator photon and electron beams are used. Electrons are more limited in use because of their lack of penetration, and photon beams more than 10 MV are not used because they can induce significant radioactivity in the sterilized product through artificial nuclide production.[37] Extremely high absorbed doses (kGy) are necessary because microorganisms are far more resistant to the effects of radiation than humans.[46]

The time required for sterilization depends on the unit's dose rate and the required absorbed dose. Packaging materials and the product contained within are sterilized. Caution must be employed in using radiation as a sterilant for medications because it may modify some medications.

An interesting student project is to check commercially prepared packages for a wide variety of single-use sterile (disposable) products to see how many were irradiated.

Radiation is used in the autosterilization of a strontium (^{90}Sr) applicator. After a strontium treatment for pterygium of the eye, the radioactive end of the applicator is wiped against a sterile alcohol pad to remove any biologic debris and then rinsed with sterile water. The surface radiation output emitted by a typical 50 mCi ^{90}Sr source is approximately 50 cGy per second, a rate high enough that it sterilizes itself with a dose of more than 4 million cGy in a 24-hour period.

Nonionizing radiations, such as ultraviolet (UV) and infrared light or microwave, are also capable of killing microorganisms, but the wavelengths are too low to allow any significant penetration. UV sources are costly and require ongoing service and maintenance; thus, they are not used for sterilization purposes except in a few extremely limited applications. Most viruses and bacteria are easily killed by UV when humidity is kept low. UV sources have been used in TB isolation areas, surgical suites, and burn units to keep microorganism concentrations down in the ambient air and general surface environment. Microwave units are not FDA cleared for sterilization purposes.[34]

Chemical Liquids

Using chemicals for sterilization or disinfection can be a relatively easy process. An item can simply be placed in a basin deep enough to completely submerge it, with care taken to ensure that the chemical can reach all inner and outer surfaces, lumens, and crevices. Caution should be exercised to ensure that the chemical will not damage the item to be processed or the basin containing the chemical itself. The most difficult part is selecting the best, most appropriate chemical. Therefore, a radiation therapist should contact a qualified CSD expert for input in choosing products and protocols for use.

Chemicals have an extremely wide range of antimicrobial action and are time sensitive. Very few can truly sterilize; the vast majority cannot, and those that can are known as *chemical sterilants*. The FDA regulates antiseptics, disinfectants, and sterilants (chemical and gaseous) used to process critical and semicritical medical devices.[34] The EPA regulates disinfectants and nonmedical chemical sterilants used on environmental surfaces (bed rails, tabletops, floors).[34]

The good news is that no data shows that antibiotic resistant bacteria (i.e., MRSA, VRE) are any harder to kill than their normal counterparts with properly used chemicals.[34] Most chemicals show that greater concentration shortens kill time.[34] Many require specific ratios when combined with water, and most achieve greater kill efficiency when combined than alone. Each chemical has its own minimal time to kill and must be followed to be effective, so read labels carefully. Many states now regulate whether healthcare disinfectants can be disposed of down drains at all or in limited concentrations, so HCWs need to be aware of disposal rules in their specific state.

The CDC cannot endorse specific products, but it can provide guidance in choosing products.[47] Other professional groups, such as the Association for Professionals in Infection Control and Epidemiology (APIC) and the Association for the Advancement of Medical Instrumentation, also publish extremely useful guidelines.[32,48] Manufacturers are also responsible for furnishing recommendations on the reprocessing of items that they produce. Thus, the chemical to be used on a specific item is based on expert guidelines, scientific literature, and manufacturer product information. Reliance on labels alone is insufficient and at times even misleading. Therefore, caution should be used with wording such as "hospital-strength disinfectant." "Hospital disinfectant" is preferred because this term indicates a higher level of disinfection.

> Seek out experts on what chemical agents should be used in your treatment and simulation areas. Always follow written procedures.

Soap's usefulness as a disinfectant is limited because of its feeble antimicrobial action. The main merit of soap is that it aids in the removal of contamination buildup. Flexible scopes used in radiation oncology examination rooms deserve a special note of caution. Written procedures, documented training, test strips, and personal protective equipment need to be in place before cleaning a flexible endoscope. Meticulous care is required to ensure that an effective quality assurance process takes place, and a log is used to indicate the procedure, patient, date, serial number or other identifier of endoscope used, and the person performing the endoscopy.[33] Another special note of caution is that liquid disinfectants and sterilants should not be used to clean brachytherapy devices, such as ovoids. These liquids are known to corrode the silver brazing that secures the ovoid to the ovoid handle.[49] Strict adherence to the manufacturer's recommendations is necessary to avoid instrument damage or cross contamination.

> Never accept responsibility for processing scopes or other medical equipment unless you have received proper, documented education for the task.

STERILITY QUALITY CONTROL MEASURES

Wide selections of mechanical, chemical, and biologic indicators are used externally and/or internally on packages subjected to a sterilization process. The purpose of the indicator is to alert the HCW that something went wrong during the sterilization process. Mechanical monitoring consists of watching pressure gauges and reviewing computer tape printouts. A review of a tape is only a first check, not a guarantee that anything was sterilized.

Chemical indicators, both external and internal, are convenient and inexpensive. They usually consist of a heat or chemical sensitive ink tape or strip that darkens or changes color if exposed to a sterilization process (Fig. 9.2).[34] External indicators do not guarantee that sterility has been achieved; they indicate only that the package was exposed to the process. Internal indicators are strategically placed inside a package at a site that is least likely to be penetrated (Fig. 9.3). Like external indicators, internal indicators do not guarantee that all microorganisms have been destroyed. Different types of external and internal chemical indicators are commercially available for the different specific sterilization processes.

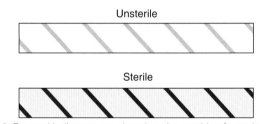

Fig. 9.2 External indicators are placed on the outside of a package to be sterilized. After exposure to the sterilization process, the tape darkens or changes color. An external indicator does not guarantee sterility; it indicates only that the package was exposed to the process. Different types of tape are used in different sterilization processes (e.g., gas, steam).

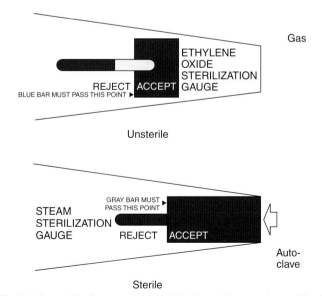

Fig. 9.3 Internal indicators are placed inside packages to be sterilized. They are placed in sites least likely to be reached by the sterilization process; internal indicators also do not guarantee sterility.

Biologic indicators are the only processes that directly monitor whether sterilization was achieved.[34] A biologic indicator consists of a specially prepared strip coated with very hard-to-kill bacterial spores and is enclosed in a small container placed inside a test package. After the test package has gone through the sterilization process with other packages, a microbiologist or another qualified expert examines the biologic indicator to determine whether all the microorganisms were killed. If not, all packages can be recalled by their processing number. Routine use of biologic indicators is required by external accrediting agencies, such as TJC.[34,50] These indicators are used daily in each sterilization unit cycle and after any repair on a particular unit. Biologic indicators, external and internal chemical indicators, and close attention to proper time and temperature combinations are all needed to ensure that products and equipment are safe for patient use.

In May 2014, TJC issued a safety report that said failure to reduce the risk of infections was one of the top five findings of noncompliance for hospitals, critical access hospitals, and ambulatory and office-based surgery facilities.[50] In fact, if they made an immediate threat-to-life discovery, the facility was immediately denied preliminary accreditation and had to take corrective action within 72 hours to eliminate the risk to patients, in addition to other actions.[50] Repercussions were bad publicity, loss of business, and a dent in reputation, even if promptly corrected. Lack of training, lack of knowledge, lack of leadership, and a lack of a culture of safety were their findings.[50] As standards change and technology advances, remember that keeping current is a responsibility for you and for whomever you work.

SUMMARY

- Standard precautions and transmission-based precautions should be used in all patient care procedures.
- The single most critical feature of avoiding disease transmission is continuous and meticulous hand hygiene.
- Radiation therapists should be well informed on sterilization and disinfection techniques that are used in their area and with the equipment/supplies that they use.
- The radiation therapist should be capable of cleaning up blood and body fluid spills safely and efficiently.
- The radiation therapist must handle and transport laundry in a manner that minimizes the transmission of pathogens.

- The radiation therapist is responsible to report unsafe work conditions to his or her supervisor or outside agencies if ever needed.
- The radiation therapist should be well informed and able to take appropriate action should he or she ever be involved in an accident, such as a needlestick or blood splash/spill event.
- The radiation therapist must wear personnel protective apparel as appropriate to the situation by properly assessing the situation and anticipating what might be needed.
- The radiation therapist will provide a clean treatment couch and treatment accessories to each and every patient on a daily basis.

REVIEW QUESTIONS

The answers to the Review Questions can be found by logging on to our website at: http://evolve.elsevier.com/Washington+Leaver/principles

1. Alcohol-based hand rubs are indicated for all of the following clinical situations except:
   a. When the hands are visibly soiled.
   b. Preoperative cleaning of hands by surgical personnel.
   c. Before inserting urinary catheters, intravascular catheters, or other invasive devices.
   d. After removing gloves.
2. What is the single most crucial way to prevent the spread of HAIs?
   a. Wearing gloves.
   b. Using universal precautions.
   c. Hand hygiene.
   d. Sterilization.
3. An inanimate object/vehicle involved in the transmission of disease is termed a _____.
   a. Vector.
   b. Fomite.
   c. Carrier.
   d. Host.
4. Standard precautions apply to all of the following except:
   a. Blood.
   b. Sweat.

   c. Nonintact skin.
   d. Bodily secretions.
5. The most reliable, available, and economical method of destroying microorganisms is:
   a. Heat.
   b. Gas.
   c. Radiation.
   d. Chemical liquids.
6. It is recommended to limit the use of lotions when using gloves.
   a. True.
   b. False.
7. It is permissible to place laundry contaminated with bodily fluid in the same laundry as noncontaminated laundry, as they are all sterilized in the washing process.
   a. True.
   b. False.
8. _____ is the gas that has been used for gas sterilization the longest.
9. _____ is a unique, infectious CNS agents composed of protein but lacking identifiable nucleic acid.
10. _____ helps provide job safety and health protection for employees by promoting safe and healthful working conditions throughout the nation.

QUESTIONS TO PONDER

1. Compare labels on various liquid chemicals used for infection control in the medical setting, and discuss what they can and cannot kill.

2. Discuss what actions should be taken when an HCW develops hypersensitivity to latex.
3. Role play "clean" hand and "dirty" hand techniques for one-person and two-person situations.

REFERENCES

1. Centers for Disease Control and Prevention. *Proceedings of the First International Conference on Nosocomial Infections.* Atlanta, GA: First International Conference on Nosocomial Infections; 1970:5–8.

2. Garner J, Simmons B. CDC Guidelines for isolation precautions in hospitals. *Infect Control.* 1983;(4):245–325.

3. Hospital Infection Control Practices Advisory Committee. Guideline for isolation precautions in hospitals. *Infect Control Hosp Epidemiol.* 1996;17:53–80.

4. Siegal JD, Rhinehart E, Jackson M, et al. *Guideline For Isolation Precautions: Preventing Transmission of Infectious Agents In Healthcare Settings. CDC Website*; 2007. https://www.cdc.gov/infectioncontrol/pdf/guidelines/isolation-guidelines.pdf. Accessed September 24, 2018.

5. Joshi SC, Diwan V, Joshi R, et al. How can the patients remain safe, if we are not safe and protected from the infections"? A qualitative exploration among health-care workers about challenges of maintaining hospital cleanliness in a resource limited tertiary setting in rural India. *Int J Environ Res Public Health.* 2018;15(9):E1942.

6. WHO guidelines on hand hygiene in health care: first global patient safety challenge, clean care is safer care 2009. World Health Organization website. http://apps.who.int/iris/bitstream/handle/10665/44102/9789241597906_eng.pdf;jsessionid=86D1700DC-46C44C808FCE973B8E1EBA4?sequence=1. Accessed September 26, 2018.

7. Kampf G, Kramer A. Epidemiologic background of hand hygiene and evaluation of the most important agents for scrubs and rubs. *Clin Microbiol Rev.* 2004;17:863–893.

8. Rotter ML, Koller W, Neumann R. The influence of cosmetic additives of the acceptability of alcohol based hand disinfectants. *J Hospital Infect.* 1991;18:57–63.

9. Bryan P, Hooton TM, Laufman GF. Guidelines for hospital environmental control. Section 1. Antiseptics, handwashing and handwashing facilities. In: CDC Prevention, ed. *Centers for Disease Control Hospital Infection Program: Guidelines for Prevention and Control of Nosocomial Infections.* Atlanta, GA: CDC; 1981.

10. Hedderwick SA, McNeil SA, Lyons MJ, Kauffman CA. Pathogenic organisms associated with artificial fingernails worn by healthcare workers. *Infect Control Hosp Epidemiol.* 2000;(8):505.

11. Salisbury D, Hutfilz P, Treen LM, et al. The effect of rings on microbial load of health-care worker's hands. *Am J Infec Control.* 1997;25:24–27.

12. Trick W, Vernon M, Hayes R, et al. Impact of ring wearing on hand contamination and comparison of hand hygiene agents in a hospital. *Clin Infect Dis.* 2003;36:1383–1390.

13. *Hand Hygiene In Healthcare Settings.* Centers for Disease Control and Prevention website; 2018. Updated. https://www.cdc.gov/handhygiene/campaign/index.html. Accessed September 24, 2018.

14. Garrett R. Bill makes hospital reveal infections. *Dallas Morning News.* March 21, 2007.

15. Chassin MR, Mayer C, Nether K. Improving hand hygiene at eight hospitals in the united states by targeting specific causes of noncompliance. *Jt Comm J Qual Patient Saf.* 2015;41:4–12.

16. McCormick RD, BUchman TL, Maki DG, et al. Double blind, randomized trial of scheduled use of a novel barrier cream and an oil-containing lotion for protecting the hands of health care workers. *Am J Infec Control.* 2000;28:302–310.

17. Centers for Disease Control and Prevention. Guidelines for hand hygiene in health-care settings. *MMWR.* 2002;51:29.

18. *Medical Glove Guidance Manual.* US Department of Health and Human Services, US Food and Drug Administration; 2008. Updated. https://www.fda.gov/downloads/MedicalDevices/DeviceRegulationandGuidance/GuidanceDocuments/UCM428191.pdf. Accessed September 25, 2018.

19. Korniewicz D, El-Masri M, Broyles J, Martin C, O'Connell K. Performance of latex and nonlatex medical examination gloves during simulated use. *Am J Infect Control.* 2002;30:133–138.

20. Occupational Safety and Health Administration. Occupational Exposure to Bloodborne Pathogens: Final Rule 29. CFR Part 1910:1030 Federal Register 1991;56:64003-64182. Revised 2001. In: Labor Do, ed. 2001:5317-5325.

21. Occupational Safety and Health Administration, US Department of Labor. Occupational Safety and Health Administration: Occupational Exposure to Bloodborne Pathogens, Final Rule 29 CFR Part 1910.1030. *Fed Reg.* 1991:64004–64182. https://www.osha.gov/pls/oshaweb/owadisp.show_document?p_id=10051&p_table=STANDARDS. Accessed November 13, 2018.

22. Respiratory fit testing. Occupational Safety and Health Administration website. https://www.osha.gov/video/respiratory_protection/fittesting.html. Accessed September 24, 2018.

23. Interim guidance for the use of masks to control seasonal influenza virus transmission. Centers for Disease Control and Prevention website. https://www.cdc.gov/flu/professionals/infectioncontrol/maskguidance.htm. Accessed September 27, 2018.

24. Emergency preparedness & response. Centers for Disease Control and Prevention website. https://emergency.cdc.gov/. Accessed September 26, 2018.

25. Guidance on personal protective equipment (PPE) to be used by health-care workers during management of patients with confirmed Ebola or persons under investigation (PUIs) for Ebola who are clinically unstable or have bleeding, vomiting, or diarrhea in U.S. hospitals, including procedures for donning and doffing PPE. Centers for Disease Control and Prevention website. https://www.cdc.gov/vhf/ebola/healthcare-us/ppe/guidance.html. Accessed September 27, 2018.

26. Laundry labeling requirements. Occupational Safety and Health Administration website. https://www.osha.gov/SLTC/etools/hospital/laundry/label.html. Accessed September 24, 2018.

27. Environmental infection control guidelines: laundry and bedding. Centers for Disease Control and Prevention website. https://www.cdc.gov/infectioncontrol/guidelines/environmental/#g. Accessed September 27, 2018.

28. Occupational Safety and Health Administration. Occupational Safety and Health Administration. Title 29, CFR, Part 1903.2. https://www.osha.gov/laws-regs/regulations/standardnumber/1903/1903.2. Accessed November 13, 2018.

29. Occupational Safety and Health Administration. Occupational Safety and Health Administration. Title 29, CFR, Part 1977.12. In: Labor Do, ed. Washington DC: Department of Labor, Occupational Safety and Health Administration; 1989.

30. Standards. Joint Commission website. http://www.jointcommission.org/accreditation/ambulatory_healthcare.aspx. Accessed September 24, 2018.

31. Accreditation guide for hospitals. Joint Commission website. https://www.jointcommission.org/assets/1/18/171110_Accreditation_Guide_Hospitals_FINAL.pdf. Accessed November 13, 2018.

32. American National Standard. Comprehensive guide to steam sterilization and sterility assurance in health care facilities, Amendment 3. In: Instrumentation AftAoM, ed. ANSI/AAMI ST79:2010/A3:20122012.

33. Rutala W. APIC guideline for selection and use of disinfectants. *Am J Infect Control.* 1996;24:313–342.

34. Rutala W, Weber J. Guideline for disinfection and sterilization in healthcare facilities. CDC website. https://www.cdc.gov/infectioncontrol/pdf/guidelines/disinfection-guidelines.pdf. Accessed September 24, 2018.

35. Block S. *Disinfections, Sterilization, and Preservation.* 5th ed. Philadelphia, PA: Lippincott Williams & Wilkins; 2000.

36. Hoeprich P, Jordan M, Infectious Diseases. *A Modern Treatise on Infectious Processes.* Philadelphia, PA: JP Lippincott; 1989.

37. Gardner J, Peel M. *Introduction to Sterilization, Disinfection and Infection Control.* 2nd ed. New York, NY: Churchill Livingstone; 1991.

38. Webster Webster. *'s New World Medical Dictionary.* Ames, IA: John Wiley & Sons; 2001.

39. Rutala W, Weber J. Guideline for disinfection and sterilization of prion-contaminated medical instruments. *Infect Control Hosp Epidemiol.* 2010;31(2):107–117.

40. Washington Post. Mad cow disease: engineered cattle avoid infection. Starr Telegram 2007.

41. CJD (Creutzfeldt-Jacob Disease), Classic. Centers for Disease Control and Prevention website. https://www.cdc.gov/prions/cjd/about.html. Accessed September 26, 2018.

42. Bartholomew A. Mixed up over mad cow: how worried should you really be? Two experts sit down to hash it out. *Reader's Digest.* 2001:104–109.

43. Ethylene oxide (ETO): hospitals and healthcare facilities must use a single chamber when sterilizing medical equipment with ETO. Environmental Protection Agency website. https://archive.epa.gov/pesticides/reregistration/web/html/ethylene_oxide_fs.html. Accessed September 27, 2018.

44. Fichtenbaum C, Gerber J. Interactions between antiretroviral drugs and drugs used for the therapy of the metabolic complications encountered during HIV infection. *Clin Pharmacokinet.* 2002;41:1195–1211.

45. Alfa M, DeGagne P, Olsen N, et al. Comparison of ion plasma, vaporized hydrogen peroxide and 100% ethylene oxide sterilizers to the 12/88 ethylene oxide gas sterilizer. *Infect Control Hosp Epidemiol.* 1996;17:92–99.

46. Kollmorgen G, Bedford J. Cellular radiation biology. In: Dalrymple G, ed. *Medical Radiation Biology.* Philadelphia, PA: WB Saunders; 1973.

47. Guideline for hand hygiene in health-care settings. Centers for Disease Control and Prevention website. https://www.cdc.gov/mmwr/PDF/rr/rr5116.pdf. Accessed November 13, 2018.

48. Rhame F. The inanimate environment. In: Bennett J, Brachman P, eds. *Hospital Infections.* 6th ed. Philadelphia, PA: Lippincott Williams & Wilkins; 2014.

49. Kubiatowicz D. *Important Safety Information (Business Letter Communication).* St. Paul, MN: 3M Health Care; 1990.

50. A growing patient safety concern: improperly sterilized or high-level disinfected equipment. The Joint Commission website. http://www.jointcommission.org/on_infection_prevention_control/growing_patient_safety_concern_improperly_sterilized_hld_equipment/. Accessed September 24, 2018.

10

Infection Control: Health and Safety

Zachary D. Smith, Charles M. Washington, Megan Trad

OBJECTIVES

- Define terms associated with epidemiology and infection control.
- Identify regulating agencies that provide oversight over public health safety.
- Describe the five transition routes in the spread of infection.
- Distinguish between specific and nonspecific defense mechanisms.
- Identify mandatory vaccinations all healthcare workers must obtain.

OUTLINE

KEY TERMS

Antibody

Antigen

Carrier

Colonization

Convalescence

Droplet nuclei

Epidemiology

Fomite

Immune serum globulin

Incubation

Mantoux tuberculin skin test

Nosocomial

Pandemic

Skin squames

Titers

Vector

Virulence

HEALTH AND SAFETY

The concept of trying to control infectious disease in medical settings has a relatively long history and is associated with famous names such as Florence Nightingale and Joseph Lister. The focus remains the same today; that is, healthcare workers (HCWs) promote the surveillance, control, and prevention of infectious disease. This chapter emphasizes measures taken to protect the HCW, the patient, and the public. Regulatory agencies and legal aspects of infection control are also briefly discussed.

DEFINITIONS

Infection involves the reproduction of microorganisms in the human body. *Disease* is the collective term used to describe related clinical signs and symptoms associated with an infectious agent or unknown etiology. A person who becomes infected typically develops specific clinical signs and symptoms that can be detected externally, and the body initiates an immune response internally. If a person develops an infection but has no clinically observable signs or symptoms, the infection is referred to as a *subclinical infection*. Note that a subclinical infection does initiate an immune response within the body. Another type of infection, which does not provoke an immune response, is known as colonization. *Colonization* involves the reproduction of an infectious microorganism, but there is no interaction between the body and the microorganism that would result in a detectable immune response. The microorganism is simply present in or on the body, and it is multiplying. A person who is colonized but not ill is known as a *carrier*. Carriers may be a source of infection on a short-term or even permanent basis.

The relevance of these sources of infection is that disease is disseminated not only by people who are obviously ill but also by those with subclinical infections and by those who are carriers. *Contamination* is defined as the presence of microorganisms on the body (commonly on hands) or on inanimate objects. It is the movement of people from one environment to another that spreads disease, either directly from the infected person or indirectly through the things that they come into contact with. By understanding the factors associated with the development of disease and its dissemination, control and prevention measures can be initiated.

Workers in the healthcare environment are especially interested in healthcare-associated infections (HAIs), also known as nosocomial infections, in the hospital setting. The term *nosocomial* was traditionally used to describe infections that developed in the hospital or to describe infections that were acquired in the hospital but did not develop until after discharge. Today, "hospital" is too restrictive and has been expanded to include outpatient care settings and other healthcare settings. HAIs may be acquired not only by patients but also by HCWs and visitors. Infections caught before a hospital admission but in which symptoms do not become apparent until after admission are not HAIs; they are community related rather than hospital related. The primary goal of the epidemiology department is to decrease all preventable HAIs. The hospital epidemiology team continuously monitors the number of infections that occur and investigates any abnormal occurrence or frequency to determine whether some action could have been taken to prevent the infection. In smaller facilities that do not have a full-time epidemiologist or team, a designated infectious disease manager (typically a registered nurse) or an outside consultant with appropriate expertise can perform some of the basic functions needed to keep the number of HAIs down.

REGULATORY AGENCIES AND PUBLIC OVERSIGHT

The Centers for Disease Control and Prevention (CDC), a federal government agency located in Atlanta, Georgia, has been actively involved in helping hospital infection control personnel investigate epidemics since the mid-1950s. Over time, this nationwide cooperative approach of hospitals and the CDC has led to the formulation of very useful standards and guidelines, changes in federal and state laws, and many studies to monitor effectiveness of infection control measures.

The CDC surveillance system for HAIs is known as the National Health Care Safety Network.[1] This agency has provided information on incidence rates of common infections for several decades.[1] Because most hospitals limit their reports to device-associated infections, selected surgical-site infections, and infections because of *Clostridium difficile* and methicillin-resistant *Staphylococcus aureus*, an accurate estimate of all types of HAIs occurring in the United States was unknown.[1]

The CDC addressed this information void by instituting a three-phase effort to develop and conduct a multistate prevalence survey of HAIs and the use of antimicrobial agents. The study began in a single city in 2009 and culminated in 2011 in a large-scale survey that estimated the prevalence of HAIs in acute care hospitals, determined the distribution of these infections according to infection site and pathogen, and generated updated estimates of the national burden of these infections.[1]

The survey method was unique in that it used trained hospital personnel to conduct a 1-day survey of randomly selected patients of all ages in small, medium, and large hospitals across the United States. The demographic and limited clinical data collected was later reviewed by CDC trained data collectors to identify HAIs active at the time of the survey. These snapshot surveys published in the *New England Journal of Medicine* showed that 4.0% of inpatients in US acute care hospitals had at least one HAI.[1,2] This equates to 1 in every 25 inpatients or about 75,000 patients with HAIs who died during their hospitalization.[1,2]

Comparisons with earlier studies have proven to be difficult or impossible because of the differences in patient populations, surveillance definitions of what constitutes an HAI, and data-collection and analytical methods.[1] The top 10 types of infection and the top 10 pathogens causing HAIs found in the CDC three-phase study are shown in Table 10.1.

The billions-of-dollar savings, which are gained by decreasing the number of HAIs, are obvious to patients, Medicare and insurance companies, hospitals, and taxpayers, and those savings are desired by

TABLE 10.1 Distribution of Top Ten Infection Types and Top Ten Pathogens Found in Healthcare-Associated Infections

Type of Infection	Rank	Pathogen	Rank
Pneumonia	1 (tie)	*Clostridium difficile*	1
Surgical-site infection	1 (tie)	*Staphylococcus aureus*	2
Gastrointestinal infection	3	*Klebsiella pneumoniae* or *Klebsiella. oxytoca*	3
Urinary tract infection	4	*Escherichia coli*	4
Primary bloodstream infection	5	*Enterococcus* species	5
Eye, ear, nose, throat, or mouth infection	6	*Pseudomonas aeruginosa*	6
Lower respiratory tract infection	7	*Candida* species	7
Skin and soft-tissue infection	8	*Streptococcus* species	8
Cardiovascular system infection	9	Coagulase-negative *Staphylococcus* species	9
Bone and joint infection	10	*Enterobacter* species	10

Modified from Magill S, Edwards J, Bamberg, W, et al. Multistate point prevalence survey of health care-associated infections. *N Eng J Med.* 2014;370:1198–1208.

all.[3,4] As consumer advocate groups speak out across the country, more external monitoring is taking place. Most states have passed laws that require hospitals to disclose how often their patients get infections, and Medicare requires that hospitals report their infection rates or face a financial penalty.[5] Public access is already providing a strong incentive for institutions to work harder to lower their HAI rate, and they are aware that HAIs are primarily caused by problems in patient care practices, such as handwashing.[6,7] As a result of financial incentives, penalties, and growing consumer awareness, healthcare systems are making great strides in providing safe, efficient, and cost-effective care.

Over the past several decades, the United States has witnessed a significant shift in healthcare delivery from the acute, inpatient hospital setting to a variety of outpatient (ambulatory care) settings. Ambulatory care is provided in hospital-based outpatient clinics, nonhospital-based clinics and surgical centers, oncology centers, and many other specialized settings. Each year, more than 1 million cancer patients receive outpatient chemotherapy, radiation therapy, or both.[8] Despite advances in surgical techniques, therapeutic medications, and radiation delivery methods, infections remain a major cause of morbidity and mortality, due mostly to treatment-related immunosuppression but also to frequent contact with HCWs and others in healthcare settings. The reality is that although treatment tools and techniques have improved, it is only when everyone caring for patients acknowledge their individual responsibility to decrease HAIs that consistent and enduring gains will be achieved.

The CDC and the Healthcare Infection Control Practices Advisory Committee (HICPAC) have released an updated version of their *Guide to Infection Prevention for Outpatient Settings: Minimum Expectations for Safe Care*.[9] This guide expands upon the information provided in the previous edition to help make infection prevention a priority away from the hospital setting.[9] The CDC and the HICPAC have recognized that ambulatory care settings typically lack both the resources and infrastructure to pursue and support infection prevention and surveillance as compared with hospitals. This evidence-based guide reflects current practices based on standard precautions and minimum infection prevention expectations for safe care. Reducing the number of HAIs is a win-win situation for all parties involved and starts with every HCW's actions.

INFECTION CYCLE AND DISEASE PHASES

Infectious disease cannot occur without the presence of an infectious agent, or *pathogen,* which is any of a wide range of small, primitive life forms. Pathogens may exist as bacteria, viruses, fungi, protozoa, algae, or lesser known agents such as Chlamydiae, Rickettsiae, and prions (Fig. 10.1).[10] Of these, bacteria and viruses are most often the sources of nosocomial infections, with fungi next, and rarely protozoa or the other forms.[11] The following terms are associated with a disease and the infectious agent.

Pathogenicity describes the ability of an infectious agent to cause clinical disease. In other words, some agents readily cause clinical disease, whereas others may be present but not cause clinical disease. The term *virulence* describes the severity of a clinical disease and is typically expressed in terms of morbidity and mortality. *Dose* refers to the number of microorganisms; thus, an *infective dose* is one in which enough microorganisms are present to elicit an infection. Microorganisms are also selective as to their host or the location at which they cause disease. The infectious agent may cause disease in animals but not in humans, vice versa, or in both. This selectivity is known as *host specificity.*

To remain viable, all microorganisms require a source and a reservoir; these may be the same or different. The *reservoir* is where the microorganism lives and reproduces. For example, the polio viral

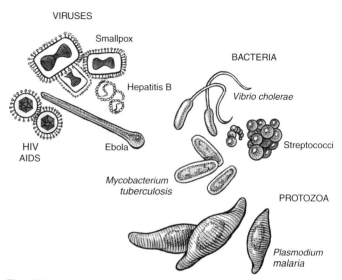

Fig. 10.1 Microorganisms that cause disease come in a wide variety of shapes and sizes.

reservoir is human, never animal, whereas the rabies viral reservoir can be human or animal. The place from which the microorganism comes is known as the *source*. From the source it moves to the host; this transfer from the source to the host may be direct or indirect.

In the case of the common cold transmitted through a sneeze, the reservoir and source are the same. An example in which the reservoir and source are not the same is histoplasmosis, which is a fungal infection. In this situation, a chicken can serve as the reservoir. The chicken's fecal droppings are deposited on soil and serve as the source. After drying, the wind carries the remains of the fecal droppings to a location where a human inhales them. Another example is hepatitis A virus (HAV); in this case, the reservoir is often a person who handles food. The food handled by the person serves as the source of the infection.

A *host* is the person to whom the infectious agent is passed. Whether the host develops clinical disease depends on the body location at which the infectious agent is deposited, and on the host's immune status and related defense mechanisms. If disease develops in the susceptible host, the host goes through three disease phases:
1. incubation
2. clinical disease
3. convalescence

Incubation is the time interval between exposure and the appearance of the first symptom. The *clinical disease stage* is the time interval in which a person exhibits clinical signs and symptoms. *Convalescence* is the stage of recovery from the illness. Depending on the specific disease, a person may be infectious to others during any or a combination of the three disease phases.

In some diseases, such as hepatitis from hepatitis B virus (HBV), in which a chronic carrier state exists, a person who is apparently well can still disseminate disease. For disease to be passed to others, a *portal of exit* is necessary. Examples include the respiratory tract, gastrointestinal tract, blood, and skin.

After an exit portal is reached, transmission can take place. *Transmission* is defined as the movement of the infectious agent from the source to the host. To cause disease, the infectious agent must gain entrance to the body. The *entrance portal* can be through normal skin such as with *Leptospira* (one form is known as Fort Bragg fever because of the number of military personnel who developed it) or through broken skin such as with a needle-stick in the transmission of human immunodeficiency virus (HIV).[11] Agents also gain access through the respiratory system, gastrointestinal tract, urinary tract,

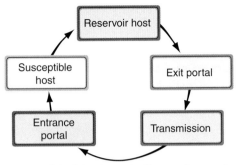

Fig. 10.2 Diagram of the infection cycle. To stop disease, the cycle can be broken at any point.

BOX 10.1 **Transmission Routes**

1. Contact
   Direct
   Indirect
2. Droplet (large)
3. Common vehicle (fomite)
4. Airborne
   Droplet nuclei
   Dust particles
   Skin squames
5. Vector borne

---

or transplantation. Transmission of an infectious agent through these entry portals is also often associated with medications or equipment such as scopes or catheters. The complete cycle of infection is shown in Fig. 10.2.

TRANSMISSION ROUTES

Transmission routes vary from one disease to another. Five transmission routes are identified: *contact, droplet, common vehicle, airborne,* and *vector borne.* Box 10.1 displays an outline of transmission routes. A specific disease may use one or more transmission modes.

Contact spread can be *direct* or *indirect.* Contact transmission is the most frequent and most important transmission route for the spread of HAIs. In *direct contact* transmission, the susceptible host makes physical contact with the source of infection, either an infected or a colonized person. Person-to-person spread can occur through simple touching such as helping a patient out of a wheelchair and onto the treatment couch. Mononucleosis, transmitted through kissing, and acquired immunodeficiency syndrome (AIDS), which is spread through sexual intercourse, also are examples of direct contact transmission. *Indirect contact* transmission involves an intervening object that is contaminated from contact with an infectious agent and then comes into contact with another individual which results in a single infective episode. An example is a needlestick to an HCW after the needle has been used in a patient infected with HIV.

Transmission by *droplet contact* involves the rapid transfer of the infectious agent through the air over short distances, such as in talking, coughing, or sneezing close to someone's face. The droplets consist of large, relatively heavy particles (larger than 5 μm) and thus are spread over short distances, typically 3 feet or less, and are deposited on the host's nasal mucosa, oral mucosa, and conjunctivae of the eye.[12] Some controversy exists over the distance infectious droplets can travel, with some experts suggesting up to 10 feet in the example of a powerful, uncovered sneeze or cough. Rubella (also known as German measles or 3-day measles), colds, and influenza are commonly transmitted in this fashion. Suctioning of a patient with a head and neck cancer is another example of how large droplets can be created. Droplet contact involves large moist droplets, and because of their weight, they do not linger in the air for long periods of time. Because of this, special air handling systems and ventilation cannot prevent droplet transmission. Droplet contact transmission should not be confused with airborne transmission. Airborne transmission is an entirely different transmission route and will be discussed later in this chapter.

Another route of transmission is *common vehicle spread.* This type of transmission involves a contaminated inanimate vehicle, known as a *fomite,* for transmission of the infectious agent to multiple persons. The number of people infected distinguishes this type of transmission from indirect contact, which involves the spread of infection to only one person.

In common vehicle spread, all the people are infected from a common fomite. Fomites include food, water, medications, medical equipment, and medical supplies. An example of historic significance is blood that was contaminated with HIV or HBV that was administered to many people before technology was developed to screen for the presence of these viruses.

Airborne transmission is spread that involves an infectious agent using the air as its means of dissemination and involves a long distance, which is typically described as 6 feet or greater, or even up to miles away. These airborne pathogens are either the remains of droplets (5 μm or smaller) that have evaporated (droplet nuclei) or the infectious agent is contained in sloughed *skin squames* (routinely shed superficial skin cells) or dust particles. In one study, skin squames were found to be the cause of several outbreaks of streptococcal wound infections and were eventually traced to hospital staff personnel.[11] These infectious microorganisms may also remain in the air for hours or even days, and may become inhaled by or deposited on a susceptible host within the same room or even miles away.[11]

Dust particles containing the infectious agent are another means of airborne transmission. One example is *Histoplasma capsulatum,* the infectious fungal agent of the disease histoplasmosis. This fungal agent grows as a mold in soil containing bird droppings, such as in a chicken coop or pigeon roost. On a windy day, the dust containing the spores of this infectious fungal agent can be carried for miles to a susceptible host.[13]

Special air handling and ventilation are required to prevent airborne transmission when infectious droplet nuclei are involved. A susceptible host can catch rubeola (measles) and varicella viruses (chickenpox and shingles) just by being in the same room with an infected person. For these two infectious viral diseases, immune HCWs can safely care for infected patients; however, if susceptible HCWs must enter the room, they should wear respiratory protection. Tuberculosis (TB) is another illness transmitted via droplet nuclei. TB has spread in hospitals because of air recirculation and low airflow rate.[14] All HCWs need to wear respiratory protection in the presence of a known or suspected infectious pulmonary TB patient.[15,16]

> Droplet contact and airborne transmission are differentiated from one another by particle size and by distance.

Vector-borne transmission involves a *vector* that transports an infectious agent to a host. An example of a vector would be a fly that transports an infectious agent on its body or legs or an *Anopheles* mosquito that carries malaria.[17] The malaria would enter the bloodstream of the human victim bitten by the mosquito. Because mosquitoes, flies, rats, and other vermin are not commonly found in US healthcare facilities, vector-borne transmission is not nearly as common as it is in other parts of the world.

DEFENSE MECHANISMS

Nonspecific Defense Mechanisms

To establish an infection, the pathogen must successfully bypass the host's defense mechanisms. The human body comes equipped with a wide variety of nonspecific defense mechanisms. For example, skin serves as a mechanical barrier and contains secretions that have antibacterial qualities. The upper respiratory system is full of cilia that facilitate the removal of pathogens. If the cilia are not successful, mucus aids in catching and removing pathogens. The respiratory system also protects against invasion through its secretions and defensive white cells that engulf and destroy pathogens. The gastrointestinal and urinary tracts are acidic and thus serve as a hostile environment to possible invaders. Even tears exhibit antibacterial activity and aid in the removal of pathogens.

Other nonspecific defense mechanisms include local inflammatory action and genetic, hormonal, and nutritional factors. Personal hygiene and behavioral habits influence the likelihood of developing disease. The age of a person also plays a role, with the extremely young and extremely old being most at risk. Alterations of any nonspecific defense mechanism through a skin break, surgery, chronic disease such as diabetes or immune deficiency disorders, standard medications, chemotherapy, and radiation all influence the host's susceptibility by lowering resistance to infectious disease processes.

Specific Defense Mechanisms

Immunity plays a critical role in reducing host susceptibility. Immunity exists in two forms: natural and artificial. Box 10.2 displays an outline of the different types of immunity. *Natural immunity* develops as a result of having acquired a specific disease. For example, children who have had rubella will never have it again. This is a general rule for most acute viral infections, and such immunity usually persists for the lifetime of the host. Natural immunity can also develop after subclinical disease in which no readily apparent disease is observed. Unfortunately, not all pathogens initiate lifelong immunity; herpes simplex virus (cold sore) is a good example. After a herpes attack, the virus lies dormant until an event triggers another outbreak.

Artificial immunity can be further subdivided into active and passive immunity. Vaccines come in several forms: killed, toxoid, and attenuated live vaccines. *Active immunization* consists of vaccination with the altered pathogen or its products. The vaccine serves as the *antigen* (foreign substance) and thereby triggers the human body's immune system to create *antibodies*. Antibodies are specific; they work against only a specific antigen. T and B lymphocytes are the key white cells in the body's immune system.

The immune response requires careful study, and its complexity is beyond the scope of this chapter; however, it is well established that the B lymphocyte transforms itself into a plasma cell. Simply put, this cell is a highly active factory that synthesizes its own genetically unique type of antibody and sets it free into the body's fluids. The antibody then seeks the specific invading antigen. With some vaccines such as tetanus, a booster is necessary after a period of time because the number of antibodies (*titers*) drops to a level insufficient to provide adequate protection.

Historically, the earliest vaccine was developed to combat smallpox in 1796 by an English country doctor named Edward Jenner.[18] Smallpox has since been eliminated from the world and exists only in such places as the CDC Level 4 research laboratories.[19] In 1981, a vaccine against HBV was released for use and began to be offered by law to all at-risk HCWs.[20] Currently, immunologists have worked for more than three decades trying to develop an effective vaccine against HIV to curtail the worldwide AIDS pandemic.

Before 1963 when almost all US children started receiving the measles, mumps, and rubella vaccines, an estimated 4 million cases, with 48,000 hospitalizations and 500 deaths, were reported annually.[21] For various reasons, there is a rising rate in some areas of the United States of intentional undervaccination. If this trend is not reversed, then the goal of complete elimination of preventable disease in the United States will not be achieved or maintained in many cases.

Passive immunity, another form of artificial immunity, is defined as the transfer of protective antibodies from one host to a susceptible host. Examples include the administration of *immune serum globulin* (e.g., a serum-containing antibody) for the prophylaxis of measles, tetanus, and infectious HAV. The transfer of maternal antibodies to the fetus through the placenta is another form of passive immunity. Other substances available for passive immunization include antiserum against rabies administered after animal bites and antibiotics in known contacts of cases of TB, gonorrhea, and syphilis. Although it protects the individual from the disease in most cases or lessens disease severity, passive immunization does not protect against future infection, nor does it prevent spread to others. Passive immunization typically has a short duration, usually several months at most, and thus, active immunization is preferable whenever possible, such as in tetanus vaccination.[11]

Environmental Factors Contributing to Healthcare-Acquired Infections

Environmental factors such as airflow, temperature, and humidity also influence links in the cycle of infection because they directly affect the pathogen and host. For example, measures directed at minimizing the risk of TB transmission within a hospital include the appropriate adjustment of airflow in designated rooms so that in any high-risk area, negative-pressure airflow occurs within the room. With the recent increase of classic TB, AIDS-related TB, and antibiotic-resistant strains of TB, the CDC has modified its guidelines. Hospitals are taking far greater protective measures to reduce the transmission of TB in the hospital environment.[22]

Many other environmental factors contribute to HAIs. A person may enjoy the comfort and beauty of carpet in a radiation oncology department, but carpeting greatly increases the microbial level when compared with linoleum-like surfaces.[23,24] Carpets also act as sponges for *C. difficile* spores, which is one of the main reasons carpets have been torn out of healthcare facilities across the United States.

Upholstered furniture should receive the same consideration as carpet. If it becomes soiled by body fluids, it should be discarded. Nonupholstered furniture should be routinely cleaned with an appropriate agent as per manufacturer's guidelines. Fresh or dried flowers, aquariums, and potted plants may enhance the beauty of surroundings, but they harbor a multitude of microorganisms such as spores and bacteria. For this reason, flowers, potted plants, and even fruit are often banned as a possible risk from high-risk areas such as bone marrow transplant wards and intensive care units.[25] Following this philosophy, flowers and fruit should be banned from any area in which immunosuppression is a concern.

BOX 10.2 Forms of Immunity

1. Natural immunity: active disease
2. Artificial immunity
   - Active immunity: vaccine
   - Passive immunity
     i. Maternal antibodies
     ii. Antibody transferred to susceptible host

Freshly laundered linen should be stored in a clean, closed closet, or cabinet or a cart that remains covered. HCWs should use caution in handling used linen or paper by making sure it is not vigorously shaken and never handling it without gloves if it is contaminated with blood or other body fluids. Soiled linen should be placed in impervious Occupational Safety and Health Administration (OSHA)–approved bags. Bags should not be filled to capacity. A second bag is to be added if there is visible leakage. Fresh linen or paper should always be used for each patient.

Items routinely used for procedures performed in a radiation oncology department should also be considered as possible infection control hazards. For instance, custom-made bite blocks should be disinfected between each use on a single patient and then dried and stored in a clean, closed container.[26] Treatment tables and slide boards for transferring patients should be cleaned between each patient.

Tattooing or placing permanent ink dots to identify treatment portal or laser alignment is a routine patient care procedure that presents risk to the radiation therapist as well as to the patient. Sterile ink vials used for more than one patient follows the same CDC guideline used for other multidose vial injectables or infusion medications: they are to be kept in areas not accessible to patients; be labeled by the manufacturer as being multidose, which typically implies they contain an antimicrobial preservative (i.e., prevents bacterial growth); are labeled with an expiration date; and are sterile. If a multidose ink vial ever enters the immediate patient treatment area (i.e., simulator table area), it can only be used once and then is to be discarded.[27] Each patient must be tattooed with a fresh syringe and needle. After being used, the needle should never be reintroduced to the ink container to avoid contaminating its sterile contents. Likewise, drawing ink into a syringe and then changing needles between the tattooing of different patients is a dangerous and unacceptable technique. A major infection hazard associated with traditional tattooing supplies was the nonsterile ink reservoir. A welcome advance over traditional methods was a tattooing device designed by a radiation therapist and marketed as SteriTatt.[28] This device incorporates sterile, nontoxic ink that is contained in a sterile ink-dispensing pouch that looks somewhat like a mixture of an eyedropper and a syringe. This device is designed for single-patient use and thus is an ideal tool for tattooing from an infection control perspective.[28,29]

> A sterile technique must be used in applying tattoos for patient alignment. Never recap a needle. The used needle should be discarded in a sharps container located in the room where used.

Ideally, bolus sheets should not be used on multiple patients. However, if bolus is to be reused, it must be wrapped in flexible plastic wrap to prevent the bolus material from being contaminated during use and then immediately and thoroughly disinfected before rewrapping for use on a subsequent patient. Pens or markers used in radiation oncology departments for drawing in a treatment port or alignment marks should also not be shared between patients The tip of the pen can become contaminated by harmful microorganisms. If the pen is then used on another patient, the contaminate can easily be spread. Radiation therapy centers have solved this problem by issuing each patient a marker and placing it in a plastic, sealable bag labeled with the patient's name.

> A pen used to apply marks on a patient's skin should never be used on multiple patients.

The use of low-temperature thermoplastics for immobilization has become a daily routine for most radiation therapists all over the world.[30] A rigid sheet of thermoplastic material can be heated until it becomes pliable enough to mold over the patient's body surface. The heating of the thermoplastic material can be accomplished in a traditional water bath or in a dry-heat oven. The use of a water bath requires the water to be heated from 145°F to 165°F. Higher temperatures will cause the thermoplastic material to become too loose and risks exposing the patient and the therapist to possible burn injury. To prevent infection, water baths must also be drained and cleaned on a regular basis according to the manufacturer's guidelines. If water baths are used, once contact has been made with the patient's skin, the thermoplastic material should never be placed back in the water reservoir because cross contamination would occur. Although reforming of the thermoplast is possible, to do so in the water reservoir is inappropriate. If reforming is necessary, it may be possible to use a separate disposable plastic container to hold the hot water for that specific patient. Some centers have also employed the use of hair dryers to reform the thermoplast when necessary, but care should be used, as this also carries burning risk for the patient.

DRUG USE AND DRUG-RESISTANT MICROORGANISMS

Antibiotics have been in use for more than 60 years and have served as the main weapon in the medical world's arsenal against disease. However, as time has passed, the efficacy of antibiotics has diminished, and attempts to reduce their inappropriate use have increased.

By changing their genetic makeup, microorganisms can resist the effects of medications. Mutations arise much faster in microorganisms than in humans because the time it takes for a new generation to be created may be a matter of minutes compared with decades in humans. If mutations develop in their relatively short evolutionary processes that are beneficial in the struggle to survive against medications, the mutants are better suited to live and reproduce. It is also possible in some circumstances for bacteria to acquire protective genes from other microorganisms[31,32] (Fig. 10.3).

Efforts are also being made to curb the use of antibiotics in the farming industry to reduce the prevalence of antibiotic-resistant bacteria in meats and poultry. Patients have also unwittingly helped in the development of drug-resistant microorganisms by not finishing prescribed medications and by demanding and receiving inappropriate antibiotics for illnesses. The tougher, remaining pathogens endure as the most fit to survive. Vaccines, like antibiotics, are challenged by mutating pathogens. This has been part of the problem in developing a successful vaccine for the continuously evolving flu and HIV viruses.

> Do not stop a prescribed antibiotic early, even if you feel much better. Doing so helps create antibiotic-resistant microorganisms.

HEALTHCARE FACILITY EPIDEMIOLOGY

The Hospital Infections Branch of the CDC was established to help hospitals minimize nosocomial infections. Today's hospitals are required to establish an epidemiology division if they wish to be accredited by and meet Joint Commission (JC) standards.[33] Even in non-JC-accredited facilities, state health department or public health codes must be met for licensure, and requirements typically include some form of epidemiologic oversight.

State laws also govern the reporting of specific infectious diseases and the disposal of medical waste. In the past three decades, the

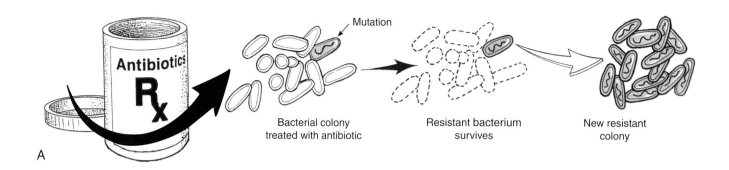

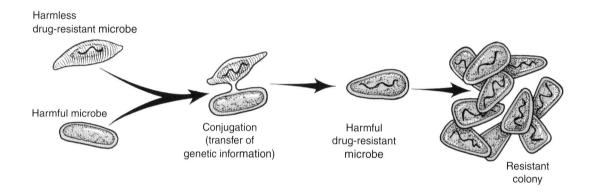

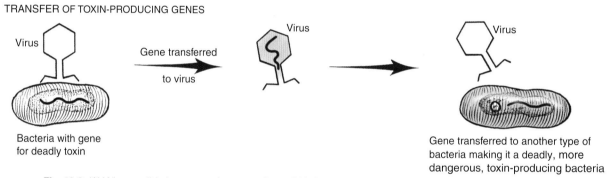

Fig. 10.3 (A) When antibiotics are used to treat a bacterial infection, most bacteria will die. However, mutated bacteria may survive and go on to produce more drug-resistant clones. (B) The transfer of a drug-resistant gene from a harmless microbe to a harmful microbe through the conjugation process. (C) A virus can carry a harmful trait to other types of bacteria, making them dangerous.

federal government OSHA has focused its attention on healthcare facilities and the HCW. In fact, OSHA mandates that employers of HCWs must offer the HBV vaccine.[34,35] Although the federal mandate only applies to paid employees, students who are not paid must meet admission criteria of their radiation therapy program, and this will include vaccinations deemed necessary to protect both them and patients. State or local laws may also stipulate what vaccination criteria a student must meet.

PERSONNEL AND STUDENT HEALTH SERVICES AND PERTINENT INFECTIOUS DISEASES

Employee or student health clinics associated with healthcare facilities have a vested interest in each individual's health because if they develop an infectious disease, they present a risk not only to themselves but also to patients, coworkers, friends, and family members. Because of

the nature of their chosen profession, HCWs have frequent and prolonged direct contact with patients who harbor a multitude of infectious pathogens and thus are at increased risk. Healthcare facilities and HCWs have a shared responsibility to optimize prevention and control programs. This responsibility includes the essential participation in a vaccination program.

Health and vaccination history of the HCW should always be reviewed before the first patient contact is made. Records should reflect whether the person has documented evidence of having the disease: documented vaccination history or serology results.[36] Records of any adverse effect after vaccination should also be documented (i.e., egg allergy for older vaccines), vaccine manufacturer and lot number, and the title of the person administering the vaccine.[36] Good records during outbreaks help in identifying HCWs who may be at risk and reduce costs and breakdown in patient care services related to absenteeism. Employees and students should also keep a permanent copy of all vaccinations for future jobs as evidence so they do not have to repeat vaccines without cause. Recommendations for HCW vaccines are broken into two categories by the CDC: (1) those routinely needed by HCWs, and (2) those needed in special circumstances.[36] A listing of recommended vaccines for HCWs is shown in Box 10.3 and described below.

Hepatitis B Virus

HBV infection is a highly infectious occupational hazard of HCWs. Transmission occurs through contact with blood and body fluids by percutaneous (i.e., skin breaks) or direct mucous membrane contact.[36] Evidence has shown that this potentially deadly virus can live on surfaces at room temperature for 7 days.[20] Vaccines to prevent HBV became available in 1981. In 1987, the CDC recommended that HCWs be vaccinated. OSHA mandated that the HBV vaccine be made available to all at-risk HCWs on December 6, 1991.[35] Workers should understand that the HBV vaccine protects against only hepatitis B, not hepatitis C, hepatitis D, hepatitis E, and so on, for which no vaccine is available at this time.[37,38] A vaccine is available for hepatitis A, a disease typically spread by fecal matter remaining on the unwashed hands of the infected individual that is commonly associated with food and drink sources. Although it is not a required HCW vaccine, it is recommended for traveling outside the United States.

BOX 10.3 Recommended Vaccines for Health Care Workers and Radiation Therapy Students Before Patient Care

Hepatitis B (HBV)

- Recombinant vaccine; three-dose series (dose #1 initial, #2 in 1 month, #3 at 5 months after dose #2). Considered protected if serologic testing shows hepatitis B (HB) surface antibody (anti-HB) to be at least 10 mIU/mL at 1–2 months after dose # 3. Given intramuscularly.
- If anti-HB is <10 mIU/mL (negative), revaccinate and retest.
- If still negative after second vaccination series, considered to be a nonresponder. If determined not to be infected, then healthcare worker (HCW) is at risk and should be counseled about precautions and the need of HB immune globulin (HBIG) postexposure prophylaxis after any known or likely exposure.
- Postvaccine testing is recommended for any HCW experiencing a work-related incident related to blood.

Influenza (Annual Flu Season)

- Preferred is the intramuscular trivalent (inactivated, i.e., killed) influenza vaccine (TIV). Available in intramuscular and intradermal (age 18–64 years) forms.
- Alternate is intranasal live, attenuated (very weakened and cannot cause flu) influenza vaccine (LAIV). Can use only if ≤49 years of age. Cannot be used in HCW caring for severely immunocompromised hospitalized patient in a protective environment (i.e., bone marrow/stem cell transplant). Also not recommended for pregnant women, diabetics, asthmatics, and others with chronic cardiovascular, pulmonary, or metabolic diseases and those living with severely immunocompromised household members (i.e., acute leukemia).
- Give one dose of TIV or LAIV annually. Is modified annually for predicted flu type.
- Effectiveness varies from year to year, depends on age and health status of person, and similarity of circulating virus's "match" to vaccine. If a vaccinated HCW still develops the flu (breakthrough influenza), they will experience a shorter and milder flu than if they had not been vaccinated.
- Some people mistakenly confuse flu symptoms with minor side effects such a minor fever and mild body aches or soreness at the injection site. True influenza symptoms are not mild. LAIV may also cause a runny nose, scratchy throat, mild cough, and headache.

Varicella (Chickenpox)

- Varicella-zoster live-virus vaccine. Two doses (28 days apart) given subcutaneously. All must show evidence of immunity through vaccination records or have serologic evidence of immunity.

- Primary infection typically confers lifetime immunity, but not always.
- Breakthrough varicella in a vaccinated person is typically milder and of shorter duration.

Pertussis, Tetanus, and Diphtheria

- All HCWs need to receive Tdap. Given intramuscularly. Tdap is an acellular pertussis vaccine first licensed in 2005. The pertussis (p) vaccine also protects against the diseases tetanus (T) and diphtheria (d). The "a" stands for "and". Tdap is a *booster* intended for those who completed their childhood vaccinations.
- Adults (and anyone else born before 2005) probably received the discontinued DTP, a whole-cell pertussis vaccine, as a child. Protection decreased with time, resulting in little to no protection 5–10 years after last dose.
- Adults who were not vaccinated as a child receive Tdap and then two additional full strength TDs.
- After receiving Tdap, it is currently recommended that a TD booster be given every 10 years thereafter, but this recommendation is expected to change to another Tdap in the near future.

MMR (Measles, Mumps, and Rubella)

- Are all live attenuated virus vaccines. Not available in the United States individually. Vaccine for all three diseases given as one. Given in two doses subcutaneously 28 days apart. Very high effectiveness rates, but not 100%.
- Immunity from each virus vaccine is believed to be long term, probably lifelong.
- HCWs need to show written documentation of two doses of *live* vaccine, lab evidence of immunity for each disease, lab confirmed evidence of having had each disease or birth before 1957. However, it is now recommended that facilities consider vaccinating the pre-1957 group.
- In the event of an outbreak of measles or mumps, all unvaccinated (i.e., pre-1957) should receive the two doses. Serologic screening is not recommended because of rapid response need.
- In the event of an outbreak of rubella, all unvaccinated (i.e., pre-1957) should receive one dose. Serologic screening is not recommended because of rapid response need.

Other vaccines are recommended for special groups of HCWs such as microbiologists and research scientists, and include hepatitis A, bacille Calmette-Guérin, meningococcal, typhoid, and vaccinia (smallpox).

Modified from Immunization of health-care personnel. Recommendations of the Advisory Committee on Immunization Practices (ACIP). Centers for Disease Control and Prevention website. http://www.cdc.gov/mmwr/pdf/rr/rr6007.pdf. Accessed November 14, 2018; Centers for Disease Control and Prevention. Epidemiology and Prevention of Vaccine-Preventable Diseases. *The Pink Book: Course Textbook, 12th Edition.* http://cdc.gov/vaccines/pubs/pinbook/index.html. Accessed November 14, 2018; Centers for Disease Control and Prevention. Prevention of measles, rubella, congenital rubella syndrome, and mumps, 2013: Summary recommendations of the advisory committee on immunization practices (ACIP). *MMWR* 2013;62.

If an HCW does not show a protective level of anti-HB titers after vaccination and posttesting, a second series should be given. The small percentage of people who still do not achieve protective levels after vaccination are either infected with HBV or are in a genetic group of nonresponders.[39,40] Hepatitis B vaccines have been shown to be safe when given to infants, children, teens, and adults, including pregnant women.[42,43] A sore deltoid muscle (injection site) and fever are the most common complaints.[41]

Hepatitis C Virus

Of increasing concern is the hepatitis C virus (HCV), which was identified in 1989.[44] As of mid-2014, HCV infection is the most common chronic bloodborne infection in the United States, with approximately 3.2 million persons chronically infected. HCV chronic infection is also the leading reason for needing a liver transplant in the United States.[45] Transmission of HCV is mostly through percutaneous exposure to infected blood. Today, most people become infected through shared-needle drug use. Before screening was implemented in 1992, HCV was commonly spread through blood transfusions and organ transplants.[44,46] Sexual exposure has also resulted in transmission, but the risk is low, and more research is needed to better understand how and when it is spread.[45] As stated earlier, no vaccine currently exists for HCV, and it is now recommended that anyone born between 1945 and 1965 be tested.[45] New treatments have been created to potentially cure HCV infection, but due to the virus's mutagenic propensity, some of those infected may not respond to therapy.

Influenza Viruses

Influenza and subsequent infections cause an estimated average of over 200,000 hospitalizations and 3,000 to 49,000 deaths annually in the United States.[47–50] The death rate is variable and depends on the type of influenza circulating in a specific year.[47] Influenza causes significant morbidity and mortality in older patients, patients with chronic underlying disease, and immunocompromised patients, all of which describe most patients seen in radiation therapy.

In the United States, flu season occurs in the fall and winter and can peak anywhere from late November through March; thus, flu vaccines should be administered to HCWs on a priority basis and as soon as that year's vaccine becomes available.[4] Protection develops in about 2 weeks.[51] Likewise, radiation therapy outpatients who are coughing or who have other upper respiratory symptoms should be provided a mask, and hand sanitizer stations at the door be made available as a safety measure for other patients and visitors.

Influenza is caused by RNA viruses of the Orthomyxoviridae family and occurs in birds and mammals. Two types exist, A and B, and different strains of A and B develop each year.[52] Influenza is spread through three major transmission modes: (1) direct contact via large droplets over a short distance; (2) airborne transmission, consisting of small-droplet nuclei that can travel longer distances than large droplet; and (3) self-inoculation after contact with contaminated materials (this usually involves the hands transferring the virus to the mucous membranes of the eye or nose).[53] Airborne transmission over much longer distances, such as from one patient room to another, has not been documented and is thought not to occur.[53] Shedding of the influenza virus from an infected individual usually lasts 5 to 7 days after the onset of symptoms. Signs and symptoms do not appear for a day or two after contracting the flu.[51] Multiple symptoms will exist at the same time and usually consist of chills and possible fever (you may or may not run fever), all-over body aches, headache, dry cough, sore throat, feeling very tired, runny or stuffy nose, and being less hungry than usual.[54] Vomiting and diarrhea may be present, but this is more common in children, and the "stomach flu" or "24-hour flu" is not influenza, which usually takes 1 to 2 weeks to feel much better.[54]

Varicella-Zoster Virus

Varicella-zoster virus (VZV) deserves special attention in a radiation oncology department. VZV is the pathogen that causes varicella zoster (chickenpox) and herpes zoster (shingles or HZ). VZV has an extremely high degree of communicability and is transmitted by the inhalation of small-droplet nuclei or by direct contact with respiratory droplets or vesicle fluid.[55,56] For children, chickenpox usually consists of a mild illness characterized by fever and a vesicular rash mainly on the body trunk. Infected persons are contagious an estimated 1 to 2 days before rash onset and remain contagious until all lesions are crusted over, usually 4 to 7 days.[55] The rash may range from one or two vesicles to hundreds; thus, extremely light or subclinical infections may go undiagnosed. The skin lesions appear in groups at different times, so late and early lesions can be seen at the same time. US childhood vaccination for varicella began in 1995 and led to dramatic declines in incidence in all age groups.[57]

In adults, chickenpox is typically more severe, and the risk of complications is higher.[36] Infection early in pregnancy is associated with neonatal complications and congenital malformations and puts both mother and baby at risk.[58] In cancer patients, chickenpox can be life-threatening in children and adults as a result of an impaired immune system. If a nonimmune cancer patient is exposed, varicella-zoster immune globulin (VZIG) can be given to minimize the disease.[55] Airborne precautions and contact precautions should be employed for patients with varicella or disseminated HZ and for immunocompromised patients with localized HZ until disseminated HZ is ruled out.[36]

Shingles is a local manifestation of a recurrent, reactivated infection by the same virus. After a person has chickenpox, the VZV is thought to remain dormant in the cells of nerve root ganglia. Shingles usually is seen in middle age; however, children and even infants occasionally develop shingles. Painful rashes of blisters appear on the skin area supplied by the affected nerve. Clinically, especially in adults, pain and severe itching occur and often last for long periods after the lesions have crusted over and healed. A significant number of transplant or cancer patients, especially those with leukemia, lymphoma, or AIDS-related cancers, develop shingles as a result of immunosuppression.[52] In 2007, the US Food and Drug Administration (FDA) approved Zostavax, a vaccine for the HZ virus.[60]

Because VZV can be life-threatening to nonimmune cancer patients, vaccination of all HCWs is recommended if not mandated by policy or law. All workers or trainees in oncology or transplant departments should have documented varicella vaccination or should be able to show serologic evidence of immunity. If a nonimmune HCW is permitted to work and is exposed to a person with chickenpox or shingles, that HCW is considered potentially communicable during the incubation period. They will have to be placed on leave beginning on the 10th day after exposure and remain on leave for the maximum incubation period of varicella, which is 21 days.[36,59] In addition, any infected worker should not return to work until all lesions have dried and crusted, which is usually 4 to 7 days from the onset of the rash.[55] VZIG can be used after exposure in nonimmune HCWs to lessen the severity of the disease if they develop it. If a nonprotected HCW receives VZIG after exposure, the incubation period is prolonged; therefore, he or she must be placed on leave for a longer time, typically 28 days after exposure.[59]

Pertussis, Tetanus, and Diphtheria Bacteria

Pertussis is a highly contagious (humans only) bacterial infection caused by Bordetella pertussis.[61] The greatest danger occurs in infants too young to be immunized and children who have not finished their vaccination series, and this danger has led to a more recent recommendation that expectant mothers be vaccinated with every pregnancy to help protect newborns until they can be immunized.[62] All HCWs who have not or are unsure if they have previously received a dose of the Tdap vaccine should receive a dose as soon as feasible and a booster every 10 years thereafter.

Pertussis is also known as whooping cough because infected children have mucous so thick it blocks their air passages to the point of cyanosis. After they have a violent coughing spell trying to expel the mucus, they take in a big breath, which makes a high-pitched "whoop" sound; infants younger than 6 months usually don't make the sound because they are too weak to breathe deeply.[63,64] The coughing lasts for weeks to months, even with antibiotics.[64] Complications include pneumonia, pneumothorax, subdural hematomas, encephalopathy, seizures, rectal prolapse, and even death. Adults typically have milder symptoms but are still known to break ribs during coughing episodes, experience urinary incontinence, and have secondary pneumonia.[64]

Tetanus, commonly referred to as lockjaw, is not a disease transmitted from one human to another but is caused by a bacteria (*Clostridium tetani*) commonly found in soil.[65] Fatalities can occur in persons never immunized or adults whose vaccine protection has lapsed. Puncture wounds (especially if contaminated with dirt, pet feces, or manure), compound fractures, crush injuries, animal bites, and other skin injuries are known causes of tetanus.[66]

Diphtheria is caused by a bacteria (*Corynebacterium diphtheriae*), which predominantly remains in the pharynx and tonsils and creates superficial necrotizing ulcerations and the formation of a grayish pseudomembrane.[52] In absence of vaccination, it starts with a sore throat, bloody watery nasal drainage, chills, and fever, and then progresses to more serious effects because of the diphtheria toxin, which causes nerve paralyses (cranial nerves), toxic myocarditis, and possible death; about 1 out of 10 adults die.[67] Children also can die of respiratory obstruction and asphyxia; in children under 5 years of age, one out of five die.[68] This disease spreads through respiratory droplets (cough, sneeze) of an infected person or by a carrier who has no symptoms.[68] If a physician thinks someone has diphtheria, they will order that antitoxin and antibiotics be started before waiting for lab results.[68]

Mumps, Measles, and Rubella Viruses

Mumps, measles (rubeola), and rubella (German measles) occurred in the vast majority of children and rarely in adolescents and adults in the prevaccine era. The first-generation vaccines became available in 1948, 1963, and 1967, respectively.[63] Newer vaccines with fewer side effects and greater safety are in use today. Revaccination is needed in those who received the first-generation versions of the vaccine and in those who are not sure what they received. This further emphasizes the need to keep a personal, permanent copy of any vaccine received.

Those born before 1957 have been exempt because they likely had these diseases as a child. However, more recent studies have shown that 2% to 9% of HCWs born before 1957 lack antibodies, and they may now be required to be vaccinated or show proof of immunity.[69–73] Complications seen with this disease include: death, pneumonia, deafness, testicular atrophy or sterility, mental retardation, fetal death, birth defects, and encephalitis. Women planning to get pregnant should not get vaccinated for 1 month before pregnancy, and pregnant women should not be vaccinated. Other health conditions may also guide an individual's vaccination with MMR.[63,74]

Other Vaccines and Considerations

If an HCW does not respond to a vaccine, they remain at risk, and if exposed, prompt prophylaxis is strongly advised. Other vaccines not specific to HCWs but recommended for many adults include human papilloma virus (HPV) and hepatitis A.[63] Still others are recommended

for travel outside the United States and are region specific. Other diseases that require exclusion from a HCW's job or training include conjunctivitis, epidemic diarrhea, streptococcus, HAV, herpes simplex of exposed skin areas such as the hands, and *S. aureus* skin lesions. The following diseases deserve special attention because there is no vaccine for them, and both have developed drug resistance and led to the death of HCWs.

Tuberculosis

At the turn of the twentieth century, TB was one of the leading causes of death. In 1882, Dr. Robert Koch presented his finding that *Mycobacterium tuberculosis*, a gram-positive, acid-fast type of bacteria, was the causative agent of TB.[75] Today, the number of deaths worldwide has dramatically decreased because of effective treatment. The United States reported 9,105 new cases in 2017.[76] Although the number has declined in the United States, TB still persists in specific populations. Current goals for control and elimination are focused on populations that are affected in disproportionate numbers.

The bacille Calmette-Guérin (BCG) vaccine has been widely used outside the United States for several decades. The BCG vaccine is used to protect infants and young children in parts of the world where TB is common, but it is not 100% effective.[77] The BCG is not recommended in the United States because of low risk of infection, variable effectiveness, and because of its potential to cause a false positive with TB skin testing. The vaccine is given in the United States only to a very select group who has high risk of exposure in select settings and with a TB expert involved in the decision. The vaccine is contraindicated in anyone who is immunosuppressed (e.g., a cancer patient undergoing chemotherapy) or if they are likely to be immunosuppressed in the foreseeable future (e.g., on kidney transplant waiting list).[78]

The primary transmission route of TB is airborne droplet nuclei. The droplet nuclei are dispersed when people sneeze, cough, or talk. Around 1985, TB made a dramatic reappearance.[79] To a large degree, its emergence was related to the AIDS epidemic, disease relapse, increased immigration, inadequate precautions being taken at healthcare facilities, and the emergence of multidrug-resistant (MDR) TB. The risk of infection of an HCW depends on the number of droplet nuclei circulating in the air and the duration of time spent breathing the contaminated air. Negative airflow rooms exhausting directly to the outside high-efficiency particulate air (HEPA) filtration, and even ultraviolet germicidal irradiation can be used to keep TB from being spread within the healthcare facility's air circulation. OSHA requires all healthcare facilities to have a TB control plan.[80]

Most healthcare facilities have some inpatient rooms that have either negative air pressure flow or have positive-pressure isolation, which keeps the airflow moving out of the room. Negative-pressure rooms are used for suspected TB and active TB cases, measles, and chickenpox, whereas positive-pressure rooms are used for stem cell transplant or other immunocompromised patients who need protection.[81]

Since the resurgence of TB between 1985 and 1992, the annual TB rate has steadily decreased.[76] However, the proportion of TB cases among foreign-born persons increased each year during 1993 to 2003 and reached 70.1% in 2017.[82,76] Racial/ethnic disparities in TB incidence persist, as do geographic disparities.[76] Four states (California, Texas, New York, and Florida) account for about half of all U.S. TB cases reported in 2017.[76] These states, except for Texas, also are among the top 15 states for highest homeless rates in 2017.[76] Strategies to address these risk factors present many challenges to control and eliminate TB in the United States.

> Multidrug-resistant tuberculosis is extremely dangerous and can be fatal.

Mandates from OSHA specify that the minimum level of respiratory protection for TB will be a National Institute for Occupational Safety and Health (NIOSH)–certified N95 half-mask respirator.[83-85] The N95 rating indicates that 95% of test particles will be stopped. OSHA also requires that HCWs who need to wear such masks be medically evaluated to wear them because of possible pulmonary or cardiac associated stresses on the user.[83-85] Individuals receiving these masks should receive training and go through face-fitting procedures before usage.[83-85] Simple surgical or isolation masks are not respirators and are not certified as such. Also of importance is that men with beards are precluded from using some of the NIOSH-approved masks because an adequate seal cannot be maintained.[83-85] Masks labeled N, R, or P meet CDC guidelines, as do those that use HEPA filters both with and without exhalation valves. Four main mask designs are available as described in Box 10.4. Symptomatic patients should wear a surgical mask during transport and should not be placed with the general population.

> Occupational Safety and Health Administration–approved masks must be provided for contact with patients with active or suspected tuberculosis.

The *Guidelines for Preventing the Transmission of Mycobacterium tuberculosis in Health-Care Settings, 2005* replaces all previous CDC guidelines (1994, 1999) for TB control in health settings and is still current as of 2018.[86,87] In 2011, the U.S. Department of Labor released a very informative, half-hour long video titled *Respiratory Protection for Healthcare Workers Training Video,* which is well suited for the radiation therapy classroom. The CDC and OSHA have released several other educational videos that address respiratory safety; all can be watched for free online.[88,89] OSHA Standard 29 CFR 1910.134 details what employers must have in place to protect HCWs from TB by law.[90]

Baseline testing for TB infection is recommended for all new HCWs (including students in healthcare education programs) and is currently conducted in the United States using either the two-step tuberculin skin test (TST) or by interferon-gamma release assay (IGRA), a blood test. Two IGRAs approved for use in the United States by the FDA are QuantiFERON-TB Gold-in-Tube test and T-SPOT TB test.[90,92] These tests are the same as those used to test the general public when indicated in an outbreak situation. The less costly TST consists of an intradermal *Mantoux TST* (purified protein derivative of tuberculin). The two-step process is shown in Fig. 10.4. Reading and interpretation of TST reactions are done 48 to 72 hours after injection and must be performed by someone specifically trained to do so.[77] If the timeline is not adhered to, the TST must be repeated on the other arm or several inches from the first site. Interpretation of TST results are based on the measurement of the reaction in millimeters, and a reaction of 5 mm, 10 mm (typical for most HCWs), or 15 mm is considered positive based on specific criteria for each reaction size.[77] TSTs should not be performed on a person who has written documentation of either a previous positive TST result or treatment for TB disease. Advantages of IGRAs are that they require a single patient visit, are not affected by perception of the reader, are more specific than skin testing, and results are available within 24 hours.[77]

> HCWs can be tested using a two-step skin test (TST) or a blood test (IGRA). A person with a positive test is at risk for developing active TB even years later; thus, treatment is highly encouraged before active TB develops.

BOX 10.4 Personal Protection Equipment for Tuberculosis and Other Infectious Airborne Diseases: Types of OSHA- and NIOSH-Approved Respirators

Disposable Particulate Respirators
Disposable, lightweight
Negative-pressure design
Half mask or half mask with face splatter shield
Can be used in sterile field area if there is no exhalation valve

Replaceable Particulate Filter Respirators
Half mask or half mask with face splatter shield
Reusable, with single or dual filters that are replaced
Negative-pressure design
Has to be disinfected and inspected
Cannot be used in sterile field area
Communication may be difficult
Also comes in full facepiece design, which provides better seal and protection

Powered Air-Purifying Respirators (PAPRS)
Battery operated
Half or full facepiece designs
Has breathing tube and uses only HEPA filters
Usually more comfortable to wear and cooler
Easier to breathe
Cannot be used in sterile field area
Is not a true positive-pressure device, can be overbreathed when inhaling
Has to be disinfected and inspected
May be bulky and noisy
Communication may be difficult
Two types: tight fit and loose fit, which does accommodate facial hair (beard)

Positive Pressure–Supplied Air Respirators
Uses compressed air from a stationary source delivered through a hose
Much more protective
Should be used when the other types do not provide adequate protection
Minimal breathing effort
Should not be worn during sterile procedures
Must be disinfected and inspected

OSHA Videos Available Online (Respiratory Protection-Training Videos—OSHA)
1. The Difference Between Respirators and Masks—2009, 6 minutes
2. Respiratory Protection for Healthcare Workers—2011, 33 minutes

HEPA, High-efficiency particulate air; *NIOSH,* National Institute for Occupational Safety and Health; *OSHA,* Occupational Safety and Health Administration.
Modified from Centers for Disease Control and Prevention. NIOSH TB respiratory protection program in healthcare facilities—Administrator's guide. In: Health NIfOSa, HHS, CDC, eds. Cincinnati, OH: Department of Health and Human Services; 1999; Respiratory Protection for Healthcare Workers Training Video. Occupational Safety and Health Administration, United States Department of Labor website. https://www.osha.gov/SLTC/respiratoryprotection/training_videos.html#video. Accessed November 14, 2018.

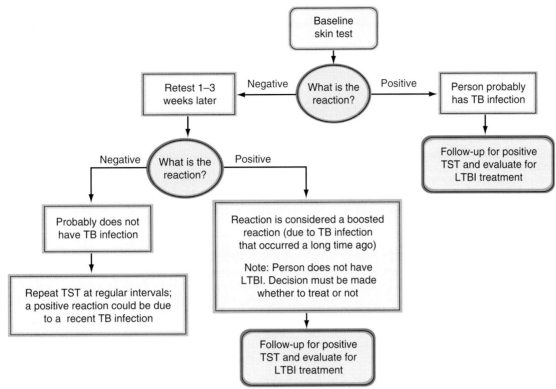

Fig. 10.4 Two-step tuberculin skin testing. *LTBI*, Latent tuberculosis infection; *TB*, tuberculosis; *TST*, tuberculosis skin test. (From United States Department of Health and Human Services: *Latent tuberculosis infection: a guide for primary health care providers, 2013.* Available at https://www.cdc.gov/tb/publications/ltbi/pdf/TargetedLTBI.pdf. Accessed August 19, 2019.)

The presence of TB can be verified by culture or nucleic acid amplification, which detects the genetic material of the infecting organism. TB can also be clinically determined by assessing symptoms plus having a positive chest radiograph if both resolve following treatment.[93] In 2013, the FDA approved a sputum test to detect DNA of the TB organism as well as genetic mutations associated with drug resistance.[94] This test allows for rapid results, which will lead to avoidance of unnecessary and costly respiratory isolation, treatment, and contact investigations.[94] Genotyping combined with epidemiologic expertise has recently enabled public health investigators to actually help track outbreaks among persons not known to be linked and to identify the probable location of TB transmission in homeless person networks, a hospital emergency department, and a public transportation hub.[95]

To determine whether treatment for latent TB infection (LTBI) or a positive conversion is indicated, HCWs should be referred for medical and diagnostic evaluation. In conjunction with the evaluation, HCWs with positive test results for *M. tuberculosis* should be considered for treatment of LTBI after TB disease has been excluded by further medical evaluation. HCWs can be compelled to take a TST, IGRA, or chest radiograph and treatment for LTBI if needed by their employer or educational institution. Persons with LTBI are not infectious and cannot spread TB infection to others, but if latent disease is not treated, it typically progresses into active TB 6 to 8 months after initial infection.[93,96] Table 10.2 shows current US Public Health Service (PHS) regimens for treating LTBI.

General symptoms of active TB include: unexplained weight loss, loss of appetite, night sweats, fever, fatigue, and chills.[77] Symptoms of lung-involved TB include: coughing for 3 weeks or longer, coughing up blood, and chest pain.[77] All persons with a history of TB or positive TB test should be alerted that they are at risk of developing the disease in the future and should promptly report any pulmonary symptoms. Table 10.3 compares LTBI with TB disease.

Over time, drug resistance has developed, and some patients are labeled as having MDR TB or extensively drug-resistant TB (XDR TB). MDR TB means that the organism is resistant to at least the two most potent TB drugs, isoniazid and rifampin.[75] XDR TB also indicates additional resistance to any fluoroquinolone and at least one of three other injectable anti-TB drugs used to treat MDR TB. MDR TB is difficult to cure and requires 18 to 24 months of treatment with drugs that cause toxic side effects. MDR TB also has a higher mortality rate than standard drug-susceptible TB. XDR TB is even more of a challenge, and clinical trials are currently underway.

HUMAN IMMUNODEFICIENCY VIRUS AND ACQUIRED IMMUNODEFICIENCY SYNDROME

Since 1983 when the first case of occupational HIV infection was documented, HCWs have been flooded with information and literature about the risk that accompanies caring for HIV-positive patients.[97] Because these patients do not always have obvious characteristics of the disease, the only logical approach that an HCW can use for self-protection is to use standard infection precautions for all patients.

Since 1995, mortality rates from HIV infection have significantly declined due primarily to the introduction of antiretroviral therapies and decreasing HIV transmission incidence. One in six of those living with HIV are unaware of their infection; thus, routine HIV testing is now recommended for all people age 13 to 64 years.[98]

Being HIV positive does not mean a person has AIDS; AIDS is the most advanced stage of HIV disease. Proper treatment can delay and possibly keep a person from progressing to full-blown AIDS.

In May 2014, the US PHS released its first clinical practice guideline aimed at giving a daily pill (brand name, Truvada) to HIV-negative people who are at substantial risk because of their unsafe sexual practices or injection drug use.[99] Consistent daily use of antiretroviral preexposure prophylaxis has been shown to reduce the risk of infection by 92%.[99]

TABLE 10.2   Drug Regimens for Latent Tuberculosis Infection[c]

Drug(S)	Age	Duration	Interval	No. of Doses (Minimum)
Isoniazid (INH)	Adults or Children	9 months[b]	Daily	270
			Twice weekly[a]	76
Isoniazid (INH)	Adults	6 months[b]	Daily	180
			Twice weekly[a]	52
Isoniazid and Rifapentine	Adults and children age 12 or older	3 months	Once weekly[a]	12
Rifampin	Adults	4 months	Daily	120

[a]Ingestion of medication must be observed by healthcare worker.
[b]Nine months is preferred over 6 months in adults for effectiveness, but choice is left to prescribing physician.
[c]Regimen choice is based on tuberculosis (TB) drug susceptibility of presumed source case (if known), coexisting medical illness, and potential for drug-TB drug interactions.
Modified from Latent tuberculosis infection: a guide for primary health care providers. United States Department of Health and Human Services website. http://www.cdc.gov/tb/publications/ltbi/pdf/TargetedLTBI.pdf. Accessed November 14, 2018.

TABLE 10.3   Differentiating Between Latent Tuberculosis Infection and Tuberculosis Disease

Latent TB	TB Disease
• No symptoms or physical findings that suggest active TB disease	• Symptoms include one or more: fever, cough, chest pain, night sweats, decreased appetite, fatigue or hemoptysis
• Testing by TST or IGRA usually are positive	• Testing by TST or IGRA usually positive
• Chest radiograph is typically normal	• Chest radiograph is typically abnormal. However, may be normal in a person with advanced immunosuppression or extrapulmonary disease
• Respiratory specimens (if done) are smear and culture negative	• Respiratory specimens are usually smear or culture positive. However, may be negative in person with extrapulmonary disease or minimal or early pulmonary disease
• Person cannot spread TB to others	• Person can spread disease to others
• Should consider treatment so infection will not progress to active TB disease	• Needs treatment for TB disease

IGRA, Interferon-gamma release assay; TB, tuberculosis; TST, tuberculin skin test.
Modified from Latent tuberculosis infection: a guide for primary health care providers. http://www.cdc.gov/tb/publications/ltbi/pdf/TargetedLTBI.pdf. Accessed November 14, 2018.

Preventing exposures to blood and body fluids is the primary means of preventing HIV infection. Appropriate postexposure prophylaxis (PEP) management is also an important element of workplace safety.[104,110] When an exposure incident occurs, the first and most urgent question is, "What actions can be taken to decrease the risk of transmission?" In 1996, the first U.S. PHS recommendations for the use of PEP after occupational exposure to HIV were published; these recommendations have been updated several times.[100–102] PEP involves the use of antiretroviral drugs after a single high-risk event to try to stop HIV from making copies of itself and spreading through the body. Sometimes the term occupational PEP is used to distinguish healthcare workplace exposure from nonoccupational PEP, which would include single-event treatment for sexual assault, consensual unprotected sex, and needle-sharing drug use.[103]

The definitions of *HCW* and *occupational exposures* have remained relatively unchanged from 1996.[104] HCW refers to all paid and unpaid persons working in healthcare settings who have the potential for exposure to infectious materials (i.e., blood, tissue, specific body fluids, or medical supplies, equipment, and environmental surfaces contaminated with these substances). An exposure that might place a HCW at risk for HIV infection is defined as a percutaneous injury (i.e., a needlestick or cut with a sharp object) or contact of a mucous membrane or nonintact skin (i.e., exposed skin that is chapped, abraded, or afflicted with dermatitis) with blood, tissue, or other body fluids that are potentially infectious. In addition to blood and visibly bloody body

fluids, semen and vaginal secretions also are considered potentially infectious.

The following fluids also are considered potentially infectious: cerebrospinal fluid, synovial fluid, pleural fluid, peritoneal fluid, pericardial fluid, and amniotic fluid. Feces, nasal secretions, saliva, sputum, sweat, tears, urine, and vomitus are not considered potentially infectious unless they are visibly bloody; the risk for transmission of HIV infection from these fluids and materials is low.[104,105] Transmission of HIV infection from a human bite has been rarely reported, but none have occurred in the healthcare setting.[106,107] To date, no additional routes of transmission have been substantiated in occupational HIV exposure, and casual contact (such as a handshake) that occurs with infected patients poses no risk to the HCW.[108,109] HCWs who are exposed or think they may have been exposed should seek expert advice immediately; never hesitate, as every hour counts. Also keep in mind that fewer than 60 cases of HCW occupational transmission of HIV have occurred in the United States and that no confirmed case has occurred since 1999, which is a testimonial to mandatory safeguards and training.[110]

The risk of acquiring HBV has been statistically calculated to be 10 to 100 times greater than the risk of acquiring HIV.[111] The risk of HBV after a needlestick or a cut exposure involving blood from an HBV-positive patient is higher than for HIV.[100,102] In studies of HCWs, the average risk for HIV transmission after a percutaneous exposure to HIV-infected blood has been estimated to be approximately 0.3%, approximately 0.1% (1 in 1000) after a mucous membrane exposure (eye, nose, mouth), and less than 0.1% on intact skin.[111,112] There have been no documented cases of HIV transmission because of exposure involving a small amount of blood (a few drops) on intact skin for a short amount of time.[112] Percutaneous exposures account for 84% of occupationally acquired HIV cases, followed by mucocutaneous exposure (13%) and combined percutaneous and mucocutaneous exposure (3%).[113] Episodes of HIV transmission after nonintact skin exposure have been documented. The risk for transmission after exposure to other body fluids or tissues that are not bloody is probably considerably lower than for blood exposures, but statistics are not known.[104]

Needlesticks account for 84% of job-related acquired HIV. There is no reason to ever recap a needle.

When an exposure incident occurs, the workplace must immediately make available to the HCW confidential medical evaluation and follow-up. The HCW should immediately be relieved from the duty they were performing, and another qualified HCW should step in; even in surgery, the surgeon should step away and be replaced. If the HCW is pregnant or breastfeeding, the decisions to offer treatment should be the same as for any other HCW; however, because unique considerations are present, counseling and discussion has to also address the child or fetus, and expert consultation is advised.[107] After an exposure, the workplace must follow all federal (such as OHSA) and state requirements for recording and reporting. The date, time, and details of the procedure being performed and details of the exposure are recorded in the exposure report and in the confidential medical record of the exposed HCW. Many big-name groups such as the American Nurses Association and the State of New York Public Health Service recommend that PEP be initiated within the first 2 hours following exposure.[115] PEP must begin within 72 hours at maximum because research has shown that PEP is possibly ineffective after 72 hours have passed.[107] Guidelines also call for the recording of the type and severity of the exposure because this information eventually provides better epidemiologic data.[112] For example, documenting the type of needle (e.g., hollow core, surgical), gauge of the needle, depth of penetration, volume of blood or body fluid, and source of fluid (e.g., blood, amniotic fluid) helps provide better analysis. Also important to PEP is whether the infective virus strain is known or suspected to be resistant to antiretroviral drugs.[112] Writing of the report should not delay an HCW in seeking a qualified provider; paperwork can be completed immediately after the expert consultation.

A true occupational exposure requires that documented seroconversion take place. This means that the HCW consented to HIV testing and tested negative for their HIV baseline shortly after an exposure then later develops clinical and/or serologic evidence of HIV infection. The documentation described above is necessary to sort out HCWs who may have unknowingly been positive for HIV at the time of exposure as a result of nonoccupational factors.

Skin and injured wound sites that have been contaminated with blood or a body fluid should be washed with soap and water. Oral and nasal mucosal surfaces should be flushed thoroughly with water. Eyes should be irrigated with water, saline, or other suitable sterile solutions. Once these steps are taken, the HCW should report the incident to their supervisor and immediately seek medical treatment. A 24-hour telephone hotline is available if a medical provider has any questions about treating an occupational exposure.[115]

If the incident involves a source individual, who is defined as any person, living or dead, whose blood or other potentially infectious body materials may be a source of exposure, the identification of the source individual will be determined except when doing so is unfeasible or prohibited by law. The HIV status of the source through medical documentation or direct testing will direct the HCW's PEP plan.

Once the HIV gains access to a living body, it seeks target cells, CD4+ lymphocytes, to replicate in. During this initial time period, the virus is not detectable in blood nor even thought to be transmitted through a blood transfusion; however, the virus would be present in the infected person's organs or even a donated organ like a kidney.[116] A short while later, low concentrations of HIV virus begin to circulate in the blood. The concentration increases exponentially with time and then plateaus before declining as the body responds by making antibodies to attack the virus.[116] The window period is the time period between when the virus begins circulation and when either the virus or the antibodies are detectable in a HIV test. There are several types of HIV tests.

One is the immunoassay, which looks for antibodies in blood or oral fluid (rubbing of mucosal gum surfaces not saliva), which can be done in a lab or as a screening *rapid test*.[117] Blood testing tends to find infection sooner. Newer lab tests can detect both antibodies and antigen (part of the virus itself), thus leading to earlier detection of infection. Follow-up diagnostic testing is performed if the first immunoassay result is positive because even though initial immunoassays are generally very accurate, it allows you and your provider to be sure the diagnosis is correct. Follow-up tests include an antibody differentiation test to distinguish HIV-1 from HIV-2: an HIV-1 nucleic acid test, which looks for the virus itself, or the *Western blot* or indirect immunofluorescence assay, which detects antibodies.[117] RNA tests are more costly and detect the virus itself and can detect HIV at about 10 days after infection.[117] HIV testing is an ever-evolving process with new testing methods and new equipment aimed at cheaper, quicker, and more accurate diagnosis.

In any facility subject to OHSA regulations, rapid HIV testing is the mandated technology for source patients. Results of FDA approved rapid tests are usually available within 20 minutes or less of testing, and have sensitivities and specificities similar to those of first- and second-generation enzyme immunoassays.[117,118] Third-generation chemiluminescent immunoassays run on automated platforms can detect HIV-specific antigens and generate test results in an hour or less.[119,107] The latest, called fourth-generation combinations p24 antigen-HIV antibody (Ag/Ab) tests, produce both rapid and accurate results, plus even allow detection in most cases in the window period.[107,119] Rapid testing of the source patient provides essential information needed to initiate and/or continue with PEP. Administration of PEP should not be delayed while waiting for test results because if the source is determined to be HIV negative, PEP can simply be discontinued. The US PHS recommends consultation with an infectious diseases specialist or another physician who is an expert in the administration of antiretroviral agents whenever possible because of the complexity of HIV PEP and evolving recommendations.[107] Consulting with an expert is especially important if the source has had prior treatment or is currently being treated for HIV, especially drug-resistant HIV.[107] Box 10.5 displays other situations requiring expert consultation. If an expert is not immediately available, another physician (such as an emergency room physician trained to handle HIV exposures) can initiate treatment with single-dose "starter packets," which are now kept on hand at any site expected to manage occupational exposures to HIV, until the exposed worker can see an expert.[107] At minimum, the physician should be capable of providing counseling and performing all medical evaluations and procedures in accordance with the most recent recommendations of the US PHS, including the administration of PEP when indicated (this is extremely unlikely to be your family doctor or the radiation oncologist with whom you work).[112]

BOX 10.5 **Situations for Which Expert Consultation for Human Immunodeficiency Virus; Postexposure Prophylaxis Is Highly Recommended**

Delayed (>72 Hours) Exposure Report
- Interval after which benefits from PEP are undefined

Unknown Source (Such Laundry or Trash)
- Use of PEP to be decided on a case-by-case basis
- Consider severity of exposure and epidemiologic likelihood of HIV exposure
- Do not test needle or sharp instrument for HIV

Known or Suspected Pregnancy in HCW
- Provision of PEP should not be delayed while awaiting expert consultation

Breastfeeding in HCW
- Provision of PEP should not be delayed while awaiting expert consultation

Known or Suspected Resistance of the Source Virus to Antiretroviral Agents
- If source person's virus is known or suspected to be resistant to one or more of the drugs considered for PEP, selection of drugs to which the source person's virus is unlikely to be resistant is recommended
- Do not delay initiation of PEP while awaiting any results of resistance testing of the source person's virus

Toxicity of the Initial PEP Regimen
- Symptoms (GI and others) are often manageable without changing PEP regimen by prescribing antimotility or antiemetic agents
- Counseling and support for management of side effects is very important, as symptoms are often exacerbated by anxiety in the HCW

Serious Medical Illness in the Exposed Person
- Significant underlying illness (renal disease and other) in HCW or HCW is already taking multiple medications that may increase the risk of drug toxicity and drug-drug interactions

See definition of expert in chapter text. Most physicians are not considered experts in HIV treatment, and an expert is preferred if immediately available. PEP HOTLINE experts are available at 888-448-4911 if a local expert is unavailable.
HCW, Healthcare worker; *HIV,* human immunodeficiency virus; *PEP,* postexposure prophylaxis.
Modified from: Kudar D, Henderson D, Struble K, et al. Updated US Public Health Service guidelines for the management of occupational exposures to human immunodeficiency virus and recommendations for postexposure prophylaxis. *Infect Control Hosp Epidemiol.* 2013;34:875–892.

> Immediately report any needlestick or body substance accidental exposure. Seek expert care quickly, because time is a critical factor. Know your rights. Discuss your situation and treatment options with a qualified physician.

The latest US PHS guideline for occupational exposure encourages the use of a PEP regimen that uses drugs chosen for optimum adherence with fewer side effects, lower toxicity, and convenient dosing schedules. This eliminates the need to assess level of risk of exposure to determine number of drugs to be used, modifies and expands the list of antiretroviral medications that can be used, and offers an option for concluding HIV follow-up testing earlier than 6 months after exposure.[107] The US PHS now recommends that exposed HCWs receive a 28-day treatment using three or more drugs.[107] Antiretroviral agents from six classes of drugs

TABLE 10.4 **Clinical Signs and Symptoms Found in Acute (Primary) Human Immunodeficiency Virus Infection**

Features	Overall (n = 375) (%)	Male (n = 355)	Female (n = 23)
Fever	75	74	83
Fatigue	68	67	78
Muscle pain	49	50	26
Skin rash	48	48	48
Headache	45	45	44
Sore throat	40	40	48
Cervical adenopathy	39	39	39
Joint pain	30	30	26
Night sweats	28	28	22
Diarrhea	27	27	21

Modified from Centers for Disease Control and Prevention, US Public Health Service: Preexposure prophylaxis for the prevention of HIV infection in the United States—2017 update: a clinical practice guideline, 2017. Centers for Disease Control and Prevention website. https://www.cdc.gov/hiv/pdf/risk/prep/cdc-hiv-prep-guidelines-2017.pdf. Accessed March 22, 2019.

are currently available to treat HIV infection.[107] The typical regimen consists of emtricitabine (FTC) plus TDF (may be dispensed as Truvada) plus raltegravir (RAL).[107] Because previous regimens showed that a substantial proportion of HCWs reported harsh side effects and many were unable to complete treatment, preemptive prescribing of drugs to combat side effects is now recommended to increase compliance.

Follow-up should consist of counseling, postexposure testing, and medical evaluation regardless of whether the HCW chooses to take PEP. At the initial meeting, the HCW should be counseled in precautions they need to take to prevent secondary transmission. Complete blood counts and renal and hepatic function tests will be conducted and repeated at 2 weeks postexposure if PEP is to be initiated to monitor for drug toxicity.[107] After the initial meeting, another meeting within 3 days is recommended to allow for anxiety levels to decrease and to allow the HCW to ask more questions and increase understanding, to increase compliance with medications, and to discuss any symptoms or side effects more effectively plus receive additional information about the source patient's results, which may alter their treatment.[107] The psychological impact of a possible or proven HIV transmission cannot be underestimated or trivialized. All results of any HIV test should be face-to-face, never by phone, text, or email. HIV testing should also be done at 6 weeks, 12 weeks, and 6 months after occupational exposure at minimum (4 months with fourth-generation testing).[107] Extended HIV follow-up (12 months) is recommended for HCWs who become infected with HCV from a source who was both HIV and HCV infected. Extended testing can also be done for HCWs with greater anxiety or for anyone developing symptoms of HIV.[107] Symptoms that are compatible with seroconversion are shown in Table 10.4. OSHA rules further state that if the worker consents to blood collection but not to an HIV test, the sample must be preserved for at least 90 days in case the HCW changes his or her mind.[120]

Counseling of the HCW should also address lifestyle changes that should be made until seroconversion occurs or until enough time has passed for the worker to be deemed free of HIV infection. Lifestyle changes include no exchange of body fluids during sex, deferment of pregnancy, cessation of breastfeeding, no intimate kissing, no sharing of razors or toothbrushes, and no donation of blood, sperm, or organs. If the HCW is involved in an accident that results in bleeding, surfaces that are contaminated should be promptly disinfected.

In general, employees should be allowed to perform their standard patient care duties following an occupational exposure. In the case of a bloodborne infection status, such as HIV or HBV positive, employers are not allowed to discriminate against the employee. Employees are protected by Section 504 of the Rehabilitation Act and the Americans with Disabilities Act, which prohibits discrimination against individuals with disabilities, including persons who are positive for HIV or HBV.[121] Employers must make every effort to maintain the employment of an individual as long as the individual is capable of performing the job and does not pose a reasonable threat of infection to others. At the same time, however, employees and students should take personal responsibility for their actions and not perform any procedure that could be dangerous to their coworkers or patients.[104]

SUMMARY

- Epidemiology is a very important component to evaluate and study HAIs.
- HAIs affect the patient, public, and HCW physically and financially.
- Radiation therapists should accept the personal responsibility of making sure that their vaccines are complete and up to date annually to protect their patients, coworkers, family, and friends.
- The radiation therapist is responsible for ensuring that proper infection control measures are practiced in the treatment area environment.

REVIEW QUESTIONS

The answers to the Review Questions can be found by logging on to our website at: http://evolve.elsevier.com/Washington/principles

1. Which of the following is a government agency that legally oversees job safety and health protection of workers?
   a. CDC.
   b. DEA.
   c. JSHP.
   d. OSHA.
2. Which of the following viruses has been shown capable of living on environmentally friendly surfaces for as long as 7 days?
   a. Human immunodeficiency.
   b. Hepatitis B.
   c. Influenza.
   d. Rubeola.
3. The term used to describe the number of antibodies present in a blood sample is:
   a. Antigen coefficient.
   b. Globulin factor.
   c. Immune serum level.
   d. Titer.
4. An employer must provide particulate respirators to HCWs who must interact with a patient diagnosed with active:
   a. HIV.
   b. Histoplasmosis.
   c. Hepatitis A.
   d. TB.
5. The concept known as universal precautions best applies to:
   a. All body fluids.
   b. All patients.
   c. All blood and other certain body fluids in all patients.
   d. All patients and all body fluids.
6. What body fluid is not considered potentially infectious under Standard Precautions?
   a. Nasal secretions.
   b. Sweat.
   c. Saliva.
   d. Urine.
7. _____ is the name for the medical science field that studies the incidence, distribution, and determinants of disease.
8. An individual who is colonized but shows no immune response is known as a(n) _____.
9. Two nosocomial infectious diseases for which no vaccine is currently available are _____ and _____.
10. The three phases that a susceptible host goes through are _____, _____, and _____.

QUESTIONS TO PONDER

1. Discuss the differences between universal precautions and body substance isolation.
2. Practice putting a mask on and taking it off using recommended infection prevention technique.
3. Compare and contrast the differences between killed, toxoid, and attenuated live vaccines.
4. Compare the actions and protective gear needed for contact, droplet, and airborne transmission.
5. Compare the major differences between large-droplet and small-droplet nuclei transmission.
6. Discuss the significance of delayed seroconversion.

REFERENCES

1. Magill S, Edwards J, et al. Multistate point prevalence survey of health care-associated infections. *N Eng J Med.* 2014;370:1198–1208.
2. Data and statistics: the 2015 national and state healthcare-associated infection data report. Centers for Disease Control and Prevention website. https://www.cdc.gov/hai/surveillance/data-reports/2015-HAI-data-report.html. Accessed November 14, 2018.
3. Umschied C, Mitchell M, Doshi J, et al. Estimating the proportion of healthcare-associated infections that are reasonably preventable and the related mortality and costs. *Infect Control Hosp Epidemiol.* 2011;32:101–114.
4. Institute of Medicine. *To Err Is Human.* Washington, DC: National Academy Press; 1999.
5. Appold K. *Medicare Penalties Make Hospital-Acquired-Infections a Priority.* The Hospitalist; 2013. https://www.the-hospitalist.org/hospitalist/article/125653/health-policy/medicare-penalties-make-hospital-acquired-infection#. Accessed November 14, 2018.

6. Haley R. The development of infection surveillance and control programs. In: Bennett J, Brachman P, eds. *Hospital Infections*. 3rd ed. Boston, MA: Little, Brown; 1992.

7. James J. A new, evidence-based estimate of patient harms associated with hospital care. *J Patient Safety*. 2013;9(3):122–128.

8. Halpern M, Yabroff K. Prevalence of outpatient cancer treatment in the United States: estimates from the Medical Panel Expenditures Survey (MEPS). *Cancer Invest*. 2008;26:647–651.

9. Guide to infection prevention in outpatient settings: minimum expectations for care. Centers for Disease Control and Prevention website; 2016. https://www.cdc.gov/infectioncontrol/pdf/outpatient/guide.pdf. Accessed November 14, 2018.

10. Gardner J, Peel M. *Introduction to Sterilization, Disinfection and Infection Control*. 2nd ed. New York, NY: Churchill Livingstone; 1991.

11. Brachman P. Epidemiology of nosocomial infections. In: Bennett J, Brachman P, eds. *Hospital Infections*. 3rd ed. Boston, MA: Little, Brown; 1992.

12. Brachman P. Epidemiology of nosocomial infections. In: Bennett J, Brachman P, eds. *Hospital Infections*. 4th ed. Philadelphia, PA: Lippincott-Raven; 1998.

13. Benenson A. *Control of Communicable Diseases in Man*. 13th ed. Washington DC: American Public Health Association; 1981.

14. Haley C, et al. Tuberculosis epidemic among hospital personnel. *Infect Control Hosp Epidemiol*. 1989;10:204–210.

15. Respiratory fit testing. Occupational safety and health administration website. https://www.osha.gov/video/respiratory_protection/fittesting.html. Accessed November 14, 2018.

16. Occupational safety and health administration, national Institute for occupational safety and health. TB study funding announcement. *Fed Reg*. 1993:148.

17. Campbell C. Malaria. In: Hoeprich P, Jordan M, eds. *Infectious Diseases*. 4th ed. Philadelphia, PA: JB Lippincott; 1989.

18. Riedel S. Edward Jenner and the history of smallpox and vaccination. *SAVE Proc*. 2005;18:21–25.

19. Smallpox: Bioterrorism. Centers for Disease Control and Prevention Website. 2016. https://www.cdc.gov/smallpox/bioterrorism/public/index.html. Accessed November 14, 2018.

20. Centers for Disease Control and Prevention. Achievements in public health: hepatitis B vaccination—United States, 1982–2002. *MMWR*. 2002;51:549–552.

21. Sugerman D, Barskey A, Delea M, et al. Measles outbreak in a highly vaccinated population, San Diego, 2008: role of the intentionally undervaccinated. *Pediatrics*. 2010;125(4):747–755.

22. Centers for Disease Control and Prevention. Guidelines for preventing the transmission of Mycobacterium tuberculosis in health care facilities. *MMWR*. 1994;43:78–81.

23. Anderson R. Biological evaluation of carpeting. *Appl Microbiol*. 1969;18:180.

24. Shaffer J. Microbiology of hospital carpeting. *Health Lab Sci*. 1966;3:73.

25. Kates S, McGinley K, Larson E, et al. Indigenous multiresistant bacteria from flowers in hospital and nonhospital environments. *Am J Infect Control*. 1991;19:156.

26. Rhame F. The inanimate environment. In: Bennett J, Brachman P, eds. *Hospital Infections*. 4th ed. Philadelphia, PA: Lippincott-Raven; 1998.

27. *Multi-dose vials*. Centers for Disease Control and Prevention website; 2011. https://www.cdc.gov/injectionsafety/providers/provider_faqs_multivials.html. Accessed November 14, 2018.

28. Matera J. Sterile tattooing: improving quality of care. *Radiat Ther*. 2001;10:165–167.

29. SteriTatt. Sterile Tattooing for Precise Radiation Delivery; 2014. https://www.steritatt.com/. Accessed November 14, 2018.

30. Guide to thermoplastics for enhanced positioning and immobilization. CIVCO website. 2013. http://www.civcort.com/ro/resources/brochures/ThermoplasticsBrochure.pdf. Accessed November 14, 2018.

31. Jacoby G, Archer G. New mechanisms of bacterial resistance to antimicrobial agents. *N Engl J Med*. 1991;324:601.

32. Lemonick M. The killers all around. *Time September*. 1994;12:183–185.

33. Infection prevention and control standards. The Joint Commission website; 2014. https://e-dition.jcrinc.com/MainContent.aspx. Accessed November 14, 2018.

34. Hepatitis B questions and answers for health professionals. Centers for Disease Control and Prevention website; 2018. https://www.cdc.gov/hepatitis/hbv/hbvfaq.htm. Accessed November 14, 2018.

35. Occupational Safety and Health Administration, US Department of Labor. Occupational safety and health administration: occupational exposure to bloodborne pathogens, final rule 29 CFR Part 1910.1030. *Fed Reg*. 1991:64004–64182.

36. Immunization of health-care personnel. Recommendations of the Advisory Committee on Immunization Practices (ACIP). Centers for Disease Control and Prevention website; 2011. https://www.cdc.gov/mmwr/preview/mmwrhtml/00050577.htm. Accessed November 14, 2018.

37. Hepatitis D Information for Health Professionals. Centers for Disease Control and Prevention website; 2018. http://www.cdc.gov/hepatitis/HDV/. Accessed November 14, 2018.

38. Hepatitis E questions and answers for health professionals. Centers for Disease Control and Prevention website; 2018. http://www.cdc.gov/hepatitis/HEV/HEVfaq.htm. Accessed November 14, 2018.

39. Alper C, Kruskall M, Marcus-Bagley D, et al. Genetic prediction of nonresponse to hepatitis B vaccine. *N Engl J Med*. 1989;321:708–712.

40. Craven D, Awdeh Z, Kunches L, et al. Nonresponsiveness to hepatitis B vaccine in health care workers. Results of revaccination and genetic typings. *Ann Intern Med*. 1986;105:356–360.

41. *GlaxoSmithKline Biologicals. Twinrix [Package Insert]*. Rixensart, Belgium: GlaxoSmithKline Biologicals; 2011.

42. Centers for Disease Control and Prevention. General recommendations on immunization: recommendations of the advisory committee on immunization practices (ACIP). *MMWR*. 2011;60.

43. Adverse effects of vaccines: evidence and causality. The National Academies of Sciences, Engineering, and Medicine: Health and Medicine Division website; 2011. http://nationalacademies.org/HMD/Reports/2011/Adverse-Effects-of-Vaccines-Evidence-and-Causality.aspx. Accessed November 14, 2018.

44. Alter M. The detection, transmission and outcome of hepatitis C virus infection. *Infect Agents Dis*. 1993;2:155–156.

45. Hepatitis C questions and answers for health professionals. Centers for Disease Control and Prevention website; 2018. https://www.cdc.gov/hepatitis/hcv/hcvfaq.htm. Accessed November 14, 2018.

46. Taylor J. FDA device clearances: hepatitis C test, laser-assisted lipolysis, percutaneous support catheter. Medscape website. 2007. https://www.medscape.com/viewarticle/559882. Accessed November 14, 2018.

47. Centers for Disease Control and Prevention. Estimates of deaths associated with seasonal influenza—United States, 1976–2007. *MMWR*. 2010;59:1057–1062.

48. Thompson W, Shay D, Weintraub E, et al. Influenza-associated hospitalizations in the United States. *J Am Med Assoc*. 2004;292:1333–1340.

49. Thompson W, Weintraub E, Dhankhar P, et al. Estimates of US influenza-associated deaths made using four different methods. *Influenza Other Respi Viruses*. 2009;3:37–49.

50. Current and past flu seasons. Centers for Disease Control and Prevention website; 2018. https://www.cdc.gov/flu/about/season/index.html. Accessed November 14, 2018.

51. Mandatory flu vaccination. Johns Hopkins Medicine website; 2012. https://www.hopkinsmedicine.org/mandatory_flu_vaccination/faq.html. Accessed November 14, 2018.

52. Cawson R, et al. *Pathology: The Mechanism of Disease*. 2nd ed. St. Louis, MO: Mosby; 1989.

53. Prevention strategies for seasonal influenza in healthcare settings. Centers for Disease Control and Prevention website; 2013. http://www.cdc.gov/flu/professionals/infectioncontrol/healthcaresettings.htm. Accessed November 14, 2018.

54. Key facts about seasonal flu vaccine. Centers for Disease Control and Prevention website; 2018. https://www.cdc.gov/flu/protect/keyfacts.htm. Accessed November 14, 2018.

55. Centers for Disease Control and Prevention. Prevention of varicella: recommendations of the advisory committee on immunization practices (ACIP). *MMWR.* 2007;56.

56. Haley R. The development of infection surveillance and control programs. In: Bennett J, Brachman P, eds. *Hospital Infections.* Philadelphia, PA: Lippincott-Raven; 1998.

57. Guris D, Jumaan A, Mascola L. Changing varicella epidemiology in active surveillance sites—United States, 1995–2005. *J Infect Dis.* 2008;197:S71–S75.

58. Riley LE. Varicella-zoster virus infection in pregnancy; 2017. https://www.uptodate.com/contents/varicella-zoster-virus-infection-in-pregnancy. Accessed November 14, 2018.

59. Centers for Disease Control and Prevention. Recommendations of the Advisory Committee on Immunization Practices: varicella-zoster immune globulin for the prevention of chickenpox. *MMWR.* 1984;33:84–100.

60. Cheney K. Skin so sad: shingles shot. *AARP.* 2007;34.

61. Pertussis (whooping cough): causes & transmission. Centers for Disease Control and Prevention website; 2013. https://www.cdc.gov/pertussis/about/causes-transmission.html. Accessed November 14, 2018.

62. Centers for Disease Control and Prevention. Updated recommendations for use of tetanus toxoid, reduced diphtheria toxoid and acellular pertussis vaccine (Tdap) in pregnant women and persons who have or anticipate having close contact with an infant 12 months of age—Advisory Committee on Immunization Practices (ACIP). In: Practices ACoI, ed. 2011.

63. Centers for Disease Control and Prevention. *Epidemiology and Prevention of Vaccine-Preventable Diseases.* 13th ed. 2015. https://www.cdc.gov/vaccines/pubs/pinkbook/downloads/table-of-contents.pdf. Accessed November 14, 2018.

64. Pertussis: clinical features. Centers for Disease Control and Prevention website; 2015. https://www.cdc.gov/pertussis/clinical/features.html. Accessed November 14, 2018.

65. Tetanus: questions and answers. Immunization Action Coalition website; 2014. https://www.immunize.org/catg.d/p4220.pdf. Accessed November 14, 2018.

66. Diseases and conditions. Tetanus. Mayo Clinic website; 2017. https://www.mayoclinic.org/diseases-conditions/tetanus/symptoms-causes/syc-20351625. Accessed November 14, 2018.

67. Diphtheria. Centers for Disease Control and Prevention Website; 2016. https://www.cdc.gov/diphtheria/vaccination.html. Accessed November 14, 2018.

68. Diphtheria. US National Library of Medicine. National Institute of health website. https://medlineplus.gov/ency/article/001608.htm. Accessed November 14, 2018.

69. Braunstein H, Thomas S, Ito R. Immunity to measles in a large population of varying age significance with respect to vaccination. *Am J Dis Child.* 1990;144:296–298.

70. Wright L, Carlquist J. Measles immunity in employees of a multihospital health-care provider. *Infect Control Hosp Epidemiol.* 1994;15:8–11.

71. Smith E, Welch W, Berhow M, Wong V. Measles susceptibility of hospital employees as determined by ELISA. *Clin Res.* 1990;38:183.

72. Kim M, LaPointe J, Liu F. Epidemiology of measles immunity in a population of healthcare workers. *Infect Control Hosp Epidemiol.* 1992;13:399–402.

73. Weber D, Consoil C, Sickbert-Bennett E, Miller M, Rutala W. Susceptibility to measles, mumps, and rubella in newly hired (2006–2008) healthcare workers born before 1957. *Infect Control Hosp Epidemiol.* 2010;31:655–657.

74. Centers for Disease Control and Prevention. Prevention of measles, rubella, congenital rubella syndrome, and mumps, 2013: Summary recommendations of the advisory committee on immunization practices (ACIP). *MMWR.* 2013;62.

75. Centers for Disease Control and Prevention. Provisional CDC guidelines for the use and safety monitoring for bedaquiline Fumarate (Sirturo) for the treatment of multi-drug resistant tuberculosis. *MMWR.* 2013;62.

76. Tuberculosis: Data and Statistics. Centers for Disease Control and Prevention website; 2018. https://www.cdc.gov/tb/statistics/default.htm. Accessed November 8, 2018.

77. Latent tuberculosis infection: a guide for primary health care providers. U.S. Department of Health and Human Services website. https://www.cdc.gov/tb/publications/ltbi/pdf/TargetedLTBI.pdf. Accessed November 14, 2018.

78. Fact sheets: TB vaccine (BCG). Centers for Disease Control and Prevention website. https://www.cdc.gov/tb/topic/basics/vaccines.htm. Accessed November 14, 2018.

79. Haley C. Drug resistant TB. *Dallas.* Lecture at Baylor University Medical Center, February 25, 1994.

80. NC TB control program policy manual. Occupational Safety and Health Administration website. https://epi.publichealth.nc.gov/cd/lhds/manuals/tb/Chapter_VIII_2016.pdf. Accessed November 14, 2018.

81. Environmental control—clinical impact EC.02.06.01. Joint Commission website. https://www.jointcommission.org/topics/ec020601_clinical_impact.aspx. Accessed November 14, 2018.

82. Centers for Disease Control and Prevention. Guidelines for preventing the transmission of Mycobacterium tuberculosis in health-care settings. *MMWR.* 2005;54:1–141.

83. Centers for Disease Control and Prevention. Guidelines for preventing the transmission of tuberculosis in healthcare settings, with special focus on HIV-related issues. *MMWR.* 1990;38:1.

84. NIOSH TB respiratory protection program in healthcare facilities—administrator's guide. Centers for Disease Control and Prevention website. https://www.cdc.gov/niosh/docs/99-143/pdfs/99-143.pdf?id=10.26616/NIOSHPUB99143. Accessed November 14, 2018.

85. Williams W, CDC. CDC guidelines for infection control in hospital personnel. *Infect Control.* 1983;4:326–349.

86. Centers for Disease Control and Prevention. Controlling tuberculosis in the United States, recommendations from the American Thoracic Society, CDC, and the infectious disease Society of America. *MMWR.* 2005;54:1–81.

87. Dooley S, Castro K, Hutton M, et al. Guidelines for preventing the transmission of TB in helath-care settings, with a special focus on HIV related issues. Center for Disease Control, December 7, 1990.

88. The difference between respirators and surgical masks. Occupational Safety and Health Administration website. https://www.osha.gov/SLTC/respiratoryprotection/training_videos.html. Accessed November 14, 2018.

89. Respiratory protection for Healthcare Workers Training Video. U.S. Department of Labor, Occupational Safety and Health Administration website. https://www.osha.gov/SLTC/respiratoryprotection/training_videos.html#video. Accessed November 14, 2018.

90. Occupational Safety and Health Administration. OSHA Standard Interpretation. CFR 1910.134 subject: tuberculosis and respiratory protection. United States Department of Labor; 2004. https://www.osha.gov/pls/oshaweb/owadisp.show_document?p_table=INTERPRETATIONS&p_id=24895. Accessed November 14, 2018.

91. Centers for Disease Control and Prevention. American Thoracic Society: Targeted tuberculin testing and treatment of latent tuberculosis infection. *MMWR.* 2000;49:1–80.

92. Snider Jr D, Ceuthen G. Tuberculin skin testing of hospital employees: infection, "boosting," and two-step testing. *Am J Infec Control.* 1984;12:305–311.

93. Centers for Disease Control and Prevention. Transmission of Mycobacterium tuberculosis in a high school-based supervision of an isoniazid-rifapentine regimen for preventing tuberculosis—Colorado, 2011-2012. *MMWR.* 2013;62:805–809.

94. Centers for Disease Control and Prevention. Availability of an assay for detecting mycobacterium tuberculosis including rifampin-resistant strains and considerations for its use—United States, 2013. *MMWR.* 2013;62:821–824.

95. Centers for Disease Control and Prevention. Notes from the field: outbreak of tuberculosis associated with a newly identified mycobacterium tuberculosis genotype—New York City, 2010-2013. *MMWR.* 2013;62:904.

96. TB infection and TB disease L. Centers for disease control and prevention website. https://www.cdc.gov/tb/topic/basics/tbinfectiondisease.htm. Accessed November 14, 2018.

97. Andrade A, Flexner C. Progress in pharmacology and drug interactions from the 10th CROI. *Hopkins HIV Rep.* 2003;15:11.

98. Center for Disease Control and Prevention. The revised recommendation for HIV testing of adults, adolescents, and pregnant women in healthcare settings. *MMWR.* 2006;55:1–17.

99. Preexposure prophylaxis for the prevention of HIV infection in the United States-2017 Update. Center for Disease Control and Prevention. https://www.cdc.gov/hiv/pdf/risk/prep/cdc-hiv-prep-guidelines-2017.pdf. Accessed October 2, 2019.

100. Centers for Disease Control and Prevention. Public Health Service guidelines for the management of healthcare worker exposures to HIV and recommendations for postexposure prophylaxis. *MMWR.* 1998;47:1–33.

101. Centers for Disease Control and Prevention. Update: provisional Public Health Service recommendations for chemoprophylaxis after occupational exposure to HIV. *MMWR.* 1996;45:468–472.

102. Centers for Disease Control and Prevention. Updated US Public Health Service guidelines for the management of occupational exposures to HBV, HCV, and HIV and recommendations for postexposure prophylaxis. *MMWR.* 2001;50(RR-11):1–52.

103. Post-exposure prophylaxis. AIDs.org website. http://aids.gov/hiv-aids-basics/prevention/reduce-your-risk/post-exposure-prophylaxis/. Accessed November 14, 2018.

104. Centers for Disease Control and Prevention. Updated US Public Health Service guidelines for the management of occupational exposure to HIV and recommendations for postexposure prophylaxis. *MMWR.* 2005;54:1–17.

105. Bell D. Occupational risk of human immunodeficiency virus infection in health-care workers: an overview. *Am J Med.* 1997;102:9–15.

106. Vidmar L, Poljak M, Tomazic J, et al. Transmission of HIV-1 by human bite. *Lancet.* 1996;347:1762–1763.

107. Kudar D, Henderson D, Struble K, et al. Updated US Public Health Service guidelines for the management of occupational exposures to human immunodeficiency virus and recommendations for postexposure prophylaxis. *Infect Control Hosp Epidemiol.* 2013;34:875–892.

108. Beekman S, Fahey B, Gerberding J, et al. Risky business: using necessarily imprecisee casualty counts to estimate occupational risk of HIV-1 infection. *Infect Control Hosp Epidemiol.* 1990;11:371–379.

109. Kozoil D, Henderson D. Risk analysis and occupational exposure to HIV and HBV. *Curr Opin Infect Dis.* 1993;6:506–510.

110. Mejicano C, Maki D. Infections acquired during cardiopulmonary resuscitation: estimating the risk and defining strategies for prevention. *Ann Intern Med.* 1998;129:813–828.

111. Owens D, Nease R. Occupational exposure to human immunodeficiency virus and hepatitis B virus: a comparative analysis of risk. *Am J Med.* 1992;92:503–512.

112. Updated U.S. Public Health Service Guidelines for the management of occupational exposures to HBV, HCV, and HIV and recommendation for postexposure prophylaxis. Centers for Disease Control and Prevention website. https://www.cdc.gov/mmwr/preview/mmwrhtml/rr5011a1.htm. Accessed November 14, 2018.

113. Centers for Disease Control and Prevention. Surveillance for occupationally acquired HIV infection - United States, 1981–1992 Personal communication update with CDC National AIDS Clearinghouse, 1995. *MMWR.* 1995;41:823–825.

114. Sharps Injury Prevention. American Nurses Association Website. https://www.nursingworld.org/practice-policy/work-environment/health-safety/safe-needles/. Accessed November 14, 2018.

115. Bloodborne infectious diseases: HIV/AIDS, hepatitis B, hepatitis C: emergency needlestick information. Centers for Disease Control and Prevention website. https://www.cdc.gov/niosh/topics/bbp/. Accessed November 14, 2018.

116. United States Department of Health & Human Services. PHS guideline for reducing human immunodeficiency virus, hepatitis B Virus, and hepatitis C virus transmission through organ transplantation. *Public Health Rep.* 2013;28:247–343.

117. HIV testing. centers for disease control and prevention website.. https://www.cdc.gov/vitalsigns/hiv-testing/. Accessed November 14, 2018.

118. How New York State's new HIV testing law affects consumers. New York State Department of Health website. http://www.health.ny.gov/diseases/aids/providers/testing/law/q_and_a_for_consumers.htm. Accessed November 14, 2018.

119. Laboratory testing for the diagnosis of HIV infection: updated recommendations. Centers for Disease Control and Prevention, Association of Public Health Laboratories website. https://stacks.cdc.gov/view/cdc/23447. Accessed November 14, 2018.

120. Occupational Safety and Health Administration. Occupational exposure to bloodborne pathogens: Final rule 29 CFR Part 1910:1030 Federal Register 1991;56:64003-64182 Revised 2001 In: Labor Do, ed.2001:5317-25.

121. Equal Employment Opportunity Commission. *Equal Employment Opportunity Commission: A Technical Assistance Manual on the Employment Provisions (Title 1) of the Americans with Disabilities Act.* Washington, DC: Equal Employment Opportunity Commission; 1992.

11

Pharmacology and Drug Administration

Charles Michael Washington, Heather Mallett

OBJECTIVES

- Recognize common terminology and nomenclature associated with medications.
- Give an example of a trade name and a generic name of a medication typically used in radiation oncology.
- Identify the various classifications of drugs.
- Identify drug resources.
- List the Six Rights of Medication Administration.
- Describe various contrast media.
- Discuss the methods of drug administration and their advantages and disadvantages.
- Prepare intravenous drugs for injection.
- Describe documentation procedures related to drug administration.
- Define abbreviations commonly used in drug administration.

OUTLINE

KEY TERMS

Allergic reactions
Anaphylactic shock
Barium sulfate
Chemical name
Contraindications
Contrast media

Cumulative effect
Drug
Drug interactions
Dyspnea
Excretion
Extravasation

Generic name
High osmolality
Hypovolemia
Idiosyncratic effects
Infiltration
Intradermal
Intramuscular
Intravenous
Ionic contrast media
Low osmolality
Medication
Metabolism

Nonionic contrast media
Parenteral
Pharmacodynamics
Pharmacokinetics
Pharmacology
Phlebitis
Standard precautions
Subcutaneous
Syncope
Tolerance
Urticaria
Venipuncture

In radiation oncology, the radiation therapist must have a general knowledge of pharmacology and specific details of each patient's medication history to provide competent patient care. The radiation therapist interacts closely with patients on a daily basis and may be the first person to notice adverse reactions or unusual symptoms when they appear. With a basic understanding of medications and their common side effects, the therapist can distinguish an expected side effect from an adverse reaction that requires medical intervention.

Although the administration of drugs is not a primary role of the radiation therapist, it is a crucial part of overall patient care.[1] The therapist may assist with the administration of medications specific to radiation therapy, such as contrast media during the simulation procedure, anesthetics, or intravenous (IV) fluids. To effectively care for the patient, it is pertinent that radiation therapists remain current with information about the drugs commonly used in their department.

This chapter discusses general principles of pharmacology and medication administration. Its purpose is not to provide detailed information about specific drugs but to identify the essential prerequisite knowledge the therapist must have to administer drugs safely to patients. Various aspects of assessment, preparation, and administration of medications are discussed. Finally, the legal aspects of medication administration are considered.

DRUG LEGISLATION AND STANDARDIZATION

Drug regulation and standardization has a long history in the United States. Before the early 1900s, medications and remedies were virtually unregulated and sold by a variety of individuals, both qualified and unqualified. These products were not required to have ingredients listed, and many people, especially infants and children, became injured, addicted, or died as a result of ingestion.[2] In 1906, the first US law regarding drug regulation, the Federal Pure Food and Drug Act, was passed and required drug companies to declare on the package label the presence of certain drugs identified as dangerous and perhaps addictive.[2] Over the years, additional legislation was passed, including the Federal Food, Drug, and Cosmetic Act of 1938 and the Controlled Substance Act of 1971, which govern the labeling, availability, and dispensation of all drugs in the United States.[3] Today, drugs are heavily controlled, and this evolution toward stringent regulation has been beneficial, resulting in safer and more effective drugs.[4] However, the development, testing, and subsequent US Food and Drug Administration (FDA) approval of new drugs is an expensive and lengthy process, requiring 10 to 15 years for completion, with costs exceeding US$1.2 billion.

DRUG NOMENCLATURE AND TERMINOLOGY

A drug is any substance that alters physiologic function? with the potential for affecting health. A medication is a drug administered for its therapeutic effects. The terms *drug* and *medication* are often used synonymously; however, there is a simple difference in these terms that

should preclude medical professionals from using them interchangeably. All medications are drugs, but not all drugs are medications.

Drug nomenclature is the systematic naming of a drug and is an important topic to discuss because it affects our ability to communicate about medications. In the majority of circumstances, drugs have three names: (1) a chemical name, (2) a generic name, and (3) a trade name. A drug's chemical name depicts the chemical composition and molecular structure of the drug and is rarely used in literature, as it can be quite long and complex. A drug's generic name (also referred to as nonproprietary or official name) is assigned by the original manufacturer in collaboration with the Food and Drugs Board and Nomenclature Committee. It is important to note that the generic name of a drug is never capitalized. A drug's **trade name** (also referred to as brand or proprietary name) is a copyrighted name given to the drug by the manufacturing and marketing company (and approved by the FDA) and is used in official publications.[5,3,6] Several manufacturers may produce the same generic drug but call that drug by different brand names; for example, acetaminophen has at least 30 trade names (Tylenol, Paracetamol, Paramol, Panadol, Capol, etc.). Radiation therapists and all health professionals need to easily access drug name information. The most commonly used sources of drug information are the *Physicians' Desk Reference, United States Pharmacopoeia,* and specific drug packaging. The *Physicians' Desk Reference* gives the accepted uses, side effects, contraindications, and doses for available drugs.

Chemical name: *N*-acetyl-*para*-aminophenol
Generic name: Acetaminophen
Brand name: Tylenol

PHARMACOLOGIC PRINCIPLES

Pharmacology is the science of drugs, including the sources, chemistry, and actions of drugs. The way in which drugs affect the body is called pharmacodynamics. Each drug has a unique molecular structure enabling it to interact with a specific enzyme or a corresponding cell type. The drug attaches itself to a target site in the body called the *receptor site* in the same way that two puzzle pieces interlock. The combined effect alters the behavior of the targeted cells or enzyme and causes physiologic changes in the patient.

The way that drugs travel through the body to their appropriate receptor sites is called pharmacokinetics. There are four basic pharmacokinetic processes: absorption, distribution, metabolism, and excretion (Fig. 11.1).[4] Many individual factors cause these processes to vary within each patient; therefore, the effectiveness of and reaction to a drug may differ greatly from one patient to another.

Absorption

Absorption is defined as the movement of a drug from its site of administration into the blood.[4] Factors affecting drug absorption include: the route of entry, the pH of the recipient environment, blood flow, the

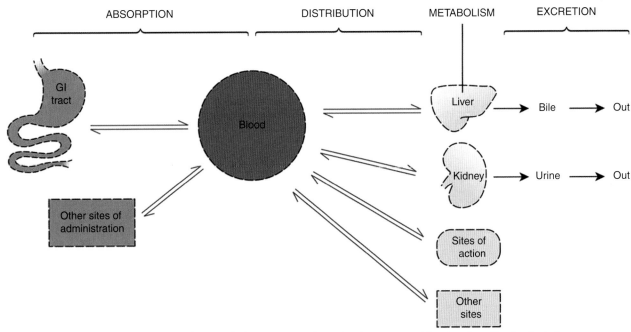

ABSORPTION   DISTRIBUTION   METABOLISM   EXCRETION

Fig. 11.1 The four basic pharmacologic processes: absorption (movement of the drug from its site of administration into the blood), distribution (drug movement from the blood to the tissues and cells), metabolism (enzymatically mediated alteration of drug structure), excretion (movement of drugs and their metabolites out of the body).[4] Dotted lines represent membranes that must be crossed as drugs move throughout the body. (From Burchum JR, Rosenthal LD. *Lenhe's Pharmacology for Nursing Care*. 9th ed. St. Louis, MO: Elsevier; 2016.)

solubility of the formula, and the drug's interaction with body chemicals while in transit.[3,6]

Distribution

Distribution is defined as the movement of drugs throughout the body, which is determined by three factors: blood flow to tissues, the ability of a drug to exit the vascular system, and the ability of a drug to enter cells. In general, as a drug travels through the circulatory system to its receptor site(s), it will connect with the molecular structure for which it was designed. Some drugs may need to bind with a certain protein or cross specific membranes to produce the desired response. The passage of drugs into the central nervous system (CNS) is tightly regulated by the blood-brain barrier (BBB), and only lipid-soluble drugs or those that have a transport system can cross. The developing fetus is also protected from many drugs, as the membranes of the placenta separate maternal and fetal circulation; however, the membranes of the placenta do not constitute an absolute barrier to the passage of drugs, and many drugs cross the placental villi and affect the fetus.

> Distribution of a drug is controlled by three factors: blood flow to the tissue, the ability of a drug to exit the blood vessel, and the capability of a drug to enter the cell.

Metabolism

"Metabolism, also referred to as biotransformation, is the process by which the body alters the chemical composition of a substance."[3] The liver detoxifies nearly all foreign substances entering the body, including drugs, and changes them into inactive, water-soluble compounds that can be excreted by the kidneys.[3] The breakdown of drugs into waste matter may also involve chemical processes and enzymatic reactions in the blood and other organs such as the gallbladder, lungs,

and intestines. If drugs accumulate or react synergistically with other substances in the body, or the organs are damaged, metabolism and excretion of the drugs may be difficult.[6]

Excretion

The body removes drugs and their by-products in a variety of ways; however, the most important organ for drug excretion is the kidney. Although the kidneys account for the majority of drug excretion, there are nonrenal routes of drug excretion including: respiration, saliva, breast milk, bile, and sweat.[4] The rate of excretion depends on the body's systems, the drug's half-life, and concentration in the tissues.

VARIABLES THAT AFFECT PATIENT RESPONSE

The caregiver must consider a variety of factors that may affect a patient's response to drugs. The following section discusses several of these factors, which also affect the optimal dose prescribed by the physician.

Patient-Related Variables

Age. Drug therapy in young children and the elderly requires careful individualization of the dosage, although for different reasons.

In children and infants, the organs are still developing, and smaller doses are required when compared with adults. Children may be hypersensitive to medications, so administration of minimal doses and close monitoring of their responses is the usual process required to decrease the likelihood of a troublesome event occurring. Determination of dosages using body weight is safer than using age, but this calculation remains imprecise because of the child's immature metabolism.[7] Administration of the prescribed dose to children can be challenging because they often have difficulty swallowing pills, spit out liquid preparations, reject suppositories, and fight injections.

Older adults may also require dose modifications, as age often decreases the efficiency of organs, which influences pharmacokinetic processes. Their circulation slows, enzymes are depleted, sensitivities develop, absorption becomes impaired, and the liver and kidneys may no longer detoxify efficiently.[5,3,6] In addition, elderly patients commonly take multiple medications that may interact negatively. Elderly patients should be monitored to ensure that the dosage of the medications they are taking is appropriate.

Weight and Physical Condition. Doses are based on the average 150-lb, healthy adult. The dose must be adjusted for heavier or lighter patients, and body mass must be considered because obesity or excessive thinness can affect circulation and organ efficiency. Liver or kidney damage, electrolyte imbalance, poor circulation, nutritional deficiency, infection, and other physiologic disorders should also be considered in the determination of the optimal dosage.[3]

Gender. Women have a lower average body weight than men and metabolize drugs differently. Women's hormone profiles and the amount and distribution of their body fat also differ greatly from those of men and influence the dosage of medications needed. The difference in fluid balance, muscle mass, and gastric fluids are all considerations when determining the optimal dosage in different genders. In women, pregnancy can also complicate the prescription and administration of drugs, as many drugs cross the placental barrier and affect the fetus.

Personal and Emotional Requirements. The effects of drugs on an individual can be unpredictable, as each person responds to drugs differently. For example, some people can ingest large amounts of caffeine and be minimally affected, whereas others cannot tolerate even small amounts of caffeine. Because of the inherent differences experienced when taking a drug, an individualized evaluation and approach is needed for each patient. Patients with negative attitudes or anxiety often require higher levels of sedation than do calm patients with positive outlooks. Healthcare professionals must relate to patients as individuals and be alert to each patient's responsiveness to the drugs administered.

Drug-Related Variables: Nontherapeutic Reactions

An important difference exists between unpleasant but expected side effects and adverse drug responses or complications. Side effects are expected reactions to medication; complications are *unexpected* reactions to medications that range from mild to severe.[3] In radiation therapy, the treatment, contrast media used for simulation, and various medications taken before and after treatment can combine to produce toxicities and discomfort for the patient.

Allergic Reactions. Allergic reactions result from the mobilization of the immune system in response to a foreign substance that the body recognizes as harmful. In a drug-related allergic reaction, the immune system recognizes the drug (to which the patient has already been sensitized) as an antigen and produces immunoglobulin E (IgE), a special class of antibody, in response. IgE circulates throughout the blood and binds to mast cells or basophils, where it triggers the release of inflammatory chemicals such as histamine.[8] Histamines cause blood vessels to leak fluid as part of the inflammatory response. The inflammatory mediators released cause contraction of smooth muscle and dilation of capillaries, resulting in the clinical symptoms of an allergic reaction, which may range from a mild rash to life-threatening anaphylactic shock. Once an allergy develops, subsequent exposures to that drug cause increasingly severe symptoms. Penicillin is a common allergenic drug. In radiation oncology, the greatest risk of an allergic reaction comes with administration of iodinated contrast media. The radiation therapist must know the emergency procedure to follow if the patient has an adverse reaction.

Tolerance. Tolerance occurs if the body adapts to a particular drug and requires increasing doses to achieve the desired effect. For example, the body develops a tolerance for narcotics/opioids when they are used for long periods of time and can develop a physical dependence, but this does not mean the individual is addicted.[9,10] Opioids given to cancer patients can include morphine and oxycodone (OxyContin) to treat moderate to severe pain. If overused, antibiotics become increasingly less effective by killing not only harmful bacteria, but also the beneficial ones. Antibiotics may also leave the patient susceptible to further infection. Bacteria that survive antibiotic use can mutate within the patient into strains that are resistant to the antibiotic during subsequent use.[6] The patient may then need to switch to a different drug if the first loses its effectiveness.

Cumulative Effect. A cumulative effect develops if the body is unable to detoxify and excrete a drug quickly enough or if too large a dose is taken.[11] Unless the dosage is adjusted, the drug accumulates in the tissues and can become toxic. Digoxin, for example, is a medication used to slow the heart rate and must be prescribed carefully because of the potential of causing a cumulative effect. The cumulative effect could cause a dangerous decrease in a patient's heart rate. In some cases, the cumulative effect is desirable, such as with medications prescribed to prevent depression.

Idiosyncratic Effects. Idiosyncratic effects are inexplicable and unpredictable symptoms caused by a genetic defect within the patient.[11] These symptoms are completely different from the expected symptoms and may occur the first time a drug is given.

Dependence. Drug dependency can result from extensive exposure to a drug or a compulsion to continue taking a drug to feel good or to avoid feeling bad. Most persons who become drug dependent do so because of physiologic or psychological problems. There are many cancer patients who fear taking pain medications because of a fear of dependency or addiction to these medications. It is important for the doctors and nurses to fully explain the rationale and benefit of taking these medications.

Drug Interactions. Drug interactions occurring between two or more drugs, or a combination of food and drugs, can create or produce positive or negative effects in patients. This interaction of drugs may result in synergism, which increases a drug's effects; interaction can also result in antagonism, which decreases a drug's effects. For example, alcohol and sedatives taken together produce a toxic synergistic reaction, whereas an antiemetic given with anesthesia can be therapeutic. Older adults commonly take many different medications, and the interactions of these drugs can cause a toxic shock situation. The person administering medications should never mix drugs without consulting a drug compatibility chart or checking with a pharmacist.

PROFESSIONAL DRUG ASSESSMENT AND MANAGEMENT

Assessment of the Patient's Medication History

Although the healthcare professional may educate, evaluate, and help the patient regarding drug use and compliance, the patient is ultimately responsible for self-medication. If the patient is forgetful, confused, depressed, taking several medications simultaneously, or has inadequate diet and exercise habits, it may be difficult to differentiate between poor compliance and additional medical needs. For example, impaired liver or kidney function may indicate toxicity from drug overuse, lack of improvement from a prior disease, poor drug distribution because of sluggish circulation, an allergic reaction, damaged organs from alcohol or drug abuse, or a negative response from drug interaction. Assessment is further complicated because the person recording the medical history must rely on the patient's verbal description and inadequate recollection.

Despite these difficulties, the therapist must assess the patient's drug use during the patient evaluation by documenting every drug that the patient is taking (including alcohol) and looking especially for overuse and underuse of prescribed drugs.[12,7,5,3,6,13] An accurate medication history is essential to proper diagnosis and treatment (see "Legal Aspects").

Application of the Seven Rights of Medication Administration

To prevent medication errors and harm, it is important that healthcare professionals systematically and conscientiously follow the seven rights[11,7,6] of medication administration. Table 11.1 identifies the seven rights of medication administration and describes how they are carried out.

Implementation of Proper Emergency Procedures

If a drug emergency occurs, the therapist (and all healthcare professionals) must follow proper emergency procedures. Each hospital and clinic has its own emergency codes and procedures. At the onset of an emergency, the therapist's first duty is to summon help by "calling a code." The therapist should know the location of emergency supplies contrast reaction kits in the simulator room and a nearby code cart. Therapists must also know the proper way to administer oxygen and perform cardiopulmonary resuscitation.

Recognizing symptoms and executing the appropriate procedure are required skills for therapists.[11] If a reaction develops while a contrast medium is administered, the therapist must stop the procedure immediately and call a code and/or the oncologist. The patient must *never* be left alone.

Types of emergencies that the radiation therapist is most likely to encounter are as follows:

- *Asthma attack,* which produces tightness or pressure in the chest, mild to moderate shortness of breath, wheezing, and coughing.
- *Pulmonary edema,* which produces abnormal swelling of tissue in the lungs because of fluid buildup with symptoms of rapid, labored breathing; cough; and cyanosis.
- *Anaphylactic shock* produces symptoms such as nausea, vomiting, diarrhea, urticaria, shortness of breath, airway obstruction, and vascular shock.
- *Cardiac arrest* is when the heart stops beating suddenly, and respiration and other body functions stop as a result.

The ability to handle medical emergencies improves with hands-on experience. All radiation therapists should seek extensive education in this area.

DRUG CATEGORIES RELEVANT TO RADIATION THERAPY

Drugs are classified into convenient groups for the sake of conformity, standardization, research, replication, and quality assurance. Oncology patients often have specific symptoms or indications for certain types

TABLE 11.1	Application of The Seven Rights of Medication Administration
Right patient	To properly identify the right patient, the healthcare professional should use two identifiers. Acceptable identifiers include: patient's full name, date of birth, assigned identification number, telephone number, hospital wristband (for inpatients), or another person-specific identifier according to The Joint Commission (TJC).[21] It is important that the therapist is vigilant when confirming patient identity because it is common for patients to mishear or nod in acknowledgment when a name, other than theirs, is called.
Right medication	Although a physician is responsible for prescribing medication, the therapist should perform a triple check of the medication's label before administration. These checks should occur when retrieving the medication, when preparing the medication, and before administering medication to the patient. It is also important to check the written order against the patient's chart, the drug label, and the pharmacy. TJC requires the use of medical reconciliation to help prevent medication errors.
Right dose	The therapist does not bear the primary responsibility for choosing the correct dose; however, as with all caregivers, the therapist must continually monitor for errors. Even if the physician or nurse (in the case of standing orders) has prescribed the drug, the therapist involved should *always* check the dosage[5,3,6] and verify that it is within the appropriate range for the patient and medication.
Right time	Administer drugs punctually, as the administration of a drug at the wrong time can have serious consequences, including poor absorption, fluctuation of blood or serum levels, increased side effects, or, in the case of contrast media, less than optimal diagnostic capability. Therapists should verify the schedule of the medication with the order and check the last dose of medication given to the patient.
Right route	Some drugs can be administered in more than one way; other drugs should be given only by a particular route. If a drug is administered incorrectly, the consequences may range from minor injury to death. The route of entry should be verified before administering and should not deviate from the route specified in the order.
Right documentation	Each time a medication is administered, it must be documented. Documentation should be punctual and should never be done before administration of the medication.
Right reason/indication	The therapist should confirm the rationale for using the ordered medication by considering the patient's history and reason he/she is taking the medication.

of drugs. In radiation therapy, for example, patients may require certain drugs (e.g., antidiarrheals and antiemetics) to relieve the symptoms of the therapy and other drugs (e.g., contrast media) to facilitate the pretherapy simulation and planning.

Pharmacologists classify drugs in the following ways: according to the effects of the drug on particular receptor sites or body systems, in terms of the symptoms that the drug relieves, or by its chemical group.[11,7,13] These categories overlap; often a single drug can be used to treat multiple conditions, and several different drugs can be used to treat a single condition. Table 11.2 identifies main drug categories and their purpose, provides examples and an explanation of how specific drugs are frequently encountered in radiation oncology, and provides information about the drug category:

CONTRAST MEDIA

In radiation oncology, many patients require contrast agents during simulation to improve the visibility of soft tissues and other areas with low natural contrast. Because the administration of contrast media is within the radiation therapist's scope of practice, it is important to discuss the specifics of contrast media.

Types of Contrast Agents

The two basic categories of contrast agents are negative (radiolucent) and positive (radiopaque).[11,7,13] Radiolucent agents have low atomic numbers and, as a result, are easily penetrated by x-rays. The spaces containing these compounds (usually in the form of gases) appear dark on radiographs and computed tomography (CT) scans. Air and carbon dioxide are the most common negative contrast media. Air alone can sometimes provide sufficient contrast for radiography of the larynx, other parts of the upper respiratory system, and the gastrointestinal system.

Radiopaque agents have high atomic numbers and absorb x-ray photons; thus, the spaces filled with these agents appear opaque (white) on a CT scan or radiograph. For some procedures, negative and positive contrast media are given together to demonstrate certain internal structures. For example, diagnostic tests of the stomach and large intestine usually use barium sulfate combined with air or carbon dioxide as the contrast media.

Heavy Metal Salt

Barium sulfate, a heavy metal salt, is the most commonly used contrast agent for gastrointestinal tract examinations.[11,7,13] This contrast agent is delivered orally or rectally in an aqueous (water-based) suspension. Barium sulfate coats the lining of the alimentary organs, and because of its high atomic number (Z = 56), it effectively absorbs x-rays, generating extremely high levels of contrast. Although barium is a heavy metal and its water-soluble compounds may be toxic, the low solubility of barium sulfate protects the patient from absorbing harmful amounts of metal. However, hazards and inconveniences do exist with the administration of barium sulfate. Barium sulfate requires additives to facilitate ingestion and prevent clumping, and it must be concentrated to coat the organs; however, if it is too thick, barium sulfate will not flow easily and may be difficult to swallow. Barium sulfate can irritate the colon and cause cramping. In rare cases, it may cause an excess of fluid volume in the blood, leading to hypervolemia or pulmonary edema. Barium sulfate is excreted with the feces but can cause constipation or peritonitis if used in patients with a gastrointestinal perforation. If preexisting conditions contraindicate the use of barium sulfate, oncologists may prescribe water-soluble agents instead.

Iodinated Contrast

As with barium sulfate, iodine has been proven to be one of the best contrast elements for imaging. Iodine-based contrast materials are typically injected into a vein (IV) and enhance the visualization of vascular organs and structures.

Iodinated contrast agents are typically classified based on their chemical composition and propensity to influence osmotic activity. Contrast agents may be ionic or nonionic (based on how they dissociate in a solution) and high or low osmolality (based on number of particles in a solution).[14] Ionic agents with high osmolality dissociate into a cation (positively charged atom) and an anion (negatively charge particle) when in a solution and displace water from the extravascular space to the intravascular space, causing an increase in intravascular pressure and dilution of the normal intravascular constituents. Because of this behavior in a solution, ionic high-osmolality contrast agents are more toxic and carry a greater risk of inducing an allergic reaction when compared with their nonionic, low-osmolality counterparts, which remain intact in a solution and have less propensity to influence fluid balance. Most of the conventional, older compounds are highly toxic ionic iodine agents; however, less toxic nonionic, low-osmolality agents have been developed over time. These agents are equally effective for imaging but are much more expensive than ionic agents, so some oncology departments reserve them for allergy-prone patients. Three common nonionic contrast agents are iopamidol, iodixanol, and iohexol. Iodine has a high atomic number (Z = 53), allowing it to absorb x-rays, which usually appear light gray to white on a CT scan or radiograph.

> The atomic number (Z) of a substance is based on the number of protons in the nucleus. The higher the Z number, the more likely it is to absorb x-rays during a radiographic exposure or CT scan.

Some contrast agents have characteristics of ionic and nonionic agents (called *ionic dimers*); they have low osmolality because the molecules are larger and do not have an osmotic (water-moving) effect, but they split and are therefore still ionic.[11,13] An example of this type of contrast agent is sodium meglumine ioxaglate.

Iodinated contrast media are generally viscous, especially at room temperature. This property causes discomfort to the patient during injection, although the discomfort can be eased somewhat by preheating the solution to body temperature. Some iodinated contrast media are so viscous that they are best delivered using a power injector.

Most iodinated contrast media, including the aforementioned agents, are aqueous (water soluble); however, contrast media can also be oil based. Oil-based agents do not dissolve in water and, therefore, stay in the body longer. They are unstable and decompose if exposed to light or heat. Although historically used for bronchography, myelography, and lymphangiograms, oil-based contrast agents are infrequently used today.[7]

ADMINISTRATION OF CONTRAST MEDIA

Each imaging procedure will likely require a unique approach in terms of type and delivery of contrast media. For example, when rapid systemic distribution is desired, bolus or power injection of contrast can be used. Direct injection of contrast media allows for optimal imaging of the organ or joint before the media are absorbed into the bloodstream and later excreted. If the intestinal tract is imaged, ionic contrast media may cause increased fluid in the intestines and increased intestinal contractions (peristalsis), thereby producing a better image.

TABLE 11.2 Main Drug Categories and Their Purpose

Drug Category	Purpose	Examples	Explanation
Analgesic	Relieves pain	Narcotics: morphine, codeine, meperidine (Demerol) Nonnarcotics: acetaminophen (Tylenol), aspirin	Narcotics are better at alleviating stronger pain; however, are associated with adverse side effects and are addictive.
Anesthetic	Suppresses the sensation of feeling by acting on the CNS.	General anesthetics: thiopental (Pentothal), Local anesthetics: procaine (Novocain) Lidocaine (Xylocaine)	General anesthetics depress the entire central nervous system, rendering the patient unconscious for major surgery. Local anesthetics act only on the nerves in a small area. For example, lidocaine is injected before taking a skin biopsy to numb the area.
Antianxiety drugs	Help calm anxious patients and relieve muscle spasms.	Lorazepam (Ativan), diazepam (Valium), Xanax (alprazolam), and chlordiazepoxide (Librium)	Antianxiety drugs can be used concurrently with radiation therapy treatments.
Antibiotics	Suppress the growth of bacteria	Erythromycin, penicillin, and tetracycline (broad-spectrum antibiotics)	Patients may develop respiratory tract infections, urinary tract infections, or any bacterial infection, which may be treated with antibiotics
Anticoagulants	Prevents blood from clotting too quickly	Warfarin (Coumadin) Heparin	Used to prevent blood clots, which reduce the risk of stroke and heart attack.
Anticonvulsants	Inhibit or control seizures	Clonazepam (Klonopin), phenytoin (Dilantin)	Clonazepam is administered orally to prevent petit mal seizures. Dilantin can be administered orally or parenterally to treat grand mal seizures.
Antidepressants	Affect neurotransmitters, which are involved in the control of mood and in other functions, such as eating, sleep, pain, and thinking	Fluoxetine (Prozac), Paxil, Lexapro, and sertraline (Zoloft). Other antidepressants, such as amitriptyline (Elavil), act on the serotonin and norepinephrine receptors	Affect communication within the cells of the brain.
Antidiarrheal	Control the gastrointestinal (GI) distress	Diphenoxylate (Lomotil) and loperamide (Imodium)	GI distress is typically from bacterial infections.
Antiemetic	Prevent nausea and vomiting	prochlorperazine (Compazine), promethazine (Phenagran), and ondansetron (Zolfran)	Most effective when given before symptoms develop. These are often used to alleviate side effects of radiation therapy and chemotherapy.
Antifungal	Treat fungal infections, such as yeast or thrush.	Ketoconazole (Nizoral), Diflucan, or nystatin	May be given to patients with head and neck cancer who have oral thrush.
Antihistamines	Treat allergies but can also be found in cold remedies and motion sickness tablets	Diphenhydramine (Benadryl), promethazine, and chlorpheniramine (Chlor-Trimeton), Claritin	Often administered to patients before surgery, as many drugs trigger allergic reactions.
Antihypertensives	Lower blood pressure	Clonidine (Catapres), metoprolol (Lopressor), and reserpine (Serpasil)	Hypertension can become a factor in many medical procedures.
Antiinflammatory drugs	Reduce inflammation	Ibuprofen (Motrin), piroxicam (Feldene), and naproxen (Naprosyn)	Do not work as quickly as corticosteroids; however, they may have fewer side effects.
Antineoplastic	Chemotherapy drugs	Alkylating agents, antimetabolites, mitotic inhibitors	Can be extremely aggressive and cause adverse side effects because chemotherapy drugs affect the entire system.
Contrast media	Enhance the visibility of internal tissues for imaging	Iodine, barium, air	Oncologists depend on these agents to pinpoint target areas for radiation treatment planning.
Corticosteroids	Reduce inflammation	Dexamethasone (Decadron) and hydrocortisone (Solu-Cortef).	Can be used to treat adrenal deficiency
Diuretics	Remove fluid from the cells	Acetazolamide (Diamox), chlorothiazide (Diuril), and furosemide (Lasix).	Used to treat edema and are often used with antihypertensives to lower blood pressure.
Hormones	Augment endocrine secretions	Estrogen (Premarin) to females; methyltestosterone to males	Sex hormones can also be used to treat neoplastic conditions in the opposite sex; that is, estrogens can be given to males and methyltestosterone can be given to females.
Narcotics	Relieve pain	Codeine, meperidine, oxycodone, methadone, and morphine.	Federally controlled substances that relax the central nervous system.
Narcotic antagonists	Used to counter the effects of narcotic drugs	Narcan and naltrexone	Narcotic antagonists bind to the opioid receptors so that the narcotic cannot bind to the opioid receptor.
Sedatives	Calm anxious patients and relax the central nervous system	Secobarbital (Seconal) and pentobarbital (Nembutal), lorazepam, diphenhydramine, and midazolam (Versed)	Can induce sleep or unconsciousness.
Skeletal muscle relaxants	Relax skeletal muscles	Cyclobenzaprine (Flexeril), baclofen, carisoprodol, and diazepam (Valium)	Treat musculoskeletal conditions such as fibromyalgia, tension headaches, and myofascial pain syndrome.

To increase efficiency and decrease toxicity of contrast media, it is important for the patient to comply with preparation instructions, which may include fasting and enemas. Compliance leads to diagnostic-quality images produced with the least possible contrast media. An accurate patient history helps to determine the optimal dose, prevent unnecessary adverse reactions, and determine the correct route so that the distribution and metabolism of the contrast media enhance the desired area.

Table 11.3 shows some of the common procedures performed with contrast media.

Taking an accurate patient history before the administration of contrast is extremely important. Most departments have some type of a contrast media administration history form. Here are some questions that are typically found on the history form:

- Have you ever had a CT scan or other examination requiring a contrast agent?
- If yes, did you have an allergic reaction following the use of a contrast agent?
- Did you ever have an allergic reaction to any medication? If so, list the details.

TABLE 11.3   Common Diagnostic Imaging Procedures That Use Contrast Media

Procedure	Route of Administration	Contrast Agent[a]
Cardiovascular	Intravascular	Diatrizoate meglumine, 60% Diatrizoate sodium, 50% Iopamidol, 61.2% Iohexol
Arthrography	Direct injection	Diatrizoate meglumine, 60% Sodium meglumine ioxaglate Air
Bronchography	Intratracheal catheter	Propyliodone oil
Cholangiography	Intravenous (IV)	Iodipamide meglumine, 10.3% Diatrizoate sodium, 50%
Cholecystography	Oral	Ipodate sodium, 500 mg Iopanoic acid, 500 mg
Computed tomography	IV injection or infusion	Ioversol, 68% Diatrizoate meglumine, 60% Iohexol
Cystography	Urinary catheter	Iothalamate meglumine, 17% Iothalamate sodium, 17% Diatrizoate meglumine, 17%
Discography	Direct injection	Diatrizoate meglumine, 60% Diatrizoate sodium, 60%
Esophagraphy	Oral	Barium sulfate, 30%–50%
Hysterosalpingography	Cervical injection	Iothalamate meglumine, 60%
Lymphography	Direct injection	Ethiodized oil
Magnetic resonance imaging	IV injection	Gadolinium and derivatives
Myelography	Intrathecal (lumbar puncture)	Iohexol
Pyelography	Instillation via catheter	Diatrizoate meglumine, 20% Diatrizoate sodium, 20% Methiodal sodium, 20%
Sialography	Catheter	Iohexol
Splenoportography	Percutaneous injection Catheter	Diatrizoate meglumine, 60% Diatrizoate sodium, 50% Sodium meglumine ioxaglate
Upper and lower gastrointestinal examination	Oral/rectal	Barium sulfate
Urography and nephrography	IV injection	Diatrizoate meglumine, 60% Iodamide meglumine, 24% Sodium meglumine ioxaglate Iohexol
Venography	IV injection	Ioxaglate meglumine Ioxaglate sodium Iohexol

[a]Some departments prefer to use nonionic contrast media on all of their patients in an effort to reduce patient reactions.

- Do you have any other allergies? If so, list the details.
- Do you have a history of asthma, hay fever, or lung disease?
- Do you have kidney disease?
- Are you taking the medications metformin (Glucophage), glyburide and metformin (Glucovance), rosiglitazone maleate and metformin HCl (Avandamet), or Metaglip?
- Are you pregnant, or is it a possibility that you are?
- List all medications you are currently taking.

Because the kidneys are responsible for eliminating contrast material after IV administration, it is important to assess kidney function before injection to minimize the risk of contrast-induced nephrotoxicity. Kidney function is typically assessed by blood work, specifically blood urea nitrogen (BUN), creatinine, and glomerular filtration rate (GFR) values. Urea nitrogen and creatinine are both waste products excreted by the kidneys, and if the levels are high, it may indicate impaired kidney function. The normal values in adults for BUN are approximately 7 to 20 mg/μL and 0.6 to 1.4 mg/dL for creatinine.[15,16,7,17] GFR is considered by medical professionals to be the best measure of kidney function. It is a test that estimates how much blood passes through the glomeruli (small microscopic filtering mechanisms) each minute, which reflects how well the kidneys are cleaning the blood. The normal GFR value in adults is approximately 120 mL/min/1.73 m². Low GFR values may indicate decreased kidney function. Each radiation oncology department will have written policies for blood work to be performed before IV contrast administration and how to proceed in cases of patients with inadequate kidney function. See Chapter 21 for more information on power injectors and the administration of contrast media.

Diabetic patients often require additional guidelines before IV contrast administration. Metformin is an antihyperglycemic agent and is indicated for individuals with type 2 diabetes mellitus and is primarily excreted by the kidneys. Administration of intravascular-iodinated contrast media to a patient taking metformin may pose a risk of metformin-associated lactic acidosis in patients with renal failure. The American College of Radiology Manual on Contrast Media suggests that patients discontinue metformin 48 hours before administration of intravascular-iodinated contrast. Each department will have a policy outlining the appropriate procedure.[15]

Distribution and Excretion of Contrast Media

After peripheral IV injection, contrast travels to the heart, the pulmonary circulation, and then reaches the central arterial system, which circulates the contrast media throughout the body.[18] As contrast circulates in the body, it is diluted by the blood and disperses as it moves downstream through the circulatory system.[18] IV contrast diffuses rapidly, and 70% of the injected dose is cleared from the blood plasma within 2 to 5 minutes, and 90% to 100% of the dose is excreted over the subsequent 24 hours.[14] The kidneys are responsible for excretion of IV contrast; generally less than 1% of contrast administered is excreted extrarenally.[14] It is important to note that the BBB largely prevents contrast media from being distributed into the CNS.[14] However, if there is a breakdown or disruption in the BBB, as in the case of high-grade brain tumors, contrast is able to penetrate the CNS.

Patient Reactions to Contrast Media

Injection of iodinated contrast media does carry a risk, and up to 54% of injected patients experience some sort of reaction,[14] which may range from mildly uncomfortable to severe. Severe, life-threatening reactions occur in only 0.1% to 0.4% of patients.[14] Some adverse reactions can be attributed to the large shift in fluid from extravascular to intravascular space that occurs with the injection of intravascular

contrast, particularly ionic, high-osmolality solutions, which may inundate the vascular system, causing **hypervolemia**. The osmotic action of ionic molecules can also cause dramatic fluctuations in kidney function, which may be counteracted by administration of IV fluids.

Iodinated contrast agents are also toxic to the kidneys. The American College of Radiology lists the following as risk factors for nephrotoxicity: age greater than 60 years, history of renal disease, history of hypertension requiring medical care, diabetes mellitus, and currently taking metformin. There is also an increased risk of adverse effects in patients with allergies, asthma, sickle cell anemia, thyroid disease, multiple myeloma, cirrhosis, and coronary disease.[14] These patients should be carefully evaluated and monitored.

> Patient history can be helpful in determining adverse effect on administering contrast media, such as: age greater than 60 years, history of renal disease, history of hypertension requiring medical care, diabetes mellitus, and the use of metformin for diabetes.

Iodinated contrast agents can also elicit allergic reactions ranging from minor to severe (anaphylactic shock) in susceptible patients. If a patient is going to react to contrast media, the reaction usually happens very quickly (i.e., within a few minutes of administration of the compound).

Classifications of the severity of adverse reactions[11] seen in contrast media administration are as follows:

- *Minor reactions* are the most common clinical manifestation and do not generally require intervention beyond routine patient care and monitoring: nausea, retching, and mild vomiting, urticaria (hives).
- *Moderate reactions* are those that require some form of treatment but involve no serious danger for the patient, and response to treatment is usually rapid: fainting, chest or abdominal pain, headache, chills, severe vomiting, dyspnea, extensive urticaria, and edema of the face and/or larynx.
- *Severe reactions* are uncommon but may be fatal in the absence of intervention. These reactions require intensive and rapid treatment: syncope, convulsions, pulmonary edema, life-threatening cardiac arrhythmias, cardiac or respiratory arrest.
- *Death.*[7]

> In evaluating a patient for a potential contrast reaction, five assessments should be made: (1) How does the patient look? (2) Can the patient speak? (3) How is the patient's breathing? (4) What is the patient's pulse? (5) What is the patient's blood pressure? For more information, see American College of Radiology at https://www.acr.org/-/media/ACR/Files/Clinical-Resources/Contrast_Media.pdf. Accessed October 19, 2019.[22]

The therapist must be ready to take immediate action if any of the previously mentioned symptoms manifest. Patients suffering a severe allergic reaction to contrast are typically treated with a combination of antihistamines, steroids, and epinephrine, although departments should have a written policy regarding the management of allergic reactions to contrast.

ROUTES OF DRUG ADMINISTRATION

Drugs may be administered via a variety of routes. General information regarding the numerous routes of administration and the effects of each can be found in clinical textbooks.[1] The following four administration routes are particularly important for radiation therapy and CT simulation imaging:

- Oral
- Mucous membrane
- Topical
- Parenteral

The remainder of this chapter discusses these methods of drug administration and related patient care issues. Table 11.4 lists a summary of the routes of administration and some of the advantages and disadvantages of each method.

Oral Administration

The oral route of administration is safe, simple, and convenient for both the patient and caregiver. Although it is the most popular method from a standpoint of convenience, oral administration has the disadvantage of being slower in onset and less potent than parenteral administration.[11,7,5,3,6,13] There is also less risk of infection for oral administration when compared with other routes. Examples of drugs given by mouth are fluoxetine (Prozac), Compazine, and dexamethasone (Decadron). Some patients are unable to take oral preparations because of vomiting or nausea, unconsciousness, intubation, required fasting before tests or surgery, difficulty swallowing, or refusal to cooperate. The latter two occurrences are especially common with children. Some drugs, such as insulin, are ineffective when given orally because they are destroyed by the secretions of the gastrointestinal tract.[22]

Whenever oral medications are given, the caregiver should do the following:

1. Wash hands.
2. Read the label and medication order before and after preparing the dose. The drug must also be reviewed by the pharmacy.
3. Identify the patient.
4. Check for allergies.
5. Assess the patient by checking and recording vital signs.
6. Prepare the medicine accurately without touching it directly.
7. Confirm the order with the physician.
8. Give water or other more palatable liquid, such as ice chips, orange juice, or a strong-tasting chaser, if indicated.
9. Elevate the patient's head if the patient is supine.
10. Observe and ensure that the medicine is swallowed and not aspirated.
11. Discard medication paraphernalia.
12. Rewash hands.
13. Confirm that medication was administered.
14. Record the medication administration in the patient's chart.

Mucous Membrane Administration

Some drugs cannot be given orally because gastric secretions inactivate the medications or because the drugs have a bad taste or odor, damage teeth, cause gastric distress, or the patient is unable to take the drug by mouth. If a drug has one of these potential side effects, it can be prepared and applied to various mucous membranes to achieve the desired effect. Methods of introducing drugs through the mucous membrane include the following:

- Insertion of suppositories into the rectum or vagina.
- Inhalation if a medicated mist.
- Direct application by swabbing.
- Gargling.
- Irrigating the target tissue by flushing with sterile or medicated fluid.

Medications can also be dissolved under the tongue for sublingual administration, a common method of nitroglycerin delivery for cardiac issues. All these methods have a systemic effect, although some affect the system more rapidly than others. Regardless of the route used, the person administering the drug must never compromise sterility by touching the drug directly.

Topical Administration

Topical administration involves placement of the drug directly on the skin. Topical applications are used for antiseptics applied preceding injections, ointments, lotions, and transdermal patches. Transdermal patches can be used to dispense medication slowly over a period of time. Scopalamine, for example prevents nauseal and vomiting, and fentanyl which is an opiod analgesic and can be dispensed via a transdermal patch. Hormones can also be

TABLE 11.4	**Routes of Administration**	
Route	**Advantages**	**Disadvantages**
ORAL	• Easy administration • Inexpensive • Economic • Safe	• Slower absorption than intravenous administration • Absorption may be highly variable • Difficult for some patients to swallow • May irritate gastric mucosa • Some medications are deactivated by gastric enzymes • Requires cooperative, conscious patients
MUCOUS MEMBRANE Rectum Sublingual	• Often preferred for pediatric patients • Rapidly absorbed • Enters blood directly	• Inconvenient • Can irritate mucous membranes • Small dose limit • Should not be used for immunosuppressed patients
TOPICAL	• Easy • Noninvasive • Lower risk of side effects	• Very slow absorption
PARENTERAL Subcutaneous Intramuscular Intravenous	• Gastrointestinal tract avoided • Rapid onset of action • Preferred in emergency situations and unconscious patients • Dependable and reproducible effects	• Injection site painful • Drug could cause local tissue damage • Increased risk of adverse effects • Suitable injection site may be hard to locate • High cost • Irreversible

dispensed through transdermal patches such as estrogen. If the caregiver is administering topical drugs, gloves should be worn to prevent absorption of the medication and introduction of infectious agents to the patient.

Parenteral Administration

Parenteral administration means that the medication bypasses the gastrointestinal tract. Taken literally, this includes the topical and some mucous membrane routes, but the colloquial meaning of the word *parenteral* is "by injection."

A drug administered parenterally is absorbed rapidly and efficiently. Because the drug is not affected by digestive enzymes, the dose is usually smaller than if given orally.[7,13] Medications may be administered parenterally in the following situations:

- The drug would irritate the alimentary tract too much to be taken orally.
- A rapid effect is needed, such as during an emergency.
- Drugs need to be dispensed through an IV during a period of time.
- The patient is unconscious or otherwise unable to take oral medications. For example, if the patient is fasting before surgery or tests, medication can be given by injection.

Parenteral administration carries with it the danger of infection from piercing the skin and an increased risk of unrecoverable error because of rapid absorption. Injections also cause genuine fear in some patients. Long-term parenteral therapy can also damage injection sites.

> The most common **parenteral** routes are subcutaneous (SC), intramuscular (IM), and intravenous (IV).

Parenteral administration is categorized by the depth of the injection and location of the injection site (Fig. 11.2). The following are the four most common parenteral routes[13]:

- **Intradermal**: a shallow injection between the layers of the skin.
- **Subcutaneous (SC)**: a 45- or 90-degree injection into the SC tissue just below the skin.
- **Intramuscular (IM)**: a 90-degree injection into the muscle used for larger amounts of mediation or a quicker systemic effect.
- **IV**: an injection directly into the bloodstream that provides an immediate effect.

Less common parenteral routes of administration include:

- Intrathecal administration: medications injected directly into the spinal canal, such as with chemotherapeutic agents.
- Intratracheal administration: medications are administered directly into the trachea.
- Intracranial administration: medications are administered directly into the brain.
- Catheterization, which includes urinary catheterization.[19]

INTRAVENOUS ADMINISTRATION

Of the four parenteral routes, therapists most often use the IV route, which places a drug directly into a vein. IV injection results in the most rapid onset of drug action. Obtaining IV access, or venipuncture, is within the scope of practice for radiation therapists in most states[1] and is best learned by hands-on experience. Every therapist should practice preparation of both the patient and IV supplies, use the appropriate equipment, and properly place an IV while maintaining a caring bedside manner.

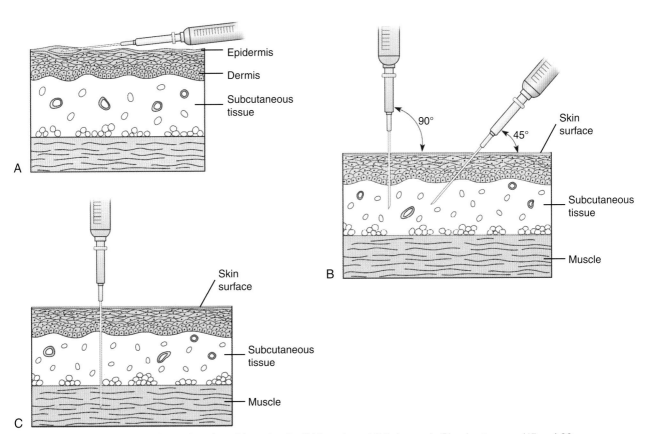

Fig. 11.2 Comparison of angles of insertion for (A) intradermal (15 degrees), (B) subcutaneous (45 and 90 degrees), (C) intramuscular (90 degrees) injections.

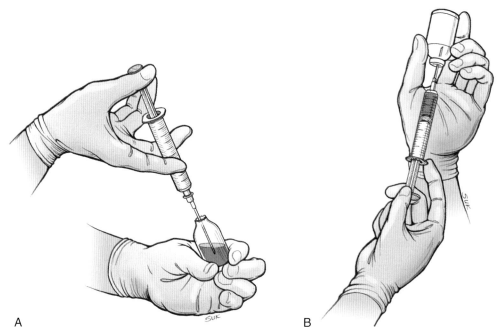

A   B

Fig. 11.3 (A) This drawing shows the way to remove the medication from an ampule. The therapist removes the medication by pulling back on the plunger of the syringe. The therapist should be careful not to contaminate the needle when inserting and removing the needle from the ampule. (B) This drawing shows the removal of medication from a vial. The rubber stopper must be cleaned with alcohol before the needle is inserted into the vial. The same amount of air must be injected into the vial as liquid will be withdrawn to equalize the pressure in the vial.

When a patient requires ongoing IV therapy, a catheter is inserted into a peripheral vein, where it can remain for a number of days. The advantage of having ongoing access is that the vein's integrity is broken only at the time of insertion. This catheter can be used for either intermittent medications, continuous infusions, or a combination of both. If continuous access is not required, the caregiver can disconnect the patient from the infusion using a heparin lock. The heparin lock has a self-seal for when it is not in use.

The therapist administering drugs through an IV route must never leave the patient alone during the procedure and must continuously monitor the patient.

Different methods of IV administration serve different purposes. The safest method is continuous infusion, in which the medication is mixed with a large volume of IV solution and given gradually over a period of time. Second, a drug can be "piggybacked" (added) onto the main IV line by means of a special valve so that the medication can be administered intermittently at prescribed levels.[5,3,6,13] During drug administration, the volume of IV fluid administered is lowered. This process usually takes less than 1 hour, after which the volume is restored to the initial level. It is important to flush the catheters with saline before and after contrast injection.

A third method of IV injection is a bolus, or push, of a concentrated dose of medication injected by a syringe directly into the vein or through the IV port. This method requires diligent observation of the patient because the effect is rapid and can be irreversible.

Two major types of IV injections pertain to radiation therapists: drugs requiring dilution and drugs requiring delivery by IV bolus. Most contrast media, if not given orally, are injected by bolus or power injection. Drugs that are diluted or solutions for the maintenance of fluid levels are administered slowly by IV drip.

Administration of Bolus and Power Injections

Certain medications, including contrast media, must be administered at full strength. If the patient has an IV line that is running a continuous infusion, the therapist must temporarily stop the infusion while the bolus is injected to avoid mixing the solutions. The IV line should remain in place because radiopaque materials are highly toxic and reactions can happen quickly. The IV line allows the patient to receive immediate remedial treatment should a adverse reaction occur.

Bolus and power injection requires the same preliminaries discussed in regard to other routes of administration (i.e., checking the medication, identifying the patient, and washing the hands). Proper preparation of the dose of contrast is required. IV contrast medication comes packaged in ampules or vials, each of which has its own specific requirements for use. An ampule contains a single dose of medicine; the tip is snapped off, and the drug is drawn into a syringe through a filter needle (Fig. 11.3A). A vial has a rubber stopper, and the needle is inserted through that stopper to draw out the medicine (Fig. 11.3B) (usually multidose vials are not used because of possible contamination, but if the vial contains more than one dose, a new needle should be used and the stopper of the vial must be wiped with alcohol before every use). The vial should be dated and initialed at the time of use. It should be discarded within 24 hours of initial use.

If the medication is not directly delivered by a vein, an IV port (Fig. 11.4A and B) may be used. The injection port of the catheter should be wiped with alcohol, or the heparin lock should be flushed with sterile saline, and then the drug may be slowly injected into the port. The correct rate for injecting the drug should be specified on the package or in the medication order. If the medication enters the vein too quickly, the body may go into speed shock, a severe, life-threatening reaction caused by the toxicity of the drug. After injection, the port should be again wiped with alcohol, or the heparin lock should be flushed and refilled with heparin solution. Only then can the IV flow be restored.

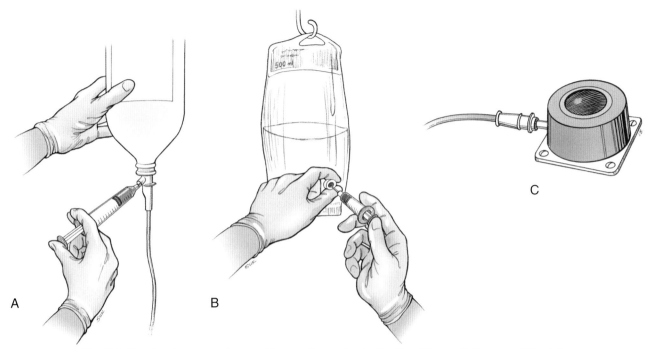

Fig. 11.4 This drawing demonstrates adding medication to a bottle (A) or (B) bag of intravenous (IV) solution. (C) Chemotherapy is often administered through a vascular access port.

Chemotherapy is often administered through a different type of vascular access port such as the Hickman, Groshong, Port-A-Cath, and PAS Port[6] (Fig. 11.4C).

Intravenous Infusion and Venipuncture Equipment

Before the actual venipuncture or injection takes place, the healthcare professional must gather all the necessary equipment. Interruption of the procedure to find missing equipment is extremely unprofessional and erodes the patient's confidence in the caregiver. The IV equipment can be prepared with the tubing capped and ready to attach before the venipuncture is performed or after the IV port is in place. The timing of the preparation depends on institutional policy or the physician's orders.

In the case of an IV drip, required equipment includes IV tubing with a clamp on it, the vacoliter or plastic drip bag, a stand on which to hang the bag of solution, an IV filter, and a meter to measure the flow rate. The most common place for sterility to be compromised is in the two ends of the tubing; neither the end going into the sterile solution nor the end connecting with the IV catheter should *ever* be touched, even with gloved hands.[12] If either end is inadvertently touched, it must be sterilized before use or discarded and replaced.

> Take time to review the procedure with the patient, answering questions and discussing signs and symptoms of intravenous (IV)-associated complications. Complications may include, swelling at the insertion site, redness around the area, and pain associated with IV fluid administration.

IV equipment varies according to the drug and dose. The equipment tray should include a tourniquet, antiseptic swabs, gloves, a syringe, a needle, cotton balls, the correct drug, and adhesive bandages. Any catheters, tubing, drip bottles, poles, and monitors required should also be in place before the procedure begins.

The type of medication and physical characteristics of the patient determine which instrument should be used for IV injection. For a one-time injection of 30 mL or less, a regular needle (i.e., 18 to 20

gauge, depending on the viscosity of the drug and size of the patient's veins) and a syringe should suffice. An infusion that takes place during a longer period of time requires a butterfly set, which is a special steel needle attached to two plastic "wings" taped to the skin. This butterfly set anchors the needle in the vein.

The use of a power injector for contrast administration should be through a flexible plastic cannula. A 20-gauge or larger catheter is more effective for flow rates of 3 mL/sec or higher. A large forearm vein is the preferred venous access site for power injections. This form of rapid administration requires careful preparation to ensure there is no air in the syringe and pressure tubing. Before injection, the catheter should be checked for venous backflow, and if there is no backflow, a saline test flush should be done.[6] Caution must be taken when preparing the power injector apparatus to ensure a reduced risk of extravasation during the injection of contrast.

Whenever the infusion requires a large volume of fluid or must be administered over an extended period of time, a plastic catheter can be inserted into the vein. Because the tubing is flexible and soft, it allows the patient to move around, and it is less irritating than a rigid metal needle. Two kinds of venous catheters exist: one is a narrow tube inserted through a hollow needle, and the other has the needle through the tube. The through-the-needle catheter is generally longer and thinner and can be inserted deeper into the vein. This type of catheter is commonly used for antineoplastic drugs. After the catheter is in place and taped down, the needle is removed.

Dosage, Dose Calculation, and Dose Response

Medication charts list standard measurements (i.e., metric or apothecary), their abbreviations, and recommended doses for commonly used medicines. Table 11.5 lists common abbreviations used for prescribing medications.[7,3] Healthcare personnel must invariably calculate individual doses for their patients if the standard packaging differs from the amount ordered. To calculate the quantity ordered, the therapist or nurse must multiply or divide the dose required by the packaged amount (make sure the two are in the same unit of measure). The math should *always* be double-checked by a second person.

TABLE 11.5 Common Abbreviations Used for Prescribing Medications

Abbreviation	Meaning
a.c.	Before meals
b.i.d.	Twice a day
c̄	With
Et	And
gm	Gram
gtt	Drop(s)
h	Hour
h.s.	At bedtime
IM	Intramuscular
IV	Intravenous
mg	Milligram
mL	Milliliter
OD	In the right eye
OS	In the left eye
p.c.	After meals
p.o.	By mouth
p.r.n.	As necessary
q.d.	Each day
q3h, q4h, etc.	Every 3 hours, every 4 hours, and so on
qh	Hourly
qid	Four times each day
qod	Every other day
Stat	At once
SQ/SC	Subcutaneous
tid	Three times a day

Doses for children should be calculated according to the child's weight or body surface area. The latter is more accurate because it also takes into account the child's height and body density.[3]

Although the specifics of dose calculation are beyond the scope of this chapter, a good nursing text will explain the way to compute the correct dose.

Whenever drugs are administered through an IV, the dosages must be calculated according to the total volume of fluid the patient receives (except in the case of a bolus injection). This calculation must be carefully monitored because flow and absorption rates can fluctuate. Also, the drug must be given in the correct dilution, at the appropriate rate, and in the correct amount. Controlling the dosage in single injections or piggyback deliveries is easier than in long-term IV treatment.

Many factors can affect the delivery rate of an IV injection. The flow can be interrupted by a kink in the tubing, a clot in the needle or catheter, the needle tip pressing against the vein wall, or a problem at the site of entry. The drip rate may depend on the patient's absorption rate, which always varies greatly from one person to another. Sudden fluctuations in flow rates happen frequently because of mechanical problems with the equipment or because the patient dislodges the catheter. All these factors influence the accuracy of delivery whenever drugs are infused IV.

Initiation of Intravenous Therapy

Patient Education. Before any IV drugs are administered, therapists should identify themselves to the patient, assess the patient's condition, and explain the procedure. Assessment involves the following:

- Taking the patient's allergy history (or reading the patient's chart if a history has already been taken).
- Taking the patient's blood pressure for a baseline reading.
- Determining whether the patient has had any medication that affects blood clotting.
- Asking the patient (not the nurse) whether the patient has been fasting.[11,3.6,13]

The physician is responsible for explaining the reason the procedure is needed; the therapist can ease any anxiety the patient may have by describing the process and answering questions. Iodinated contrast media can produce adverse reactions within minutes after administration, so the therapist must ask the patient to report any symptoms that he or she may experience before administering the drug. It may help the patient to know some common sensations related to the medication and whether they are serious.

Site Selection for Venipuncture

The site chosen for venipuncture depends on the drug to be administered and the length of time that the IV line will be in place (Fig. 11.5A). The large antecubital vein in the arm is convenient for drawing blood or for injecting a single dose or viscous solution, but this vein is inappropriate for long-term IV therapy because it hinders the patient's mobility. The best choices for long-term infusion include sites above the anterior wrist (lower cephalic, accessory cephalic, and basilic veins) or veins on the posterior hand (basilic, metacarpal, and cephalic veins)[3] (Fig. 11.5B). If the patient is right-handed, putting the IV line into the left arm allows the patient to maintain use of the dominant arm.

Certain contraindications at a specific venipuncture site mean that a different site should be chosen. These contraindications include scar tissue or hematoma that necessitates injection above the site, infection, skin lesions that could introduce infection into the bloodstream, burns, collapsed veins, or veins too small for the chosen gauge of the needle. Special techniques apply if a patient has rolling veins, has phlebitis, is on dialysis, or is extremely obese. If the patient is taking blood thinners, extra compression is needed.

Venipuncture Technique

The venipuncture may be performed after the preliminaries, such as collection of supplies, patient identification, informing the patient of the procedure, and patient assessment, are completed. The procedure[13] is as follows:

1. Position the patient. The patient should be sitting or lying down, and the arm should be placed in a relaxed position. The arm may need to be anchored to an arm board if the patient is extremely active.
2. Determine the best site for the venipuncture.
3. Wash your hands and put on gloves. All standard precautions should be followed because of potential contact with body fluids. These precautions include utilizing proper personal protective equipment, properly handling needles, and disposing of used equipment into the proper receptacle. Many institutions use syringes with retractable needles, which reduces the risk of a needle stick.
4. Apply the tourniquet tightly so that it can be removed with one hand. The tourniquet should be approximately 2 to 4 inches above the puncture site. Never leave a tourniquet on for more than 2 minutes.
5. It may be necessary to tap or stroke the vein or to have the patient make a fist to enhance distention of the vein (Fig. 11.6).
6. Cleanse the skin with an antimicrobial solution (tincture of iodine 2%, 10% povidone-iodine, 70% isopropyl alcohol, or chlorhexidine) in small concentric circles outward to a radius of

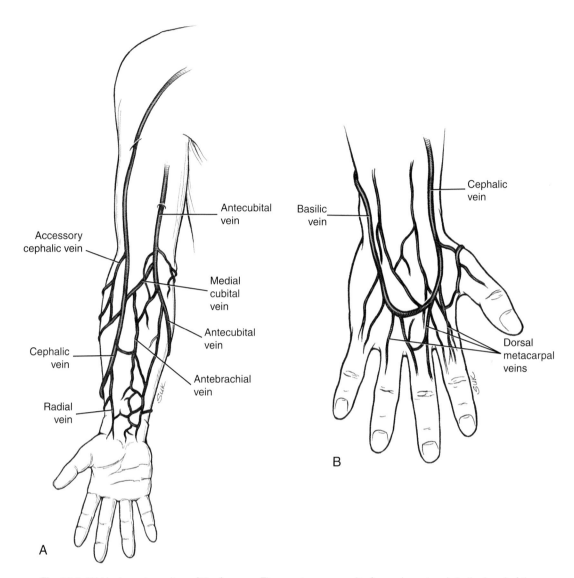

Fig. 11.5 (A) Venipuncture sites of the forearm. The most common site for venipuncture is in the bend of the elbow, an area called the antecubital fossa. The medial cubital vein is usually selected, as it is very superficial and easier to see and feel. (B) Venipuncture sites of the wrist and hand.

approximately 2 inches. Do not touch the cleansed area with a nonsterile object. If local anesthetic is used, inject it intradermally at this time.

7. Verify that you have the proper medication.
8. Anchor the vein firmly below the puncture site with the thumb of your free hand. This will prevent the vein from "rolling."
9. Insert the needle parallel to the vein, bevel side up, at a 30-degree angle, and then flatten the needle to a 10- to 15-degree angle. If the angle is too shallow, the needle will skim between the skin and vein; if the angle is too deep, the needle will penetrate the posterior wall of the vein and cause bleeding into the tissues. When blood flows back into the syringe or hub of the cannula, the needle is in the vein. Allowing the blood to fill the hub before attaching tubing ensures that air bubbles are not trapped in the line.
10. Remove the needle from the catheter. Release the tourniquet and push the catheter deeper into the vein and up to the hub, if possible.
11. Attach IV tubing and place an antiseptic swab or patch over the puncture site, and fix the catheter in place with adhesive tape or, if injecting contrast media with a butterfly needle and syringe,

proceed with the injection after securing the butterfly needle in place.
12. If the venipuncture is unsuccessful, withdraw the needle or catheter and immediately apply light pressure to the insertion site and remove the tourniquet.

Infusion of Medication

The procedure[11,7,5,6] for starting a drip infusion after venipuncture has been performed, and an IV line is in place is as follows:

1. Wash your hands.
2. Double-check the patient's name. Assess the patient. Ask the patient about allergies to drugs.
3. Triple-check the physician's orders against the solution label.
4. Check the bag or vacoliter for an expiration date, signs of contamination (such as discoloration, cloudiness, or sediment), and cracks or leaks.
5. Put on gloves and follow all standard precautions according to institutional policy.
6. Remove the metal cap and rubber diaphragm from the bottle or bag without touching the rubber stopper.

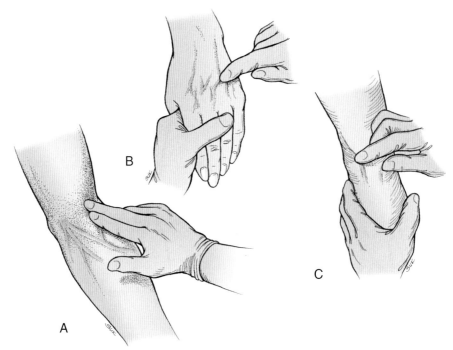

Fig. 11.6 Techniques to distend veins include tapping the vein (A), gently stroking the vein (B), and having the patient make a fist (C).

7. Close the clamp on the tubing, attach the inline filter, and insert the spike of the drip chamber into the rubber stopper without touching the sterile end.
8. Invert the fluid container and hang it on an IV pole 18 to 24 inches above the vein.
9. Remove the cap covering the lower end of the tubing, release the clamp, and allow the fluid to flow through the tube to get rid of air bubbles (if air is left in the tubing, it will be forced into the vein). Close the clamp. Attach the tubing to the IV line.
10. Monitor the flow until the desired rate is established.
11. Monitor the condition of the patient.
12. Discard used materials and gloves according to institutional policy.
13. Rewash hands.
14. Record the medication procedure in the patient's chart.

Hazards of Intravenous Fluids

Perhaps the biggest challenge of administering drugs IV is to get the drug into the vein without introducing foreign microorganisms that can cause infection. Individuals should avoid touching fluid ports, needle, ends of tubing, or any other part of the equipment through which germs could pass into the bloodstream. Diligent observation of the venipuncture site allows the caregiver to recognize symptoms of sepsis at its earliest stage.

IV infusion involves unique hazards. Any swelling around the injection site accompanied by cool, pale skin and possibly hard patches or localized pain is a sign of infiltration.[13] This can occur if the catheter is improperly placed or dislodged resulting in fluid seeping into adjacent SC tissue. Infiltration can also occur if the IV bottle is hung too high and the hydrostatic pressure is so great that the vein cannot absorb the fluid quickly enough, causing it to saturate the surrounding tissue. If the therapist mistakenly misses the vein and injects a vesicant drug into the tissues surrounding the vein, the result is a similar condition called extravasation, which is not only painful, but can cause severe tissue damage.[5,3,16] The difference between an infiltration and

extravasation is the type of medicine or fluid that has escaped the vein into the SC tissue.

Other hazards of IV infusion include an allergic reaction to the drug, an air embolism caused by failure to eliminate air bubbles in the equipment, a metabolic or an electrolyte imbalance, edema caused by the dressing being too tight at the site or too much fluid, speed shock from too rapid a delivery, drug incompatibility, thrombus (blood clots), and phlebitis. Phlebitis can be prevented if the needle is a small enough gauge that the blood can flow around it. A "keep vein open" drip keeps the blood from clotting at the site; likewise, the heparin in a heparin lock prevents the injection site and bloodstream from developing clots.

Sudden increases in fluid volume introduced by IV equipment can accidentally occur. If the patient is extremely frail or has a head trauma, a sudden overload can be fatal. Any time fluid is infused too quickly, the excess can collect in the lungs, thereby causing pulmonary edema. Rapid infusion can also result in an overdose of the medication. Too little fluid may result in dehydration or an insufficient dose of the required medication. These are only a few of the reasons that monitoring IV lines closely is crucial.

Discontinuation of Intravenous Therapy

Because the potential for contamination is so high in IV therapy, the infusion set should be changed every 24 to 48 hours. If IV therapy must be continued for a longer period, changing to a new venipuncture site may be necessary, depending on the condition of the original site. Most of the drugs that therapists administer are infused over a short period of time, through a single site.

To remove the IV line, the therapist must gather the following supplies: sterile gauze pads, gloves, and tape. After the patient has been properly identified and informed of the procedure, these steps should be followed to discontinue IV therapy[1,3]:
1. Wash your hands.
2. Clamp off the IV tubing and remove the tape holding the catheter in place.

3. Put on gloves and follow standard precautions according to institutional policy.
4. Apply a folded gauze sponge over the insertion site and hold it down with your thumb. Grasp the needle or catheter and withdraw in one smooth motion.
5. Before taping the gauze, inspect the site.
6. Tape the gauze pad in place and elevate the patient's arm. Apply direct pressure for 1 to 2 minutes.
7. Dispose of the used IV materials properly.
8. Rewash the hands.
9. Record the appropriate information in the patient's chart.

LEGAL ASPECTS

When considering legal aspects, the radiation therapist's scope of practice must be reviewed. The scope of practice for radiation therapists includes the delivery of radiation to treat disease, providing patient care (including comfort, dignity, and education) monitoring, and documentation.[1] Increasingly, the practice of venipuncture and the administration of IV medications and contrast media are also included.

The therapist may not legally diagnose, interpret images, reveal test results to patients or family members, prescribe drugs, admit or discharge patients, or order tests, as those duties belong to the physician. The therapist, like every healthcare professional, is legally required to report incidents or errors and is allowed to act without liability in an emergency if no other care is available (the Good Samaritan laws).

> Good Samaritan laws provide basic legal protection for those who assist a person who is injured or in danger. In all 50 states and the District of Colombia, Good Samaritan laws protect the person who acts in good faith in assisting an injured or ill stranger from liability if unintended consequences result from their assistance.

The therapist is legally liable for administering competent treatments and accurately communicating with the patient. The two most common complaints leading to malpractice suits in radiology and oncology are false-negative or false-positive diagnoses of fractures or cancers and the misadministration of contrast media.[20] The oncologist does not bear these risks alone. The radiation therapist is part of the team and on the frontline of patient care.

Although radiation oncology team members cannot be held accountable for poor health results, they are liable if they act negligently or cause injury. Because the profession can be so hazardous, it is in everyone's best interest that efforts be taken to communicate *all* risks before any procedure or treatment takes place. Every precaution must be taken in the actual treatment of each patient.

Different states have different laws regulating the radiation therapist's scope of practice. You must adhere to state laws and institutional policies and procedures regarding venipuncture and the administration of medication.

Documentation of Administration

The medical record is a legal document and is evidence for the caregiver and patient in the event of confusion or litigation.[11] Therefore, it is in the therapist's best interest to make sure the information in the chart is thorough and accurate. For example, if the patient verbally informs the therapist of a sensitivity to iodine and the therapist fails to pass on the information or record it in the chart, the therapist could be held liable for adverse reactions. A previously documented sensitivity should be clearly stated in the patient's permanent record, and in this situation, the therapist is responsible for noticing and making sure the physician is also aware of the sensitivity.[17]

The patient's chart or medical record is often the primary means of communication among the members of a healthcare team. Oncology patients are likely to be treated by various members of the healthcare team, all of whom require clear, unambiguous patient information to perform their jobs effectively.

Accurate documentation protects the patient from errors in treatment; it also protects the caregivers from making procedural, ethical, or legal errors. Every medication, every treatment procedure, every diagnostic test, and even verbal communication should be documented in the patient's permanent medical record.

Although each medical institution is allowed to develop its own system of recordkeeping, certain standards are required by the various accrediting bodies in the medical profession; these include the following[11,7]:

1. Patient identification and demographic information.
2. Medical history, including family history, allergies, and previous illnesses.
3. Nature of the current complaint and a report of examinations and treatments.
4. Orders for and results of any tests or procedures.
5. Record of all medications, whether self-administered, prescribed, or professionally administered. The information should include, but is not limited to, time, route, dosage, site of administration, and caregiver's signature.
6. Physician's notes, instructions, and conclusions.
7. Informed consent form.

Documentation of any complications or adverse reactions to a medication is especially critical to the medical record of any patient.[11,7,3] A sensitivity to any medication must be prominently displayed in the patient's record. Remedial action taken to counteract the complication must also be recorded.

The therapist is responsible for interpreting the chart accurately and entering information in the record.

Medical records are confidential and may not be released without the patient's consent. Orders of any kind must be signed by the attending health care professional.

Informed Consent

Radiation therapy and diagnostic imaging require informed consent from the patient. In addition to the general consent form the patient signs when entering a healthcare facility, each radiation therapy procedure requires a separate entry in the patient's record.[13]

Especially in cases of radiation administration and ionic contrast media in which the potential risk is so high, a gray area exists about what constitutes "informed" consent. If a patient agrees in writing to receive ionic contrast media but suffers a reaction, the oncologist could be held liable if that oncologist failed to inform the patient that nonionic agents were available. The issue of cost (e.g., nonionic media costs considerably more than ionic media) should not determine how much the physician tells the patient. Open communication about risk and cost are part of the patient's legal rights.

Informed consent expectations and documentation vary by state and institution. Informed consent generally include the name of the authorized physician; a description of the procedure and associated medications; an assurance that the purpose, benefit, risk, and any alternative options have been imparted and understood; an area where patients can add in their words what the procedure entails; and a disclaimer, which does not always hold up in court, releasing the caregiver and facility from liability if complications develop or the treatment fails.

SUMMARY

- The content in this chapter do not qualify a radiation therapist to perform those actions but is intended to provide only an overview of pharmacology and drug administration.
- The technique of venipuncture and assisting in the administration of IV drugs and contrast media are crucial skills required for the practice of radiation therapy.
- The therapist must study the principles of pharmacology and must have hands-on experience before performing these techniques on patients.
- The therapist who is knowledgeable in all pertinent aspects of drug administration contributes an invaluable service to the success of the radiation therapy team.
- Pharmacologic principles include absorption, distribution, metabolism, and excretion.
- Patient-related variables that affect response include age, weight, physical condition, gender, and personal and emotional requirements.
- Drug-related variables are allergic reaction, tolerance, cumulative effect, dependence, and drug interactions.
- The Seven Rights of Medication Administration are to identify the right patient, select the right medication, give the right dose, give the right medication at the right time, give the medication by the right route and for the right reason, and document what you have done.
- Routes of drug administration are oral, mucous membrane, topical, and parenteral.
- Parenteral drug administration routes include intradermal, SC, IM, and IV.
- Patient assessment is imperative before the initiation of any IV therapy and should include an allergy history, baseline blood pressure reading, determination of whether the patient is taking any medication that could affect blood clotting, and, if applicable, asking the patient whether he or she has been fasting.

REVIEW QUESTIONS

The answers to the Review Questions can be found by logging on to our website at: http://evolve.elsevier.com/Washington/principles

1. Which of the following is not one of the seven rights of drug administration?
   a. Right patient.
   b. Right route.
   c. Right time.
   d. Right syringe.
2. Barium sulfate is a contrast agent that would be used to enhance the:
   a. Blood vessels.
   b. Gastrointestinal tract.
   c. Genitourinary tract.
   d. Gynecologic structures.
3. The way in which drugs affect the body is called:
   a. Pharmacokinetics.
   b. Metabolism.
   c. Pharmacodynamics.
   d. Drug effectiveness.
4. Which of the following is *not* a parenteral route of administration for medications?
   a. SC.
   b. Instillation.
   c. IV.
   d. IM.
5. The type of drug given to cancer patients to relieve nausea and vomiting is a(n):
   a. Antacid.
   b. Emetic.
   c. Cathartic.
   d. Antiemetic.
6. The abbreviation "qod" stands for:
   a. Once daily.
   b. Once every other day.
   c. Daily.
   d. None of the above.
7. Which of the following is the correct category for the drug Imodium?
   a. Analgesic.
   b. Antidiarrheal.
   c. Antianxiety.
   d. Anticoagulant.
8. Which drug would be given to a patient who needs a blood thinner?
   a. Dilantin.
   b. Decadron.
   c. Heparin.
   d. Zoloft.
9. The escape of fluid from a vessel into the surrounding tissue, which can cause localized vasoconstriction, is termed:
   a. Anaphylaxis.
   b. Extravasation.
   c. Edema.
   d. Hematoma.
10. Which of the following is a parenteral route of administration?
    a. IV.
    b. Topical.
    c. Oral.
    d. Inhalation.

QUESTIONS TO PONDER

1. Why is following standard precautions during drug administration important?
2. Discuss the advantages and disadvantages of parenteral drug administration.
3. Compare the absorption of medications in different genders.
4. Describe the differences between ionic and nonionic contrast media.

REFERENCES

1. American Society of Radiologic Technologists. *Radiation Therapy Practice Standard*. Albuquerque, NM: The American Society of Radiologic Technologists; 2009

2. McKenry LM, Tessier EG, Hogan MA. *Mosby's Pharmacology in Nursing*. 22nd ed. St. Louis, MO: Elsevier Mosby; 2006.

3. Potter PA, Perry AG. *Fundamentals of Nursing*. 9th ed. St. Louis, MO: Elsevier Mosby; 2016.

4. Burchum JR, Rosenthal LD. *Lenhe's Pharmacology for Nursing Care*. 9th ed. St. Louis, MO: Elsevier; 2016.

5. Perry AG, Potter PA. *Clinical Nursing Skills and Techniques*. 9th ed. St. Louis, MO: Elsevier/Mosby; 2017.

6. Taylor C, Lillis C, Lynn P. *Fundamentals of Nursing: The Art and Science of Nursing Care*. 8th ed. Alphen aan den Rijn, Netherlands: Wolters and Kluwer; 2014.

7. Ehrlich RA, Coakes DM. *Patient Care in Radiography With an Introduction to Medical Imaging*. 9th ed. St. Louis, MO: Elsevier/Mosby; 2017.

8. Janeway Jr CA, Travers P, Walport M, et al. *Immunobiology: The Immune System in Health and Disease*. 5th ed. New York, NY: Garland Science; 2001.

9. National Library of Medicine. Substance use disorder. National Institutes of Health website. http://www.nlm.nih.gov/medlineplus/ency/article/001522.htm. Accessed November 15, 2018.

10. Acute pain management in the opioid-tolerant individual. Medscape Nurses (website) http://www.medscape.org/viewarticle/581948. Accessed October 16, 2019.

11. Adler AM, Carlton RR, eds. *Introduction to Radiologic Sciences and Patient Care*. 6th ed. St Louis, MO: Elsevier/Saunders; 2016.

12. Beebe RO, Funk DL. *Fundamentals of Emergency Care*. Albany, NY: Delmar; 2001.

13. Dutton A, Ryan, T. *Torres' Basic Medical Techniques and Patient Care in Imaging Technology*. 9th ed. Alphen aan den Rijn, Netherlands: Wolters and Kluwer; 2019

14. Matthews EP. Adverse effects of iodine-derived intravenous radiopaque contrast media. *Radiol Technol*. 2015;86(6):623–637.

15. ACR manual on contrast media, version 10.3, 2018 ACR Committee on Drugs and Contrast Media website. https://www.acr.org/-/media/ACR/Files/Clinical-Resources/Contrast_Media.pdf. Accessed November 15, 2018.

16. Dugdale D. Creatine Blood Test. National Institutes of Health, U.S. National Library of Medicine, MedlinePlus website; 2013. http://www.nlm.nih.gov/medlineplus/ency/article/003475.htm. Accessed November 15, 2018.

17. Exploration of lab values. Dialysis Clinic, Inc. website. www.dci-inc.org/values.php. Accessed November 15, 2018.

18. Bae KT. Intravenous contrast medium administration and scan time at CT: considerations and approaches. *Radiology*. 2010;256(1):32–56.

19. Holleb A, Fink DJ, Murphy GP. *Clinical Oncology: A Multidisciplinary Approach for Physicians and Students*. 8th ed. Atlanta, GA: American Cancer Society; 2001.

20. Brice J. Imaging and the law: simple tactics to minimize exposure to malpractice. *Diagn Imaging*. 1992;14(3):43–46.

21. Kienle P, Useton J. Maintaining compliance with Joint Commission medication management standards. Patient safety and quality healthcare website. http://www.psqh.com/julaug08/medication.html. Accessed November 15, 2018.

22. Asperheim MK, Favaro J. *Introduction to Pharmocology*. 12th ed. St. Louis, MO: Elsevier Saunders.

Applied Mathematics Review

Charles M. Washington, E. Richard Bawiec Jr.

OBJECTIVES

- Explain why mathematics is involved in radiation therapy and explain its significance in conducting treatments.
- Compare and contrast the differences between direct proportionality and inverse proportionality.
- Describe the three most common trigonometric functions associated with a right triangle, and describe instances when they are used in treatment.
- Understand when to use linear interpolation in treatment.

- Explain how natural logarithms and exponential factors are inverses of each other.
- Compare and contrast the three categories of uncertainty in measurements.
- Explain two differences between accuracy and precision and how they are used in radiation therapy treatment.
- Describe why errors occur in radiation therapy.

OUTLINE

KEY TERMS

Adjacent
Algebraic equation
Base
Cosine
Dimensional analysis
Direct proportionality
Exponent
Hypotenuse
Inverse proportionality
Linear interpolation

Logarithm
Opposite
Proportion
Ratio
Right triangle
Scientific notation
Significant figures
Sine
Tangent

The practice of radiation therapy requires the use of exact quantitative measurements for the accurate delivery of a therapeutic dose. Patient simulation, treatment planning, and quality assurance have a strong functional dependence on mathematics. Because of this, the radiation therapist and the medical dosimetrist must have a good working knowledge of both basic and advanced mathematical skills to accurately perform their duties. This chapter serves as a review of the principles of the mathematical concepts that are important in the delivery of ionizing radiation in cancer management. The emphasis is on practical application, not on teaching theoretical principles. This chapter also reviews ratios and proportions, exponential functions, logarithms, basic units, uncertainty, and dimensional analysis. Appropriately, practical applications are emphasized. The initial sections are structured as a review of math concepts, and the reader is presumed to have a working knowledge of basic entry-level college algebra.

REVIEW OF MATHEMATICAL CONCEPTS

Algebraic Equations With One Unknown

In many situations, an algebraic equation is used to describe a physical phenomenon based on the interaction of several factors. For example, the dose to any point from a brachytherapy source requires knowledge of the source activity, source filtration, distance from the source to the point of calculation interest, and several other factors. The ability to solve an equation for the value of an unknown variable is important. The following "rules" of algebra are helpful in remembering how do to this:

- When an unknown is multiplied by some quantity, divide both sides of an equation by that quantity to isolate the unknown.
- When a quantity is added to an unknown, subtract that quantity from both sides of the equation to isolate the unknown. When the quantity is subtracted from the unknown, add it to both sides.
- When an equation appears in fractional form, that is, the unknown is divided by some quantity, cross multiply both sides by that quantity, then solve for the unknown.[1]

Algebraic manipulation is commonly used in radiation therapy, so the radiation therapist and medical dosimetrist should be comfortable solving these types of equations. An example of a typical algebraic manipulation scenario is shown in the practical examples at the end of this chapter.

Ratios and Proportions

A ratio is the comparison of two numbers, values, or terms. The ratio denotes a relationship between the two components. Often these relationships allow the radiation therapist to predict trends. The notation for writing a ratio of a value or term, x, to another value or term, y, is most often written as

$$x / y \text{ or } x : y$$

One important property of a ratio is that any ratio, x/y, remains unchanged if both terms undergo operations by the same number. For example, the ratio $32/80$ can be simplified to the ratio $2/5$ by dividing both the numerator and the denominator by 16, a common factor of both numbers.

If two ratios are equal, this is known as a proportion. A proportion can also be looked at as an equation relating two ratios. This principle can assist in solving for an unknown factor in a proportion. For example, examine the following proportion:

$$5 : 7 = n : 49$$

This can be rewritten in a more recognizable form as follows:

$$5/7 = n/49$$

By cross multiplication, this proportion can be solved for n:

$$(49 \times 5) = 7n \text{ or } 7n = (49 \times 5)$$
$$7n = 245$$
$$n = 35$$

In the clinical radiation therapy environment, inverse and direct proportions can occur in various ways. The concepts of inverse and direct proportionality are pertinent in the management of cancer with ionizing radiation, so a brief review of these concepts is beneficial.

Inverse Proportionality

Consider a hypothetical situation in which a number of aircraft must complete a trip of 1000 miles. Each aircraft travels at a different velocity. The time required for each plane to make the trip depends on that plane's velocity. Table 12.1 lists the times and velocities for each aircraft.

TABLE 12.1 Aircraft Velocities and Times to Complete Trip

Aircraft	Velocity (Miles/Hour)	Time (Hours)
A	500	2.0
B	400	2.5
C	250	4.0
D	200	5.0
E	125	8.0

What simple relationship can we determine from these data? By examining the table, the following conclusions can be made:

- When velocity increases, time decreases.
- When velocity is doubled, time is halved.
- When velocity is quadrupled, time decreases by a factor of 4.

This example illustrates the concept of inverse proportionality. Velocity (v) is inversely proportional to time (t). Mathematically, this concept is written as follows:

$$v \alpha 1/t \text{ or } v = k / t$$

where k is a constant of proportionality. We can also relate two different aircrafts' velocities and times as an inverse proportion:

$$v_1 : v_2 = t_2 : t_1 \text{ or } v_1/v_2 = t_2/t_1$$

Example 2 in the practical examples section demonstrates inverse proportionality while solving for an unknown.

Inverse proportionality is commonly seen in radiation therapy. For example, depth and percentage depth dose are inversely related (while depth increases, percentage depth dose decreases), as are beam energy and penumbra width (while energy increases, the width of the beam's penumbra decreases). Another good example of inverse proportionality is the inverse square law, which states that the intensity of radiation from a point source varies inversely with the square of the distance from the source. This is especially important in brachytherapy and when applying radiation protection principles.

Direct Proportionality

The distance traveled by an aircraft moving at a constant velocity depends on the length of time that the aircraft is airborne. Suppose we consider an aircraft traveling at a constant velocity of 400 miles per hour. The time required for this aircraft to travel 100 miles is 0.25 hours; for 200 miles, the time is 0.5 hours; and so forth. Table 12.2 lists several distances and the time required by the aircraft to complete each distance.

Like the inverse proportionality example, conclusions can be reached from the data in this table, as follows:

- While time increases, distance increases.
- While time doubles, distance doubles.
- While time triples, distance triples.

Therefore we say that distance (D) is directly proportional to time (t). Mathematically, that is written as follows:

$$D \alpha t \text{ or } D = kt$$

where k is the constant of proportionality. We can also relate two different distances and times as a direct proportion:

$$D_1 : D_2 = t_1 : t_2$$

or

$$D_1/D_2 = t_1/t_2$$

TABLE 12.2 Distance and Time Values for Aircraft	
Distance (Miles)	**Time (Hours)**
0	0.00
100	0.25
200	0.50
300	0.75
400	1.00

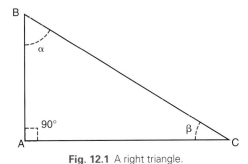

Fig. 12.1 A right triangle.

Example 3 in the practical examples section demonstrates direct proportionality while solving for an unknown.

Direct proportionality is also commonly seen in radiation therapy. For example, field size and percentage depth dose are directly proportional (while field size increases, percentage depth dose increases), as are beam energy and tissue air ratio (TAR) or tissue maximum ratio (TMR) (while energy increases, TAR and TMR increase). These relationships assume that all other related factors are constant.

Trigonometric Ratios and the Right Angle Triangle

Calculation of angles, such as collimator and gantry angles, and depths and lengths that are related to these angles, is common in setups during patient simulation and treatment. In many of these cases, a solution is derived by using the properties of a right triangle. A right triangle is a three-sided polygon on which one corner measures 90 degrees. The three most common functions associated with the right triangle are the sine, cosine, and tangent. Fig. 12.1 diagrams these quantities. There are six quantities that describe a right triangle: the three angles (a, b, and the 90-degree angle) and the three lengths (line segments AB, AC, and BC). The sine, cosine, and tangent of an angle on a right triangle are defined mathematically (by using the angle α, for example), as follows:

$$\sin(\alpha) = \frac{\text{Opposite}}{\text{Hypotenuse}} = \frac{AC}{BC}$$

$$\cos(\alpha) = \frac{\text{Adjacent}}{\text{Hypotenuse}} = \frac{AB}{BC}$$

$$\tan(\alpha) = \frac{\text{Opposite}}{\text{Adjacent}} = \frac{AC}{AB}$$

In these equations, opposite refers to the length of the side of the right triangle that is opposite the specified angle, hypotenuse refers to the length of the longest side of the triangle, and adjacent refers to length of the side of the right triangle that is close, or adjacent, to the specified angle.

To solve for any unknown quantity on a right triangle, only specific combinations of two of the five remaining quantities (excluding the 90-degree angle) must be known. One other characteristic of the right triangle is that the all angles equal 180 degrees. Expressed mathematically, this is simply: $\alpha + \beta + 90 = 180$. Example 4 in the practical example section illustrates how one can determine unknown quantities in a right triangle.

Sine, **cosine**, and **tangent** are the primary trigonometric knowledge required of the radiation therapist and are used frequently for specific clinical functions, such as matching the divergences of two abutting treatment fields or measuring the angle or thickness of a chest wall. Values of specific trigonometric functions can be determined either by looking them up in tables or by using a handheld scientific calculator. Because of the simplicity and common use of such calculators, this method for calculating the sine, cosine, or tangent of an angle is used here.[2]

Scientific calculators use the SIN, COS, and TAN keys. To obtain the specific trigonometric value desired, enter the known angle into the calculator in degrees and press the desired trigonometric function key. For example, to find the tangent of 30 degrees, type in the following:

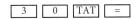

The calculator should display 0.57735. This means that the ratio of the opposite side of the 30-degree angle to the side adjacent to the 30 degrees is 0.57735. It is also possible to determine the measure of an angle by knowing the ratio between the two sides. If the ratio of the opposite side to the hypotenuse is 0.6, then the angle associated with this ratio can be calculated. Remember that the ratio opposite of the hypotenuse defines the sine of the angle. Therefore sin α = 0.6. To calculate the angle, one simply needs the inverse sine of 0.6. This is obtained on most scientific calculators by pressing either the inverse sine button or the button followed by the sine button. For the example, the inverse sine of 0.6 is 36.87 degrees. Therefore $\alpha = 36.87$ degrees.

Success in understanding trigonometric functions and identities depends, to a large degree, on the clinical application. Trigonometric functions are the most difficult type of mathematical problems for many therapy practitioners. Practice through didactic work or experience with these problems firsthand can aid the radiation therapist and medical dosimetrist in recognizing these problems and solving them when they occur.

Linear Interpolation

To determine many of the factors that are often used in the practice of radiation therapy, one must find values from tables that contain these needed factors. Field-size dependence factors, TARs, TMRs, percentage-depth doses, and so forth, are conveniently listed in easy-to-read tables. For example, a radiation therapist or medical dosimetrist can easily look up the TAR for a 10- × 10-cm field size at a 10-cm depth. However, the tables list the factors only in incremental values. What happens if the exact depth of calculation and/or field size is not listed in the table or lies between two table values? In this case, the radiation therapist or medical dosimetrist can use an approximate evaluation for the intermediate point. The process of calculating unknown values from known values is called linear interpolation. Linear interpolation assumes that the following statements are true[3]:

1. Two values are known.
2. The rate of change between the known values is constant.
3. An unknown data point must be found.

The rate of change can be assumed as constant between the values typically used when finding the unknown value. To minimize any inherent rate of change and be more precise, it is important to use known values that are close together. In most tables used in radiation therapy dose calculations, algebraic ratios can be used to assist the radiation therapist and medical dosimetrist in finding the intermediate number. If a desired point is directly between two known points, a simple average of the two factors for the two respective points is all that is required to determine the new value. When the desired point is not directly between the two known points, the new value must be determined by simple ratios. The ratio of the difference between the unknown value and the upper and lower known values equals the ratio of the difference between the desired point and the upper and lower points in the table. In some cases, the number that we need may require a double interpolation where the unknown value is between known values in two different directions. A TAR may be needed for a field size of 11×11 cm at a depth of 8.5 cm. In this case, values for the field size and depth needed are not listed in a TAR table, and it is necessary to find values for one of the unknowns before the other can be calculated. Example 5 in the practical example section demonstrates how factors are interpolated from a table when the known values lie "above" and "below" the unknown value. Relationships are established between the known values, and these relationships must be maintained throughout the calculation to arrive at the correct factor.

Working with Exponents

An exponent, or power, is a shorthand notation that represents the multiplication of a number by itself a given number of times. For example, $4^3 = 4 \times 4 \times 4 = 64$. In this case, the superscript 3 represents the exponent, and the 4 represents the base. The 3 is also said to be the power. One could verbally express 4^3 as "four raised to the third power." The following simple rules are important to remember when working with exponents:

$$x^0 = 1$$
$$x^a \times x^b = x^{a+b}$$
$$\left(x^a\right)^b = x^{ab}$$
$$(xy)^a = x^a y^a$$
$$[x/y]^a = x^a/y^b$$
$$X^{-a} = [1/x^a] \text{ and } [1/x^{-a}] = x^a$$

Scientific notation is a special use of exponents that uses base 10 notation. It is used to represent either very large or very small numbers.[4] Numbers written in scientific notation are written in the following form:

$$n.nnn \times 10^P$$

where *n.nnn* indicates the first four numeric values of the specified number. The power to which the base of 10 is raised *(p)* depends on the size of the specified number. For example, 2657.89 can be written in scientific notation as 2.65789×10^3; it can also be written as 26.5789×10^2. However, in the scientific community, placing only one number to the left of the decimal point is the preferred style. Example 6 in the practical example section illustrates the use of exponents.

Significant Figures

All measurements are approximations; no measuring device can give perfect measurements without some experimental uncertainty. In most radiation oncology physics measurements, this uncertainty is typically very small. The number of significant figures in a measurement or calculation is simply the number of figures that are known with some degree of reliability. The number 10.2 is said to have 3 significant figures. The number 10.20 is said to have 4 significant figures.

There are several rules for deciding the number of significant figures in a measured quantity.

1. All nonzero digits are significant: 1.234 cm has 4 significant figures, and 1.2 cm has 2 significant figures.

2. Zeroes between nonzero digits are significant: 1002 kg has 4 significant figures, and 3.07 mL has 3 significant figures.

3. Zeroes to the left of the first nonzero digits are not significant; such zeroes merely indicate the position of the decimal point: 0.001°C has only 1 significant figure, and 0.012 g has 2 significant figures.

4. Zeroes to the right of a decimal point in a number are significant: 0.023 mL has 2 significant figures, and 0.200 g has 3 significant figures.[5,6]

When a number ends in zeroes that are not to the right of a decimal point, the zeroes are not necessarily significant: 190 miles may be 2 or 3 significant figures, and 5040 centigray (cGy) may be 3 or 4 significant figures.

The last rule can be made clearer by the use of standard exponential, or scientific, notation. For example, depending on whether 3 or 4 significant figures is correct, we could write 5040 cGy as follows:

$$5.04 \times 10^3 \text{ cGy} \quad (3 \text{ significant figures})$$

or

$$5.040 \times 10^3 \text{ cGy} \quad (4 \text{ significant figures})$$

When combining measurements with different degrees of accuracy and precision (different number of significant figures), the accuracy of the final answer can be no greater than the least accurate measurement. This principle can be translated into the following rules:

- When measurements are added or subtracted, the answer can contain no more decimal places than the least accurate measurement.
- When measurements are multiplied or divided, the answer can contain no more significant figures than the least accurate measurement.[5,6]

Natural Logarithms and the Exponential Function

A logarithm operates as the reverse of exponential notation. Although the example 4^3 is considered "four raised to the third power" in exponential notation and equals 64, the logarithm base 4 of 64 equals 3. In mathematical notation, the logarithm is written as follows:

$$\log_b (N) = x$$

where *b* is the base, *N* is the desired product, and *x* is the power. In exponential notation, this is written as follows:

$$b^x = N$$

Certain physical processes have been discovered in nature that obey a special type of logarithmic, and thus exponential, behavior. A radioactive substance is said to decay exponentially.[2,1,7,8] This simply means that the physical process that occurs can be described by exponential notation. However, rather than the base being an integer, the base is a special number that was discovered by Euler, a mathematician. This special number is represented by the letter *e* and is called Euler's constant or the "base of the natural logarithms." Numerically, *e* is equal to 2.718272. Logarithms based on *e* are called natural logarithms. Exponential function is the terminology used to describe *e* raised to a power and is written as follows:

$$e^x = N$$

A special notation is also given to the natural logarithm. The symbol *ln* is shorthand for "(natural) logarithm base *e*" and can be written as follows:

$$\ln (N) = x$$

These two equations can be combined to yield an important identity:

$$\ln (e^x) = x$$

In other words, the natural logarithm and the exponential functions are inverses of each other. The exponential function has the following important properties that can be beneficial to the radiation therapy practitioner:

- If the power *(x)* is greater than 0 (meaning the power is positive), then the value of e^x is greater than 1.
- If the power is less than 0 (meaning the power is negative), then the value of e^x is a number greater than 0 and less than 1.
- If the power is exactly 0, then the value of e^x is exactly equal to 1.

To summarize:

$$e^x > \text{if } x > 0$$

$$0 < e^x < 1 \text{ if } x < 0$$

$$e^x = 1 \text{ if } x = 0$$

Example 7 in the practical example section demonstrates how to use the exponential function.

Basic Units

The system of basic units used most commonly in radiation therapy clinics is the metric or International System of Units system. This system is the world standard for scientific and technical work. The metric system is based on fundamental units of time, distance, mass, and electrical current, and several derived units that are combinations of the four fundamental units. In addition, prefixes may be added to the four fundamental units to represent large or small quantities of the fundamental units.[1,4,6,7]

The four fundamental units in the metric system are the second (time), the meter (distance), the kilogram (mass), and the ampere (electrical current). These units are defined internationally by standards kept at a laboratory near Paris, France. However, secondary standards are kept in national laboratories in most countries. In the United States, the National Institute of Standards and Technology maintains the secondary standards.[4] Commonly used prefixes and their meanings are listed in Table 12.3.

Special units have been defined for the radiologic sciences. The roentgen (R) is the unit of radiation exposure that represents a measure of the amount of ionization created by radiation in the air. A derived unit for exposure is the coulomb/kilogram (C/kg). Thus the relationship between these two quantities is $1 R = 2.58 \times 10^{-4}$ C/kg.

The accepted unit of absorbed dose is the gray (Gy). Absorbed dose describes the amount of radiation × energy absorbed by a medium. The Gy can be expressed in units as joule/kilogram (J/kg). An outdated unit that was replaced by the Gy is the rad. A rad is equal to 0.01 Gy or, restated, 100 rad = 1 Gy. Therefore 1 rad = 1 cGy.[1]

The accepted unit of energy is the joule (J), which is equal to 1 kg-meter^2 per second^2 ($1 \text{ kgm}^2/\text{s}^2$). A joule of energy is a rather large amount of energy, relative to the energies associated with radiation therapy. Therefore another special derived unit is the electron volt (eV). The relationship between the electron volt and the joule is as follows:

$$1 \text{ eV} = 1.602 \times 10^{-19} \text{ J}$$

The kiloelectron volt (keV = 10^3 eV) and the megaelectron volt (MeV = 10 eV) are the most common energy units used in the radiation therapy clinic.[1]

Measurements and Experimental Uncertainty

During the course of a program in radiation therapy, a student eventually becomes familiar with certain quantities such as source-to-axis distance and source-to-skin distance (SSD) measurements, as well as certain units such as absorbed dose (cGy), exposure (roentgen), and

TABLE 12.3 Numeric Prefixes Used With International System of Units

Prefix	Symbol	Multiplier
pico	P	10^{-12}
nano	N	10^{-9}
micro	M	10^{-6}
milli	M	10^{-3}
centi	C	10^{-2}
deci	D	10^{-1}
kilo	K	10^{3}
mega	M	10^{6}
giga	G	10^{9}

activity (millicurie).[1,4,7,8] Different instruments can be used to measure these and various other quantities. The process of taking a measurement is basically an attempt to determine a value or magnitude of known quantity.

For example, the quantity of SSD is a physical measurement of distance. Suppose an SSD of 93.5 cm was measured from the source of radiation to the chest wall of a patient during the treatment simulation process. This measurement indicates that the centimeter was used as a unit of length and that the distance to the skin surface was 93.5 times larger than this unit. Stated differently, a measurement is a comparison of the magnitude (how large or small) of a quantity with that of an accepted standard. In this measurement and in other measurements, such as determining the temperature by using a thermometer, the barometric pressure by using a barometer, or the exposure rate by using an exposure rate meter, an amount of uncertainty is inherent. Therefore the measuring process requires that the person taking the measurement have the knowledge that this uncertainty exists. Referring to the SSD measurement, the distance of 93.5 cm will contain error that is introduced not only by the measuring device but also by the fact that the patient will most probably be moving as a result of inhalation and exhalation. This inherent or built-in uncertainty in making a measurement is a characteristic of almost all of science. Uncertainties can be grouped into three categories: systematic errors, random errors, and blunders.

Systematic Errors. A systematic error is an error or uncertainty inherent within the measuring device. A systematic error always affects the measurement in the same way: the measurement will either be too large or too small, depending on the device. These errors are commonly obtained, for example, from one or more of the following: human biases such as vision inaccuracies; imperfect techniques that may occur, for example, during experimental setup; and unacceptable instrument calibrations. Stem leakage of an ionization chamber and the inaccuracy of reading an analog temperature meter on an annealing oven are examples of systematic errors.

Although computer-controlled treatment plans reduce the rate of random treatment delivery errors, they may be susceptible to systematic errors, which may be hard to detect. New technology can create new types of errors when staff do not have proper knowledge or understanding regarding new equipment, which can result in the use of workarounds when encountering system errors.[9] Adequate education on new techniques and technology must be part of an implementation plan to limit this occurrence.

Random Errors. Random errors, as the name implies, are a result of variations attributed to chance that are unavoidable. Random errors can either increase or decrease the result of a measurement. To correct for this type of error, a common practice is to take several measurements and average them. Random errors can also be reduced by making improvements in the measuring device and/or technique. An uncontrolled rapid change in temperature or barometric pressure, accidental movement of a patient during setup, and electronic noise are all examples of random errors.

Blunders. Blunders during measurement are errors that occur as a result of human error in algebraic or arithmetic calculations or from improper use of a measuring device. Errors in judgment can also be classified as a blunder. These errors can be avoided by properly educating the individuals who will be making the measurements. They can also be avoided by comparing the measurements taken to previous measurements that are known to be correct, or even by comparing them with theoretical values. If large discrepancies exist between the correct values and the values that the individual is obtaining, then something must have been done incorrectly, and retracing the setup and procedure can be an easy way to remedy the error.

Uncertainty can be directly related to human errors, which are caused by interrelationships between individuals, the tools they use, and the environment in which they live and work.[10] Education, training, familiarity, and accountability are essential to limit the amount of uncertainty in any instance.

Accuracy and Precision of Measurements. Another facet of measurements that must be discussed is the importance of and the difference between the accuracy and precision of a measurement. When measurements are made, the individual must be concerned with how close the measurements are to the true value. Although the true value cannot be known exactly, theoretical calculations can define a value that is accepted as a true value. How close a measurement comes to this true value is referred to as accuracy. The precision of a measurement indicates the reproducibility of a particular measurement or the consistency of the measurement.

Fig. 12.2 illustrates the difference between accuracy and precision. The bull's-eye represents the true value. The arrows represent measurements. In the first picture, the measurements are neither precise nor accurate. The arrows (measurements) did not hit the bull's eye, nor did they land close to each other. In the second picture, the arrows were precise but inaccurate. They all hit close to the same location but were not close to the bull's eye. In the third picture, the arrows were precise and accurate, because they were grouped together close to the bull's eye.

As another example, consider the output measurement of a linear accelerator as performed by three therapists as part of the daily quality assurance program. After setting up the necessary apparatus and following the policy and procedure outline, the following data were gathered. Each therapist made four measurements with the ionization chamber to obtain an average value for the output and thereby eliminate random errors.

	Therapist A	Therapist B	Therapist C
	2.702	2.650	2.738
	2.701	2.660	2.578
	2.702	2.655	2.737
	2.702	2.651	2.579
Average	2.702	2.654	2.657

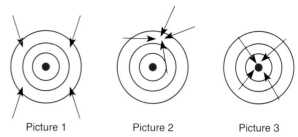

Picture 1   Picture 2   Picture 3

Fig. 12.2 Representation of the contrast between accuracy and precision. *Picture 1* is neither accurate nor precise. *Picture 2* demonstrates precision but not accuracy. *Picture 3* illustrates both precision and accuracy.

The accepted value for the output for that accelerator was 2.658. A number of questions could be asked about the values obtained by the radiation therapists. Which therapist had the most accurate values? Which therapist had the most precise values? Which therapist had the best overall results? The measurements made by Therapist A were more consistent and more precise because the values do not differ by more than 0.001. However, the average results obtained by Therapists B and C were closer to the accepted value. Apparently, Therapists B and C were more accurate than Therapist A, although Therapist A was the most precise. By comparing the individual values that were obtained by Therapists B and C, one can see that Therapist C's values had a large range. Therefore, although Therapist C's average value was the closest to the accepted value, it was obtained through imprecise readings. Therefore the values obtained by Therapist B are deemed the most acceptable because they were precise and accurate.

From this example, it is apparent that a measurement can be precise without being accurate and vice versa. Radiation therapy practitioners should be concerned not only with accuracy but also with precision. Discerning between the two is a function of analytical judgment and critical thinking skills, both very important in the practice of radiation therapy.

Experimental Uncertainty. Because it is impossible to eliminate all systematic errors, random errors, and blunders, an absolutely accurate and precise measurement cannot be achieved. Although this seems disheartening to the scientist, there is a method that is accepted by the scientific community to handle this experimental uncertainty. It is common practice to measure the percent relative error in a measurement to discover the degree of accuracy. The percent relative error can be thought of as the percentage of error in a measurement relative to the accepted value. It is calculated by using the following equation:

$$\% \text{ Relative error} = \left[\frac{\text{Experimental value} - \text{Accepted value}}{\text{Accepted value}} \right] \times 100$$

Look at the measurement result of Therapist A. The percent relative error in that result can be calculated as follows by using the previous equation:

$$\% \text{ Relative error} = \left[\frac{2.702 - 2.658}{2.658} \right] \times 100 = 1.65\%$$

The percent relative error in the result obtained by Therapist A was +1.65%. This means that the result was 1.65% higher than the accepted value. The percent relative errors in the results obtained by Therapists B and C can be calculated by the reader as −0.15% and −0.04%, respectively. Both of these values were low.

Dimensional Analysis

A technique that can be very useful in radiation therapy (as well as in many other branches of science) is dimensional analysis. Dimensional analysis is a process that involves the careful assessment of the units of measurement used in calculating a specific quantity. This technique involves canceling common units that appear in the numerator and denominator of an equation. When one or more quantities are manipulated to obtain a specified quantity, the units of the known quantities when combined must be equivalent to the unit of measurement of that specified quantity. For example, to obtain the specific quantity of velocity, one must divide distance by time. In other words, velocity is measured in meters per second, distance is measured in meters, and time is measured in seconds.[1]

When an equation is used, ensure that all of the units when combined equate to the units desired. There are a few "rules of thumb" that can be used when analyzing the dimensions of an equation. First, any quantity divided by 1 is equal to the quantity itself. Next, any quantity divided by itself is equal to 1. In addition, the process of division is equivalent to multiplying the numerator by the inverse of the denominator.[4,1] Using these facts, one can cancel units in any equation until no cancellation possibility remains. The units that remain should be equivalent to the desired units. If this is not true, then an error must have occurred.

PRACTICAL EXAMPLES OF MATHEMATICS IN RADIATION THERAPY

Mathematical theories must be put into practice for the radiation therapist to really understand the concepts and what it means to radiation therapy practice. Several examples have been used throughout this chapter to help focus the content into useful information. This section of the chapter provides more in-depth analysis of practical application examples of mathematical principles as seen in radiation therapy.

Example 1: algebraic equations. For the value of an unknown to be determined, it is necessary to use the rules of algebra. For example, if a radiation therapist knows the total dose that a patient is to receive and the dose per fraction, then the number of treatments can be determined. Assume that the total dose is 5000 cGy and the daily dose is 200 cGy. The number of fractions can be determined from the following equation:

$$200 \text{ cGy/fraction} \times N \text{ (fraction)} = 5000 \text{ cGy}$$

where *N* represents the number of fractions. To isolate the unknown (*N*), the value of 200 can be divided out of both sides of the equation without disturbing the equality:

$$200 \text{ cGy/fraction}/200 \text{ cGy/fraction} \times N =$$
$$5000 \text{ cGy}/200 \text{ cGy/fraction}$$

The first term in this equation is equal to 1, and any value multiplied by 1 equals that number. In addition, because the unit cGy appears in both the numerator and the denominator of the fraction on the right side of the equation, it can be canceled. The resulting equation is thus:

$$N = 5000/200 \times 1/1/\text{fraction}$$

At this point, one other algebraic rule can be applied. Any fraction that appears in the denominator of a fraction can be written as the reciprocal of that fraction. Therefore our final answer becomes the following:

$$N = 5000/200 \text{ fraction} = 25 \text{ fractions}$$

Thus the radiation therapist knows that the patient has 25 fractions prescribed.

As already stated, values can be subtracted from both sides of an equation to find an answer. Suppose that a radiation therapist knows that the physician wants to deliver 200 cGy on a particular day and knows that on the previous day the patient received 250 cGy. Therefore the unknown can be determined from the following equation:

$$250 \text{ cGy} - X = 200 \text{ cGy}$$

Obviously, this is a simple problem, but it is used to illustrate a principle. From this point, one can subtract 250 cGy from both sides of the equation, as follows:

$$250 \text{ cGy} - X - 250 \text{ cGy} = 200 \text{ cGy} - 250 \text{ cGy}$$

Subtracting 250 from itself equals 0, and 0 added to any value simply equals that value. In addition, one can multiply both sides of an equation by the same value without disturbing the equality. Therefore if both sides of the equation are multiplied by −1, the following results:

$$-X = 200 \text{ cGy} - 250 \text{ cGy} = -50 \text{ cGy}$$

$$(-1) \ x - X = (-1) \ x - 50 \text{ cGy}$$

$$X = 50 \text{ cGy}$$

Thus the radiation therapist knows that the daily dose was reduced by 50 cGy.

Example 2: inverse proportionality. A radiation therapist just learned from a medical physicist that the therapy unit would be running at a dose rate of 400 cGy/min on a given day. The radiation therapist knows that the normal dose rate is 300 cGy/min and wonders how this new dose rate will affect the patient's treatment times. This example illustrates inverse proportionality. If a particular patient's treatments took 1.2 minutes with the normal dose rate of 300 cGy/min, then what would it be with the new dose rate? This can be solved by the following equation:

$$300 \text{ cGy/min} \times 1.2 \text{ minutes} = 360 \text{ cGy}$$

$$360 \text{ cGy}/400 \text{ cGy/min} = 0.9 \text{ minute}$$

Therefore, while the dose rate increases, treatment times decrease, which demonstrates the concept of inverse proportionality.

Example 3: direct proportionality. A radiation oncologist wants to increase the dose that a patient receives per fraction but does not want to change the total number of fractions. Assume that originally, the physician had planned to give 200 cGy per fraction for 25 fractions, then decided that 230 cGy would achieve better results. Initially, the total dose would have been as follows:

$$230 \text{ cGy/fraction} \times 25 \text{ fractions} = 5750 \text{ cGy}$$

But because the dose per fraction was changed to 230 cGy, the total dose would also change:

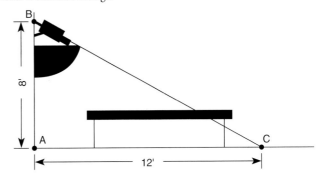

$$230 \text{ cGy/fraction} \times 25 \text{ fractions} = 5750 \text{ cGy}$$

Therefore note that while the dose per fraction increases, the total dose increases. This is an example of direct proportionality.

Example 4: unknown quantities and the right triangle. A medical physicist wants to know at what angle a wall-mounted laser is directed at the floor. Assume that she also wants to know the distance from the laser to its intersection point on the floor. First, she measures the distance from the wall to the intersection point on the floor (Segment AC measures 12 ft). Then she measures how far up the wall the laser is mounted (Segment AB measures 8 ft).

From the trigonometric identities outlined in the text, the physicist knows that the tangent of the angle is equal to the length of the opposite side divided by the length of the adjacent side. That can be stated in mathematical form as follows:

$$\tan \beta = \text{opposite/adjacent}$$

$$\tan \beta = \text{Segment AC/Segment AB} = 12 \text{ ft/8 ft}$$

$$\tan \beta = 1.5$$

$$\tan \beta = \tan^{-1}(1.5)$$

$$\tan \beta = 56$$

Therefore angle β is equal to 56 degrees. In addition, the physicist knows that the sine of β is equal to the length of the opposite side divided by the hypotenuse. This can be written as follows:

$$\sin \beta = \text{Opposite/Hypotenuse} = \text{Segment AC/Segment BC}$$

Because the length of segment BC is desired, the equation can be rewritten and solved for that length:

$$\text{Segment BC} = \text{Opposite/} \sin\beta = 12 \text{ft/sin} (56°)$$
$$= 12/0.829 = 14.5 \text{ ft}$$

Therefore the distance from the laser's position on the beam wall to the point where the beam intersects the floor is 14.5 ft.

Example 5: linear interpolation. A medical dosimetrist wants to determine the output of a cobalt machine for two different field sizes for one specific date from the following output table. The field sizes are 12 × 12 cm and 19 × 19 cm. The desired date is March 30. Assume that this date is exactly halfway between March 15 and April 15.

Because the 12 × 12 cm field size is listed on the table, the only step required to determine the output for that field size is to determine the intermediate value between the March 15 and April 15 outputs for that field size. The outputs for a 12 × 12 cm field size for March 15 and April 15 are 216.18 and 213.82 cGy/min, respectively. Therefore the output

for the 12 × 12 cm field size for March 30 is the simple average of the two outputs:

$$\frac{216.18 + 213.82}{2} = \frac{430.0}{2} = 215.00 \text{ cGy/min}$$

The first step to determine the desired output for the 19 × 19 cm field size is to determine the intermediate values of the output for March 30 for the field sizes nearest to 19 × 19 cm. These values would be the 15 × 15 cm and 20 × 20 cm field sizes. The outputs for March 15 and April 15 for the 15 × 15 cm field size are 219.60 and 217.21 cGy/min, respectively, whereas the outputs for March 15 and April 15 for the 20 × 20 cm field size are 223.24 and 220.80 cGy/min, respectively. To determine the intermediate values for March 30 for each field size, the simple averages are calculated and can be shown to be 218.41 cGy/min for the 15 × 15 cm field size and 222.02 cGy/min for the 20 × 20 cm field size. The next step is to determine the ratio of how "far" the 19 × 19 cm field size is from either the smaller or the larger field size. For this example, we will choose the smaller field size. The 19 × 19 cm field size is 4 cm greater than the 15 × 15 cm field size. The difference between the 15 × 15 cm and 20 × 20 cm field sizes is 5 cm. Therefore the 19 × 19 cm field size is four-fifths of the "distance" between the two known values, and thus the output for the 19 × 19 cm field size must also be four-fifths of the "distance" between the two intermediate outputs that we just determined previously. It should be noted that the direction one would move on the table in going from a 15 × 15 cm² field size to a 20 × 20 cm² field size will be the same direction one would move on the table to determine the output as well. Now, to calculate the desired output, one must know the distance between the two intermediate values and then multiply that distance by the field size distances ratio. This will give the desired output of 221.30 cGy/min:

$$222.02 \text{ cGy/min-}218.41 \text{ cGy/min} = 3.61 \text{ cGy}$$

$$3.61 \text{ cGy/min} \times 4/5 = 2.89 \text{ cGy/min}$$

$$218.41 \text{ cGy/min} + 2.89 \text{ cGy/min} = 221.30 \text{ cGy/min}$$

Therefore the output for March 30 for the 19 × 19 cm field size was 221.30 cGy/min. Although the use of cobalt-60 continues to decrease in clinical use, the concepts demonstrated here are still pertinent for the radiation therapist's understanding, particularly in understanding the mathematical relationship described.

Example 6: exponents. A brief example of the use of exponents is all that is demonstrated here. The primary use of exponents in the field of radiation therapy is in scientific notation. If one must calculate the product of two numbers that are represented in scientific notation, some of the rules outlined in this chapter can be useful. For example, assume that a radiation physicist desires to determine the total amount of exposure produced by ionizing radiation in a specified mass of air. She knows that 1 R is equal to 2.58×10^{-4} C of charge liberated per

Output (cGy/min) for Theratron 780 at 80 cm in air (source-to-axis treatment) (15th of month).

Field size	January 15	February 15	March 15	April 15	May 15
5 × 5 cm	210.71	208.41	205.13	203.88	201.66
10 × 10 cm	218.58	216.19	213.83	211.50	209.19
12 × 12 cm	220.98	218.57	216.18	213.82	211.49
15 × 15 cm	224.48	222.03	219.60	217.21	214.83
20 × 20 cm	228.19	225.70	223.24	220.80	218.39

kilogram of air present. She measured 3.23×10^{-2} C in 1 kg of air mass. Mathematically, this is written as follows:

$$\text{Exposure } (x) = \frac{3.23 \times 10^{-2} \text{ C}}{1 \text{ kg air}} \times \frac{1 \text{ R}}{2.58 \times 10^{-4} \text{ C/1 kg air}}$$

$$\text{Exposure } (x) = \frac{3.23 \times 10^{-2} \text{ C/1 kg air}}{2.58 \times 10^{-4} \text{ C/1 kg air}} \times 1 \text{ R}$$

$$\text{Exposure } (x) = 1.25 \times \frac{10^{-2}}{10^{-4}} \text{ R}$$

If a number with a negative exponent is in the denominator of a fraction, then that is the same as the same number with the equal positive exponent moved to the numerator of the equation:

$$\text{Exposure } (x) = 1.25 \times 10^{-2} \times 10^{4} \text{ R}$$

$$\text{Exposure } (x) = 1.25 \times 10^{(-2+4)} \text{ R}$$

$$\text{Exposure } (x) = 1.25 \times 10^{2} \text{ R} = 125 \text{ R}$$

Example 7: exponential functions. The decay of a radioactive substance behaves in an exponential manner. Therefore if one wishes to calculate the amount of activity of a particular substance that remains after a specific amount of time, the following equation can be used:

$$A_t = A_0 \times e^{-\lambda t}$$

where A_t is the activity after time t, A_0 is the initial activity, and λ is the decay constant that is specific to the particular radioactive substance being used. As an example, assume that the activity of a sample of iridium-131 is known exactly 2 days after it was received from a manufacturer. Assume that we would like to know what the activity was when it arrived. The activity at the present is 5 Curies (Ci). Therefore we know that $t = 2$ days and $A_t = 5$ Ci. In addition, the decay constant for iridium-131 is 8.6×10^{-2}/day. So, plugging these values into the decay equation gives the following results:

$$5 \text{ Ci} = A_0 \times e^{-\left(8.6 \times 10^{-2}/\text{day}\right) \times (2 \text{ days})}$$

$$A_0 = 5 \text{ Ci}/e^{-0.172} = 5 \text{ Ci}/0.842$$

$$A_0 = 5.94 \text{ Ci}$$

Therefore the activity on arrival 2 days earlier was 5.94 Ci. One can also determine the activity of the substance 2 days after the present date by using the same equation. The reader can calculate this independently.

SUMMARY

- Although treatment planning and calculation checking are, for the most part, performed by a member of the dosimetry or physics team, it is imperative that every member of the radiation therapy staff know how to perform basic treatment calculations.
- With a basic knowledge of the calculations, a radiation therapist can determine whether a treatment dose looks correct for what is about to be treated. If something looks suspicious, the therapist can have another member of the treatment planning team verify the dose and possibly avoid a mistreatment.
- Emergent situations demand that therapists have a good working knowledge of treatment planning. These situations often occur outside of clinic hours or when radiation needs to be delivered very quickly, so it is up to the radiation therapists to calculate and administer the dose, often without a treatment plan.

REVIEW QUESTIONS

The answers to the Review Questions can be found by logging on to our website at: http://evolve.elsevier.com/Washington/principles

1. $(10^3)^5$ equals:
   a. 10^8.
   b. 10^2.
   c. 10^{15}.
   d. 10^{-2}.
2. Convert 190,600,000 to scientific notation.
   a. 1.906×10^8.
   b. 1.906×10^7.
   c. 19.06×10^8.
   d. 1906×10^7.
3. If an instrument positioned 1 m from a point source is moved 50 cm closer to the source, the radiation intensity will be:
   a. Increased by a factor of 4.
   b. Increased by a factor of 2.
   c. Decreased by a factor of 4.
   d. Decreased by a factor of 2.
4. While the depth in tissue increases, the percentage depth dose values decreases. This is an example of:
   a. Inverse proportionality.
   b. Direct proportionality.
   c. Interpolation.
   d. None of the above.
5. What is the ratio of 100 cGy to 500 cGy?
   a. 5:1.
   b. 1:5.
   c. Both a and b.
   d. Neither a nor b.
6. How many significant figures are there in 780,000,000?
   a. 2.
   b. 3.
   c. 6.
   d. 9.
7. How many significant figures are there in 0.0101?
   a. 2.
   b. 3.
   c. 4.
   d. 5.
8. Errors that occur because of human error in algebraic or arithmetic calculations or from improper use of a measuring device are:
   a. Systematic errors.
   b. Random errors.
   c. Blunders.
   d. Precision.

9. $\ln(e^x) = x$ is:
   a. True.
   b. False.

10. $\dfrac{10^x}{10^y} = 10^{x+y}$
   a. True.
   b. False.

REFERENCES

1. Harris M. *Radiation Therapy Physics Handbook*. Houston, TX, 1992: The University of Texas M.D. Anderson Cancer Center.
2. Christian PE, Waterstram-Rich KM. *Nuclear Medicine and PET/CT Technology and Techniques*. 7th ed. St. Louis, MO: Elsevier Mosby; 2017.
3. Linear interpolation (website): http://en.wikipedia.org/wiki/Linear_interpolation. Accessed November 7, 2018.
4. Bushong SC. *Radiologic Science for Technologists: Physics, Biology, and Protection*. 11th ed. St. Louis, MO: Elsevier Health Sciences; 2017.
5. Significant figures (website). http://www.chem.tamu.edu/class/fyp/mathrev/mr-sigfg.html. Accessed November 7, 2018.
6. Significant figures (website). http://www.chem.sc.edu/faculty/morgan/resources/sigfigs/sigfigs3.html. Accessed November 7, 2018.
7. Khan FM, Gibbons JP. Khan's *The Physics of Radiation Therapy*. 5th ed. Philadelphia, PA: Lippincott Williams & Wilkins.
8. Stanton R, Stinson D. *Applied Physics for Radiation Oncology*. 2nd ed. Madison, WI: Medical Physics Publishing.
9. Amols HI. New technologies in radiation therapy: ensuring patient safety, radiation safety and regulatory issues in radiation oncology. *Health Phys.* 2008;95(5):658–665.
10. Ford EC, Fong-de Los Santos L, Pawlicki T, et al. Consensus recommendations for incident learning database structures in radiation oncology. *Med Phys.* 2009;39:7272–7290.

13

Introduction to Radiation Therapy Physics

Narayan Sahoo

OBJECTIVES

- Identify and describe the different sources of ionizing radiation.
- Discuss the units and measurements often needed in the field of radiation therapy.
- Identify types of forces responsible for interactions between particles.
- Define binding energy, excitation, and ionization and relate them to the field of radiation therapy.
- Differentiate and describe the different forms of radioactive decay.
- Identify and describe the different forms of photon interaction used in radiation therapy.

OUTLINE

KEY TERMS

Atom
Atomic mass number
Atomic mass unit
Atomic number
Auger electron
Binding energy per nucleon
Bohr atom model
Bremsstrahlung
Characteristic radiation
Characteristic x-rays
Electrical charge
Electromagnetic radiation
Electron's binding energy

Excitation
Excited nuclear energy level
Frequency of the wave
Gamma rays (γ-rays)
Gravity
Ground state
Half-value layer
Heavy charged particles
Ionization
Mass equivalence
Neutron
Nuclear binding energy
Nuclear energy level

Radiation is transmitted energy in the form of electromagnetic (EM) waves, charged particles and neutral particles from different sources such as the sun and atoms. Radiation therapy involves the use of ionizing radiation that can ionize the medium it passes through to deliver a lethal dose to target cells while keeping the dose delivered to normal tissue below its tolerance level as much as possible. This ionizing radiation can be from different sources such as x-rays, gamma rays, electrons, protons, other heavy charged particles, or neutron beams, which are produced by accelerators and radioactive sources. The process of dose deposition in tissue involves a complex interaction between the ionizing source and the molecules of the tissue. A good understanding of the source and nature of radiation, as well as the processes involved in the transport or interaction of the radiation in tissue, will help the radiation therapy practitioner to plan the radiation dose delivery to the target volume in the patient. The objective of this chapter is to describe some of the basic principles of radiation therapy physics.

RADIATION QUANTITIES AND UNITS

Four major quantities that are important in radiation physics are: (1) radioactivity, (2) radiation exposure, (3) radiation-absorbed dose, and (4) radiation dose equivalent. Every physical quantity is characterized by its magnitude and unit. Units are agreed-on standard quantities of measurements such as meters, seconds, and grams. From these fundamental units, the units of other quantities can be derived. Two systems of units existed before 1977, namely, the foot-pound-second system and the meter-kilogram-second system to express measurements of length, mass, and time. In 1977 a new Système Internationale d'Unités (International System of Units [SI]), was adopted to create a uniform worldwide standard.

In the International System of Units (SI) system, the seven basic physical quantities are assigned the following units.

Length (l): meter (m)

Mass (m): kilogram (kg)

Time (t): second (s)

Electrical current (E): ampere (A)

Temperature (T): kelvin (K)

Amount of substance: mole (mol)

Luminous intensity: candela (cd)

All other physical quantities and their units can be derived from the above seven quantities and units. More information on SI units is available at http://physics.nist.gov/cuu/Units/index.html.

Example: Speed is the rate of change of position and is given by the ratio distance/time. Thus, it is quantified by l/t and its unit is m/s.

Practice: What will be the unit of momentum, which is mass multiplied by velocity?

The original units for each of the important radiation quantities of interest are given in Table 13.1, along with the new SI units and the conversion factors to change the original unit to the new one.

It is often necessary to convert between various systems and magnitudes of units.

Example:

1. How many minutes are in 2 hours and 14 minutes?

$$2\ hr \times \frac{60\ min}{1\ hr} + 14\ min = 134\ min$$

2. How many meters are in 5.5 miles?

$$5.5\ miles \times \frac{5280\ ft}{1\ mile} \times \frac{12\ in}{1\ ft} \times \frac{2.54\ cm}{1\ in} \times \frac{1\ m}{100\ cm} = 8851.4\ m$$

Throughout this chapter and this text, you will find the opportunity to convert many types of units.

ATOMIC PHYSICS

Subatomic Particles

The smallest unit of an element that retains the properties of that element is called an atom. It is well known that an atom consists of electrons and a nucleus made of protons and neutrons. The electrons, protons, and neutrons are called *subatomic particles*.[1-3] The electrons are considered to be elementary particles belonging to the class of particles called *leptons*. The neutrons and protons are composite particles and belong to the *hadron* group of particles. Hadrons are considered to be made up of constituent quarks bound together by gluons. Many types of subatomic particles have been discovered or postulated since the discovery of electrons in 1897 by JJ Thomson.[2] The subatomic particles are classified into two groups: leptons and hadrons. There are four types of forces, which are responsible for the interaction between different particles:

1. Gravity: The force responsible for interaction between particles with nonzero mass and has infinite range.
2. EM: This force is responsible for interaction between electrically charged particles and particles with nonzero magnetic moments. It has infinite range. This force is responsible for the binding of the electrons and the nucleus to form the atoms, the binding of atoms to form molecules, and the binding of atoms and molecules to form liquids and solids. Production of light or EM radiation is a process associated with EM interactions.
3. Strong force: This is a short-ranged force that is responsible for interaction between neutron and proton and other particles belonging to the hadrons family.
4. Weak force: This is a short-ranged force that is responsible for interaction between elementary particles involving neutrinos or antineutrinos. This force is also responsible for radioactive decay of a neutron to a proton, an electron, and an antineutrino, called *beta decay*.

The strong force is the strongest among the four forces, followed by EM force, the weak force, and the weakest being gravity. The particles affected by the strong force are called *hadrons*, and all others are grouped as *leptons*.

The subatomic particles important for radiation therapy are electrons, positrons, protons, neutrons, and photons. Rest mass and electrical charge are the properties of these particles with which we will

TABLE 13.1 Radiation Activity, Exposure, and Dose Units of Measurement

Measured Property	Old Unit	New SI Unit	Conversion Factor
Radioactivity	curie (Ci) = 3.73×10^{10} dps	becquerel (Bq) = 1 dps	1 Ci = 3.7×10^{10} Bq 1 Bq = 2.7×10^{-11} Ci
Radiation exposure	roentgen (R) = 2.58×10^{-4} C/kg	coulomb/kg (C/kg)	1 R = 2.58×10^{-4} C/kg 1 C/kg = 3.88×10^3 R
Radiation absorbed dose	rad = 100 erg/g	gray (Gy) = 1 J/kg	1 rad = 0.01 Gy 1 Gy = 100 rad
Radiation dose equivalent	rem = QF × rad	sievert (Sv) = QF × Gy	1 rem = 0.01 Sv Sv = 100 rem

dps, Disintegrations per second; *QF*, quality factor; *SI*, International System of Units.
(From Waterstram-Rich KM, Gilman D, eds. *Nuclear Medicine PET/CT: Technology and Techniques*. 8th ed. St. Louis, MO: Elsevier; 2017.)

be concerned. The rest mass refers to the mass (weight) of the particle when it is not moving. Einstein's theory of special relativity states that subatomic particles moving at high speeds will have increased mass. At this point, we will not need to concern ourselves with this theory, other than to know of it.

The mass of subatomic particles can be measured in terms of the standard metric system mass unit, the kilogram. For those more familiar with US units of measure, 1 kg is equivalent to approximately 2.2 lbs. Because of the very small masses of these particles, expressing them in kilograms would make these values very cumbersome to handle. Therefore, a quantity called the *atomic mass unit (amu)* was defined.

> The atomic mass unit is defined such that the mass of an atom of carbon-12 is exactly 12.00 amu. As you may remember, the number of atoms in 12 grams of carbon-12 is equal to 6.022×10^{23}, which is Avogadro's number. Thus, the mass of each carbon-12 atom = $12/(6.022 \times 10^{23})$ grams = $1.99 \times 10^{-23}/1000$ kg = 1.99×10^{-26} kg, which is equal to 12.00 amu. Thus 1 amu = $1.99 \times 10^{-26}/12$ kg = 1.66×10^{-27} k

$$1 \text{ amu} = 1.66 \times 10^{-27} \text{ kg}$$

This relationship can be used to convert from one mass unit to another.[2]

Example: The mass of a proton is equal to 1.00727 amu. Express this mass in terms of kilograms.

$$(1.00727 \text{ amu}) \times \frac{1.66 \times 10^{-27} \text{ kg}}{(1 \text{ amu})} 1.672 \times 10^{-27} \text{ kg}$$

The electrical charge is a fundamental property or character of subatomic particles. It determines the strength of their EM interaction just as the mass of particles determines the strength of their gravitational interaction. A particle can have a positive, negative, or zero charge. By definition or convention, the electron is assigned a negative charge and the proton a positive charge. The electron and the proton have the same amount of electrical charge, 1.6×10^{-19} coulomb (C) (the C is the metric unit of electrical charge). The neutron, as the name implies, carries no electrical charge. Photons are quanta of EM energy of different frequencies and have zero rest mass and electrical charge. Two particles with an electrical charge of the same sign experience a repulsive EM force, whereas this force is attractive when the charges are of the opposite sign.

The radiation energy is transferred to any medium through its interaction with the atomic electrons and nucleus. A good understanding of the atomic structure will be helpful to understand the radiation interaction with matter.

Model of the Atom

Historically, JJ Thomson proposed the first model of the atom, known as the *raisin bread* or *plum pudding model*. According to this model, the positive charges and negatively charged electrons are uniformly distributed in the spherical volume of the atom with a radius of a few angstroms. However, Geiger-Marsden's alpha particles scattering from a metal foil experiment proved this to be wrong by observing an unexpected large scattering probability at angles greater than 90 degrees, contrary to the prediction by Thomson's plum pudding model. It led Rutherford to propose a new model in 1911. According to the Rutherford model, the positive electrical charge (+Ze) in an atom is not uniformly distributed over the whole area of the atom but is localized in a small area with a diameter in the order of 10^{-14} m, called the *nucleus*. The negatively charged electrons are distributed in the remaining space of the spherical atomic volume with a diameter in the order of 10^{-10} m and are postulated to be rotating around the nucleus like the planets in the solar system. This model could explain very well the backscattering of the alpha particles from the metal foil as the result of repulsion of the positively charged alpha particle from the localized positively charged nucleus. However, this model could not explain the stability of the atom. While the electrons are rotating around the nucleus, they will experience the centripetal acceleration, will continuously lose energy, and will eventually collapse to the nucleus. The Rutherford model also could not explain the discrete spectra of emitted radiation from atoms. In 1913, Neils Bohr attempted to explain the observed atomic spectra by combining the Rutherford atomic model with the newly postulated quantum theories of Einstein and Planck. This model, known as the *Bohr atom*, has since been replaced with complex quantum mechanical models of the atom; however, it is still an excellent way to derive a mental picture of the atom's structure. The Bohr atom seen in Fig. 13.1 consists of a central core, called the *nucleus*, and the electrons in fixed orbits. The Bohr atom model is based on the following four assumptions or postulates:

1. Electrons surrounding the nucleus exist only in certain energy states or orbits.[1,4]
2. Electrons do not lose energy when they reside in any of the allowed orbits.
3. When an electron moves from one orbit with higher energy to a lower-energy orbit, the atom emits radiation. The lost energy is seen as the atomic spectra.
4. In any allowed orbit, the angular momentum (L) of the electron, which is the product of electron mass, its velocity, and the radius of its orbit, can have only quantized or fixed values and are given as an integer multiple of a fundamental constant, called *Planck's*

constant (h). The model was successful in predicting the energy levels of hydrogen and other hydrogen-like atoms and ions with single electrons (e.g., singly ionized helium and doubly ionized lithium). The energy of the orbiting electron was derived to be as follows:

$$E_n = -13.6 \text{ eV } (Z/n)^2$$

where Z is the number of protons in the nucleus, and n is an integer known as the principal quantum number, which is related to the different available orbits for the electron to occupy. The ground state or the lowest energy state is n = 1; n > 1 corresponds to the excited states. Some energy has to be given to the atom for the electron to move from the ground state to different excited states. Similarly, when the electron moves from a higher n excited state to a lower n excited state or to the ground state with n = 1, some energy has to be given up, leading to discrete observed spectra for these atoms and ions.

The Bohr atom model can also be used to predict qualitatively the binding energy of the electrons and the transition of electrons between the possible electron orbits or levels leading to the emission or absorption of photons for multielectron atoms and ions. For multielectron atoms, the electrons are assigned to different shells. The proton number Z in the equation is replaced by Z_{eff}, which is the effective proton number seen by the electrons in the outer shell to account for the screening of the net nuclear charge by electrons in the inner shells. The Bohr model, which was based on postulates without a solid physical foundation, has many limitations and could not explain many observed phenomena in atomic physics. It was replaced by the quantum mechanical model of atoms, in which the electron in an atom or a molecule is described by its characteristic wave function and quantum numbers. The wave function or the atomic orbital gives a probabilistic description of the position of the electron around the nucleus under the influence of its attractive force and effect of the presence of other electrons. The wave function and the associated quantum numbers are obtained by solving the quantum mechanical many-body Schrödinger equation. The quantum numbers reflect the symmetry of the potential energy function of the electron and the restrictions imposed by the boundary conditions on the solution of the many-body equation. At present, the electronic structure of any atom can be computed with a high level of accuracy because of the use of quantum mechanics and high-speed computers. The energy and spatial distribution of an electron in an atom depend on its four quantum numbers: principal quantum number *(n)*, azimuthal or orbital angular momentum quantum number *(l)*, magnetic quantum number *(m_l)*, and spin quantum number *(m_s)*. The three-dimensional nature of the orbital requires three quantum numbers *n, l,* and *m* to distinguish each orbital from the other, and m_s is associated with the spinning nature of the electron. The principal quantum number determines the energy and size of the atomic orbital, has only nonzero positive integral values (n = 1, 2, …), and electrons with the same n are considered to belong to the same shell. Shells with n = 1, n = 2, n = 3, n = 4, n = 5, n = 6, and n = 7 are designated as K, L, M, N, O, P, and Q shells. The energy of the shell increases with the increase in the value of n. The *l* quantum number determines the angular shape of the orbital and determines the angular momentum of the electron because of its orbital motion. The value of *l* depends on the n value of the orbital and can have integer values only between 0 and n − 1. For example, if n = 1, then *l* = 0. For n = 4, the allowed values of *l* are 0, 1, 2, and 3. The energy of the electron is also determined by the value of *l* of its orbital, and it increases with the increase of *l*. Electrons in an atom with the same value of *l* are considered to belong to the same subshell. The subshells are designated as s, p, d, and f for *l* = 0, 1, 2, and 3, respectively. The magnetic quantum number *(m_l)* is used to differentiate the orientation of the orbital in each subshell. It is used to describe the change in the energy of the electron under the influence of the external magnetic field. The energy of the electron with no external magnetic field is not affected by m_l. The allowed values of m_l are integers between −*l* and

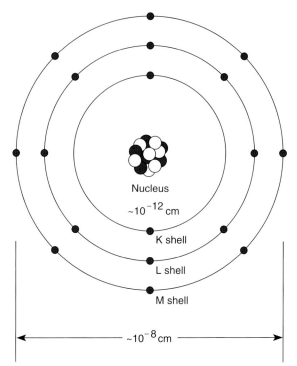

Fig. 13.1 The Bohr atom model with central nucleus surrounded by the electron orbits. (From Waterstram-Rich KM, Gilman D, eds. *Nuclear Medicine PET/CT: Technology and Techniques.* 8th ed. St. Louis, MO: Elsevier; 2017.)

+*l*. Thus m_l can have 2*l* + 1 values. For example, with *l* = 0, m_l = 0, for *l* = 2, m_l has five values: −2, −1, 0, 1, and 2. The number of allowed m_l values determines the number of possible orbitals within a subshell. Every elementary particle-like electron has an intrinsic spin angular momentum. This can be thought of as a consequence of its own spinning motion similar to that of the earth around its own axis. This can have two values to describe either the clockwise or counterclockwise direction of electron spin. The two values are +1/2 or −1/2.

The electronic configuration or occupation of different allowed orbitals is governed by the principle that every electron would like to occupy an orbital that would lead to the lowest energy state of the atom called the *ground state.* Electrons also obey the Pauli exclusion principle, which states that no two electrons in an atom can have the same four quantum numbers.

The orbital occupation of electrons in different atoms in the periodic table can be worked out with the aid of these principles, and allowed values of different quantum numbers are as discussed previously.

As seen in Fig. 13.1, electron shells are numbered and are given letter names that represent, in increasing order, their distance from the nucleus.

The maximum number of electrons in any shell is determined by the formula $2n^2$, where n is the shell number. As the atomic number increases, the number of electrons needed to keep the atom electrically neutral also increases. The rules by which the electrons fill the shells are as follows:

No shell can contain more than its maximum number of electrons.

The outermost shell can contain no more than eight electrons.

Example: Describe the electron shell configuration of an atom of stable nitrogen (Z = 7).

The first two electrons will fill the K shell. The five remaining electrons will fill five of the eight electron positions in the L shell.

Example: What is the electron configuration of an atom of electrically neutral cobalt (Z = 27)?

The K and L shells contain 10 electrons. The remaining 17 electrons would be spread between the M and N shells, even though the M shell can hold 18 electrons. This results from the second rule, which states that only 8 electrons can be in the outermost shell. Predicting the exact configuration of the electrons will involve using chemical principles, which we are not concerned with here. The important fact is that the electrons will be in four shells.

Practice: How many electronic shells are occupied in a neutral atom of oxygen with eight electrons?

> To learn more about structure of atoms, visit: http://education.jlab.org/qa/atom_idx.html

Atomic Energy Levels

An electron's binding energy is the amount of energy required to remove that electron from the atom. The binding energy is different for each shell and depends on the makeup of the nucleus. The larger the number of positive charges in the nucleus, the greater the attraction of the electrons toward it, and thus the higher the binding energy. The electron binding energy has a negative value and is usually measured in kiloelectron volts (keV). It represents the amount of energy that must be added to the electron's total energy before the electron can begin to move away from the atom.

The electrons in the outermost shell of the atom are called *valence electrons* and are responsible for chemical reaction and bonding of the atom with other atoms. When some energy is imparted to the electrons of the atom, the electrons will move to higher-energy empty states, called *excited states,* and the atom will then reach an unstable state. This process is called excitation. Eventually, the excess energy will be given up as radiation by the electron to return to its ground state. The excitation of valence electrons will require less energy as compared with that for tightly bound core electrons. If sufficient energy is given to the atom, one or more electrons of the atom can overcome its (their) binding energy and can be completely removed from the atom. This process is called *ionization.* When a core electron is ionized, a vacancy in its shell is created. An electron from one of the higher-energy orbitals immediately fills this vacancy or hole. This transition is accompanied by emission of excess energy in the form of photons, known as characteristic x-rays. The energy of these photons is equal to the difference in the energy of the two orbitals involved in the transition. The excess energy can also knock out one of the outer electrons from the atom. Such an ejected electron is known as an Auger electron (pronounced "O-zhey").

> When atoms of any material are exposed to radiation, the electrons of the atom can get excited and ionized, leading to the energy transfer from the incident radiation to the medium.

Atomic Nomenclatures

The atom consists of a nucleus and the orbiting electrons. The nucleus consists of protons and neutrons tightly bound together by a force known as the *strong nuclear force.* This force is strong enough at the extremely small distances found within the nucleus that it can hold together the positively charged protons that are trying to repel each other. Outside the nucleus, the strong nuclear force quickly becomes ineffective. The number of protons and neutrons within the nucleus defines the physical and chemical properties of the atom. Elements are substances made up entirely of atoms of a single kind. Some familiar substances that are elements include oxygen, carbon, helium, aluminum, and cobalt. All other substances are called *compounds* and are made up of various combinations of elements. As previously stated, each element contains a unique number of protons in its nucleus: carbon has six, oxygen has eight, and so forth. If a nucleus gains or loses protons, its elemental identity changes. For example, if a carbon atom gains a proton, it becomes a positive ion of nitrogen (which has seven protons). The number of protons in the nucleus is known as the atomic number of the atom. The number of protons and neutrons in the nucleus is termed the atomic mass number.

> The symbol used to identify an atom (X), its atomic number (Z), and atomic mass number (A) is as follows:
> $$^A_Z X$$

The periodic table in Fig. 13.2 is a listing of the elements and their symbols.

Nuclear Forces

The nucleus of the atom consists of protons and neutrons, which are together called *nucleons.* The protons are positively charged particles, and neutrons are neutral with no electrical charge. As you can imagine, the electrostatic force between the positively charged protons will repel each other. To hold a nucleus together, another force must be present. This force must be strong enough to overcome the electrostatic force that is attempting to break up the nucleus. This particular binding force is called the nuclear force. The nuclear force comes into play only over very short distances (10^{-14} m). The nature of this force and others within the nucleus to hold the nucleus together is complex. This is not discussed in detail here, but the major force that holds the nucleus of an atom together is the nuclear force.

Nuclear Structure, Stability, and Isotopes

The arrangement of nucleons in the nucleus is described by the nuclear shell model. The nucleons occupy different shells in the nucleus with discrete energy levels like that in the atomic shell model. The total amount of energy that it takes to hold a nucleus together is called the nuclear binding energy and is measured in megaelectron volts (MeV). To compare the binding energy of one nucleus with another, one must calculate the binding energy per nucleon. The binding energy per nucleon is the binding energy divided by the atomic mass number. It should be noted that a peak at an atomic mass number of approximately 56 represents the most stable state of iron (Fe). A nucleus can have more energy than is required for stability; to illustrate this, one can think of a staircase. The ground state is the minimum amount of energy needed to keep the nucleons together. The bottom step represents the ground state of the nucleus. Higher and higher steps of the staircase represent higher and higher energy states of the nucleus. As in a staircase, the steps have finite levels. The energy levels of a nucleus do not have transition zones between the steps, so the energy level of the nucleus must be one step or the other, not between. Each of the higher steps is called an excited nuclear energy level. As with an atom, if energy is imparted to the nucleus, some of the nucleons can move to higher-energy shells. Unstable nuclei or atoms are those that are not at their ground states. Similar to an atom, an excited nucleus tends to lose the excess energy and return to its ground state. This can be achieved in a number of ways, including radioactivity. Radioactivity is the emission of energy from the nucleus in the form of EM radiation or energetic particles.[4]

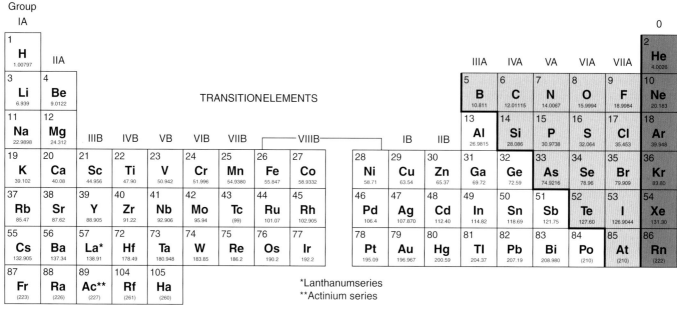

Fig. 13.2 Periodic table of elements. (From Waterstram-Rich KM, Gilman D, eds. *Nuclear Medicine PET/CT: Technology and Techniques*. 8th ed. St. Louis, MO: Elsevier; 2017.)

TABLE 13.2 Nuclear Configurations

Name	Z	A	N
Isotope	Same	Different	Different
Isobar	Different	Same	Different
Isotone	Different	Different	Same
Isomer	Same	Same	Same

A, Atomic mass number; *N*, number of neutrons; *Z*, atomic number.

As can be imagined, any element can have different nuclear configurations. Atoms with the same atomic number but different atomic mass numbers are called *isotopes* of that atom.[2,4] Other nuclear configurations, related to the various combinations of atomic number and number of neutrons, are summarized in Table 13.2. An easy way to remember this table is to recall the next to last letter of the configuration—isoto**p**e, isoba**r**, isoto**n**e, and isom**e**r—which tells the value that remains constant (one must assume that **e** stands for everything). For example, when looking at isotopes, the Z, or atomic number, remains the same. Thus the number of protons that define the element remains constant. In that case, the *p* (second from the end) becomes a quick reminder. The same is true for the others as well.

Particle Radiation

Radiation can be considered to consist of both waves and particles. In 1925, de Broglie hypothesized the dual nature of matter. According to his principle, waves can behave similar to particles, and every particle can have a wavelike character. Thus, EM waves sometimes act as particles. These particles are termed *photons*, and they have momentum similar to other particles. This is important to the definition of particle radiation, because the propagated energy has a definite rest mass, a definite momentum (within limits), and a position at any time. This hypothesis is discussed in more detail later.

Radiation therapy uses radiation that can create ionization in the medium by removing electrons from the atomic shells of the target, which can then lead to breaking of chemical bonds and other damages leading to cell death. This radiation is classified as ionizing radiation, and all others are known as nonionizing radiation. Ionizing radiation is divided into two groups, namely, directly ionizing radiation and indirectly ionizing radiation. The directly ionizing radiation, as the name indicates, produces the ionization itself: the group consists of charged particles such as electron, proton, and alpha particles and other heavy charged particles. The indirectly ionizing radiation group consists of neutral particles such as photons and neutrons, and the ionization by this group involves two steps. In the first step, their interactions with the electrons and nuclei of the target create charged particles such as electrons, positrons, protons, and other heavy ions in the medium. These released charged particles then create the actual ionization of the target atoms in the second step.

ELECTROMAGNETIC RADIATION

Radiation is defined as energy that is emitted by an atom and travels through space. This energy can take the form of EM radiation or can be transferred to subatomic particles such as electrons and cause the particles to move away from the atom. This section covers the phenomenon of EM radiation.

Photons

A photon is any "packet" of energy that travels through space at the speed of light, 3×10^8 m/sec (in a vacuum). Although a photon

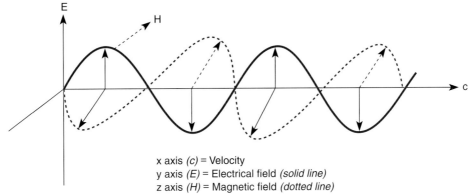

x axis (c) = Velocity
y axis (E) = Electrical field (solid line)
z axis (H) = Magnetic field (dotted line)

Fig. 13.3 Electromagnetic wave component energy fields. (From Waterstram-Rich KM, Gilman D, eds. *Nuclear Medicine PET/CT: Technology and Techniques*. 8th ed. St. Louis, MO: Elsevier; 2017.)

can be envisioned as a particle, it has no mass of its own, nor does it have an electrical charge. It has only its energy, which is a fixed quantity for that particular photon. Thus, high-energy photons can pass through miles of dense material unscathed, because they have no mass with which to "bump" into atoms and no electrical charges to attract or repel other particles that might interfere with their travels.

The nature of photons puzzled physicists until early in the twentieth century, when a new branch of physics called *quantum mechanics* burst into prominence. This field of study was an attempt to explain atomic and nuclear phenomena on their own level rather than trying to make the physics of these extremely small and special bits of matter correspond to the physics of large objects such as automobiles or planets. One of the discoveries of the new science was that photons can be viewed in one of two ways, depending on the situation: either as massless particles, as described previously, or, alternatively, as waves, similar to the movements of a violin string or the human voice. Photons are a special case of a type of wave called an *EM wave*, which consists of an electrical field and a magnetic field traveling through space at right angles to each other[1] (Fig. 13.3).

Photons exhibit the characteristics of a particle at times and the characteristics of a wave at other times. This phenomenon is known as *wave-particle duality.*

Both of these manifestations of the photon and how they are associated in a single equation are discussed in the following sections.

Physical Characteristics of an Electromagnetic Wave

An EM wave has three major distinguishing physical characteristics, which are closely interrelated. They are as follows:

1. The frequency of the wave, which is represented by the Greek letter ν (read as nu), is the number of times that the wave oscillates or cycles per second and is measured in units of cycles per second. Because the term "cycles" does not really have a unit, but is simply a number, the unit for frequency is 1/sec, called the *Hertz (Hz)*.

2. The wavelength of the wave is the physical distance between peaks of the wave. Wavelength is represented by the Greek letter lambda (λ) and is measured in meters (m). Usually the waves that we will be working with have wavelengths of approximately one-billionth of a meter, so to avoid having to constantly write very small numbers,

TABLE 13.3 Electromagnetic Spectrum

Radiation	Average λ (m)	Average ν (Hz)
Gamma rays	10^{-12}	10^{20}
Ultraviolet light	10^{-8}	10^{17}
Visible light	10^{-6}	10^{14}
Infrared light	10^{-5}	10^{13}
Microwaves	10^{-2}	10^{10}
Radio and television waves	10^{2}	10^{6}

(From Waterstram-Rich KM, Gilman D, eds. *Nuclear Medicine PET/CT: Technology and Techniques*. 8th ed. St. Louis, MO: Elsevier; 2017.)

we will express wavelengths in terms of the nanometer (nm), which is equal to 10^{-9} m. Another unit of wavelength seen frequently is the angstrom (Å), equal to 10^{-10} m, or 0.1 nm.

3. The final important wave characteristic is the velocity of the wave while it travels through space. For our purposes, we will assume that all EM waves travel at the same speed, which is the speed of light in a vacuum, represented by the letter "c" and equal to 3×10^8 m/sec.

The relationship between these three quantities is as follows:

$$c = \nu\lambda$$

Note that if you rearrange the variables, there are two other forms of this equation:

$$\nu = c / \lambda$$

$$\lambda = c / \nu$$

Looking closely at these equations, you can see that the frequency ν and wavelength λ of an EM wave are inversely related. As one gets larger, the other gets smaller. Table 13.3 lists some of the frequencies and wavelengths present in the range of known EM waves.

Example: Calculate the wavelength of an EM wave that has a frequency of 4.5×10^{14} Hz.

To calculate wavelength from frequency, we can use the equation $\lambda = c / \nu$:

$$\lambda = c/\nu = \frac{3 \times 10^8 \,m/s}{4.5 \times 10^{14} \,Hz} = 6.67 \times 10^{-7} m$$

This answer could also be expressed in nanometers and angstroms:

$$\left(6.67 \times 10^{-7} \text{m}\right)\left(1 \text{ nm} / 10^{-9} \text{m}\right) = 667 \text{ nm, or } 6670 \text{ Å}$$

Example: An FM radio station broadcasts at a wavelength of 3.125 m. At what frequency will you find this station on your radio dial?

$$\nu = c / \lambda = \frac{3 \times 10^8 \text{m/s}}{3.125 \text{ m}} = 96,000,000 \text{ Hz, or } 96 \times 10^6 \text{ Hz}$$

This station broadcasts at 96 megahertz (MHz).

Photon Energy

As stated previously, the energy of a photon is its major characteristic, especially from the viewpoint of radiation therapy physics. Fortunately, there are ways to calculate the energy of the wave when its other properties are known. The energy can, for example, be calculated when the frequency (ν) of the wave is known by using the following equation:

$$E = h\nu$$

where E is the energy of the wave, and h is a constant called *Planck's constant,* which has the value 6.626×10^{-34} J • s; this is equivalent to 4.15×10^{-15} eV • s. Either value can be used, depending on whether you want the resultant energy in joules (J) or electron volts (eV).

A joule (J) is the metric system, or SI, unit of energy and is equivalent to 1 kg • m²/sec². This unit is typically used for applications involving "real-world" objects, such as billiard balls, cans of light beer, and space shuttles. However, the energies of EM waves are usually much smaller than the energies involved in these situations (with the possible exception of light beer), so another smaller unit is used. This unit is the eV and represents the amount of energy that one electron would pick up as it passed through an electrical field, the potential difference of which was 1 V. This unit will be the standard unit for photon energy in this text and is related to the joule as follows:

$$1 \text{ eV} = 1.6 \times 10^{-19} \text{ J, or } 1\text{J} = 6.25 \times 10^{18} \text{ eV}$$

Example: If an EM wave has a frequency of 1.8×10^{20} Hz, what are its wavelength and energy (in eV)?

$$\lambda = c / \nu = \frac{3 \times 10^8 \text{m/s}}{1.8 \times 10^{20} \text{Hz}} = 1.667 \times 10^{-12} \text{m}$$

$$E = h\nu = \left(4.15 \times 10^{-15} \text{eV•s}\right)\left(1.8 \times 10^{20} \text{ Hz}\right)$$

$$= 747,000 \text{ eV} = 0.747 \text{ MeV}$$

Example: The photon emitted from the decay of the radioisotope ^{99m}Tc has an energy of approximately 142 keV. What are the frequency and wavelength of this photon?

Because we know that E = 142 keV = 142,000 eV, we can find ν by the following:

$$\nu = E / h = \frac{142,000 \text{ eV}}{4.15 \times 10^{-15} \text{ eV•s}} = 3.422 \times 10^{-19} \text{ Hz}$$

Now λ can be found:

$$\lambda = c / \nu = \frac{3 \times 10^8 \text{m/s}}{3.422 \times 10^{-19} \text{ Hz}} = 8.77 \times 10^{-12} \text{ m}$$

Another interesting fact about photons can be discovered by using Einstein's theories of relativity, in which he postulated the famous equation for relating the mass of any object to the amount of energy that it can be converted into:

$$E = mc^2$$

where E represents the energy, m represents the mass of the object, and c represents the speed of light. Note that because c^2 has units of m²/sec², it is necessary to express the mass of the object in kilograms so that we obtain an answer in joules whenever we use this equation.

This equation gave the first indication to the scientific world that matter and energy are actually different aspects of the same phenomenon and that one can be directly converted into the other. This discovery has drastically changed the world in which we live by increasing our understanding of the universe and giving us the ability to harness the power of the stars in nuclear fusion reactions, which convert a small amount of matter directly into a huge amount of energy. Unfortunately, the only current use of this knowledge in any viable sense is the stockpile of hydrogen bombs present in our defense arsenals.

If you set this equation for E equal to the Planck equation and solve, you find that:

$$m = h\nu / c^2$$

With this equation, it is possible to calculate the mass equivalence of a photon. Although the photon has no actual mass, the equation allows one to treat the photon as if it actually had mass of its own—the more energy, the greater the mass equivalence. Thus, the previous equation neatly combines the particle and wave natures of the photon into a single, tidy equation.

Example: Calculate the mass equivalence of a photon of green light, with a nominal wavelength of 520 nm.

First, calculate the energy of this wave, letting $\nu = c / \lambda$:

$$E = hc / \lambda = \frac{\left(6.626 \times 10^{-34} \text{ J•s}\right)\left(3 \times 10^8 \text{ m/s}\right)}{520 \times 10^{-9} \text{ m}} = 3.823 \times 10^{-19} \text{ J}$$

Note that to keep the units consistent, we have used the value for Planck's constant in joules. The SI unit of meters present in the photon wavelength will cancel out along with the seconds in others. Having found the energy, we can now calculate the mass equivalence by solving Einstein's equation for the mass:

$$m = E / c^2 = \frac{\left(3.823 \times 10^{-19} \text{ J}\right)}{\left(3 \times 10^8 \text{ m/s}\right)^2} = 4.248 \times 10^{-36} \text{ kg}$$

RADIOACTIVITY

Unstable atomic nuclei tend to seek their ground state, meaning that they tend to give off their excess energy until they reach a point at which the energy in the nucleus is just enough to maintain nuclear stability. The process by which they lose this energy is called radioactivity. Radioactivity may involve the emission of particles, EM radiation (photons), or a combination of the two. This section discusses the processes by which atoms rid themselves of this excess nuclear energy and the mathematical methods used to describe them.

Nuclear Stability Curve

The nuclear stability curve is shown in Fig. 13.4. The vertical axis represents the atomic number (Z) of the atom, that is, the number of protons in the nucleus. The horizontal axis represents the number of neutrons (N) in the nucleus. The straight line represents the condition $\frac{N}{Z} = 1$, that is, atoms with the same number of neutrons and protons in the nucleus. The curved line shows the "line of stability"; atoms whose proton/neutron combinations place them on this line are stable and will not undergo radioactive decay because they have no excess energy. The two lines are coincident at low values of Z; for example, Z less than 20, indicating that these atoms have identical numbers of protons and neutrons. While Z increases, however, the curve begins to diverge from the ideal line, curving to the right. This indicates that while the number of protons grows larger, more neutrons than protons are required to maintain stability, and the required neutron/proton ratio increases while Z increases. Atoms that do not meet this criterion appear at other positions on the graph, away from the stability curve; these represent unstable atoms. While these atoms lose energy, they will move closer to the stability curve, finally reaching a stable state.

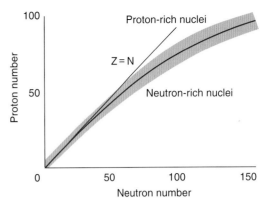

Fig. 13.4 Nuclear stability curve. (From Waterstram-Rich KM, Gilman D, eds. *Nuclear Medicine PET/CT: Technology and Techniques*. 8th ed. St. Louis, MO: Elsevier; 2017.)

You may recall that the combinations called isotope, isobar, and isotone refer to different arrangements of nuclear particles. Similarly, the terms isotopic, isobaric, and isotonic refer to types of transformations that change the atom to an isotope, isobar, or isotone of itself. For example, an isotopic transition is one in which the Z of the atom remains constant, but the atomic mass number (A) increases or decreases. Similarly, during an isobaric transition the A of the atom remains the same, and the Z and N change appropriately; during an isotonic transition, the N remains constant, and Z (and therefore A) changes. By undergoing as many of these transitions as necessary, atoms can move from an unstable to a stable state.

Types of Radioactive Decay

Alpha Decay. An alpha particle, symbolized by the Greek letter α, consists of two neutrons and two protons bound together; this is equivalent to a helium atom (Z = 2) that has been stripped of its two electrons.[1-4] Large, unstable atoms that have a large amount of excess energy tend to undergo radioactive decay by the emission of α particles, which eliminates four nuclear particles and therefore a substantial amount (in nuclear terms) of excess energy. The equation for radioactive decay is as follows:

$$^A_Z X \rightarrow ^{A-4}_{Z-2} Y + ^4_2 \alpha + Q$$

where Q represents the excess energy shed by the nucleus. This energy often appears in the form of photons, which, because of their nuclear origin, are called gamma rays (γ-rays).

Examine this equation carefully. Its written meaning is that a nucleus X with a known A and Z decays to a new atom with atomic mass number A−4 and atomic number Z−2; the two missing protons and two missing neutrons appear as an α particle emitted from the nucleus. In addition, a certain amount of energy is given off, either in the form of kinetic energy (i.e., speed of the α particle) or as γ-rays or, more commonly, as a combination of the two. A key feature of this equation is that the numbers of protons, neutrons, and electrical charges on both sides of the arrow are equal. This is a critical feature of all radioactive decay equations: the two sides of the arrow must balance exactly in terms of number of particles, electrical charges, and energy. The most important thing to note, however, is that the

original atom has now changed into a new element by the loss of two nuclear protons.

Example: An atom of uranium, U, undergoes α decay. What is the result?

$$^{238}_{92} U \rightarrow ^{234}_{90} Th + ^4_2 \alpha + \gamma$$

The atom of uranium has been transformed into an atom of thorium.

Alpha decay occurs when the $\frac{N}{Z}$ ratio is too low, that is, when the atom falls "underneath" the stability curve on the $\frac{N}{Z}$ graph. By eliminating two neutrons and two protons, plus the associated energy, this transition increases the $\frac{N}{Z}$ ratio, attempting to correct for the too low $\frac{N}{Z}$ ratio that existed before the transition.

The energies of the α particles emitted by a given isotope are fixed and discrete. Even though an isotope may emit more than one α particle, each α particle will have one of a selection of fixed energies. This contrasts with beta (β) decay, described in the next two sections, in which essentially infinite numbers of particle energies are possible.

Beta-Minus Decay. Recall that a beta-minus (β−) particle is the same as an electron. The difference in name stems from the difference in place of origin. An electron is found orbiting in the electron shells, whereas a β− particle is emitted as the result of a nuclear decay. To understand β− decay, think of a neutron as a "mixture" of a proton plus an electron:

$$n^0 \rightarrow p^+ + e^-$$

What essentially happens during a β− decay is that a neutron in the nucleus "decays" into a proton plus an electron, as shown. The proton remains in the nucleus, and the electron is ejected and leaves the atom; this ejected electron is called the β− *particle*. The equation for β− decay is as follows:

$$^A_Z X \rightarrow ^A_{Z+1} Y + ^0_{-1} \beta + \nu_a$$

where the symbol ν_a represents the emission of a tiny particle called the *antineutrino*. This particle carries away the energy that is left over when the β− does not carry away all of the atom's excess energy. You can see that when undergoing β− decay, the atom increases its Z by one while maintaining the same A (having lost a neutron but gained a proton), making this an isobaric transition. Because of this property, the ratio $\frac{N}{Z}$ of this atom will decrease. Usually, the daughter nucleus of a β− decay is itself radioactive and can undergo radioactive decay in many ways, typically by giving off its

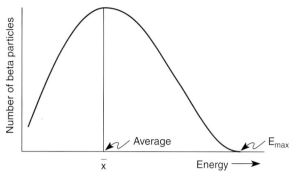

Fig. 13.5 Beta particle energy spectrum. (From Waterstram-Rich KM, Gilman D, eds. *Nuclear Medicine PET/CT: Technology and Techniques.* 8th ed. St. Louis, MO: Elsevier; 2017.)

excess energy as γ-rays. In fact, there are very few isotopes that emit only β⁻ particles; the majority are accompanied by γ-ray emission from the daughter nucleus.[1-4]

Example: Cobalt-60 decays by β⁻ decay to an excited state of ^{60}Ni, which then decays by the emission of two high-energy γ-rays as follows:

$$^{60}_{27}\text{Co} \rightarrow {}^{60}_{28}\text{Ni} + {}^{0}_{-1}\beta + \nu \rightarrow {}^{60}_{28}\text{Ni} + 2\gamma$$

Beta-emitting isotopes do not give off β⁻ particles of fixed energy as do alpha emitters. Instead, the emitted β⁻ particles possess energies between 0 and a given maximum (E_{max}), creating what is called a *beta spectrum* (Fig. 13.5). The average energy of the β⁻ particle in the spectrum is approximately one-third of E_{max}. The extra energy between E_{max} and the actual energy of the β⁻ particle is carried away by the antineutrino (ν_a).

β-plus decay. There is a subatomic particle that has exactly the same characteristics as an electron, except that it possesses a positive electrical charge rather than a negative charge. This particle is called a *positron* and is represented by the symbol β⁺. In addition, similar to a β⁻, it is ejected from an atomic nucleus. In this case, a nuclear proton decays into a neutron and a positron:

$$p^+ \rightarrow n^0 + \beta^+$$

Thus, the equation for β⁺ decay is as follows:

$$^{A}_{Z}\text{X} \rightarrow {}_{Z-1}{}^{A}\text{Y} + {}^{0}_{+1}\beta + \nu$$

Because of the loss of a proton but the gain of a neutron, the atom retains the same A, but the Z of the atom decreases by 1 and the N/Z ratio of the atom increases, making this an isobaric transition.[1]

Sodium-22 (^{22}Na$_{11}$) is a common radioactive isotope of natural sodium. It decays by β⁺ decay to a stable isotope of the gas neon, with the emission of a β⁺ particle and a γ-ray, as follows:

$$^{22}_{11}\text{Na} \rightarrow {}^{22}_{10}\text{Ne}^* + {}^{0}_{+1}\beta \rightarrow {}^{22}_{10}\text{Ne} + \gamma$$

As with β⁻ decay, a spectrum of energies is emitted, with an average energy of one-third E_{max}; the remainder of the energy is carried off by the neutrino (ν), as in β⁻ decay.

Electron capture. Although the Bohr model of the atom depicts the electrons in fixed orbits outside of the nucleus, according to theories of quantum mechanics, it is possible that the electrons may, at some time, come very close to the nucleus. An electron that strays too close to the

nucleus may be captured and combined with a proton, reversing the process for β− decay:

$$p^+ + e^- \rightarrow n^0 + \nu$$

This process is known as *electron capture* and has the same result as β⁺ decay; in other words, the Z of the parent nucleus decreases by 1, and the $^N/_Z$ ratio of the atom increases.

Because of the proximity of the K shell to the nucleus, it is most likely that the captured electron will be taken from this shell, although it is possible to capture an electron from the L or M shell. When an electron is taken from one of the electron shells, it leaves a "hole" in the shell; this will place the atom in an unstable configuration in terms of energy, because an inner shell electron has lower energy than an outer shell electron. As a result, one of the electrons from an outer shell will "fall" toward the nucleus, moving from a higher energy state to a lower one, and this excess energy, no longer needed to maintain stability, will be given off in the form of an x-ray. This type of radiation is called characteristic radiation and is an important part of many radioactive decay schemes and radiation/matter interactions.

Isomeric transition or gamma decay. An isomer is an atom with the identical Z and A of another atom but which is currently in what is called a *metastable state*. This represents a daughter product of some other kind of decay that is itself in an excited state, but instead of instantly decaying by γ emission (see the example for β⁻ decay), it remains in this excited state for a given period of time and then decays. Such a nucleus is represented by a small "m" next to its atomic mass number, as in ^{99m}Tc. A nucleus that has no metastable state but decays instantly has an asterisk to the right of its chemical symbol (^{60}Ni*). Metastable isotopes, or isomers, usually decay by emitting the excess energy as a γ-ray.

^{99m}Tc is an isotope used daily in nuclear medicine procedures. It is a daughter product of ^{99}Mo, and the decay equation appears as follows:

$$^{99}_{42}\text{Mo} \rightarrow {}^{99m}_{43}\text{Tc}^* + {}^{0}_{-1}\beta + \nu \rightarrow {}^{99}_{43}\text{Tc} + \gamma$$

Specification of Radioactivity

To quantify the amount of radioactivity present in a given sample, in the early 20th century, the curie (Ci) was defined as the activity of 1 g of ^{226}Ra, the most well-known isotope in use at that time. Unfortunately, while measurement techniques improved, disputes arose as to exactly what the activity of 1 g of ^{226}Ra meant in terms of the number of radioactive atoms present. Thus, eventually the unit of radioactivity, the curie, was defined as follows:

$$1 \text{ Ci} = 3.7 \times 10^{10} \text{ } dis/\sec$$

where *dis/sec* stands for nuclear disintegrations per second, that is, the number of atoms that undergo some kind of radioactive decay every second. Because disintegration is merely a quantity and does not have a unit, the curie is numerically equal to 1/sec or sec⁻¹. In fact, the SI unit of radioactivity, the becquerel (Bq), is equal to 1 *dis/sec*. Because many disintegrations per second are present in even a small sample of radioactive material, the becquerel is a much smaller unit than the curie. You can easily see that 1 Ci = 3.7 × 10¹⁰ Bq = 37 billion Bq. For this reason, the curie still remains the popular unit of radioactivity, although we are supposed to use the SI units.

For various amounts of radioactive material, multiples of the curie, such as the millicurie (mCi, 10⁻³ Ci) and the microcurie (μCi, 10⁻⁶ Ci), are used. A typical nuclear medicine procedure uses amounts of radioactivity in the range of hundreds of millicuries, whereas a cobalt teletherapy machine uses a source of cobalt-60 of an activity in the range of 5000 to 6000 Ci.

Exponential Decay of Radioactivity

The amount of radioactivity present in a given sample is never a constant quantity, but rather is reduced continuously by the decay of the radioactive atoms in the sample.[2,4] This decay process follows a mathematical pattern known as *exponential behavior*. Any value that increases or decreases exponentially will double or halve its value within a certain amount of time. When that time interval passes again, the value will have further reduced by half or increased by two times. Although it is impossible to say exactly which atoms in a radioactive sample will decay at any given time, it is reasonably straightforward to determine what percentage of the atoms will remain after a given amount of time.

The equation of exponential decay of radioactivity is as follows:

$$A_t = A_0 e^{-\lambda t}$$

where A_t is the activity at time t, A_0 is the activity at time zero (when the activity was measured), and λ is a value known as the *exponential decay constant*, which is discussed in more detail later. The symbol e represents the base of the natural logarithms, which governs exponential behavior; it has the value $e = 2.718282\ldots$.

According to the rules of logarithms, e to any negative power will always be less than 1.000, e to a very small negative number power will be very close to 1.000, and many hand calculators will give the value of 1.000 in this case. However, the number should never be greater than 1.000; if this is the case, you have made a mathematical error, because radioactive decay will always result in a decrease in the amount of radioactivity present.

To make this point clear, we will use a little algebra to rearrange the previous equation:

$$A_t/A_0 = e^{-\lambda t}$$

This equation states that the final amount of radioactivity divided by the initial amount is equal to the exponential side of the equation, which will always be between 0 and 1.

Another important principle in working with natural logarithms is that the inverse of the exponential function e is the natural logarithm *ln*, which makes

$$\ln\left(e^{anything}\right) = anything$$

or in this case:

$$\ln\left(e^{-\lambda t}\right) = -\lambda t$$

Example: A radioactive sample is measured to contain 100 mCi of radioactivity. If the decay constant of this isotope is 0.115 hr^{-1}, how much activity will remain after 24 hours?

$$A_t = A_0 e^{-\lambda t} = (100 \text{ mCi}) e^{(-0.115)(24)} = 6.329 \text{ mCi}$$

Note the units on λ, which are time^{-1}. Because the units of t are in time and the units of λ are time^{-1}, these must cancel out, leaving the exponent of e with no units. To accomplish this, λ and t must be in the same unit of time, that is, minutes, hours, days, years, and so forth.

The λ is a constant for a given isotope; that is, all atoms of a given isotope will decay with the same λ, which will not change no matter what environmental conditions persist. You cannot change the λ of an isotope with heat, pressure, or any other known factors.

How can we use the exponential decay equation to derive the useful quantity, known as the *half-life* of an isotope? The half-life is the time required for the activity of any sample of a particular radioisotope to decay to half of its initial value. Thus the quantity we seek to solve for is t, the time, which we will give the special symbol t_h to represent half-life.

How do we solve the equation for half-life? We know that the activity after one half-life will be half of the initial activity, by definition. Thus, we can write the following:

$$A_t/A_0 = 0.5$$

Knowing this, solve for t_h:

$$A_t/A_0 = e^{-\lambda t}$$

$$0.5 = e_h^{-\lambda t}$$

$$\ln(0.5) = \ln\left(e_h^{-\lambda t}\right)$$

$$-0.693 = -\lambda_h^t$$

We now divide and cancel the minus signs to get the final solution:

$$t_h = \frac{0.693}{\lambda}$$

We can, if needed, rearrange this equation:

$$\lambda = \frac{0.693}{t_h}$$

You should go through this derivation several times and try it yourself so that the method is clear. These equations are used frequently in calculations involving radioactive isotopes.

Example: A sample of an isotope with a half-life of 8.0 days is measured to have an activity of 25.0 mCi on Monday at noon. What would the activity be on Friday of that week, at noon?

Find λ by using the previous equations with 4.0 days as the value for t:

$$\lambda = \frac{0.693}{t_h} = \frac{0.693}{8.0 \text{d}} = 0.087 \text{d}^{-1}$$

Activity after 4 days = 25.0 mCi x $e^{-(0.087 \times 4)}$ = 17.7 mCi.

The exponential decay equation is powerful because it can be solved algebraically in a number of ways, depending on the results required. For example, if you take two activity readings from an isotope sample, you can call these A_0 and A_t, and the elapsed time between the two readings will be t. You can now find the decay constant and half-life of this isotope by rearranging the exponential decay equation into a new form:

$$\frac{A_t}{A_0} = e^{-\lambda t}$$

$$\ln\frac{A_t}{A_0} = \ln e^{-\lambda t} = -\lambda t$$

$$\ln\frac{A_t}{A_0} \times \frac{-1}{t} = \lambda$$

Note that we have made use of the relationship between ln and e; that is, that the natural log function and the exponential function are inverse functions. One will cancel the effect of the other. This allows us to find any unknown quantities that may exist in the exponent of the exponential function, such as λ or t. The previous equation can be used to find λ and therefore the half-life of the isotope.

Two readings of the activity of a radioactive sample are taken 40 hours apart. The first reading is 125.0 mCi; the second one is 1.232 mCi. Calculate the half-life of this isotope.

Find λ, then find t_h:

$$\ln\frac{A_t}{A_0} \times \frac{-1}{t} = \lambda$$

$$\ln\frac{1.232\ mCi}{125.0\ mCi} \times \frac{-1}{40.0\ hr} = \lambda$$

$$(-4.620)\,(-0.025) = 0.116\ hr^{-1} = \lambda$$

$$t_h = \frac{0.693}{0.116\ hr^{-1}} = 6.0\ hr$$

Activity of an isotope with a decay constant $\lambda = 0.043\ hr^{-1}$ was measured after 24 hours of decay. The measured activity at the end of this period was 17.8 mCi. What was the initial activity?

$$A_t = A_0 e^{-\lambda t}$$

$$17.8 = A_0 e^{(-0.043)(24)}$$

$$17.8 = A_0\,(0.356)$$

$$A_0 = 50\ mCi$$

A quantity called the *mean life* $(\bar{t})$ of the isotope is sometimes used in brachytherapy calculations involving short-lived isotopes (i.e., isotopes with short half-lives). The mean life of $\bar{t}$ is related to the half-life and decay constant of the isotope as follows:

$$\bar{t} = 1.44 t_h = \frac{1}{\lambda}$$

Radioactive Equilibrium

It is common for some radioisotopes, especially high Z isotopes, to decay to daughter products that are themselves radioactive. An example of this process is ^{226}Ra, which is one of a number of isotopes along a "chain" of daughter products created when ^{238}U, found in nature, decays to ^{206}Pb during the course of millions of years. When parent and daughter isotopes exist in this manner, it is possible that a condition of equilibrium (i.e., balance) will be established in this system—the daughter and parent isotopes will begin to appear to decay with nearly the same half-lives and with the same activities.

To illustrate this, consider the case of the decay of ^{226}Ra to ^{222}Rn via α decay:

$$^{226}_{88}Ra \rightarrow\ ^{222}_{86}Rn + ^{4}_{2}\alpha + Q$$

^{226}Ra has a half-life of more than 1600 years, whereas the half-life of the daughter ^{222}Rn is only approximately 3.8 days. A sample that starts out as pure radium begins to decay to radon, causing a buildup of radon. However, the radon decays with a shorter half-life and so will have a higher activity (number of disintegrations per second). Eventually the daughter product is so active that it essentially equals the activity of the parent. This condition is called *secular equilibrium* and can occur only when the half-life of the

parent is much greater than the half-life of the daughter isotope, that is, when

$$t_{hparent} >> t_{hdaughter}$$

If the differences in parent and daughter half-life are not as dramatic, but the parent is still longer lived than the daughter, the daughter activity will actually grow slightly larger than the parent activity and then appear to decay at the same rate (with the same half-life). This condition is called *transient equilibrium* and occurs when

$$t_{hparent} > t_{hdaughter}$$

In the case of $t_{hparent} < t_{hdaughter}$, no equilibrium can exist.

Radioactive equilibrium conditions can be exploited to provide a steady source of some radioisotopes used in nuclear medicine procedures. An excellent example of this is the use of "generators" that contain a source Mo, which decays by β^- decay to the metastable isotope *Tc. The parent half-life of 67 hours is greater than the daughter half-life of 6 hours, so transient equilibrium is reached. Each week a fresh generator is delivered to the nuclear medicine department. At the beginning of each day, the technologist adds a solvent to the generator, which chemically separates the ^{99m}Tc from the ^{99}Mo, and the ^{99m}Tc is drawn off. ^{99m}Tc can then be used as a radioactive injection in a number of diagnostic studies. Of course, because the ^{99}Mo is decaying away, at the beginning of each day, less ^{99m}Tc is available than the day before. Thus, at the end of the week, the generator is stored for further decay and then returned to the manufacturer when radiation levels reach acceptable levels.

> You can learn more about basic nuclear physics by visiting http://www.lbl.gov/abc/.

PHOTON INTERACTIONS

When a beam of radiation from any source strikes some material, a number of processes can occur that lead to transfer of energy from the radiation to the medium; this energy can then affect the medium in many ways. Biologic tissue, for example, may suffer damage to the nucleic acid structures (deoxyribonucleic acid) and lose its ability to reproduce itself, thereby damaging the organism as a whole. Other materials may undergo physical or chemical changes as a result of the energy transfer, such as heating or disruption of crystal structures. This section discusses the ways in which photons (x-rays or γ-rays) interact with matter.

Inverse Square Law

The intensity of flux of a radiation beam is defined as the number of photons in the beam per square centimeter. Note that this definition does not take into account the energy of the radiation in the beam, only the number of photons present in the beam at a given instant per square centimeter. Thus, a beam can be called "low intensity" if it has just a few photons per square centimeter, even if the photons are very high energy; similarly, a "high-intensity" beam may consist entirely of a large number of very-low-energy photons. For practical purposes, the intensity of a radiation beam is usually measured in terms of the exposure rate ($\dot{X}$, mR/h) or dose rate ($\dot{D}$ cGy/min) of the beam at that point, rather than the number of photons present.

Often in radiation therapy physics, we are interested in describing the intensity from a point source of radiation. A point source is a source that is so small (from the viewpoint of the observer) that it appears to have no area, and all photons coming from it appear to originate at the same point. In reality, most radiation sources have some finite area; however, if the distance from the source is large, it will appear to be a point. For example, a coin viewed from a distance of 3 meters will appear to be a point. Thus, if the distance from the source to the point of interest is at least five times the physical size of the source, the source can be treated as a point source. This assumption greatly simplifies most radiation therapy calculations; because the distance from a radiation therapy source to the point of interest is rarely shorter than five times the source size, most sources can be considered point sources for our purposes. This is not always true in the case of internally implanted radioisotopes.

Given that we are working with a point source, the intensity of the radiation beam coming from this source can be determined first by assuming that the radiation is emitted isotropically from the source—that is, it is emitted evenly in all directions from the point source. If this is the case, the intensity of the beam at any distance from the source is calculated by dividing the number of photons coming from the source by the area of the sphere surrounding the source at that distance. If we let Δp represent the number of photons emitted by the point source in any instant, we can say that the intensity of the beam at distance d_1 from the point source is equal to the following:

$$I_1 = \text{number of photons} / \text{area of sphere} = \Delta p / 4\pi d_1^2$$

where $4\pi d_1^2$ is the area of the sphere of radius d_1.

How does the intensity change while we move closer to or farther away from our point source? If we assume that none of the photons are attenuated (taken out of the beam), then Δp will remain the same; only d, the distance from the point source, will change. If we call the new distance d_2, then the intensity at this point is equal to the following:

$$I_2 = \Delta p / 4\pi d_2^2$$

Thus, the change in intensity moving from distance d_1 to distance d_2 is the ratio of I_1 to I_2:

$$\frac{I_1}{I_2} = \left(\frac{\Delta p / 4\pi d_1^2}{\Delta p / 4\pi d_2^2}\right) = \left(\frac{d_2^2}{d_1^2}\right) = \left(\frac{d_2}{d_1}\right)^2$$

When we solve this equation for I_2, we get the following result:

$$I_2 = I_1 \left(\frac{d_1}{d_2}\right)^2$$

This is one statement of the inverse square law, an important principle in radiation therapy physics.

The basic idea of the inverse square law is that the intensity of a radiation beam in a nonabsorbing medium decreases or increases as the inverse of the square of the distance.[1]

A few examples should clarify the use of this principle.

Example: The intensity of a radiation beam is measured at 10.0 mR/h at a distance of 10 cm. What will be the intensity of this beam at 20.0 cm?

Let $I_1 = 10$ mR/h, $d_1 = 10.0$ cm, and $d_2 = 20.0$ cm. The intensity at d_2 will be as follows:

$$I_2 = (10.0 \text{ mR/hr}) (10.0 \text{ cm} / 20.0 \text{ cm})^2 = 2.5 \text{ mR/hr}$$

The intensity at twice the distance is one-fourth of the original intensity.

If, in the preceding example, d_2 is equal to 5 cm (i.e., the new distance is closer to the source than the original), what will be the change in beam intensity?

With d_2 now equal to 5 cm, the solution becomes:

$$I_2 = (10.0 \text{ mR/hr}) (10.0 \text{ cm} / 5.0 \text{ cm})^2 = 40.0 \text{ mR/hr}$$

Because the distance change was in the opposite direction of the previous example, the intensity increased by four times.

The inverse square law, as indicated earlier, is an important factor in radiation therapy dose calculations.

Exponential Attenuation

The inverse square law is strictly correct only when certain conditions are met. For example, the size of the radiation source must be small enough to be treated as a point source. In addition, we have assumed that none of the radiation emitted from the source is removed from the beam, but rather continues outward from the source undisturbed. When working with photons in air, this condition is met well enough that the inverse square law can be said to apply in most of these cases. For high-energy medical accelerators, the inverse square law applies to a limited degree when the photons are traveling in some material such as water or a patient. In most cases of photon interactions with material, however, the photons will indeed interact with the atoms of the material, giving up their energy and being removed from the beam. This process is called *attenuation*.

Earlier we saw that the decay of a radioactive source is an exponential function, described by the following equation:

$$A_t = A_0 e^{-\lambda t}$$

where λ is a constant for a given radioisotope, and t is the time between measurements A_0 and A_t. This represents a statistical view of the problem; it is impossible to say exactly when each individual atom will decay, but large numbers of atoms can be described with high precision. The attenuation of radiation by a medium can also be described in this way. For this purpose, we define a quantity called the *linear attenuation coefficient* with the symbol μ. This describes the probability that each photon in the beam will interact with the medium and lose its energy, per centimeter of material that the photons pass through, and has units of cm^{-1}. It is not a constant like λ, but instead depends greatly on the energy of the photon beam and the medium in which the interaction is taking place.

The extent of attenuation of a photon beam by a medium is then calculated by the following equation:

$$I_x = I_0 e^{-\mu x}$$

where I_0 is the intensity of the beam before it strikes the medium, I_x is the intensity after it passes through the medium, μ is the linear attenuation coefficient for this beam energy and medium, and x is the thickness of the medium (in cm). Note that this equation is in exactly the same form as the equation for radioactive decay, indicating that the two processes are similar to each other because they are statistical in nature, rather than exact.

Similar to the radioactive decay equation, the equation of attenuation can be used in many ways. Some examples are given subsequently.

Example: A beam of cobalt-60 photons is incident on a lead sheet 1.0 cm thick. If the initial dose rate of the cobalt beam (I_0) was 50 cGy/min, what will the dose rate be after the beam passes through the lead sheet if the value of μ for this beam in lead is 0.533 cm^{-1}?

$$I_x = I_0 e^{-\mu x}$$

$$I_x = (50) e^{(-0.533)(1.0)}$$

$$I_x = (50) (0.587)$$

$$I_x = 29.35 \text{ cGy/min}$$

Example: With the data from the previous example, calculate the initial dose rate if the dose rate after the beam passes through the lead sheet is measured to be 15.0 cGy/min.

From the previous example, $\mu = 0.533 \text{ cm}^{-1}$ and $x = 1.0 \text{ cm}$:

$$I_x = I_0 e^{-\mu x}$$

$$15.0 = I_0 e^{(-0.533)(1.0)}$$

$$15.0 = I_0 (0.587)$$

$$I_0 = 25.55 \text{ cGy/min}$$

The values of μ for materials and photon energies important in radiation therapy are provided in Table 13.4.

$$HVL = 0.693 / \mu$$

The exponential radioactivity decay equation can be used to derive a special quantity, the half-life, that describes the amount of time required for the isotope to decay to half of its original activity. In the same manner, we can define a quantity, called the half-value layer (HVL), that is, the thickness of some added material required to reduce the beam intensity to half of its original value:

TABLE 13.4 Linear Attenuation Coefficients (μ)(cm−1)

Energy (MeV)	Water	Tissue	Aluminum	Copper	Lead
0.010	5.0660	5.360	71.1187	1964.0300	1507.4720
0.050	0.2245	0.2330	0.9803	22.9466	88.7330
0.100	0.1706	0.1760	0.4604	4.0759	62.0370
0.200	0.1370	0.1412	0.3306	1.4067	11.2612
0.500	0.0969	0.0998	0.2281	0.7500	1.8040
0.662	0.0857	0.0883	0.2013	0.6496	1.2314
0.800	0.0787	0.0810	0.1846	0.5914	0.9906
1.000	0.0707	0.0729	0.1660	0.5277	0.7963
1.250	0.0632	0.0651	0.1482	0.4704	0.6600
1.500	0.0575	0.0593	0.1352	0.4301	0.5873
2.000	0.0494	0.0510	0.1169	0.3763	0.5146
3.000	0.0397	0.0409	0.0955	0.3226	0.4737
4.000	0.0340	0.0350	0.0839	0.2975	0.4714
5.000	0.0303	0.0312	0.0767	0.2840	0.4805
8.000	0.0242	0.0249	0.0713	0.2715	0.5157
10.00	0.0222	0.0229	0.0626	0.2778	0.5544
20.00	0.0182	0.0186	0.0586	0.3055	0.6952
30.00	0.0171	0.0176	0.0594	0.3324	0.7952
50.00	0.0167	0.0172	0.0623	0.3692	0.9168
80.00	0.0169	0.0173	0.0656	0.4005	1.0122
100.0	0.0172	0.0177	0.0677	0.4184	1.0544

Because μ depends on the energy of the beam and the material with which the radiation interacts, HVL values must be defined by both energy and attenuating material. This procedure is fairly straightforward if the photon beam is monoenergetic, that is, if it consists of only a single-photon energy. Unfortunately, this is not the case with photon beams produced by most modern radiation therapy equipment, which produce polyenergetic beams consisting of a wide spectrum of photon energies. Therefore, the HVL is usually simply measured for a given machine and beam energy and, in the case of low-energy x-ray units, is used to describe the characteristics of the treatment beam.

We know that exponential decay data plotted on a semilogarithmic graph paper yields a straight line. This technique can also be applied to exponential attenuation by plotting the percentage of radiation that passes through a material as a function of the material thickness. By plotting data such as these and drawing in the straight line formed by the data, the HVL of the beam can be determined experimentally. Once the graph is done, the thickness of material required to reduce the beam intensity to any fraction of its initial value can be found simply by reading the graph. If a large number of attenuation readings are taken, the curve may not actually display a single line but a series of line segments of decreasing slope. This effect results from the "hardening" of the beam, explained in the next section.

X-Ray Beam Quality

The HVL is an important quantity for photon beams and can be used as a description of "beam quality." Photon beams can be classified as "hard" or "soft" beams, depending on their HVL.[4] Although there are no strict rules to determine the hardness or softness of a radiation beam, a hard beam will have a higher HVL and higher penetrating ability than a soft beam.

This concept of beam hardness becomes more important when one considers the various factors involved. Softer beams have less penetrating ability and therefore will tend to deposit their energy in a medium fairly quickly. If the medium in question is actually a radiation therapy patient, this means that the skin dose to that patient will be increased. In some situations, this is desirable; in many situations, however, it is not. Consider, for example, a conventional radiation therapy simulator (or any diagnostic x-ray device). A soft beam will not penetrate adequately through the patient to the imaging device but will instead leave a large amount of dose inside the patient without contributing any quality to the final image. In this setting, the therapist should attempt to reduce the softness of the beam (and therefore the patient dose) without requiring a large increase in radiation exposure to take the image.

To understand one solution to these problems, consider a polyenergetic beam of radiation striking a medium such as lead. The beam consists of a large variety of x-ray energies—some low, some more energetic. While the beam passes through the lead, the softer x-rays (those with the lower energy) tend to be absorbed by the lead, whereas the harder x-rays, whose μ value is lower, are not as likely to be absorbed and may pass through the lead untouched. Thus, if you examine the various energies in the beam before and after it passes through the lead, you can see that the beam exiting from the lead will have a higher average energy (i.e., fewer low-energy x-rays) and a larger HVL than the initial beam. By passing the beam through this lead attenuator, we have actually increased the overall HVL of the beam, although the intensity of the beam has been decreased. This effect is called *beam hardening* and is very important in the design and use of diagnostic and radiation therapy equipment.[2-4]

Low-energy x-ray units (diagnostic and superficial therapy) usually have a certain amount of "inherent filtration;" that is, some filtration material is built into the machine. Usually this consists of the metal window where the radiation beam exits the inside chamber of the tube, where it is produced, with a small amount of added filtration (usually aluminum) to harden the beam for use in patient diagnosis and treatment. High-energy x-ray units (i.e. linear accelerators) have several devices in the treatment head that harden the beam, in addition to changing the distribution of the radiation within the field so that the dose delivered across the patient's body is uniform. These devices assist in improving the uniformity of dose within the treatment volume while eliminating excessive dose in areas where tissue sparing is desirable.

Types of Photon Interactions

The exact mechanisms of the interactions of photons with the atoms of the irradiated medium are known to a large extent from the work performed in the late nineteenth and early twentieth centuries by Thomson, Einstein, Compton, Rutherford, and many others. There are five photon interaction processes that occur in the energy range of concern in radiation therapy:

1. Rayleigh (coherent) scattering
2. Photoelectric scattering
3. Compton (incoherent) scattering
4. Pair production
5. Photodisintegration

Rayleigh (coherent) scattering. In Rayleigh scattering, the incident photon is of very low energy, not energetic enough to ionize the atom. The photon, coming into the region close to the atom, is absorbed, but because not enough energy is present to cause the release of any electrons, the atom re-emits a second photon of exactly the same energy as the incident photon but headed in a new direction. So, from the outside, it appears that the photon bounced off of the atom into another direction. In this case, no damage is done to the atom, so this interaction has no biologic effect. The interaction is called *coherent* because the wavelength and energy of the emitted photon are identical to those of the incident photon, a condition known in physics as *coherency*.

Photoelectric scattering. The photoelectric effect was first described in detail by Einstein, who was awarded the Nobel Prize in physics for the discovery (his other theories were believed to be too controversial and far out for serious consideration at the time). This interaction occurs exclusively at low photon energies (≤1 MeV) and is more relevant to diagnostic radiology than to radiation therapy.

In a photoelectric interaction (Fig. 13.6), the incident photon interacts with an electron in the inner shells of the atom—usually the K or

L shell—leading to transfer of all the energy of the photon to the electron. When the energy received by an electron in the shell is sufficient to overcome its binding energy, this electron is ejected from the atom with energy equal to the following:

$$E^{electron} = E^{photon} - E^{binding}$$

where $E^{electron}$ is the kinetic energy of the electron leaving the atom (related to its mass and speed), E^{photon} is the energy of the incident photon, and $E^{binding}$ is the binding energy of the involved electron shell. After ejection of the electron, there is a "hole" in the electron shell, which is then filled by outer shell electrons "falling" into it, losing energy in the process. The energy lost by these outer shell electrons usually appears as low-energy x-rays, called *characteristic radiation*.[1-4]

Whenever characteristic radiation is produced, there is a possibility that the characteristic x-ray photon may be absorbed by an orbital electron rather than leaving the atom. The electron, now having an excess of energy, will be ejected from the atom in place of the photon. An electron that leaves the atom in this manner is called an *Auger electron* and is capable of causing biologic damage on its own.

Compton (incoherent) scattering. Compton scattering is the most common photon interaction that occurs in the energy range used in radiation therapy.[4] In a Compton interaction, as shown in Fig. 13.7, the incident photon interacts with an outer shell electron; that is, an electron very loosely bound to the atom (sometimes called a *free electron* because the binding energy of the electron is much less than the incident photon). This electron absorbs some of the photon's energy and is ejected from the outer shell, making an angle with the direction of the incident photon. The photon is scattered from its incident path and has different energy and wavelength than the incident photon. This interaction is also called *incoherent scattering*.

The ejected electron, also known as a *Compton electron,* and the scattered photon travel away from the atom at different angles, which can be calculated by using several complex equations relating the angles and energies of the particles involved both before and after the interaction takes place. The equations for energy of the scattered photon (hv′) and the kinetic energy of the Compton electron (E_k) can be derived by using the physics principles of conservation of energy and momentum and are given below.

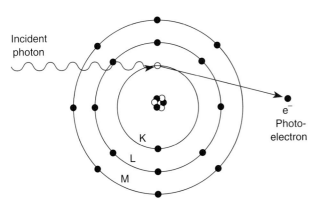

Fig. 13.6 In the photoelectric effect, the incident photon is totally absorbed and transfers all of its energy to the resultant photoelectron. (From Waterstram-Rich KM, Gilman D, eds. *Nuclear Medicine PET/CT: Technology and Techniques.* 8th ed. St. Louis, MO: Elsevier; 2017.)

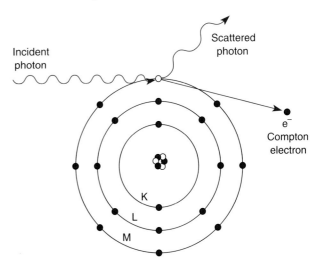

Fig. 13.7 Compton scattering occurs in outer electron shells. The atom is left ionized. (From Waterstram-Rich KM, Gilman D, eds. *Nuclear Medicine PET/CT: Technology and Techniques.* 8th ed. St. Louis, MO: Elsevier; 2017.)

$$h\nu' = h\nu \frac{1}{1 + \varepsilon\,(1 - \cos\theta)} \ , \ E_k = h\nu \frac{\varepsilon\,(1 - \cos\theta)}{1 + \varepsilon\,(1 - \cos\theta)}$$

In the previous equation, $h\nu$ is the energy of the incident photon, θ is the angle between the paths of the incident and scattered photons, and ε is equal to $h\nu/m_e c^2$, where m_e is the rest mass of the electron and $m_e c^2 = 0.511$ MeV.

The relation between the scattering angle (θ) of photon and scattering angle (ϕ) of the Compton electron with respect to the direction of the incident photon is given by the following equation:

$$\cot\phi = (1 + \varepsilon)\,\tan(\theta/2)$$

Although the mathematics of this process is complex, a few examples can show the effect of angle on the results of a Compton interaction:

1. *Direct hit on the target atom.* If the incident photon makes a direct hit on the atom, the Compton electron will go straight forward (in the same direction the incident photon was traveling) and carry away most of the energy, whereas the scattered photon will travel backward from the atom and carry away a minimum of energy. This effect is called *backscatter*. At high photon energies (such as those from a typical therapy accelerator), the energy of the secondary photon approaches a maximum value of 0.255 McV, and the number of photons that scatter directly back is very small.
2. *Grazing hit on the target atom.* A grazing hit on the atom by the incident photon will cause very little energy loss; most of the energy will be carried away by the scattered photon, which, as a result, will have nearly the same energy as the incident photon.
3. *90-degree scatter.* It is important for radiation protection purposes to look at what takes place when the scattered photon emerges at an angle 90 degrees to the incident photon. It turns out that the energy of this photon reaches a maximum value of 0.511 MeV and is essentially independent of the energy of the incident photon, even at very high photon energies.

Pair production. Pair production interactions occur at high energies; in fact, they are physically impossible when the energy of the incident photon is less than 1.022 MeV.[1–4] In the pair production interaction (Fig. 13.8), the incident photon passes close to the nucleus of the atom. When the photon interacts with the EM field of the nucleus, it is absorbed, and instantly the energy is re-emitted as an electron-positron pair (β^-, β^+), which is then ejected from the atom. If you use Einstein's equation $E = mc^2$, viewing m as equal to

the mass of an electron, you can calculate that the rest energy of an electron or positron (i.e., the energy needed to create one during an interaction) is equal to 0.511 MeV. Because two such particles are created, this explains why at least two times that energy ($2m_e c^2$), or 1.022 MeV, must be present for pair production interaction to occur. The leftover energy of the incident photon, after the 1.022 MeV has been used for creation of the electron-positron pair, is divided between the electron and positron. Electron-positron pair production can also occur under the influence of the EM field of the electrons in the target material and is called *triplet production*. The electron-positron pair and the electron with which the photon interacts share all the photon energy. The triplet production has a threshold energy of $4m_e c^2$, or 2.044 MeV, and has a relatively small probability of occurrence compared with other photon interactions in the target medium.

The electron created usually begins to interact with other atoms outside of the original atom until it loses its excess energy and is absorbed. The positron, however, suffers a more interesting fate. When it has undergone several interactions and is moving somewhat more slowly than when it left the atom where the pair production interaction took place, it will collide with a free electron, creating an annihilation reaction. The positron is called an "antimatter" version of the electron, and when the two meet, both are destroyed, with the energy of the two being emitted as two photons of 0.511 McV each, traveling at 180 degrees to each other (i.e., in opposite directions). These two photons will have further interactions with the atoms of the medium.

Photodisintegration. A photodisintegration reaction is one in which the photon strikes the nucleus of the target atom directly and is absorbed. The sudden absorption of this energy causes the nucleus to emit both neutrons and γ-rays in an attempt to maintain stability. This interaction occurs mainly in high Z materials and at usually higher energies (>7 MeV), depending on the material. Thus it is a very unimportant interaction in tissue, where the Z_{eff} is approximately 7.42 (in other words, very low Z). However, it is extremely important when working with high-energy medical accelerators, those with photon or electron beam energies of 10 MeV or greater. Because of the high energies of these beams, combined with the massive amounts of high Z materials such as lead and tungsten in the beam production systems of these accelerators, a substantial neutron hazard to patients or personnel can occur. If you look at the inside of the treatment head of a high-energy linear accelerator, you will probably see some neutron shielding in the form of a borated plastic that slows down ("moderates") the neutrons so that they can be captured.

Effects of combined interactions. When a radiation beam interacts with a medium, no single type of photon interaction occurs; instead, the result is usually a combination of two or more of the previous interactions. The factor μ, discussed earlier, actually represents the combined effects of all of the possible interactions for a given energy and material:

$$\mu = \sigma_{coh} + \tau + \sigma_{inc} + \pi + II$$

where σ_{coh} represents Rayleigh (coherent) scattering; τ, photoelectric interactions; σ_{inc} the Compton (incoherent) interactions; π, the pair production interactions; and II, the photodisintegration and other high-energy reactions that were not discussed here. Each of these symbols represents a probability that the photon, when it interacts with the medium, will undergo that type of reaction; μ describes the total probability of an interaction. Table 13.5 shows the relative importance of the three interactions of greatest concern in radiation

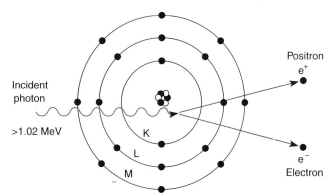

Fig. 13.8 In the pair production interaction, the incident photon passes close to the nucleus of the atom and creates a positron-electron pair. The positron will undergo annihilation with another electron. (From Waterstram-Rich KM, Gilman D, eds. *Nuclear Medicine PET/CT: Technology and Techniques.* 8th ed. St. Louis, MO: Elsevier; 2017.)

TABLE 13.5 Relative Importance of Photon Interactions in Water (the Number of Each Type that Occurs Per 100 Photons)

Photon Energy (MeV)	τ	σ_inc	π
0.010	95	5	0
0.026	50	50	0
0.060	7	93	0
0.150	0	100	0
4.000	0	94	6
10.00	0	77	23
24.00	0	50	50
100.0	0	16	84

therapy physics: the photoelectric, Compton, and pair production interactions.

As you can see from the table, at low energies, most photon interactions taking place are photoelectric (τ) interactions. However, while energy increases, the Compton (σ_inc) interaction quickly takes precedence and is itself slowly replaced by the pair production (π) and other interactions as the energy continues to increase. Average energies of most of the photon beams used in radiation therapy fall into the range of 1 to 5 MeV, where Compton predominates. You can also see this trend in Table 13.4, especially for lead: the values of μ start extremely high, drop to a minimum at energies around 4.0 MeV, then begin to climb again while the pair production interactions begin to produce more and more interactions as energy increases. You should keep this behavior of μ in mind when thinking about exponential attenuation problems.

> The relative importance of different photon interactions with an attenuator depends on the energy of the photon, the atomic number (Z), and the electron density of the attenuating material.
>
> The coherent scattering is important only for photons with energy less than 10 keV and high Z materials and has no significance in radiation therapy. The photoelectric interaction is known to dominate at low photon energies in keV ranges and in high Z materials. The Compton interaction plays the leading role for photon energies in the low MeV range, and the probability of this interaction is independent of Z but depends on the electrons per gram of the attenuating material. The pair production dominates for photon energies greater than 10 MeV in high Z material, with a threshold of 1.02 MeV. The photodisintegration usually occurs for a photon with energy in the MeV range and has a threshold energy that depends on the nuclei present in the material. The probability of this interaction is much smaller than that for pair production, but this interaction is the major source of neutron production in high-energy accelerators used for radiation therapy. As you can imagine, Compton interaction of photons plays an important role in imaging and radiation therapy and is responsible for the loss of contrast in diagnostic and megavoltage beam portal images. It is also the major process responsible for megavoltage therapeutic photon beam dose deposition in tissue.

OTHER PARTICLE INTERACTIONS

The interactions of nonphoton particulate radiation with matter differ considerably from those of photons because of the different nature of this particulate radiation. Although photons have no mass and no electrical charge, particles do have mass, and most have some amount of electrical charge as well. As a result, interactions between particles

and atoms tend to resemble "billiard ball" interactions, familiar to us on an everyday level. This section examines some of the interactions that take place in the cases of particle radiations used in radiation therapy, namely, electrons, protons, heavy charged particles, and neutrons. Among these, electron beam radiation therapy is widely used, proton beam therapy is also available in many centers in the United States and outside, and heavy charged particle beam therapy and neutron beam therapies are available in a small number of radiation therapy centers in the world. The electrons, protons, and heavy charged particles such as carbon-12 are charged particles, and they interact with the orbital electrons and nuclei of the atoms in the material, which are also charged entities, through the coulomb force. The collision or interaction of the particulate radiation with the atomic electrons of the material leads to excitation and ionization of the atoms. The interaction of charged particles with the nuclei can lead to their radiative energy loss through a process called bremsstrahlung (German for "braking radiation"). Heavy charged particles can also have a nuclear reaction with the nuclei of the material and can make them radioactive.

A neutron is electrically neutral with zero charge. The collision of neutrons with the nuclei of the atoms of the material produces protons or other heavy charged particles. These protons and heavy charged particles then deposit their energy in the material by different processes discussed previously. The neutron is thus an indirectly ionizing particle similar to a photon.

Elastic and Inelastic Collisions

The collisions of particle radiations can be likened to the collisions between large-scale objects such as billiard balls. Each ball can be described as possessing kinetic energy, that is, energy caused by its motion through space. When the balls collide, their directions and speeds will change depending on the conditions of the collision, and thus, each ball may lose or gain kinetic energy; the total kinetic energy, however, may or may not remain the same before and after the collision. If no kinetic energy of the system is lost in the collision, the collision is elastic; if kinetic energy is lost from the system, the collision is inelastic.

Example: Two balls with kinetic energies equal to 10 J each collide. After the collision, one ball has a kinetic energy of 15 J, and the other has a kinetic energy of 5 J. Because the total kinetic energy in the system has not changed (20 J = 20 J), the collision was elastic.

If, in the same example, the kinetic energies of the two balls after the collision had been measured as 12 J and 6 J, this would have been an inelastic collision, because kinetic energy was lost during the collision (20 J > 18 J). The remaining 2 J of energy were converted into other forms of energy, such as vibrational energy or heat.

> Note that whether or not kinetic energy is conserved, the total energy of the system (which includes all other forms of energy such as heat) must remain the same. In the second example, the 2 J of kinetic energy lost to the billiard balls did not disappear but rather were converted into another form of energy. This concept is called the *principle of conservation of energy* and is one of the basic concepts of physics and chemistry.

The interactions between atoms and particle radiations can be classified in the same manner. If the total kinetic energies of the particle and atom are the same after the interaction, then an elastic collision has taken place; if not, the collision was inelastic. We next look at how these definitions apply in the cases of interactions of electrons, protons, heavy charged particles such as carbon-12 ion, and neutron radiations with a medium.

Electron Interactions

Electron-electron interactions. When electrons from a radiation source interact with the electrons in different shells of the atoms in the medium, they give up energy to those atomic electrons and are then deflected away from the atom in a new direction. Because they have given up energy to the atomic electron, the original electron is now moving at a slower speed (and therefore has less kinetic energy). The target electron in the atomic orbit may be "kicked up" to a shell farther from the nucleus (excitation) or may be ejected completely from the atom (ionization) if the energy gained from the incident electron is high enough for the process to occur. Remember that a "collision" between two particles does not necessarily mean that actual physical contact between the particles has occurred; a collision can also result if the EM fields of the two particles come close enough to interact with each other, a distance that may be several times larger than the physical size of these particles.

Recall from our study of the Compton interaction that outer shell electrons are considered to be "free" electrons because their binding energies are very low compared with the energy of the incoming photons. If one of these free electrons is involved in the electron-electron interaction just described, the binding energy of the target electron is so small that it may be ignored; therefore, the total kinetic energy of the incident and target electrons before and after the collision is taken to be same. In this case, the collision can be considered elastic. If, however, the interaction involved an electron in a shell close to the nucleus, the binding energy must be taken into account. In this case, because of the principle of conservation of energy already discussed, some of the kinetic energy of the original electron will be lost to overcome the binding energy of the target electron before the target electron can change shells or leave the atom, making this an inelastic collision because the final total kinetic energy of the particles is reduced from its initial value.

When the electron's energy is finally depleted by a series of collisions, an atom in its vicinity captures it.

Elastic electron-nuclei collisions. In materials heavier than hydrogen (Z = 1), electrons with certain energies are more likely to undergo elastic scattering with the nuclei of atoms than with the atomic electrons. As with an electron-electron elastic collision (already described), the incident electrons lose a small amount of energy to the nucleus of the atom and bounce away with reduced energy. Because the nuclei are so much heavier than electrons, the electron will retain a larger percentage of its energy than if it had collided with an electron and is more likely to bounce straight backward from the atom after the collision. This effect diminishes quickly while the energy of the incident electrons is increased, and, at energies in the range usually used in radiation therapy (4–25 MeV), the electrons interact mainly by electron-electron scattering (discussed previously) or inelastic nuclear scattering (discussed later).

Inelastic electron-nuclei collisions. High-energy electrons can pass close to the nucleus of a target atom, as seen in Fig. 13.9, and be so strongly attracted by the charges in the nucleus that they will slow down, losing some of their kinetic energy; this energy will be emitted from the atom as a photon with energy (hv) equal to the energy lost by the electron when it slowed down.[1] This process, bremsstrahlung, is the most important method of producing x-ray beams in therapy units.

The photon created in the bremsstrahlung process can be of any energy from zero to the energy of the incident electron, and can emerge from the atom in any direction. Thus similar to β decay, bremsstrahlung produces not a single-energy x-ray, but rather a spectrum of x-ray energies ranging from zero to the energy of the incident electron beam.

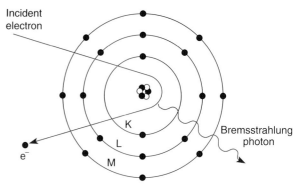

Fig. 13.9 Deceleration of a charged particle passing near the nucleus results in a release of energy in the form of bremsstrahlung radiation. (From Waterstram-Rich KM, Gilman D, eds. *Nuclear Medicine PET/CT: Technology and Techniques*. 8th ed. St. Louis, MO: Elsevier; 2017.)

The average energy of the bremsstrahlung spectrum is approximately one-third of the maximum possible energy (E_{max}).

When the electron beam is in the lower-energy range (50–300 keV), the photons are emitted in a wide range of angles. While the electron beam energy increases, the photons tend to be emitted closer to the direction of the incident electron, a phenomenon known as *forward peaking* of the photon beam. This effect is very important in the design and use of high-energy photon machines such as linear accelerators and betatrons, because for the high-energy electron beams that hit the targets used in these machines, the bremsstrahlung photon beam is highly forward peaked.

Bremsstrahlung production is more likely in high Z materials such as lead or tungsten than in low Z materials such as water or tissue. For this reason, high Z materials can be bombarded with a beam of high-energy electrons to produce high-energy photon beams in radiation therapy machines. For low Z materials such as water or soft tissue, the bremsstrahlung production from electron beams is very small. The energy loss of electrons is mostly by ionization and excitation, leading to energy deposition in the medium. The electrons lose approximately 2 MeV/cm in water or soft tissue.

X-rays are photons produced by the interaction of electrons with any material. The x-ray tubes and high-energy radiation therapy accelerators use a high-voltage power supply and the necessary technology to generate a narrow or focused high-energy electron beam, which then hits a high Z target to produce the x-ray beam for imaging and radiation therapy. The two atomic processes responsible for production of x-rays are (1) bremsstrahlung, and (2) characteristic x-ray emission by atomic electrons. The physics of these processes were discussed earlier in this chapter. The x-ray energy spectra consist of the continuous bremsstrahlung photon energies between zero to the value of energy of the incident electron superimposed with the peaks at discrete energies of the characteristic radiation of the target. The efficiency of the x-ray production by this process is proportional to both the atomic number (Z) of the target and the strength of the applied high voltage. Usually, less than 1% of the kinetic energy of the electron is converted to x-rays or photons, and the rest of it is converted to heat, thus requiring a good cooling system for the target to remove this heat. The direction of the x-ray beam emission depends on the energy of the incident electrons. In the keV energy range, most of the x-rays are emitted at a direction perpendicular to the path of the incident electron beam. In the MeV energy range, x-rays are emitted in the same direction as the incident electrons. Therefore, a reflectance target is used in diagnostic energy x-ray tubes, whereas a thick transmission-type target is used in therapy accelerators. The thick target not only stops the electrons but also hardens the beam by filtering out the low-energy components of the x-ray spectra. Suitable filters are also added to diagnostic and superficial kilovoltage therapy units to remove the unnecessary low-energy x-ray photons to harden the beam and reduce the skin dose to patients.

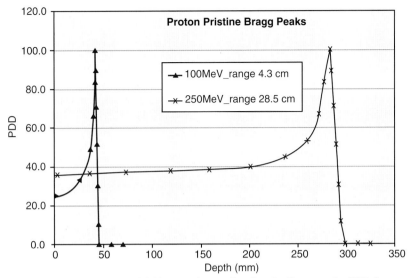

Fig. 13.10 Depth dose curve of a 250-MeV proton beam showing the Bragg peak. *PDD*, Percentage depth dose. (From N. Sahoo, MD Anderson Cancer Center, Houston, TX, private communication.)

You can learn more about the physics of x-ray production by visiting https://physics.info/x-ray/.

Heavy Charged Particle Interactions

Protons, alpha particles (helium nucleus with two protons and two neutrons), and heavier charged particles, such as carbon-12 ions, lose their energy by C interactions with atomic electrons and nuclei. In addition, they also undergo nuclear reactions with the nuclei. Similar to electrons, the heavy charged particles undergo multiple scattering resulting from elastic collisions with electrons and the nuclei without loss of energy. Because of their heavy mass, they undergo less multiple scattering compared with electrons. They deposit their energy in the medium mostly by ionization and excitation resulting from the inelastic collision with the atomic electrons. The inelastic collision of heavy charged particles with the nuclei of the medium creates nuclear fragments. These fragments usually deposit their energy locally. Unlike electrons, radiative bremsstrahlung energy loss is not significant for heavy charged particles. The rate of energy loss per unit path length is proportional to the square of the charge of the particle and inversely proportional to the square of the velocity of the particle. While the heavy charged particle slows down, the rate of energy loss increases, leading to higher deposition of dose in the medium. Thus, these particles deposit the maximum dose when they are very close to being stopped in the medium or near the end of their range of travel, giving rise to a Bragg peak, as shown in Fig. 13.10. The dose beyond the Bragg peaks falls to zero very rapidly. This is one of the most attractive and useful features of the dose distribution of heavy charged particles. These peaks can be broadened to any desirable width by combining the Bragg peaks of heavy charged particles with different energies

with the help of range-modulating wheels or other energy modulation schemes. The existence of Bragg peaks allows one to use these beams to deposit the maximum dose inside the target volume while reducing the dose beyond the target to a very small value.

Neutron Interactions

The neutron has zero electrical charge similar to the photon but has a large mass relative to the electron. The neutron interacts with the nucleons of the atomic nucleus of the medium through the nuclear force. The neutrons cannot create any ionization by removing the atomic electrons themselves. However, when neutrons have a head-on collision with an atomic nucleus, it leads to generation of other charged particles, such as protons and alpha particles. These secondary charged particles deposit their energy through inelastic collision with atomic electrons and the atomic nuclei. The transfer of energy from neutrons to the secondary particles is very high when they collide with the nuclei of a hydrogen atom, which is a proton with almost equal mass as a neutron. Thus a neutron beam will deposit a higher dose to fatty tissue because of the high concentration of hydrogen atoms. A neutron loses very little energy when it collides with heavier nuclei. A nuclear reaction of a neutron with nuclei in the medium can lead to nuclear disintegration, giving rise to more neutrons, heavy charged particles, and γ-rays. As mentioned earlier, these secondary particles then deposit their energy in the medium. The dose distribution of the neutron beam is similar to that of γ-rays from a cobalt-60 source.

You can learn about heavy particle therapy from: http://www-bd.fnal.gov/ntf/reference/hadrontreat.pdf.

SUMMARY

To understand the discipline of radiation physics, one must be familiar with the developments, theories, and technologic advances that have taken place since Roentgen discovered the x-ray in 1895. From the Curies, who discovered radioactivity and determined the activity of 1 g of radium (^{226}Ra), to Bohr's attempt to explain the atom, to Einstein's work that earned him the Nobel Prize for photoelectric effect, the areas of atomic physics and nuclear physics have significantly contributed to development and advances in diagnostic and therapeutic radiology. The knowledge of the interactions of radiation with subatomic particles is critical to understanding the scientific basis and intelligent use of radiation therapy. This chapter introduces the following concepts to provide the foundation for understanding the discipline of radiation physics.

- **Structure of the atom:** An atom consists of negatively charged electrons distributed in specific orbitals around a positively charged nucleus made of protons and neutrons. The laws of quantum mechanics determine the occupation of orbitals. The electrons play the vital role in determining the structure and properties of materials important to radiation therapy physics. The protons and neutrons are bound together in the nucleus by a strong nuclear force. Atoms and nuclei are stable only when they are in their lowest-energy ground state configurations. When they are in excited states, they tend to return to their respective ground states by emitting the excess energy as different kinds of radiation.

- **Radiation:** Radiation can be in the form of EM waves or particles. According to de Broglie's principle of wave particle duality, every particle has a wavelike character and vice versa. The characteristic wavelength (λ) of a particle is expressed by the equation $\lambda = h/p$, where h represents Planck's constant, and p represents the momentum of the particle, which is equal to m $\times$ v, the product of the mass (m) of the particle with velocity (v). According to Einstein's mass-energy equivalence principle, any mass (m) has an equivalent energy (E) and vice versa, and their relationship is expressed by the formula E = mc^2. Some radiation can ionize the matter by removing the electrons from atomic shells of the target and are known as *ionizing radiation*. Ionizing radiation can be either directly ionizing, such as electrons, protons, and heavy charged particles, which are charged particles, or indirectly ionizing, such as photons and neutrons, which are neutral. Radiation therapy involves the use of ionizing radiation only.

- **Photon:** The photon is the particle associated with an EM field, and its energy is expressed by the formula E = hv. The frequency v of the photon is related to the wavelength of the EM wave by $\lambda = c / v$.

- **Radioactivity:** Radioactivity is the process in which the unstable nuclei give up the excess energy in the form of radiation to move toward their stable ground state. Radioactive nuclei decay by emitting alpha particles (He-4 nucleus), beta particles (electrons or positrons), and gamma rays (photons), and these are known as alpha, beta, and gamma decay, respectively. Characteristic x-rays and Auger electrons are also produced from electronic shells of the atom during the radioactivity. Gamma rays are emitted from the nuclei, whereas x-rays are from electrons, and both consist of photons. Radioactivity can also be classified as isotopic, isotonic, isobaric, or isomeric transitions in which either the number of protons or neutrons or their sum or both remains unchanged, respectively, after the decay. All radioactivity is statistical in nature and follows an exponential decay law, with the activity (A) at any time (t) being determined from the initial activity A0 from $A = A_0 e^{-\lambda t}$. The half-life of decay (t_h) = $0.693/\lambda$, λ being the decay constant. The SI unit of activity is the becquerel (Bq) or disintegrations per second, but the curie (Ci) is the old and widely used practical unit: 1 Ci = 3.7×10^{10} Bq.

- **Photon interactions:** When a beam of x-ray and gamma-ray photons strikes a target, some of the photons will:
    1. pass through the target without any interaction,
    2. change the direction of motion without losing any energy by coherent Rayleigh scattering with electrons,
    3. change direction and lose some energy by the incoherent Compton scattering with electrons, or
    4. lose all their energy
        a. by photoelectric effect or triplet production while interacting with the atomic electrons, or
        b. by pair production or photodisintegration while interacting with the nuclei of the target.

- The probability of various photon interactions with the atomic electrons and nuclei of the target depends on the energy of the photon and atomic number Z of the target material. Among the interactions in which the photon loses some or all of its energy, the photoelectric effect is dominant at low photon energies in keV ranges, the Compton effect in the high keV to low MeV range, and the pair production in the high MeV range. The photonuclear interaction is responsible for neutron production in high-energy linear accelerators used in radiotherapy. The attenuation of a photon beam with an initial intensity of I_0 while it passes through a target follows the exponential law, $I_x = I_0 e^{-\mu x}$. I_x is the intensity after the photon beam passes through a thickness of x cm in the medium, and μ is the linear attenuation constant of the medium. The quality of the photon beam or penetrating power of a photon beam can be specified by the beam's HVL, which is the thickness of the attenuator that reduces the beam intensity to half of its initial value. HVL is related to μ by the equation HVL = $0.693/\mu$. Tenth value layer (TVL) is the thickness of the attenuator that reduces the beam intensity to 10% of its initial value and is related to μ by the equation TVL = $\ln(10)/\mu$.

- **Electron and heavy charged particle interaction:** Charged particles lose their energy while passing through the target medium, predominantly through excitation and ionization of the atomic electrons. In addition, interaction with the nuclei of the target atoms results in energy loss through emission of bremsstrahlung x-ray photons by electrons and production of nuclear fragments by heavy charged particles. The electrons also undergo multiple scattering without losing any significant amount of energy. Electrons lose approximately 2 MeV per cm of travel in water. Unlike photons, charged particles have finite ranges in the medium, and their intensity falls to zero after this range. In addition, energy loss of heavier charged particles such as protons, alpha particles, and carbon-12 ions exhibit Bragg peaks at certain depths depending on their initial energy, making them attractive for conformal radiation therapy.

- **Neutron interaction:** Neutrons interact with the nuclei of the atoms in the target and lose their energy to the target nuclei by billiard ball–like collision processes. These collisions lead to production of charged particles such as protons, alpha particles, and gamma rays, which then deposit the energy by their interaction with the electrons and nuclei of the target medium. The dose distribution of neutrons in water is very similar to that of the photons from a cobalt-60 source.

- **Inverse square law:** According to the inverse square law, in a nonabsorbing medium such as air, the intensity of radiation from an effective point source at any distance d from the source is inversely proportional to the square of d. Thus the intensity I_2 at a distance d_2 can be calculated from the intensity I_1 at a distance d_1 from the equation, $I_1/I_2 = d_2/d_1$.

REVIEW QUESTIONS

The answers to the Review Questions can be found by logging on to our website at: http://evolve.elsevier.com/Washington/principles

1. How many seconds are there in 2.54 minutes?
   a. 174.0.
   b. 114.0.
   c. 152.4.
   d. 92.4.
   e. 254.

2. Calculate the wavelength of an EM wave that has a frequency of 3.95×10^{14} Hz.
   a. 1.32×10^6 m.
   b. 13.2×10^6 m.
   c. 7.59×10^{-8} m.
   d. 7.59×10^{-7} m.
   e. 7.59×10^{-6} m.

3. An FM radio station broadcasts at 102.0 MHz on your radio dial. What is the wavelength of the station's signal?
   a. 34.0 m.
   b. 3.40 m.
   c. 2.941 m.
   d. 2.941×10^6 m.
   e. 29.41 m.

4. An EM wave has a frequency of 2.1×10^{21} Hz. What is the energy of the wave?
   a. 3.355×10^{54} eV.
   b. 1.39×10^{12} eV.
   c. 5.060×10^{35} eV.

   d. 8.250 MeV.
   e. 8.715 MeV.

5. If an EM wave has energy of 6 MeV, what would its wavelength be?
   a. 50 m.
   b. 3.313×10^{-32} m.
   c. 2.075×10^{-13} m.
   d. 2.075×10^{-12} m.
   e. 2.075×10^{-7} m.

6. A sample of an isotope has a half-life of 74 days and is measured to have an activity of 8.675 Ci at noon on that day. What will the activity of the isotope be 94 days later at 6 PM?
   a. 4.338 Ci.
   b. 3.588 Ci.
   c. 3.596 Ci.
   d. 5.034 Ci.
   e. 2.37 Ci.

7. The intensity of a radioactive beam is measured at a distance of 100 cm and found to be 250 mR/min. What will the intensity of this beam be at 105 cm?
   a. 226.8 mR/min.
   b. 238.1 mR/min.
   c. 205.7 mR/min.
   d. 275.6 mR/min.
   e. 262.5 mR/min.

8. A 6-MeV photon beam is incident on a 1.5-cm-thick lead sheet. If the initial dose rate of the beam is 300 cGy/min, what will the dose rate be after it passes through the lead sheet if the linear attenuation coefficient for this beam in lead is 0.4911 cm^{-1}?
   a. 79.0 cGy/min.
   b. 183.6 cGy/min.
   c. 147.33 cGy/min.
   d. 143.6 cGy/min.
   e. 221.0 cGy/min.

9. What is the HVL of the beam in question 8?
   a. 2.72 cm.
   b. 4.07 cm.
   c. 0.941 cm.
   d. 1.386 cm.
   e. 1.411 cm.

10. In the problem given in question 8, what minimal thickness of lead is needed to reduce the dose rate to less than 9 cGy/min?
   a. 2 cm.
   b. 10 cm.
   c. 100 cm.
   d. 7.0 cm.
   e. 7.5 cm.

QUESTIONS TO PONDER

1. A portal image is taken with a high-energy photon beam (MeV range). Why is the image inferior in diagnostic quality when compared with an image taken on a simulator (keV range)?

2. Explain the difference between the TVL of a material and its linear attenuation coefficient.

3. Explain the reason for the use of lead as a shielding material for x-ray rooms and/or vaults.

4. Explain the concept of the exponential decay constant and how it relates to half-life.

5. What feature of proton dose distribution makes it more attractive than electron and photon dose distribution.

REFERENCES

1. Byme P, Nielsen C. Physics in Nuclear Medicine. In: Waterstram-Rich KM, Gilman D, eds. *Nuclear Medicine PET/CT: Technology and Techniques.* 8th ed. St. Louis, MO: Elsevier; 2017, 223–244.

2. Hendee WR, Ritenour R. *Medical Imaging Physics.* 4th ed. New York, NY: Wiley-Liss; 2002.

3. Johns HE, Cunningham JR. *The Physics of Radiology.* 4th ed. Springfield, IL: Charles C Thomas; 1983.

4. Khan FM. *The Physics of Radiation Therapy.* 4th ed. Baltimore, MD: Lippincott Williams & Wilkins; 2010.

14

Aspects of Brachytherapy

Gil'ad N. Cohen

OBJECTIVES

- Discuss the importance of brachytherapy as an option for treatment.
- List advantages and disadvantages of brachytherapy.
- Identify the different types of brachytherapy treatments.
- Recognize the most commonly used isotopes, their half-lives, and their energy classifications.
- Describe how remote afterloading decreases the exposure to radiation of staff and patients.
- Compare and contrast high-dose brachytherapy and low-dose brachytherapy.
- Describe the different types of intracavitary applicators.
- Compare and contrast different imaging modalities in brachytherapy.
- Identify and explain the role of surrogate markers used in brachytherapy.

OUTLINE

KEY TERMS

Activity
Afterloading
Brachytherapy
Decay constant
Half-life
High-dose rate
Interstitial brachytherapy
Intracavitary brachytherapy
Intraluminal brachytherapy
Intravascular brachytherapy
Low-dose rate

Mean life
Medium-dose rate
Milligram-radium-equivalent
Ovoid
Pulsed dose rate
Remote afterloading
Source activity
Specific activity
Surface brachytherapy
Tandem

HISTORIC OVERVIEW

The discovery of x-rays by Roentgen in the late nineteenth century has had, more than any other innovation, a dramatic effect on modern medicine. Shortly after the discovery of x-rays, Henri Becquerel and Pierre Curie began investigating the existence of similar rays produced by known fluorescent materials. Curie, in his experimentation, deliberately produced an ulcer on his arm and described in detail his experience of the various phases of a moist epidermitis and his recovery. At that point, he gave a small radium tube to a colleague and suggested he insert it into a tumor. Subsequently, several physicians began investigating the effects of these rays on malignant tumors and thus began the therapeutic use of ionizing radiation. The initial experience gained with the therapeutic use of radium sources is referred to as *classic brachytherapy*. Despite technological and computational advances, classic brachytherapy is still the basis for many brachytherapy procedures performed today.

Today, brachytherapy is a standard treatment modality for a large number of malignancies, including those of the uterus and uterine cervix, lung, prostate, and breast. Brachytherapy use in cancer therapy is increasing and is paralleled by the increasing desire for improved organ preservation and cosmetic results. In current oncology practice, there are many opportunities for medical dosimetrist and radiation therapist involvement in the practical application of brachytherapy. The scopes of practice for the medical dosimetrist and radiation therapist require an intimate understanding of key concepts and critical thinking in their application in the brachytherapy clinic.

WHAT IS BRACHYTHERAPY?

The term brachytherapy is derived from the Greek words "brachy," meaning short, and "therapy," meaning treatment. Brachytherapy, treatment at short distance, refers to radiotherapy in which sources of radiation are placed at close proximity to, or directly in the target volume. Teletherapy, on the other hand ("tele" is the Greek word for long), refers to radiotherapy treatment in which the source of radiation is located away from the patient.

Sources used for brachytherapy are usually sealed sources, in which the radioactive isotope is encased and sealed within a small metal structure, usually titanium or stainless steel tubes that are welded shut at the ends (Fig. 14.1). Recently, some new sources have been introduced in which the isotope is embedded in plastic or similar material.

Of particular interest is electronic brachytherapy (EB). Introduced into clinical practice in the last few years, it makes use of miniature x-ray devices instead of radioactive sources. The radiation safety advantages of this emerging technology are obvious. However, because the x-ray generator requires cooling, the source assembly is still too large to fully replace traditional sources in all clinical applications. Although EB appears promising, its use is still limited.

Brachytherapy dose distributions are characterized by islands of very high dose at close proximity to the radiation sources. As the distance from a brachytherapy source of radiation increases, the dose absorbed in tissue decreases (and can be predicted by using the inverse square law for high-energy photons: see discussions below), or, conversely, the closer the point of interest to the source of radiation, the higher the dose absorbed at that point. Brachytherapy dose distributions are therefore inherently inhomogenous. In contrast to external beam treatment in which hot spots are typically minimized, in the practice of brachytherapy, physicians use these hot spots to increase the therapeutic ratio of the treatments. By strategically placing the radiation sources in or at close proximity to the treatment volume and away from normal tissue, very high tumoricidal doses of radiation can be delivered to the target area while sparing surrounding tissue and organs at risk. Brachytherapy may be used alone, as monotherapy, or as adjuvant therapy, often referred to as a *boost*, to external beam irradiation. A combination treatment provides the benefits of localized high-dose brachytherapy and the treatment of more distal but well-defined volume of disease by using external beam irradiation. For example, in the treatment of cervical cancer, brachytherapy used to treat the cervix and uterus contributes a small dose to pelvic nodes that are located 5 cm or more from the sources; hence a complementary treatment of the whole pelvis with external beam is administered as well. Finally, because brachytherapy often involves invasive surgical procedures, some patients may not be ideal candidates for this therapeutic approach.

SOURCE SPECIFICATION

Source Activity and Source Strength

The amount of radiation emitted from a source is directly proportional to the absorbed dose around it. Before a brachytherapy treatment can be devised, the quantity of radiation emitted from the source to be used must be known. This quantity, used to describe the strength of a source, is activity.

Source activity is defined as the number of disintegrations per unit of time for a particular source. Note, therefore, that the activity of any radioactive source changes with time as source decays. The historic unit of activity is the curie (Ci), named after Marie Curie and assigned the activity of 1 g of radium. One curie equals 3.7×10^{10} disintegrations per second. The unit for activity, recommended by the International System of Units is the Becquerel (Bq), named after the French scientist, Henri Becquerel. One Becquerel is one disintegration per second. Thus:

$$3.7 \times 10^{10} \, \text{Bq} = 1 \, \text{Ci}$$

Although the Becquerel is the unit recommended for use, old habits are hard to change, and the curie is still commonly used in practice.

A source's activity, although easy to calculate, is difficult to measure because some of the emitted radiation interacts with the source material and encapsulation. For this reason, the measure of activity is poorly suited for dose calculations, and, for photon sources, the American Association of Physicists in Medicine (AAPM) Task Group 43 (TG-43)[1] recommends the use of source strength instead. The unit recommended for source strength specification, air kerma strength, is denoted by the symbol S_K, and has the units of U, where:1 U = 1 cGy/hr·cm^2.

The formalism introduced by TG-43 has been applied to all photon radiation sources and is the basis for current dose calculations in clinical brachytherapy treatment planning systems.

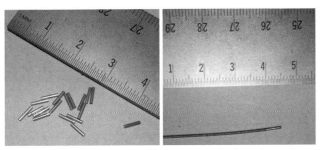

Fig. 14.1 Interstitial seeds used for permanent implantation and some temporary application *(left)* and a high-dose-rate source *(right)*. High-dose-rate sources are inserted into and retracted from catheters and applicators through the use of a metal cable to which the source is welded. Note the similar size of the sources despite the large difference in source activity.

TABLE 14.1   Photon-Emitting Isotopes

Isotope	E_{ave} (MeV)	$T_{1/2}$	Γ	Roentgen·cm² / mCi·hr
Radium-226	0.830	1622 years	8.25	
Cobalt-60	1.25	5.27 years	13.1	
Cesium-137	0.662	30.0 years	3.26	
Iridium-192	0.380	73.83 days	4.69	
Gold-198	0.412	2.7 days	2.33	
Iodine-125	0.028	59.4 days	1.51	
Palladium-103	0.021	17 days	1.48	
Cesium-131	0.034	9.7 days		

TABLE 14.2   Beta-Emitting Isotopes

Isotope	E_{max} (MeV)	$T_{1/2}$	Max Range H_2O (cm)
Strontium-90/ yttrium-90	2.27	28.9 years	1.1
Phosphorus-32	1.71	14.3 days	0.7
Ruthenium-106/ rhodium-106	3.55	367 days	1.8

Energy of Emitted Radiation

The average energy (E_{ave}) of photon-emitting isotopes determines the dose profile around the source. In general, the higher the energy of the photons, the more penetrating they are. Photon-emitting brachytherapy sources are typically divided into high- and low-energy groups. The photons emitted from sources in the high-energy group interact with matter, primarily via Compton scatter. Sources in this group are similar to the classic radium sources in that the dose profile associated with them approximates the inverse square law. In contrast, photons emitted from sources in the low-energy group interact with matter primarily via photoelectric absorption. This results in a much steeper dose profile than is seen with the high-energy sources. Table 14.1 lists the average energy for photon-emitting isotopes commonly used in brachytherapy.

Beta (electron)-emitting isotopes have also been used in brachytherapy. ^{90}Sr has been in use for many years in the treatment of pterygium. ^{32}P, used for many years in colloid form for injections, has been recently investigated in a new solid source for treatment of the spinal dura and other localized tumors. ^{106}Ru, mostly used in Europe for the treatment of ocular melanoma, is available in the United States as well.

Compared with photon emitters, the dose profile for beta sources is steeper than the profile observed with low-energy photons. The range of beta particles depends strongly on the particles' energy. Because the energy spectrum of the electrons is continuous, the maximum energy and the maximum range are often tabulated. Table 14.2 lists data for the abovementioned isotopes.

RADIOACTIVE DECAY

Radioactive decay is a stochastic process. If we were able to pick a single radioactive atom of a known isotope, we would not be able to say when exactly it would decay. However, from observations of a large number of atoms, we would know the probability that it will decay within a certain time interval, Δt. This probability is the decay constant, λ, of

the isotope and has units of sec^{-1}. Consider now a large quantity, N, of atoms of this isotope. The fraction of atoms, $\Delta N / N$, that will disintegrate (or the probability that N atoms will disintegrate) during the time interval, Δt, is:

$$\frac{-\Delta N / N}{\Delta t} = \lambda$$

where the negative sign is added because the number of atoms, N, is decreasing with time. This equation can be rewritten to define mathematically the activity, A, of a given source with N atoms, as follows:

$$\frac{-\Delta N}{\Delta t} = \lambda N = A$$

The reader should compare this definition to the description of activity above. As expected, the activity of the source is directly proportional to the total number, N, of isotope atoms present.

Consider again the equation for activity (the delta sign in the previous equation is replaced here with the letter "d" to denote a very small change in time):

$$\frac{dN}{dt} = -\lambda N$$

Rearranging and integrating over t (readers with knowledge of calculus may attempt this as an exercise), one obtains the exponential expression for radioactive decay:

$$N_t = N_0 e^{-\lambda t}$$

where N_0 represents the initial number of atoms of the isotope present in the source, and N_t represents the number of atoms remaining after time t has elapsed. Multiplying both sides of the equation by the decay constant, one obtains a similar relationship for activity:

$$A_t = A_0 e^{-\lambda t}$$

where A_0 represents the initial activity of the source, and A_t represents the activity of the source after time t has elapsed.

Let us reconsider now the definition of the decay constant, λ, namely, the probability that an atom will decay within a certain time Δt, or the fraction of atoms within a sample that will decay within a certain time Δt. The inverse of this quantity, $1/\lambda$, is the average time it will take atoms within the sample to decay. This is the mean life of the isotope:

$$T_{Avg} = \frac{1}{\lambda}$$

or

$$\lambda = \frac{1}{T_{Avg}}$$

Substituting for λ in the exponent of the equation for activity above, one obtains the following:

$$A_t = A_0 e^{\frac{-t}{T_{Avg}}}$$

Example 1: The mean life of iodine-^{125}I is 85.5 days. How long will it take for a sample of ^{125}I to decay to exactly one-half its original activity?

Answer: If A_0 is the initial sample activity, then we wish to solve for the time, t, after which the sample activity, A_t, will equal $0.5A_0$. Therefore we can write the following:

$$1/2 A_0 = A_0 e^{\frac{-t}{T_{Avg}}}$$

or

$$\frac{1}{2} = e^{\frac{-t}{T_{Avg}}}$$

Taking the natural logarithm of both sides and solving for t, we find that

$$\ln(0.5) = \frac{-t}{T_{Avg}}$$

or

$$t = \ln(2)\ T_{Avg}$$

Finally, solving for t:

$$t = \ln(2) \times 85.5 = 0.693 \times 85.5 = 59.4 \text{ days}$$

The quantity calculated in the example above is the half-life of ^{125}I. Half-life, the time it takes for a sample of a radioactive isotope to decay to half its initial activity, is denoted by $T_{1/2}$, and is often favored over mean life. From the example above, the expression for $T_{1/2}$ is

$$T_{1/2} = \ln(2)\ T_{Avg} = \frac{\ln(2)}{\lambda}$$

and the equation for radioactive decay can then be written as the following:

$$A_t = A_0 e^{-\frac{\ln(2)\,t}{T_{1/2}}}$$

Tables 14.1 and 14.2 list isotopes commonly used in radiation therapy with their half-lives.

Example 2: A ^{137}Cs source was assayed on March 15, 1996, when the activity of the source was determined to be 69.5 mCi. What would be the activity for this source on June 15, 2020?

Answer: Calculating the elapsed time (in years to keep units the same) and using the equation for radioactive decay:

$$A_t = A_0 e^{-0.693\frac{t}{T_{1/2}}} = 69.5 e^{-0.693\frac{24.25}{30}}$$

$$A = 39.7 \text{ mCi}$$

Example 3: Because of its long half-life, a cesium source can be used for many years. How often would the activity of the source need to be determined if the resulting dose calculations are to be within approximately ±1%?

Answer: The key to answering this question is in the direct relationship between dose and activity. In other words, we wish to determine the activity of the source to within approximately ±1%, or the difference between A_t and A_0, to be approximately 2%. Therefore:

$$0.98 = \frac{A_t}{A_0} = e^{-0.693\frac{t}{T_{1/2}}}$$

and solving for t:

$$t = \frac{\ln(0.98)}{-0.693}\,30y = 0.86y$$

or approximately 1 year.

Although thinking of the amount of activity and the rate of decay in terms of the isotopes' half-life is convenient, the mean life of an isotope remains a useful quantity in dose calculations. Consider the following exercise.

Example 4: In a permanent implant, ^{125}I seeds are left to decay in the patient's prostate. The initial dose rate for the implant is 7 cGy/hr. What is the total dose for the implant?

Answer: The mean life of ^{125}I is:

$$T_{Avg} = 1.44 \times (59.4 \text{ days}) \times (24 \text{ hours / day}) = 2057 \text{ hours}$$

The total dose delivered to the prostate is:

$$D = 7 \text{ cGy / hr} \times 2057 \text{ hours} = 14{,}400 \text{ cGy}$$

Example 5: In this case, a temporary implant with ^{192}Ir is planned so its duration is exactly 5 days (120 hours). However, because of clinical reasons, the implant is postponed by 3 days. How long will it take to deliver the prescribed dose if the original plan is used?

Answer: The half-life of ^{192}Ir is 73.83 days (see Table 14.1). In 3 days, the source will decay by the following:

$$e^{-0.693\frac{t}{T_{1/2}}} = e^{-0.693\frac{3}{73.83}} = 0.972$$

Because the dose rate is directly proportional to the source activity and implant duration is inversely proportional to the source activity, the implant duration will be the following:

$$\frac{5 \text{ days}}{0.972} = 5.14 \text{ days} = 123.4 \text{ hours}$$

TEMPORAL CONSIDERATIONS

From these examples, one can readily see that brachytherapy may be delivered by using various temporal patterns. Let us discuss some of these. Permanent brachytherapy, or seed implantation, refers to the placement of small radioactive sources directly in the targeted tissue where they are left to decay. These sources, or seeds, deliver the dose to the tumor during a period of several weeks or months. The most common use of permanent brachytherapy today is for the treatment of prostate cancer. Temporary brachytherapy, as its name implies, refers to the placement of radiation sources in or next to a target volume for a limited amount of time before they are removed from the patient. In delivering temporary implants, practitioners usually use what are known as afterloading techniques, in which the applicator or catheters are first placed in the patient (often with the patient under anesthesia).[2] When the treatment plan and the sources are readied and checked, the treatment is delivered. In the classic application of brachytherapy temporary implants, the source would be placed manually into the applicator or catheters by the physician. At the completion of the treatment, the sources and the applicator would be removed from the patient. This approach meant that the patient would be "radioactive" while the treatment was in progress. Thus the patient would be required to stay in isolation in the hospital, and hospital staff would be exposed to radiation when attending to the patient and when inserting or removing the implant. Therefore radiation safety precautions would have to be enforced to minimize these exposures, including protection for staff and other patients and limits on patient visitors. Remote afterloading techniques eliminate the radiation exposure associated with manual brachytherapy. With this approach, a highly radioactive source is housed in a treatment unit (Fig. 14.2) that is programmed to send the source into the applicator or catheters according to a predetermined treatment plan. Each treatment fraction delivered in this manner takes a few minutes to complete, after which the source is retracted back into the shielded position in the remote afterloader. Temporary implant treatment schedules may involve a single or multiple treatment

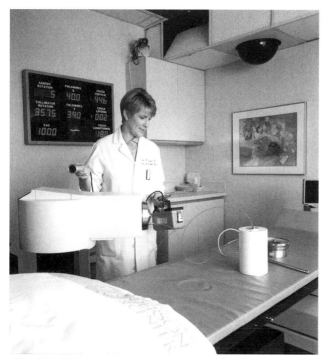

Fig. 14.2 High-dose-rate unit undergoing quality assurance tests.

TABLE 14.3	**Examples of Typical Dose Prescriptions in Brachytherapy**	
	Low-Dose Rate	**High-Dose Rate**
Prostate	I-125 permanent implant of 144 Gy Pd-103 permanent Implant of 125 Gy Cs-131 permanent Implant of 115 Gy	4 fractions of 9.5–10 Gy = 38–40 Gy
Cervix	Two implants of 20 Gy = 40 Gy	5 weekly fractions of 6 Gy = 30 Gy 4 weekly fractions of 7 Gy = 28 Gy
STS/breast	Single implant to deliver 45-50 Gy	10 BID fractions of 3.4 Gy = 34 Gy Single IORT treatment: 15–20 Gy

BID, Twice per day; *IORT,* intraoperative radiation therapy; *STS,* soft tissue sarcoma.

fractions. Less invasive temporary implants may involve several applicator placements separated by a few days or weeks.

The widely varying treatment durations require different dose rates and corresponding total dose to achieve the desired clinical effect. Depending on the dose rate used to deliver the treatment, temporary implant treatments may be delivered in as short a time as a few minutes or as long as a few days.

Dose rates used in brachytherapy are categorized as follows: low-dose-rate (LDR) treatments refer to dose rates under 2 Gy/hr, medium-dose-rate treatments refer to dose rates ranging from 2 Gy/hr to 12 Gy/hr, and high-dose-rate (HDR) brachytherapy treatments refer to dose rates greater than 12 Gy/hr. The categorization of these dose rates is not arbitrary. Rather, it is based on the relationship between the treatment duration and the rate of tumor cell proliferation and DNA repair. That is, if the duration of the treatment is long in comparison to the rate of cell proliferation (as is the case with permanent implants, for example), the implant would be considered an LDR procedure. If, on the other hand, the treatment duration is short in comparison to the repair times (as is the case in intraoperative radiation therapy procedures in which the full dose is delivered in minutes), the implant is considered a HDR procedure.

Furthermore, because the biologic effect increases with dose rate, the total prescribed should be reduced accordingly. Table 14.3 lists some common dose prescriptions for LDR and HDR treatments.

Of course, to be able to deliver an HDR treatment, a high-activity source is also required. With the use of such high-activity sources, some radiation safety risks are also introduced. Incidents involving HDR brachytherapy are often catastrophic in nature. A qualified physician and a qualified physicist must be present during the delivery of HDR treatments. Special precautions are taken, and emergency procedures must be in place to handle radiation emergencies. All staff involved with the delivery of HDR treatments, including therapists, must be properly credentialed for the procedures, be familiar with their institution's emergency procedures, and undergo yearly refresher training.

Remote afterloaders are expensive. Initial investment may include the additional cost of installation and shielding. Ongoing maintenance

costs, in addition to increased staffing requirements, may all seem prohibitive. However, the ability to reduce costs through outpatient treatment, the benefits of consistent customized treatments, and the reduction of medical personnel radiation exposures have made this modality part of today's standard of care in brachytherapy.

Practitioners who wish to reproduce the biologic effectiveness of LDR treatments with remote afterloading technology have done so with pulsed dose rate brachytherapy. With this modality, a remote afterloader, similar to HDR brachytherapy afterloaders, is used to deliver very short radiation treatments. With such radiation pulses delivered approximately once per hour, the pulsed dose rate hyperfractionation scheme seeks the lower toxicity attributed to the slow treatment pattern of LDR brachytherapy and take advantage of the radiation safety advantages of HDR brachytherapy.

Sources used for HDR brachytherapy must have a high specific activity, defined as the activity per unit mass of a radioactive material (e.g., Ci/g). The specific activity dictates the maximum activity that a source of a given mass can have. Although several radionuclides are suitable for implantation, not all are suitable for HDR brachytherapy because their specific activity may not be high enough.

Food for thought: Describe the necessary criteria for a radioisotope to be used as a permanent implant.

BRACHYTHERAPY APPLICATIONS

Yet another way to classify brachytherapy procedures follows the method of source placement. Interstitial brachytherapy refers to the placement of radioactive sources directly into a tumor or tumor bed. Rigid needles or flexible tubes may be used in the actual placement of the sources. Interstitial brachytherapy is commonly used in treatments of the neck, breast, prostate, and soft tissue sarcomas.

Intracavitary implants are placed within a body cavity for treatment. An applicator is placed in the cavity, and the radiation sources are then inserted into the applicator. This type of brachytherapy has been the mainstay in treatment of cervical cancer for more than 50 years.

Intraluminal brachytherapy refers to the placement of sources of radiation within body tubes such as the esophagus, trachea, and bronchus via catheters and various centering applicators. Closely related to intraluminal brachytherapy is intravascular brachytherapy. Widely used in the past to reduce the rate of restenosis after angioplasty and the placement of stents in blood vessels, it has ceded its popularity to drug alluding stents. Intravascular brachytherapy today is limited in practice and is reserved for selected recurrent cases.

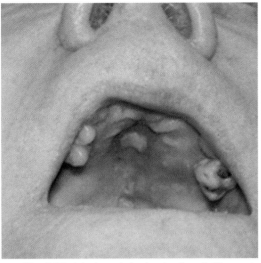
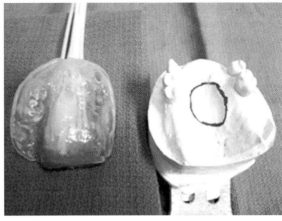

Fig. 14.3 A lesion of the hard palate (*left*) was treated with a mold (*right*). An impression of the patient's mouth was made from which a mold was designed. Note the lead shield used to protect the oral tongue. The mold was used for high-dose-rate treatments, with the source traveling through the catheters to deliver the treatment.

Surface brachytherapy places the radioactive sources on top of the area to be treated. Most commonly used for the treatment of nonmelanoma skin cancer, a custom mold of the body part treated may be taken and prepared to place the sources in definite arrangements to deliver the prescribed dose. Other areas commonly treated with external applicators include oral cavity, nasal cavity, hard palate, and orbital cavity, to name a few. Ingenuity and creative thinking are typically used in creating applicators for treatment of these superficial lesions. These molds can be designed to incorporate shielding for adjacent sensitive structures so that they do not receive as high a dose as the lesion (Fig. 14.3). For smaller skin lesions, Leipzig and Valencia applicators have been widely used. Eye plaques are used in the management of ocular tumors such as uveal melanoma and retinoblastoma (Fig. 14.4).

In the past, enucleation (the surgical removal of the eye) was the main option in the treatment of ocular melanomas. The Collaborative Ocular Melanoma Study (COMS) compared surgery, the gold standard, with eye plaque radiotherapy by using ^{125}I seeds. The study showed that eye plaque brachytherapy can be used for small- and medium-sized tumors with similar survival results with the added benefit of partial vision preservation and improved cosmetic results. To describe the procedure briefly, ^{125}I seeds are placed in a cup-shaped gold plaque that sits directly on the eye. A dose of 8500 cGy is delivered during the course of a few days. The reader may find it of interest that the first treatments of ocular cancer were, in fact, done with radium needles. Today, ^{103}Pd seeds are also used in COMS eye plaques. Other plaque designs have been introduced, including plaques that use ^{106}Ru beta-emitting isotope as a source. These ocular treatments with brachytherapy have also been competing with proton beam and stereotactic radiotherapy.

EXPOSURE FROM A RADIOACTIVE SOURCE

Most radiation measurements are performed in air. Exposure is defined as the charge deposited per unit mass in air:

$$X = \Delta Q / \Delta M$$

The unit for exposure is roentgen, denoted by R:

$$1\ R = 2.58 \times 10^{-4}\ C / kg\ of\ air$$

For example, when physicists place an ion chamber in a linac beam, they measure exposure to the air in the chamber cavity. The radiation safety officer uses a survey meter to measure exposure or exposure rate to determine an area is safe. Similarly, a well chamber is used in brachytherapy to confirm the strength of a source (see Fig. 14.2).

In brachytherapy, we are often interested in predicting the exposure from a particular source. The exposure rate constant, Γ, has been measured for various isotopes (see Table 14.1) and is defined as:

$$\Gamma \equiv \dot{X}\ \frac{d^2}{A}\ \frac{R \cdot cm^2}{mCi \cdot hr}$$

where $\dot{X}$ is the exposure rate from the source, d is the distance from the source at which the measurement is done, A is the activity of the source, and the units are as indicated. The exposure rate form a known source is then given by:

$$\dot{X} = \Gamma A \frac{1}{d^2}$$

And the total exposure from a known source during a period of time (t), assuming decay during that time is negligible, is:

$$X = \Gamma A \frac{1}{d^2} t$$

Example 6: During a radiation emergency, the therapist is assisting the physician removing a 9.5 Ci ^{192}Ir HDR source from the patient. Calculate the exposure to the therapist if it took 15 minutes to get the source to a shielded safe. Assume a 20-cm distance from the therapist to the source.

Answer: Given Γ of Ir-192 = 4.69 R·cm²/mCi/hr, d = 20 cm, A = 9.5 Ci, and t = 15 minutes, the following can be stated:

$$X = 4.69 \frac{Rcm^2}{mCi.h} 9500mCi \frac{1}{20^2 cm^2} 0.25h \cong 28R$$

Radium Substitutes

Extensive clinical experience gained with the use of radium led to the development of implant protocols, referred to as *classical systems*, in

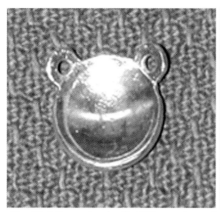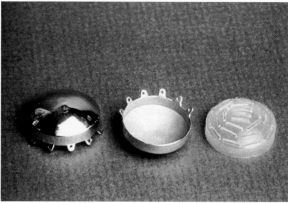

Fig. 14.4 Example of a Ru-106 eye plaque (left) and a Collaborative Ocular Melanoma Study plaque (*right*) used in topical brachytherapy of the eye. The thin gold shielding on the back of the plaque is sufficient to block more than 99% of low-energy photons of ^{125}I and ^{103}Pd used.

which the physician prescribes milligram hours of radium. When radium was replaced with other, safer isotopes, clinicians needed to estimate the equivalent amount of activity needed to achieve the same clinical results achieved with radium sources. They wanted to continue and use classic implant systems and reproduce their clinical results with the new isotopes. In other words, clinicians wanted to know what amount of the new isotope would have the same exposure as 1 mg (or 1 mCi) of radium. To calculate this, we use the definition of exposure above and set equal the exposure of the two sources:

$$X = \Gamma_{Ra} A_{Ra} \frac{1}{d^2} t = \Gamma A \frac{1}{d^2} t$$

Therefore we can state the following:

$$\Gamma_{Ra} A_{Ra} = \Gamma A$$

Rearranging this equation, we can now define an equivalent activity, milligram-radium-equivalent (mg-Ra-eq, or mRe) as follows:

$$A_{eq} = \frac{\Gamma}{\Gamma_{Ra}} A$$

where A is the activity of the new isotope, and A_{eq} is the radium equivalent of that isotope.

Example 7: To see how this works, consider a 25.0-mCi ^{137}Cs source exposed at 10 cm for 1 hour. Calculate (1) the exposure from the source, (2) the milligram radium equivalent of the source, and (3) the exposure for the equivalent activity calculated in part 2 (compare the results obtained in 1 and 3).

Answer:

1. The exposure rate constant for ^{137}Cs is 3.26 R·cm²/mCi/hr. Therefore we can state the following:

$$X = 25 \cdot 3.26 \cdot \frac{1}{10^2} \cdot 1 = 0.815 R$$

2. Using the ratio of dose rate constants for Cs (3.26 R·cm²/mCi/hr) and Ra (8.25 R·cm²/mCi/hr):

$$A_{eq} = \frac{3.26}{8.25} 25 = 9.879 mRe$$

3. Because we are using a radium equivalent activity, exposure is calculated as if the isotope used were radium.

$$X = 9.879 \cdot 8.25 \cdot \frac{1}{10^2} \cdot 1 = 0.815 R$$

CLASSICAL SYSTEMS

Dose distribution from radium-226 is the basis of all dose calculations in classic brachytherapy. As seen earlier, knowledge of the relationship of radium substitutes and radium allows the radiation therapy practitioner to deliver an accurate dose to a patient. A keen knowledge of anatomy and adherence to a few rules will provide the medical dosimetrist and radiation therapist with the ability to develop optimized treatment plans for patients. This section provides a generalized discussion of dosimetry and dose distribution for interstitial implants. Three systems are discussed: the Paterson-Parker (also known as the Manchester system), Quimby, and Paris systems.

Paterson-Parker (Manchester) System

With use of the gamma factor of radium, it is possible to perform radium dosimetry calculations, assuming the point source approximations stated previously. However, for patient dosimetry, a number of sources are typically used, and the accurate calculation of the dose distributions from these implants before the use of computers was a complex procedure. In addition, it required that the radioactive sources be implanted in the patient before the calculations are done, so the physician, medical physicist, and medical dosimetrist have no idea of how the patient is being treated until after the sources are already in place. In the 1930s at the Manchester Hospital in England, R. Paterson and H. M. Parker developed a series of guidelines and dosimetry methods known as the *Paterson-Parker*, or *Manchester*, system of radium dosimetry to circumvent these difficulties.[3,4]

The Paterson-Parker implantation philosophy strives to deliver a uniform dose to a plane or volume. To achieve this goal, the system uses a nonuniform distribution of radioactive material to produce a uniform distribution of dose. A set of source distribution guidelines was established that, if followed, would result in a dose of ±10% within the targeted area or volume. The system assumes that linear radium sources are implanted in tissue in planes or other geometric shapes and gives rules for placing the radium sources in each case. Designed before computers were available, the system provides tables that, along with distribution rules, are used to calculate the desired treatment time and activity (milligram-hours) to deliver the desired dose to the target. These rules, established for both planar and volume implants, can

TABLE 14.4   Manchester Planar Implant Source Distribution Rules

Area (cm²)	Fraction of peripheral activity
Area < 25	⅔
25 < Area < 100	½
Area > 100	⅓

Prescription plane

H

Source plane

easily be adapted for use with modern brachytherapy sources and are still useful tools in the clinic today.

Planar arrangement of sources is summarized, as an example, in Table 14.4 for square and rectangular implants. In this scenario, the prescription plane is defined at a distance H from the source plane so that the target tissue is between the plane of the sources and the prescription plane. That is, the tissue to be treated is meant to receive at least the prescription dose, with the tissue closest to the sources receiving the highest dose. The prescription distance is usually 0.5 or 1 cm. But the tables have been designed to accommodate other treatment distances, as well as two plane implants in cases in which the prescription distance is excessively large, resulting in too high a dose to tissue adjacent to the source plane.

If the geometry of the implanted volume resembles a three-dimensional shape more than a plane, it is called a *volume implant*. Shapes defined by the Paterson-Parker system include cylinders, ellipsoids, spheres, and cubes. Similar distribution rules as those shown for planar implants have been devised for volume implants as well. Interested readers are encouraged to review the reference list at the end of the chapter.

In general, it has been shown that the source arrangements and milligram-hours values predicted by the Manchester system closely approximate computer-optimized plans. This similarity is caused by our efforts to achieve the most uniform dose possible to a treatment volume. This makes the Manchester system an effective tool to assist in the independent verifications of brachytherapy treatment plans.

Quimby/Memorial Dosimetry System

The Quimby system is similar in concept to the Paterson-Parker system. It provides a set of tables used to calculate the required milligram-hours for radium, given a number of implant parameters such as area or volume and dose prescribed.[5,6] However, in the Quimby system, the distribution of activity within the implant is uniform, resulting in a nonuniform distribution of dose. One of the rationales behind the Quimby system was that when implanting a solid tumor, cells at the center of the tumor are hypoxic and therefore more radioresistant than the rest of the tumor cells, requiring a higher dose at the middle of the implanted volume. It was recognized, however, that for planar implants, in which the tumors are usually resected, the dose at the center of the implant should be lowered, and rather than prescribed at the edge of the target (as was done for volume implants), the prescription for the planar implant should be defined at the center of the target.

The Quimby system is used less frequently than the Paterson-Parker system but has been adapted into a system called the *Memorial system*, whose tables are based on computer calculations that account for filtration at all angles, modern units of activity, and dose. The dose computation system developed at Memorial Hospital formed the basis for the modern AAPM TG-43 formalism used today.

Food for thought: Why does a uniform activity distribution result in a nonuniform dose? Where is the hot spot?

More food for thought: To compare the Quimby and the Paterson-Parker systems, consider as an example a 4 cm × 4 cm planar implant, with a total of 25 sources of equal activity. How many sources would be at the periphery, and how many at the center according to each system? For this particular implant, what is the difference between the two implant systems?

Paris System

The Paris system[7] is based on clinical work done by Dr. Pierquin and Dr. Chassange in the 1960s. It follows the development of remote afterloading technology and the introduction of ^{192}Ir sources into clinical practice a decade earlier by Dr. Henschke at the Memorial Hospital in New York.

Similar to the Quimby system, the Paris system uses uniform distribution of the radiation sources. Newly introduced here are the basal reference points, located on the midplane of the implant, equidistant from adjacent source lines, where dose gradients are relatively low and dose calculations are more reliable (Fig. 14.5). The Paris system attempts to avoid the toxicity associated with high doses at the center of the implant by ensuring the dose to the basal points is limited.

The well-defined geometry and the definition of basal dose points in the Paris system means it can be easily implemented in modern computer-based treatment planning systems.

DOSE CALCULATIONS IN BRACHYTHERAPY

The following is a brief explanation of key terms and definitions used for dose calculations in brachytherapy. Earlier, we introduced exposure (this is the charge per unit mass in air that we measure). The charge we measure is the result of ionizations produced by the incident radiation. As it turns out, the average charge per ion pair produced is constant. Denoted W/e, the charge per ion pair produced is 33.97 J/coulomb (J/C).

Let us introduce a new quantity, the *kinetic energy released to the medium, kerma* (where the letter "a" is added for phonetic reasons). As will be shown below, by using kerma, we will calculate the dose in tissue. AAPM recommends we specify the strength of a source in a unit of air kerma rate resulting from the source at a standard distance.

To convert measured exposure to kerma in air, we use the average energy required to create one ion pair, W/e:

$$K_{air} = \frac{W}{e} X$$

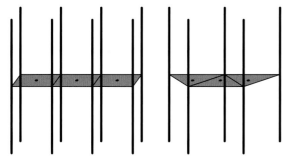

Fig. 14.5 A schematic of Paris system rectangular (*left*) and triangular (*right*) implant geometry is shown. Basal points are located on the midplane of the implant and are equidistant from the source lines.

For clinical calculations, we wish to know the kerma in tissue rather than the kerma in air. This conversion is calculated by using the ratio of mass attenuation coefficients of tissue to air, as follows:

$$K_{tissue} = K_{air} \left(\frac{\mu_{en}}{\rho} \right)_{air}^{tissue}$$

Now, extending this to a point a distance, r, from the source, one obtains:

$$K_{tissue}(r) = K_{air} \left(\frac{\mu_{en}}{\rho} \right)_{air}^{tissue} \phi(r)$$

where φ(r) accounts for the transmission through a distance, r, in the medium.

As already mentioned, source strength specification is based on the measurement of exposure in air. Using the formalism above, we can calculate the dose to tissue from any source with known air kerma strength. Remembering that source strength analogous to source activity, air kerma rate, $\dot{S}_K$, is specified as:

$$\dot{S}_K = \dot{K}_{air} r_0^2$$

and is assigned the unit U $\left(1\,U = 1\,cGy/hr\,cm^2 \right)$, where r_0 is the reference distance (in this case, 1 cm).

To keep things simple, let us assume a point source. The dose rate from a source of strength, $\dot{S}_K$, at a point at distance, r, from the source is:

$$\dot{D}(r) = \dot{S}_K \left(\frac{\mu_{en}}{\rho} \right)_{air}^{tissue} \varphi(r) \frac{1}{r^2}$$

Using TG-43 parlance, the ratio of mass attenuation coefficients corresponds to the dose rate constant (Λ), and the transmission factor is associated with the radial dose function (g[r]):

$$\dot{D}(r) = S_k \Lambda g(r) \frac{1}{r^2}$$

A more detailed formulation of this equation that accounts for source geometry and anisotropy is used for dose calculations in modern brachytherapy treatment planning systems. However, by using the basic formulation shown above, one can approximate the dose rate from brachytherapy sources in water. Although efficient and easy to implement in treatment planning software, this formalism has some limitations, stemming from the approximation that the sources are in an infinite water medium. In fact, the body is a finite and complex medium. New advances in dose calculation algorithms are beginning to introduce model and Monte Carlo–based dose calculations to account for tissue

inhomogeneities, air cavities, and dose perturbations from applicators and shields.[8] However, at the writing of this chapter, the latter are still in their infancy, and the TG-43[1] formalism is still used in clinics worldwide.

CLINICAL EXAMPLES

Although similar in concept, the details of brachytherapy procedures vary from one clinic to another. In some clinics, therapists may be responsible for the maintenance of the applicators and ancillary equipment, as well as the preparation and operation of imaging systems including ultrasound, fluoroscopy, and computed tomography (CT), used during brachytherapy procedures. These are highly dedicated devices and systems, and general hospital staff may not have sufficient training to handle them. Radiation therapists involved with brachytherapy procedures are expected to have a high level of competency. This competency includes an understanding of the clinical procedures, the operation of the imaging systems and remote afterloading unit, as well as of the applicators and accessories used for each procedure. A description of the various procedures and systems used is beyond the scope of this chapter. Instead, the section that follows attempts to provide the readers with an inkling of the type of procedures they may encounter.

Permanent Implants

Most permanent brachytherapy implants today are used for the treatment of prostate cancer. Iodine-125, palladium-103, cesium-131, and gold-198 have all been used for permanent implants, although ^{125}I and [103]Pd are the most commonly used isotopes. The tumor volumes to be treated commonly require placement of many sources, which, in turn, requires a rapid and accurate means of source application.

In the simplest application, seeds embedded in suture or polyglactin 910 (Vicril) mesh can be placed onto a surgically exposed area to treat microscopic disease after resection of a tumor. This technique has been used in tumors of the lung, neck, and brain. However, to implant deep-seated target volumes such as the prostate, image guidance is needed. The introduction of transrectal ultrasound (TRUS) revolutionized prostate brachytherapy because it enabled visualization of the prostate; critical organs such as the urethra, rectum, and bladder; as well as the needles inserted. With TRUS imaging, practitioners can plan the implant to ensure therapeutic doses are delivered to the target and that organs at risk are spared. Two methods are used in conjunction with TRUS for prostate implantation. In the first method, needles preloaded with seeds or strands of seeds prepared either according to a standard protocol or a patient-specific treatment plan are used to place the seeds or strands in the target volume. Depending on the hospital's protocol, the seeds can be preloaded by the manufacturer according to a plan prepared a week or two before the procedure, or built in the operating room in what is referred to as *intraoperative technique* with an intraoperatively designed treatment plan. In the second approach, a gunlike applicator is used for seed placement according to the treatment plan. Here, too, either preoperative plans or intraoperative plans may be used. This device, known as a *Mick applicator*, allows the practitioners to make on-the-fly adjustments to the seed loading to achieve optimal implants. This may be especially important when preoperative planning is used, because the patient anatomy and organ positioning may change between planning and treatment. After a needle is pushed through the skin into the target area where seeds are to be deposited, the applicator is attached to the hub of the needle and is then used to push sources through the needle into the tumor. In a repetitive process, the needle is withdrawn a specified distance, and a source is inserted into tissue at the tip of the needle until the planned treatment length and the desired sources are applied. Although TRUS provides superior visualization of the prostate and is now universally used to guide the implantation procedure, it is sometimes difficult to visualize the seeds because of artifacts from hemorrhage, calcifications in the gland, needles, or other neighboring seeds.

An important step in any permanent implant is the postimplant assessment to verify the seeds were placed correctly, and that the patient receives an adequate treatment. These postimplant evaluations can be done directly after the implant so that practitioners may have an immediate assessment of the implant quality, but many prefer to have the patient return later, when procedure-related edema subsides (usually a few weeks after the implant). These evaluations are typically done by using CT imaging, although magnetic resonance imaging (MRI)–based evaluations have been conducted for improved delineation of the prostate gland (Fig. 14.6).

Absorbable Hydrogel Spacer

Because the rectum is located adjacent to the prostate, it is considered an organ at risk in both external beam radiotherapy and brachytherapy procedures used to treat prostate cancer. With the use of an absorbable hydrogel spacer, about 11 mm of space can be created between the posterior prostate capsule and the anterior wall of the rectum.[14] PEG hydrogel (SpaceOAR System, Augmenix, Inc., Bedford, MA) is widely used today for both internal or external radiation procedures in treating prostate cancer. Other materials have been used in the past to create space between the prostate and rectum with less success. The spacer material has been shown to reduce rectal dose and results in long-term reductions in rectal toxicity, as well as improvements in bowel, urinary, and sexual function.[9]

The procedure takes about 30 minutes and is usually performed in a hospital, surgical center, or doctor's office. The spacer material, using TRUS guidance, is injected through the perineum into the tissue space posterior to the prostate and anterior to the rectum, forming a soft gel within 10 seconds (Fig. 14.7). The resulting hydrogel spacer maintains its shape for about 3 months while radiation treatment is delivered, and then gradually is absorbed by the body over several months. Fig. 14.8 compares two MRI images, 3 and 6 months postimplant.

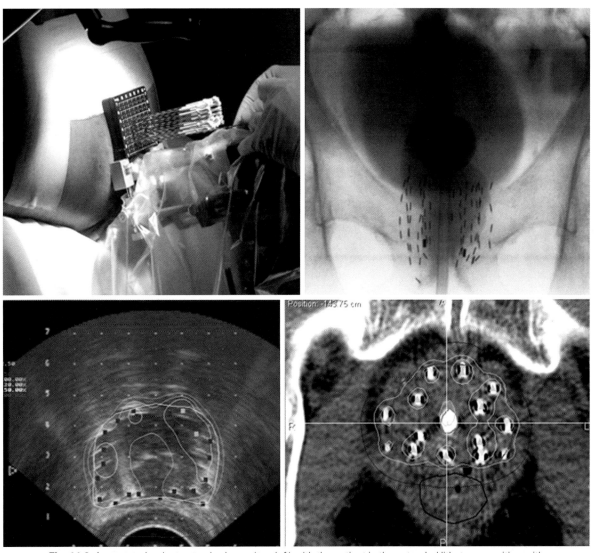

Fig. 14.6 A prostate implant setup is shown (*top left*) with the patient in the extended lithotomy position with needles positioned in the gland. The transrectal ultrasound probe is used to visualize the prostate, urethra, and needles/seeds. A typical transverse ultrasound image is shown (*bottom left*). While the implant progresses, fluoroscopy imaging (*top right*) may be used to verify seeds placement (note the dark gold markers and Foley catheter that are used as surrogates for the superior and inferior borders of the prostate). After completion of the implant, a computed tomography scan is used to evaluate the final dosimetry of the implant (*bottom right*).

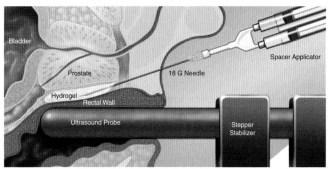

Fig. 14.7 Illustration of transperineal polyethylene glycol hydrogel spacer injection. The needle is placed and the hydrogel is injected at the midprostate level between the posterior capsule of the prostate and rectal wall. The ultrasound probe is used to guide the placement of the spacer material. (From Karsh LI, Gross ET, Pieczonka CM, et al. Absorbable hydrogel spacer use in prostate radiotherapy: a comprehensive review of Phase 3 clinical trial published data. *Urology* 2018;115:39–45.)

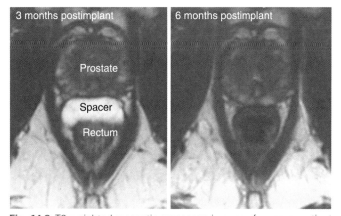

Fig. 14.8 T2-weighted magnetic resonance images of a spacer patient showing hydrogel persistence through completion of radiation therapy *(left)*, and absorption 6 months after implantation *(right)*. (From Karsh LI, Gross ET, Pieczonka CM, et al. Absorbable hydrogel spacer use in prostate radiotherapy: a comprehensive review of Phase 3 clinical trial published data. *Urology* 2018;115:39–45.)

High-Dose-Rate Prostate Implants

Similar to permanent implants, HDR implants (Fig. 14.9) of the prostate are performed in the operating room under ultrasound guidance. HDR implants of the prostate are used most commonly as adjuvant treatment to external beam intensity-modulated radiation therapy. However, primary definitive and salvage treatments (to address post–radiation therapy local recurrence) are also under investigation. Implantation and planning techniques are wide-ranging: implants have been done in one insertion and several treatment fractions, two insertions performed a week or two apart with one treatment fraction per insertion, as well as a single-insertion, single-fraction treatment. Planning can be done intraoperatively by using ultrasound alone or postoperatively by using CT or MRI. Ultrasound may be favored for hospitals with a shielded operating theatre in which the patient may be implanted and treated while still under anesthesia. For clinics with access to MRI, the benefits of visualization of the prostate with this modality may be attractive. However, with CT widely available, it is the most commonly used imaging modality for this type of treatment.

Intracavitary Implants

Insertion of radioactive sources into body cavities has been a viable component of radiation therapy for many years. Several applicators have been designed and used, most for the treatment of gynecologic tumors. The designs of newer applicators allow practitioners to take advantage of three-dimensional imaging modalities such as CT and MRI for treatment planning to obtain customized dose distributions that maximize the dose to the tumor and spare adjacent, sensitive structures.

By far, the most common intracavitary implants are performed for treatment of cervical cancer. Cervical cancer is usually treated with a combination of external beam and intracavitary brachytherapy. The external beam portion precedes the brachytherapy portion of the treatment, and serves two purposes: (1) to treat parametrial disease and pelvic lymph nodes that cannot be treated with brachytherapy, and (2) to reduce the tumor volume, thereby reducing the treatment volume and the toxicity associated with the brachytherapy treatment that follows. Gynecologic brachytherapy insertions for either LDR or HDR applications often use tandem and ovoid-style applicators. These applicators have been used for many years with good clinical results. Briefly, a tandem, a long,

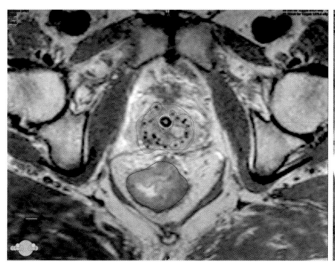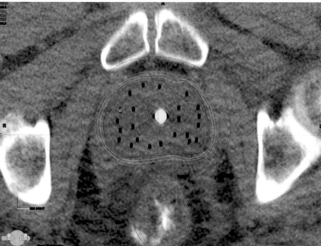

Fig. 14.9 Examples of a computed tomography *(left)* and a magnetic resonance imaging *(right)* of a prostate high-dose-rate implant.

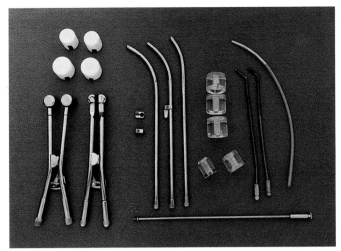

Fig. 14.10 A Fletcher Suit, Delclos manual afterloading system is shown. From left to right: small colpostats with additional caps for conversion to medium and large; microcolpostats; intrauterine "tandems;" Delclos and cylindrical colpostats (selected); colpostats carriers; and tandem carrier. Bottom, horizontal: Anderson marker needle. (From Fletcher GH. *Textbook of Radiotherapy*. Baltimore, MD: Williams & Wilkins; 1980.)

narrow tube, is inserted through the cervix into the uterus. The two ovoids (or colpostats), cylindrical or semispherical shaped, are inserted into the lateral vaginal fornices (Fig. 14.10). These applicator sets come with various tandem lengths and curvatures as well as several ovoid sizes and ovoid caps to accommodate the variances in patient anatomy.

In classic applicators, all ovoids, with the exception of the smallest ones, have small shields placed anterior and posterior to the sources. This was done to protect the urinary bladder and rectum while maximizing dose to the cervix (located medially and superiorly between ovoids and tandem) as well as boosting parametrial disease (located laterally to the implant). Early versions of these applicators made for HDR afterloading still incorporated the shields in the ovoids. However, while new CT and MR imaging modalities became available, designs of these applicators omitted the shields to avoid undesirable image artifacts. Doing so paved the way for new applicator design such as the tandem and ring, and split-ring applicators in which the ring (as the name implies) replaces the ovoids (Fig. 14.11).

Tandems and ovoids are placed into the female anatomy and stabilized with packing. This vaginal packing (sterile gauze) not only stabilizes the apparatus during its placement, but also serves to displace the rectum and bladder from the sources. This packing can be substituted by specialized balloons or retractors, as seen in Fig. 14.10.

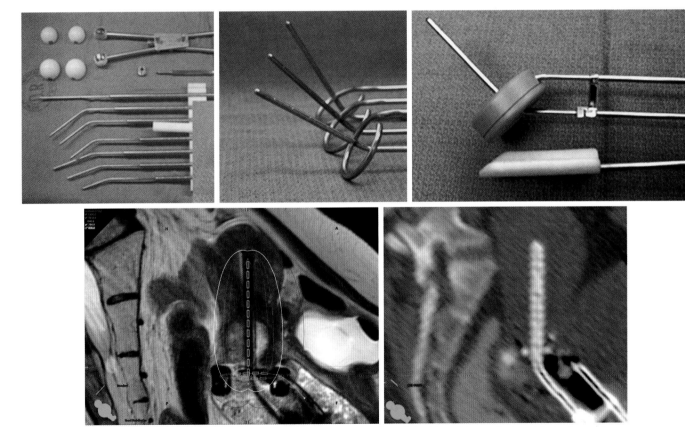

Fig. 14.11 Clockwise from top left: a high-dose-rate version of the Henschke applicator with tandems of varying lengths and angles and ovoid caps. The tungsten shields in the anterior and posterior aspects of the ovoids are visible (inset); tandem and ring applicators with various angles and a 6-cm tandem; a tandem and ring applicator is assembled with a buildup cap and an optional rectal retractor (note the slim applicator design and lack of shields); a computed tomography reconstruction in a sagittal plane of a tandem and ring application (note the placement of the tandem in the uterus and the location of the rectum and bladder with respect to the implant); a sagittal T2 magnetic resonance imaging sequence of a tandem and ring applicator (note that although anatomy visualization is superior to computed tomography, plastic and metallic applicator components and air cavities generate no signal and appear black).

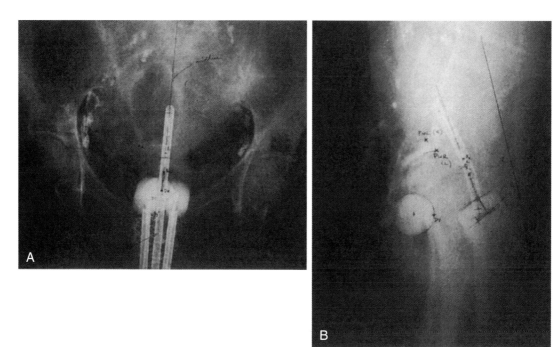

Fig. 14.12 Orthogonal radiographs of tandem and ovoids localization. (A) Anterior-posterior, and (B) left-lateral. Note the packing that serves to stabilize the placement of the applicators as well as "push" the urinary bladder and rectum away from the applicator. (From Cox JD. *Moss' Radiation Oncology*. 7th ed. St. Louis, MO: Mosby; 1994.)

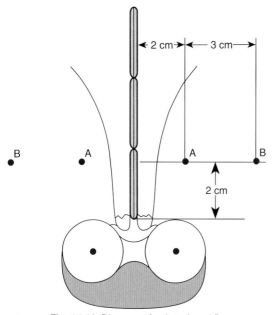

Fig. 14.13 Diagram of points A and B.

Historically, treatment planning for afterloading implants was based on planar films. Planning in this manner visualized the applicator as well as fiducial markers and imaging contrast placed in the patient, but soft tissue could not be seen directly. The applicators and radiographic markers in the patient were therefore used as surrogates for the target and organs at risk. Gynecological (GYN) intracavitary implants were no exception. A typical localization film set of a tandem and ovoids applicator used for implant geometry reconstruction and treatment planning dose calculations is shown in Fig. 14.12.[10]

The anatomic points historically used for cervical and uterine treatment are points A and B. Point A, where the prescription dose is specified, is located 2 cm superior to the top of the ovoids along the tandem

and 2 cm lateral to the tandem in the plane of the applicator. It approximates the location where the uterine arteries and the ureters intersect and is chosen to ensure that the cervix located between point A and applicator receives at least the prescription dose. Point B, located 2 cm superior to the top of the ovoids and 5 cm lateral to the patient midline, represents the parametria. Fig. 14.13 shows a schematic of points A and B with respect to an applicator. An important part of implant reconstruction and planning is the localization of organs at risk. Here, the Foley balloon is used as a surrogate for the bladder, and rectal markers and vaginal packing are used as surrogates for the anterior rectal wall.

Although these points of dose specification have been used for years, their use for dose prescription in modern treatment planning is slowly being replaced as accurate target delineation on MRI is introduced in the clinic. However, their function as robust dose calculation points makes them useful tools in treatment planning quality assurance (QA). Yet, even as three-dimensional imaging modalities replace planar film for treatment planning, planar films remain a common and useful of pretreatment verification, used to ensure accurate treatment geometry is maintained from the time of placement and planning through actual treatment. MRI is the imaging modality of choice for GYN implants. With the use of MRI for planning GYN implants, clinicians are able to ensure gross tumor volumes are treated appropriately. Furthermore, with the ability to customize the treatment volume to the actual target, the overall treatment volume can be reduced as the tumor volume decreases, which results in reduced toxicity as critical organs are spared.

Vaginal Cylinders

One other common GYN brachytherapy application is the prophylactic treatment of posthysterectomy endometrial cancer. The applicators are of different lengths and diameters and may incorporate shielding. Usually, standard single-channel vaginal cylinders are used, but customized multichannel applicators designed to give a high dose to vaginal lesions without delivering an excessive dose to the urinary bladder or rectum are also available.

These treatments are relatively simple: they do not require anesthesia and can be performed on an outpatient basis. Such endometrial treatments are typically administered in three fractions, 1 week apart. Treatment is usually prescribed 5 mm from the applicator surface (Fig. 14.14), but care should be taken not to overdose the vaginal surface and genitalia.

Temporary Interstitial Implants

Building on the clinical experience of classic brachytherapy described above, plastic catheters or metallic needles introduced in tissue accommodate placement of the radioisotopes. Iridium-192 is used in most applications. True to the classic experience, the catheters are often spaced 1 cm apart; several catheter planes or volume geometry may be used, depending on the tumor size and shape. Dummy source wires (nonradioactive radiopaque markers that can be seen on a radiographic image) are used when planning is based on planar x-rays. The dummy sources are aligned and spaced just as the radioactive seeds would be. This is done to enable visualization of source placement, to ensure that the implants are positioned correctly, and for treatment planning and dose calculation without unnecessary radiation exposure to the patient and personnel. Here, too, the reconstructed dummy wires serve as surrogates to the target volume that cannot be directly visualized on planar images (Fig. 14.15). This is especially true when the tumor has been resected, and the target volume consists of the tumor bed only.

Fig. 14.16 demonstrates the catheter placement and CT plan for an HDR implant of a postresection lateral neck cancer. In this case, although critical structure can be accurately delineated, even with three-dimensional imaging, the target volume can only be defined by surrogate markers, prior knowledge of the practicing physician about the tumors' prior location, and the placement of the catheters.

Temporary Breast Implants

Motivated by the desire to reduce toxicity in the treatment of breast cancer, clinicians have devised various methods for treating only a portion of the breast. These approaches, known generally as partial breast radiation therapy, include both external beam and brachytherapy. The implants are placed either at the time of lumpectomy or soon after. In these approaches, the target volume comprises the lumpectomy cavity surrounded by a 1-cm margin, except where critical structures are present. Critical structures to avoid are primarily the skin and chest wall. Brachytherapy implants fall into three categories: interstitial catheter–based implants, balloon-based implants, and intraoperative radiation therapy–based treatments.

In the United States, the balloon-based approach has gained popularity for its simplicity, favorable cosmetic results, and patient comfort. Here, a balloon with one or multiple catheters is placed in the lumpectomy cavity. Positioning of the balloon applicator within the cavity as well as its proximity to critical structures is assessed by using CT images obtained after insertion. This CT study is also used for treatment planning and is used as a reference for daily treatments.

When used as a primary treatment, patients are treated to the equivalent of a 45Gy LDR implant (see Table 14.3). In general, these techniques are reserved for low-risk patients.

RADIATION SAFETY AND QUALITY ASSURANCE

The safe handling of radioactivity has been a matter of concern in hospitals for many years. Those small, seemingly harmless ribbons and tubes can cause a great panic if not dealt with appropriately. The subject of practical radiation safety of brachytherapy merits a few general thoughts concerning this important aspect of therapeutic administration.

The storage of the sources should facilitate source identification by type and strength. Appropriate documentation should be kept for source control from initial receipt through calibration, inventory, treatment, and disposal.

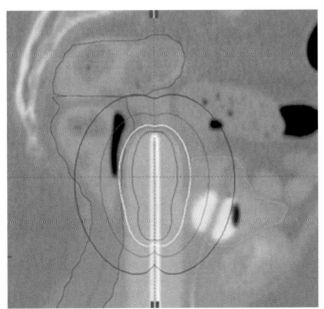

Fig. 14.14 Sample sagittal reconstruction of a computed tomography plan for the treatment of endometrial cancer with a vaginal cylinder is shown. This particular applicator allows the source to reach the very tip of the applicator and is known as a stump vaginal cylinder. Note the proximity of the bladder and rectum to the vaginal cuff.

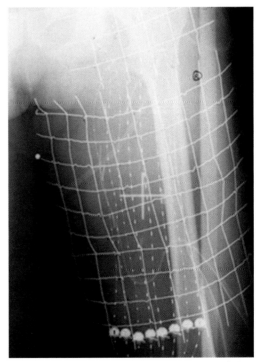

Fig. 14.15 A simulation film of an interstitial implant of the thigh for the treatment of soft tissue sarcoma. Dummy source wires are used to identify actual source locations. The rectangular grid of radiopaque wires was placed on the skin to help ensure that the skin doses are maintained at acceptable tolerance levels.

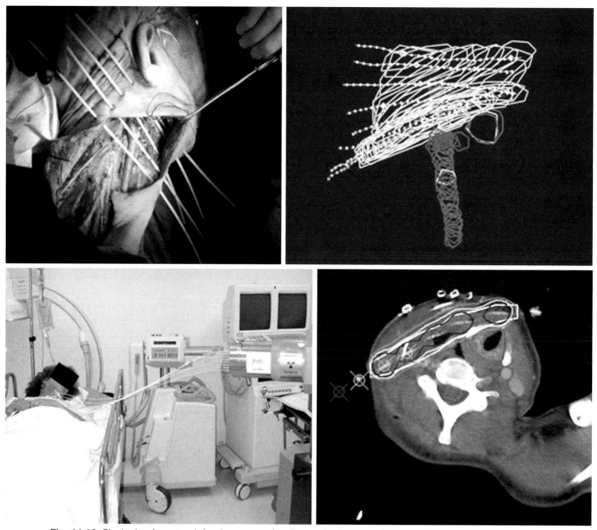

Fig. 14.16 Clockwise from top left: placement of catheters in the operating room (note the proximity of the catheters to the carotid artery); three-dimensional implant reconstruction includes outline of the target with use of the catheters as surrogates, and outlines of organs at risk; computed tomography base planning showing a typical isodose distribution; setup of a high-dose-rate treatment.

All treatment plans and dose calculations should also be double-checked. A QA program can be the difference between safe administration of radiation and a massive radiation disaster.

All treatments should be verified before the administration of radiation. For HDR treatments, this will require verification before each treatment fraction. New treatment platforms may offer a record and verify system to assist in this task.

Finally, the use of HDR requires special precautions.[11,12] A malfunction of the HDR unit may leave the patient and staff exposed to the source with potentially catastrophic results. Each HDR clinic has emergency procedures in place, designed to handle the various scenarios that may be encountered. These procedures, rehearsed on a yearly basis by all staff involved with HDR treatments, require the active intervention of a physicist and a physician should a radiation emergency occur. An authorized radiation oncologist and a qualified medical physicist must be physically present for each HDR treatment delivery.

Many brachytherapy procedures are performed in the intraoperative setting. For cases that are implanted, planned, and treated in sessions, this means that time is limited. In such a high-pressure environment, the radiation therapists' familiarity with the hardware and clinical procedures of their respective clinics goes a long way to ensure the safe delivery of HDR treatments.

Food for thought: Compare the exposure to staff that results from LDR and HDR brachytherapy applications. Refer to example 6. What is the exposure in terms of LD50? (LD50 represents the individual dose [lethal dose] required to kill 50% of a test population.)

ELECTRONIC BRACHYTHERAPY

Electronic Brachytherapy (EB), a "method of radiation therapy using electrically generated x rays to deliver a radiation dose"[13] to a nearby target area, is characterized by the low energy of the x-rays generated. Reduced shielding requirements, and the portability of some the treatment units, means that (unlike Ir-192 base afterloaders) they could be installed in regular clinics and operating rooms. This, together with the prospect of highly conformal treatment afforded by such low-energy beams, triggered much interest in the application of this new technology to various clinical indications. Indeed, applications of EB are wide ranging and most commonly include superficial skin lesions, GYN intracavitary cervix, intravaginal cuff brachytherapy, and partial breast brachytherapy. Yet initial clinical results have mixed results.

The low-energy beams' steep dose gradients result in highly inhomogeneous dose distributions, often forcing clinicians to compromise target coverage in order to keep safe dose limits close to the source/applicator. The American Brachytherapy Society's recently published consensus statement[14] recommends that EB be used within prospective studies or clinical trials to better assess their efficacy in comparison to traditions radiotherapy and isotope-based brachytherapy, and to gather longer follow-up data.

SUMMARY

- Brachytherapy is an art and a science that has evolved throughout the years into a specialized aspect of malignant disease management.
- Today, brachytherapy is a standard technique used to treat a large number of malignancies through various means.
- Through the use of radioisotopes, a very high dose may be delivered to a tumor while sparing normal tissues, adhering to the basic tenets of disease management with ionizing radiation.
- Because of the highly conformal nature of brachytherapy, it is reserved for the treatment of localized disease.

- Many of the conveniences offered by brachytherapy in general, and HDR brachytherapy in particular, require highly trained personnel and diligent QA for safe and accurate treatment delivery.
- Brachytherapy has become the preferred course of treatment for many early-stage cancers such as breast, cervical, and prostate cancers, and with continued research, the future is constantly looking brighter.

REVIEW QUESTIONS

The answers to the Review Questions can be found by logging on to our website at: http://evolve.elsevier.com/Washington/principles

1. Afterloading techniques were developed primarily to reduce:
   a. The possibilities of loading errors.
   b. The time required for an implant.
   c. Exposure to personnel.
   d. Exposure to nearby dose-limiting structures.
2. Which of the following statements about radioactivity is true?
   a. The change in the number of atoms per unit time is proportional to the number of atoms present.
   b. The change in unit time per change in the number of atoms is proportional to the number of atoms present.
   c. The change in the number of atoms per unit time is equal to the number of disintegrations per second.
   d. The change per unit time per change in the number of atoms is proportional to the number of disintegrations per second.
3. The decay constant describes:
   a. The half-life of a particular radionuclide.
   b. The number of ionizations produced in tissue per unit time.
   c. The fraction of the number of atoms that decay per unit time.
   d. None of the above.
4. The average lifetime of radioactive atoms is the definition of:
   a. Half-life.
   b. Decay constant.
   c. Specific activity.
   d. Mean life.
5. The dose profile (depth dose curve) around a brachytherapy source depends on the source's:
   a. Activity.
   b. Strength.
   c. Energy.
   d. Half-life.
6. A new batch of iridium-192 wire has arrived, and its calibration must be checked. The supplier states that the activity of the material was 0.351 U/seed 10 days earlier. What is the expected activity of the iridium-192 today?
   a. 0.002 U.
   b. 0.320 U.
   c. 0.386 U.
   d. 0.910 U.
7. The most commonly used isotopes for permanent implants are:
   a. I-125 and Pd-103.
   b. Au-198 and I-125.
   c. Cs-137 and Pd-103.
   d. Ra-226 and Ir-192.
8. Packing in gynecologic implants serves which of the following purposes?
   I. Spaces sources to even out dose distributions.
   II. Aids in pushing dose-sensitive structures farther from the sources.
   III. Provides stability of applicator placement.
   A. I and II.
   B. I and III.
   C. II and III.
   D. I, II, and III.
9. A source's activity is:
   a. Inversely proportional to the particle energy.
   b. Inversely proportional to treatment time.
   c. Inversely proportional to dose rate.
   d. Inversely proportional to exposure rate.
10. At 15 cm from an ^{192}Ir source, the exposure rate is 313 mR/hr (0.313 R/hr). What is the activity of this source?
    a. 1.0 mCi.
    b. 15.0 mCi.
    c. 48.0 mCi.
    d. 70.5 mCi.

REFERENCES

1. Rivard MJ, Coursey BM, DeWerd LA, et al. Update of AAPM Task Group No. 43 Report: a revised AAPM protocol for brachytherapy dose calculations. *Med Phys.* 2004;31:633–674.
2. Henschke UK. Afterloading applicator for radiation therapy of carcinoma of the uterus. *Radiology.* 1960;74:834.
3. Paterson R, Parker HM. A dosage system for interstitial radium therapy. *Br J Radiol.* 1938;11:252–266.
4. Meredith WJ, ed. *Radium Dosage: The Manchester System.* Livingston: Edinburgh, 1967.
5. Quimby EH. Dose calculation in radium therapy. *Am J Roentgenol Radium Ther.* 1947;57:622–627.
6. Quimby EH, Castro V. The calculation of dosage in interstitial radium therapy. *Am J Roentgenol Radium Ther Nucl Med.* 1953;70:739–759.
7. Marinello G. Paris system for interstitial brachytherapy. In: Lemoigne Y, Caner A, eds. *Radiotherapy and Brachytherapy. NATO Science for Peace and Security Series B: Physics and Biophysics.* Dordrecht: Springer; 2009.
8. Beaulieu L, Tedgren AC, Carrier JF, et al. Report of the Task Group 186 on model-based dose calculation methods in brachytherapy beyond the TG-43 formalism: current status and recommendations for clinical implementation. *Med Phys.* 2012;39(10):6208–6236.
9. Hwang ME, Black PJ, Elliston CD, et al. A novel model to correlate hydrogel spacer placement, perirectal space creation, and rectum dosimetry in prostate stereotactic body radiotherapy. *Radiat Oncol.* 2018;13(1):192. https://doi.org/10.1186/s13014-018-1135-6. Published 2018 Oct 1.
10. International Commission of Radiation Units: Measurements: dose and volume specification for reporting intracavitary therapy in gynecology therapy, Bethesda, 1985, ICRU. ICRU Report No. 38.
11. Kubo HD, Glasgow GP, Pethel TD, et al. High dose-rate brachytherapy treatment delivery: report of AAPM Radiation Therapy Committee Task Group No. 59. *Med Phys.* 1998;25:375–403.
12. American College of Radiology. ACR-AAPM technical standards for the performance of high-does-rate brachytherapy physics, Revised 2015 (resolution 50). Available at https://www.acr.org/-/media/ACR/Files/Practice-Parameters/HDR-BrachyTS.pdf, Accessed date: 9 October 2019.
13. Report No. 152: the 2007 AAPM response to the CRCPD request for recommendations for the CRCPD's model regulations for electronic brachytherapy. AAPM Reports website. https://www.aapm.org/pubs/reports/detail.asp?docid=157. Accessed January 26, 2019.
14. Tom MC, Hepel JT, Patel R, et al. The American Brachytherapy Society consensus statement for electronic brachytherapy. *Brachytherapy.* 2019;18(3):292–298.

BIBLIOGRAPHY

Thomadsen BR, Rivard MJ, Butler WM. *Brachytherapy Physics.* 2nd ed. Madison, WI: Medical Physics Publishing; 2005.

Williamson JF, Thomadsen BR, Nath R. *Brachytherapy Physics.* Madison, WI: Medical Physics Publishing; 1994.

15

Advanced Procedures

Lisa DiProspero, Laura D'Alimonte

OBJECTIVES

- Describe new radiation therapy practices that address some of the limitations of conventional radiation therapy: image-guided, stereotactic, respiratory motion management, magnetic resonance–guided, and heavy charged particle therapy.
- Identify the options available for treatment unit imaging, including kilovoltage and megavoltage.
- Define cone-beam computed tomography.
- Compare ultrasound imaging with kilovoltage imaging.
- Identify the advantages and disadvantages of fiducial-guided treatment.
- Name the core elements of stereotactic guided treatments.
- Describe four-dimensional computed tomography imaging.

- Discuss the basic concept of gated treatments.
- Identify the advantages and disadvantages of mechanical methods of motion management.
- Describe magnetic resonance–guided therapy and state the potential advantages.
- Discuss proton therapy and state the potential advantages.
- Describe carbon ion therapy and state the potential advantages.
- Describe radiomics and explain its potential impact on radiation therapy.
- Explain what microbubbles are and their potential impact on radiation therapy.
- Discuss the potential impact of artificial intelligence on the practice of radiation therapy.

OUTLINE

KEY TERMS

Artificial intelligence
Carbon ions
Computed tomography-on-rails
Cone-beam computed tomography
Electronic portal imaging devices
Fiducial
Four-dimensional computed tomography
Gated treatments
Image registration
Image-guided radiation therapy (2D vs. 3D)
Information flow
Intensity-modulated proton therapy

Kilovoltage
Magnetic resonance imaging
Megavoltage
Microbubbles
Personalized medicine
Protons
Radiomics
Respiratory cycle
Robotic couch
Stereotactic
Ultrasound
Volumetric imaging

INTRODUCTION

Radiation therapy is a therapeutic treatment for cancer whereby a set dose is delivered to a specified area of the body. The goal of radiation therapy is the eradication of the tumor cells by delivering the maximum dose to the target volume. To do this requires accurate daily positioning of the patient to minimize the chances of a geographical miss of the target and overexposure of surrounding dose-limiting critical structures. Before the era of image-guided radiation therapy (IGRT), radiation therapy treatments were delivered conformally using external marks and tattoos on the patients' body surfaces as a representation of internal anatomy.[1,2] Before treatment, orthogonal electronic portal images (EPIDs) using MV photon beams were acquired to visualize bony internal anatomy.[3] Using these pretreatment images, the position of the internal bony anatomy was compared with reference images acquired during the radiation planning process.[3] Because most tumors are not directly correlated with bones,[3] and knowing that soft tissues move, larger planning target volume margins were used to account for these uncertainties. Unfortunately, these uncertainties resulted in larger treatment margins at the cost of treating greater volumes of normal surrounding tissues. The introduction of intensity-modulated radiation therapy (IMRT) for cancer treatment has enabled highly conformal dose distributions to be delivered to the target while minimizing the dose to surrounding normal structures. To ensure dose distributions are delivered as originally planned, and to take advantage of the dose gradients created, precise patient positioning, setup accuracy, and target localization are required. Imaging plays an important role in assuring the accurate delivery of the radiation therapy treatment.[4] In the past, highly sensitive and automated on-board EPIDs acquired low-dose portal images to adjust patient position relative to bony anatomy before treatment.[4] However, the drawback of portal imaging is the reduced soft tissue and three-dimensional (3D) geometric visualization as EPIDs are a two-dimensional (2D) projection of 3D anatomy.[4] This limitation motivated the development of 3D imaging with the patient in the treatment position in the treatment room. Over the last decade, computed tomography (CT) based IGRT has afforded the safe and effective delivery of dose escalated treatments to the targets.

This chapter reviews the evolution of IGRT, from 2D to 3D volume-based cone-beam imaging, and provides a look ahead at magnetic resonance (MR)–guided radiation therapy, the next evolution of IGRT. In addition, the benefits and limitations of specialized IGRT techniques, including stereotactic radiation therapy (SRT), the management of respiratory motion, and the basic principles of proton therapy and carbon ion treatments, are discussed. All of these developments are offered at an increasing number of institutions. Finally, a review of recent radiation therapy innovations, including artificial intelligence (AI), radiomics, and microbubbles, is presented.

IMAGE-GUIDED RADIATION THERAPY

In the treatment room, IGRT has been available for decades. Kilovoltage (kV) x-ray units were mounted at an angle to the side of cobalt-60 units. The kV images produced by such devices provided the healthcare team with more information (better resolution, higher-contrast images) to make clinical decisions regarding patient positioning with the patient in the treatment position. Fig. 15.1 is an image of a kV x-ray tube mounted on the side of a Theratron 780-C cobalt unit.

Ultrasound imaging was commercially introduced approximately one decade ago for localization of the prostate, with the use of 2D B-mode approach to image a thin slice of anatomy.[5–8] Ultrasound imaging involves sending high-frequency sound waves into the body and recording the echo waves while the sound bounces back from various tissue interfaces. Generally, the therapist positions the linear phased-array ultrasound transducer on the patient's anterior pelvic surface and views the ultrasound image on an in-room monitor. Fig. 15.2 shows a therapist holding the transducer in the pelvis of a male patient and acquiring either a sagittal or an axial image. These systems are designed to compare the position of the prostate and surrounding anatomy (bladder and rectum) with the patient on

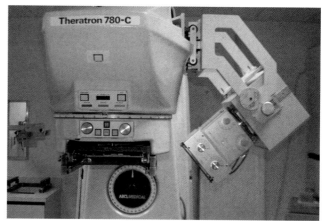

Fig. 15.1 An x-ray tube and housing mounted on the side of a Theratron 780-C cobalt-60 unit.

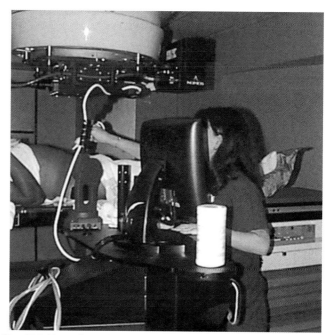

Fig. 15.2 Therapist positioning the ultrasound probe to locate the prostate with the patient in the treatment position.

the treatment table with the position of these structures at the time of simulation. To obtain better agreement between the planned and delivered treatment, the ultrasound device must be registered (image registration) with the treatment delivery unit to know where in space its images of the prostate are (i.e., to register the images with respect to the isocenter of the accelerator). Axial and sagittal ultrasound images are obtained and then overlaid with the contours of structures defined in the treatment planning process. Fig. 15.3 displays an axial ultrasound image, together with contours of the bladder, prostate, and rectum, which were generated from the CT simulation images. The therapist can digitally move the ultrasound images to a position in which there is reasonable coincidence between the two data sets: the contours from the planning system and the ultrasound images appear to overlay each other. The treatment couch can then be shifted by these increments that have just been determined. The American Association of Physicists in Medicine (AAPM) Task Group 154 describe quality assurance procedures for US-guided external beam prostate radiotherapy.[8]

The greater use of ultrasound and related new devices in the radiation treatment of prostate cancer has increased the confidence of the healthcare team that the patient's daily setup truly replicates the patient's position during simulation. For example, the introduction of the bladder scanner, a handheld device that digitally reads how many milliliters of urine are in the bladder, allows the therapist to be confident that the patient's bladder fullness at the time of treatment most closely represents the bladder status at the time of simulation and aids in patient readiness for treatment. If not, the patient can continue to drink while the therapist moves on to another patient, saving everyone time.

Such B-mode ultrasound systems have been widely accepted. They are available from several different manufacturers, with many generations of such devices available from a single vendor. There is general agreement that the added time required to image the patient, which can be several minutes, is justified by more precise patient setups as a best practice.

Beam's-eye-view MV planar imaging with a linear accelerator (linac) has been common for decades. The small focal spot size of the linac is capable of providing high-resolution images, but the soft tissue contrast was poor because of the use of x-rays produced by MV sources. Special films, which required a small number of monitor units, were developed for MV imaging. The films may have been placed in lead-lined cassettes or in paper cassettes. **EPIDs** replaced films in many clinics within the last decade.[9] There are at least two different basic designs for EPIDs. One design obtains images by using a scintillation screen and a television camera. The other design uses an amorphous silicon flat-panel detector, which consists of an array of photodiodes that detect light from an x-ray–stimulated scintillator. Both approaches produce clinically useful MV images in a digital format. One great advantage of the digital format is that the images can be reviewed from multiple locations, as opposed to being available only on a piece of film, which must be carried to the review location, benefitting the efficiency and accessibility of the treatment delivery process pathway.

The introduction of kV in-room planar x-ray systems as an integral part of a linac treatment delivery system is well established commercially. Oncologists, therapists, and others are generally more comfortable reviewing kV images because they provide better soft tissue contrast compared with MV images. Thus in theory, kV images should provide an easier tool to ensure proper patient positioning on the treatment table. kV imaging systems have been implemented in several different ways. The kV x-ray system is generally only used to view anatomy because it has a different geometry than the treatment geometry. The AAPM Task Force Group 142 report on quality assurance of medical accelerators[10] provides comprehensive quality assurance recommendations, including kV imaging systems on treatment devices.

One commercial planar image product, the Varian On-Board Imager, mounts the x-ray unit and image receptor system by using robotic arms on the accelerator gantry at 90 degrees from the MV x-ray beam with its EPID system. This arrangement is shown in Fig. 15.4. Thus kV, MV, or both planar images can be taken with the patient in the treatment position. The gantry can be rotated, and two perpendicular kV images can be obtained. Reference images (e.g., digital reconstructed radiographs) can be downloaded from the treatment planning systems and used as the gold standard to compare with the kV images taken with the patient on the treatment table. Software tools are available to register the two different image sets and calculate the couch shifts to align the patient by superimposing the bony anatomy. Elekta offers a similar kV product for their linacs. This equipment is shown in Fig. 15.5.

Another commercial example of a planar image-guided x-ray system, the ExacTrac from BrainLAB, is not attached to the accelerator and uses two floor-recessed x-ray units and two ceiling-mounted

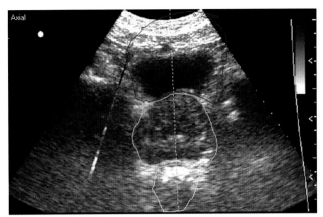

Fig. 15.3 Axial ultrasound image with contours of the bladder (red), prostate (blue), and rectum (yellow), which were generated in treatment planning.

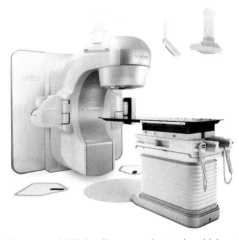

Fig. 15.4 A new-model Varian linear accelerator in which various functions are integrated. (From Varian Medical Systems, Palo Alto, CA. With permission.)

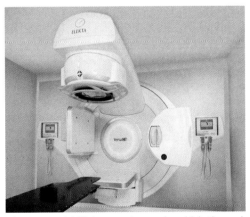

Fig. 15.5 A new-model Elekta accelerator in which the various functions are integrated. (From Elekta, Stockholm, Sweden. With permission.)

amorphous silicon flat-panel detectors. Images from this system can be analyzed and couch corrections calculated to position the patient before treatment. An infrared tracking system is used to track the patient during treatment.

In the treatment room, volumetric imaging (3D imaging vs. 2D imaging) with use of a CT unit, which is separate from the accelerator

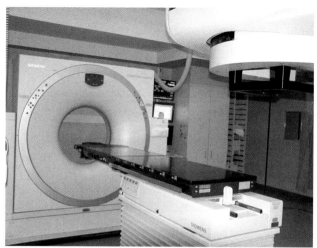

Fig. 15.6 A computed tomography-on-rails system with the treatment couch rotated to the imaging position. Note the treatment unit head is in the foreground.

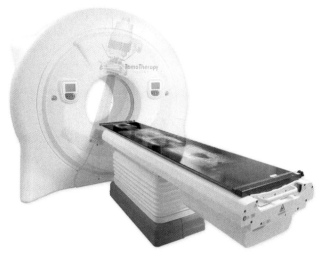

Fig. 15.7 TomoTherapy Hi-Art imaging and treatment system, which uses the same MV source for computed tomography and for treatment. (From TomoTherapy, Madison, WI. With permission.)

but shares a registration system, has been available for more than 10 years. The first report by Uematsu et al[11] was designed for frameless SRT. The treatment couch has two rotation axes: one for rotation about the accelerator's isocenter and the other to rotate between the accelerator and the CT scanner. Fig. 15.6 shows the treatment couch in the imaging position within the treatment room CT device. Another approach placed a CT simulator in the treatment room and used a sliding couch top to transport the patient between the CT scanner and the accelerator treatment table. There are at least two different commercial versions of the **CT-on-rails** approach with systems provided by General Electric and Siemens.[12–14] The accelerator treatment table is rotated 180 degrees, and the CT unit moves on rails while the patient is imaged with the couch in a stationary position. This is the opposite of the normal CT imaging technique in which the CT unit is stationary and the couch moves the patient into the imaging position. Such CT-on-rails systems, if used and maintained properly, can provide very accurate patient localizations with uncertainties of less than 1 mm. The images obtained with the moving CT unit have almost the same quality as those obtained from a stationary CT unit, but the low-contrast resolution is worse compared with couch-moving CTs. Organizations and departments have had to write their own software to calculate couch corrections for these systems, which represents a potential weakness of this approach. However, these systems can be used to deliver very precise treatments (e.g., metastasis to the vertebral body within 1 to 2 mm of the spinal cord).

One commercial product combines CT imaging and treatment delivery by using the same x-ray source, namely, TomoTherapy, which is shown in Fig. 15.7.[7] A continuous 360-degree ring gantry geometry, which is the CT scanner geometry, is used to support a straight-through 6-MV waveguide, which is used for both MV CT imaging and MV treatments. MV images have poor low-contrast resolution compared with kV images but are able to define the position of the patient on the treatment table. One benefit of MV images is that they avoid the metal artifacts that are present in kV images (e.g., from hip prostheses). Helical intensity-modulated radiation treatments are delivered after the patient is imaged. The treatment can be adjusted to match the position of the patient. This unit is designed to deliver only helical IMRT, as opposed to customized or rectangular fields, and the patient is moved through the imaging/treatment section in a manner similar to diagnostic CT imaging. This self-contained approach has a certain aesthetic appeal.

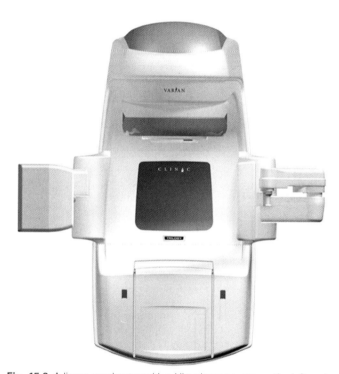

Fig. 15.8 A linear accelerator with a kilovoltage source on the left and a flat-panel detector on the right. The gantry rotates 360 degrees around the patient while a series of radiographs are taken. These radiographs are constructed into a three-dimensional computed tomography data set.

In the treatment room, volumetric imaging using an integrated accelerator with an x-ray system has recently become available using several different approaches. **Cone-beam CT** (CBCT) differs from fan beam CT in that the CT detector is an area detector (a 2D extended digital array) (Fig. 15.8).[15] At certain degree intervals during the rotation of the gantry, single-projection images are acquired, for example, at every 1 degree. These different gantry angle images are slightly offset one from another and are the basis upon which a 3D volumetric data set is generated. The net result is a 3D reconstruction data set, which can project images in three orthogonal planes (axial, sagittal, and coronal). The rotation speed of the gantry remains at 1 revolution per minute, which is a standard specification for safety purposes and may result in patient motion during this 1-minute revolution, resulting in positioning discrepancies. In addition, x-rays, which are scattered in the patient, may degrade the resultant images, especially when imaging thick body parts such as the pelvis. However, the final product is a 3D CT data set with the patient in the treatment position.

CBCT permits registration of two different 3D data sets. Registration is the process of aligning multiple data sets into a single coordinate system so that the spatial locations of corresponding points coincide. As a simple example of the rigid body registration of two images, consider the image of a penny on a table and a second image of the same penny on the same table that has been moved in the X and Y (lateral and longitudinal) directions. To register these two images, a calculation must be performed that determines the amount of displacement in the X and Y directions of the two images of the penny. This can be described as a geometric transformation. Rigid body registration is routinely performed with medical images (e.g., the positron emission tomography [PET] image is registered with the CT image in a display of both data sets superimposed on each other). It is possible to register 2D image sets to address translational setup differences between the reference images and the daily image set. Examples of such images are shown in Fig. 15.9. Three-dimensional volumetric data sets can address both translational and rotational differences. In a radiation oncology application, the CT reference data set is taken at the time of simulation and is the basis of the treatment plan. The other 3D volumetric data set, which can be from CBCT or CT-on-rails, is taken with the patient on the treatment table before treatment.

The IGRT approaches, which have been described previously, rely on rigid body image registration (i.e., registration of bony anatomy). Rigid body registration restricts the searched transformation to a combination of translations in the X, Y, and Z directions and rotations, which are sufficient to describe the movement of solid objects. Many therapy treatment tables have rotation capabilities, which are limited to rotation about the isocenter and do not provide for rotation about the long axis of the couch (pitch) or the short axis of the couch (roll). Robotic couches with 6 degrees of freedom are now commercially available and are beginning to be placed into routine clinical use.

Deformable image registration is a more difficult problem than rigid body registration. Consider an image of a dish of ice cream with candy embedded in the ice cream. Now consider a second image of this dish of ice cream and candy after this combination has melted and is almost liquid. Deformable registration is transformation that maps the current position of the candy in the deformed ice cream volume to the original position of the candy in the ice cream. One initial application of deformable image registration was the correlation of functional images in the brain, which have well-defined neuroanatomy, with images of a diseased brain. For model-based deformable registration, a surface in the 3D image data set is defined and then warped (bent and twisted) into alignment with features in the target image data set. There is also a pixel approach that maps on a pixel-by-pixel basis. Image warping is an active field of image processing in which an image is geometrically distorted to conform to a given specification. In most interactive warping systems, the user specifies the warp in a general way, and then the software automatically interpolates this specification to produce the mapping. In radiation oncology, deformable image registration defines a transformation that deforms an image template, such as the daily CBCT image set, into alignment with the target image of interest, the 3D reference image set. Clinically, it can be used to track radiation doses in the target and surrounding tissue during the 5 to 8 weeks of treatment while the patient's anatomy changes. This permits the development of adaptive radiation therapy.[16]

In summary, today it is possible to image and analyze the patient's position on the treatment table and compare this in-room image set

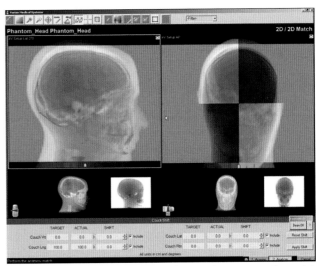

Fig. 15.9 Two-dimensional reference images (anteroposterior and lateral) and daily images have been registered and fused. The couch shifts, which are designed to bring these two data sets into better alignment, are about to be calculated.

with the image set used for treatment planning as part of daily treatment delivery. This should result in a more focused treatment, which avoids more normal tissue and limits toxicity. There will be changes in current practice while daily information on the patient is obtained and reviewed. As an example of the potential use of image-guided therapy, Barker et al[17] reported on CT imaging performed on 15 head and neck patients three times per week. These patients demonstrated significant anatomic changes during the course of their treatment. The location of the center of the mass of the tumor changed during the course of treatment, and the parotid glands shifted in the medial direction. The opportunity to adjust to these changes in the patient now awaits the development of clinical understanding of what to do to change the treatment plan and when to do it during the course of treatment.

RESPIRATORY MOTION MANAGEMENT

The systems described previously are designed to address interfraction motion, or the differences in the patient position between the treatment planning imaging study or the first day of treatment imaging study, the reference images, and the daily images. However, even if the patient position is in perfect agreement with the reference image data set, there remains the issue of intrafraction motion. Patients breathe, and, as a consequence, many organs change their location. Organs whose locations are affected by the breathing process may include the lungs, breast, esophagus, liver, and pancreas. The breathing pattern of a patient can change significantly during treatment in reaction to the sequelae of the radiation treatment and medical oncology treatments. Physiologically, a healthy adult at rest breathes in and out, one respiratory cycle, approximately 12 to 16 times per minute, or approximately 1 cycle every 4 seconds. Under normal circumstances, an adult inhales and exhales approximately 0.5 L of air in each respiratory cycle. In addition to respiratory motion, peristaltic motion (esophagus) is also addressed to limit the volume of normal tissue irradiated.

The management of respiratory motion has become an important topic in radiation oncology. There are at least five different strategies to reduce respiratory motion effects, namely, breath hold, respiratory gating, abdominal compression, integration of motion into treatment planning, and tracking. The AAPM published a report, "The Management of Respiratory Motion in Radiation Oncology Report of AAPM

Task Group 76."[18] The magnitude of respiratory motion, which is a 3D process, is very patient specific. Although generalizations may not be accurate, Ekberg et al[19] found, for lesions in the lower lobe of the lung, respiratory motion as much as 12 mm in the superoinferior direction and as much as 5 mm in the anteroposterior and left and right lateral directions. However, respiratory motion is not a significant issue for every patient. In a study of 22 patients, Stevens et al[20] reported that 10 patients showed no tumor motion in the superoinferior direction. The range of superoinferior motion of the remaining 12 patients was from 3 to 22 mm.[20]

A simple approach to managing motion is provided by abdominal compression. A commercial device is designed to compress the abdomen and thus limit motion by limiting the amount of air that the patient can inhale. This forced shallow breathing technique was initially designed to manage motion for stereotactic lung and liver treatments. This device includes a rigid stereotactic body frame with an attached vacuum bag. A pressure plate is attached to the frame. The amount of abdominal compression is controlled by the position of the plate, which can be adjusted by a screw mechanism. Published reports describe the accuracy and reproducibility of this mechanical system. Other mechanical systems used include pressure or compression belts.[21,22]

Given the emergence of the CT simulator as a common device within radiation oncology, CT is now widely used to study respiratory motion in addition to its role in imaging. MR and PET are also used, but less frequently than CT.[23] There are at least three different CT approaches: slow CT scanning, two breath-hold CT studies with the patient at inhalation and at exhalation, and four-dimensional (4D) CT. The slow CT scanning technique involves operation of the scanner at a low number of revolutions per second (one revolution per second or greater) so that multiple respiration phases are recorded on the same axial image. The inhalation and exhalation breath-hold technique requires the patient to hold his or her breath in a reproducible manner while these two independent CT studies are performed. The data sets are then registered, and the target volume defined on one set is fused with the target volume on the second set. A typical 4D CT method uses an oversampled spiral CT with a pitch of 0.5, a scanner rotation time of 1.5 seconds, and an external respiratory signal. (*Pitch* is defined as the ratio of the table feed in millimeters per 360-degree rotation divided by the product of the number of detector rows multiplied by the slice collimator in millimeters. A pitch of 0.5 indicates that the same location in the body is in more than one axial image.) Each image obtained through a 4D CT study can be sorted into a bin that corresponds to the phase of the respiratory cycle at which the image was acquired. A complete set of such respiratory cycled images, the 4D CT data set, would display target motion during the breathing cycle. If 10 different image sets were acquired, then images would be available from peak inhale through midexhale to peak exhale to midinhale and back to peak inhale in 10 different complete image sets. One clinically useful approach to tracking lung tumors is to use the maximum intensity projection, which is the maximum CT number found in a given voxel in the 4D CT data set, to visualize the volume encompassed by motion of the tumor. With a modern multislice CT scanner, a 4D CT scan can be obtained within 1 to 2 minutes. The consensus is that any approach that defines targets while considering motion is better than ignoring the effects of motion.

After treatment planning has been performed on a 4D CT study, the patient can be treated, accounting for respiratory motion that occurs during treatment delivery. One simple approach is to define an internal target volume, which encompasses the maximum extent of the target through the breathing cycle. This is a conservative approach, which may include more normal tissue than is absolutely necessary.

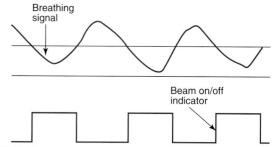

Fig. 15.10 The *top trace* displays the breathing pattern of a patient. The *bottom trace* indicates when the accelerator is turned on and off. Note that the accelerator is on during the exhalation portion of the respiratory cycle.

Another approach is **gated treatments**; that is, the radiation is turned on when the target is within the treatment volume, and the radiation is turned off when the target is outside the target volume. This approach is demonstrated in Fig. 15.10. With the linac turned on and off, the length of time required to deliver the treatment will increase significantly; however, the cost of accuracy outweighs the cost of efficiency.[24]

Although it is of benefit to account for movement during treatment delivery, complete accuracy will account for the location. At this point in time, one treatment system can simultaneously image and treat, namely, ViewRay. This system uses a split-magnet MR imaging (MRI) for volumetric and multiplanar imaging and three cobalt-60 sources, each with its own multileaf collimator for treatment. Multiplanar images are available in approximately 500 msec intervals.[25]

MAGNETIC RESONANCE–GUIDED RADIATION THERAPY

MR-guided radiation therapy (MRGRT) represents the next evolution of IGRT with the potential toward even more conformal high-dose volumes. MRI provides superior tissue contrast for tumors and the surrounding soft tissue. Currently, there are three configurations of MR-guided radiotherapy systems: (1) the radiation therapy beam is parallel to the main magnetic field (B_0), (2) the radiation therapy beam is perpendicular to the B_0, and (3) MR-on-rails allowing for the MR to move in and out of a radiotherapy treatment unit.[26] There are five different MR treatment delivery systems currently documented in the literature: Aurora RT Viewray MRIdian, MRgRT Suite, Elekta Unity, and Australian MRI-Linac. The use of high-precision MRI-guided radiotherapy systems holds the promise for dose escalation and further margin reduction, leading to higher cure rates and less toxicity.[27]

Common current approaches to motion management involve the use of commercial devices that can provide the external respiratory signal. They are all surrogate methods in that an external device is used to track the internal target motion. One such device is the Varian Real-time Position Management system, in which an infrared reflective plastic box is placed on the patient's upper anterior abdominal surface. Motion is tracked by in-treatment room cameras, which detect the reflective markers. This device can be used for monitoring respiratory motion during both imaging and treatment. This approach assumes that this device, which is placed on the patient's upper abdomen, appropriately tracks the motion of the target in the patient's lung. Other vendors have their own approaches to gating their treatment devices, such as Elekta's Active Breathing Coordinator system, which helps the patient hold their breath. A recent review article[a] by Giraud and Houle[22] discusses the main technical aspects and clinical benefits of respiratory gating.

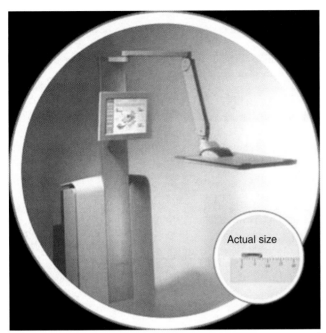

Fig. 15.11 An electromagnetic array localization system, which can be used to determine the position of a transponder, which is shown in the *inset*. The photon radiation beam passes through this system. (Courtesy Varian Medical Systems, Palo Alto, CA.)

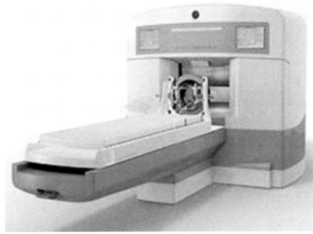

Fig. 15.12 A Gamma knife without a patient on the treatment table. The dose is delivered through a series of locations. When the patient is to be treated, the shielding doors open, and the patient is moved to a position so that the focused sources irradiate a small volume in the patient's head. The patient is then moved out of the beam, and the shielding doors close. A new location is defined on the frame, and the process repeats itself.

A completely different approach for both interfraction and infrafraction motion management involves the implantation of an electromagnetic transponder in or near the treatment site. (A transponder is a radio transmitter and receiver that is activated for transmission by the reception of a predetermined signal.) The electromagnetic transponders, glass-encapsulated circuits 8.5 mm in length and 1.85 mm in diameter, are placed in the target by using an invasive technique. The position of the target can be determined based on signals received from the transponders by use of an electromagnetic array localization system that is placed above the patient. This is shown in Fig. 15.11. Real-time feedback is provided because the target isocenter can be monitored as much as 10 times per second. Litzenberg et al[28] have reported on the use of this approach for prostate localization with a commercial system. The use of this technology for other treatment sites, including the lung, is under development.

STEREOTACTIC RADIATION THERAPY

Cranial stereotactic treatments have become a routine treatment approach during the past several decades. The stereotactic approach, first reported in 1951, has led to the development of dedicated treatment units (e.g., the Gamma knife, which contains as many as several hundred individual cobalt-60 sources that are focused on a single point). Such a unit is shown in Fig. 15.12. Both malignant and nonmalignant conditions, such as arteriovenous malformations, have been managed with this approach.

How does a stereotactic treatment differ from a normal treatment? Stereotaxis is a method used in neurosurgery, neurologic research, and radiation oncology to locate points within the brain by using an external 3D frame of reference, usually based on the *X, Y, Z* Cartesian coordinate system. The position of the target in the brain is correlated with an external fiducial system. (*Fiducials* are a standard of reference in a number of disciplines, including surveying. *Fiduciary,* a term in general use, relates to the holding of something in trust for another or a system of ranking in the field of view of an optical instrument that

is used as a reference point or measuring scale.) In radiation therapy, fiducials are used to define a coordinate system in the treatment planning and delivery process, which can be the basis to target the tumor by using an external 3D frame of reference. SRT can be thought of as a high-precision targeting technique, which, in conjunction with 3D treatment approaches, produces a focused dose distribution with rapid dose falloff. Cranial SRT generally involves the invasive fixation of the fiducial system to the skull, followed by imaging, treatment planning, and treatment delivery. The fiducial system remains on the patient for this entire process, which may last for 3 to 8 hours.

The management of brain metastases with SRT generally involves a single fraction and is called *stereotactic radiosurgery.* Fractionated stereotactic treatments are generally called *FSRT.*

Stereotactic body radiation therapy (SBRT) has been defined as a "radiation therapy treatment method to deliver a high dose of radiation to the target, utilizing either a single dose or a small number of fractions with a high degree of precision within the body."[29] The goal of SBRT is to deliver the treatment encompassing the target with great accuracy and with rapid dose falloff to spare surrounding tissue. SBRT treatments are delivered by using as many as five fractions.

After approximately 50 years of experience with cranial stereotactic treatments, this approach was expanded to treat extracranial sites. Why did this development of a highly focused, precise, limited field treatment approach for targets in the body take such a long time? Two important technologic advances were required to permit body stereotactic treatments. One advance is **image guidance**: the extent of the target needs to be precisely defined to lower the possibility of geometric misses, and the patient needs to be set up by using images taken with the patient in the treatment position. The other technologic advance is **motion management**: large treatment fields treated by using a single fraction result in significant acute and long-term side effects. For stereotactic treatments, the target should be mostly the tumor, and its motion must be well controlled because the patient will be on the treatment table for a period of time that is much longer than for routine treatments.

To take advantage of the stereotactic precision in the targeting and treatment delivery, the reference frame and the patient must be properly registered. There are a number of different approaches to register the patient with the frame, including the use of an invasive frame and vacuum-based patient immobilization system. The frame of reference is present for patient simulation, planning, and treatment. The location of target isocenter, which uses the coordinates defined by the frame of reference, can be defined in the planning process and used in treatment delivery. The stereotactic technique evolved from the dedicated unit to the common linac, with use of the same basic concepts of stereotactic frame-based, high-precision small-field treatments. One early approach to increasing the accuracy of linac-based stereotactic treatments involved a separate support device, independent of the treatment couch, for the patient's head. With the advent of high-quality in-room imaging and tighter mechanical specifications for the accelerators, the need for such elaborate patient supporting devices has been lessened. The American College of Radiology has published a practice guideline for the performance of SBRT.[30] This guideline states that the radiation therapy delivery treatment should have mechanical tolerances for radiation therapy of ±2 mm. Section II of this document describes the qualifications and responsibilities of personnel participating in these procedures, including the radiation oncologist, the medical physicist, and the radiation therapist. AAPM Task Group 101 has published a report on SBRT, which outlines the best practice guidelines for SBRT.[31] Section V of this report includes subsections on immobilization, image-guided localization, localization, tumor tracking and gating techniques for respiratory motion management, image-guided techniques, optical tracking techniques, respiratory gating techniques, and delivery data reporting. This report emphasizes the need for everyone involved in the SBRT program participate in continuing education as this technology changes.

The American Society for Therapeutic Radiology and Oncology (ASTRO) has published a white paper on the quality and safety considerations in SBRT.[32] The ASTRO report provides a potential list of responsibilities for the radiation therapist for SBRT. These responsibilities include "preparing the treatment room, performing patient positioning/immobilization and assisting the treatment team by answering any questions about the patient's set up, and operating the treatment unit after the radiation oncologist and the medical physicist have approved the clinical and technical aspects for beam delivery."

The CyberKnife is another radiosurgery system that is designed to treat anywhere in the body with high accuracy using a nonisocentric treatment approach. This is an integrated system that combines an accelerator on an industrial robot and two ceiling-mounted x-ray tubes (Fig. 15.13). The robot moves the accelerator to predefined positions and delivers relatively small-field radiation beams. Image guidance is obtained in almost real time, using a combination of external infrared

fiducial markers and radiographs. Fiducial-free spine and lung tracking treatment is being offered. Treatment can be conducted within 30 to 90 minutes after the patient is first brought into the treatment room. Yu et al.[33] report that for the treatment of relatively stationary spinal lesions, which are targeted with fiducial tracking, this system is capable of submillimeter accuracy. This system positions itself in the marketplace as an alternative to surgery for many different clinical situations.

There have been important upgrades in the standard linac that enable fast and accurate SBRT treatments. Volumetric-modulated arc therapy is an example of a new treatment approach that may increase the speed of treatment. The treatment is delivered with the gantry rotating over one or more arcs of as much as 360-degree rotation for each arc. The dose rate and the field size are changed while the gantry rotates, which results in a modulated conformal dose distribution. Flattening filter-free photon delivery systems are another example of faster treatments through higher dose rates. The flattening filter is moved out of the beam, resulting in a high dose rate (1400 cGy/min to 2500 cGy/min), nonflat photon beams. Such beams may result in shorter treatment times for SBRT-type treatments. Six-degrees-of-freedom treatment couches have been recently introduced with the goal of increasing the accuracy of patient positioning. In addition to the standard X, Y, and Z motions (up/down, left/right, toward gantry/away from gantry), rotational motions over a limited arc are now available. Pitch is the motion that rotates by using the short axis of the couch so that the head or the feet pitch higher or lower. Roll is the motion about the long axis of the couch so that the body rolls from left to right. Yaw is the rotation of the entire couch about an axis, such as the axis of the couch support stand. The ability to perform small rotations, as well as translational motions, should result in more precise patient setups, especially because there are good image analysis tools available.

A well-established application for stereotactic extracranial treatments is the management of metastasis to the spine. The University of Pittsburgh reported their experience with radiosurgery for 500 cases of spinal metastases.[34] Long-term tumor control was obtained in 90% of the lesions treated with radiosurgery as a primary treatment modality by using a mean intratumoral dose of 20 Gy. Many other institutions are also offering this important palliative therapy.

There is substantial interest in hypofractionated stereotactic treatments for cancer of the lung, as well as for primary and secondary liver tumors. Some lung cancer patients with early-stage lung disease are medically inoperable. Timmerman et al[35] reported a phase I three-fraction-regimen dose-escalation study in which patients were enrolled in three different groups based on tumor size. For the smaller tumors, less than 5 cm, greater than 90% local control was observed by using a 20 Gy × 3 fraction regimen. Patients who receive this treatment course are at risk for adverse events, including fatal toxicities. However, there are also substantial benefits to be gained, including short treatments with high local control. To state the obvious, SBRT treatments must be simulated, planned, and delivered with great care.

The National Cancer Institute–funded cooperative group, NRG Oncology, which includes the Radiation Therapy Oncology Group, is conducting or planning a number of protocols to study this stereotactic treatment approach, especially for lung tumors. The studies include centrally located lung tumors in inoperable patients and patients with tumors that can be approached surgically. These protocols require the use of a fixed 3D coordinate system defined by fiducial markers. The position of the target within the patient is defined by using this coordinate system. A number of different fiducial systems are permitted in these protocols, including metallic seeds, which are invasively placed in the lung near the tumor. Typical doses being studied by such protocols are 45 to 60 Gy, which is delivered in 5 fractions during a 2-week period. Well-defined normal tissue dose-volume limits are required

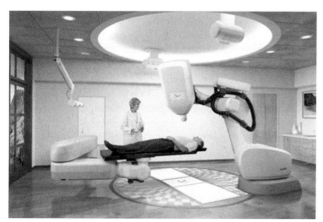

Fig. 15.13 An accelerator on a robotic arm. The two ceiling-mounted x-ray tubes are clearly shown.

by such a treatment approach. These protocols require that the effect of internal organ motion, resulting from breathing, be accounted for and that localization images be obtained with the patient on the treatment couch for each fraction. The potential exists that this treatment approach will offer patients high local control with less toxicity than traditional treatments. This treatment approach may increase the number of patients receiving radiation to manage their early-stage lung cancers.

The evolution of radiation oncology toward greater precision in target definition and in patient positioning, including internal organ motion, raises the question of greater precision in dose distributions. IMRT is one approach to obtaining this greater precision. Another approach is heavy charged particles, such as protons or carbon ions.

HEAVY CHARGED PARTICLE TREATMENT

Protons are heavy charged particles. Electrons are also charged particles but are approximately 2000 times lighter than protons. The range of the proton beam can be defined to within 1 mm in a water phantom. In addition to the limited range, protons have a very sharp falloff, which is the great clinical advantage of protons. This is demonstrated in Fig. 15.14. The limited range/sharp falloff has the potential to be a major pitfall. The allure of protons is the ability to deposit the dose in the target and to spare normal tissue that is located distally from the target. Consider a target volume in a patient, the spinal cord in a patient with meduloblastoma that is to be treated with a posterior radiation beam. A posterior photon beam will treat the target but exit through the patient's chest and abdomen. A posterior proton beam will stop at the end of range. If the maximum depth of the target is 5.0 cm and the proton beam stops at 5.3 cm, then the patient is well served. If, however, the maximum depth of the target is 5.0 cm and the proton beam stops at 4.7 cm, then the patient is not well served. Proton therapy requires a greater dedication to managing the details of patient simulation, treatment planning, and treatment delivery than photon therapy. DeLaney and Kooy[36] provide a comprehensive review of proton radiotherapy.

Protons have been used in radiation oncology for decades. A 1957 article in *Cancer* reported on the irradiation of the pituitary gland with protons.[37] The number of organizations offering protons has increased, with more than 32 institutions offering this type of treatment in the United States at the end of 2019, an increase of more than 150% (tripling) in 5 years. The number of institutions that offer the use of protons or other heavy particles is expected to grow dramatically in the next decade. Proton facilities are expensive to build, on the order of 10 to 100 or more times than a photon unit, and expensive to maintain, on the order of 10 times more expensive than a photon unit. The clinical conditions that may benefit from this expensive and demanding delivery therapy are being defined. Clearly, the conditions include pediatric patients who are receiving radiation therapy and, possibly, patients for whom the acute and long-term toxicities limit the therapeutic options available to them.

The most common design of proton facilities involves one proton accelerator for three to five treatment beamlines or treatment rooms, although one-room proton systems have now begun to be used to treat patients. After acceleration to the desired energy, the protons are extracted from the cyclotron and directed to the treatment rooms using electromagnets, which can be turned on or off. The proton beam that exits from the cyclotron is monoenergetic and is described as having a pristine Bragg peak. Most beamlines today use a passive scattering technique to modulate the proton beam—spread out the proton beam along the direction that the beam is traveling. For passive modulation, a rotating modulation wheel or similar device is used to absorb energy, and thus a spread-out Bragg peak (SOBP) is produced. Typically, the widths of the SOBPs can be varied, such as from 2 to 16 cm. Scanning proton beam treatments are now available at multiple institutions. Scanning beam treatments paint the dose distribution by changing the location of the beam spot and the beam energy. Changing the location of the beam spot is easy to do, given the fact that protons are charged particles and can be magnetically steered. Changing the energy of the proton beam, and thus its range, may be relatively easy to do, using a modern proton clinical accelerator. Scanning beams enable intensity-modulated proton therapy (IMPT). There are several approaches to dose optimization with scanning proton beams. In one approach, each field is optimized individually to deliver a fraction of the prescribed dose to the entire volume, single-field optimization. Single-field optimization also permits a simultaneous integrated boost treatment. In the other approach, the weights of all spots in all fields are simultaneously optimized, and the prescribed dose to the entire volume is delivered after all fields have been treated. The multifield planning and delivery is described as IMPT, although consensus on the exact definitions has yet to be reached. Treatment sites that may benefit from IMPT include the oropharynx and lung. The complex nature of both distributions is easily observed. The final dose distribution is the sum of multiple fields. Many believe that the scanning beam approach is the future of proton therapy. Some proton centers, which are currently under construction, will only offer scanning beams.

The promise of protons is their limited range (i.e., protons stop). Assuming that uncertainties are addressed appropriately, there should be no exit dose into normal tissue. Limiting the dose to normal tissue may result in less toxic radiation treatments, even for very high doses. Carefully defined studies and time will be required to conclude that the promise of protons can be fulfilled.

The proton treatment room has much in common with a photon treatment room. For example, there is a gantry that can rotate 360 degrees, a patient treatment couch, and various in-room imaging systems to define the patient treatment position. The gantry supports the beam nozzle, which contains beam-scattering foils and the rotating modulation wheel, both of which are used for passive modulation. The nozzle also contains the transmission ion chamber and a system that is designed to hold the aperture; the custom block or aperture,

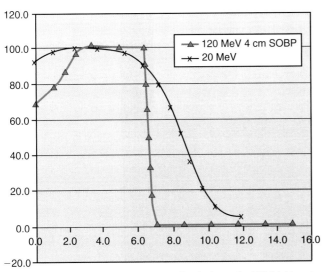

Fig. 15.14 The central axis percentage depth dose of a 120-MeV proton beam with a 4-cm spread-out Bragg peak and a 20-MeV electron beam in water. The distal 90% dose is the same for both beams. Note that the 90% to 10% falloff of dose requires several millimeters for a proton beam and several centimeters for an electron beam.

which defines the treatment field; and the compensator, a low–atomic number device that compensates for the fact that the patient has air spaces and bones. Tissue heterogeneities affect the range of protons in the patient.

Proton therapy is image-guided therapy. After positioning the patient on the treatment couch, the therapists produce a set of perpendicular radiographs. The oncologists and the therapists review these images and adjust the patient position appropriately. Just as with photon therapy, reference images can be downloaded from the electronic medical record and used for comparison with the daily images. The daily in-treatment room images can be uploaded to the electronic medical record. Some proton treatment nozzles do not have light fields or reticules, which are traditionally used in photon therapy for aiding in the patient setup.

Retinoblastoma is an uncommon tumor (approximately 200 cases per year) that occurs in very young children. There is substantial experience in the management of this disease with external beam radiation therapy, despite the known sequelae. Protons have been used at Massachusetts General Hospital for several decades.[38] Massachusetts General Hospital is treating these patients under a protocol that is designed to study both local control and adverse effects from the radiation. The ability to stop the proton from entering the brain should limit the consequences of the radiation treatment. This effect is demonstrated in Fig. 15.15 for a 16-month-old patient treated at University of Texas MD Anderson Cancer Center.

Carbon ion therapy is a similar to proton beam therapy and can be used to treat a broad spectrum of cancers with minimal side effects. There are several physical and biological advantages of carbon ion therapy over traditional photon-based treatments.[39] First, given their physical charge, mass, and high initial energy, carbons ions deposit very little ionization energy at or very near the surface with almost all dose deposited at a defined depth.[39] In addition, carbon ion beams have less Coulomb interactions, which allows for sharper lateral penumbra compared with proton beams.[40] These two physical characteristics are believed to have the ability to deliver higher energies to deep-seated tumors while sparing surrounding radiosensitive organs at risk.[41] Radiobiologically, carbon ion beams have increased linear energy transfer compared with both photons and protons, which results in

increased damage to the DNA of cancer cells.[39,41] The downside of carbon ion treatments is that the facilities are extremely expensive; however, carbon ion beam centers are growing in numbers. A carbon ion facility will typically include a dedicated and highly specialized synchrotron machine, which is a machine similar to a particle accelerator, a beam transport system, a beam delivery system, isocentric gantries, and a patient alignment and imaging systems.[41]

INNOVATION TO PRACTICE: A PERSPECTIVE OF THE FUTURE[a]

Ultrasound-Mediated Microbubble Radioenhancing Agents and Measuring Radiation Response Using Radiomic Markers

The tumor vasculature plays an important role in the development and progression of malignancies by delivering nutrients and enabling cell-cell communication, and it facilitates metastasis by evading immunological signals.[42,43] Unlike blood vessels in normal tissue, the vascular architecture in solid tumors is aberrant and immature and exhibits endothelial cell gaps, which result in a "leaky" vessel matrix. These characteristics are a major therapeutic challenge for the following reasons[44]: (1) poor perfusion leads to hypoxia, which is a major radiation resistance factor; and (2) leaky blood vessels cause inefficient transport of cytotoxic agents into the tumor stroma. The interdependence between blood vessels and tumor cells have been the focus of intense research, and novel treatment strategies are exploiting ***antivascular agents*** to maximize the therapeutic ratio in oncology. There is recent evidence to suggest that antivascular agents using ***ultrasound-driven microbubbles*** can address these challenges associated with abnormal tumor blood vessels and tumor progression.

Microbubbles are gas-filled microspheres (5–10 μm) that have a lipid, protein, or biopolymer shell, and their relative diameter to red blood cells permit intravenous injection and passage into veins, arteries, and capillaries. Thus microbubble particles were initially developed for use

[a] Special contribution by William T. Tran and Caitlin Gillan.

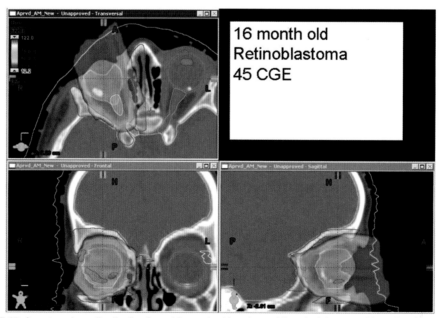

Fig. 15.15 A proton dose distribution for a 16-month-old patient with retinoblastoma. Note the limited dose to normal tissue, such as the brain. *CGE,* Cobalt gray equivalent.

in diagnostic radiology, particularly for contrast-enhanced sonography of cardiac and hepatic blood vessels.[45,46] Under lower acoustic pressures, microbubbles vibrate, resonate, and produce echoes.[47,48] Sonographic contrast enhancement is achieved by detecting the increased acoustic backscatter from ultrasound-microbubble interactions.

It was later discovered that microbubbles exposed to a high **mechanical index** (MI), relating to the acoustic peak negative pressure and frequency, resulted in greater inertial cavitation (i.e., bubble oscillations), perturbing structures within the particle's proximity.[49] The bioeffects from inertial cavitation were previously studied by Kobayashi et al, who demonstrated that endothelial cells that constitute the microvascular lumen were impacted by oscillating microbubbles.[50] It is now understood that shear stress on the endothelial cell surface activates *sphingomyelin* on the plasma membrane.[51] Consequently, activated sphingomyelin initiates a biochemical cascade in the cytoplasm that leads to apoptotic cell death.[52] Preclinical experiments by Czarnota et al. have shown that in xenograft mouse models for breast, prostate, and bladder cancers, vascular disruption using ultrasound-stimulated microbubbles (MI >0.8) in combination with radiation (single dose, 8 Gy) resulted in a 10-fold increase in tumor cell death.[53–55] Studies from the same research group have also reported using imaging biomarkers, such as quantitative ultrasound, power-Doppler ultrasound, and photoacoustic imaging to evaluate treatment efficacy and tumor response in their experimental work.[55-57] The acquisition of data from medical imaging, mining of imaging biomarkers, and subsequent analysis using computer-assisted algorithms is termed *radiomics*.

Indeed, medical imaging plays an important role in patient care; it is primarily used as a tool to identify anatomical structures and determine their morphological characteristics. Radiomics is a rapidly developing field that is focused on extracting high-dimensional, quantitative data from medical images that are clinically meaningful, in essence, to be used as a decision-support tool for clinicians.[58] Attaining radiomics data constitutes a discrete workflow, which involves the following steps: (1) images are acquired using standardized settings; (2) regions of interest are selected; (3) features are extracted from the image-sets based on computational analysis; and last (4) data mining and modeling.[58,59] Data output is usually large; thus the term "big data" is used interchangeably to refer to radiomics analyses in the same way as it is referred for other "*omics*"-type sciences (e.g., genomics). These scientific approaches contain immense datasets that represent the underlying biology of tumors. Importantly, the data are minable and computationally expansive. Radiomics analysis has the potential for developing robust diagnostic, predictive, ad prognostic models that can be used for validating therapeutic efficacy in experiments (e.g., US-mediated microbubble antivascular agents) or as a clinical tool to monitor the patient's response to treatment after validation.

In oncology imaging, radiomic features represent the spatial, temporal, and biological properties of tumors associated with metabolism, cellularity, and tissue composition. Recent reports have used radiomic attributes (features) derived from imaging signals to model prognostic and treatment-response outcomes after therapy.[60,61] Taken together, the ultimate goal for radiomics is to provide *actionable insight* from quantitative imaging data, that is, to give scientists, clinicians, and patients meaningful information about disease, treatments, and outcomes.

ARTIFICIAL INTELLIGENCE

As society becomes increasingly aware of the potential of artificial intelligence (AI), medicine is beginning to consider how to harness related innovations to improve care. AI encompasses a spectrum of technologies, the common thread being the use of a computer system to process information in such a way as to determine and enact a rational response.[62] It encompasses technology designed to perform tasks regularly attributed to intelligent beings, such as human reasoning and the ability to generalize and learn from experience.[63] Such technologies include radiation therapy–specific innovations such as automated target contouring or treatment planning algorithms[64] and technical equipment[65,66] quality control programs, which can serve to augment the ability and efficiency of radiation therapists, dosimetrists, and other colleagues to provide high-quality care. Also under the AI umbrella are other societal innovations that can be put to use in radiation therapy: automated speech-to-text and language translation devices for dictating and for communicating with patients who do not speak the same language as staff, wearable monitoring devices that can track vitals and other parameters, and staff and patient scheduling optimization algorithms.

The common input required by many of these AI strategies, collectively termed "machine-learning" technologies, is data. By capitalizing on the computational power of a machine to manipulate data, AI technologies can make sense of massive amounts of data inputs—big data—that would be beyond human cognitive capacity to manage, flagging patterns and performing designated actions based on those patterns. In medicine, big data might include patient demographic data, imaging and laboratory data, information on radiation treatments and outcomes, and even patient satisfaction data, culled systematically from electronic health records or other primary databases.

Such innovations could generate major efficiencies and improvements in care. Time-consuming, repetitive tasks such as delineating targets, generating treatment plans, and quality assurance could be offloaded to AI, freeing time to increase patient throughput and/or explore more adaptive and personalized treatment techniques. Insights from past radiation therapy patient outcomes could be better incorporated clinical decision-making.[67] To make the most of AI, there are many considerations that require attention in diverse but related areas: industry research and development, privacy policy, healthcare human resources, and professional practice and advocacy.[67]

▌ SUMMARY

- Radiation is an effective modality in the management of many different types of cancer.
- Radiation is not selective; it can damage both malignant tissue and normal tissue.
- The maturation of radiation oncology as a therapeutic modality has included better targeting through improved diagnostic studies, in-treatment room imaging, motion management, and stereotactic techniques.
- This maturation has also included more conformal treatment delivery through the use of IMRT, which, in the past decade, has become a standard treatment technique. This treatment has also included the expanded use of protons and carbon ions.
- MR-guided therapy appears to be increasing as a standard technique in the next decade.
- Innovative techniques such as radiomics and microbubbles are gaining interest as radiation therapy becomes more adaptive and personalized to respond to changes in tumor response.
- AI will increasingly be integrated into practice to offer radiation oncology clinicians the opportunity to learn from patient outcome data that can aid in better clinical decision-making.

REVIEW QUESTIONS

The answers to the Review Questions can be found by logging on to our website at: http://evolve.elsevier.com/Washington+Leaver/principles/Megan Trad

1. Modern photon radiation treatment units may:
   a. Be one device on the hospital network receiving treatment-specific information.
   b. Have both kV and MV imaging capabilities.
   c. Be controlled by multiple computer systems.
   d. Be designed to deliver nonisocentric treatments.
   e. All of the above.
2. Image-guided radiation therapy:
   a. Has been available only in the 21st century.
   b. Permits a faster patient positioning process.
   c. Must use registered images of the treatment position with the simulation position.
   d. Requires an x-ray tube mounted on the accelerator C-arm.
3. MV images differ from kV images in that MV images have:
   a. Better soft tissue contrast.
   b. Higher spatial resolution.
   c. Smaller amounts of metal artifacts.
   d. Lower radiation dose to the patient.
4. Four-dimensional CT:
   a. Requires the patient to hold his or her breath.
   b. Can be used to define the extent of respiratory motion.
   c. Would not display the target motion during the respiratory cycle.
   d. Images an anatomic location in the patient only once.
5. CBCT differs from regular CT in that CBCT:
   a. Uses a 2D x-ray detector.
   b. Must use a kV source of x-rays less than 10 kV to reduce scattering.
   c. Produces images that have a smaller amount of scatter.
   d. Must be produced with a megavoltage source.
6. The respiratory cycle of a normal resting adult is approximately:
   a. 1 second.
   b. 4 seconds.
   c. 10 seconds.
   d. 15 seconds.
   e. 20 seconds.
7. Stereotactic treatments require:
   a. A dedicated treatment unit, such as a Gamma knife.
   b. That the site of treatment be in the brain.
   c. A frame of reference that is used for imaging and treatment.
   d. A large-dose, single-fraction treatment.
8. Managing the patient's respiratory motion can be accomplished by:
   a. Asking the patient to hold his or her breath for more than 1 minute.
   b. Using vacuum bags to position the patient on the treatment table.
   c. Abdominal compression.
   d. Respiratory gating.
   e. Both c and d.
9. One significant advantage of protons compared with photons is that:
   a. Protons are less expensive to produce than photons.
   b. Energy is deposited only to malignant tissue and not to normal tissue.
   c. Protons have limited range in the patient.
   d. Image guidance is not required.
10. An advantage of fiducial marker–guided treatments is that fiducial markers:
    a. Emit electromagnetic waves.
    b. Are easily imaged with ultrasound.
    c. Contain radioactive material and can be located with a Geiger counter.
    d. May be easy to track with x-rays.
11. MRI-guided radiotherapy systems are beneficial because they offer:
    1. Dose escalation
    2. Margin reduction
    3. Potential of less toxicity
    4. Faster treatments
       A. 1, 2, and 3 only.
       B. 2, 3, and 4 only.
       C. 3 and 4 only.
       D. 1, 2, 3, and 4.
12. A carbon ion facility will usually include all of the following except:
    a. Synchrotron.
    b. Beam transport system.
    c. Patient alignment system.
    d. Multileaf collimation.

QUESTIONS TO PONDER

- What are the most important hardware characteristics of an external beam treatment delivery system that facilitate accurate and precise treatments?
- What are the most important software characteristics for an external beam treatment delivery system that facilitate accurate and precise treatments?
- What are the advantages of dedicated treatment units versus general purpose treatment units?
- What are the disadvantages of dedicated treatment units versus general purpose treatment units?
- What will standard radiation therapy treatment units look like in the next 10 years? Is MR-guided therapy going to be standard of care?
- How will personalized medicine influence how we care and treat our patients?
- How will AI influence radiation therapy practice as it becomes more integrated within healthcare?

REFERENCES

1. Bental G. *Patient Positioning and Immobilization in Radiation Oncology.* New York, NY: McGraw Hill; 1999.
2. Misfeldt J, Chessman L. Advances in patient positioning. *J Oncol Manag.* 1999;8:14–16.
3. Dawson L, Jaffray D. Advances in imaged guided radiation therapy. *J Clin Oncol.* 2007;25(8):938–946.
4. Morin O, Gillis A, Chen J, et al. Megavoltage cone beam CT: system description and clinical applications. *Med Dosim.* 2006;31(1):51–61.
5. Chandra A, Dong L, Huang E, et al. Experience of ultrasound-based daily prostate localization. *Int J Radiat Oncol Biol Phys.* 2003;56:436–447.

6. Langen KM, Pouliot J, Anezinos C, et al. Evaluation of ultrasound-based prostate localization for image-guided radiotherapy. *Int J Radiat Oncol Biol Phys.* 2003;57:635–644.

7. Forrest LJ, Mackie TR, Ruchala K, et al. The utility of megavoltage computed tomography images from a helical tomotherapy system for setup verification purposes. *Int J Radiat Oncol Biol Phys.* 2004;60:1639–1644.

8. Molloy JA, Chan G, Markovic A, et al. Quality assurance of U.S.-guided external beam radiotherapy for prostate cancer: report of AAPM Task Group 154. *Med Phys.* 2011;38:857–871.

9. Boyer AL, Antonuk L, Fenster A, et al. A review of electronic portal imaging devices (EPIDs). *Med Phys.* 1992. 191-16.

10. Klein EE, Hanley J, Bayouth J, et al. Task Group 142 report: quality assurance of medical accelerators. *Med Phys.* 2009;36:4197–4212.

11. Uematsu M, Fukui T, Shioda A, et al. A dual computed tomography linear accelerator unit for stereotactic radiation therapy: a new approach without cranially fixated stereotactic frames. *Int J Radiat Oncol Biol Phys.* 1996;35:587–592.

12. Chang EL, Loeffler JS, Riese NE, et al. Phase I clinical evaluation of near-simultaneous computed tomographic image-guided stereotactic body radiotherapy for spinal metastases. *Int J Radiat Oncol Biol Phys.* 2004;59:1288–1294.

13. Court L, Rosen I, Mohan R, et al. Evaluation of mechanical precision and alignment uncertainties for an integrated CT/LINAC system. *Med Phys.* 2000;30:1198–1210.

14. Wong JR, Grimm L, Uematsu M, et al. Image-guided radiotherapy for prostate cancer by CT-linear accelerator combination: prostate movements and dosimetric considerations. *Int J Radiat Oncol Biol Phys.* 2005;61:561–569.

15. Jaffray DA, Siewerdsen JH, Wong JW, et al. Flat-panel cone-beam computed tomography for image-guided radiation therapy. *Int J Radiat Oncol Biol Phys.* 2002;53:1337–1349.

16. Brock KK, Dawson LA, Sharpe MB, et al. Feasibility of a novel deformable image registration technique to facilitate classification, targeting and monitoring of tumor and normal tissue. *Int J Radiat Oncol Biol Phys.* 2006;64:1245–1254.

17. Barker Jr JL, Garden AS, Ang KK, et al. Quantification of volumetric and geometric changes occurring during fractionated radiotherapy for head and neck cancer using an integrated CT/linear accelerator system. *Int J Radiat Oncol Biol Phys.* 2004;59:960–970.

18. Keall PJ, Mageras GS, Balter JM, et al. The management of respiratory motion in radiation oncology report of AAPM Task Group 76. *Med Phys.* 2006;33:3874–3900.

19. Ekberg L, Holmber O, Wittgren L, et al. What margins should be added to the clinical target volume in radiotherapy treatment planning for lung cancer? *Radiother Oncol.* 1998;48:71–77.

20. Stevens CW, Munden RF, Forster KM, et al. Respiratory-driven lung tumor motion is independent of tumor size, tumor location, and pulmonary function. *Int J Radiat Oncol Biol Phys.* 2001;51:62–68.

21. Cole AJ, Hanna GG, Jain S, O'Sullivan JM. Motion management for radical radiotherapy in non-small cell lung cancer. *Clin Oncol (R Coll Radiol).* 2014;26:67–80.

22. Giroud P, Houle A. Respiratory gating for radiotherapy: main technical aspects and clinical benefits. *ISRN Pulmonol.* 2013:1–13.

23. Ghani MNHA, Ng WL. Management of respiratory motion for lung radiotherapy: a review. *J Xiangya Med.* 2018;3:27.

24. Yorke E, Rosenzweig KE, Wagman R, et al. Interfractional anatomic variation in patients treated with respiration-gated radiotherapy. *J Appl Clin Med Phys.* 2005;6:19–32.

25. Green O, Goddu S, Mutic S. SU-E-T-352: Commissioning and quality assurance of the first commercial hybrid MRI-IMRT system. *Med Phys.* 2012;39(6):3785.

26. Eccles CL, Campbell M. Keeping up with the hybrid magnetic resonance linear accelerators: how do radiation therapists stay current in the era of hybrid technologies? *J Med Imaging Radiat Sci.* 2019;50(2):195–198.

27. Pollard J, Wen Z, Sadagopan R, Wang J, Ibbott GS. The future of image-guided radiotherapy will be MR guided. *Br J Radiol.* 2017;90:1.

28. Litzenberg DW, Willoughby TR, Balter JM, et al. Positional stability of electromagnetic transponders used for prostate localization and continuous, real-time tracking. *Int J Radiat Oncol Biol Phys.* 2007;68:1199–1206.

29. Potters L, Steinberg M, Rose C, et al. American society for therapeutic radiology and oncology and american college of radiology practice guidelines for the performance of stereotactic body radiation therapy. *Int J Radiat Oncol Biol Phys.* 2004;60:1026–1032.

30. ACR-ASTRO practice parameter for the performance of stereotactic body radiation therapy. American College of Radiology website. Revised 2014. https://www.acr.org/-/media/ACR/Files/Practice-Parameters/s-brt-ro.pdf. Accessed October 9, 2019.

31. Benedict SH, Yenice KM, Followill D, et al. Stereotactic body radiation therapy: the report of AAPM Task Group 101. *Med Phys.* 2010;37:4078–4101.

32. Solberg TD, Balter JM, Benedict SH, et al. Quality and safety considerations in stereotactic radiosurgery and stereotactic body radiation therapy: executive summary. *Pract Radiat Oncol.* 2012;2:2–9.

33. Yu C, Main W, Taylor D, et al. An anthropomorphic phantom study of the accuracy of Cyberknife spinal radiosurgery. *Neurosurgery.* 2004;55:1138–1149.

34. Gerszten PC, Burton SA, Ozhasoglu C, et al. Radiosurgery for spinal metastases: clinical experience in 500 cases from a single institution. *Spine.* 2007;32:193–199.

35. Timmerman R, Papiez L, McGarry R, et al. Extracranial stereotactic radioablation: results of a phase I study in medically inoperable stage I non-small cell lung cancer patients. *Chest.* 2006;125:1946–1955.

36. Delaney TF, Kooy HM, eds. *Proton and Charged Particle Radiotherapy.* Philadelphia, PA, 2008: Lippincott Williams & Wilkins.

37. Lawrence JH. Proton irradiation of the pituitary. *Cancer.* 1957;10:795–798.

38. Krengli M, Hug EB, Adams JA, et al. Proton radiation therapy for retinoblastoma: comparison of various intraocular tumor locations and beam arrangements. *Int J Radiat Oncol Biol Phys.* 2005;61:583–593.

39. Mohamad O, Yamada S, Durante M. Clinical indication for carbon ion radiotherapy. *Clin Oncol.* 2018;30:317–329.

40. Durante M, Paganetti H. Nuclear physics in particle therapy: a review. *Rep Prog Phys.* 2016;79:37–43.

41. Mohamad O, Sishc BJ, Saha J, et al. Carbon ion radiotherapy: a review of clinical experiences and preclinical research, with an emphasis on DNA damage/repair. *Cancers (Basel).* 2017;9(6):66.

42. Jain RK, Duda DG, Willett CG, et al. Biomarkers of response and resistance to antiangiogenic therapy. *Nat Rev Clin Oncol.* 2009;6(6):327–338.

43. Condeelis J, Pollard JW. Macrophages: obligate partners for tumor cell migration, invasion, and metastasis. *Cell.* 2006;124(2):263–266.

44. Dudley AC. Tumor endothelial cells. *Cold Spring Harb Perspect Med.* 2012;2(3):a006536.

45. Claudon M, Dietrich CF, Choi BI, et al. Guidelines and good clinical practice recommendations for contrast enhanced ultrasound (CEUS) in the liver – update 2012. *Ultrasound Med Biol.* 2013;39(2):187–210.

46. Cosgrove D, Harvey C. Clinical uses of microbubbles in diagnosis and treatment. *Med Biol Eng Comput.* 2009;47(8):813–826.

47. Harvey C. Ultrasound with microbubbles. *Cancer Image.* 2015;15(suppl 1):O19.

48. Unnikrishnan S, Klibanov AL. Microbubbles as ultrasound contrast agents for molecular imaging: preparation and application. *Am J Roentgenol.* 2012;199(2):292–299.

49. Haar G. Safety and bio-effects of ultrasound contrast agents. *Med Biol Eng Computer.* 2009;47(8):893–900.

50. Kobayashi N, Yasu T, Yamada S, et al. Endothelial cell injury in venule and capillary induced by contrast ultrasonography. *Ultrasound Med Biol.* 2002;28(7):949–956.

51. El Kaffas A, Al-Mahrouki A, Hashim A, Law N, Giles A, Czarnota GJ. Role of acid sphingomyelinase and ceramide in mechano-acoustic enhancement of tumor radiation responses. *J Natl Cancer Inst.* 2018;110(9):1009–1018.

52. Al-Mahrouki A, Giles A, Hashim A, et al. Microbubble-based enhancement of radiation effect: role of cell membrane ceramide metabolism. *PLoS One.* 2017;12(7):e0181951.

53. Czarnota GJ, Karshafian R, Burns PN, et al. Tumor radiation response enhancement by acoustical stimulation of the vasculature. *Proc Natl Acad Sci U S A.* 2012;109(30):E2033–E2041.

54. Kim HC, Al-Mahrouki A, Gorjizadeh A, Karshafian R, Czarnota GJ. Effects of biophysical parameters in enhancing radiation responses of prostate tumors with ultrasound-stimulated microbubbles. *Ultrasound Med Biol.* 2013;39(8):1376–1387.

55. Tran WT, Iradji S, Sofroni E, Giles A, Eddy D, Czarnota GJ. Microbubble and ultrasound radioenhancement of bladder cancer. *Br J Cancer.* 2012;107(3):469–476.

56. Kwok SJ, El Kaffas A, Lai P, et al. Ultrasound-mediated microbubble enhancement of radiation therapy studied using three-dimensional high-frequency power Doppler ultrasound. *Ultrasound Med Biol.* 2013;39(11):1983–1990.

57. Tran WT, Sannachi L, Papanicolau N, et al. Quantitative ultrasound imaging of therapy response in bladder cancer in vivo. *Oncoscience.* 2016;3(3–4):122–133.

58. Gillies RJ, Kinahan PE, Hricak H. Radiomics: images are more than pictures, they are data. *Radiology.* 2016;278(2):563–577.

59. Lambin P, Leijenaar RTH, Deist TM, et al. Radiomics: the bridge between medical imaging and personalized medicine. *Nat Rev Clin Oncol.* 2017;14(12):749–762.

60. Kumar V, Gu Y, Basu S, et al. Radiomics: the process and the challenges. *Magn Reson Imaging.* 2012;30(9):1234–1248.

61. Vallières M, Kay-Rivest E, Perrin LJ, et al. Radiomics strategies for risk assessment of tumour failure in head-and-neck cancer. *Sci Rep.* 2017;7(1):10117.

62. Russell S, Norvig P. *Artificial Intelligence: A Modern Approach.* 3rd ed. Essex, UK: Pearson Education Ltd; 2009.

63. Copeland BJ. Artificial Intelligence. https://www.britannica.com/technology/artificial-intelligence. Accessed January 18, 2018.

64. Valdes G, Chan MF, Mutic S, et al. IMRT QA using machine learning: a multi-institutional validation. *J Appl Clin Med Phys.* 2017;18:279–284.

65. Hoisak JDP, Pawlicki T, Kim G-Y, Fletcher R, Moore KL. Improving linear accelerator service response with a real-time electronic event reporting system. *J Appl Clin Med Phys.* 2014;15:4807.

66. Purdie TG, Dinniwell RE, Letourneau D, Hill C, Sharpe MB. Automated planning of tangential breast intensity-modulated radiotherapy using heuristic optimization. *Int J Radiat Oncol Biol Phys.* 2011;81(2):575–583.

67. Thompson RF, Valdes G, Fuller CD, et al. Artificial intelligence in radiation oncology: a specialty-wide disruptive transformation? *Radiother Oncol.* 2018;129(3):421–426.

REFERENCES FOR MRI LINAC UNITS COMMERCIALLY AVAILABLE: ACCESSED MAY 28, 2019

Elekta Unity. https://www.elekta.com/radiotherapy/treatment-delivery-systems/unity/?utm_source=unity&utm_medium=redirect&utm_campaign=redirects.

Magnetic Resonance-Guided Radiation Therapy (MRgRT) Suite, Princess Margaret Cancer Centre. https://www.uhn.ca/PrincessMargaret/Health_Professionals/Programs_Departments/RMP/Pages/mrgrt.aspx.

MagnetTx Oncology Solutions. AuroraRT. https://magnettx.com/origin/aurora-rt/.

MRIdian Linac by ViewRay. https://viewray.com/discover-mridian/.

The Australian MRI-Linac for Cancer Treatment, Ingham Institute for Applied Medical Research. https://inghaminstitute.org.au/where-we-work/ingham-institute-mri-linac/.

16

Particle Therapy

Matthew B. Palmer

OBJECTIVES

- Define particle therapy and its role in radiation therapy.
- Describe the differences between conventional radiation therapy and particle therapy.
- Describe the types of particle therapy delivery systems.
- Explain the importance of understanding the uncertainties in particle therapy.

- Compare and contrast passively scattered particle therapy and intensity-modulated particle therapy.
- Discuss the advances and benefits that particle therapy provides compared with conventional photon radiation therapy.

OUTLINE

KEY TERMS

Particle therapy
Passively scattered protons
Pencil beam scanning protons
Intensity-modulated proton therapy
Bragg peak
Cyclotron
Range modulator wheel
Synchrotron
Nozzle
Spread-out Bragg peak
Compensator
Smearing
Apertures
Uniform scanning

Nonuniform scanning
Relative biologic effectiveness
Linear energy transfer
Water equivalent thickness
Range uncertainty
Relative stopping power
Robust analysis
Beam-specific planning target volume
Repainting
Robust optimization
Edge effect
Patch planning
Distal blocking

INTRODUCTION

The goal of radiation therapy is to deliver as large a dose possible to cancer cells while avoiding radiation to nearby normal tissue. To achieve the maximum dose to the tumor, photon therapy requires multiple beams, which expose the normal tissue to high volumes of low doses of radiation. The exposure of normal tissue to unnecessary radiation when an attempt is made to maximize the dose to the target is the primary reason why radiation dose escalation for some types of cancers is not feasible. On the other hand, particle therapy has the ability to reduce the exposure of normal tissue beyond the targeted cancer cells because the maximum energy can be focused to a specific range within each patient. Particle therapy is a form of external beam therapy that uses particles accelerated to high energies. The most common particles used therapeutically are protons and carbon, but others, such as neutrons, helium, neon, and silicon, have been used. The properties of these particles make it possible to deliver the maximum energy at a finite and defined depth. The maximum energy can be spread out, thus making it possible for a single beam to cover the tumor three-dimensionally, which is not feasible with photon therapy. This reduction in normal tissue dose increases the probability of dose escalation and, in turn, the probability of tumor control.

The trade-off for additional precision and dose fall-off are a number of uncertainties, such as range uncertainty, computed tomography (CT) density conversion uncertainties, and the relative biologic effectiveness (RBE) at the distal range of the particle beam. Particle therapy has been used clinically to treat a wide range of cancers, including tumors located in the base of skull, head and neck (HN), liver, lung, prostate, breast, spine, as well as uveal melanomas and pediatric cancers.

Proton therapy represents approximately 88% of the particle therapy market and 100% of the United States market; therefore the majority of this chapter will be focused on protons.[1] Proton therapy has been traditionally treated with passively scattered particle therapy (PSPT). PSPT delivers monogenergetic protons, and apertures and compensators are used to shape the dose uniformly throughout the tumor. Advancements in proton delivery systems provide the ability to treat with pencil beam scanning (PBS), otherwise known as intensity-modulated proton therapy (IMPT), which delivers protons by scanning multienergy protons as discrete or continuous spots with magnets throughout the tumor. IMPT can now match the high-dose conformality of intensity-modulated radiation therapy (IMRT) with the added benefit of low-dose sparing to the normal tissue. Proton therapy accelerator design and other technological advances have accelerated the market in the United States and the world. This chapter will explain the benefits and uncertainties with particle therapy, primarily proton therapy.

HISTORIC PERSPECTIVE

Protons were discovered by Ernest Rutherford in the early nineteenth century. He named them after the Greek word "protos," which means "first." His initial tests concluded that protons have a definable range. The peak dose is deposited at a depth correlated to the proton's energy, and there is no dose beyond this peak. The Bragg peak phenomenon was discovered by William Bragg (Fig. 16.1).[2]

Ernest O. Lawrence, an American physicist, and his team invented the first cyclotron in 1930 that could accelerate protons with sufficiently high energy for the treatment of cancer. A cyclotron accelerates charged particles by alternating electric fields in a circular magnetic field. They were able to generate 340-megaelectron volt (MeV) protons through a 184-in. diameter synchrocyclotron a decade later.

The first scientist to propose proton therapy for the treatment of cancer was Dr. Robert Rathburn Wilson, a physicist at Harvard

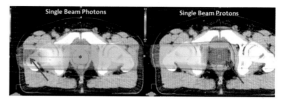

Fig. 16.1 Protons versus photons: one beam.

University, in 1946.[3] He emphasized that the fundamental property of protons, the Bragg peak, could be controlled within millimeters and the maximum energy could be spread out with the use of a range modulator wheel. A modulator wheel is made of absorbers of multiple thicknesses that rotate in the path of the beam to change the range of the maximum energy needed to reach the most distal end of the target. The first patient with a pituitary tumor was treated at the University of California, Berkeley, in 1954.[4] Thirty patients were treated at this facility from 1954 to 1957.

The particle therapy industry continued to slowly grow in the 1950s and 1960s, with the establishment of the particle beam facility in Upssala, Sweden in 1957, the Massachusetts General Hospital-Harvard Cyclotron Laboratory in 1961, and the Institute for Theoretical and Experimental Physics in Moscow in 1967. Most of the early facilities were not primarily used for patient care, and the primary tumors treated were intracranial or ocular tumors. The particle therapy field was advanced in the 1970s and 1980s, mainly through clinical data published for ocular, brain, skull base, and pediatric tumors. Technologies that aided in the delineation of tumors and normal tissue as well as the calculation algorithms for proton treatment planning were advanced during this time. The world's first hospital-based proton therapy facility opened in 1990 in Loma Linda, California, with a 250-MeV passively scattered synchrotron with three rotating gantries and one fixed beam. A synchrotron accelerates charged particles within an electric field and has an increasing magnetic field for increasing energy.

The number of particle therapy centers worldwide, primarily in the United States, Asia, and Europe, has almost quadrupled since 2005 from 20 centers (1954–2005, 0.6 centers/year) to 54 centers in 2014 (2006–2014, 3.8 centers/year) and 98 in 2019 (2015–2019, 8.8 centers/year), because of the increasing body of clinical evidence of their efficacy in treating many different types of tumors. In addition, commercial solutions and recent advancements in accelerator design are resulting in significantly lower facility requirements and costs. A comprehensive list of current and proposed particle beam facilities in the world is available on the Particle Therapy Co-operative Group website.[1]

GENERAL PARTICLE THERAPY PRINCIPLES

Accelerators

The accelerators typically used for the treatment of cancer are typically cyclotrons or synchrotrons. Both cyclotrons and synchrotrons are used worldwide. In general, synchrotrons achieve a continuously variable energy through a clean methodology, whereas cyclotrons create a higher dose rate with a uniform intensity.

Although cyclotrons are reliable, compact, and easy to operate, synchrotrons have the ability to generate the energies needed to treat the patient. The extraction of the desired energy eliminates the need of energy degraders downstream. The energy degraders add extra interactions with the pencil beam, which increases the creation of secondary neutrons. The increase in neutrons in turn increases the amount of shielding that is needed near the beam exit.[5] This design also causes the metal in the energy degrading system to become more radioactive. This can affect the time before maintenance begins because the metal

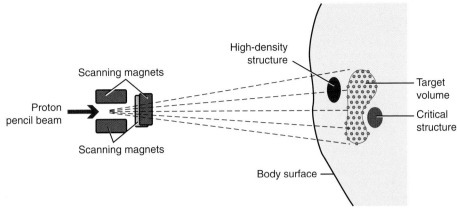

Fig. 16.2 Spot scanning for conformal proton therapy. (Courtesy MD Anderson Cancer Center website.)

needs time to "cool down." A disadvantage of a synchrotron is the complex system necessary to extract the precise energy needed. In addition, the current is less than a cyclotron, which could produce longer treatment times.[6] This issue has been addressed by recent advances in the synchrotron designs so that it produces similar dose rates to cyclotrons.[6] For example, both accelerators can produce dose rates between 1 and 2 Gy per minute for a 30 × 30-cm field.[5]

Therapeutic protons are accelerated to high energies, typically in the range of 50 to 250 MeV. The accelerated protons are transported in a vacuum through a series of strong magnets, which focus the pencil beam through the transport system into each room. There are multiple options for the type of beam delivery into a proton therapy treatment room. The beam can be delivered through a fixed horizontal, fixed vertical or specific angle, 360-degree gantry, or partial gantry, (i.e., 185 degrees.) The largest facility in the world has five rooms, and most centers have different beam delivery options.

The nozzle houses devices to further focus and shape the proton beam. The devices are specific to the type of accelerator and proton delivery technique (i.e, passively scattered particle therapy [PSPT] versus PBS).

Passively Scattered Particle Therapy

The PSPT approach is currently the most common method of delivering proton beam therapy worldwide, but PBS is rapidly growing. PSPT uses devices to scatter the proton beam laterally and distally. Single or double scattering devices within the nozzle spread out the focused proton pencil beam to the lateral edges of the field.[7] A range modulator wheel is used to create the spread-out Bragg peak (SOBP) so that the maximum energy can treat the entire tumor from the most distal edge to the most proximal edge.[8] The distal dose is conformed to the tumor shape with the use of an acrylic or wax compensator.[9] The treatment planning system (TPS) creates the compensator design based on the water equivalent thickness (WET) between the patient's skin surface and the distal surface of the target. The compensator is then smeared. Smearing is a process that modifies the compensator design to take into account the internal motion of the tumor and setup uncertainties.[10,11] Smearing is used to ensure that the target dose is not compromised when uncertainties are introduced. The compensator also takes into account tissue heterogeneities and the external shape of the patient.

PSPT beams use collimation through the use of multileaf collimators (MLCs) or brass apertures, with brass apertures more commonly used. These collimating devices shape the dose laterally. Clinically insignificant results were found in dose distributions between MLCs and brass apertures.[12,13] Although MLCs provide an efficient and cost-effective alternative to brass for proton beams, some clinicians

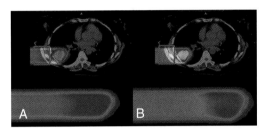

Fig. 16.3 Images of lung cancer treated with passively scattered particle therapy (A) and pencil beam scanning (B).

caution against using a tungsten alloy because it produces more secondary neutrons and increased radiation exposure for patients and staff.[13,14]

Pencil Beam Scanning Particle Therapy

PBS uses the charge of the protons and two magnets to focus and direct the protons throughout the tumor in a scanning fashion (Fig. 16.2). A cyclotron delivers scanning beam therapy through an energy selection system after beam extraction and before the nozzle because only the maximum energy can be extracted in a cyclotron. The lateral scanning is achieved by a raster or discrete spot scanning system.[15] A synchrotron achieves scanning beam therapy by extracting the required energy at each range, and the protons are spread laterally by a lateral spot beam scan.[15] Beam-shaping devices are not needed with PBS; therefore the dose distribution is more conformal on the proximal and distal ends. This also reduces the amount of potential neutrons in the field.

There are two types of PBS, uniform scanning and nonuniform scanning. Uniform scanning delivers a uniform dose distribution throughout the tumor with each beam. If multiple beams are used, each beam could treat the tumor to the full dose if treated independently. On the other hand, nonuniform scanning delivers a nonuniform dose per beam to make the composite dose uniform (Fig. 16.3). The nonuniform scanning technique applies similar modulation techniques to IMRT, its photon counterpart. Hence nonuniform scanning is also called *IMPT* because it shares similar optimization techniques with its photon counterpart.

Radiobiology

Particle therapy has important radiobiologic considerations that must be taken into consideration more than conventional photons. The RBE is higher for charged particles than for photons; therefore less radiation is needed to achieve the same biologic effect.[16] RBE is the test of the biologic effectiveness of one type of radiation compared with a reference radiation.

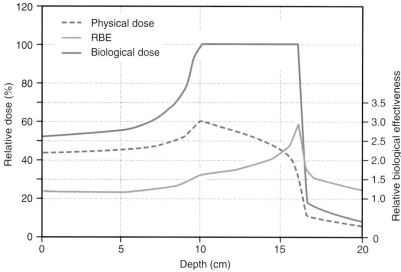

Fig. 16.4 An image that shows the differences between biologic and physical dose. *RBE*, Relative biologic effectiveness. (From Suit H, DeLaney T, Goldberg S, et al. Proton vs carbon ion beams in the definitive radiation treatment of cancer patients. *Radiother Oncol.* 2010;95:3–22.)

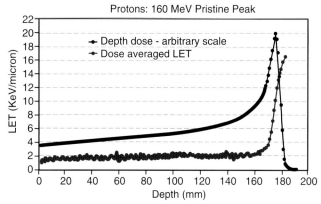

Fig. 16.5 Linear energy transfer *(LET)* of a proton beam shows how the average energy of the beam is deposited along the beam path. Note how the profile peaks at a certain depth, which is determined by the energy level. (From Suit H, DeLaney T, Goldberg S, et al. Proton vs carbon ion beams in the definitive radiation treatment of cancer patients. *Radiother Oncol.* 2010;95:3–22.)

Protons have a lower RBE than carbon because they have a lower linear energy transfer (LET) value. LET is the average energy loss of a charged particle to a medium within a defined distance.[17] Protons have an accepted RBE value of 1.1, whereas carbon's RBE can range between 3 and 5 in the Bragg peak region.[18,19] Although these accepted values are used, the RBE can vary depending on the physical and biologic characteristics in the path of the beam.[20] The 1 to 2 mm beyond the Bragg peak, the area with the highest uncertainty and the maximum dose, could potentially extend into a critical structure when a beam is directed at such a structure (Fig. 16.4).[21] This is an important consideration during treatment planning, and attention should be given to beams directed at sensitive normal tissues, especially while the RBE value increases (Fig. 16.5).

SIMULATION

Image Acquisition

CT imaging is primarily used for treatment planning in radiation therapy. The three dimensional information is used to delineate the tumor and normal tissue structures. The immobilization techniques have been well established in radiation therapy. The goal of immobilization is to create a reproducible setup for the patient on a day-to-day basis. Custom-designed immobilization devices and/or body molds made of thermoplastics, polyurethane-foaming agents, and vacuum-forming molds are created during the simulation. Table extensions and extended head holders are commonly used for HN and intracranial targets to increase the number of available beams that can be selected for treatment. The particle therapy market has grown significantly, and vendors are providing particle therapy-specific solutions. It is important to note for facilities with multiple modalities (i.e., protons and photons) that particle therapy–specific immobilization devices can be used for photon therapy, but the opposite is not always true.

Extra considerations must be given to the following: immobilization device uncertainty, day-to-day variability, edge effects with the patient and immobilization device, anatomic changes, device uncertainty, and target motion.[22] The type of immobilization is site specific and is chosen to maximize the anatomy for optimal beam entry. Beam selection and direction are an important component of particle therapy; therefore daily setup must be consistent and reproducible because the Bragg peak depth can be significantly altered with slight internal or external changes. This could result in less tumor coverage or a higherdose to a critical structure. Immobilization devices should be indexed when possible relative to the treatment couch. Indexing will streamline patient setup and minimize large variations in the initial position of the patient before imaging.[23] Immobilization devices, primarily head holders, without sharp density changes along the edges should be used if possible.

Special attention must be given to the type and thickness of the material used in the immobilization device. Minimizing the WET is important because it affects the penumbra and range uncertainty.[22] WET is the water equivalent thickness of the material a beam traverses. The beam is attenuated more while the WET value increases. The WET of each device must be known and accurately modeled in the TPS so that the range can be accurately calculated.[22]

Immobilization Device Uncertainty

It is important to properly evaluate custom-made immobilization devices before using them in the clinic. Nonuniformity in the thickness

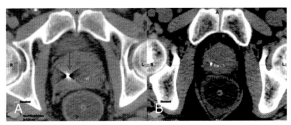

Fig. 16.6 Fiducial images that show too much streaking (A) and an acceptable level of streaking (B).

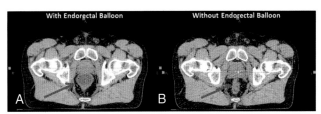

Fig. 16.7 An image with (A) and without (B) rectal balloon.

or pockets of inhomogeneities can impact the range uncertainty when they are shifted relative to the patient interfractionally, intrafractionally, or the simulation CT scan. Also, verify that molds and body casts do not change over time. External stimuli (e.g., heat, cold, or humidity) could potentially change the shape of the device relative to shape at simulation. Not only could these changes reduce the stability of the immobilization, but also the range uncertainty of the particle beam. This highlights the importance of doing a thorough evaluation of a new, customizable immobilization device for consistency, shape, and reliability over time.[22]

Communication about what devices were used during the simulation is very important between the simulation and treatment rooms because all immobilization devices used during treatment must have the same size, shape, composition, and WET as those during simulation. Interchangeability must be thoroughly evaluated before one device is used in place of another. Variation in any of the parameters without evaluation could introduce additional range uncertainties.[22] Standardization of the immobilization devices for each treatment site and provision of access by staff to these devices in each room can help eliminate potential setup and immobilization errors.

Anatomic Changes

Consistency of the patient's external anatomy is also very important. Changes in external anatomy, whether it is the result of weight loss or shifting tissue in obese patients, can change the WET of the originally calculated particle beam. Changes in the WET of the target can lead to underirradiation of the target and/or overirradiation of structures beyond the distal edge. Body molds are commonly used for obese patients so that the skin surface can be more reproducible on a daily basis. Weight loss, especially in patients with HN cancers, is a major area of concern because it can decrease the stability and reproducibility of the immobilization device.

Motion Management

Internal motion management concepts for particle therapy are very similar to the techniques for conventional photon therapy. Inadequately accounting for tumor motion can result in missing the tumor or overdosing normal tissue beyond the tumor. It is recommended that sites affected by respiratory motion use four-dimensional CT scans, a breath-hold gating, or respiratory gating to account for the motion of the tumor relative to other internal structures such as the ribs, sternum, clavicles, and shoulders. Insertion of low z-material fiducial can help with tumor tracking and patient setup. Fiducials in particle therapy are commonly used for lung, liver, and prostate tumors, but it is important to use a fiducial that has the lowest density possible so that artifact streaking through the CT is minimized (Fig. 16.6).

Internal changes such as bowel gas, rectal gas, or bladder filling can also affect tumor motion daily. Endorectal balloons filled with water or air improve internal setup uncertainties on a daily basis for prostate cancer. Wang et al. demonstrated a 40% reduction in the symmetrical internal margin for prostate cancer. The endorectal balloon also

reduces unpredictable uncertainties in the prostate position resulting from rectal gas (Fig. 16.7).[23]

Immobilization and patient setup play an important role in particle therapy. Taking all of the considerations into account will decrease the potential impact from immobilization devices to tumor coverage and normal tissue dose because of range uncertainty.

TREATMENT PLANNING CONSIDERATIONS

The ability of particle therapy to maximize the dose delivered to the tumor and reduce the dose delivered to healthy tissue is its major benefit versus its photon counterpart. A reduction of normal tissue doses makes dose escalation more feasible, reduces the chances of toxicities, and lowers the risk for secondary malignancies in younger patients.

Treatment Planning Uncertainties

The benefits of particle therapy come at the expense of extra uncertainties that are manageable but warrant special consideration during treatment planning. The following are treatment planning considerations that will be reviewed: range uncertainties, RBE, setup errors, immobilization devices, organ motion, anatomic variations, and artifacts.

Range Uncertainties. Multiple factors can impact the range uncertainty of the particle therapy beam, such as dose calculations, setup, organ and anatomic variations, and biologic considerations.[24] Range uncertainty can be defined as the calculated uncertainty added to the expected end of the proton beam range.

The CT images are acquired with kilovoltage (kV) x-ray energies, and the information is used to calculate the attenuation and scatter of radiation. The original linear attenuation coefficient information in the CT is converted into Hounsfield units (HU), which gives the material in each pixel a value relative to that of water. The HU then have to be converted to relative electron densities for particle therapy relative stopping power (RSP). The conversion of HU values to RSP for proton therapy has been discussed in the literature.[25-27] The accepted value for range uncertainty caused by the CT number/HU to stopping power conversion accepted value is 3.5%, based on calculations done by Moyer et al.[28] The calculation of proximal and distal margins are well established for PSPT by using the RSP conversion method mentioned above, but this method has not been effectively adapted to PBS because the delivery and modulation techniques differ from PSPT. Proximal and distal margins are additional margins added to the clinical target volume (CTV) of the beam path to take into account setup, motion, and range uncertainties.

A proton tomography unit is one method to eliminate the uncertainties associated with RSP conversion because the image generated will calculate the proton stopping powers directly inside the body. Proton tomography was created in 1981, but it has not been made available for commercial use to date.[29] Dual-energy CT scans (DECT) have also been proposed to reduce uncertainties related to RSP because of its properties. There is ongoing research to determine the true benefits of DECT for proton therapy treatment planning. Therefore it is extremely

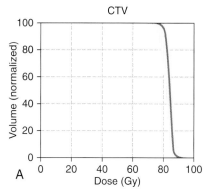
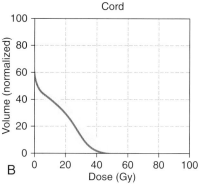

Fig. 16.8 An image of a robust analysis dose volume histogram. *CTV,* Clinical target volume. (Courtesy Dr. Mohan and Dr. Liu, MD Anderson Cancer Center.)

important to calibrate the CT correctly and apply the appropriate conversion tables for RSP so that the uncertainty in the distal range of the particle beam can be minimized.

Additional range uncertainty exists because of the uncertainties in calculating the end of the Bragg peak. The Bragg peak can be degraded; the amount of degradation is dependent on the proton energy and the heterogeneities in the path of the beam relative to that Bragg peak. The conclusion was made that there is a positional difference of approximately 2 mm in the 80% to 20% falloff for a 220 MeV beam and approximately 1.5 mm for the 90%.[30–32] Treatment planning algorithms cannot account for the end of range degradation; thus additional margins must be added to the 3.5% CT number to RSP conversion.[32–35] The amount of extra margin added depends on the institutional policies, but they range from 1 mm to 3 mm.[24]

There is a high degree of caution with the use of beams that distally range into a critical structure, because there is the possibility that the range can travel farther than calculated in the TPS. This may be difficult for some cases; therefore if a beam ranging toward a critical structure has to be used, it is recommended that the other beams used in the plan avoid distally ranging into the same critical structure.

Robust analysis is commonly performed on cases that may have a large degree of uncertainty. This analysis is performed by scaling the CT number to RSP conversion curves by the same degree of expected range uncertainty (i.e, ±3.5%) and creating a verification plan with frozen parameters. The analysis will sum the total uncertainty effects for both the tumor coverage and critical structure doses. The treatment plan can be reoptimized if the robust analysis is unfavorable. Isocenter displacements (i.e, ± 3 mm) can also be simulated in the robust analysis, and the worst-case scenario of all verification plans can be displayed on a dose volume histogram (DVH). This analysis tool helps add a degree of confidence that the treatment plan is safe and robust (Fig. 16.8).

Relative Biologic Effectiveness. RBE is another important factor that should be considered when particle therapy planning is performed. The clinically accepted RBE value for proton therapy is 1.1.[36] Carbon therapy has an RBE range between 3 and 5.[17,18] The RBE at the distal end of a proton beam can be as much as an additional 25% higher than the 10% added clinically because the LET increases with depth in an SOBP.[32] The distal range, a 90% depth dose, can be an extra 2 mm or more when the range is corrected for RBE.[36–39] Theoretically, an extra 2 mm or more should be added to the proton beam to take into account the changes in LET through the SOBP and the increased RBE at the end of the range. Similar to the range uncertainty, TPSs do not take into account the effective RBE, especially at the end of the range, where it is usually higher. Therefore it is up to the clinical team to estimate the potential effects of the RBE for each treatment plan.

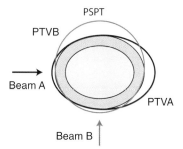
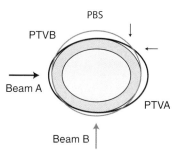

Fig. 16.9 Differences in contouring techniques. *PBS,* Pencil beam scanning; *PSPT,* passively scattered proton therapy; *PTVA,* planning target volume A; *PTVB,* planning target volume B.

Setup Errors. Setup errors can significantly impact the coverage to the CTV because of the misalignment of the beam and the target. The PTV is a geometric concept used in photon therapy to determine the lateral margins so that the CTV receives the prescribed dose in the event of potential setup errors.[40] Setup errors not only affect the lateral margins for particle therapy but also in the depth direction. Therefore the PTV concept is not used for proton therapy because additional margins must be considered in the depth direction to account for range uncertainties, which are typically different than the lateral margins. If the setup error is in the plane of the beam entry without a change in the WET, then the impact on the tumor coverage will be minimal. Photons, on the other hand, would potentially be impacted significantly. The International Committee on Radiation Units and Measurements Report 78 on prescribing, recording, and reporting proton-beam therapy is a guideline that should be used to address specific issues related to range uncertainties for proton therapy.[41] Each beam will have different distal and proximal margins from the CTV because of the distal range and the properties of the material in the path of the beam. Therefore a uniformly expanded margin (i.e, PTV) is not applicable (Fig. 16.9).

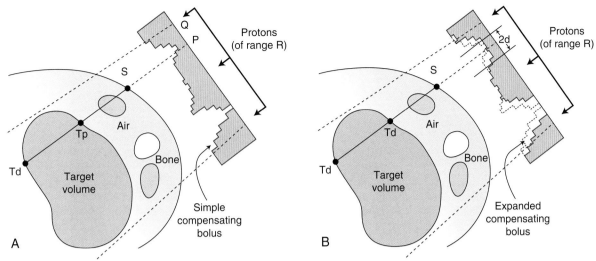

Fig. 16.10 Design of a bolus for protons of range R to compensate for surface and target irregularities and tissue heterogeneities. (a) Sample line ray along which a line integral is performed to obtain the water equivalent areal density between the skin (S) and the proximal (T,) and distal (Td) target volume surfaces. (b) Expansion of the bolus to ensure target volume treatment within positioning and motion uncertainties of distance d. (From Urie M, Goitein M, Wagner M. Compensating for heterogeneities in proton radiation therapy, *Phys Med Biol.* 1984;29:553–566.)

In the PSPT approach, the maximum energy is calculated by using the pencil beam calculation. The broad proton beam is scattered into small pencil beamlets, and each one is ray traced to determine the WET required for the treatment field. The compensator is designed based on the ray tracing results so that the dose is conformal on the distal end of the tumor. For example, the compensator thickness will be thinner where the ray tracing detects bone and thicker where the ray tracing detects low-density lung tissue. Patient motion, internal or external, or setup errors can change the relative spacing of the patient to the compensator, creating a misalignment of the compensator and the original WET calculations. If a bone is moved relative to the compensator because of internal organ motion, the beamlet may pass through an area in the compensator that is thicker or thinner, causing it to stop before the distal end of the tumor or stop beyond the distal end of the tumor, respectively. Common examples of internal motion that can cause issues are shoulder placement, rib motion, and pelvic rotation. Evaluating the motion of the structures around the tumor is a concept that is not commonly applied in photon therapy, but it is an important aspect of particle therapy treatment planning. To evaluate effects of organ motion, weekly four-dimensional CTs, CT-on-rails, or cone-beam CTs (CBCTs) are common for patients treated in or near the lungs or diaphragm, whereas patients with inconsistent organ motion, such as bladder filling or bowel gas, may only require verification CTs or CBCTs during the course of treatment on a case-by-case basis.

Urie and colleagues proposed the concept of smearing to account for these potential changes in WET resulting from setup error or organ motion. The thinner part of the compensator is modified by a given radius, smearing margin, which is equal to or larger than the potential setup errors or organ motion (Fig. 16.10).[10]

At the expense of tumor coverage in the event of a setup error or organ motion, application of smear to the compensator reduces the overall thickness, which causes more of the dose to travel beyond the tumor and into the healthy tissue.

The technique of smearing does not apply to PBS because the approach does not use a compensator, and the delivery technique is more complex because the dose is painted layer by layer with small spots. One proposed concept to account for range uncertainties for PBS uniform scanning is called the beam-specific planning target volume (bsPTV).[42,43] Uniform scanning techniques lack physical compensators that account for unexpected shifts in the range; therefore the standard uniform PTV may not be adequate to account for these range uncertainties. On the other hand, a bsPTV for proton beams is created by modifying the ray tracing to account for potential misalignments caused by setup error or organ motion. Systematic range uncertainties are added to the proximal and distal margins from the CTV, and then an extra margin is added for potential range errors.

Significant research efforts toward finding a technique to account for setup errors and organ motion for IMPT, nonuniform scanning, are ongoing. The interplay between the delivery of thousands of spots in multiple layers relative to the organ motion makes this a complex problem to address. WET changes can result in the spots delivered in other layers, which causes hot areas at the overlap and cold areas where the spots were expected to go. All of these potential uncertainties are not accounted for in conventional treatment planning. Studies have shown that the delivery errors can be significant per fraction for multiple sites, for instance, 34% in a single fraction and 18% in 30 fractions for a lung treatment, and 33% for one fraction for a liver treatment.[44–46] Motion management techniques, such as gating, breath-hold gating, and fiducial tracking, should be considered when there is a significant chance for organ motion for an IMPT treatment so that the dosimetric effects are minimized. Repainting, the process of delivering a fraction in portions of the fractional dose multiple times throughout the treatment volume, for IMPT delivery has been suggested.[45,47] The drawback of repainting is a proportional increase in treatment delivery time to the number of repaints that are applied.

Robust optimization, a treatment planning approach to minimizing uncertainties for PBS by incorporating them into the optimization process, is also in development. One approach uses the "worst case" out of nine plans that include ± setup errors in each plane (A-P, R-L, S-I), ± range uncertainty plans, and the baseline optimized plan. The optimizer assigns the lowest dose to each voxel inside the CTV and the highest dose per voxel outside of the CTV based on all nine plans and then optimizes this plan to meet the objectives.[48] This technique has demonstrated more robustness to setup errors and range uncertainties compared with a PTV-based plan. In addition, the doses to the healthy tissue were reduced.

Immobilization (External Edge Effects). Edge effect can be defined as a particle beam passing through the edge of an immobilization device or boundary (i.e., a table edge or head holder clips). The particle beam range can be significantly impacted when the patient is shifted in his/her positioning relative to this edge if a beam passes through it.

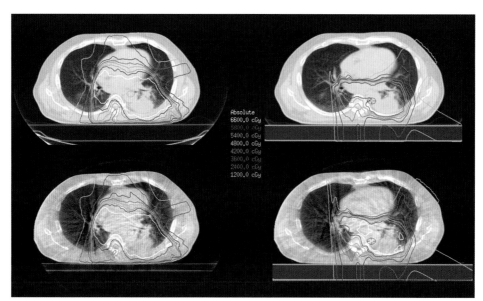

Fig. 16.11 Cone-beam computed tomography versus off-line computed tomography. (Courtesy Dr. Joey Cheung, MD Anderson Cancer Center.)

Setup differences in positioning relative to these edges not only affect the range but also the heterogeneity of the dose around the edge.

Selected beams during the treatment planning process should avoid these areas if these immobilization devices are needed to ensure stable immobilization. The edge of the treatment couch can cause significant problems when a beam is treating through this area because the patient will not lie in the same exact location laterally each day. A study at University of Texas MD Anderson's Proton Center found that the daily lateral couch shifts can be more than 1 cm in positioning relative to the patient.[49]

Organ Motion (Internal Edge Effects). Sharp changes in the WET of anatomy within the patient can significantly affect the dose distribution for particle therapy when translational or rotational setup errors or organ motion occurs. These changes can be accounted for in the smear of the compensator but at the expense of more heterogeneities. It is therefore recommended that beams parallel to high-gradient WET areas should be avoided.

Anatomic Variations. Anatomic changes, including in the tumor, are common for HN and lung tumors, but any tissue in the path of any proton beam can affect dosimetry. The anatomy for HN tumor changes are primarily the result of tumor shrinkages and weight loss. Lung tumors, especially big and bulky ones, are suspect to larger changes. Anatomic changes can be caused by immobilization devices (i.e., vacuum bags), which can introduce unwanted changes in the soft tissue around the chest wall.[50] Vacuum bags or body molds may be beneficial when posterior beams are needed because they can shape the tissue consistently so that the WET remains constant. The reproducibility of breast tissue is hard to manage; therefore careful consideration should be taken for the beam-angle selection in or around the breast tissue.

Weekly off-line CTs are an effective technique to evaluate anatomic changes throughout the course of treatment. The weekly CTs can be used to generate a verification plan on the new anatomy. Adaptive planning can be implemented during the course of treatment to minimize the effects of anatomic changes on the dose distribution. Off-line CTs are typically used for verification plans because they have the correct CT number to RSP conversion compared with CBCT (Fig. 16.11).

A study done at MD Anderson showed that an adaptive plan for HN IMPT treatment plans done during the fourth week of treatment with off-line CT and implemented in the fifth week of treatment approximately 10 fractions out of 33 fractions, was the most effective time to maintain CTV coverage and minimize the increase in the parotid doses. The study showed that adaptive planning is indicated if the patient loses 10 pounds or 5% body weight or more within the first 4 weeks of treatment.[51]

A similar study was done by Shi et al for lung cancer. They reported that without adaptive replanning for a lung cancer case after significant tumor shrinkage, the lung V20 would have increased by 20% or more, the spinal cord by 150%, and the esophagus by 200% more than the original plan.[52,53] Other published studies have shown the benefits of adaptive planning for lung, craniopharyngiomas, spinal tumors, retroperitoneal sarcomas, pancreas, liver tumors, and rectal filling for prostate patients.[54–61]

The benefits of adaptive planning to compensate for anatomic changes are evident for IMPT, but guidelines, frequency, and timing of adaptive planning for most treatment sites have not been firmly established. This is an active area of evaluation for the proton therapy industry because it is evident that IMPT is susceptible to significant changes when there are anatomic changes in the treatment volume. For example, Beltran et al. suggest that replanning should be considered for IMPT, IMRT, and PSPT for craniopharyngiomas when there is a 5%, 10%, and 25% change to the PTV volume, respectively.[57]

Metal and Artifacts. Implanted high z-material and devices into the body can cause uncertainties for proton beam dose calculations because the highest CT numbers that can be calculated in most CT scanners is 4095.[24] Therefore any high z-material that has a value greater than 4095 will be assigned an incorrect value of 4095 by the CT scanner. The metal and the scattered higher- and lower-density streaks it causes must be delineated and assigned the correct CT number. The CT number overrides for high z-material are very important so that the correct stopping power is assigned, thus preventing incorrect dose calculations during treatment planning (Fig. 16.12).

Passively Scattered Particle Therapy Versus Pencil Beam Scanning Therapy

The dosimetric benefits of both delivery techniques are similar, but each has its own unique characteristics that makes it preferred for

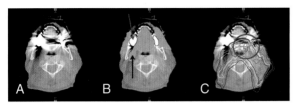

Fig. 16.12 Images with streaking and metal. Image A shows a CT scan as acquired with high Z material. Image B shows the streaks delineated out, while image C shows the two images fused together with the treatment plan.

certain types of cases. Most of the new centers in development will only have PBS, so it will be important for them to translate some of the PSPT benefits into clinical practice with PBS. No matter what technique is selected, all the uncertainties and considerations previously mentioned must be considered.

In general, the PSPT approach works well for most cases because it is more robust when there are setup errors, organ motion, or anatomic changes. PSPT are preferred for simple tumor shapes, shallow tumors, and cases with expected organ or tumor motion. However, PBS is preferred for concave tumors that wrap around a critical structure, complex tumor shapes, or simultaneous integrated boosts.

A couple of PSPT approaches have been used to treat complex tumor shapes. One technique is called patch planning, and the other technique uses distal blocking. Patch planning uses two beams to treat the tumor, each beam treating a partial volume of the tumor.[62] A "thru" beam treats the majority of the tumor, and the patch field matches the sharp distal margin fall-off at the end of the SOBP with the 50% isodose line of the "thru" field. This planning technique typically requires junction fields to homogenize the match line. One junction technique is to use three patch fields during the course of treatment. This technique changes the patch field match from the 50% isodose line of the patch field to the 50% of the thru field to the 25% isodose line of the patch field to the 75% of the thru field after a specific number of fractions and then the 12.5% and 87.5% after a specific number of fractions. This technique modulates the "hot" spots so that they are not in the same location for the entire treatment.[63] Incorrect calculation or setup of the patch field could cause the distal range of the patch field to travel into the "thru" field or end before the match line. Both scenarios could have significant compromises, such as increasing the dose to nearby critical structures or losing tumor coverage, respectively. This technique is very difficult and requires extreme precision for both treatment planning and delivery.

Distal blocking is a technique that adds thickness to the compensator to achieve additional sparing of a critical structure distal to the tumor volume. This technique can be used when the tumor wraps around a critical structure. Modification of the compensator may affect the end of range uncertainty. In addition, setup error or motion may cause misalignment of the added thickness and the critical structure, which will void the sparing. Clinicians in the process of beam selection for particle therapy should take into consideration the treatment planning technique, tumor location, nearby critical structures, external and internal edge effects, heterogeneities in the beam path, distal range uncertainties, and clearance. Similar to electron planning, the proton pencil beam penumbra is smaller the closer the snout and devices are to the patient. The nozzle and snout housing can be big and bulky and sometimes hard to model during the treatment planning process. The TPSs do not accurately model the treatment room or devices, so either the snout positions should be verified before treatment or conservative snout position should be selected to avoid collisions with the patient. Beam selection is often a difficult task for proton therapy compared with photon therapy because of the considerations and limitations listed above.

TABLE 16.1 Scanning Comparisons	
Uniform Scanning	**Nonuniform Scanning**
Always consider before nonuniform scanning is performed	Considered intensity-modulated proton therapy
Each beam covers the tumor volume, similar to passively scattered protons.	Fields are patched to create uniform dose
Works well for simple volumes	More versatile to get better plan
Less sensitive to uncertainties	More sensitive to uncertainties
May have superficial range limits, depending on lowest energy	Robust optimization or analysis should be considered during planning or evaluation
Can incorporate simultaneous integrated boost	Can incorporate simultaneous integrated boost

PBS can be divided into two different delivery types, uniform scanning and nonuniform scanning. Table 16.1 highlights the considerations to take into account.

The properties of the spots and the delivery system can impact plan quality. The TPSs algorithms are designed to enable placement of the spots for PBS as effectively as possible based on the delivery system. Delivery systems that can deliver smaller spots can create tighter dose gradients around the tumor edges than a delivery system with larger spots. This is beneficial for cases in which tighter dose gradients are needed (i.e., intracranial tumors). On the other hand, larger spot sizes may be more beneficial for cases with organ motion or anatomic changes. A study done at MD Anderson's Proton Center evaluated the dosimetric effects of the interplay of PBS with uniform and realistic breathing motions.[64] The researchers concluded that the interplay effect may not be of concern with use of their delivery system with larger spots and an isolayer repainting style. The authors commented that the observations of their study were based on spot sizes that may be considered large compared with cases at other institutions, so the recommendations should be cautiously followed. Another study that evaluated the interplay of motion and spot size for PBS also concluded that bigger spots are more robust than smaller spots.[65] On the other hand, a benefit of smaller spots noted in this study was that they reduced the doses to normal tissue because of the sharper dose gradient. Most delivery systems have one or the other, but in the future, it might be possible to select the spot size based on the type of case that is being treated.

Plan Evaluation

Because of the range of uncertainties associated with particle beam therapy, each beam has unique properties and should be analyzed independently along with the composite dose distribution. Evaluating each beam's dose distribution can help show potential range issues, heterogeneities, and interactions between the beam and the tissue in the path of the beam. Independent modification of each beam versus composite dose distribution is a good systematic approach to help minimize as many uncertainties as possible.

IMPT's significant flexibility in comparison with PSPT offers much promise because it is considered to be the equivalent of IMRT with photons. Unlike IMRT, IMPT has a third dimension, depth, which needs to be addressed. The extra dimension makes it more susceptible to degradation than IMRT with photons.[66] The potential treatment plan degradation results can be best displayed through a robust analysis. A robust analysis shows the DVH for the target and normal tissue structures for nine different plans, six with setup errors introduced in the A-P, R-L, and S-I planes, two range uncertainty plans with scaled

CT number curves, and the proposed, optimal treatment plan. The DVH bands represent the potential error on a given day. This analysis is a valuable tool, but it does not explain all of the uncertainties in the plan; therefore it is important to use this as a value-added tool with all of the other considerations mentioned in this chapter.

While technology advances, not only will more robust analysis tools be available, but with advances such as robust optimization, DVHs with range uncertainties, and RBE, biologic optimization will improve during the treatment planning process so that each plan can be delivered as safely as possible.

TREATMENT DELIVERY

Delivery Systems

Treatment delivery rooms of particle therapy centers have some similarities but significant differences versus conventional photon treatment rooms. The ability to concurrently treat patients in multiple rooms is not feasible for multiroom centers that share the same linear accelerator. Rooms that are waiting on the beam must go through proper safety checks before they are added to the queue. The room in which the patient is treated will lose the beam to another room that is in the queue; therefore there may be longer treatment delivery times because of this logistical issue. Sophisticated control rooms are designed to maximize efficiency and switch times between the rooms based on the queue. The control rooms have the ability to prioritize a room for a specific patient or a block of time when there is a complicated case that needs a short delivery time, but this feature is more commonly used for pediatric patients under anesthesia.

Beamline Types

There are operational benefits to the use of a fixed beam, but patient setup, imaging, and applications can be limited. Beam angles are limited to one direction; therefore creative setup techniques sometimes must be used to achieve desired directions. Careful consideration should be given to the immobilization techniques to achieve these patient positions so they are reproducible and safe. Other centers have installed incline beams or limited arc beamlines. This delivery technique gives more flexibility than the fixed horizontal beam, but beam-angle selection is still limited. Isocenter gantries can rotate around the patient who is typically in the supine position, which provides a higher degree of freedom in beam selection. The gantry systems have one major problem: they require a large cable system with large magnets to bend the beam with precision and large facilities. For example, the gantries at the MD Anderson Proton Center weigh 220 tons and span three stories in height.

Small footprint gantries are a recent development for centers that are considering proton therapy but do not have the capital or patient volume to build a large facility with multiple rooms and the traditional gantry system. This design has been achieved because of advancements in the cyclotron or synchrocyclotron design. The advancements have significantly reduced the accelerators' size so that they are mounted in the head of the gantry. Other small footprints are equipped with their accelerator in a nearby room. The small footprints have isocentric diameters that are approximately 25% of a traditional gantry system.[67] Small-footprint proton systems typically do not have a full 360-degree rotational system. Most of them are designed with approximately 185 to 190 degrees of rotational flexibility, but they are equipped with six dimensional robotic couches, giving them the same degrees of freedom as a full gantry system. These systems have accelerated the growth of the proton therapy industry because they are more affordable and offered by multiple vendors.

Passively Scattered Particle Therapy Versus Pencil Beam Scanning Therapy Treatment Delivery

PSPT delivery systems are more involved than PBS because they require the use of multiple devices, such as range shifters, brass apertures, range compensators, and range modulator wheels, in the path of the beam that are beam and energy specific. Some of these devices have to be changed out before the next beam is delivered, but the device exchange time is slightly mitigated because plans typically have only one to three beams per treatment. In addition, a treatment room typically loses the beam to another room, inherently giving the radiation therapist enough time to make the device changes without adding any time to the total delivery time. Clearance issues are more common for PSPT because the compensator typically hangs outside of the nozzle and the size increases while the SOBP increases. This can limit the selection of beams and may require the snout position to be retracted more than desired to obtain clearance. Centers with PSPT typically have three different snout sizes: small, medium, and large. The snouts are very large and heavy and are usually changed by a group of engineers with a hydraulic system. Snout changes can take between 20 to 40 minutes, so patients with similar snout sizes are scheduled together to improve efficiency.

The primary advantage of PBS compared with PSPT is the ability to treat the patient without additional devices in the path of the beam. Eliminating the brass or other collimating devices from the path of the beam also reduces the potential radiation exposure, protons and neutrons, to the staff and patient that results from activation of the devices from the high-energy proton beams. Some proton therapy systems have added the ability to add static or dynamic collimation in imaging.

Image-guided radiation therapy is an integral part of proton therapy because of the steep falloffs of the proton beam and high degree of precision that is needed. Most centers are equipped with three x-ray tubes for kV imaging and an imaging room within the treatment vault. Some centers have implemented setup rooms because imaging can represent a large percentage of the overall setup time.[67] Patients are set up on a table that can be transferred to the treatment couch by a manual or robotic trolley. Proximity of the setup room to the treatment rooms is vital to minimize transport time. In one study, the authors concluded that the use of an external setup room can improve patient throughput as much as 30% based on their computer simulations.[67] In another study, Monte Carlo simulations were calculated with standard input parameters for one, two, and three treatment rooms and variable transporter and imaging and correction speeds. The Monte Carlo simulations show a decreasing advantage of a setup room from one to two treatment rooms, and there was no benefit for three treatment rooms in all simulations (Fig. 16.13).[68]

Volumetric imaging has not been historically included in most rooms of particle therapy centers, so off-line verification CTs are typically done in most centers to verify the patient's anatomy and tumor size. CBCT has been incorporated into second-generation proton therapy systems and is now more commonly used with proton therapy. The CBCT quality is suboptimal compared with traditional CT; therefore the added benefit of imaging the patient in the treated position with CBCT may be diminished by the imaging quality needed to accurately define the tumor and critical structures relative to the dose distribution. Some systems have incorporated dual-energy CBCTs into their systems, which have increased the quality of the CBCT and improved visualization of the soft tissue. CT-on-rails setup is another option that could provide a center with a high-resolution CT image while the patient is in the treatment position. The inclusion of in-beam positron emission tomography (PET) into proton centers may be a future development that would add the ability to see the dose deposition per fraction.[69]

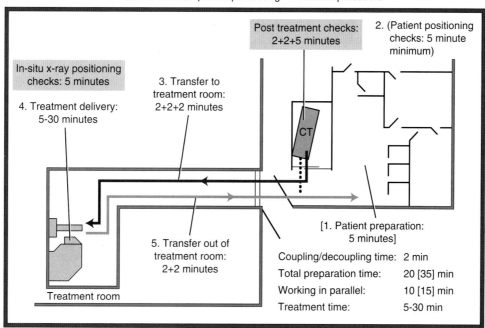

Fig. 16.13 Remote positioning setup for Paul Scherrer Institute for Proton Therapy, Switzerland. *CT*, Computed tomography.

QUALITY ASSURANCE

Many levels of quality assurance (QA) are performed throughout the entire process, from simulation through treatment. The following QA procedures are both formal and best practice recommendations.

Simulation

The QA required for the CT scanner is a very important part of the QA process because it verifies that CT scanner properties are accurate for dose calculations. It is also important to establish standards for patient immobilization. Verification of the correct proton-compatible immobilization devices is good procedure for the physicist or dosimetrist before treatment planning. Correct documentation of the setup is very important so that the treating radiation therapist uses the correct devices.

Treatment Plan Quality Assurance

All treatment plans are quality assured by a physicist before treatment. All of the treatment planning parameters in the final, physician-approved plan are cross checked in the TPS, on the printed treatment plan, and in the record and verify (R&V) software for consistency. The treatment plan is also dissected thoroughly to make sure all of the uncertainties and margins were accurately added to each beam. As discussed, one tool that is used is the robust analysis report, which shows the worst-case scenarios when setup and/or range uncertainties are applied to the plan.

Beam clearance is another check during this procedure. Most TPS software does not include a three-dimensional model of the treatment room with the selected beams, isocenter, snout position, nozzle, and treatment devices in the treatment plan. Manual verification, otherwise called a dry run, is one method to ensure that all of the selected beams clear the treatment couch, treatment devices, and patient. This reduces the risk of having to replan and delay the patient's start date, but it can be labor intensive if it has to be done for most treatment plans. Some centers have developed three-dimensional models of their treatment rooms into a software that can read the treatment plan parameters. This is a more efficient method for verifying the treatment planning parameters during the treatment planning process, but this technique also has limitations because it is not always 100% accurate. For example, it is typical that CT scans do not include the entire patient and immobilization devices; therefore the software has to make estimations in the areas that are cut off.

Device Quality Assurance

QA of the compensator and aperture design and fabrication are important for PSPT. The three-dimensional pattern for the compensator and the two-dimensional pattern for the apertures are sent electronically to a machine shop from the TPS. The software and milling machines are able to read the files and generate the appropriate "cut" patterns required for the devices. There are many different ways that the devices can be milled to achieve the same end product. The higher the resolution, the longer it takes to manufacture the device. The compensators are typically milled with tapered drill bits that cut the acrylic by plunging in and out of the compensator until it achieves the desired shape. Some of the internal patterns can be difficult to mill, especially if the compensator is very thick with extreme changes in depth. It is important to develop a technique to verify that the final design for the compensator and aperture match the TPS. There are multiple techniques that can be used. The simplest technique is to randomly select 10 points in the compensator and manually measure the depth with a special ruler. This depth is compared with the depth from the files sent from the TPS. An additional verification tool for this technique is to overlay a transparency with the compensator pattern and aperture border to visually inspect the isodepth lines match the design of the compensator. Another technique uses a CT scan of the compensator, which is then registered to the reference depth map from the TPS. Further developments are needed to make this technique more efficient and clinically acceptable.[70,71] One other technique proposed in the literature was the use of a fluoroscopic electronic portal imaging device for the verification of compensator thicknesses. The fundamental philosophy is based on the ratio of the transmission of the portal dose with and without the compensator in the beam to determine the thickness of the compensator.[72]

Dosimetric Verification

Dosimetric verification that the measured dose matches the calculated dose from the TPS is very important for particle therapy because there are so many uncertainties, especially the distal range uncertainty, that need to be considered. Formal QA procedures have not been well documented because of the variability in delivery systems and vendors and the relative infancy of the particle therapy industry. QA techniques will also differ for PSPT and PBS techniques and also between uniform scanning versus nonuniform scanning PBS. Because of the complexity of PBS dosimetric verification, it can be very time-consuming to take the measurements and analyze the data. The following publications can be referenced for an in-depth look at proton therapy QA.[73–77]

Daily Quality Assurance

Daily QA procedures are very similar to the procedures used for photon therapy. Daily QA ensures that everything inside the room is mechanically working and that the proton beam is delivering the dose with the correct output, range, and symmetry. This is very important for a facility to implement. Ding et al. list all of their QA parameters that are checked on a daily basis. The parameters are categorized based on safety, mechanical, imaging, and dosimetry, and their tolerances are included.[78]

Treatment Delivery

The treatment plans for proton therapy have unique parameters that are not conventional compared with photon therapy. Electronic medical records with R&V functionality have been adapted to treat proton therapy. This system has been more complicated to implement because there are only a small number of proton centers, and all of the vendors have similar but different parameters. Many of the accelerator vendors have created their own R&V software that records the delivered dose and verification images and then transfers this information into commercial R&V software. This process requires more information technology involvement and checks to make sure that the information between the two R&V systems is correct. The parameters should be checked daily before treatment and during the weekly QA chart checks.

Particle therapy centers use similar imaging techniques that are used for photon therapy. A set of orthogonal setup images are sent to the R&V software and are used as a standard to compare the daily portal images that are used to verify the patient's setup. The setup images are reconstructed so that metal clips or fiducials can be seen on the image. This helps the therapist verify that the isocenter is in the correct location. The delineation of setup structures can be burned into the image for additional information.

Weekly Quality Assurance

Off-line weekly or scheduled CT scans are common for patients who may have immobilization concerns, potential anatomic changes because of weight loss or tumor shrinkage, or who have significant motion in the treated area. Verification CTs are important because they help evaluate the robustness of the plan currently under treatment. The original treatment plan parameters are set to static and are applied to the weekly CTs. The resultant dose distribution is displayed on the current anatomy and compared with the original treatment plan. The treatment plan is typically changed if the target has lost significant coverage or if a critical structure dose has increased beyond comfortable levels. If a new plan is needed, then the whole treatment planning and QA process must be repeated for the new plan. The adaptive planning rate for particle therapy is higher than photon therapy because it is more sensitive to the changes listed above.

Weekly chart checks are also part of the QA process. This procedure verifies that the parameters on the first day of treatment are the same throughout the course of treatment.

SUMMARY

- Particle therapy has unique properties that give it several advantages versus conventional photon therapy.
- Its major advantage is its ability to define the maximum dose at a desired depth within the tumor with reduced entrance dose and no exit dose.
- The reduction in dose to healthy tissue near the target makes dose escalation more feasible. Dose escalation increases the likelihood of better control rates.
- The conformality of particle therapy dose distribution is achieved by apertures and compensators for PSPT and small pencil beam spots that are modulated for PBS.
- The development and advancement of the PBS technology has given particle therapy centers a highly conformal technique similar to IMRT, except the doses to healthy tissues are significantly lower.

- These benefits come at the risk of additional uncertainties. It is important for any center that implements particle therapy to fully understand these uncertainties and address them during the treatment planning process.
- The particle therapy industry is growing rapidly because of the potential of this technique, and while it grows, more technology will be developed to help address the uncertainties and make the therapy safer.
- The entire clinical team, from the simulation process through treatment delivery, plays an important role in particle therapy.

REVIEW QUESTIONS

The answers to the Review Questions can be found by logging on to our website at: http://evolve.elsevier.com/Washington/principles

1. What is the name of the peak of maximum dose for particle therapy?
   a. Rutherford peak.
   b. Lawrence peak.
   c. Proton peak.
   d. Bragg peak.
2. What device is used to spread out the maximum dose?
   a. Synchrotron.
   b. Range modulator wheel.
   c. Cyclotron.
   d. Energy absorber.
3. What is created at the end of the beam for cyclotrons, which is more than synchrotrons?
   a. Neutrons.
   b. Alpha particles.
   c. Beta particles.
   d. Electrons.

4. Why is the compensator "smeared?"
   a. To make the design more smooth.
   b. To make the compensator easier for quality assurance.
   c. To modify the design so that it can take into account internal motion and setup error.
   d. To reduce the impact of the compensator on the dose distribution.
5. What is the most common device used for collimating the dose for passive scattered particle therapy?
   a. Cerrobend.
   b. Brass.
   c. Tin.
   d. Aluminum.
6. What is the relative biologic effectiveness for proton therapy?
   a. 1.1.
   b. 5.0.
   c. 1.6.
   d. 0.5.
7. What margins are added to the target to take into account the range uncertainty of particle therapy beams?
   a. Anterior and posterior margins.
   b. Uniform margins.
   c. Superior and inferior margins.
   d. Proximal and distal margins.
8. What analysis can be generated to test the treatment plan with range uncertainties and setup errors applied?
   a. Security analysis.
   b. Robust analysis.
   c. Simulated analysis.
   d. Delivery analysis.
9. What is the term to describe the passively scattered proton therapy approach to treat complex tumor shapes by matching two fields together based on their penumbra?
   a. Squaring.
   b. Circling.
   c. Ranging.
   d. Patch planning.
10. Are all particle therapy beams treated with a rotational gantry?
   a. Yes.
   b. No.

QUESTIONS TO PONDER

1. What are the advantages of particle therapy for each treatment site compared with photon therapy?
2. What treatment areas should be investigated that have not already been done?
3. How do you envision the role of particle therapy in radiation oncology while the industry continues to grow?

REFERENCES

1. Particle therapy facilities in operation. Particle Therapy Co-Operative Group (PTCOG) website. http://ptcog.web.psi.ch/ptcentres.html. Accessed April 18, 2019.
2. Brown A, Suit H. The centenary of the discovery of the Bragg peak. *Radiother Oncol.* 2004;73:265–268.
3. Wilson RR. Radiological use of fast protons. *Radiology.* 1946;47:487–491.
4. Levy RP, Blakely EA, Chu WT, et al. The current status and future directions of heavy charged particle therapy in medicine. *AIP Conf Proc.* 2008;1099:410–425.
5. Coutrakon GB. Accelerators for heavy-charged-particle radiation therapy. *Technol Cancer Res Treat.* 2007;6(suppl 4):49–54.
6. Peach K, Wilson P, Jones B. Accelerator science in medical physics. *Br J Radiol.* 2011;84(1):S4–S10.
7. Koehler AM, Schneider RJ, Sisterson JM. Flattening of proton dose distributions for large-field radiotherapy. *Med Phys.* 1977;4:297–301.
8. Koehler AM, Schneider RJ, Sisterson JM. Range modulations for protons and heavy ions. *Nucl Instrum Methods.* 1975;131:437–440.
9. Wagner MS. Automated range compensation for proton therapy. *Med Phys.* 1982;9:749–752.
10. Urie M, Goitein M, Wagner M. Compensating for heterogeneities in proton therapy. *Phys Med Biol.* 1983;29:553–566.
11. Moyers MF, Miller DW, Bush DA, et al. Methodologies and tools for proton beam design for lung tumors. *Int J Radiat Oncol Biol Phys.* 2001;49:1429–1438.
12. Daartz K, Bangert M, Bussiere MR, et al. Characterization of a mini-multileaf collimator in a proton beamline. *Med Phys.* 2009;36(5):1886–1894.
13. Moskvin V, Cheng CW, Das IJ. Pitfalls of tungsten multileaf collimator in proton beam therapy. *Med Phys.* 2011;38(12):6395–6406.
14. Diffenderfer ES, Ainsley CG, Kirk ML, et al. Comparison of secondary neutron dose in proton therapy resulting from the use of a tungsten alloy MLC or a brass collimator system. *Med Phys.* 2011;38(11):6248–6256.
15. DeLaney T, Kooy H. *Proton and Charged Particle Radiotherapy.* Philadelphia, PA: Lippincott Williams & Wilkins; 2008, 1–320.
16. Wambersie A. RBE, reference RBE and clinical RBE: applications of these concepts in hadron therapy. *Strahlenther Onkol.* 1999;17(suppl 2):39–43.
17. Paganetti H. Significance and implementation of RBE variations in proton beam therapy. *Technol Cancer Res Treat.* 2003;2:413–426.
18. Weyrather WK, Kraft G. RBE of carbon ions: experimental data and the strategy of RBE calculation for treatment planning. *Radiother Oncol.* 2004;73(suppl 2):S161–S169.
19. Dale RG, Jones B, Carabe-Fernandez A. Why more needs to be known about RBE effects in modern radiotherapy. *Appl Radiat Isot.* 2009;67(3):387–392.
20. Robertson JB, Williams JR, Schmidt RA, et al. Radiobiological studies of a high-energy modulated proton beam utilizing cultured mammalian cells. *Cancer.* 1975;35(6). 166-1677.
21. Washington C, Leaver D. *Principles and Practice of Radiation Therapy.* 4th ed. 2016, St. Louis, MO: Elsevier.
22. Wroe AJ, Bush DA, Slater JD. Immobilization considerations for proton radiation therapy. *Technol Cancer Res Treat.* 2014;13. 217-216.
23. Wang KK, Vapiwala N, Deville C, et al. A study to quantify the effectiveness of daily endorectal balloon for prostate intrafraction motion management. *Int J Radiat Oncol Biol Phys.* 2012;83(3):1055–1063.
24. Paganetti H. Range uncertainties in proton therapy and the role of Monte Carlo simulations. *Phys Med Biol.* 2012;57:R99–R117.
25. Mustapha AA, Jackson DF. The relation between x-ray CT numbers and charged particles stopping powers and its significance for radiotherapy treatment planning. *Phys Med Biol.* 1983;28:169–176.
26. Schneider U, Pedroni E, Lomax A. The calibration of CT Hounsfield units for radiotherapy treatment planning. *Phys Med Biol.* 1996;41:111–124.

27. Schaffner B, Pedroni E. The precision of proton range calculations in proton radiotherapy treatment planning: experimental verification of the relation between CT-HU and proton stopping power. *Phys Med Biol.* 1998;43:1579–1592.

28. Moyers M, Sardesai M, Sun S, et al. Ion stopping powers and CT numbers. *Med Dosim.* 2010;35(3):179–194.

29. Hanson KM, Bradbury JN, Cannon TM, et al. Computed tomography using proton energy loss. *Phys Med Biol.* 1981;26(6):965–983.

30. Petti PL. Differential-pencil-beam dose calculations for charged particles. *Med Phys.* 1992;19:137–149.

31. Petti PL. Evaluation of a pencil-beam dose calculation technique for charged particle radiotherapy. *Int J Radiat Oncol Biol Phys.* 1996;35:1049–1057.

32. Urie M, Goitein M, Holley WR, et al. Degradation of the Bragg peak due to inhomogeneities. *Phys Med Biol.* 1986;31:1–15.

33. Sawakuchi GO, Titt U, Mirkovic D, et al. Density heterogeneities and the influence of multiple Coulomb and nuclear scatterings on the Bragg peak distal edge of proton therapy beams. *Phys Med Biol.* 2008;53:4605–4619.

34. Goitein M. The measurement of tissue heterodensity to guide charged particle radiotherapy. *Int J Radiat Oncol Biol Phys.* 1977;3:27–33.

35. Goitein M, Sisterson JM. The influence of thick inhomogeneities on charged particle beams. *Radiat Res.* 1978;74:217–230.

36. Paganetti H, Goitein M. Radiobiological significance of beam line dependent proton energy distributions in a spread-out Bragg peak. *Med Phys.* 2000;27:1119–1126.

37. Carabe A, Moteabbed M, Depauw N, et al. Range uncertainty in proton therapy due to variable biological effectiveness. *Phys Med Biol.* 2012;57:1159–1172.

38. Robertson JB, Williams JR, Schmidt RA, et al. Radiobiological studies of a high-energy modulated proton beam utilizing cultured mammalian cells. *Cancer.* 1975;35. 1664–1177.

39. Wouters BG, Lam GKY, Oelfke U, et al. RBE measurement on the 70MeVproton beam atTRIUMFusingV79 cells and the high precision cell sorter assay. *Radiat Res.* 1996;146:159–170.

40. International Commission on Radiation Units & Measurements. Prescribing, recording, and reporting photon beam therapy (ICRU Report 50). Available at: https://icru.org/home/reports/prescribing-recording-and-reporting-photon-beam-therapy-report-50. Published 1993. Accessed April 18, 2019.

41. International Commission on Radiation Units & Measurements. Prescribing, recording, and reporting proton beam therapy (ICRU Report 78). Available at https://icru.org/home/reports/prescribing-recording-and-reporting-proton-beam-therapy-icru-report-78. Published 2009. Accessed April 18, 2019.

42. Park P, Zhu R, Lee A, et al. A beam-specific planning target volume (PTV) design for proton therapy to account for setup and range uncertainties. *Int J Radiat Oncol Biol Phys.* 2012;82(2):e/.

43. Rietzel E, Bert C. Respiratory motion management in particle therapy. *Med Phys.* 2010;37:449–460.

44. Kraus KM, Heath E, Oelfke U. Dosimetric consequences of tumor motion due to respiration for a scanned proton beam. *Phys Med Biol.* 2011;56. 6563–6381.

45. Seco J, Robertson D, Trofimov A, et al. Breathing interplay effects during proton beam scanning: simulation and statistical analysis. *Phys Med Biol.* 2009;54:N283–N294.

46. Zhang Y, Boye D, Tanner C, et al. Respiratory liver motion estimation and its effect on scanned proton beam therapy. *Phys Med Biol.* 2012;57:1779–1795.

47. Zenklusen SM, Pedroni E, Meer D. A study on repainting strategies for treating moderately moving targets with proton pencil beam scanning at the new Gantry 2 at PSI. *Phys Med Biol.* 2010;55:5103–5121.

48. Liu W, Zhang X, Li Y, et al. Robust optimization of intensity modulated proton therapy. *Med Phys.* 2012;39:1079–1091.

49. Ma C, Lomax T. *Proton and Carbon Ion Therapy.* 2012, Boca Raton, FL: CRC Press.

50. Li Z. Toward robust proton therapy planning and delivery. *Transl Cancer Res.* 2012;1(3):217–226.

51. Palmer MB. The optimal timing for off-line adaptive planning for head and neck intensity modulated proton therapy (IMPT) is week 4. Presentation at the meeting of American Society for Radiation Oncology. Boston, MA; 2012.

52. Shi W, Nichols RC, Flampouri S, et al. Tumour shrinkage during proton-based chemoradiation for non-small-cell lung cancer may necessitate adaptive replanning during treatment. *Hong Kong J Radiol.* 2011;14:190–194.

53. Shi W, Nichols RC, Flampouri S, et al. Proton-based chemoradiation for synchronous bilateral non-small-cell lung cancers: a case report. *Thoracic Cancer.* 2012;4(2):198–202.

54. Hui Z, Zhang X, Starkschall G, et al. Effects of interfractional motion and anatomic changes on proton therapy dose distribution in lung cancer. *Int J Radiat Oncol Biol Phys.* 2008;72:1385–1395.

55. Koay EJ, Lege D, Mohan R, et al. Adaptive/nonadaptive proton radiation planning and outcomes in a Phase II trial for locally advanced non-small cell lung cancer. *Int J Radiat Oncol Biol Phys.* 2012;84(5):1093–1100.

56. Beltran C, Naik M, Merchant TE. Dosimetric effect of target expansion and setup uncertainty during radiation therapy in pediatric craniopharyngiomas. *Radiother Oncol.* 2010;97:399–403.

57. Beltran C, Roca M, Merchant TE. On the benefits and risks of proton therapy in pediatric craniopharyngiomas. *Int J Radiat Oncol Biol Phys.* 2012;82:e281–e287.

58. Albertini F, Bolsi A, Lomax AJ, et al. Sensitivity of intensity modulated proton therapy plans to changes in patient weight. *Radiother Oncol.* 2008;86:187–194.

59. Swanson EL, Indelicato DJ, Louis D, et al. Comparison of three-dimensional (3D) conformal proton radiotherapy (RT), 3D conformal photon RT, and intensity-modulated RT for retroperitoneal and intra-abdominal sarcomas. *Int J Radiat Oncol Biol Phys.* 2012;83:1549–1557.

60. Nichols Jr RC, Huh SN, Prado KL, et al. Protons offer reduced normal-tissue exposure for patients receiving postoperative radiotherapy for resected pancreatic head cancer. *Int J Radiat Oncol Biol Phys.* 2012;83:158–163.

61. Vargas C, Mahajan C, Fryer A, et al. Rectal dose-volume differences using proton radiotherapy and a rectal balloon or water alone for the treatment of prostate cancer. *Int J Radiat Oncol Biol Phys.* 2007;69:1110–1116.

62. Hug EB, Adams J, Fitzek M, et al. Fractionated, three-dimensional, planning-assisted proton-radiation therapy for orbital rhabdomyosarcoma: a novel technique. *Int J Radiat Oncol Biol Phys.* 2000;47(4):979–984.

63. Li Y, Zhang X, Dong L, et al. A novel patch-field design using an optimized grid filter for passively scattered proton beams. *Phys Med Biol.* 2007;52:N265–N275.

64. Li Y, Kardar L, Li X, et al. On the interplay effects with proton scanning beams in stage III lung cancer. *Med Phys.* 2014;41:021721.

65. Grassberger C, Dowdell S, Lomax AJ, et al. Motion interplay as a function of patient parameters and spot size in spot scanning proton therapy for lung cancer. *Int J Radiat Oncol Biol Phys.* 2013;86:380–386.

66. Lomax AJ, Pedroni E, Rutz HP, et al. The clinical potential of intensity modulated proton therapy. *Med Phys.* 2004;14:147–152.

67. Bolsi A, Lomax AJ, Pedroni E, et al. Experiences at the Paul Scherrer Institute with a remote patient positioning procedure for high-throughput proton radiation therapy. *Int J Radiat Oncol Biol Phys.* 2008;71(5):1581–1590.

68. Fava G, Widesott L, Fellin F, et al. In-gantry or remote patient positioning? Monte Carlo simulations for proton therapy centers of different sizes. *Radiother Oncol.* 2012;103(1):18–24.

69. Enghardt W, Parodi K, Crespo P, et al. Dose quantification from in-beam positron emission tomography. *Radiother Oncol.* 2004;73(suppl 2):S96–S98.

70. Li H, Zhang L, Dong L, et al. A CT-based software tool for evaluating compensator quality in passively scattered proton therapy. *Phys Med Biol.* 2010;55:6759–6771.

71. Yoon M, Kim J, Shin D, et al. Computerized tomography-based quality assurance tool for proton range compensators. *Med Phys.* 2008;35(8):3511–3517.

72. Pasma K, Kroonwijk M, van Dieren E, et al. Verification of compensator thicknesses using a fluoroscopic electronic portal imaging device. *Med Phys.* 1999;25(8):1524–1529.

73. Arjomandy B, Sahoo N, Ciangaru G, et al. Verification of patient specific dose distributions in proton therapy using a commercial two-dimensional ion chamber array. *Med Phys*. 2010;37(11). 5831–5387.

74. Pedroni E, Scheib S, Böhringer T, et al. Experimental characterization and physical modelling of the dose distribution of scanned proton pencil beams. *Phys Med Biol*. 2005;50:541–561.

75. Boon N, Van Luijk P, Schippers M, et al. Fast 2D phantom dosimetry for scanning proton beams. *Med Phys*. 1998;25:464–475.

76. Arjomandy B, Sahoo N, Ding X, et al. Use of a two-dimensional ionization chamber array for proton therapy beam quality assurance. *Med Phys*. 2008;35(9):3889–3894.

77. Zhu R, Poenisch F, Song X, et al. Patient-specific quality assurance for prostate cancer patients receiving spot scanning proton therapy using single-field uniform dose. *Int J Radiat Oncol Biol Phys*. 2011;81(2):552–559.

78. Ding X, Zheng Y, Ziedan O, et al. A novel daily QA system for proton therapy. *J Appl Clin Med Phys*. 2013;14(2):115–126.

17

Radiation Safety and Protection

Lawrence T. Dauer

INTRODUCTION

The importance of awareness of radiation protection is paramount for professionals who work in the field of radiation oncology. Concerns about exposure to doses of radiation are deeply rooted in the early history of our field. Many of the early pioneers developed radiation-associated diseases, some of which were fatal, in part because the deleterious effects of radiation on human tissue were not completely understood. Marie Curie herself suffered from the effects of the doses she received during her early work with radium-226 (^{226}Ra) and her work with x-ray equipment on the battlefield in World War I.[1] Since that early experience, we have continued to refine our understanding and methods. This chapter will discuss the general principles of radiation protection within the environment of a radiation oncology facility, but the principles outlined are not a substitute for an understanding of the individualized program for a facility.

UNITS

Exposure

The unit exposure is the oldest unit used to describe the interactions of radiation. Exposure is only applicable to photons (i.e., x-rays and gamma rays while they interact in air). Exposure is defined as the amount of ionization produced by photons in air per unit mass of air. The unit of exposure is the roentgen (R). The unit of charge is the coulomb (C).

$$1 \text{ R} = 2.48 \times 10^{-4} \text{ C/kg of air}$$

For practical reasons, the use of exposure is limited to photons with energies below 3 MeV.

Absorbed Dose

The unit absorbed dose is defined as the amount of energy absorbed per mass of any material while radiation interacts in the material. Unlike exposure, absorbed dose is not limited to air. The traditional unit of absorbed dose is the **rad**. Both the erg and the joule are units of energy. In the Système International (SI) nomenclature, the unit of absorbed dose is the gray (Gy).

$$1 \text{ rad} = 100 \text{ erg/g}$$

$$1 \text{ Gy} = 1 \text{ J/kg}$$

Because 1 Gy = 100 rad or 1 rad = 1 cGy, the current standard also includes the use of cGy to describe the absorbed dose.

Equivalent Dose

The unit **equivalent dose** is an attempt to account for the biologic effects of different types of radiations as they interact in tissue. Radiations such as alpha particles and neutrons deposit more energy per unit path length than photons. The energy deposited per unit path length is called **linear energy transfer (LET)**, with units of keV/ μm. For alpha particles, the LET may be 100 keV/μm, whereas for photons, the LET may be 1 keV/μm. To account for these differences, the absorbed dose is multiplied by a **radiation weighting** factor (w_R) to produce a new unit called equivalent dose. The traditional unit of is the rem or, in the SI nomenclature, the Sv.

$$\text{rem} = \text{rad} \times w_R$$

$$\text{Sv} = 100 \text{ rem} = \text{gray} \times w_R$$

Activity

The unit **activity** defines the number of radioactive disintegrations (transformations) per unit of time. This unit was originally based on the disintegrations measured from 1 g of radium in equilibrium with its daughter products. Using the instrumentation available at the time, 1 g of radium was equal to 1 **curie (Ci)** of activity. More modern methods have shown this statement to be slightly incorrect. However, in some therapeutic applications described in older texts, activity is defined in terms of milligrams of radium.

$$\text{curie} = 3.7 \times 10^{10} \text{ disintegrations / second}$$

This is a very large amount of activity, and typically smaller subdivisions of the curie are used (e.g., the millicurie [mCi] and the microcurie [μCi]). In the SI nomenclature, the unit of activity is the **becquerel (Bq)**.

$$1 \text{ Bq} = 1 \text{ disintegration / second}$$

$$1 \text{ Ci} = 3.7 \times 10^{10} \text{ Bq}$$

Table 17.1 provides a summary of the traditional and SI units.

NATURAL BACKGROUND RADIATION

Radiation is a part of our natural environment. Among the contributions to natural background are radiations that reach our planet from high-energy photon emissions beyond our atmosphere, chiefly from our sun. These radiations are the so-called "cosmic radiation." The earth's atmosphere absorbs some of these emitted radiations before

TABLE 17.1 Traditional and International System of Units

Quantity	Traditional Unit	SI Unit
Exposure	roentgen (R)	2.58×10^{-4} C/kg
Activity	Curie (Ci)	becquerel (Bq)
Absorbed dose	rad	gray (Gy)
Dose equivalent	rem	sievert (Sv)
Linear energy transfer	keV/μm	

SI, International System of Units.

TABLE 17.2 Sources of Natural Background Radiation[2]

Source	Dose/Year
Cosmic radiation	33 mrem; 0.33 msv
Terrestrial radiation	21 mrem; 0.21 msv
Internal exposure	29 mrem; 0.29 msv
Radon and Thoran	228 mrem; 2.1 msv

Modified from National Council on Radiation Protection and Measurements. *Ionizing Radiation Exposure of the Population of the United States.* Report 160. Bethesda, MD: National Council on Radiation Protection and Measurements; 2018.

they reach the planet's surface. The contribution to natural background radiation varies according to location on the earth (latitude and longitude), sun-spot cycles, and height above sea level. In the United States, the amount of cosmic radiation in Denver is approximately twice the amount at sea level.

The soil and mineral elements in the earth itself contain small amounts of naturally occurring radioactive materials. As might be expected, areas that have a high mineral content have higher amounts of these radioactive materials and higher background radiations. Across the United States, these contributions may vary by a factor of four. Because we too are made of elements, some of those are radioactive. The largest contribution to internal exposure is from potassium-40 (^{40}K), which amounts to approximately 20 mrem or 0.2 mSv/year. Radon, a radioactive gas, is found in the atmosphere and in areas rich in granite formations. The average concentration in the United States is approximately1 pCi/L (37 mBq/L), which results in a dose of approximately 200 mrem (2 mSv)/year. The usual value quoted for natural background dose to the US population is 300 mrem or 3 mSv total.

See Table 17.2 for a summary table for natural background radiation.

Medical Exposures

In addition to natural background radiation, the population is also exposed through medical applications of radiation, primarily through diagnostic x-rays. This dose has been steadily increasing as a result of the greater availability of computed tomography (CT) technology. The medical exposure to the population reported in 1987 contributed approximately 15% to individual radiation exposure totals; the medical exposure rate in 2009 was 48%.[2] The National Council on Radiation Protection and Measurements (NCRP) now estimates that doses from medical CT applications may be approaching the amount that the population receives from the natural background.

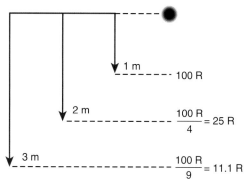

Fig. 17.1 Inverse square law relationship. Radiation exposure from a small source is dependent on the inverse square of the distance from the surface. For example, if the distance is doubled, the exposure is reduced to one fourth of the original value. *m*, Meter; *R*, roentgen.

FOUNDATIONS

The principles of "time, distance, and shielding" are usually considered the cornerstones of radiation protection. The paragraphs below discuss some applications of these principles.

Time

It would seem obvious that the less time one is exposed to radiation or is in the vicinity of radiation sources, the lower the dose received. From a practical view, the application of this maxim is seldom possible in the radiation oncology department. Although few are still in operation in the United States, the concept of "time" is important in the use of cobalt-60 (^{60}Co) teletherapy units. Because the source is never "off" in these treatment units, it would seem logical to spend as little time as possible in the treatment room. Similarly, patients treated with interstitial implants (see Chapter 14) may have measurable exposure rates because of radioactive sources on their person, and time spent in their vicinity should be limited.

Distance

An increase in distance from a source of radiation will dramatically reduce radiation exposure. The inverse square law is generally applicable to sources approximating a point source. Doubling the distance from a source will reduce the dose rate by a factor of four. If the distance is tripled, the dose rate will decrease by a factor of nine (Fig. 17.1).

Even for larger sources, the falloff of the dose rate with an increase in distance will be dramatic.

Shielding

In the radiation oncology department, shielding is used for many applications. Its application for facility design is discussed in another section of this chapter. The choice of shielding material depends on the energy of the radiation. Lead is often thought of as the preferred shielding material because of its weight and density. This application is true at lower energies in the diagnostic region because the primary interaction is photoelectric events. However, although the energy increases into the region where Compton events are the predominant interaction, other materials such as concrete or steel may be used based on space and cost. The thicknesses required will be different for each material. For new installations with no space restrictions, large rooms and concrete barriers may be the most economic choices.

REGULATORS

The use of radiation is one of the most regulated of the professions. To help sort out the alphabet soup, the various groups will be sorted by category.

Federal Agencies

The most prominent and important of all federal regulators is the Nuclear Regulatory Commission (NRC). Originally established as the Atomic Energy Commission in 1954, the role of the current NRC has evolved during several decades. The Commission initially controlled the by-products of atomic fission and products produced by irradiation in a reactor. Examples of such materials include iodine-131 (^{131}I), strontium-90 (^{90}Sr), and ^{60}Co. More recently, the Commission has expanded its role to include radioactive materials made in accelerators, such as cyclotrons (e.g., fluorine-18 [^{18}F]) and naturally occurring radioactive materials (e.g., ^{226}Ra and radon-222 [^{222}Rn]). The regulations of the NRC are published in Title 10 of the Code of Federal Regulations.[3] The medical uses of radiation are published as Part 35 of Title 10, 10CFR35, and the standards for dose limits are published as Part 20, 10CFR20.[4]

Regulations governing the shipment of radioactive materials are contained in the regulations of the US Department of Transportation, Title 49.[5] These regulations specify the packaging of materials, information to be placed on the package, information for the shipper, and the allowable means of transportation. As an example, shipments of radioactive materials may be transported by passenger and cargo aircraft where regulations specify the allowable dose rates for these packages.

The US Food and Drug Administration (FDA) also plays a role with regard to radiopharmaceuticals and radiation-producing equipment. X-ray machines, including linear accelerators, cannot be offered for sale unless the FDA has reviewed the claims made by the manufacturer and the electrical safety of the unit. The regulations of the FDA concerning radiopharmaceuticals are found in Title 21 of the Code of Federal Regulations.[6] These regulations delineate the routine and investigational use of radioactive materials and the pharmacy restrictions for these uses.

State Agencies

The role of state agencies has also evolved. State regulations specify the parameters for diagnostic x-ray equipment. The regulations may vary from state to state, but in general, they specify the frequency with which certain measurements must be performed, the limits these measurements must meet, and, in some states, who is qualified to perform these measurements. In most states, simulators, which are not intended for diagnostic applications, do not need to meet the dose limits for diagnostic equipment. For cases in which positron emission tomography/CT units are used for simulation, the units must meet the state requirements for radioactive materials and for the CT portion of the exam. Accreditation of these units is discussed below.

State agencies also have jurisdiction over radioactive materials. Certain states are designated as "agreement states." Agreement states have entered into contracts or agreements with the NRC that give them the authority to license and inspect by-products, sources, or special nuclear materials used or possessed within their borders. Under these agreements, the NRC has relinquished regulatory control over certain by-product, source, and special nuclear material uses in the state. NRC periodically assesses the compatibility and adequacy of the state's program for consistency with the national radioactive materials programs.

Accrediting Agencies

The Joint Commission. The Joint Commission (TJC), formerly The Joint Commission on the Accreditation of Health Care Organizations, accredits healthcare facilities, including hospitals and clinics, which meet the standards established by the Commission.[7] Surveyors from the Commission, including at least a physician, a nurse, and an administrator, conduct a site visit to each facility on a periodic basis (e.g., once every 3 years). Part of their site visit includes a review of practice standards in radiation oncology and radiology. Without accreditation from TJC, facilities cannot receive Medicare or Medicaid reimbursement. Most recently, TJC has begun to accredit practices in radiology and to issue requirements regarding the radiation dose to patients from CT and interventional radiology procedures. More information can be found on the TJC website at www.jointcommission.org.

American College of Radiology. The American College of Radiology (ACR) is a sponsor of the American Board of Radiology, which certifies physicians and physicists in therapeutic radiology and in radiation oncology physics, respectively. The ACR also accredits practice in ultrasound, mammography, magnetic resonance imaging, and molecular imaging.[7,21] An accreditation is given in radiation oncology to facilities that meet ACR standards. This accreditation is typically given for a 3-year period, with site visits for the initial accreditation and renewal of accreditation. Site visitors include both physicists and radiation oncologists. The ACR accreditation is required for Medicare and Medicaid reimbursement.

Facilities may also be accredited by the American College of Radiation Oncology,[8] which has established standards for the practice of radiation oncology. Depending on the individual state, either accreditation by the ACR or by the American College of Radiation Oncology may be acceptable.

Recently, the American Society for Radiation Oncology (ASTRO)[9] has announced that it intends to establish an accreditation process for radiation oncology practice, separate from the accreditation process of the ACR.

Voluntary Organizations

Various scientific organizations offer voluntary standards through a series of reports. Some of these voluntary standards eventually find their way into regulation.

National Council on Radiation Protection and Measurements. Possibly the most influential organization that issues reports is the NCRP. Their reports cover all the radiation-associated industries from nuclear power to space travel to medicine. Their reports are referenced later in this section. The NCRP issues reports that are available in pamphlet form or online.[10]

American Association of Physicists in Medicine and American Society for Therapeutic Radiology. Both the American Association of Physicists in Medicine and ASTRO issue reports covering a variety of topics including quality assurance and performance improvement. These reports may be published in their journals or online. The reports are intended to establish the standards for good practice.[11]

DOSE LIMITS

The evolution of dose-limiting recommendations extends from the discovery of radiation. Initially, there were no limits for persons working with either radioactive sources or radiation-producing equipment, and the biologic effects of radiation on persons administering radiation treatment were not well understood. Many of the early pioneers suffered from cancers and radiation-induced deterministic effects. Because the application of radium and radiation treatments were regarded as a panacea, secondary cancers and radiation effects were seen in patients treated for skin diseases such as ringworm, deformities such as alkylosing spondylitis, and other noncancer problems. By the time the Manhattan project was carried out in the 1940s, dose limits had been implemented. The Japanese populations of Hiroshima and Nagasaki were and remain a living laboratory for the study of radiation damage in humans. The reports of the United Nations Subcommittee on the Effects of Atomic Radiation[12] continue to be issued and to document radiation effects on the second and third generations of survivors. These reports and others of human experiences of radiation have been incorporated into the Reports of the National Academy of Science, the so-called BEIR (Biological Effects of Ionizing Radiation) reports, which periodically review the human experience of radiation damage and recommend radiation risk values to be used in deriving dose limits.[13]

Radiation effects can be divided into nonstochastic and stochastic effects. Nonstochastic effects have a threshold for induction and the severity of the effect increases with dose. Examples of these effects include erythema, epilation, and cataract formation. Stochastic effects have no induction threshold and are proportional to the dose received. Examples of these effects include cancer induction, genetic effects, and teratogenic effects. The radiobiology of these effects and dose modeling are discussed in Chapter 4. Regardless of which model is used, it is generally agreed that the smaller the dose of radiation, the lower the risk.

As Low As Reasonably Achievable

In general, the term **ALARA** (as **l**ow as **r**easonably **a**chievable) is used to describe the philosophy of dose-limiting principles. The dose to be received must be as low as can reasonably be achieved with normal dose-limiting precautions. The term "reasonable" assumes that there is a benefit to be derived from the dose that can be achieved at a nominal or reasonable cost. Comparisons for radiation workers are made with workers in so-called "safe industries" in which the risk of injury is approximately 1 in 10,000 per year. Because radiation-induced effects may exhibit a latent period (i.e., a time before the injury is expressed), these comparisons are difficult. The reports of the NCRP review and recommend dose limits for both radiation workers and the general public.[14,6] The limits recommended by the NCRP are shown in Table 17.3. The dose for occupational workers is higher than that for the general public because the number of radiation workers is relatively small in comparison to the population as a whole. It is believed that the risk to this group is offset by the benefits to the entire population. However, it is also believed that the risks incurred are within acceptable limits. The recommended dose limits exclude doses from the natural background and from medical and dental procedures.

The developing cells of young children and embryos have been shown to be more sensitive to the effects of radiation than the cells of adults. Therefore the dose limits for these groups are lower than the limits for occupational workers. The dose limits for the general public are even lower because the entire population would be affected by these doses. There are also lower limits for pregnant women, which are essentially one-tenth of the occupational limit. The declaration of pregnancy by a woman is voluntary. Once a pregnancy is declared, the woman should discuss her work environment with the radiation safety officer (RSO). The RSO may recommend modifications to the work environment and may issue a special monitor to be worn by the woman during her pregnancy.

TABLE 17.3 Radiation Weighting Factors for Various Ionizing Radiations

Type of Radiation	Radiation Weighting Factor
Photons	1
Electrons and muons	1
Protons and charged pions	2
Neutrons	2.5–20 (depending on energy)
Alpha particles, fission fragments, heavy ions	20

Genetically Significant Dose

The term **genetically significant dose (GSD)** is a measure of the genetic risk to the population as a whole from exposure to ionizing radiation to some or all members of the population. The GSD is the dose that, if received by every member of a population, would be expected to result in the same total genetic effect on the population as the sum of the individual doses actually received. Not everyone contributes equally to the GSD. Doses received by persons beyond child-bearing potential have no effect on the GSD. A dose received by a young person (e.g., a teenager) has a higher weighting factor because younger people have a longer reproductive life. NCRP report number 93 discusses the GSD for the US population.

PERSONNEL MONITORING

In general, persons entering areas in which radiation-producing equipment or radioactive materials are used are issued personnel monitors. The decision of whether to issue monitors is left to the judgment of the facility RSO and may vary from facility to facility.

The general purpose of personnel monitoring is to estimate the doses received by individuals working in or entering radiation areas. The monitor also allows administrative staff to confirm the radiation environment present and provides a permanent record of doses received. In general, personnel monitors are required to be worn by persons who have the potential to receive 10% of the occupational dose limits.

Film Monitors

The "traditional" personnel monitor relied on the use of a film in a light-tight wrapper approximately smaller than the size of a dental film pack. The film was placed in a holder with a clip and assigned on an individual basis. Film is inherently energy dependent and subject to heat and humidity artifacts. To assess the radiation energy responsible for an exposure, individual filters were added to the film holder. After the film was developed, it was read by a person using a light densitometer. The optical density under each filter was compared with an unfiltered portion of the film, and an estimation of the dose and energy of the radiation responsible for the dose was given. One other major problem with film is that it ages within a relatively short period and the information on the film could not be retrieved after a period of time, approximately 6 months. If the film monitor was stored in a high heat or high humidity environment, artifacts affecting the accuracy of the reading might also result. Film was relatively inexpensive, but it is gradually being replaced as a primary monitor in many facilities.

Thermoluminescent Dosimeters

Thermoluminescent dosimeters (TLD) are small in size and have found a variety of applications in radiation oncology, including measurements on patients under treatment. The dosimeter consists of a crystal substance that when irradiated has electrons displaced in its crystal lattice. A typical crystalline substance used for personnel monitoring is lithium fluoride (LiF). When the crystal is heated, the electrons return to their normal locations (i.e., they return to the original energy states [original valence bands]), with the emission of characteristic energy that can be seen as light by using a detector, a photomultiplier tube, coupled to a reader. The dose received is proportional to the radiation damage in the crystal. This reading can only be done once, which is a limiting factor. The TLD badge also contains filters to account for different energies or types of radiation. Although small numbers of TLD badges can be read by an individual institution, the requirements for standardization and calibration generally require a commercial service.

Optically Stimulated Luminescence Dosimeters

One of the newest technologies available for personnel monitoring is the use of badges containing optically stimulated luminescent dosimeters (OSL). These badges also contain crystals, but are read by laser technology. They can be read for as long as 1 year after irradiation and do not exhibit heat or humidity artifacts. Filters are used in these badges as well to estimate the quality of the radiation responsible for the reading. Because of the small size of the OSL itself, the dosimeters are also finding increasing applications in patient measurement in radiation oncology.

> Optically stimulated luminescent dosimeters (OSL) have, for the most part, replaced film-badge dosimeters for personnel monitoring.

RADIATION MEASUREMENT

Although the interactions of radiation in matter cannot ordinarily be seen or felt by human senses, instruments have been developed which can detect radiation interactions. Some of these instruments are specialized, and not every instrument is suitable for all purposes. An instrument called an "ionization chamber" detects the ionizations produced by the interactions in a gas, usually air, in a contained volume of the gas. An ionization chamber can, therefore be used to measure exposure directly. Specialized ion chambers may be used to measure the output (i.e., the dose rate) at the isocenter of a linear accelerator. This same instrument would not be suitable for radiation safety applications such the measurement of transmitted dose rate and exposure rate through a wall of a shielded room or the exposure rate from a patient implanted with iodine-125 (^{125}I) seeds. In this section, we will discuss the various types of instruments used as survey devices in radiation protection and some of their applications.

Ionization Chamber Survey Meters

Portable ionization chamber survey meters are used to give a measurement of exposure in specific situations. In this case, the detector and the electronics are contained in one device that can be moved easily from place to place (Fig. 17.2). The device reads directly in exposure per unit of time (e.g., milliroentgen/hour). There are a variety of scales available that increase or decrease the sensitivity of the device. If an ion chamber "pegs" (i.e., goes to the highest point on the scale and remains there), the radiation field is larger than the ability of the instrument to give a reading. Such situations need to be evaluated by a radiation safety professional.

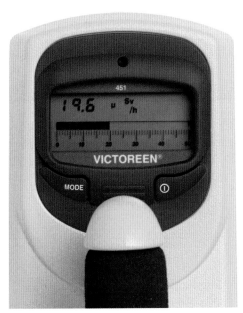
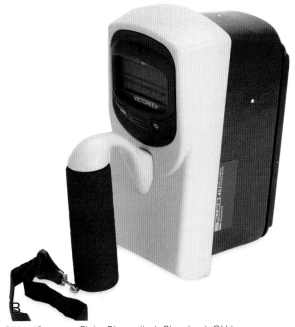

Fig. 17.2 A 451B Ion Chamber Survey Meter with Beta Slide. (Courtesy Fluke Biomedical, Cleveland, OH.)

Geiger-Müller Detectors

The Geiger-Müller (GM) detector is the classic radiation survey instrument. When people think of the detection of radioactivity, they picture this "clicking" detector. The detector is a gas-filled tube. The tube has walls that are more or less thick, depending on the energy of the radiation to be detected. Once an ionizing event occurs in the tube, a phenomenon known as gas multiplication makes the single event appear to be multiplied by a factor as high as 10^6. The result is a very large pulse, which is more easily detected than the initial single event. Most Geiger counters are, therefore, very sensitive and can even detect background radiation. GM tubes are also less expensive to manufacture than ion chambers. A common GM application includes detection of contamination (i.e., detecting the presence of radioactive materials in areas or on surfaces where they are not wanted). The source position indicators used in high-dose-rate (HDR) rooms or in teletherapy rooms are GM detectors. In these applications, these devices indicate the presence of radiation (e.g., a source is outside a safe level), but do not provide quantitative information.

> Because of their sensitivity, the Geiger-Müller detectors are best for locating contamination and other low levels of radiation.

Scintillation Detectors

Scintillation detectors do not rely on gases. Crystals are used for the detection of the ionizing events. The most commonly used scintillation crystal is sodium iodide (NaI). These devices are very sensitive radiation detectors and, in large sizes, are used in nuclear medicine imaging because of their sensitivity. As with GM counters, the sole requirement is that the ionizing event be detected in the crystal. The scintillation detector uses an electronic tube, called a *photomultiplier tube*, which enhances the originating event so that a very large pulse is available for analysis. Scintillation counters can be used in applications such as finding lost or misplaced sources and detecting the presence of low levels of contamination.

Both Geiger counters and scintillation detectors are "event" or pulse detectors. In very large radiation fields, the detectors can become swamped (i.e., the number of events is too large for the detector to function). If a detector continuously gives no indication of the presence of radiation, two things are possible: the batteries are not functional, or there is a large radiation field present and personnel should be removed from the location until the situation is assessed by the RSO.

BRACHYTHERAPY

Brachytherapy, literally, therapy at short distances, is a technique that dates back at least to the 1890s, which was the dawn of radiation treatment. The original therapy was performed with radium sources and seeds containing radon and its daughter products. The use of this form of therapy continued into the 1950s until it was recognized that radium substitute sources were needed because the doses received by technical personnel were close to the accepted dose limits. At that time, cesium-137 (^{137}Cs) was proposed as a substitute for ^{226}Ra for intracavitary procedures, and iridium-192 (^{192}Ir) and ^{125}I were proposed as substitutes for radon seeds. Some of the important properties of photon-emitting brachytherapy sources include photon energy, half-life, specific activity, cost of production, toxicity, and safety of the radionuclide and its decay products. Photon energy is less important in brachytherapy than in external beam radiation therapy. For sources emitting photons with energies greater than 100 keV, the inverse-square law predicts transverse-axis dose falloff to within 5% greater than the therapeutically significant distance range from 0 to 5 cm. Low-energy photon sources, such as ^{125}I and palladium-103 (^{103}Pd), produce dose-rate distributions that significantly deviate from inverse-square law approximations, depend significantly on the atomic composition of the surrounding tissue, and are sensitive to small changes in photon spectrum. Even though penetration in tissue is essentially independent of photon energy greater than 100 keV, the half-value layer in lead rises steeply with energy. Because they have nearly identical depth-dose characteristics, artificial brachytherapy radionuclides with mean photon energies in excess of 100 keV are often referred to as "radium substitutes." A summary of NCRP recommendations is listed in Table 17.4.

Intracavitary Applications

One form of brachytherapy treatment is intracavitary insertions. This modality involves the positioning of applicators and the bearing of

TABLE 17.4 Summary of National Council on Radiation Protection and Measurements recommendations

Recommendation	Limit
Occupational whole body	50 mSv (5 rem) annual
Occupational lens of eye	50 mSv (5 rem) annual
Occupational skin	500 mSv (50 rem) annual
Public whole body	1 mSv (100 mrem) annual
Embryo-fetus exposures (declared pregnant)	0.5 mSv (50 mrem) monthly

appropriate sources into a body cavity in proximity to the target tissue. Intracavitary treatment is almost universally used in definitive radiation therapy of locally advanced cervix cancer and other gynecologic treatment procedures. All intracavitary implants are temporary implants that are removed from the patient as soon as the prescribed dose has been delivered. The vaginal cylinder is the most commonly used intracavitary surface-dose applicator in gynecologic brachytherapy. Transluminal brachytherapy consists of the insertion of a single-line source into a body lumen to treat its surface and adjacent tissues.

The other common form of brachytherapy treatment is interstitial implantation, which consists of surgical placement of small radioactive sources, also called "seeds," directly into target tissues. Temporary interstitial implants place radioactive sources into steel needles or plastic catheters inserted in the target tissue. The sources are removed at the end of a precalculated treatment, or "dwell" time. A permanent interstitial implant remains in place for the lifetime of the individual. The initial source strength is chosen so that the prescribed dose is fully delivered only when the implanted radioactivity has decayed to a negligible level.

Remote Afterloading (High-Dose-Rate Afterloading)

High-Dose-Rate (HDR) brachytherapy blends traditional intracavitary, interstitial, and transluminal dose delivery strategies with external beamlike instantaneous dose rates, outpatient treatment orientation, and dose-time-fractionation philosophy. A remote afterloading system consists of a pneumatically or motor-driven source transport system to robotically transfer radioactive material between a shielded safe and each treatment site. The applicators or catheters are connected to a shielded safe by means of transfer tubes. Most remote afterloaders are equipped with a timer that automatically retracts the sources when the programmed treatment time, corrected for gaps and interruptions, has been delivered. A common model of a remote afterloader uses a single cable-driven, 370-GBq ^{192}Ir source that sequentially treats each dwell position in each catheter.

Because HDR brachytherapy is mostly an outpatient modality, patient convenience is enhanced, and the method has the potential to reduce costs by eliminating the need for hospitalization. Radiation exposure to personnel is almost completely eliminated. Finally, HDR brachytherapy offers the ultimate in technical flexibility because each dwell position can be placed anywhere along the catheter track and its dwell time can be programmed individually. Treatment planning software capable of optimizing target volume coverage or dose uniformity through automated manipulation of the dwell-time distribution is offered by all major vendors.

The increased complexity, compression of time for planning and treatment delivery processes, and rapid delivery of high-dose fractions that are characteristic of HDR brachytherapy, create opportunities for serious treatment delivery errors. This modality requires a well-organized procedure, a large technical staff, and a complex quality assurance program. Typical locations for HDR units include treatment rooms or specialized facilities with dedicated brachytherapy suites.

At a minimum, four essential participants should be on the treatment team: the radiation oncologist, the radiation oncology physicist, the dosimetrist, and the treatment unit operator (usually a radiation therapist). A successful program requires a well-qualified and integrated treatment delivery team with substantially more expertise than is gained by formal certification processes. The additional expertise, required above and beyond board certification, is usually acquired through focused self-study, careful planning and preparation, extensive practice with the devices, and visits to established HDR brachytherapy programs.

Despite the low probability of an emergency event, all institutions that practice HDR brachytherapy should design and train staff in appropriate emergency procedures to rapidly bring an unretracted source under control. Such procedures should also address emergency removal of the applicator system. Section 4 and Appendix C of NCRP Report No. 155 discuss quality assurance in HDR therapy.[15]

Interstitial Implantation

Virtually any surgically accessible body site with a well-defined target volume can be treated with localized interstitial brachytherapy. Common sites for the use of this technique include localized tumors of the breast, head and neck, gynecologic and genitourinary systems, extremities, brain, and various body lumina including the esophagus, biliary duct system, and bronchi. Currently, longer-lived but very low-energy photon emitters are used for permanent implantation, namely, ^{125}I and ^{103}Pd. The patient's own tissues or a thin lead foil are sufficient to limit external exposure rates to very low levels. Use of these sources reduces the exposure to the radiation oncologist's hands and fingers and eliminates the need to hospitalize patients solely for radiation protection purposes. Interstitial implants require strict inventory controls to minimize any potential for loss of seeds. Seeds may be kept in a separate controlled and locked space or be kept in a "hot lab" within a controlled, secure area.

The low initial prescription dose rates characteristic of low-energy seed implants, typically 3 to 20 cGy/h, require delivery of doses ranging from 100 to 145 Gy for definitive treatment versus doses between 60 to 80 Gy for classic seed implants. The most common permanent implant procedure is the transperineal prostate implant with the use of transrectal ultrasound guidance.[16,17] A template with a rectangular array of holes is used to guide the perineal implant needles. The template may be rigidly mounted to the ultrasound probe. Usually, a pretreatment ultrasound examination, or "volume" study, of the patient in treatment position has been performed. The transverse images are contoured to form a three-dimensional model of the target volume, anterior rectal wall, and urethra. These data are then downloaded into a treatment planning computer. Treatment planning is used to optimize the needle locations and depths and loading sequence of radioactive seeds and spacers needed to achieve acceptable dosimetric coverage of the prostate and normal tissue sparing. Under ultrasound guidance, the needles are positioned to approximate as closely as possible the preoperative treatment plan. After completion of the procedure, CT imaging is used to localize the seeds and delineate the prostate. The dose distribution is then recalculated to evaluate the technical success of the procedure. Transrectal ultrasound–guided perineal implant procedures require meticulous attention to quality assurance and accuracy of treatment planning and delivery to avoid large dose delivery errors.

The term "half-value layer" is used to describe the amount of material necessary to reduce the radiation intensity by a factor of 2. The half-value layer is typically provided in the thickness of lead and is a function of the radiation energies emitted by the various sources.

TELETHERAPY

The term "teletherapy," or treatment over long distances, was originally applied to the use of ^{60}Co units for external beam therapy. Cobalt-60 machines were developed for commercial use in the 1960s, but have gradually been replaced with the use of linear accelerators. The reasons for this are many: sources need to be replaced approximately every 5 years, the dose rates achieved are lower than those of accelerators, and the sources pose a security risk to the facilities. Typically, moving the source from a shielded to an unshielded position requires the use of a hydraulic system, and there have been rare failures of a retracting source, which have required the therapist to manually push the source back to a shielded position and remove the patient from the treatment room.

Cobalt-60 sources continue to be used in so-called "Gamma knife" facilities for treatment of head tumors, both benign and cancerous. These machines are available in specialized facilities and require specialized training to operate.

SHIELDING DESIGN

The dose rate in beams produced by radiation-producing equipment intended for radiation therapy is more intense than the dose rates from diagnostic x-ray equipment. In addition, the energy of the therapeutic beams is much higher than the diagnostic energies. For these reasons, extra concern is required in the design of the barriers and precautions designed to limit the dose to operators and the public at large.

The accelerator manufacturer will supply a design or installation package to the facility or to the owner, which contains specifications for the placement of the accelerator and room layout. These packages may include typical shielding designs and show the minimum room dimensions required to place the machine in a treatment room. Such shielding designs typically carry a disclaimer that the design for a facility must be evaluated individually by a qualified expert and that the design supplied by the manufacturer is only a template to be considered for further evaluation.

The term "qualified expert" is defined as a medical physicist or health physicist who is competent to design radiation shielding in radiation therapy facilities, and who is certified by the American Board of Radiology, American Board of Medical Physics, American Board of Health Physics, or the Canadian College of Physicists in Medicine. Such an expert may work at the facility, be hired as a consultant to the facility, or be hired by the architectural firm to oversee the design. A number of states specify in their regulations the qualifications of such experts, and they may require that these experts be registered or licensed.

A "controlled area" is defined as a limited-access area in which the occupational exposure of personnel to radiation-producing equipment or radioactive materials is supervised by an individual in charge of radiation protection.[18,19] For radiation oncology facilities, such areas typically include the treatment room, control console, and any adjacent treatment rooms. An "uncontrolled area" would include any other area in the environment. Examples include lobbies, offices, waiting areas, examining rooms, restrooms, and outside areas. Doses suitable for the general public would apply in these areas.

Employees in controlled areas are trained in radiation protection techniques. NCRP Reports 147 and 151 recommend an annual dose limit of 50 mSv/year for individuals in radiation areas, with the cumulative dose not to exceed the product of 10 mSv times the worker's age in years.[18,19] That dose limit notwithstanding, NCRP recommends that for the design of new facilities, the total dose in a year should be a fraction of 10 mSv.

Radiation within the treatment room arises from the machine itself, from leakage radiation transmitted through the head of the treatment unit, and from radiation scattered from objects in the path of the primary beam. The primary beam, alternately called the "useful beam," is emitted directly from the accelerator and is "aimed" at the patient (i.e., at the treatment field). Barriers that intercept the primary beam are called primary barriers. Typically, the accelerator will rotate in a 360-degree circle with the isocenter as the central point of the circle. Portions of the floor, ceiling, and side walls will generally receive the primary beam and are primary barriers. Leakage radiation arises from radiation interactions in the treatment head. The amount of leakage radiation transmitted is regulated and is only slightly degraded from the energy of the primary beam. The remaining radiations found in the treatment room arise from scattered radiation from the patient and other objects in the path of the primary beam. Barriers that receive only the leakage radiation from the treatment head and/or scattered radiation from the patient are called "secondary barriers."

Workload

The most important factor used to calculate shielding is the evaluation of the **workload (W)** anticipated in the facility. The workload is defined as the time integral of the absorbed dose rate (cGy/minute or rad/minute) determined at the depth of maximum absorbed dose, 1 m from the "source" (NCRP 151).[19] Typically, the workload is specified during a period of 1 week. The values for W are usually taken as the absorbed dose from photons delivered to the isocenter in 1 week. The value chosen must necessarily be a function of the amount of time that the beam is "on" (i.e., in a treatment mode). For machines capable of operating at more than one photon energy (e.g., 6 MV, 10 MV, 15 MV, or 18 MV), the shielding calculation for the higher-energy mode will usually determine the required shielding. However, in some cases, it may be desirable to calculate the shielding separately for each treatment modality. The introduction of intensity-modulated radiation therapy and image-guided radiation therapy techniques will increase the workload.

Use Factor and Occupancy Factor

The definitions of use factor (U) and occupancy factor (T) are given in the NCRP reports (NCRP 151).[19] Both of these factors are intended to modify the workload so that the person performing the calculations can more realistically estimate the actual radiation doses likely to be delivered in the areas to be shielded. The **U** requires that one know the fraction of the "beam-on" time (i.e., the workload) that the beam is pointed toward the area to be shielded. Use factors only apply to the primary beam. It is normal for the physicist to assume that the beam points at the lateral walls approximately 25% of the total beam-on time. It is essential that the overall treatment pattern for the room be evaluated.

The **occupancy factor (T)** refers to the fraction of time that the space that is shielded is occupied. This is the typical reason that treatment vaults are placed in the lowest floor of buildings; specifically, there is no occupancy below, and, in most cases, no shielding may be required, only structural material. The occupancy factor for controlled areas must always be 1. In considering occupancy around the vault, the designer may wish to consider future use of the space above and around the vault. For example, if a garden or public space is placed above the ceiling, is it likely or possible that another building or space

TABLE 17.5	Sample Values for Accelerator Shielding Thicknesses	
X-Ray Energy (MV)	Primary Barrier (Feet of Concrete)	Secondary Barrier (Feet of Concrete)
6	6–9	3–4
15	7–12	4–5

Values shown are for concrete with a density of 2.35 g/cm³ or 147 lb/ft³. These values should not be quoted or used for specific installations. Considerations for each installation need to be calculated separately and reviewed by a qualified expert.

may be built by using the shielding walls as foundation for that building? Occupancy above the shielded vault, if it is located on the lowest level of the facility, may have a public access area such as a lobby, cafeteria, or other uncontrolled area directly above.

Distance

Rooms should be designed to take the maximum advantage of the inverse square reduction in radiation intensity. The manufacturer's packages will recommend minimum distances (d) required for placement of the machine, access to the machine controls inside the treatment room, and requirements for couch movement. In addition, the package will specify the minimum distances required to get the machine into the room, including the minimum dimensions and weight of the machine as it is delivered. Typical clear dimensions would include a door frame height of 7 ft and a clear width of 4 ft. Because of the weight of the accelerator and its associated shielding, it is usually necessary to provide rigging to place the accelerator. Advice from a structural engineer may be necessary to plan the delivery route, because it may traverse locations where the floor loading may need to be enhanced.

Reduction of radiation intensity by increases in distance are always more effective than additional shielding. Architects often use English units, thus conversion to metric units will be necessary to use the shielding paradigms in the NCRP reports. Treatment accessories such as molds, blocks, and electron applicators will be stored in the treatment room as well as alignment devices, cameras, and other items. These items will add to the overall interior space needed.

See Table 17.5 for examples of sample shielding barrier thicknesses in radiation oncology installations.

SAFETY DEVICES

In radiation treatment rooms, certain safety devices are mandated by regulation and practice. These devices include the items discussed below.

Door Interlocks

Door interlocks are required to turn off the radiation beam when the circuit is interrupted. These devices are required for all installations that use therapeutic equipment. Once an interlock is activated, a deliberate action by the operator is required to allow treatment to resume.

Safety Edges

Safety edges or electronic type protective beams are required for all doors for treatment rooms. These edges cause the door to retract when activated. The edges should be present on both sides of the door and run the horizontal and vertical lengths of the door. There have been accidents that occurred, for example when a therapist attempted to enter a door while the door was closing. This is a very dangerous practice, and safety systems ensure that if touched by a body part, the door will not close on the object.

Warning Lights

Warning lights are required at the entrances to treatment facilities. These lights indicate when the beam is "on," or, in the case of HDR or ^{60}Co units, when the source is out of its safe position. A warning light may also be inside the treatment room so that someone unknowingly left in a treatment room is aware that the beam is activated.

Visual and Auditory Communication

All treatment rooms are required to have a means for the operator to hear any communication from inside the treatment room (e.g., a cry from a patient or someone unknowingly left inside the room). The operator must also be able to see the patient during treatment. Most installations require at least two television monitors, a near field of the patient and a far-field view of the areas immediately around the patient.

Emergency Power-Off Switches

Emergency power-off switches are usually supplied with the accelerator on the treatment couch and on the gantry. These switches turn off all power to the machine and the couch. It is also recommended that these switches be placed on the walls of the treatment room and that drills be conducted on all emergency procedures.

SUMMARY

- There are two main types of radiation treatment: external beam radiation therapy and brachytherapy.
- It is universally agreed that the less radiation dose received, the lower the risk.
- Every means should be taken to reduce the individual dose.

- Practical radiation protection continues to include the principles of time, distance, and shielding.
- The use of brachytherapy in all its forms requires the radiation oncology practitioner to develop and maintain a comprehensive knowledge of radiation safety practices and protection.

REVIEW QUESTIONS

The answers to the Review Questions can be found by logging on to our website at: http://evolve.elsevier.com/Washington/principles

1. Activity is defined as:
   a. The rest mass of a proton
   b. Rate of nuclear decay
   c. Ionization per unit mass by photons
   d. Product of absorbed dose and quality factor

2. The source of radiation that contributes the most dose to the general population in the United States is:
   a. Medical procedures
   b. Nuclear power
   c. Natural background
   d. Cosmic radiation

3. A dose to which of the following persons is most likely to contribute to the genetically significant dose to the population?
   a. A 70-year-old person
   b. A 50-year-old person
   c. A 20-year-old person
   d. All doses count

4. The annual effective dose equivalent for radiation workers is:
   a. 0.5 mSv
   b. 5 mSv
   c. 50 mSv
   d. 500 mSv

5. The most significant factor influencing the shielding design for an accelerator is the:
   a. Use factor
   b. Occupancy factor
   c. Workload
   d. Energy of the accelerator

6. A measurement of exposure rate is made at 1 m from a point source of radiation. At 2 m, the exposure rate would be reduced by a factor of:
   a. 2
   b. 4
   c. 8
   d. 16

7. Which of the following units is not an SI unit?
   a. Gray
   b. Becquerel
   c. rem
   d. Sievert

8. Which of the following radiation detectors does not rely on crystal technology?
   a. TLD
   b. OSL
   c. Scintillation detector
   d. Ionization chamber

9. Brachytherapy techniques include all of the following except:
   a. HDR units
   b. ^{125}I seed implants
   c. Intraluminal treatments
   d. Stereotactic radiosurgery

10. All of the following are required in an external beam facility except:
    a. Warning lights
    b. Interlocks
    c. Television monitors
    d. Transportation

QUESTIONS TO PONDER

1. Is it possible or reasonable to attempt to shield or protect the general population from natural background radiation?

2. Is it important that regulatory agencies oversee the use of radiation for patient treatment?

3. What are some of the specific challenges that accompany the increasing emphasis on quality assurance?

4. How does the ALARA concept influence radiation protection practice?

5. How do increasing workloads with intensity-modulated radiation therapy and image-guided radiation therapy techniques influence room design?

REFERENCES

1. Curie E. *Madame Curie*. Garden City, NY, 1937: Doubleday, Doran and Company.

2. National Council on Radiation Protection and Measurements. *Ionizing Radiation Exposure of the Population of the United States*. Report 160. Bethesda, MD: National Council on Radiation Protection and Measurements; 2018.

3. US Nuclear Regulatory Commission. Title 10, Code of Federal Regulations: Energy, Standards for Protection Against Radiation. Chapter 1, Part 20. https://www.nrc.gov/reading-rm/doc-collections/cfr/part020/. Accessed October 25, 2019.

4. US Nuclear Regulatory Commission. Title 10, Code of Federal Regulations: Energy, Part 35, Medical Use of By-Product Material. https://www.nrc.gov/reading-rm/doc-collections/cfr/part035/. Accessed October 25, 2019.

5. US Department of Transportation. Title 49, Code of Federal Regulations. www.usdot.gov. Accessed September 26, 2018.

6. US Food and Drug Administration. Title 21, Part 361, Code of Federal Regulations. www.fda.gov. Accessed October 25, 2019.

7. The Joint Commission website. www.jointcommission.org. Accessed September 26, 2018.

8. American College of Radiation Oncology website. www.acro.org. Accessed September 26, 2018.

9. American Society for Therapeutic Radiology website. www.astro.org. Accessed September 26, 2018.

10. National Council on Radiation Protection and Measurements website. www.ncrponline.org. Accessed September 26, 2018.

11. American Association of Physicists in Medicine website. www.aapm.org. Accessed September 26, 2018.

12. United Nations Subcommittee on the Effects of Atomic Radiation. Sources, Effects and Risks of Ionizing Radiation. www.unscear.org; 2013. Accessed September 26, 2018.

13. National Research Council Committee on the Biological Effects of Ionizing Radiation. *Health Effects of Exposure to Low Levels of Ionizing Radiation: BEIR V*. Washington, DC, 2004: National Academy Press.

14. National Council on Radiation Protection and Measurements. *Limitation of Exposure to Ionizing Radiation* Report 116. Bethesda, MD: National Council on Radiation Protection and Measurements; 1993.

15. National Council on Radiation Protection and Measurements. *Management of Radionuclide Therapy Patients* Report 155. Bethesda, MD: National Council on Radiation Protection and Measurements; 2006.

16. Blasko JC, Radge H, Schumacker D. Transperineal percutaneous iodine-125 implantation for prostatic carcinoma using transrectal ultrasound and template guidance. *Endocurie Hypertherm Oncol*. 1987;3:131–139.

17. Dauer L, Zelefsky M, Horan C, et al. Assessment of radiation safety instructions to patients based on measured dose rates following prostate brachytherapy. *Brachytherapy*. 2004;3:1–6.

18. National Council on Radiation Protection and Measurements. *Structural Shielding Design for Medical X-Ray Imaging Facilities* Report 147. Bethesda, MD: National Council on Radiation Protection and Measurements; 2004.

19. National Council on Radiation Protection and Measurements. *Structural Shielding Design and Evaluation for Megavoltage X- and Gamma Ray*

Radiotherapy Facilities, Report 151. Bethesda, MD: National Council on Radiation Protection and Measurements; 2006.

20. National Council on Radiation Protection and Measurements. *Guidance on Radiation Dose Limits for the Lens of the Eye*. Commentary 26.

Bethesda, MD, 2006: National Council on Radiation Protection and Measurements.

21. American College of Radiology website. www.acr.org. Accessed September 26, 2018.

18

Culture of Safety in Radiation Oncology

Lukasz M. Mazur, Robert D. Adams

OBJECTIVES

- Discuss the current challenges for developing and managing continuous quality improvement (CQI) programs in radiation oncology.
- Compare and contrast the best practices adopted from high reliability and value creation organizations designed to enhance quality and safety in radiation oncology centers.

- Describe how to implement infrastructures to drive continuous improvements in quality and safety in radiation oncology centers.
- Define important radiation safety terms.

OUTLINE

KEY TERMS

Behavior (or quality/safety behavior)
Burnout
Crew resource management
Continuous quality improvement
Human error
Event (or safety event)
Good catch
High-reliability organization
Improvement cycles

Plan-Do-Study-Act
Safety mindfulness
Situational awareness
Standard work procedures
Toyota Production System
Transformational leadership
Time-out
Transactional-transformational leadership
Workload

MOTIVATION

In 2010, the radiation oncology community was rocked by Walt Bogdanich's articles in the *New York Times*; his writings took an in-depth look at leadership, radiation dose, and patient safety.[1-4] For the first time in its history, the radiation oncology community was accused of being unsafe and lacking in leadership (Table 18.1). In response to these articles, the American Society for Radiation Oncology (ASTRO), American Association of Physicists in Medicine (AAPM), Society of Radiation Oncology Administrators (SROA), American Association of Medical Dosimetrists (AAMD), and American Society of Radiologic Technologists (ASRT) all issued leadership statements regarding patient safety; moreover, the presidents of ASTRO and the AAPM were called to a congressional hearing in Washington, DC, entitled *Medical Radiation: An Overview of the Issues*.[5-8] The statements released by the societies mentioned above, combined with the testimonies at the congressional hearing, resulted in stronger leadership by radiation therapy professional societies in instituting change and increasing patient safety in clinical practice.

For example, ASTRO has initiated a new accreditation program aimed at improving accountability of radiation therapy practices. Its mission statement is "to recognize facilities by objectively assessing the radiation oncology care team, the facility itself and it policies and procedures." There are currently 16 standards that they will use in their accreditation process. Of particular interest is number 7, the "culture of safety."

Of standard 7, ASTRO says, "Modern radiation therapy is complex and rapidly evolving. The safe delivery of radiation therapy requires the concerted and coordinated efforts of many individuals with varied responsibilities." The rapidly evolving nature of radiation oncology requires that processes and workflows be continually reassessed. One of the most crucial activities in a quality radiation oncology department is the organized review and monitoring of all aspects of safety, errors, and

TABLE 18.1   Examples of Radiation Therapy Treatment Errors

Patient Name	Age	Location of Incident	Type of Error	Result of Mistreatment
Scott Jerome-Parks	43	St. Vincent's Hospital in Manhattan, New York City	Multileaf collimator shaping lost when computer rebooted several times during transfer of head and neck plan from planning system to treatment machine. Multileaf collimator positions were erased, leaving open fields for his treatment. He received seven times the planned amount of radiation.	Short-term complications included lots of swelling of head and neck, severe pain, nausea, loss of taste, and difficulty swallowing. Long term, he lost most of his vision, and his hearing degenerated, along with his balance. He eventually needed to be fed with a gastric tube and took a plethora of medications. Two years after the misadministration of his radiation treatment, he died.
Alexandra Jn-Charles	34	Downstate Medical Center's University Hospital of Brooklyn	Wedge not used for treatment for breast cancer. Patient received 3.5 times amount of planned radiation during the course of 27 fractions.	It took more than a year for her wound to heal; during much of her convalescence, the wound exposed her ribs and smelled strongly. She was unable to do anything for herself or her family. Eventually after multiple surgeries, the wound did heal. The incorrect use of the wedge in her treatment meant that, in addition to the grievous injury that resulted, her tumor was not adequately treated. She died several months later.
Frederick Stein	71	Veterans Affairs Medical Center, East Orange, New Jersey	An intensity-modulated radiation therapy plan was approved for him without proper quality controls in place. Department personnel signed off on various parts of intensity-modulated radiation therapy plans that should have been signed by a medical doctor.	A sore throat that worsened while treatment continued. A rash followed, concurrent with other skin problems. Difficulty swallowing developed, and the patient lost weight as a result. His pain increased to the point that he needed morphine; other pain medication followed. Two therapists treating him told their manager they thought he was being overdosed. They were fired shortly thereafter.

quality. Creating a "culture of safety" depends on guidance, direction, and financial means from the leadership of the institution and of the radiation therapy department, on individual effort by every member of the department, and on organized support for quality and safety at every level of the institution. It is critical that a culture that appropriately manages change exists; ensuring that change facilitates safety and quality. Furthermore, all team members must be open to having any member of the team (whether in leadership positions or not) raise concerns about safety as well as suggesting and considering change. Indeed, it is often the frontline staff who are more likely to understand the limitations of current procedures and suggest improvements. Thus an ideal open environment with a safety-minded culture only exists where staff are permitted and encouraged to suggest and lead change to improve safety, quality, and efficiency.[9]

This is a major shift in terms of the focus on a culture of safety. Until now, the quality and safety of radiation oncology centers have been overseen mostly by a selected group of stakeholders (mostly physicians and physicists), with a goal of meeting a predefined set of quality and safety indicators. Upon meeting those quality and safety indicators, the improvements were considered to have served their purpose, and it was assumed that virtually no further improvement in the culture of safety was necessary. This is no longer the status quo that can be considered the goal. The intended culture of safety requires virtually all members of the organization to participate to be effective. Why? The field of radiation oncology is rapidly evolving, mostly because of technological innovations. These new technologies present not only novel ways to treat cancer; they also provide new challenges for established practices. The pace of this change means that it is now necessary to make a shift in the focus of the culture of safety, from an undertaking that occurs perhaps as much as a couple times a year via dedicated interventions, to an ongoing commitment that needs constant effort to keep pace and continue to provide an efficient and safe workplace for both employees and patients.

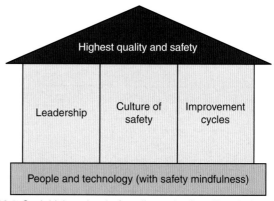

Fig. 18.1 Goal: highest level of quality and safety. Foundation: people (staff members). Pillars: engaged and strong leadership, organizational shift to a culture of safety mindfulness, and improvement cycles supported by reliable methods and tools.

This paradigm shift takes a lot of effort to put into practice. To successfully make this organization-level change, radiation oncology centers must focus on developing safety mindfulness in people, as previously shown by high reliability and value creation organizations[10–13] (Fig. 18.1). To achieve this change requires many elements, and the most important is leadership. The overhaul of an organizational culture requires a tremendous amount of leadership effort. Maintaining reliable practices, while constantly making changes to processes and workplaces, requires a handful of dedicated and trained people to oversee the various projects that facilitate this change. Next, you need to continuously support a culture of safety. As a discipline, radiation oncology has grown considerably since its inception, and it will need to continue to grow to keep providing a high standard of care for patients. A culture of safety is a shift away from organizational norms of punishment or ridicule for making errors, to a culture that allows people to report and challenge the errors and inefficiencies they see so that everyone can benefit from the improvements that are subsequently made. These improvements come out of a system of improvement cycles, the final piece of the puzzle. Such a system, supported by reliable methods and tools, ensures that improvements made to processes can be sustained with time.

LEADERSHIP

Strong leadership is essential to make a change of this magnitude. Each organization is established to work a certain way and develops its own patterns of interaction. These patterns have long since accrued a kind of momentum. This is not only useful, but necessary to maintain any organizational system. It is this momentum, however, that makes it difficult to implement drastic changes. As a result, leaders will need to identify staff members who are able to help them guide the rest of the staff through this process. These people begin the process of identifying which improvements are relevant and appropriate for the organization. The leaders regularly remind the other staff of the improvement goals that have been set, and also of the various methods that have been chosen to meet those goals. While progress is made, these leaders keep everyone up to date on which processes are showing improvement and which still need work.

Leading Change

Implementing change in radiation oncology centers is more than just a technical challenge; it is also a challenge to change management. Successful change to management requires strong leadership.[14–18]

Kotter suggests that to successfully implement change, leadership must first develop a high sense of urgency for the change effort.[17,18] Next, a powerful guiding coalition needs to be established to lead the change from the top. Subsequently, vision and strategy need to be drafted and clearly communicated. This is followed by acts of empowerment for broad-based action to generate and consolidate short-term wins that anchor new approaches in the culture (Fig. 18.2).

At the organizational level, research shows that leadership actions and styles that vary from Kotter's change management recommendations have contributed to rigid divisions of labor in many areas of healthcare, especially between nursing and management, in addition to nursing and physicians. These divisions negatively affect healthcare innovations and improvements.[19–21] Weingart and Page,[20] based on the conclusions from Minnesota Executive Sessions on Patient Safety,[21] emphasize that little is known about how leaders should implement effective organizational and managerial structures and systems that could produce the necessary changes in patient safety. Ramanujam and Rousseau[22] suggest that the desired changes can be potentially achieved via dedicated leadership and an organizational structure for patient safety that promotes continuous improvement. McFadden and colleagues[23] tested the following seven improvements strategies proposed by the Agency for Healthcare Research and Quality (AHRQ): partnership with stakeholders, reporting errors free of blame, open discussion of errors, cultural shift, education and training, statistical analysis of data, and system redesign. The authors concluded that creation of a cultural shift toward patient safety should be a top priority for hospital leaders.[23] Beyond the healthcare industry, findings in a variety of other industrial settings note that successful change requires strong and effective leadership.[24] This is particularly true for the multiprofessional change effort needed in radiation oncology departments, where physicians, physicists, dosimetrists, therapists, nurses, and administrators each have specific needs and challenges to be addressed. According to change management experts, if organizational change is to be

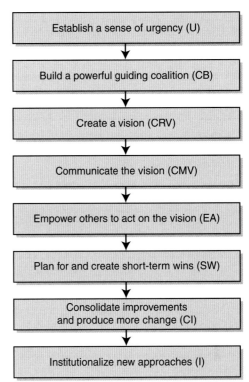

Fig. 18.2 An example of a value stream map of the process of computed tomography simulation at the University of North Carolina. (From Chera BS, Jackson M, Mazur L, et al. Improving quality of patient care by improving daily practice in radiation oncology. *Semin Radiat Oncol.* 2012;22:77–85.)

successful, leadership must be exerted at all levels via a blend of transactional-transformational leadership (TTL).[25] TTL focuses on the relationship and interactions of the leader and follower. Transactional leadership defines the leader-follower relationship through a series of transactions or exchanges. Followers receive rewards or positive recognition when they comply with the wishes of the leader. Conversely, if they act against the leader's wishes or expectations, followers receive punishment and negative reinforcement. Transactional leadership is a task-oriented command-and-control approach to leading, where the emphasis is on what needs to be done and how to do it. Alternatively, transformational leadership focuses on the relationship between the leader and follower. It is concerned with motivating and inspiring followers to do more than expected and is contingent on followers having strong levels of trust, admiration, loyalty, and respect for the leader. Transformational leaders may be charismatic or highly inspirational, conveying a vision of the future that their followers can believe in. They may also exhibit strong consideration for the professional or personal needs of followers, or intellectually excite followers to strive above and beyond the norm. Whereas transactional leadership focuses more on what to do and how to do it, transformational leadership focuses on why it needs to be done.

TTL has received a great amount of attention in the leadership research literature. Bass and Bass provide a comprehensive review of the concepts and general research findings during the past few decades.[14] Transformational leadership has been shown to result in greater employee job satisfaction, higher likelihood of staff helping others in the organization, higher trust in the leader, and higher organizational citizenship behaviors.[26] More specifically, TTL has been used in healthcare to examine leader effectiveness of hospital chief executive officers, community health center medical directors, and nursing leaders.[27–29] Note that both transactional and transformational leadership behaviors may be appropriate, depending on the context and the nature of the leadership challenge.[30] Research suggests that there is a dynamic interrelation between leadership style and the nature of the objective to be accomplished, whether it is geared toward exploration or exploitation.[31,32] When organizations operate within existing constraints and structures and seek to exploit efficiencies for gain, there is value in transactional leadership behaviors. On the other hand, when organizations attempt to adapt, innovate, and change to address new opportunities and new challenges, there is value in transformational leadership behaviors. TTL can be assessed through the use of the Multifactor Leadership Questionnaire.[33]

Practical Implications

At the heart of the initiative to spearhead a culture of safety lies a possible leadership paradox. Radiation oncology centers are required to embrace process innovation that alters how staff members will perform their jobs, but this may be a difficult change for employees to accept. This might suggest that transformational leadership is a more appropriate style to use, in which leader effectiveness depends on building trust, motivation, and internal commitment in the change target population. Yet, to the degree that the culture of safety is accepted and implemented in the radiation oncology centers, it will move staff members toward job actions that promote less variability, higher repeatability, and more standardization. In other words, jobs may become oriented more toward exploiting efficiencies for gain. This might suggest that transactional leadership is a more appropriate style to use, in which leader effectiveness depends on clearly defining the change required and monitoring performance against these expectations. Effective radiation oncology center leaders (e.g., department chair, quality, and safety directors) must be able to respond dynamically to all portions of the organization and provide the leadership behavior that fits the task at hand.

An example of a leadership change is found in a white paper ASTRO produced on clinical peer review. In the past, all ASTRO white papers addressed advances in technology and treatments. For the leadership to mandate a white paper on peer review was a huge cultural change. The ASTRO white paper on peer review had explicit peer review concepts, not just for radiation oncologists and medical physicists, but also for medical dosimetrists and radiation therapists.[34,35] It should be noted that at the time of writing of this white paper, neither the medical dosimetrists nor radiation therapists had any mention of peer review in their professional standards.

The *New York Times* articles marked the first instance in the history of the radiation therapy profession wherein all five professional societies (ASTRO, AAPM, SROA, AAMD, and ASRT) issued concurrent public statements about leadership and patient safety. The *New York Times* articles were a defining point in our 40-year-old profession: what had been considered the norm for leadership was no longer relevant. As a result of the pace of change in our industry and the increase in public scrutiny, the levels of leadership also needed to become greater and take on a different impetus. The radiation oncology profession had progressed to a multimillion dollar industry with larger public responsibilities and increased levels of accountability to its communities of interest. Probably the greatest reaction to the *New York Times* articles has been the recent creation by ASTRO of its own professional accreditation program, with standards created by ASTRO. All of this has led to the need for leadership within the community of physicians, physicists, dosimetrists, and radiation therapists, all working together in creating a culture of safety.

Leaders must actively work together to promote safety and efficiency. Successful change management in healthcare requires trusted physicians with high levels of urgency for change, charisma, and vision. Physicians must act as transformational leaders, knowing that it is crucial to promote, encourage, motivate, and coach staff towards safety and quality mindfulness. All of this is contingent on staff having strong levels of trust, loyalty, and respect for leaders. Leaders must be: good listeners, which allows for constructive two-way communications; persistent and determined to reach patient safety and quality goals; and unafraid of criticism. These qualities do not necessarily come naturally, and leaders need to be consistent in their promotion of these principles. Leaders' behaviors, actions, and words can carry great weight because others will emulate them. A leader who does not consistently and overtly espouse these principles may inadvertently discourage others from embracing these concepts. Leaders need to continuously inspire people to go beyond their regular duties and identify ways to improve quality and safety.

CULTURE OF SAFETY

The pace of innovation and advancement in radiation oncology has reached a point where common sense approaches to problem-solving are no longer able to keep up and maintain a high level of patient care and clinical practice. An organizational infrastructure supportive of a high reliability and value creation is necessary to create a culture of safety. We could learn from the aviation industry. The following are some of the key measures that the commercial aviation industry adopted to implement a culture of safety.[10–13]

- Training: First, there is a need for training initiatives that focus on mitigating secondary catastrophic incidents that may result from human errors (slips, lapses, and mistakes). For example, most commercial airline carriers encourage, reward, and pay staff to ensure that they receive the quality/safety training required. If an employee misses or fails training/proficiency checks, they usually face restrictions until their underperformance has been rectified. One popular training program for pilots is called crew resource management (CRM). CRM is a training program focused on culture, teamwork, communication, and the inevitability of errors. It also covers ways to avoid, trap (i.e., contain), and mitigate hazards resulting from errors before they lead to serious or catastrophic harm.

- Policies and procedures that enforce safe operations: There must always be two physiologically and psychologically sound pilots to fly a plane. This minimum safety requirement applies with no exceptions. This requirement is often audited by random drug and alcohol tests. Furthermore, during the safety-critical phases of a flight, such as flying below an altitude of 10,000 feet, the pilots and cabin crew must adhere to strict standard operating procedures and refrain from all nonessential activities (e.g., reading newspapers or chatting idly). This safety requirement is known as the "sterile cockpit rule." Crew members are taught how to call, without awkwardness, for the sterile cockpit rule to be implemented at additional times when particular concentration becomes necessary. The entire crew is informed about when the rule is in force through warnings or alert systems. Adoption of comparable policies in radiation oncology centers would be controversial, but they might better ensure patient safety.

- Flight recorders: These recorders, also known as "black boxes," monitor key flight parameters throughout each flight, and these data are analyzed by computers after every flight. Readings outside of predetermined acceptable ranges trigger warning signals that can initiate an investigation. The full exploration of flight recording is only conducted in catastrophic circumstances, but pilots and staff know that all their actions and conversations are monitored and recorded.

So, how do we begin to build an infrastructure to support a culture of safety in radiation oncology centers? Where do we start? The new philosophies and methodologies to battle against the emerging threats to patient safety within radiation oncology departments will require organizations to develop and maintain a high level of urgency toward change and innovation. Perhaps the first step is to recognize the symptoms of employee burnout that have been present in our industry for a long time but have not been approached proactively. Second, we might want to apply robust and validated methodologies to move toward a more prominent culture of psychological safety, and not spend more time "reinventing the wheel."

Psychological Safety and Burnout

Psychological safety and dominance of short-term approaches to address problems in the healthcare industry are often major barriers to change implementation.[36–40] Edmondson showed that psychological safety enables a willingness to engage in "second-order" problem-solving behavior because improvement efforts are inherently risky and can have negative consequences for the person who raises the concerns. Second-order problem-solving behavior occurs when a worker takes action to address underlying causes, in addition to patching the problem, so that the immediate task at hand can be completed. Being associated with problems and change efforts can result in damage to one's reputation,[38] so workers are more likely to engage in improvement efforts if they feel they have some protection from such backlash. Nembharth and Edmondson showed that leader inclusiveness—words and actions exhibited by leaders that invite and appreciate others' contributions—can help healthcare workers and teams overcome the inhibiting effects of psychological safety, allowing members to collaborate in process improvement.[41] Tucker and Edmondson suggested that nurses are likely to engage in improvement efforts if managers are physically present on the nursing floor, have a reputation for safety and improvement, and have the time needed to devote to problem-solving efforts. Such managerial presence and support can often increase the feeling of gratification and, at the same time, prevent the feelings of burnout from frontline healthcare professionals. Studies of organizations with a strong track record of high reliability and safety have shown that psychological safety and vigilance by frontline workers is essential to detect threats to safety before they actually become errors, adverse events, or both.[10,42] Furthermore, researchers have shown that psychological safety and autonomy is linked to higher satisfaction and productivity and therefore higher improvement efforts by promoting self-management.[43,44]

This, in turn, increases worker motivation by empowering them to make decisions that affect their productivity.[45,46]

It is apparent that what has always been assumed to be a stressful occupation, working with cancer patients, has become increasingly stressful in the face of rapidly changing paradigms for radiation therapists. Clinical radiation therapists are forced to provide more patient care despite dwindling social, economic, and technological resources.[47] Radiation therapists are also required to provide more patient care services because of changes both in reimbursements and the increased needs of cancer patients and their families.[47] Because of their specialized type of work, stressors for radiation therapists may be very different than the stressors associated with other members of the radiation therapy treatment team.

Occupational stress and burnout are separate constructs. Theoretically, when individuals experience increased occupational stress over a period of time, they may develop symptoms of burnout; accordingly, stress can lead to burnout. Gillespie defines burnout as "a reaction to chronic, job-related stress characterized by physical, emotional, and mental exhaustion that results from conditions of work, job strain,

worker strain, and defensive coping."[48] The origin of burnout was discovered by Dr. Harold Freudenberger, a German born American psychologist Freudenberger identified the physical signs of burnout as exhaustion, headaches, fatigue, gastrointestinal problems, and insomnia.[49] For radiation therapists, the reasons for the potential of increased burnout are many. Radiation therapists deliver very high doses of radiation to a cancer site while simultaneously trying to minimize doses to the surrounding tissue.[50] Approximately 1.7 million people in the United States will be treated for cancer each year, and, of these, approximately 1 million cancer patients will receive radiation therapy treatments.[51] The incidence of cancer naturally increases with age (approximately two-thirds of all cancer patients are older than 65 years of age), and because the demographics of the United States are changing to an aging population, the need for radiation therapy services is most likely to increase in the future.[52]

It is important for the radiation therapist to understand that burnout occurs in a linear fashion. There are three levels of burnout[53]: emotional exhaustion, depersonalization, and a decreased sense of personal accomplishment.[53] These phases occur sequentially, with the radiation therapist more likely to be a victim of burnout while time progresses. In the first state of burnout, emotional exhaustion, the radiation therapist experiences physical and emotional exhaustion, sleeps poorly, and is prone to headaches and colds. The person becomes overinvolved emotionally and feels overwhelmed by the demands of other people. Once emotional exhaustion sets in, the individual feels he or she no longer can "give" to others.[53] During the second stage of burnout, depersonalization, the radiation therapist becomes cynical toward coworkers, clients, and themselves. This sets the stage for detached and dehumanized behaviors.[53] During the final stage of burnout, reduced personal accomplishment, the individual feels disgust with everyone and everything. This stage is rarely encountered because such individuals usually have already left the radiation therapy profession.[53]

The original studies in radiation therapist burnout in the United States were done by Adams and Akroyd.[54–57] Their studies indicate that radiation therapists have higher levels of emotional exhaustion and depersonalization as compared with other types of healthcare professionals (doctors, nurses, and radiographers). Moreover, the studies on radiation therapists have been replicated in Great Britain and Australia with almost identical results.[58–60] Research in three countries indicates that radiation therapists have high levels of burnout. It is important for radiation therapists to recognize the symptoms of burnout and act accordingly to alleviate those symptoms and maintain a very high level of patient care and safety.[1,62]

Learning From Toyota

The Toyota Production System (TPS) is perhaps the most powerful model devised to date for the efficient design and management of large-scale operations.[63] This system helped propel Toyota Motor Corporation from a small, struggling truck maker in the aftermath of World War II to one of the world's largest automakers in 2019. Research by Spear and Bowen uncovered a number of fundamental principles by which Toyota's "lean" management process operates.[64] They observed that Toyota experts define processes in terms of "connections" and "pathways" and then redesign the processes to streamline pathways and make direct connections with simple, binary communications. They also learned that every piece of the process is predicated on a testable hypothesis of the operation's expected results, such that results that are different than expected are made readily visible and countermeasures can be taken. This process explains why standardized work is so critical to the system. Every time an improvement is proposed, the proposal explicitly states the expected outcome (i.e., a hypothesis), which can be verified or refuted through experimentation. Every employee is trained in this method of improvement.

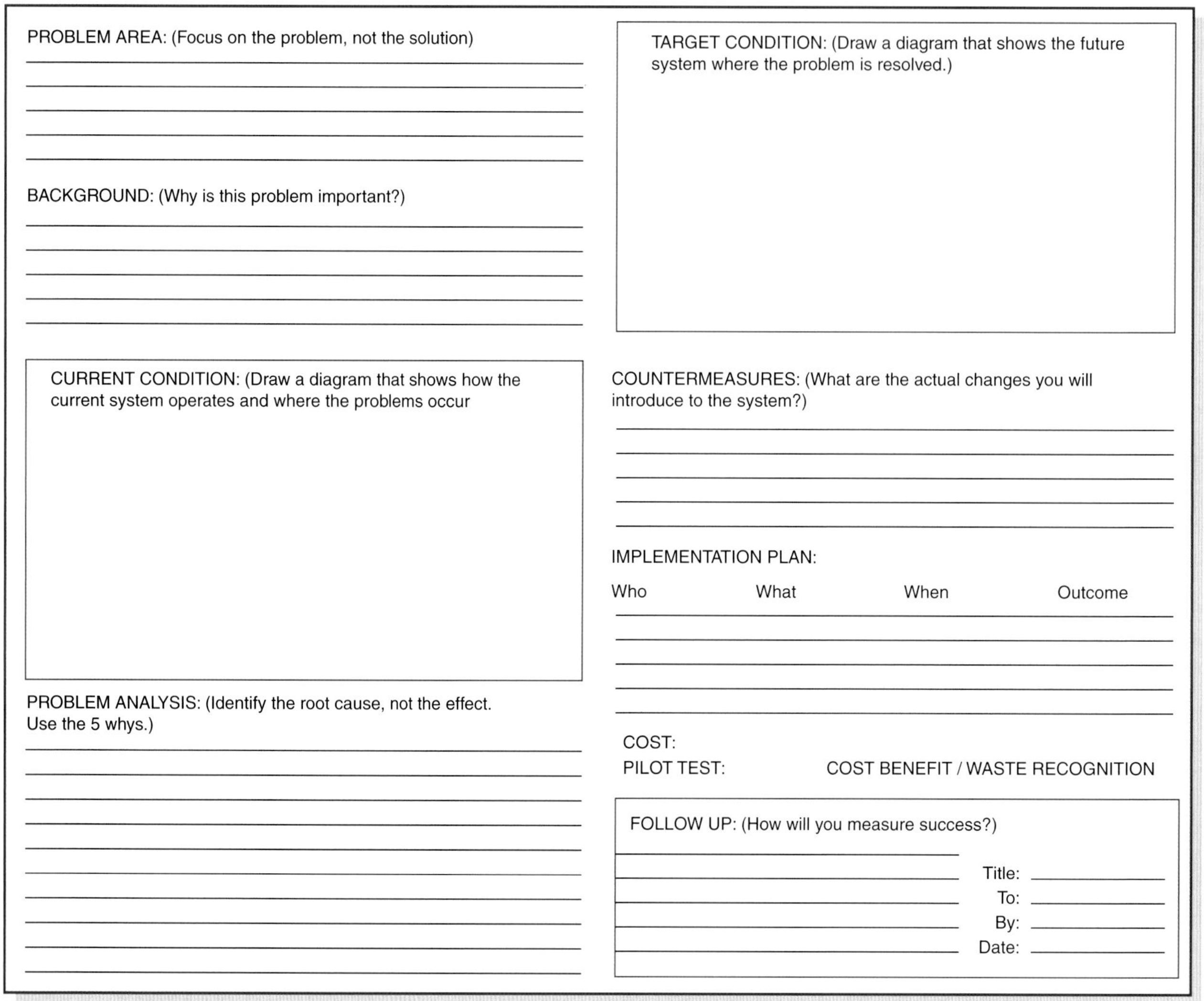

PROBLEM AREA: (Focus on the problem, not the solution)

TARGET CONDITION: (Draw a diagram that shows the future system where the problem is resolved.)

BACKGROUND: (Why is this problem important?)

CURRENT CONDITION: (Draw a diagram that shows how the current system operates and where the problems occur

COUNTERMEASURES: (What are the actual changes you will introduce to the system?)

IMPLEMENTATION PLAN:

Who	What	When	Outcome

PROBLEM ANALYSIS: (Identify the root cause, not the effect. Use the 5 whys.)

COST:
PILOT TEST: COST BENEFIT / WASTE RECOGNITION

FOLLOW UP: (How will you measure success?)

Title: _____
To: _____
By: _____
Date: _____

Fig. 18.3 A3 template. The A3 tool consists of four stages that the investigator must go through to get from "problem faced" to "problem solved." In summary, at each stage the investigator performs the following activities. Stage 1: Plan (P) to improve your operations by identifying the problems and the ideas to solve these problems. Stage 2: Do (D) changes that are designed to solve the problems on a small or experimental scale. Stage 3: Study (S) whether the experimental changes are achieving the desired result or not. Stage 4: Act (A) to implement changes on a larger scale if the experiment is successful. If the experiment is not successful, the investigator skips the Act (A) stage and goes back to the Plan (P) stage to develop new ideas to solve the problem and repeats the cycle. This iterative process makes A3 thinking robust and explains why it was chosen for use in the department.

The Institute for Healthcare Improvement believes that lean principles can be and are already being successfully applied to the delivery of healthcare.[53] Thus it makes sense to take a closer look at Toyota's experience with development of a culture of safety.

Academics and practitioners who espouse the virtues of TPS (or "lean") typically describe lean on two levels. At the conceptual level, lean is a philosophy, a perspective that relentlessly strives to eliminate defects and waste, and continually attacks both in a never-ending pursuit of perfection.[65,63] The term *lean* has become popular recently and, like many buzzwords, has taken on various shades of meaning and implementation, some of which stray from the true intentions of its inventor. Most descriptions of lean therefore quickly move beyond the philosophical to an interrelated set of practices that range from overall material flow in the factory to detailed work and equipment design and human resource practices.

At the operational level, lean is equipped with two basic tools, *value stream mapping* (see Fig. 18.2) and the *A3 problem-solving tool*[66,67] (Fig. 18.3). Value stream maps graphically represent the key people, material, and information required to deliver a product or service. They are designed to distinguish value-adding from nonvalue-adding steps. As a problem-solving method used by Toyota, the term *A3* derives from the paper size used for the report, which is the metric equivalent to 11×17 in paper.

Two healthcare organizations that deserve particular recognition for their work with the lean system are Virginia Mason Hospital in Seattle, led by Dr. Gary Kaplan, and ThedaCare, Inc., a health delivery system in Wisconsin, formerly led by Dr. John Toussaint. Virginia Mason, by working to eliminate waste, created more capacity in its existing programs and practices so that planned expansions were scrapped, saving significant capital expenses: US$1 million for an additional hyperbaric

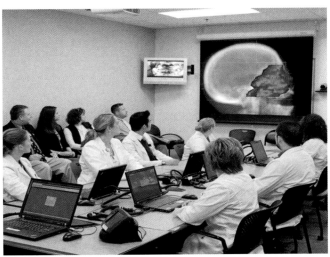

Fig. 18.4 Morning simulation review from the Department of Radiation Oncology at the University of North Carolina. This review involves radiation oncologists, dosimetrists, nurses, physicists, and radiation therapists, among others. The purpose is to maximize the opportunity to reduce any errors in the treatment plan as well as to ensure the highest level of patient care.

chamber that was no longer needed, US$1 to US$3 million for endoscopy suites that no longer needed to be relocated, and US$6 million for new surgery suites that were no longer necessary.[68] Working closely with lean master level experts to eliminate defects, the heart attack rate at ThedaCare was reduced from 91,471 defects per million opportunities to 7000 defects per million opportunities in just 4 years.[54]

Practical Implications

The term "culture of safety" could be considered to encompass the entirety of the changes suggested, from the level of the organization as a whole down to the level of each work area, including nursing, dosimetry, therapy, and the rest of the organization. However, what we are actually referring to when we use this phrase is the individualized approach that has been created by each organization's leaders. This may include a morning simulation review, an online "good-catch" (or error reporting) system, as well as other improvement processes that encourage staff members to take part in the system. None of these tools create this culture individually. Instead, they show the intention of the organization is to listen to anyone with an idea about how to improve the system, and then to take action, based on those ideas, to make needed improvements. When these mechanisms are paired with leaders who reinforce those tenets, then the cultural momentum can begin its shift away from its starting point to one of safety mindfulness.

There are various additional practices that can facilitate a positive cultural shift toward safety mindfulness in radiation oncology. The following are a few of those practices.

- *Good catch:* A good catch system is a way to allow department members to quickly report various issues they notice during the course of their day. This ranges from small workarounds, all the way up to incidents that reach the patients. Ideally, the system allows for both anonymous and nonanonymous submissions so that staff members are not anxious about reporting issues and errors they have seen or committed. Allowing submissions to be submitted in this way can also encourage those who like recognition when undertaking improvement efforts with organizational support.[69–71]
- *Morning simulation review* (Fig. 18.4): For many years now, radiation oncology departments have recognized the value in having each patient's treatment plan reviewed and discussed by as many

members of the team as possible. This involves radiation oncologists, dosimetrists, nurses, physicists, and radiation therapists, among others. The purpose is to maximize the opportunity to reduce any errors in the plan, as well as to ensure the highest level of patient care. Ideally, this review should occur before the patient receives his or her first treatment so that the likelihood of errors affecting the patient is decreased as much as possible. Traditionally, this review has occurred at some point after the start of treatment, but modern changes in the way we deliver radiation to patients have resulted in less ability to correct for errors in patient treatment. The previously discussed change to the timing of this review is meant to address that lessened ability.[69,72,70,73]

- *Safety rounds:* A method for the departmental leaders to speak with frontline employees about ways to make their work areas safer and more efficient. The goal of safety rounds is to ensure workers have the needed tools to perform reliably in their respective environments. This allows staff to discuss problems or resources needed to do their work successfully. Safety rounds can be held monthly or quarterly.[72–75]
- *Huddles:* Brief meetings to improve communication flow among the various departmental work teams. The innovative ideas that come out of the daily huddles have the potential to quickly improve both the quality and safety of the workday. The huddles can also help improve interpersonal and organizational communication, and break down unnecessary hierarchies.[69,72,74,75]
- *Peer review:* Also known as the evaluation of creative work or performance by other people in the same field to enhance the quality of work or the performance. Questions such as the following are welcomed: "Is this the correct patient?" "Are we treating the correct site?" "Is there overlap with a previously irradiated field?" "Do the fields and monitor units make sense given all of the above?"[69,76,35,77,78]
- *Workload optimization:* The increased complexity of linear accelerators has led to the placement of two or more therapists per machine, at least in part to distribute workload, optimize situational awareness, and to check each other's work. However, many therapist groups and pairs sometimes use a "divide and conquer" approach. Each therapist performs different tasks for speed and efficiency and forgets to double-check one another. This situation only gets more complex while additional systems (e.g., image-guided radiation therapy, motion management, and gating) become more commonplace. Understanding and optimizing workloads for all staff members involved in the radiation therapy process should be one of the central efforts for leaders.[79–82]
- *Time-out:* A time-out is a standardized approach to help review the most crucial aspects of a radiation treatment delivery process (something like a presurgery checklist in an operating room). For example, patient setup is a qualitative action because positioning of the human body in a reproducible and precise way is a matter of tolerances and decisions rather than specific right and wrong actions. The use of a daily time-out by therapists to perform a peer review for critical information is likely to improve the quality of the decisions made during the patient setup process.[83–86]

Such practices and many others can be found in high-reliability organizations. A consistent theme is that high-reliability organizations have a strong safety mindfulness that bolsters their high levels of reliability. Along with the creation and implementation of practices to improve the patient safety culture, new instruments had to be created to measure progress in improving the culture. Colla and colleagues reviewed nine survey instruments that measured the patient safety climate in hospitals.[87] Only one of the nine instruments, the AHRQ Survey on Patient Safety, examined the relationship between patient outcomes and patient safety, which seems especially important for radiation oncology centers.

Cultural changes spread through an organization via its social connections. Social connectedness is different from the organization's formal structure in which the reporting relationships and hierarchy of the organization are defined. Instead, it is the rich network of relationships, or links, within which leaders, change agents, middle management, and frontline professionals are embedded. Understanding social connectedness has been used to reveal the topology and intensity of these organizational relationships, as well as the types of information exchange within networks. These can include knowledge sharing, seeking or giving advice, influencing, problem solving, and decision making.[88,89] There is value in understanding the social networks of the various types of individuals active in transformation efforts in radiation oncology centers. For the change leaders, their social networks are expected to have a significant influence on the implementation process. Bono and Anderson examined the advice and influence networks of transformational leaders to determine whether transformational leaders were relied on more for advice and had greater influence on organizational decision making than nontransformational leaders.[90] They found a positive association between transformational leadership and the degree to which these leaders were centrally located in advice and influence networks. This association suggests that transformational leaders may be particularly able to lead change efforts throughout organizations by utilizing their extensive social networks. In a similar vein, Balkundi and Kilduff developed a framework for linking leadership to social networks, noting that appropriate leadership style and the use of social capital through well-developed networks are both supportive of effective leadership.[92] Beyond the change leaders, identify those people in each organization that frontline professionals and middle management turn to for advice and support for change initiatives.[92]

IMPROVEMENT CYCLES

To spearhead change, we need improvement cycles. This is the engine that drives change forward and ensures that proposed improvements are implemented and sustained over time. Often, this cycle is referred to as Plan-Do-Study-Act (PDSA). Radiation oncology departments are highly complex entities that require numerous subsets of employees who work simultaneously to achieve the common goal of treating patients safely, effectively, and efficiently. Within each of these groups there are numerous opportunities to improve workflow and outcomes. Although any improvement may have a positive effect within its specific group, there is a real possibility that other groups will develop unforeseen problems as a result of changes made to achieve that improvement. The PDSA cycle, when correctly implemented, takes into account the complexity of the interrelationships between these groups, and considers the unintended consequences suggested improvements might have on the system as a whole instead of just one part. The major steps in the cycle are:

- *Plan:* This is the start of the cycle. In the planning stage, a problem within the system is identified and described in detail so that a set of goals and expected outcomes can be determined.
- *Do:* This is the initial implementation stage. Corrections that come out of the planning step are put into place, and data are collected that relate to the efficacy of these corrections.
- *Study:* This is the stage of the cycle that takes the data collected in the previous step and analyzes how well everything is working. This stage is where one determines whether the outcomes of the changes match the expectations. Analyses made here are carried forward into the next stage.
- *Act:* This is sometimes said to be the "adjust" phase of the cycle. The point is to take the analyses from the study phase and determine what adjustments can or should be made to better address the problem that is the topic of focus.

The choice of PDSA as a theoretical foundation for continuous improvement is grounded in a belief that improvement effort is a form of experiential learning in which effectiveness depends on the ability to change human behavior.[93] As such, factors associated with PDSA improvement efforts are grounded in how individuals self-regulate their actions.[94] This approach was used by the National Health Services in England to explore individual and organizational learning and the characteristics of the organizational cultures needed to underpin such learning.[95,96]

Individuals who engage in improvement efforts place importance on fundamental values that govern organizational behaviors that propel peoples' actions from the outset.[97,86] A question of obvious importance is, "What are the critical behaviors and factors that might guide or drive the improvement cycles in radiation oncology centers?"

Mazur and colleagues found that when the system is compromised by defects, individuals will try to either quickly fix the problems without addressing the underlying root causes or try to identify and initiate efforts to eliminate the root causes of problems.[98] Alternately, when the system is not compromised by defects, individuals engage in one of the following three behaviors: continue to conform to standard procedures and processes, deviate from standard procedures and processes by taking shortcuts to get work done without explicitly degrading operating performance or patient safety, or seek to make permanent enhancements to work processes and activities in the spirit of continuous improvement.[20] Fig. 18.5 and the following bullet points depict the categories of improvement behavior.[98]

- *Quick fixing:* Detection and correction of defects. Although the defect is recognized, the focus is on fixing what is wrong and moving on.
- *Initiating:* Formal reporting of defects and the initiation of an improvement effort (such as PDSA) to improve the system. This also involves formal acknowledgment and action by the organization to correct the documented defects.
- *Conforming:* Compliance with standard procedures and processes under the conditions of a system free of defects.
- *Expediting:* Noncompliant procedures performed to complete the work under the conditions of a system free of defects.
- *Enhancing:* Efforts to make long-lasting system improvements with regard to work efficiency, effectiveness, or patient safety, although the system is not overtly defective.

The consequences to the organization of each of the five behaviors are quite different. When defects occur, quick-fixing behavior is effective at resolving immediate crises, but not necessarily effective at preventing recurrences of the underlying root causes of the defects. In the absence of defects, individuals can conform, expedite, or enhance. The most desirable behavior is enhancing because this type of individual focuses on growing the organization's capabilities for efficient, high-quality healthcare delivery. Thus the challenge for the radiation oncology centers is to promote, support, and sustain initiating and enhancing behaviors. In contrast, expediting and conforming behaviors should be virtually eliminated because they involve shortcuts and deviations from standard operating procedures and do not motivate individuals to make continuous quality improvement efforts. The next sections offer actionable recommendations for making progress to guide individuals to initiating and enhancing behaviors.

Transforming Behaviors

This challenge is one of how radiation oncology professionals will respond to defects when they occur, not whether they will respond at all. By and large, radiation oncology professionals are dedicated

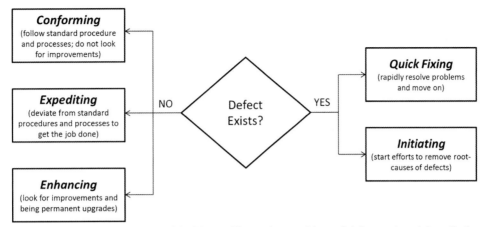

Fig. 18.5 Categories of behaviors and decision-making under conditions of defect and no defect. Preferred behaviors are enhancing and initiating because they promote individual and organizational learning toward high reliability and value creation. The remaining three behaviors, conforming, expediting, and quick fixing, lead to systems decay and unusable knowledge and learning. (From Mazur LM, McCreery J, Chen G. Quality improvement in hospitals: what triggers behavioral change? *J Healthc Eng.* 2012;4:621–648.)

BOX 18.1   Summary of Key Driving Forces and Restraining Forces That Affect The Individual While Developing Initiating and Enhancing Behaviors

Driving Forces	Restraining Forces
• Standard operating procedures	• Low staffing levels and high work loads
• Positive feedback	• Load efficiency requirements
• Role models	• Burdensome defect reporting systems
• Job-related autonomy	• Concerns related to psychological safety
• Support for direct supervisor	• Gratification and burnout
• Individualized attributes of the employee	• Suboptimal training on improvement philosophy
• Organizational accountability	• Lack of knowledge of improvement methods/tools
	• Lack of employee's social network for personal improvement

---

employees who take pride in safety of their patients. Developing initiating and enhancing behaviors is the responsibility of both the individual and the organization, in addition to supportive and engaged leadership and a strong culture of safety. Box 18.1 presents additional key driving forces *(left column)* and restraining forces *(right column)* that affect the individual while the organization attempts to develop employee initiating and enhancing behaviors.

- *Standard operating procedures:* To support employees with detection of defects. When standard operating procedures continuously "fail," this should cause a conflict with the desire to conform to existing ways of operating. This, in turn, should spur individual motivation for change.
- *Positive feedback:* Employees need to know their improvement efforts are valued, even under circumstances of suboptimal final results. If this feedback is positive, employees are more likely to invest in future improvement efforts.
- *Role models:* Employees need to see that initiating and enhancing behavior are rewarded. The exact nature of the reward, whether it be money or job title or other nonmonetary recognition, is not as important as the fact that the reward was meaningful to the

recipient and valued by the members of the organization. This creates tangible examples for others to emulate.

- *Job-related autonomy:* Without a sense of autonomy, employees will tend to follow the rules, especially if the rules are perceived to be good enough and not openly causing harm. Without autonomy, conformance is seen as a safe choice.
- *Support from direct supervisor:* This is needed to create an appealing work environment for initiating and enhancing behaviors. Employees must be empowered by supervisors to take action.
- *Individualized attributes of the employee:* Employees with a strong sense of care and concern for patients, coworkers, and the organization are more likely to break free from the status quo to take improvement actions based on initiating and enhancing behaviors.
- *Critical thinking skills:* Employees must be trained to skillfully conceptualize and assess situations, question assumptions, determine options for responding to the situation, apply improvement tools, and make intelligent decisions.
- *Organizational accountability:* This accountability refers to becoming a continuous improvement organization. In the presence of defects, it is leadership's role to set improvement expectations at a high but attainable level. In the absence of defects, leadership must develop this sense of urgency to improve and communicate its importance.

Although understanding, developing, and promoting the driving forces for positive change is of high importance, careful consideration must also be given to restraining forces that can act as barriers to the transition to initiating and enhancing behaviors.

- *Low staffing levels and high work efficiency requirements:* If employees are to become initiators or enhancers, they first must have the time in their workdays to take the necessary actions for improvements. If staffing levels are low and the demands for efficiency and productivity are high, the perception is that there is not sufficient time to institute real improvements. Thus making quick fixes, expediting, or conforming is more likely to happen.
- *Burdensome defect reporting systems:* When reporting systems are too administratively burdensome, then employees will not be inclined to report a defect, which, in turn, decreases an organization's ability to learn.
- *Concerns related to psychological safety:* Employees' ability to think and act freely without fear of negative consequences to self-image, status, or career is repeatedly identified as a significant restraining

force. As mentioned earlier, prior research has demonstrated that higher psychological safety increases the willingness of individuals to engage in defect reporting and improvement behaviors, even though such efforts are inherently risky and can have negative personal and career consequences.[37,38]

- *Gratification and burnout:* Naturally, initial reactions to quickly fixed problems or procedural shortcuts under time pressure can bring some satisfaction. This feeling of instant gratification can be a powerful motivator for continuing to use quick fixing and expediting to get rapid resolution of problems. Such firefighting behavior becomes the norm, and the desire for true improvement is dampened. However, in the long run, when employees find themselves solving the same problems, a more insidious restraining force arises over time because of personal burnout. This can lead to undesired conforming behaviors.

- *Culture of conforming to work procedures:* When organizational pressure to conform to standard work procedures is strong, employees will not be motivated to engage in process improvement efforts. Note that this force does not imply abandoning efforts to develop standard operating procedures. Rather, it implies that the desire to comply with work procedures might motivate employees to keep doing their jobs the same way as they have always done them.

- *Suboptimal training on improvement philosophy:* If employees have not been exposed to an improvement philosophy at work, they are less likely to know the mechanics of how to continuously improve. The specialized methods, tools, and mindset required to succeed at initiating and enhancing behaviors must be disseminated to frontline workers. This requires dedicated training and a sustained commitment by the leadership team.

- *Lack of dedicated improvement time:* Without the time to invest in initiating and enhancing behavior, employees will find it difficult to sustain this type of behavior over the long run.

- *Lack of knowledge of improvement methods/tools:* Those who are effective at initiating and enhancing need to be trained in these areas and build experience over time in applying tools and methods.

- *Lack of operational visibility:* Radiation oncology centers are tightly coupled systems, where the actions of one professional group tend to affect or be affected by actions in other professional groups. The lack of visibility of how their local work areas are connected to the larger operating system can limit employees' ability to be effective at initiating and enhancing behaviors. Without sufficient visibility and understanding, it is difficult for employees to identify sources of defects and make system-wide improvements.

- *Lack of employee's social network for improvement:* Outside of senior leadership, direct supervision, and explicit continuous improvement role models, potential initiators, and enhancers need a support system of colleagues. Employees who strive to enhance will have inevitable setbacks and challenges along the way. The support and encouragement of colleagues can prove to be invaluable to staying the course.

Practical Implications

Those with formal power in the radiation oncology centers can take positive actions in many of the areas described above to increase initiating and enhancing behaviors and reduce quick-fixing, conforming, and expediting behaviors. Researchers found that a psychologically safe climate must be cultivated by leaders and managers if frontline employees are to begin to report defects and initiate improvements.[84,94,99,100,101,102,103] Accordingly, as stated by Mazur and colleagues, "management involvement, style, and explicit behavior play important roles in organizational change. Perhaps here lies a critical step in the journey of developing highly reliable organizations: the need for leaders and managers to 'look in the mirror' and admit that that they are responsible for developing improvement behaviors, and therefore they must build organizations with values and a purpose beyond quick fixing, conforming, and expediting."[98]

Leadership teams can only do so much. It is also up to each individual to make the internal commitment to become a valuable contributor in the face of defects and deep-seated problems with processes and ways of performing work. Such work occurs over a prolonged period of time and depends upon each employee's understanding, motivation, abilities, and desire to make constructive changes in his/her work environment. Because initiating and enhancing behaviors are usually difficult if attempted by one isolated employee, a good example of a coordinated, collaborative activity that helps employees accomplish such behaviors is the multiday, multidisciplinary rapid improvement event. Participation in these events and other improvement activities will build a sense of confidence in employees that they can make a difference. There are various basic tools that can facilitate employees' transformation during improvement efforts. The following are a few of those tools:

- *Ishikawa (fishbone) diagram:* An Ishikawa diagram is created to figure out what factors lead to an error or undesirable outcome. The error is listed at the "head" of the fish, and the bones are the factors leading up to the error. These factors are grouped together by type. Common groupings are people, methods, machines, materials, measurements, and environment.

- *Histogram:* It is often important to know more than just the average occurrence of a particular problem. The ability to see the range of entries for a data set will often help determine ways to make improvements. A histogram is a graph that shows this range so that those improvements can be made.

- *Pareto chart:* A style of bar graph where the more important factors are highlighted. It often allows users to visualize the "80/20" rule of cause-and-effect relationship.

- *Scatter diagram:* A scatter diagram plots data points on a set of *x*- and *y*-axes to determine if there is a relationship between the two variables used for the *x*- and *y*-axes.

- *Control charts:* These are graphs that visually depict how different processes change while time goes on, allowing a department to determine whether a change is effective in its current implementation.

SUMMARY

- The challenge for radiation oncology centers is to develop a culture of safety, one that can effectively and efficiently spearhead positive changes in quality and safety.

- Leadership is the most important component to accomplishing this monumental task, because without it, virtually no significant organizational change can succeed. Leaders in radiation oncology must have a vision and a clear set of goals for quality and safety. They need to continually empower and support their staff during improvement efforts. Leaders must send this message overtly, verbally, and implicitly through their actions and behaviors. Second, continuous support for a culture of safety is vital, because it must be maintained to allow staff members to begin to see their work differently, no longer accepting workarounds and frustrations. Instead, staff members must realize that they have two roles: to do their job and to improve the manner in which they do their job. Finally, departments need to develop a systematic manner in which problems and potential solutions are considered. We offered the PDSA cycle as a dependable approach, especially if broad participation of staff is achieved to help ensure that all aspects of a particular problem are being adequately considered.

- The power of the culture of safety lies in its systematic nature rather than in its specific structure. Scholars studying high-reliability and value-creation industries such as commercial automobiles, aviation, or nuclear plants speculate that their long-term organizational effectiveness depends on their continuous and never-ending efforts towards safety mindfulness, which requires interaction between leadership, a culture of safety, and improvement cycles. Some well-known approaches that provide structure to this end goal include lean, Six Sigma, and change management programs.

REVIEW QUESTIONS

The answers to the Review Questions can be found by logging on to our website at: http://evolve.elsevier.com/Washington/principles

1. The field of radiation oncology is rapidly evolving mostly because of:
   a. Cultural changes.
   b. Educational requirements.
   c. Technological advancements.
   d. Accreditation requirements.
2. As stated in standard 7 of the ASTRO accreditation document, a culture of safety depends on:
   a. Guidance, direction, and financial means from the leadership of the institution and of the radiation therapy department.
   b. Individual effort by every member of the department.
   c. Organized support for quality and safety at every level in the institution.
   d. All of the above.
3. Which of the following elements are crucial in creating an organization-wide transformation to a culture of safety?
   I. Leadership.
   II. Higher-level technology.
   III. Culture of safety.
   IV. Improvement cycles.
      a. I, II, and III.
      b. I, II, and IV.
      c. I, III, and IV.
      d. All of the above.
4. What are the desired characteristics of leaders promoting a culture of safety?
   I. Being a good listener.
   II. Persistence and determination.
   III. Lack of empathy.
   IV. Ability to work within economic constraints.
      a. I, II, and III.
      b. I, II, and IV.
      c. I, III, and IV.
      d. All of the above.
5. In 2010, the radiation oncology community was confronted by articles in the *New York Times*, which examined:

   I. Leadership.
   II. Radiation dose.
   III. Patient safety.
   IV. Environmental factors.
      a. I, II, and III.
      b. I, II, and IV.
      c. II and IV.
      d. III and IV.
6. What is a problem-solving tool used by Toyota that has been adapted to healthcare delivery?
   a. A2.
   b. A3.
   c. B3.
   d. B2.
7. What is the goal of safety rounds in a radiation oncology practice?
   a. Workers have the needed tools.
   b. Workers can learn about safety.
   c. Workers can perform higher-level physics quality assurance.
   d. Workers have a chance to practice continuing education.
8. What are the desired improvement behaviors?
   a. Conforming.
   b. Initiating and enhancing.
   c. Expediting.
   d. Quick fixing.
9. What is the PDSA cycle?
   a. Plan, Do, Safety, Act.
   b. Plan, Do, Study, Act.
   c. Prepare, Do, Study, Act.
   d. Perform, Discuss, Simplify, Accept.
10. Which of the following are tools of the PDSA process?
   I. Ishikawa diagram.
   II. Pareto chart.
   III. Scatterplot.
   IV. Venogram.
      a. I, II, and III.
      b. I, II, and IV.
      c. I, III, and IV.
      d. All of the above.

QUESTIONS TO PONDER

1. What is culture?
2. What is culture of safety?
3. What are the critical factors needed to develop culture of safety? Why?
4. What is safety mindfulness?
5. Can practices from TPS, or lean, be adapted to radiation oncology centers to develop culture of safety? Why?
6. What other improvement cycles beside PDSA could be used in radiation oncology centers?
7. How will you contribute to continuous quality improvement efforts at your organization?

REFERENCES

1. Bogdanich W. Radiation offers new cures, and ways to do harm. *New York Times*. 2010. https://www.nytimes.com/2010/01/24/health/24radiation.html. Accessed January 25, 2019.

2. Bogdanich W. As technology surges, radiation safeguards lag. *New York Times*. 2010. https://www.nytimes.com/2010/01/27/us/27radiation.html. Accessed January 25, 2019.

3. Bogdanich W. At hearing on radiation, calls for better oversight. *New York Times*. 2010. https://www.nytimes.com/2010/02/27/health/policy/27radiation.html. Accessed January 25, 2019.

4. Bono JE, Anderson MH. The advice and influence networks of transformational leaders. *J Appl Psychol*. 2005;90:1306–1314.

5. ASTRO. *Hearings Before the Subcommittee on Health of the House Committee on Energy and Commerce*; 2010. Testimony of Michael Herman, PhD, American Association of Physicists in Medicine. https://www.govinfo.gov/content/pkg/CHRG-111hhrg76012/pdf/CHRG-111hhrg76012.pdf. Accessed January 20, 2019.

6. ASTRO. *Hearings Before the Health Subcommittee of the House Energy and Commerce Committee*; 2010. Testimony of Tim Williams, MD, Chairman of the Board of Directors on Behalf of ASTRO. https://www.govinfo.gov/content/pkg/CHRG-111hhrg76012/pdf/CHRG-111hhrg76012.pdf. Accessed January 20, 2019.

7. Medical Dosimetry News Archives (website). www.MedicalDosimetry.org. Accessed January 25, 2019.

8. Odle TG, Rosier N. Radiation therapy safety: the critical role of the radiation therapist (white paper). https://www.asrt.org/main/news-publications/research/white-papers. Accessed January 25, 2019.

9. ASTRO. *Accreditation program for excellence (APEX)* Washington; 2014. https://www.astro.org/Daily-Practice/Accreditation. Accessed October 15, 2019.

10. Colla JB, Bracken AC, Kinney LM, Weeks WB. Measuring patient safety climate: a review of surveys. *Qual Saf Health Care*. 2005;14:364–366.

11. LaPorte T. High reliability organizations: unlikely, demanding and at risk. *J Contingencies Crisis Manag*. 1996;4:60–71.

12. Perrow C. *Normal Accidents: Living With High-Risk Technologies*. New York, NY: Basic Books; 1999.

13. Roberts KH, Bea R. Must accidents happen? Lessons from high reliability organizations. *Acad Manag Exec*. 2001;15:70–79.

14. Bass BM, Bass R. *The Bass Handbook of Leadership: Theory, Research, and Managerial Applications*.4th ed. New York, NY: Free Press; 2008.

15. Judson A. *Changing Behavior in Organizations*. Hoboken, NJ: Cambridge: Blackwell Publishing; 1991.

16. Kotter JP. Accelerate!. *Harv Bus Rev*. 2012;44–52:149.

17. Kotter JP. *Leading Change*. Boston, MA: Harvard Business School Press; 1996.

18. Kotter JP. *Our Iceberg Is Melting*. 1st ed. New York, NY: St. Martin's Press; 2006.

19. Institute of Medicine. *To Err Is Human: Building a Safer Health System*. Washington, DC: National Academies Press; 1996.

20. Weingart SN, Page D. Implications for practice: challenges for healthcare leaders in fostering patient safety. *Qual Saf Health Care*. 2004;13:ii52–ii56.

21. Weingart SN, Weissman JS, Zimmer KP, et al. Implementation and evaluation of a prototype consumer reporting system for patient safety events. *Int J Qual Health Care*. 2017;29(4):521–526.

22. Ramanujam R, Rousseau DM. The challenges are organizational, not just clinical. *J Organ Behav*. 2006;27:811–827.

23. McFadden KL, Towell ER, Stock GN. Implementation of patient safety initiatives in US hospitals. *Int J Oper Prod Manag*. 2006;26:326–347.

24. Galpin T. *The Human Side of Change: A Practical Guide to Organization Redesign*. San Francisco, CA: Jossey-Bass; 1996.

25. Bass BM. *Leadership and Performance Beyond Expectations*. New York NY: Free Press; 1985.

26. Podsakoff PM, MacKenzie SB, Bommer WH. Transformational leadership behaviors and substitutes for leadership as determinants of employee satisfaction, commitment, trust, and organizational citizenship behaviors. *J Manag*. 1996;22:259–298.

27. Spinelli RJ. The applicability of Bass's model of transformational, transactional, and laissez-faire leadership in the hospital administrative environment. *Hosp Top*. 2006;84:11–18.

28. Stordeur S, Vandenberghe C, D'hoore W. Leadership styles across hierarchical levels in nursing departments. *Nurs Res*. 2000;49:37–43.

29. Xirasagar S, Samuels ME, Stoskopf CH. Physician leadership styles and effectiveness: an empirical study. *Med Care Res Rev*. 2005;62:720–740.

30. Bass BM. *Transformational Leadership: Industry, Military, and Educational Impact*. Mahwah, NJ: Erlbaum; 1998.

31. Eisenbeiss SA, van Knippenberg D, Boerner S. Transformational leadership and team innovation: integrating team climate principles. *J Appl Psychol*. 2008;93:1438–1446.

32. Jansen JP, Vera D, Crossan M. Strategic leadership for exploration and exploitation: the moderating role of environmental dynamism. *Leadersh Q*. 2009;20:5–18.

33. Avolio BJ, Bass BM. *Multifactor Leadership Questionnaire*. Redwood City, CA: Mind Garden; 1965.

34. Adams RD, Marks LB, Pawlicki T, et al. The new radiation therapy clinical practice: the emerging role of clinical peer review for radiation therapists and medical dosimetrists. *Med Dosim*. 2010;35:320–323.

35. Chera BS, Mazur L, Adams RD, Marks LB. The promise and burden of peer review in radiation oncology. *J Oncol Pract*. 2016;12:e61–e69.

36. Aiken LH, Clarke SP, Sloane DM. An international perspective on hospital nurses' work environments: the case for reform. *Policy Polit Nurs Pract*. 2001;2:255–263.

37. Edmondson A, Moingeon B. Learning, trust and organizational change. In: Easterby-Smith M, Araujo L, Burgoyne J, eds. *Organizational Learning and the Learning Organization*. London, UK: Sage; 1999.

38. Edmondson AC. Psychological safety and learning behavior in work teams. *Adm Sci Q*. 1999;44:250–282.

39. Tucker AL, Edmondson AC. Why hospitals don't learn from failures: organizational and psychological dynamics that inhibit system change. *Calif Manage Rev*. 2003;45:55–72.

40. Uribe CL, Schweikhart SB, Pathak DS, et al. Perceived barriers to medication-error reporting: an explanatory investigation. *J Healthc Manag*. 2002;47:263–279.

41. Nembharth IM, Edmondson AM. Making it safe: the effects of leader inclusiveness and professional status on psychological safety and improvement efforts in health care teams. *J Organ Behav*. 2006;27:941–966.

42. Reason J. *Human Error*. Cambridge, UK: Cambridge University Press; 1990.

43. Institute of Medicine. *Quality Through Collaboration: The Future of Rural Healthcare*. Washington, DC: National Academies Press; 2005.

44. Scott JG, Cohen D, Dicicco-Bloom B, et al. Understanding healing relationships in primary care. *Ann Fam Med*. 2008;6(4):315–322.

45. Chassin MR, Loeb MJ. The ongoing quality improvement journey: next stop, high reliability. *Health Affairs*. 2011;30:559–568.

46. Hackman JR. The design of work teams. In: Lorsch J, ed. *Handbook of Organizational Behavior*. Englewood Cliffs, NJ: Prentice-Hall; 1987.

47. Fratt L. The new economics of radiation oncology. *Health Imaging*. 2013. https://www.healthimaging.com/topics/healthcare-economics/new-economics-radiation-oncology. Accessed January 25, 2019.

48. Gillespie D. Burnout among health service providers. *Adm Policy Ment Health*. 1991;18:161–171.

49. Frederberger H. The staff burnout syndrome in alternative institutions. *Psychother Theory Res Pract*. 1975;12:73–82.

50. Kahn F. *The Physics of Radiation Therapy*. 4th ed. Madison, WI: Medical Physics Publishing; 2009.

51. Annual report of cancer facts and figures Atlanta. American Cancer Society; 2019 (website). https://www.cancer.org/research/cancer-facts-statistics/all-cancer-facts-figures/cancer-facts-figures-2019.html. Accessed December 19, 2019.

52. Gunderson L, Tepper J. *Clinical Radiation Oncology*. 4th ed. Philadelphia, PA: Saunders/Elsevier; 2016.

53. Maslach C, Jackson S. Burnout in health professions: a social psychological analysis. In: Sanders G, Suls J, eds. Social *Psychology of Health and Illness*. Hillsdale, NJ: Erlbaum; 2019:227–251.

54. Akroyd D, Adams R. Examining stress and burnout. *Industry Insider*. 1999;1:4–7.

55. Akroyd D, Adams R. The cost of caring: a national study of burnout in radiation therapists. *Radiat Ther J Oncol Sci.* 2000;9:123–130.

56. Akroyd D, Caison A, Adams R. Burnout in radiation therapists: the predictive value of selective stressors. *Int J Radiat Oncol Biol Phys.* 2002;52:816–821.

57. Akroyd D, Caison A, Adams R. Patterns of burnout among US radiographers. *Radiol Technol.* 2002;73:215–223.

58. Probst H, Griffiths S, Adams R, et al. Burnout in therapy radiographers in the United Kingdom. *Br J Radiography.* 2012;85:e760–e765.

59. Schneider ME, Knight K, Luc D, et al. Sustainability, productivity, and efficiency in health workforce education and training: occupational burnout among Australian medical radiation science health professionals-the impact of a quality workforce. Presented at: People in Health Summit-Developing Victoria's Health Workforce; Melbourne, Australia; 2005.

60. Schneider ME, Wright CA, Church JA, et al. Occupational burnout among radiographers and radiation therapists in Australia. Presented at the ASMMIRT 10th Annual Scientific Meeting; Hobart, Tasmania, Australia; 2005.

61. Passmore G. Burnout in radiation therapy: examining the six leading influences. https://dune.une.edu/theses/98/. Accessed October 15, 2019.

62. Singh N, Knight K, Wright C. Occupational burnout among radiographers, sonographers and radiologists in Australia and New Zealand: findings from a national survey. *J Med Imaging Radiat Oncol.* 2017;61(3): 304–310.

63. Womack JP, Jones DT, Roos D. *The Machine That Changed the World.* New York, NY: Rawson Associates; 1990.

64. Spear SJ. Fixing health care from the inside, today. *Harv Bus Rev.* 2005;83(9):78–91.

65. Liker JK. *The Toyota Way: Fourteen Management Principles from the World's Greatest Manufacturer.* New York, NY: McGraw-Hill; 2005.

66. Mazur LM, Johnson K, Pooya P, Chadwick J, McCreery J. lean exploration loops into healthcare facility design: programming phase. *Health Environ Res Des J.* 2017;10(3):116–130.

67. Mazur LM, Chen S-J, Prescott B. Pragmatic evaluating of Toyota Production System (TPS) analysis procedure for problem solving with entry-level nurses. *J Ind Eng Manag.* 2008;1:240–268.

68. Institute for Healthcare Improvement. *Going Lean in Health Care.* Innovation Series white paper. Cambridge, MA: Institute for Healthcare Improvement; 2005.

69. Adams R, Church J, Chang S, et al. Fostering a culture of patient safety. Presented at: University of North Carolina Hospitals Poster Sessions; Chapel Hill, NC October 19, 2010.

70. Davidoff F. Heterogeneity is not always noise: lessons from improvement. *JAMA.* 2009;302:2580–2586.

71. Herzer K, Mirrer M, Xie Y. Patient safety reporting systems: sustained quality improvements using a multidisciplinary team and 'good catch' awards. *Jt Comm J Qual Patient Saf.* 2012;38:339–347.

72. Adams R. Improving patient safety through lean techniques in radiation oncology. Presented at: The National Medical Dosimetrist Conference of the American Association of Medical Dosimetrists (AAMD); June, 2013; San Antonio, TX.

73. Frankel A, Grillo SP, Pittman M, et al. Revealing and resolving patient safety defects: the impact of leadership walkrounds on frontline caregiver assessments of patient safety. *Health Serv Res.* 2008;43:2050–2066.

74. Fine B, Golden B, Hannam R, Morra D. Leading lean: a Canadian healthcare leader's guide. *Healthc Q.* 2009;12:26–35.

75. Montgomery V. Impact of staff-led safety walk rounds (website). http://www.ahrq.gov/downloads/pub/advances2/vol3/advances-montgomery_42.pdf. Accessed January 25, 2019.

76. Adams R, Church J, Chang S, et al. Quality assurance in clinical radiation therapy: a quantitative assessment of the utility of peer review in a multi-physician academic practice. Presented at: The American Society for Radiation Oncology (ASTRO); October, 2009; Chicago, IL.

77. Grol R. Quality improvement by peer review in primary care: a practical guide. *Qual Health Care.* 1994;3:147–152.

78. Toohey J, Shakespeare T, Morgan G. RANZCR peer review audit instrument. *J Med Imaging Radiat Oncol.* 2008;52:403–413.

79. Mazur LM, Mosaly P, Hoyle L, Jones E, Chera B, Marks LB. Relating physician's workload with errors during radiotherapy planning. *Pract Radiat Oncol.* 2013;4(2):71–75.

80. Mazur LM, Mosaly P, Moore C, et al. Towards a better understanding of task demands, workload, and performance during physician-computer interactions. *J Am Med Inform Assoc.* 2016;23(6):1113–1120.

81. Mazur LM, Mosaly P, Hoyle L, et al. Subjective and objective quantification of physician's workload and performance during radiotherapy planning tasks. *Pract Radiat Oncol.* 2013;3(4):e171–e177.

82. Mosaly P, Mazur LM, Jones E, et al. Quantification of physician's workload and performance during cross-coverage in radiation therapy treatment planning. *Pract Radiat Oncol.* 2013;3:e179–e186.

83. Gawande A. *The Checklist Manifesto: How To Get Things Right.* 1st ed. New York, NY: Metropolitan Books; 2011.

84. Marks LB, Adams RD, Pawlicki T, et al. Enhancing the role of case-oriented peer review to improve quality and safety in radiation oncology: executive Summary. *Pract Radiat Oncol.* 2013;3:149–156.

85. Marks LB, Hubbs JL, Light KL, et al. Improving safety for patients receiving radiotherapy: the successful application of quality assurance initiatives (abstract). *Int J Radiat Oncol Biol Phys.* 2008;72:S143.

86. Tucker AL, Edmondson AC, Spear S. When problem solving prevents organizational learning. *J Org Change Manag.* 2002;15:122–137.

87. Das P, Johnson J, Hayden S, et al. Rate of radiation therapy events in a large academic institution. *J Am Coll Radiol.* 2013;10(6):452–455.

88. Brass DJ, Galaswiewicz J, Greve HR, et al. Taking stock of networks and organizations: a multilevel perspective. *Acad Manag J.* 2004;4:795–817.

89. Brass DJ. Social capital and organizational leadership. In: Zaccaro SJ, Klimoski RJ, eds. *The Nature of Organizational Leadership: Understanding the Performance Imperatives Confronting Today's Leaders.* San Francisco, CA: Jossey-Bass; 2001;132-152.

90. Borgatti SP, Foster PC. The network paradigm in organizational research: a review and typology. *J Manag.* 2003;29:991–1013.

91. Balkundi P, Kilduff M. The ties that lead: a social network approach to leadership. *Leadersh Q.* 2006;17:419–439.

92. McCreery J, Aiman-Smith L. Organizational boundary spanners: identifying competencies and gaps. Proceedings of 2008 PICMET Conference; Cape Town, South Africa; 2008: 2416-2428.

93. Davies HT, Nutley SM. Developing learning organizations in the new NHS. *Br Med J.* 2000;320:998–1001.

94. Tucker AL. An empirical study of system improvement by frontline employees in hospital units. *Manuf Serv Oper Manag.* 2007;9:492–505.

95. Dutton JE. The making of organizational opportunities: an interpretive pathway to organizational change. In: Cummings LL, Staw BM, eds. *Research in Organizational Behavior.* Greenwich, CT: JAI Press; 2017:195-226.

96. Ferlie EB, Shortell SM. Improving the quality of health care in the United Kingdom and the United States: a framework for change. *Milbank Q.* 2001;79:281–315.

97. Huq Z, Martin TN. Workforce cultural factors in TQM/CQI implementation in hospitals. *Health Care Manage Rev.* 2000;25:80–93.

98. Mazur LM, McCreery J, Chen S-J. Quality improvement in hospitals: what triggers behavioral change? *J Healthc Eng.* 2012;4:621–648.

99. Kerfoot K. Staff engagement: it starts with the leader. *Medsurg Nurs.* 2008;17:64–65.

100. Koys D. The effects of employee satisfaction, organizational citizenship behavior, and turnover, on organizational effectiveness: a unit-level, longitudinal study. *Pers Psychol.* 2001;54:101–114.

101. Mazur LM, Chen SJ. An empirical study for medication delivery improvement based on healthcare professionals' perceptions of medication delivery system. *Health Care Manag Sci.* 2009;12:56–66.

102. McAlearney AS. Leadership development in healthcare: a qualitative study. *J Organ Behav.* 2006;27:967–982.

103. Runciman W, Hibbert P, Thomson R, et al. Toward an international classification for patient safety; key concepts and terms. *Int J Qual Health Care.* 2009;21:18–26.

19

Quality Improvement in Radiation Oncology

Lisa Bartenhagen, Jana Koth

OBJECTIVES

- Discuss the evolution and purpose of quality improvement in radiation oncology.
- Discuss the components of a quality management program in the development of a culture of safety in radiation oncology.
- Describe the roles of accreditation and regulatory agencies, as well as professional organizations, in the development of a quality improvement plan for radiation oncology.
- Delineate the responsibilities of the quality improvement team members in radiation oncology.

- Differentiate among quality control, quality assurance, and quality management.
- Identify quality indicators in radiation oncology.
- Highlight quality control procedures and recommended tolerances for which a radiation therapist is responsible.
- Explain the importance of a quality audit.
- Defend the rationale for voluntary error reporting.

OUTLINE

KEY TERMS

Action levels
Continuous quality improvement
FMEA, failure mode and effects analysis
Healthcare quality
Near miss
Outcomes
Plan-do-check-act (or plan-do-study-act)
Quality
Quality assessment

Quality assurance
Quality audit
Quality control
Quality improvement
Quality indicators
Radiation oncology quality improvement team
Regulatory agency
Joint Commission

INTRODUCTION

Over the years, organizations have taken various approaches to ensure quality. These approaches are dependent on the needs of the industry, the definition of quality, and the management of the process. For improvement to occur in any system, one must define what constitutes quality and how it should be measured. This chapter follows the American Society of Radiologic Technologists (ASRT)'s recommended curriculum for radiation therapy education. The authors discuss the role of quality improvement (QI) in radiation oncology and illustrate how a facility can implement an effective program to ensure the best of care.

EVOLUTION OF QUALITY IMPROVEMENT

Finding an all-encompassing definition of quality can be difficult. A radiation oncologist might define quality as the ability to offer the most sophisticated treatment technologies, whereas the radiation therapist might define quality as the expertise involved in precise treatment delivery. From a patient's point of view, quality may be short wait times and minimal side effects. The National Academy of Medicine (NAM), formerly the Institute of Medicine (IOM), broadly defines healthcare quality as the degree to which health services for individuals and populations increase the likelihood of desired health outcomes and are consistent with current professional knowledge.[1] Outcomes can be described as the anticipated benefits or results from the planned implementation of a process. The NAM includes six aims for a healthcare system:

1. Safe: The care that is intended to help patients should not harm them.
2. Effective: Use knowledge to provide services to those it will benefit and avoid misuse to those who may not benefit.
3. Patient-centered: All clinical decisions are based on patient needs and values.
4. Timely: Reduce waits and delays for both patients and those providing care.
5. Efficient: Avoid any type of waste.
6. Equitable: Do not vary quality of care to any individual.[2]

The concept of quality evolved from the industrial revolution in the United States to ensure uniform manufacturing processes, such as the assembly line implemented by Henry Ford. At that time, quality was associated with inspection. Individuals who expanded on the concept of quality during the twentieth century were Joseph M. Juran and W.E. Deming. Juran added the human dimension to quality management by advocating for education and training of individuals with the philosophy of the 80/20 rule from Italian economist Vilfredo Pareto. The 80/20 rule was applied toward quality management in that 80% of the problems are caused by 20% of the defects.[3] W.E. Deming introduced total quality management (TQM) in 1950 to the Japanese Union of Scientists and Engineers, who went on to establish the QI model of **plan-do-check-act** (PDCA), or plan-do-study-act (PDSA), which is a model widely used in healthcare today.[4–5] See Box 19.1 for a summary of Deming's principles.[6]

QUALITY IMPROVEMENT MODELS

Lean

A methodology for process improvement is Lean Management, or simply Lean. It was developed by Toyota to become more efficient and eliminate waste.[7] The goal of Lean is to add value to a service, and if any resources are used for reasons other than adding value, they are considered waste and should be eliminated from the process.[8] Lean management focuses on eight guiding principles. The first is that all staff must be respected and valued. If staff feels valued, then moving from compliance, where they do something because they "have to,"

BOX 19.1 W.E. Deming's 14 Points of Management

1. Create constancy of purpose toward improvement of product and service, with the aim to become competitive and stay in business and provide jobs.
2. Adopt a new philosophy.
3. Cease dependence on mass inspection to achieve quality. Build quality into the product in the first place.
4. End the practice of awarding business on the basis of price alone. Instead, minimize total cost. Move toward a single supplier for any one item because of a long-term relationship built on loyalty and trust.
5. Improve constantly and forever the system of production and service to improve quality and productivity and thus constantly reduce costs.
6. Institute training on the job.
7. Institute leadership to help people do the job better.
8. Drive out fear so that everyone can work effectively for the good of the organization.
9. Break down barriers among departments.
10. Eliminate slogans, exhortations, and targets for the work force.
11. Eliminate work quotas. Substitute leadership.
12. Eliminate merit rating systems.
13. Institute a vigorous program of education and self-improvement.
14. Involve everyone in the organization in the transformation of total quality improvement (TQI).

From Deming WE. *Out of the Crisis.* Cambridge, MA: Center for Advanced Educational Services, MIT Press; 1986; Papp J. Introduction to quality management. In: Papp J, ed. *Quality Management in the Imaging Sciences.* 6th ed. St. Louis, MO: 2011 Elsevier.

TABLE 19.1 The Eight Wastes of Lean Management[9,10]

Type of Waste	Example of Waste in Radiation Oncology
Overproduction	Too many images being taken daily
Transportation	Patients transported inefficiently by the inappropriate staff
Inventory	Space costs money, excessive stock occupies space
Motion	Personnel transferring from facility to facility
Defects	Improper imaging techniques or protocols
Overprocessing	3D reconstructions performed unnecessarily
Waiting	Treatment unit is idle while others are delayed
Skills	Underutilizing staff capabilities

3D, Three-dimensional.

transforms to a commitment of adding value. This leads to change that is sustainable.[9] Second is observing the process where it takes place. This allows workers to show leadership where the inefficiencies exist and suggest improvements. Next is eliminating the waste. Table 19.1 identifies eight waste examples in the lean approach. Having a machine sit idle while another is overbooked illustrates waste.[10] Step 4 involves standardization. This decreases variation and increases efficiency. The use of a pretreatment checklist is an example of standardizing a process. Value stream mapping is useful in finding variations to a process. This includes mapping out the entire process from start to finish.[11] The next two steps involve communicating and updating everyone during the process with the use of visual tools such as reports and storyboards. Last, but no less important in the lean process, is adding value for the customer. Feedback should be collected to ensure that value is being added.[8] Patient satisfaction surveys are useful for collecting feedback.

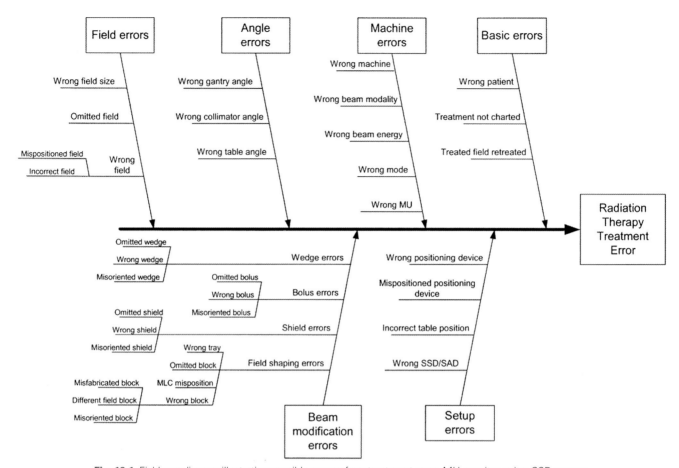

Fig. 19.1 Fishbone diagram illustrating possible causes for a treatment error. *MU,* monitor units; *SSD,* source-skin-distance; *SAD,* source-axis-distance; *MLC,* multi-leaf collimator. (From Patton GA, Gaffney DK, Moeller JH. Facilitation of radiotherapeutic error by computerized record and verify systems. *Int J Radiat Oncol Biol Phys.* 2003;56(1):50–57.)

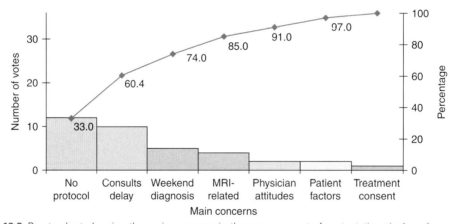

Fig. 19.2 Pareto chart showing the main concerns in the management of metastatic spinal cord compression. (From Lee K, Tsou I, Wong S, et al. Metastatic spinal cord compression as an oncology emergency—getting our act together. *Int J Qual Health Care.* 2007;19(6):377–381.)

As mentioned, it is important to display the process, communicate progress, and serve as efficient dialogue for the organization. Fig. 19.1 is an example of a fishbone chart, which is one way to display a process. It is a visual tool used to look at cause and effect. The problem or effect is displayed at the head, and the possible causes are the bones of the fish.[12–13] Another way to display data is with a Pareto chart. This is used to summarize the relative importance or frequency of things that may be causing problems. Fig. 19.2 displays a Pareto chart showing the main concerns in the management of metastatic spinal cord compression.[14]

Plan, Do, Check, Act

Strategies used to improve long-lasting, effective change in a process include the PDCA model. This process should be iterated over and over for continuous improvement. The four-step process includes:

1. Plan: Recognize and plan a change.
2. Do: Carry out the change on a small-scale study.
3. Check: Monitor the change, analyze the results. and identify areas for improvement in the next cycle.
4. Act. Take action based on the change.[5]

The benefits of performing PDCA are that the steps are simple and can be done in small increments. On the other hand, because it is an incremental process, the improvement may result slowly, and it is necessary to have buy-in from everyone affected by the process.[15] An example of the PDCA methodology in radiation oncology was demonstrated by Gillian et al, who investigated head and neck patient start times from simulation to the first day of radiation treatment. From consult to the start of treatment, the department wanted to decrease wait times from 15 to 10 days. Below is the process followed:

Plan: Implement a process of prebooking magnetic resonance imaging (MRI) and positron emission tomography (PET) appointments to be within one day of the computed tomography (CT) simulation.

Do: The plan was implemented and monitored. Outcomes collected reasons for unexpected delays, the impact on other scheduling, and the changes in wait times.

Check: The collected data was analyzed.

Act: If the small change in practice met the goal of decreasing wait times, then a new standard of practice could be documented. If the goal was not met, then a modified plan could be put into place during the next iteration.[15]

A3

A tool developed again by Toyota is the A3. The name is derived from the paper size used for the report (11" × 17"). The A3 outlines the process from "problem faced" to "problem solved" and often incorporates PDCA.[16] There are variations of the A3 tool, but it generally includes 10 sections.[9,16 17]

Step 1: Issue: A clear statement identifying the problem.

Step 2: Background: Useful baseline information and metrics.

Step 3: Current condition: Drawing that completely describes the current situation so improvements can be discovered (process mapping is useful here).

Step 4: Goal: A statement that quantifies how improvement is measured. Goals need to be SMART (specific, measurable, attainable, relevant, timely).[17]

Step 5: Root cause analysis: Five whys, fishbone, Pareto, and histograms can be used for a retrospective analysis.[8]

Step 6: Target condition: What is necessary to meet the goal, and what the situation will look like after the improvement.

Step 7: Countermeasures: Improvements needed.

Step 8: Implementation and cost analysis: A complete list of tasks to achieve the improvement with who is responsible for the actions, timelines for completion, and the expected outcome. This section will also include the cost for completing the plan, the savings incurred, and what waste was eliminated.

Step 9: Test: Start with a small pilot project of a couple weeks, and see if initial results align with goal.

Step 10: Follow up/audit: Audit plan is described, results of audit, lessons learned, and recommendations for next A3.

Generally, steps 1 to 7 fall into the "Plan" of PDCA, step 8 is the "Do" component, "Check" falls into step 9, and step 10 incorporates "Act."[17] A basic example of an A3 can be found in Fig. 19.3.

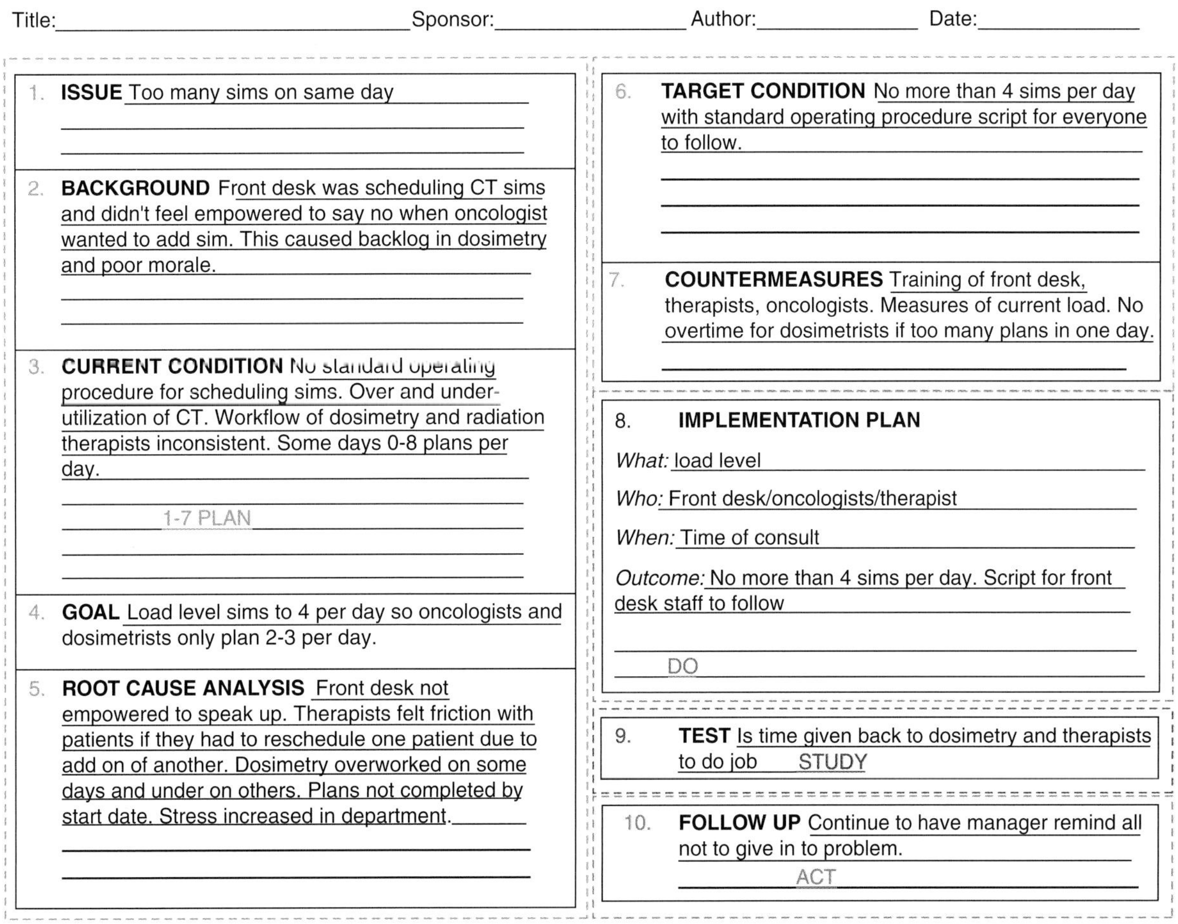

Title:_____ Sponsor:_____ Author:_____ Date:_____

1. **ISSUE** Too many sims on same day

2. **BACKGROUND** Front desk was scheduling CT sims and didn't feel empowered to say no when oncologist wanted to add sim. This caused backlog in dosimetry and poor morale.

3. **CURRENT CONDITION** No standard operating procedure for scheduling sims. Over and under-utilization of CT. Workflow of dosimetry and radiation therapists inconsistent. Some days 0-8 plans per day.

1-7 PLAN

4. **GOAL** Load level sims to 4 per day so oncologists and dosimetrists only plan 2-3 per day.

5. **ROOT CAUSE ANALYSIS** Front desk not empowered to speak up. Therapists felt friction with patients if they had to reschedule one patient due to add on of another. Dosimetry overworked on some days and under on others. Plans not completed by start date. Stress increased in department.

6. **TARGET CONDITION** No more than 4 sims per day with standard operating procedure script for everyone to follow.

7. **COUNTERMEASURES** Training of front desk, therapists, oncologists. Measures of current load. No overtime for dosimetrists if too many plans in one day.

8. **IMPLEMENTATION PLAN**

What: load level

Who: Front desk/oncologists/therapist

When: Time of consult

Outcome: No more than 4 sims per day. Script for front desk staff to follow

DO

9. **TEST** Is time given back to dosimetry and therapists to do job   STUDY

10. **FOLLOW UP** Continue to have manager remind all not to give in to problem.

ACT

Fig. 19.3 Sample improvement process using an A3 tool. (From Bassuk JA, Washington IM. The A3 problem solving report: a 10-step scientific method to execute performance improvements in an academic research vivarium. *PLoS One.* 2013;8(10):e76833.)

Six Sigma

Six Sigma, on the other hand, is a statistically driven improvement process. Sigma refers to the number of standard deviations a process is from average performance. If a process is within six standard deviations of the average performance, then it is said to be in Six Sigma. At this point, the process results in approximately 3.4 errors per million opportunities, or it is 99.99996% error free.[18] The framework of Six Sigma includes: define, measure, analyze, improve, and control (DMIAC). The model is ideally used to improve a process, product, or service by eliminating variation and errors in the process. See Box 19.2 for details of the DMAIC framework.

As illustrated from the discussed process improvement models, the goal of a quality management program is still to provide the best care possible, but the culture of how to accomplish that is changing. Although it is important that all equipment perform according to specifications and operate within tolerances, a better understanding of the interaction of the people, clinical processes, and the potential failures associated with treatment outcomes is necessary. For example, there are more than seven intensity-modulated radiation therapy (IMRT) delivery methods (e.g., step and shoot, physical compensators, volumetric arc therapy, etc.), so it is unlikely to develop a quality management protocol for every treatment technique and delivery equipment.[19] Moving from a reactive approach of quality and safety to a prospective approach is discussed in the following section.

Whatever model a facility chooses, it must be patient centered. Data-driven decisions and a willingness to change by working as a team are needed for continuous QI (CQI).

REGULATING AGENCIES

A regulatory agency establishes mandates with authorization from Congress to write standards and regulations that explain the technical, operational, and legal details necessary to implement laws. Regulations are mandatory requirements that can apply to individuals, businesses, state or local governments, nonprofit institutions, and others. These standards and regulations provide the cornerstones for the radiation oncology facility's QI plan. A radiation oncology facility must be familiar with all national, state, and professional regulations that affect the facility's operation. This process is ongoing because new guidelines and practice standards must be followed with the development and use of new equipment and treatment techniques.

Federal and state government, professional, and accreditation agencies mandate standards to ensure not only that equipment is functional and operates within acceptable limits but also that operators of this equipment are truly qualified individuals.

BOX 19.2   Six Sigma Tools

Define	Define the Project, Goals, and Other Parameters
Measure	Use tools to determine quality, identify variation, validate measuring process, and collect data.
Analyze	Identify underlying causes for an issue, testing statistical significance from the population sampled.
Improve	Solutions are implemented to improve a process so it will be efficient, economical, and safe.
Control	Systems are in place to ensure improvements are sustained.

From Varkey P, Kollengode A. Methodologies for quality improvement. In: Pawlicki T, Dunscombe P, Mundt AJ, eds. *Quality and Safety in Radiotherapy*. Boca Raton, FL: CRC Press, Taylor & Francis Group; 2010.

Federal Agencies

Nuclear regulation became the responsibility of the Atomic Energy Commission (AEC) when Congress passed the Atomic Energy Act of 1946. The AEC's programs sought to ensure public health and safety from the hazards of nuclear power but hesitated to impose excessive requirements that would deter growth in the industry. After great scrutiny, the US Nuclear Regulatory Commission (NRC) was created as an independent agency by Congress in 1974. Its mission is to ensure the safe use of radioactive materials for beneficial civilian purposes while protecting people and the environment.[20] The scope of the Commission's responsibility includes regulation of nuclear power plants, research reactors, and other medical, industrial, and academic licensees for the use and storage of radioactive materials in a way that eliminates unnecessary exposure and protects radiation workers and the public.

The NRC regulates the use of radioactive materials through the Code of Federal Regulations, Title 10 Part 20, specifically the Standards for Protection Against Radiation.[21] The agency's requirements include the following:

- dose limits to radiation workers and members of the public
- exposure limits for individual radionuclides
- monitoring and labeling of radioactive materials
- posting of signs in and around radiation areas
- reporting of theft or loss of radioactive material
- penalties for noncompliance with NRC regulations

Although the NRC is the major federal regulating agency for ensuring adequate protection of public health and safety in the use of radioactive materials, other federal agencies assist the NRC in fulfilling its mission. One such agency is the US Environmental Protection Agency (EPA). The EPA was established in 1970 to establish standards for human and environmental protection from radioactive materials. The EPA's primary responsibilities are to set limits on levels of radioactivity found in water, soil, and air.[22] They also develop technical reports to standardize dose and risk assessment as well as aid state and local agencies responding to radiological emergencies.

The transportation of hazardous materials is monitored and regulated through the Department of Transportation (DOT). The DOT's effort is coordinated through the Pipeline and Hazardous Materials Safety Administration, which is responsible for regulating and ensuring that hazardous materials are moved safely by all forms of transportation. To achieve this, the administration establishes national policy and enforces set standards.[23]

Another federal agency responsible for radiation protection is the US Food and Drug Administration (FDA). This agency regulates the manufacturing and use of devices that generate isotopes; however, the operation of the actual equipment or device is monitored by the state. The FDA also heads the Center for Devices and Radiological Health program to protect the public from unnecessary exposure from radiation-emitting electronic products.[24] Examples of some of the devices regulated can be found in Box 19.3. The program promotes radiation safety by ensuring manufacturers' designs of products are safe. The regulators collect and disseminate information on the use of these products and act when necessary.

The Electronic Product Radiation Control Program, which is part of the Federal Food, Drug and Cosmetic Act, holds the manufacturers responsible in the reporting of safety issues regarding radiation-producing electronic products. The Safe Medical Devices Act of 1990 (SMDA) requires medical facilities to report to the FDA any medical device that has caused death or injury of a patient or employee. In addition to the SMDA, in 1996, the FDA began the Medical Device Reporting (MDR) regulation to help monitor significant adverse events involving medical devices. The goal of the MDR is to correct any problems in a timely manner.[25]

BOX 19.3 Devices Regulated by the Center for Devices of Radiological Health

Medical Diagnostic
- General radiography
- CT, MRI, ultrasonography

Medical Therapeutic
- Linear accelerators
- Low-level laser therapy

Business, Commercial, Security
- Baggage x-ray
- Suntan parlors

Consumer
- Video monitors
- Microwave ovens

From Radiation-emitting products. US Food and Drug Administration website. https://www.fda.gov/Radiation-EmittingProducts/RadiationEmittingProductsandProcedures/default.htm. Accessed November 14, 2018.

For the protection of healthcare providers, the US Congress passed the Occupational Safety and Health Act of 1970. With provisions of this Act, the Occupational Safety and Health Administration (OSHA) was created to ensure safe and healthful working conditions for working men and women by setting and enforcing standards and by providing training, outreach, and education.[26]

In the mid-1980s, OSHA mandated a policy on bloodborne pathogens that stated that an exposure control plan must be in place for all industries in which workers may come in contact with blood and other infectious materials. This plan must contain precautionary procedures, educational programs for employees, and proper disposal procedures.[27] The policy on bloodborne pathogens is part of the radiation oncology facility's policy and procedures manual.

Although OSHA has set standards for exposure to cadmium and lead that primarily cover industrial work environments, these standards also apply to mold rooms in radiation oncology centers where Cerrobend (shielding) blocks are constructed. The personnel working in mold rooms must be aware of and follow the safety standards outlined by OSHA.

> Regulation standards for Cerrobend block rooms can be found at www.osha.gov/Publications/3136-08R-2003-English.html.

State Agencies

Section 274b of the Atomic Energy Act of 1954 provides a basis for the NRC to relinquish to the states portions of its regulatory authority relating to licensing and regulating by-product materials (radioisotopes), source materials (uranium and thorium), and certain quantities of special nuclear materials.[28] The first agreement state was established in 1962 with the Commonwealth of Kentucky. Currently, 37 states have entered into agreements with the NRC.[28] See Fig. 19.4 for a listing.

In such agreements, the NRC aids the states with review of the agreement request, training courses and workshops, and evaluation of technical licensing and inspection issues.

Institutional Agencies

The movement of quality in healthcare has caused facilities to reflect on the care they provide and to fabricate strategies to optimize quality care. One such strategy is identification of evidence-based quality indicators. Indicators are generally quantitative variables; quality metrics quantify the degree of adherence a facility has to its quality indicators.[29] Quality indicators are discussed subsequently in the chapter. Numerous agencies have developed over the years to address and improve quality of healthcare. These agencies include the National Committee for Quality Assurance, the Agency for Healthcare Research and Quality, the Centers for Medicare and Medicaid Services (CMS), and The Joint Commission (TJC).

TJC is a nonprofit organization that accredits and certifies more than 21,000 healthcare organizations in the United States.[30] Accreditation and certification by TJC symbolizes an organization's commitment to quality with certain performance standards. Accreditation by TJC is important to an organization in that it provides professional advice and education to staff regarding best practices; it is recognized by insurers and third parties, and certification may fulfill regulatory requirements in some states. Without TJC accreditation, an institution may not receive reimbursement from CMS, have a physician residency program, or receive malpractice insurance. TJC is dedicated to improving quality patient care. A standard developed to promote this is the requirement for hospitals to conduct a proactive risk assessment, at least every 18 months, on a process considered to be high risk.[31] Available resources to conduct a thorough risk assessment include:

- Institute for Safe Medication Practices Medication Safety Risk Assessment: This tool is designed to help reduce medication errors. https://www.ismp.org/selfassessments/default.asp.
- Contingency diagram: This uses brainstorming to generate a list of problems that could arise from a process. https://healthit.ahrq.gov/.
- Potential problem analysis is a method for determining what could go wrong while developing a plan. https://healthit.ahrq.gov/
- Process decision program chart systematically identifies errors with a plan during its creation. https://healthit.ahrq.gov/

The American College of Radiation Oncology (ACRO) was founded in 1991 to meet challenges facing radiation oncologists. The ACRO Accreditation Program was developed in 1995 to accredit radiation oncology centers. An extensive review was completed in 2010 to improve the process and resulted in changes that included the ability to submit cases for review online.[32] The accreditation process includes a peer review of the specifics of a practice outlined as follows;

1. Practice demographics. This includes things such as number of consultations, simulations, and patients treated.
2. Process of radiation therapy. A facility is evaluated for appropriateness of care.
3. Clinical performance measures. This looks at the patient's record and lists what should be included. Specific criteria can be found in Table 19.2.[33]
4. Policies and procedures. Policy manuals must be current and updated annually.
5. Physical plant. The environment must be clean and safe for patients and staff. Aspects include adequate parking, waiting rooms, and treatment rooms.
6. Radiation therapy personnel. Each department develops a staffing plan to meet the needs of the facility. For the therapist, they must be certified and registered by the American Registry of Radiologic Technologists (ARRT) and hold a state license, if applicable. Two therapists must be available for each unit at all times to ensure patient safety.

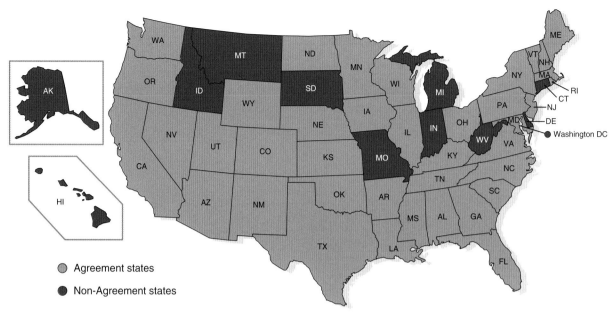

Fig. 19.4 Nuclear Regulatory Commission agreement and nonagreement states. (From Agreement state program. US Nuclear Regulatory Commission website. https://www.nrc.gov/reading-rm/doc-collections/maps/agreement-states.html. Accessed October 18, 2019.)

TABLE 19.2   Required Clinical Documents in Patient Record ACRO Accreditation

Clinical Documents	√ Included in Chart
Histopathologic diagnosis	
Site of disease (or ICD-9 code)	
Stage of disease	
Pertinent history and physical examination performed by a radiation oncologist	
Treatment plan	
Documentation of informed consent to treatment	
Simulation record, when applicable	
Dosimetry calculations	
Graphic treatment plan (e.g. isodose distribution and DVH), when applicable	
Daily/weekly/total radiation therapy dose and treatment volume records	
Weekly record of radiation oncologist's treatment management	
Continuing weekly medical physics review	
Port image(s) documenting each treatment field, when applicable	
Record of brachytherapy or radionuclide therapy procedure(s), when applicable	
Treatment summary note	
Follow-up plan	

These documents must be included in the patient record, and they will be reviewed as part of the chart audit.
DVH, Dose-volume histogram; *ICD,* International Classification of Disease.

7. Radiation therapy equipment. Use of megavoltage equipment and CT simulation. A record and verify (R&V) system for all linear accelerators is required.
8. Radiation therapy physics. A radiation safety program is required, which includes morning quality assurance (QA) procedures following American Association of Physicists in Medicine (AAPM) protocols.
9. CQI. Chart checks will be performed regularly, and all incident reports will be reviewed.
10. Safety program. A safe environment is mandatory. The facility must comply with American Disability Act of 1990 (ADA), OSHA, and fire safety requirements.
11. Education program. All members of the team must have access to continuing medical education.

These examples, in addition to others, are listed in the ACRO Accreditation Manual.[33]

Hospital/critical care accreditation may also be obtained through DNV Healthcare, a part of Det Norske Veritas, a foundation focused on promotion of safety of life, property, and the environment. It was given accrediting authority in 2008 by the CMS, and integrates CMS Conditions of Participation with the International Organization for Standardization 9001: quality management requirements.[34]

The CMS is a medical assistance program for those who qualify, and was established in 1965. CMS sets a standard payment for services based on diagnosis and clinically comparable resource consumption. The federal government pays states a percentage of program expenditures called Federal Medical Assistance Percentage based on a state's per capita income. The average percent reimbursement in the United States is 50%.[35] This percentage can leave an organization with considerable uncovered costs, thus reinforcing the importance of a good quality control (QC) program.

Professional Organizations

Several professional organizations provide resources and practice standards to guide appropriately educated professionals within their organizations. Professional practice standards establish the role of the practitioner and create criteria used in performance evaluation. The American College of Radiology (ACR), with more than 37,000 members, is the primary organization of radiologists, radiation oncologists, medical physicists, and allied health professionals in the United States. The ACR devotes its resources to making imaging accessible to those who need it in a safe and effective manner. They also collaborate with the CMS and the Physician Quality Reporting System by encouraging physicians to submit outcome information.[36]

The AAPM, a professional organization for medical physicists, has been a forerunner in the development of minimum standards to guide medical physicists in the development of a QA program as it relates to treatment planning and delivery. Several reports have been produced by special task groups of the AAPM relating to the development of a comprehensive QA program in radiation oncology, such as the AAPM Task Group (TG) 40 and TG142, TG158, and TG53 reports, which outline a comprehensive QA program for radiation therapy treatment planning.[37] These reports have emphasized the technical performance of treatment planning and delivery equipment. A recent report by the AAPM (TG100) states that major disruptions in quality are a result of variations and weaknesses in the radiation therapy process.[19] This report will be addressed later in the chapter.

In 1995, the professional organization for radiation therapists, the ASRT, developed practice standards for radiation therapists. The professional practice standards are divided into six sections:

- Introduction: Defines the practice and minimum qualifications required.
- Scope of practice: Delineates the parameters within which to work.
- Clinical performance standards: Defines the activities of the individual in terms of patient care and treatment delivery.
- Quality performance standards: Outlines individual safety standard assessment and technical performance activities.
- Professional performance standards: Defines the individual's activities in regard to interpersonal relationships, ethics, and self-assessment.
- Advisory Opinion Statements: Interpretation of the standards for guidance and clarification.[38]

To be effective, the QI plan must incorporate all practice standards for each member of the QI team.

The American Society for Radiation Oncology (ASTRO) was founded in 1958 and now has more than 10,000 members, including radiation oncologists, medical physicists, radiation therapists, and other members of cancer care teams. ASTRO offers continuing education for its professional members, and it also serves as a practice accrediting agency known as the Accreditation Program for Excellence (APEx). APEx is grounded by five pillars of excellence, which include:

1. The process of care.
2. The radiation oncology team.
3. Safety.
4. Quality management.
5. Patient-centered care.[39]

The accreditation process includes a peer-review site visit and evaluation with the goal of recognizing high-quality oncology centers. It ensures accountability by establishing standards from evidence-based guidelines. Currently, ASTRO offers a 4-year accreditation. The standards followed by the APEx program can be found in Box 19.4.

The radiation therapist may keep current with the regulations and guidelines created by various relevant agencies by visiting the following websites:

National:
  NRC: www.nrc.gov
  NAM: https://nam.edu/
  DOT: www.transportation.gov
  OSHA: www.osha.gov
  CMS: www.cms.gov
Consider Professional/Certifying:
  ARRT: www.arrt.org
  ACR: www.acr.org
  AAPM: www.aapm.org
  ASRT: www.asrt.org
  ASTRO: www.astro.org
Accrediting:
  JC: www.jointcommission.org
  ACRO: www.acro.org
  ASTRO: www.astro.org

BOX 19.4   American Society for Radiation Oncology's Accreditation Program for Excellence Standards

1. Patient evaluation, care coordination, and follow-up
2. Treatment planning
3. Patient-specific safety interventions and safe practices in treatment preparation and delivery
4. Staff roles and accountabilities
5. Qualifications and ongoing training of staff
6. Safe staffing plan
7. Culture of safety
8. Radiation safety
9. Emergency preparation and planning
10. Facility and equipment
11. Information management and integration of systems
12. Quality management of treatment procedures and modalities
13. Peer review of clinical processes
14. Patient consent
15. Patient education and health management
16. Performance measurement and outcomes reporting

From *APEx: accreditation program for excellence.* American Society for Radiation Oncology website. www.astro.org/Practice-Management/Practice-Accreditation/Index.aspx. Accessed October 17, 2109.

DEFINITIONS

Multiple definitions exist regarding the various components of **QI**.

Quality, as defined by Merriam-Webster, is the standard of something as measured against other things of a similar kind, the degree of excellence of something.[40] In reference to radiation oncology, it is defined as "the totality of features and characteristics of a radiation therapy process that bear on its ability to satisfy stated or implied needs of the patient."[41] For determination of whether quality standards are met, each feature or characteristic of the radiation therapy process must be identified and measured and the results analyzed.

BOX 19.5   Joint Commission Criteria to Identify Quality

- Research: Strong scientific evidence demonstrates that performing the evidence-based care process improves health outcomes (either directly or by reducing risk of adverse outcomes).
- Proximity: Performing the care process is closely connected to the patient outcome; there are relatively few clinical processes that occur after the one that is measured and before the improved outcome occurs.
- Accuracy: The measure accurately assesses whether or not the care process has actually been provided. That is, the measure should be capable of indicating whether the process has been delivered with sufficient effectiveness to make improved outcomes likely.
- Adverse effects: Implementing the measure has little or no chance of inducing unintended adverse consequences.

(© Joint Commission Resources: Specifications Manual for Joint Commission National Quality Measures (v2016A). Oakbrook Terrace, IL: Joint Commission on Accreditation of Healthcare Organizations, 2016. Reprinted with permission.)

QA is defined as "all those planned or systematic actions necessary to provide adequate confidence that a product or service will satisfy given requirements for quality."[41] QA in oncology represents the actions taken to ensure that a radiation therapy facility consistently delivers high-quality care in the treatment of patients to lead to the best outcomes with the least amount of side effects. All the aspects of a QA program can be checked with use of a quality audit. The quality audit is equivalent to peer review of a program with evidence-based criteria for good practice. Auditors do not have authority to enforce sanctions, and the audit does not carry any regulatory authority; it is meant to give recommendations for QI.[42]

QC is defined as "the operational techniques and activities used to fulfill requirements for quality."[41] The term typically refers to those procedures and techniques used to monitor or test and maintain the components of the radiation therapy QI program, such as the tests that measure the mechanical integrity of the treatment units. Quality assessment is the systematic collection of data, and QI encompasses the activities directed to improve the quality of a system by reducing error or variation in that system.[43] Synonymous terms include **CQI** and TQM. TQM is a customer-centered approach that is driven by data and long-term strategies for improvement. This approach was made popular by Deming, as previously discussed. In comparison, CQI's principle is based on a system-level approach, and that, instead of identifying the shortcomings of an individual, an organization should focus on process improvement through perpetual improvement processes.[15] It integrates QA, QC, and assessment into a system-wide improvement program that revolves around the healthcare organization's mission and goals.

STANDARDS

Measurement of patient outcomes is now required by TJC for accreditation. In 1987, TJC introduced its Agenda for Change. This agenda includes a set of standardized core measurements into the accreditation process. In 1999, the ORYX initiative was implemented to include a more standardized set of valid, reliable, and evidence-based quality measures.[44] The core performance measures were categorized into accountability and nonaccountability measures in 2010. The four criteria identify the measures that have the greatest impact on patient outcomes when improvement is demonstrated[45] (Box 19.5).

The use of target analysis, in addition to a control chart, is a key feature of TJC's analytic methods. In control chart analysis, the norm is determined from an organization's own historic data so that one may assess the organization's internal process stability. In target analysis, the norm is obtained based on multiple organizations performance data to evaluate relative performance level. The use of two perspectives can provide a more comprehensive assessment of an organization's overall performance level.[44]

Safety Recommendations in Radiation Oncology

Increasing demands have been placed on all members of the radiation oncology team. Changes in national healthcare, both structurally and financially, and changes in billing and reimbursement levels add to the burden of healthcare professionals. Documentation requirements have exponentially increased along with the complexity of treatment planning and delivery. A culture that manages change must exist to ensure quality and safety with a more efficient process. Consider deleting ASTRO, in 2019, published *Safety Is No Accident: A Framework for Quality Radiation Oncology and Care.* It states that radiation therapy departments must satisfy numerous requirements of quality. The following list is a summary of the suggested framework.[45]

1. Quality management of the facility itself. Design of treatment rooms must include appropriate shielding, patient monitoring capabilities, and electronic cables for dosimetric verification. Each department must have access to CT or MRI for planning and electronic access to patient information systems and a picture archiving and communication system.
2. Radiation oncology program requirements. The program should be accredited by a radiation oncology–specific accrediting body and implement well-described policies and procedures. Capability requirements include machine calibration equipment, a preemptive program for maintenance and repair of equipment, and a peer-review process.
3. Radiation safety. The AAPM guidelines for handling radioactive sources must be followed, and a monitoring program for all personnel must be used.
4. Monitoring of safety, errors, and medical quality. A culture of awareness and safety is important to establish in radiation therapy. To ensure this goal, each department should have a review committee to evaluate near misses (good catches), events (errors), and procedural issues that could lead to errors.

Terms established by TG100 to help define the new culture of quality and safety in reporting include the following:

1. Errors: acts of commission or omission then execute an action incorrectly
2. Mistakes: incorrect intentions or plans that lead to failure
3. Violations: intentionally not following procedure resulting in either sabotage or attempting to achieve the goal by introducing a shortcut
4. Event: the entire clinical process, with the failure resulting in diminished quality
5. Near event: an occurrence that, if not have been detected and corrected, would result in a failure (also known as a close call, near miss, or good catch)[19]

Safety issues that result from time constraints can be avoided with the development of processes with adequate time allotments. See Table 19.3 for an example of a time allocation process.

Along with the importance of quality and safety, the treatment planning and delivery process must have an evaluation of patient-specific issues. For proper coordination of a patient's care, multidisciplinary case conferences or tumor boards should occur regularly. In 2018, the ACR and ASTRO revised the "ACR Practice Parameter Guidelines for Radiation Oncology." Radiation therapy is a complex process, so it is important to carry out recognized activities

TABLE 19.3 Sample Process Sheet for Safety Issues

Process Step	Minimum Process Time Required for Saftey
After imaging: target volumes identified, plan defined, normal tissue volumes and anatomy approved	X days

After anatomy approval:
    Planning: 3D conformal radiation therapy
    Planning: 3D IMRT, VMAT
    Planning: 3D SBRT
    Planning: SRS
	X days
	X days
	X days
	X hours

IMRT QA and analysis	To be completed X hours before treatment
Treatment preparation: transfer from planning system to treatment system	Allow X hours
Final checks before treatment	X minutes or hours
Treatment setup and delivery: varies with complexity of treatment	X minutes

ACR, American College of Radiology; *CMD,* certified medical dosimetrist; *IMRT,* intensity-modulated radiation therapy; *QA,* quality assurance; *SBRT,* stereotactic body radiation therapy; *SRS,* stereotactic radiosurgery; *TJC,* The Joint Commission; *VMAT,* volumetric modulated arc therapy; *3D,* three-dimensional.
From Safety is no accident: a framework for quality radiation oncology and care, 2012. American Society for Radiation Oncology website. www.astro.org/uploadedFiles/Main_Site/Clinical_Practice/Patient_Safety/Blue_Book/SafetyisnoAccident.pdf. Accessed November 21, 2018.

BOX 19.6 Radiation Therapy Prescription

1. Anatomically specific target volumes including specific names of boost volumes, as appropriate, with their associated total doses
2. Treatment technique (includes, but is not limited to: anteroposterior [AP], posteroanterior [PA], right and/or left laterals, en face electrons, intensity modulated radiation therapy [IMRT], volumetric modulated arc therapy [VMAT], stereotactic radiosurgery [SRS], stereotactic body radiation therapy [SBRT])
3. Beam-modifying devices (e.g., bolus thickness)
4. Radiation modality
5. Energy(s)
6. Dose per fraction
7. Total number of fractions
8. Fractionation schedule
9. Total dose
10. Prescription point/isodose line
11. Reference to image guidance when appropriate

From https://www.acr.org/-/media/ACR/Files/Practice-Parameters/RadOnc.pdf.

to ensure quality patient care can be provided. Steps in this process include thorough clinical evaluation of the patient, including a history and physical. Weighing risk versus benefit and establishing goals are important and should be communicated with all involved in the care of the patient. Obtaining informed consent and educating the patient should be thorough and documented. All aspects of simulation and treatment planning should have electronic orders as well as a completed prescription. Items to be included in the radiation therapy prescription can be found in Box 19.6. Multidisciplinary review takes place for coordination of services; then the CT simulation, contouring, and plan evaluation steps follow. On-treatment visits, chart rounds, and follow-up visits are scheduled for assessment of tumor response and radiation-induced side effects.[46]

Outcomes are the driving force of cancer care. A patient's performance status before, during, and after treatment is a good measure of outcomes, as is tumor response. Tumor registries, such as the Surveillance, Epidemiology and End Results (SEER) program, provide clinicians with population data stratified by age, gender, race, year of diagnosis, and geographic areas. This information can identify variations in treatment, process of care, and other variables that can improve a physician's methods of cancer management.[47]

Staffing in Radiation Oncology

Although radiation therapists work under the supervision of a radiation oncologist, their responsibilities continue to expand. Operating complex equipment, reviewing protocols and prescriptions, and monitoring and assessing patients on a daily basis all take time and resources. The staffing needs of a radiation oncology department vary from facility to facility, depending on patient load, complexity of treatment, and accreditation requirements. In ASRT's white paper, "Radiation Therapy Safety: The Critical Role of the Radiation Therapist," best practice is documented as having all radiation therapy treatments delivered by an ARRT-certified and registered therapist and as having all sites staff at least two therapists per machine.[48] One therapist focuses on monitoring the patient, and the other operates the treatment console. Some facilities recommend having a third therapist per machine to attend to finding documents, performing QA, or communicating with other professionals (Fig. 19.5).[49] Guidelines are also set by accrediting agencies.

Figure 19.6 outlines the roles and responsibilities of the radiation oncology clinical care team; including the radiation oncologists, medical physicists, radiation therapists, medical dosimetrists, oncology nurses and others.[45]

The number of therapists in a department is important, but so is their competence. Currently, 12 states do not regulate licensing of radiation therapists.[50] Despite the lack of regulation, facilities that set minimum qualifications and recommendations include that therapists be certified and registered by the ARRT.

Quality Improvement Team

An effective QA program requires commitment from everyone in the radiation oncology department. The radiation oncology QI team includes radiation oncologists, medial physicists, radiation therapists, medical dosimetrists, nurses, engineers, and other support staff.[33,51] Every member must understand the principles, concepts, and operations of the QA program so that comprehensive improvement is attained.

Common practice is for the medical director of a radiation oncology center to be responsible for the establishment and continuation of a QI program. The director may appoint a QI committee to develop and monitor the program, collect and evaluate the data, determine areas for improvement, implement changes when areas for improvement have been identified, and evaluate the results of the actions taken.

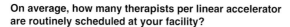

On average, how many therapists per linear accelerator are routinely scheduled at your facility?

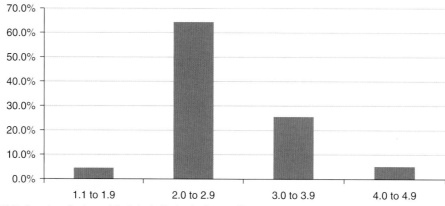

Fig. 19.5 American Society of Radiologic Technologists staffing survey shows number of therapists per machine. (From American Society of Radiologic Technologists: Radiation therapy staffing and workplace survey, 2018. https://www.asrt.org/main/news-publications/research/staffing-surveys. Accessed October 17, 2019).

			Relative FTE factor		Required FTE		Required total FTE	
	Services - # of units or licenses	No. of systems	Physicist	Dosimetrist	Physicist	Dosimetrist	Physicist	Dosimetrist
Equipment, sources and systems	Multi energy accelerators	4	0.25	0.05	1	0.2		
	Single energy accelerators	0	0.08	0.01	0	0		
	Tomotherapy, CyberKnife, GammaKnife	1	0.3	0.03	0.3	0.03		
	Cobalt Units, IMRT, PACS, EMR and Contouring	0	0.08	0.03	0	0		
	Orthovoltage and superficial units	0	0.02	0.01	0	0		
	Manual brachytherapy; LDR seed implants	1	0.2	0.03	0.2	0.03		
	HDR brachytherapy	1	0.2	0.02	0.2	0.02		
	Simulator, CT-Simulator, PET, MRI Fusion	1	0.05	0.02	0.05	0.02		
	Computer planning system (per 10 workstations)	1	0.05	0.02	0.05	0.02		
	HDR planning system	1	0.2	0.01	0.2	0.01		
						Subtotal	2.0	.033
	Annual # of patients undergoing procedures	No. of patients						
No. patient procedures	External beam RT with 3D planning	500	0.0003	0.003	0.15	1.5		
	External beam RT with conventional planning	200	0.0002	0.002	0.04	0.4		
	Sealed source brachytherapy (LDR & HDR)	100	0.008	0.003	0.8	0.3		
	Unsealed source therapy	25	0.008	0.005	0.2	0.125		
	IMRT, IGRT, SRS, TBI, SBRT	400	0.008	0.005	3.2	2		
						Subtotal	4.39	4.33
	Estimated total (Phys & Dosim) FTE effort	FTE effort						
Nonclinical - estimated total FTE effort	Education & training (FTE)	0.1	0.667	0.333	0.0667	0.00333		
	Generation of internal reports (FTE)	0.1	0.667	0.333	0.0667	0.00333		
	Committees & meetings; inc. rad. safety (FTE)	0.1	0.667	0.333	0.0667	0.00333		
	Administration and management (FTE)	0.5	0.667	0.333	0.0667	0.00333		
						Subtotal	0.53	0.27
						Total	6.92	4.92

Fig. 19.6 Roles and Responsibilities of the Radiation Oncology Clinical Care Team. The team, including the radiation oncologists, medical physicists, radiation therapists, medical dosimetrists, oncology nurses, and others work together to provide every patient with the needed medical, emotional, psychological and nutritional care before, during and after treatment[45]. (From Safety is no accident: a framework for quality radiation oncology care, 2019. American Society of Radiation Oncology website. https://www.astro.org/Patient-Care-and-Research/Patient-Safety/Safety-is-no-Accident. Accessed October 18, 2019).

The director is also responsible for ensuring that all employees are qualified to carry out their duties. Job descriptions must clearly state the qualifications, credentials or license required, continuing education requirements, and scope of practice for each position. Institutional requirements regarding maintenance of qualifications in cardiopulmonary resuscitation, attendance at infectious disease seminars, fire and safety seminars, and observance of all radiation safety standards are monitored.

Staff physicians are required to actively participate in departmental QI activities, and documentation of participation is reviewed as part of the medical staff recredentialing process. The radiation oncologists participate in these activities during chart review, morbidity and mortality conferences, review and development of departmental policies and procedures, portal film review, patient and family education, and the completion and review of incident reports.

Members of the physics division (physicists, dosimetrists, and engineers) develop and carry out the QC program to meet the needs of the department and to comply with national, state, and professionally accepted or mandated standards. They also conduct weekly and final physics reviews of the treatment records.

The radiation therapists perform warm-up procedures on the treatment units, perform QC tests on the simulation and treatment units, verify the presence of completed and signed prescription and consent forms, review the prescription and treatment plan on each patient before the initiation of treatment, deliver accurate treatments that adhere to the prescription, accurately record treatment delivered, take initial and weekly portal images, evaluate the health status of the patient daily before treatment delivery to ensure there are no adverse reactions to treatment or other impending physical or psychologic problems that require assistance, participate in patient and family education, and provide care and comfort to meet the needs of the patient.[52]

The oncology nurses perform a nursing assessment on each new patient to determine overall physical and psychologic status; evaluate the educational needs of each patient and family to determine any barriers to education; develop an educational program to meet the needs of the patient and family; evaluate the effectiveness of the entire educational program, including the education given to the patient by the radiation oncologist, nurses, and radiation therapists; monitor the patient's health status on a routine or as-needed basis throughout the course of treatment; and order, evaluate, and record blood counts and weights according to departmental policy.

The departmental support staff gathers pertinent information and prepares the treatment chart before the patient's initial visit; contacts the patient or family to set up appointments and give instructions regarding information or diagnostic studies to be brought with the patient; greets and assists the patient and family daily; informs the radiation oncologists, nurses, or radiation therapists of the patient's arrival; answers the patient's questions and gives assistance whenever possible or refers the patient to an individual who can help; completes and files treatment records; and sets the tone for the entire radiation therapy treatment encounter.

Development of a Quality Improvement Plan

The QI plan must be comprehensive enough to encompass the entire radiation process so that uncertainties can be determined. Also included in the plan is a quality audit mechanism. A quality audit is an independent, external evaluation, assessment, or peer review.[53]

Quality indicators are tools used to measure, over time, a department's performance of functions, processes, and outcomes.

With the development of quality indicators, the purpose of the measure is important to identify. A universal set of indicators is unlikely to be developed for all purposes because of the diversity of the potential users, but the demands for measurements used for benchmarking, accreditation, credentialing, and reimbursement are increasing.

Quality indicators used can be categorized as structure, process, and outcome measures.[54] Structure indicators looks at the setting of where the care occurs and the capacity of that setting to produce quality. Examples of structure indicators are a hospital maintaining TJC accreditation or a therapist earning and maintaining certification and registration. Process indicators looks at adherence to guidelines and how the care is delivered. Indicators include consultation, imaging studies, and therapeutic procedures (Table 19.4) Last are indicators of outcomes, some of which measure overall survival, disease-free survival, patient satisfaction, and quality of life.[55] These capture the effectiveness of the process.[54]

Quality outcomes have been the focus of the National Cancer Institute and TJC, but in radiation oncology, these sometimes are hard to measure. Ultimate outcomes in radiation therapy are often not immediately apparent, such as 5-year survival rates.[56] Also, patients receive different combinations of care, which makes comparisons difficult. Because of these complexities, much of the work in healthcare improvement focuses on the process measures associated with improved outcomes. The benefits of measuring a process rather than a direct outcome include:

- Direct feedback to aid QI initiatives.
- Less dependence on risk adjustment.
- Usefulness for benchmarking.
- Less follow-up time needed for measures.[56]

As previously mentioned, the quality indicators must be defined. It needs to be reliable and feasible and should include a standard. The standard is a statistical value based on a comparison of some sort. A sentinel event is an example of an indicator that should carry a zero threshold; one occurrence warrants immediate action.[56]

An established, robust QA program is validated by the quality audit. As mentioned, the quality audit is a peer review of a facility. TJC requires an annual appraisal of oncology departments.[44]

Review of personnel, the facility, and all services provided, including treatment units and brachytherapy, physics measurement tools and calibration, and proper NRC or state licenses, is conducted during the site visit.[57] Audits can be performed on a smaller scale as well. An example is the ACR-recommended monthly review of patient charts. This review needs to be performed by someone not directly responsible for this task. Another example is mailing of thermoluminescent dosimeters (TLDs) to an external service for verification that treatment unit calibration is consistent with national standards.[58]

Quality Improvement Moving Forward

Healthcare in general has learned so much from the initiators of QA. As previously discussed, the PDCA model and Lean management

TABLE 19.4 Process Indicators

Indicator	Example
Documentation of clinical stage	TNM staging documentation
Informed consent	Signed consent in chart before treatment
Appropriate use of radiation therapy	Sequence of therapy after surgery/chemotherapy
Appropriate evaluation of recurrence	PSA, DRE, mammography

DRE, Digital rectal examination; *PSA*, prostatic specific antigen; *TNM*, tumor-node-metastasis staging system.
From Donabedian A. The quality of care: how can it be assessed? *JAMA* 1988;260:1743–1748.

revolutionized the definition of quality. More specifically, radiation therapy has also made changes in how quality and safety are measured. The publication of the IOM's *To Err Is Human: Building a Safer Health System* in 1993 has made QA in healthcare a top priority.[59] The CDC compiles a list of the most common causes of death annually. It is created from using the International Classification of Disease (ICD) code information on death certificates. Unfortunately, deaths because of human error or system failures are not captured, leading to underreporting of deaths because of accidents.[60] According to the CDC's National Vital Statistics report from 2019, unintentional accidents is suggested to be the third most common cause of death in the United States behind heart disease and cancer.[61]

Radiation oncology began using a process the airline industry uses to identify and resolve safety issues. The Air Safety Reporting System is a national error reporting system in which the Commercial Aviation Safety Teams use to "design the risk out of airplanes."[62] Internationally, the Radiation Oncology Safety Information System exists, and in the United States, ASTRO and the Radiation Oncology Institute are currently developing the National Radiation Oncology Registry. The goal of the registry is to allow comparison of treatment modalities, outcomes, quality and safety, and cost.[63] This resource will be promoted through education and outreach programs.[64] Other agencies established include the Agency for Healthcare Research and Quality and, more recently, the Hospital Quality Alliance.

The Radiation Oncology Incident Learning System, or RO-ILS, was developed in 2011 through a collaboration between the AAPM and ASTRO. It allows for secure reporting of patient safety events, including near misses, unsafe situations, and events that reached the patient with or without harm. In addition to an open-ended question about the event, other required information includes patient positioning, prescription, treatment site, and method. Users are also asked to enter details about workflow, type of equipment and software used, the severity of the event, and the possible causes. One of the most important factors is how the event was found and what was implemented to prevent it from occurring again.[65]

Reports are reviewed three to four times per year by the Radiation Oncology Healthcare Advisory Council, a group of radiation oncology professionals. They look at the reported data to determine the level of importance and interest. A statistical summary is generated that includes trends, details of the most important reports, and lessons learned. Report summaries are available on the website and are sent to contributing institutions. Descriptive statistics are used to show the number of events and severity and how they were originally found during the treatment process.[65]

In a recent published report from July to September 2017, there were 365 reported events. Of these, 34% were reported as an operational or process improvement. A near miss made up 22% of the total events, and unsafe conditions were the least reported. The most common workflow step in which the event occurred was treatment planning, and the majority of events were discovered during treatment delivery or the imaging process. Of all the treatment techniques, three-dimensional treatment was the most likely to be associated with a reported event. Of the dose deviations reported, the majority were less than or equal to 5% maximum dose deviation to the target.[66]

All of these committees and agencies share one important goal: they highlight the importance of reporting, analyzing, and improving processes to lead to systems that provide safe procedures and fewer errors.[59] Kalapurakal and associates[67] began a voluntary error reporting system in their department with the goal of studying causative factors of errors, analyze their clinical consequences, and develop broad consensus recommendations to reduce or prevent their occurrence. Many of the QA strategies include the use of checklists and time-outs.

Fig. 19.7 shows how this system can be incorporated.[67] Results of the Kalapurakal study included:

1. The total number of errors, with the introduction of checklists and time-outs, decreased from 221 errors in 126 patients to 35 errors in 13 patients.
2. Of the self-reported errors that included treatment of the wrong patient, wrong site, or wrong dose, the incidence rate went from 23 errors in 14 patients to zero during the reporting period with the use of checklists and time-outs.[67]

The culture of radiation oncology is moving from a reactive approach that is implemented when a failure occurs, such as a sentinel event, to a more prospective approach to identify a failure before it happens. TG100 recommends a team-based approach and includes everyone in analysis and process mapping. A strategy they highly recommend for process improvement is failure modes and effects analysis (FMEA). FMEA is a proactive risk assessment that studies a process to reduce the incidence of an adverse event by understanding the contributing factors to a failure.[68] The number of steps in a FMEA process may vary by the complexity of the task. The first step is to identify a process to review and establish the stakeholders. Next, the team will develop a process map. Fig. 19.8 illustrates a process map for a radiation oncology department using FMEA to mitigate risks in using organ-sparing targeted marrow irradiation (TMI) as an alternative to total body irradiation. For each step in the process, a failure mode describing what specifically could happen and what the result could be is identified.[15] In the TMI example, a postanesthesia care unit nurse may be needed for transport but not available at the time. Each failure mode is ranked by severity, frequency of occurrence, and detection, and then assigned a risk prioritization number (RPN).[15] A high RPN could be assigned to an incorrect patient shift during the first treatment. All attempts are then made to build safety around those risks so they do not occur. A recommended action for the TMI patient would be to capture the couch parameters before treatment. Team members will share the recommended actions with everyone who needs to know; this leads to implementation and eventually project completion. For the couch copy to be implemented, the lead therapist will send out an email to all therapists and have face-to-face communication before treatment. All members involved need to feel empowered for the process to be successful.

A QI program is only as good as the QC procedures that are performed. The next section discusses specific procedures that are recommended to be performed on equipment and processes to ensure a quality outcome.

> Continuous quality improvement is important to the operation of a radiation oncology facility. The Safety Radiation Oncology Stakeholders Initiative (RO-SSI) collaborative group has recently been formed by stakeholders independent of organizations and agencies. Their mission is to facilitate safety improvements by addressing challenging issues. More information can be found at: info.radoncssi.org.

CLINICAL ASPECTS OF QUALITY CONTROL AND IMPROVEMENT

Devices Needed for Quality Control Procedures

A major component of the QI plan focuses on QC procedures that are routinely performed, documented, and evaluated on the simulator, imaging equipment, immobilization devices, accessory equipment, treatment planning computer systems, and treatment units. These procedures ensure that all is in proper working order according to manufacturer, department, and national specifications. Instrumentation used in performing QC checks include ion chambers used for equipment

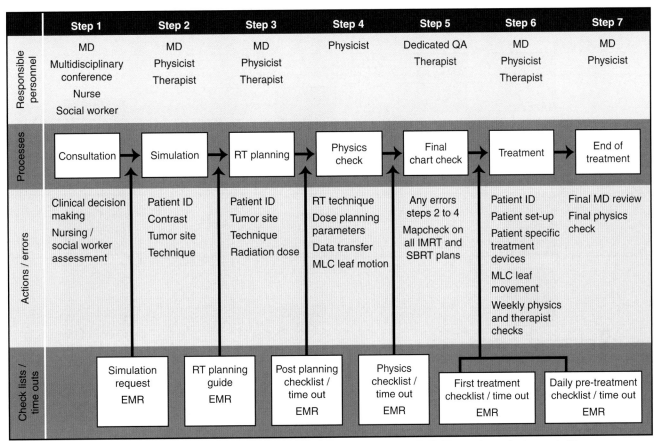

	Step 1	Step 2	Step 3	Step 4	Step 5	Step 6	Step 7
Responsible personnel	MD Multidisciplinary conference Nurse Social worker	MD Physicist Therapist	MD Physicist Therapist	Physicist	Dedicated QA Therapist	MD Physicist Therapist	MD Physicist
Processes	Consultation	Simulation	RT planning	Physics check	Final chart check	Treatment	End of treatment
Actions / errors	Clinical decision making Nursing / social worker assessment	Patient ID Contrast Tumor site Technique	Patient ID Tumor site Technique Radiation dose	RT technique Dose planning parameters Data transfer MLC leaf motion	Any errors steps 2 to 4 Mapcheck on all IMRT and SBRT plans	Patient ID Patient set-up Patient specific treatment devices MLC leaf movement Weekly physics and therapist checks	Final MD review Final physics check
Check lists / time outs	Simulation request EMR	RT planning guide EMR	Post planning checklist / time out EMR	Physics checklist / time out EMR	First treatment checklist / time out EMR	Daily pre-treatment checklist / time out EMR	

Fig. 19.7 Checklists and time-outs incorporated in radiation oncology. *EMR,* Electronic medical record; *ID,* identification; *IMRT,* intensity-modulated radiation therapy; *MLC,* multileaf collimation; *QA,* quality assurance; RT, radiation therapy; *SBRT,* stereotactic body radiation therapy. (From Kalapurakal JA, Zafirovski A, Smith J, et al. A comprehensive quality assurance program for personnel and procedures in radiation oncology: value of voluntary error reporting and checklists. *Int J Radiation Oncol Biol Phys.* 2013;86:241–248.)

calibration and QA measurements for treatment planning systems, as well as miscellaneous dosimetry devices such as TLDs and film for absolute dose measurement. Devices to verify machine output and consistency include geometric and anthropomorphic phantoms.[69] Each radiation oncology center determines the frequency of these QC checks based on the stability of equipment performance and recommendations set by the AAPM. Regular intervals (e.g., daily, monthly, or annually) are usually established for the QC procedures. Daily tests include those that could seriously affect patient positioning, such as lasers and the optical distance indicator (ODI), and procedures to verify accurate patient dose delivery, such as output constancy. Safety equipment such as emergency switches, door interlocks, and communication devices are included in daily QC checks.[70] Daily quality checks are best performed in the morning before the first patient undergoes simulation or treatment. An example of a morning QA procedure is shown in Box 19.7. Mechanical and electrical devices such as override switches, emergency off switches, limit switches, and collision rings are devices that the therapist should check regularly. Also known as a dead-man switch, the hand pendant/couch controls rely on this switch for safety of the machine and the patient. The following is the procedure for testing override switches.

1. Check that adequate clearance exists for the test and for a malfunction without injury or damage.
2. Turn on the primary switch, but do not depress the override switch. There should be NO motion.
3. With the primary switch in the on position, depress the override switch. Motion should begin.
4. Release the override switch. Motion should stop.

This spot check should be performed daily, and the tolerance is pass/fail.

> All mechanical and electrical safety checks are pass/fail. If tests are passed, the machine is suitable for use. If any tests fail, a physicist or engineer should be notified immediately and the machine not used. Follow-up action to verify the corrections have been made should be documented in a permanent log.

Monthly testing consists of more refined testing of parameters that either have a lesser impact on the patient or have conditions that are less likely to change in a month's time.[70] Monthly checks include treatment couch indicators, field light/radiation congruency, and beam flatness. The QC procedures and tolerances are established and managed by the physicist; however, the radiation therapist plays a major role in obtaining this information because of the therapist's familiarity with, and knowledge of, the equipment. Therefore the therapist must be familiar with commonly performed QC procedures and recommended tolerances for all equipment and procedures in the department.

General Conditions of Patient Care Areas

Without attention to the details of general conditions, care of the patient is diminished and may, in some circumstances, be hazardous. The treatment room should be clean and orderly with the lights, heat, and temperature controls operating properly. Routine supplies for treatment setup should be available, as should ample linens, emesis

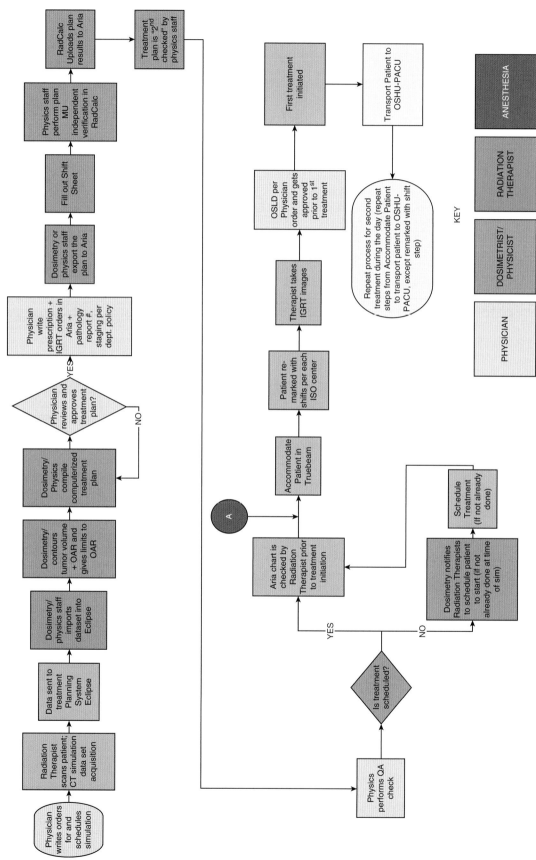

Fig. 19.8 Process map for targeted marrow irradiation (TMI).

BOX 19.7   Daily Quality Assurance Example for Varian TrueBeam

I. Power up from standby
   A. Unlock the turnkey at control console
   B. Select "machine QA" on the major mode screen
   C. Log in to power on
II. Mechanical checks
   A. Under the "cooling" tab in service, check the following:
      1. Gas pressure
      2. Water level (at least ¾ full)
      3. Water temp
   B. In the treatment room, check the following:
      1. Water pressure
      2. Laser Guard activation (wave hand over collimator)
      3. Collision interlock activation (wave hand in front of kV source)
III. Output checks
   A. QA mode
      a. Select open plan
      b. Go to appropriate network drive and select the daily QA file
      c. If the motion management device appears, select 'none' under devices
      d. File will show all photon and electron energies and Winston Lutz angles
      e. Power on the QA device
      f. Center the QA device with the crosshairs and light field
      g. Set to 100 cm SSD

   h. Launch the QA software and log in
   i. The software will search for the device and do a background correction
   j. Select the first energy and click start
   k. Deliver the beams
      a. Accept or reject after each beam
      b. Output tolerance should be less than 3%
      c. Close the software and power off the QA device
IV. MLC preparation
   A. Preview, add imaging, MV during dosimetry
   B. Extend imagers and capture image
   C. Measure lateral, should measure between 17.7–17.9cm
   D. Save image
      I. Daily imaging QA
   A. kV CBCT
      a. Align white box to small cross hair
      b. Verify enough clearance for gantry rotation
      c. At console on any available beam, click add imaging, CBCT, before
      d. Deliver the kV CBCT
      e. Manipulate images by selecting region of interest and auto match
      f. Verify seed alignment
      g. Save and apply shifts
      h. If Winston Lutz is required (SBRTs), do that now. Otherwise, verify isocenter with a kV pair.

CBCT, Cone beam computed tomography; *kV CBCT*, kilovolt CBCT; *MLC*, multileaf collimation; *QA*, quality assurance; *SBRT*, stereotactic body radiation therapy; *SSD*, source-to-skin distance.

---

basins, emergency supplies, intravenous poles, marking instruments, and a flashlight, to name a few. The rationale for having rooms in good condition is patient care, safety, and hygiene. Frequency of checking general conditions should be daily, at the start or at the end of each day. Documentation is important if any corrective action is needed. Service engineers and medical materials staff should be contacted for corrective actions. A checklist of all necessary items should be maintained for all rooms.

Communication

Ensuring communication devices are functioning properly in the treatment room is important because patient movement may result in missing the treatment volume and radiating normal tissue. The patient may also need assistance, or the therapist may need to communicate instructions or reassurance to the patient. Both audio and visual communications are necessary, and functionality should be documented daily. Mechanical and electrical malfunctions can occur. If the communication devices malfunction, the engineer or physicist should be notified immediately.

Mold/Block Fabrication

Although the use of Cerrobend has declined with the advent of multileaf collimation (MLC), a QC process is still important to have in place. The AAPM recommends that block cutting systems be checked monthly with fabrication of a block outline and comparison of the aperture of the block cutter with a treatment machine.[70]

The block room itself should be assessed annually with an air sample analysis that follows OSHA guidelines.[71] Dust collector floor mats and high-efficiency particulate arrestance vacuums should be used as protective measures of exposure to metallic oxide fumes. Proper documentation should be kept in a log, with all corrective actions noted.

Accessory Devices

Treatment accessories are used to indicate beam direction, modify beam attenuation, and aid in positioning and immobilization. These devices should be checked for physical integrity and reliability. Latching mechanisms for interlocking accessories, such as electron cones, wedges, trays, and compensators, should be checked monthly.[72] Methods for checking devices include manipulation, visualization, and radiography. Examples of each method include:

- Visualization: Check wedges for dents and chips and trays for excessive cracks.
- Manipulation: Check that breast boards firmly lock into position and head holders do not sag under pressure.
- Radiography: Image wedges or Cerrobend blocks to check for variations in density.[70]

The record of results should include date of check, device evaluated, condition of device, person notified of defect, corrective actions taken, and follow-up dates and information. Good QA of treatment accessories leads to better outcomes in patient safety, precision of setup, and treatment delivery and in financial savings for the department.

Treatment Chart

The treatment chart documents every aspect of the patient's care. Whether the documentation is a paper chart or an electronic medical record, it should contain the following components: patient identification; initial physical evaluation of patient, including clinical information; treatment planning; treatment execution; and QA checklists (Table 19.5). The daily treatment record is of special importance to the radiation therapist. Items the therapist records daily are:

- Date
- Time-out performed
- Daily and cumulative doses to all prescription, critical structure, and anatomic reference points

TABLE 19.5 Components of the Treatment Chart

Component of Treatment Chart	Material Included
Patient identification	Patient name
	Identification
	Digital image
Initial evaluation	Histologic diagnosis of disease
	Stage
	Grade
	History and physical
Treatment planning	Simulator and setup instructions
	Beam and patient parameters
	MU or time setting
	In vivo dosimetry results
	Special physics calculations
Treatment execution	Signed consent form
	Prescription
	Daily record
	Time-out documentation
	Chronology of changes in treatment
	Treatment field documentation: both graphic portal imaging and digital images of field markings
	Description of setup, treatment devices and modifiers, field parameters
	On-treatment clinical assessment
	Treatment summary and follow-up
QA checklist	Chart check

MU, Monitor unit; *QA,* quality assurance.
Modified from Kutcher GJ, Coia L, Gillin M, et al. *Comprehensive QA for Radiation Oncology: Report of AAPM Radiation Therapy Task Group 40*; 1994. www.aapm.org/pubs/reports/RPT_46.PDF. Accessed October 17, 2019.

- Fraction number and elapsed days
- Treatment aids
- Verification imaging

Once the treatment chart has been established, QA of the chart is ongoing. A chart check protocol should be performed several times. The first time is before treatment delivery. The treatment plan should be checked against the prescription with verification that all data were properly transferred to the treatment machine. The second time is weekly chart checks by both the radiation therapist and physicist. This check is to identify any modifications since the previous check or any upcoming changes. A final review of the chart is performed at treatment completion to verify department policy was followed.[70] Table 19.6 shows a sample chart check protocol.

With the implementation of CMS's meaningful use or Electronic Health Record Incentive program, the majority of care is generated and delivered electronically.[73] The therapist can review the plan and data in the R&V system to ensure they are correct. QC procedures on the R&V system should be conducted at specific times. One example is with software updates to the R&V system or to treatment planning software that shares information directly with the system.[74] Any time modifications to the machine library are calibrated, verification that beam data are correct is important. All unexpected values or messages displayed by the R&V system should be documented and followed up on by facility engineers or physicists.[74]

TABLE 19.6 Radiation Therapist Chart Checklist

Date of initial chart check	
ISO	Right acoustic neuroma
Verify consult note and stage	Complete in one chart
Pathology report	Benign
Prescription approved	Yes
Primary or secondary physician attached to all relevant appointments	Yes
Physics second check completed	Yes
Computer plan	Complete
Simulation sheet	Approved
Field setup	Yes
Face photo	Yes
Consent approved	Yes
Mus, energy, wedges, bolus	Checked initial
Machine verification	Yes, Edge
Patient shift	No
IMRT QA complete	Yes
Virtual simulation sheet started	Yes
Control points and check multiisocenter cals	<Select>
Notes	
Therapist initials	

IMRT, Intensity-modulated radiation therapy; *ISO,* Isocenter; *QA,* quality assurance.

Portal/Onboard Imaging

Image-guided radiation therapy (IGRT) has emerged in radiation therapy because of stereotactic radiosurgery (SRS), dose escalation, and organ motion.[75] QA recommendations on electronic imaging equipment are somewhat generic but are based on the themes of safety, geometric accuracy, image quality, and dose.[75] For technologies such as kilovolt cone beam CT (kV-CBCT), megavolt CBCT, and CT on rails, geometric accuracy is important because of the spatial relationship between the imager and the linear accelerator's radiation isocenter.[76] Table 19.7 summarizes QC recommendations for CT-based IGRT systems.

For planer imaging with an electronic portal imaging device (EPID) or onboard imager, QA recommendations are similar to that of CT-based imagers. The functionality of interlocks should be verified daily, as should imaging and treatment field coincidence. The tolerance for the coincidence test should be 2 mm or less.[52] Monthly QA procedures for both kV and MV imagers look at uniformity and noise, which should fall into baseline tolerance. Annually, the imaging dose is calculated for imagers; this, too, should be recorded at baseline levels.[52]

Simulators

CT produces images of high spatial resolution and fidelity to define anatomy in three dimensions. When properly calibrated, CT images can also provide electron density information that, in turn, is used in heterogeneity-based treatment plans and dose calculations.

Improvements in detector configurations, scanner geometry, and reconstruction algorithms occur regularly. Thus aspects of QA of CT simulators are more complex. A typical QA program includes evaluation of:
1. Radiation and patient safety: Safety interlocks and emergency off switches.
2. CT dosimetry: Dose index comparison.

TABLE 19.7 Quality Assurance Recommendations for Kilovolt and Megavolt In-Room Computed Tomography Imagers

Quality Check	Frequency	Tolerance	Person Responsible
Collision/door interlocks	Daily	Functional	Therapist
Warning lights and sounds			
Laser/image/treatment isocenter coincidence		±2 mm	
Phantom localization and couch shift			
kV/MV/laser alignments	Monthly	±1 mm	Therapist or physicist
Accuracy of couch shift motion			
High-contrast spatial resolution		≤2 mm	Physicist
CT number accuracy		Baseline	
Noise and uniformity			
Imaging dose	Annually	Baseline	
X-ray generator performance (kV only)			

CT, Computed tomography; kV, kilovolt; MV, megavolt.
From Song WY: Linear accelerator-based MV and kV imaging systems. In: Pawlicki T, Dunscombe P, Mundt AJ, eds. *Quality and Safety in Radiotherapy*. Boca Raton, FL: CRC Press, Taylor & Francis Group; 2010, and from Bissonnette JP, Balter PA, Dong F, et al. Quality assurance for image-guided radiation therapy utilizing CT-based technologies: a report of the AAPM TG-179. *Med Phys.* 2012;39(4):1946–1963.

3. Electromechanical components: Checking of x-ray generator parameters (kVp, mAs) and couch/laser alignment.
4. Image quality: Resolution and contrast.[77]

Table 19.8 gives a complete listing of QC procedures recommended by the AAPM.

Some daily checks performed by the radiation therapist may include measurement of image noise and alignment of gantry lasers with the center of the imaging plane.[78] AAPM guidelines recommend CT number accuracy be checked as follows: daily with water, monthly with four to five different density materials, and annually with the electron density phantom. The purpose is to check for uniformity, accuracy, and electron density conversion. The procedure involves scanning a water phantom with 110 kV and 130 kV photons. Hounsfield units (HU) are measured at five regions of interest, and the homogeneity results must be within 5 HU as recommended by the AAPM.[78]

Not only should the equipment be evaluated, so should the simulation process. Tasks performed in one aspect of the simulation can affect the accuracy and efficiency of the entire process, so improvement of the entire process should include the following:
- Patient positioning and immobilization.
- Scan limits and protocol.
- Contrast or special instructions, including pediatrics and anesthesia cases.
- Data acquisition.
- Localization and marking.
- Virtual simulation.
- Digitally reconstructed radiograph and setup documentation.[78]

Fusion imaging is becoming more commonplace in radiation therapy. Along with CT imaging, modalities like MRI, nuclear medicine

TABLE 19.8 Quality Assurance of Computed Tomography Simulators

Procedures	Tolerances (±)
Daily	
Alignment of gantry lasers with center of imaging plane	2 mm
Monthly and After Laser Adjustments	
Orientation of gantry lasers with respect to the imaging plane	2 mm over the length of laser projection
Spacing of lateral wall lasers with respect to lateral gantry lasers	2 mm and scan plane
Orientation of wall lasers with respect to the imaging plane	2 mm over the length of laser projection
Orientation of the ceiling laser with respect to the imaging plane	2 mm over the length of laser projection
Monthly or When Daily Laser QA Tests Reveal Rotational Problems	
Orientation of the CT scanner tabletop with respect to the imaging plane	2 mm over the length and width of the tabletop
Monthly	
Table in vertical and longitudinal motion	1 mm over the range of table motion
Semiannually	
Sensitivity profile width	1 mm of nominal value
Annually	
Table indexing and position	1 mm over the scan range
Gantry tilt accuracy	1 degree over the gantry tilt range
Gantry tilt position accuracy	1 degree or 1 mm from nominal position
Scan localization	1 mm over the scan range
Radiation profile width	Manufacturer specification
After Replacement of Major Generator Components	
Generator tests	Manufacturer specification or AAPM report 39 recommendations

AAPM, American Association of Physicists in Medicine; CT, computed tomography; QA, quality assurance.
From Mutic S, Palta JR, Butker EK, et al. Quality assurance for computed-tomography simulators and the computed-tomography simulation process: report of the AAPM Radiation Therapy Committee Task Group No. 66. *Med Phys.* 2003;30(10):2762–2792.

imaging with single photon emission computed tomography, and especially PET, are being used in the planning process. Both anatomic and biologic information aids are used in design of the optical course of radiation therapy for patients. PET/CT manufacturers are developing QA tests to assess the steps involved in generating a PET/CT image and QC tests to evaluate the final image itself. Generally, on a daily basis, the performance of the detectors should be evaluated to include signals, coincidences, timing, and energy drifts of all detectors in the system.[77] Detector normalization and well counter correction should be performed quarterly, and scanner alignment, along with a full drift analysis, should be an annual procedure.[77]

MRI simulation QA focuses on the safe and accurate operation of MRI equipment. It should include daily and weekly tests performed by a MR technologist or therapist, with additional tests performed by the

TABLE 19.9 **MRI Simulator QA Protocol**[80]		
Weekly QA (Technologist/ Therapist)	**Monthly QA (Medical Physicist)**	**Annual QA (MRI Physicist)**
Transmitter gain constancy	Patient safety (monitors, intercom, emergency off, signage)	RF coil integrity check
Center frequency constancy	Patient comfort (bore lights, bore fan)	B0 constancy
Signal to noise ratio constancy	Percent signal ghosting	B1 + constancy
Slice thickness accuracy	Percent image uniformity	Gradient linearity constancy
Slice position accuracy	High/low contrast constancy	
	Laser alignment	
	Couch position accuracy	
	Image artifacts	

MRI, Magnetic resonance imaging; *QA,* quality assurance; *RF,* radiofrequency.

TABLE 19.10 **Daily Quality Assurance Procedures for Medical Accelerators**			
	MACHINE TYPE AND TOLERANCE		
Procedure	**NON-IMRT**	**IMRT**	**SRS/SBRT**
Dosimetry	3%		
X-ray output constancy (all energies)			
Electron output constancy (if not equipped, then weekly)			
Mechanical			
Laser localization	2 mm	1.5 mm	1.0 mm
Distance indicator (ODI) at isocenter	2 mm	2 mm	2 mm
Collimator size indicator	2 mm	2 mm	1 mm
Safety			
Door interlock (beam off)	Functional		
Door closing safety			
Audio/visual monitors			
Stereotactic interlocks (lockout)	NA	NA	Functional
Radiation area monitors (if used)	Functional		
Beam on indicator			

IMRT, Intensity-modulated radiation therapy; *ODI,* optical distance indicator; *SBRT,* stereotactic body radiation therapy; *SRS,* stereotactic radiosurgery.
From Levy L. Radiation therapy equipment and quality assurance. In: Levy L, ed. *Mosby's Radiation Therapy: Study Guide and Exam Review.* St. Louis, MO: Mosby; 2010.

medical physicist on a quarterly and annual basis. Image QC includes geometric, slice thickness and slice position accuracy, and signal intensity uniformity.[79] A sample MRI QA protocol can be found in Table 19.9.[80]

Linear Accelerators

Quality assurance is performed on linear accelerators to ensure that characteristics of the machine do not vary significantly from the time of acceptance and commissioning. Acceptance testing involves measurement of output and performance of the linac against manufacturer specifications. Commissioning of a linac establishes baseline values that are used in future dosimetric measurements and verifies that the machine operates within certain tolerances and with mechanical integrity.[52] Before 2009, quality of linear accelerators followed AAPM TG40 recommendations. Since TG40 was published, numerous technologies have become commonplace in clinical practice. These technologies include MLC, EPID, SRS, stereotactic body radiation therapy (SBRT), and IMRT. In 2009, the AAPM published TG142 to build on previous recommendations for these newer technologies.

As mentioned previously, the goal of linac QA is to keep deviation from baseline values within set tolerance levels. Variance could result from machine malfunction or mechanical breakdown. Replacement of components such as the waveguide or bending magnet may alter machine performance and overall aging of the equipment.[52] AAPM TG142 has increased the scope of testing performed on linacs and the number of variables. Procedures are broken down into daily, monthly, and annual timeframes, and incorporate machine-type tolerances for non-IMRT, IMRT, and SRS/SBRT treatment capabilities. Along with the equipment QA, patient and process QA is also needed for IMRT, SRS, and SBRT treatments. For example, before the first or only fraction, the target construction must be validated, image guidance strategies established, and monitor units (MUs) validated; also necessary is assurance that adequately trained personnel are familiar with the individual setup. Increased demands for QA also increase the time needed to perform it. Tests should be simple, rapid, and reproducible.[81] Each member of the QA team has responsibilities; Table 19.10 shows the therapists primarily responsible for daily QA.[72]

X-ray and electron output constancy fall into the daily testing procedures, as do laser localization and checking that the interlocks are functioning properly. Tables 19.11 and 19.12 illustrate some of the

procedures performed monthly and annually.[52] These responsibilities generally fall on the medical physicist. A complete listing of procedures is found at www.aapm.org/pubs/reports/RPT_142.pdf.

If measurements fall outside the allowed deviation, machine adjustments are needed to bring the values back into compliance. Action levels are set by the medical physicist to determine when intervention is needed, depending on how far and how often values fall outside the tolerance levels. Action levels are categorized as levels 1 to 3. Level 1 is an inspection action. Treatment may continue during this time, but the cause of the deviation should be investigated. A scheduled action falls into level 2. Treatment in this case may continue as well, but an intervention should be scheduled within 1 to 2 working days. For example, when a machine's dose rate consistency is slightly outside the tolerance but will not cause a significant clinical impact, then within a day or two, scheduled maintenance should take place.[52] A level 3 action requires immediate action or corrective action. Treatments should be stopped during this time. Examples of a level 3 action are a significant error in flatness of the beam or a nonfunctioning door interlock.[52]

Multileaf Collimation

MLC has become a primary component of a linear accelerator. Movement of each leaf is monitored with a charge coupled device (CCD). A CCD is an integrated circuit etched onto a silicon surface. Photons incident on this surface generate charge that can be read with electronics and turned into a digital copy of the light patterns falling on the device.[82] QA concerns for MLCs fall into two main categories: attenuation properties and positional precision.[83] According to the AAPM TG142, qualitative

TABLE 19.11 Monthly Quality Assurance of Medical Accelerators

Procedure	Non-IMRT	IMRT	SRS/SBRT
		MACHINE-TYPE TOLERANCE	
Dosimetry			
X-ray output constancy		2%	
Electron output constancy		2%	
Backup monitor chamber constancy		2%	
Typical dose rate output constancy	NA	2% (@ IMRT dose rate)	2% (@ stereo dose rate)
Photon beam profile constancy		1%	
Electron beam profile constancy		1%	
Electron beam energy constancy		2% or 2 mm	
Mechanical			
Light/radiation field coincidence		2 mm or 1% on a side	
Light/radiation field coincidence (asymmetric)		1 mm or 1% on a side	
Distance check device for lasers compared with front pointer		1 mm	
Gantry/collimator angle indicators		1 degree	
Accessory trays (port film graticule)		2 mm	
Jaw position indicators (symmetric)		2 mm	
Jaw position indicators (asymmetric)		1 mm	
Cross-hair centering		1 mm	
Treatment couch position indicators	2 mm/1 degree	2 mm/1 degree	1 mm/0.5 degree
Wedge placement accuracy		2 mm	
Compensator placement accuracy		1 mm	
Latching of wedges, blocking trays		Functional	
Localizing lasers	±2 mm	±1 mm	±1 mm
Safety			
Laser guard interlock test		Functional	
Respiratory Gating			
Beam output constancy		2%	
Phase, amplitude beam control		Functional	
In-room respiratory monitoring system		Functional	
Gating interlock		Functional	

Refer to American Association of Physicists in Medicine Task Group 142 (AAPM TG142) report for further information.
IMRT, Intensity-modulated radiation therapy; *SBRT,* stereotactic body radiation therapy; *SRS,* stereotactic radiosurgery.
From Klein EE, Hanley J, Bayouth J, et al. *Quality Assurance of Medical Accelerators: Report of the American Association of Physicists in Medicine Task Group 142;* 2009. www.aapm.org/pubs/reports/RPT_142.pdf. Accessed November 21, 2018.

tests should be performed weekly on linacs that perform IMRT and volumetric modulated arc therapy. An example of this test is known as the picket fence test that looks at deviations in interleaf transmission.[52]

Monthly procedures should include verification of the MLC setting versus the radiation field. For non-IMRT treatments, the tolerance is 2 mm; leaf position accuracy for IMRT fields is 1 mm at four gantry angles to account for the gravitational pull on the leafs. Fig. 19.9 shows a pattern used in leaf position verification.[83] Annual QC procedures include checking that the average of leaf and interleaf leakage for all energies is ±0.5% from baseline values established during commissioning.[52] The AAPM Practice Guideline 2.a includes commissioning and QA protocols for IGRT systems. Information can be found at: https://www.ncbi.nlm.nih.gov/pmc/articles/PMC5711227/.[84]

Particle Accelerators

Some aspects of QA testing for particle accelerators are mandated by the NRC or state regulations, so specific frequencies and tolerances of tests must be followed for state compliance. When referring to a proton therapy unit, QA procedures should primarily focus on safety of personnel and constancy of beam parameters.[72] Daily checks generally performed by the radiation therapist include ensuring that door interlocks and that radiation room monitors and audiovisual monitors are all functioning properly. Room lasers and the ODI have a daily tolerance of 2 mm.[70]

Most proton therapy accelerators have very structured QA recommendations and protocols. A system established by Ding and associates[85] implemented a process that is carried out daily by the radiation therapist, with the total time to complete the procedures comparable with that of a linac. Four categories (safety, mechanical, imaging, and dosimetry) are evaluated. Parameters that fall in the safety category are verification of functionality of door interlocks and the proton beam on light. Couch movement and image panel positioning fall into the mechanical category and have tolerance levels of less than 1 mm.[85] Tolerance levels for dosimetry measurements of proton beam output and beam symmetry are less than 3%. Three task forces addressing proton-related issues are TG156, which is looking

TABLE 19.12 Annual Quality Assurance of Medical Accelerators

	MACHINE-TYPE TOLERANCE		
Procedure	NON-IMRT	IMRT	SRS/SBRT
Dosimetry			
X-ray flatness change from baseline		1%	
X-ray symmetry change from baseline		±1%	
Electron flatness change from baseline		1%	
Electron symmetry change from baseline		±1%	
X-ray/electron output calibration		±1%	
X-ray beam quality (PDD_{10} or $TMR_{10/20}$)		±1% from baseline	
X-ray MU linearity	±2% ≥ 5 MU	±5% (2–4 MU)	±5% (2–4 MU)
		±2% ≥5 MU	±2% ≥5 MU
Mechanical			
Collimator rotation isocenter		±1 mm from baseline	
Electron applicator interlocks		Functional	
Coincidence of radiation and mechanical isocenter	±2 mm from baseline	±2 mm from baseline	±1 mm from baseline
Tabletop sag		2 mm from baseline	
Table angle		1 degree	
Safety			
Follow manufacturer test procedures		Functional	
Respiratory Gating			
Beam energy constancy		2%	
Calibration of surrogate for respiratory phase/amplitude		100 ms of expected	
Interlock testing		Functional	

Refer to American Association of Physicists in Medicine Task Group 142 (AAPM TG142) report for further information.
IMRT, Intensity-modulated radiation therapy; *MU,* monitor unit; *PDD,* percentage depth dose; *SBRT,* stereotactic body radiation therapy; *SRS,* stereotactic radiosurgery; *TMR,* tissue maximum ratio.
From Klein EE, Hanley J, Bayouth J, et al. *Quality Assurance of Medical Accelerators: Report of the American Association of Physicists in Medicine Task Group 142*; 2009. www.aapm.org/pubs/reports/RPT_142.pdf. Accessed November 21, 2018.

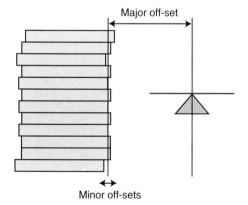

Fig. 19.9 Leaf calibration test. (From Hounsell AR, Jordan TJ. Quality control aspects of the Philips multileaf collimator. *Radiother Oncol.* 1997;45:225–233)

at calibrating the passively scattered proton beam; TG185, which deals with commissioning of systems; and TG183, which is focusing on nomenclature, specifications, safety, and acceptance testing.[86] The AAPM and the ACR have published technical standards for the performance of proton beam radiation therapy. They list daily machine checks for scattered and uniform scanning beams, which include:

- Output consistency
- Range and modulation verification for a subset of field parameter configurations

- X-ray and laser alignment
- Interlocks
- Beam-on and x-ray on indicator lights
- Two-way audio-visual patient and accelerator-control communication systems
- Door-opening beam-interrupt interlocks[87]

Brachytherapy

Brachytherapy is the use of radioactive isotopes to deliver a high dose of radiation over a short distance. The radiation therapist may or may not directly participate in a brachytherapy procedure, but an understanding of how QA can help ensure accuracy and precision is important. Aspects of a good QA program for brachytherapy include testing of source calibration and calibrators, treatment planning and dosimetric evaluation, brachytherapy devices, and also radiation safety.[70] The AAPM recommends that sources be calibrated with direct or indirect traceability to national standards and that the mean batch of sources fall within 3% of the manufacturer's value.[70] The integrity of the sources should be evaluated as well, with physical inspection and performance of leak tests every 6 months.

Source inventories are required for all brachytherapy programs. Both long and short half-life sources have an active inventory located in the hot laboratory and in a permanent file located with the medical physicists. Some items included in the active inventory include the number of sources, their activity, and identification methods such as engraving or color coding. The permanent file contains information results from leak and wipes tests and the institution's verification of calibration.[70]

TABLE 19.13 Quality Assurance of Remote Afterloading Brachytherapy Units

Test[a]	Tolerance
Room safety: door interlocks, lights, and alarms	Functional
Console functions: switches, batteries, printer	Functional
Visual inspection of sources guides	Free of kinks and firmly attached
Verify accuracy of ribbon preparation	Autoradiograph

[a]Each test is performed before each treatment day.
From Kutcher GJ, Coia L, Gillin M, et al. *Comprehensive QA for Radiation Oncology: Report of AAPM Radiation Therapy Task Group 40.* www.aapm.org/pubs/reports/RPT_46.PDF, 1994. Accessed November 21, 2018.

Verification of the dose calculations is recommended to be done in a timely fashion so that any errors may be corrected before the completion of treatment. For each implant, a minimum of one critical point must be independently calculated. Agreement between the independent check and the dose calculation should be within 15%.[70] Remote afterloaders used in high-dose-rate (HDR) brachytherapy should be maintained with proper performance. A list of tests performed on each day the unit is used can be found in Table 19.13, and all AAPM recommendations are located at www.aapm.org/pubs/reports/RPT_46.PDF.[70]

Whether the brachytherapy procedure is performed with HDR or low dose rate, the principle of ALARA (as low as reasonably achievable) applies. The rules of time, distance, and shielding aid in keeping exposure to a minimum. Categories that require radiation safety measures include:

- Facility: Inventory, storage, transporting.
- Maintenance: Identification, cleaning, disposal.
- Clinical application: Preparation of sources, patient discharge, and personnel monitoring.
- Emergencies and special precautions: Contamination, lost source, GM Counter testing and education and training of all personnel.[70]

Treatment Planning Systems and Medical Dosimetry

Unlike errors in treatment delivery, which are usually random in nature (e.g., forgetting to place a bolus for a treatment), errors with treatment planning computers tend to be systematic.[88] Planning a treatment with a 30-degree wedge instead of a 45-degree wedge could lead to serious overdosing of the patient. QA of treatment plans and systems is a significant part of the overall goal for CQI. All beam data are recommended to be acquired by a medical physicist using a water tank with an automated dose acquisition system. Computer software should be commissioned for each treatment machine and energy and checked when purchased and updated on an annual basis.[70] Daily QA procedures for treatment planning systems include verification that input and output devices, such as a digitizer, fall within a 1-mm tolerance of the initial planning reference set. MU checks should be performed at commissioning and annually. The tolerance for this QA procedure is 2% accuracy.[70]

Once a treatment plan and dose calculations have been performed, there is QA for individual patients as well. The entire radiation therapy team plays a part in individual patient QA. The treatment plan should be reviewed by the oncologist and the physicist before treatment. Specific day 1 verification methods may include; patient identification, portal imaging, SSD measurements, and prescription check.[45] When therapists implement the plan, they too should verify that all accessories and doses are entered into the treatment machine properly. Recommendations are that the oncologist be present for the first fraction and review pretreatment images on all curative or complex palliative treatments. The International Commission on Radiation Units and Measurements recommends that the radiation dose that is delivered be within 5% of the prescribed dose,[89] which means that each step of the treatment process, including simulation, planning, imaging, and delivery, must be less than 5% each to meet the goal. With advanced technologies such as IMRT, respiratory gating, biologic optimization, and adaptive radiation therapy on the rise, the time commitment for an effective QA program is increasing as well. The recommendation of TG53 is that a facility concentrates its efforts on the issues that are a high priority for that institution so the best individual outcome can be met.[37]

For the QA program to be effective, an annual QA report should be documented. Items to be included in the report follow the tolerances set by the AAPM, which can be categorized as:

- Dosimetry
- Mechanical
- Safety
- Imaging
- Special devices and procedures

This report should be verified by the medical physicist and incorporated into the larger QI process.[52]

CONTINUOUS QUALITY IMPROVEMENT IMPLEMENTATION

Countless indicators can be improved upon in radiation therapy. Another example of how the PDSA model has been implemented follows. The treatment planning and delivery process has many components, each with their own uncertainties. One such uncertainty is the interobserver variation of normal tissue contouring.[90] Deviations in maximum doses to organs at risk (OAR) have been documented ranging from −22% to +35%.[82] These variations in normal tissue delineation can be reduced following an effective PDCA model implemented by Breunig and colleagues.[91]

Plan: Reduce variation while producing high-quality normal tissue contours.

Do: Have numerous dosimetrists contour normal anatomy on the case image.

Check: Compare contours with the gold standard of the oncologist's contour; provide instruction.

Act: Perform additional contours and reevaluate as training reduces variability.

The results of the Breunig study reported that of 30 OAR contoured, 19 achieved a passing score based on the study's analysis. At that time, the dosimetrists compared their results with the gold-standard contours and were allowed to recontour structures with magnetic resonance fusion images when needed. Retesting showed that of the 11 OAR recontoured, improvement was shown in 10 of the cases.[91] From this point, new objectives can be identified, the cycle continuously repeats, and the process continuous to improve. For this process, further objectives are to include written guidelines and pictorial examples to aid the dosimetrists and feedback provided by the oncologist on a case-by-case basis.

QI in healthcare has stemmed from the knowledge of other industries. Simulation in aviation, checklists in the auto industry, and CQI that focuses on the process and not the person fit well into a radiation therapy department. Quality indicators and the outcomes achieved continue to be monitored. These outcomes effect reimbursement for services and accreditation of facilities. The cycle is never-ending, so a diligent QA program that includes a voluntary error reporting system and a culture of patient safety and care is essential. Quality cannot be adjunct to the process but must be integrated in the design phase and continued throughout the entire process.[3]

> Statistical analysis of the data collected in assessment of a QI process is vital to the selection of the appropriate solution or response. These data should be organized in a format that is easy to understand. Learn more about different types of charts or graphs that may be used to display data by visiting the American Society for Quality at www.asq.org.

SUMMARY

- QI in healthcare is a systematic approach to the continuous study and improvement of the process of providing healthcare services to meet the needs of patients and others. Synonymous terms include CQI and TQM. It is premised on Dr. W.E. Deming's 14 principles of management. These principles emphasize CQI through proactive employee participation in a customer-responsive environment. QI involves doing things right and doing things well.
- Regulatory agencies set mandates for quality and safety. National agencies include the NRC, the FDA, and the OSHA. Individual states can be an agreement state with the NRC, and facilities follow the regulations set forth by their state agency.
- Institutional agencies award accreditation (TJC) and guide quality through reimbursement, as with the CMS.
- Quality is attained through QC procedures outlined in a QA program to ensure QI.
- Because of the diversity of healthcare organizations, the organization may choose to use a variety of management methods to implement the CQI plan. These methods may include the adoption of system-wide programs such as Six Sigma or PDSA.

- The complexity of radiation therapy treatments is increasing. Thus recommendations are for two therapists per machine and participation as part of the QI team headed up by the medical director.
- Quality indicators have been established for diseases with high incidence and mortality rates. QIs can be measured, and performance of a quality audit ensures best practices.
- Clinical aspects of QC are a major responsibility of the radiation therapist. Daily QC should be performed on all equipment used in the treatment process. Monthly and annual testing is primarily conducted by a medical physicist. Communication and documentation are key with QC tests.
- Action levels are designated 1 to 3 to indicate when intervention is needed for a piece of equipment. A level 3, action should terminate the use of the equipment until corrective measures have been taken.
- A successful QI plan is the end result of total commitment and involvement from all healthcare providers at all times. Linked to cost containment, increased quality of care, professional practice standards, and TJC criteria, CQI has become routine practice in the delivery of healthcare.

REVIEW QUESTIONS

The answers to the Review Questions can be found by logging on to our website at: http://evolve.elsevier.com/Washington/principles

1. The QI model PDSA stands for:
   a. Plan-document-study-assess.
   b. Process-develop-study-act.
   c. Plan-do-study-act.
   d. Prepare-develop-structure-analyze.
2. A culture of safety should be encouraged in radiation oncology. The best way to do this is to:
   a. Report all errors and near misses.
   b. Support continuing education activities for therapists.
   c. Include competency evaluations in all employee performance evaluations.
   d. Prosecute employees who make an error.
3. TJC is an example of a(n):
   a. Federal regulatory agency.
   b. Institutional accrediting body.
   c. Professional society for oncologists.
   d. State peer-review agency.
4. The EPA regulates:
   a. A facility's use of radioactive materials.
   b. A facility's handling and disposal of isotopes.
   c. The use of devices that generate isotopes.
   d. Contamination procedures.
5. What is QA?
   a. Peer-review evaluation of quality.
   b. The operational activities used to fulfill quality.
   c. The planned actions to satisfy quality requirements.
   d. A process to satisfy the needs of a patient.

6. It is the responsibility of the _____ to establish a QI program.
   a. Head medical physicist.
   b. Medical director.
   c. Radiation safety officer.
   d. Department manager.
7. Which is an example of a structure quality indicator in a QI plan?
   a. Staff competency.
   b. Informed consent.
   c. Quality of life.
   d. All of the above.
8. Which is considered a nonfunctional audio/visual communication?
   a. Level 1 action.
   b. Level 2 action.
   c. Level 3 action.
   d. Level 4 action.
9. What are the frequency and tolerance of checking image/treatment isocenter coincidence on a kVCT imager?
   a. Daily and ±2 mm.
   b. Daily and baseline.
   c. Monthly and ±1 mm.
   d. No check needed.
10. The therapist performs a laser localization check daily on a linac that delivers IMRT treatment. What is the tolerance of this spot check?
    a. 1.0 mm.
    b. 1.5 mm.
    c. 2.0 mm.
    d. 2.5 mm.

QUESTIONS TO PONDER

1. Explain why the phrase "If it ain't broke, don't fix it" cannot be applied in a QI program.
2. An initial step in improving a process is defining those activities used in completing the process. Develop a process map that outlines the steps necessary to complete a simulation in the radiation oncology department.

3. Referring to Deming's principles of management, what suggestions would you give a coworker who consistently complains about a specific problem relating to the treatment delivery process in radiation oncology?
4. Describe how uncertainties in a radiation oncology department can affect outcomes.
5. How will the efforts of TG100 and TG142 change how a radiation oncology department functions?

REFERENCES

1. Institute of Medicine. *Crossing the Quality Chasm: A New Health System for the 21st Century*. Washington, DC: National Academy Press; 2001.
2. Quality and patient safety: the six domains of healthcare quality. Agency for Healthcare Research and Quality website. www.ahrq.gov/professionals/quality-patient-safety/talkingquality/create/sixdomains.html#_ftn1. Accessed November 2, 2018.
3. Carrigan M. Quality management: an overview. In: Pawlicki T, Dunscombe P, Mundt AJ, eds. *Quality and Safety in Radiotherapy*. Boca Raton, FL: CRC Press, Taylor & Francis Group; 2010.
4. Sun GH, MacEachern MP, Perla RJ, et al. Health care quality improvement publication trends. *Am J Med Qual*. 2014;29(5):403–407.
5. Plan-Do-Check-Act. Quality resources. American Society for Quality website. asq.org/learn-about-quality/project-planning-tools/overview/pdca-cycle.html. Accessed November 2, 2018.
6. Papp J. Introduction to quality management. In: Papp J, ed. *Quality Management in the Imaging Sciences*. 6th ed. St. Louis, MO:2011 Elsevier.
7. Toyota Production System. https://www.toyota-global.com/company/vision_philosophy/toyota_production_system/. Accessed November 2, 2018.
8. Kelly AM, Cronin P. Practical approaches to quality improvement for radiologists. *Radiographics*. 2015;35:1630–1642.
9. Kruskal JB, Reedy A, Pascal L, Rosen MP, Boiselle PM. Quality initiatives: Lean approach to improving performance and efficiency in a radiology department. *Radiographics*. 2012;32(2):573–587.
10. Vallejo B. Tools of the trade: lean and six sigma. *J Healthc Q*. 2009;31(3): 3–4.
11. Lee E, Grooms R, Mamidala S, Magy P. Six easy steps on how to create a lean sigma value stream map for multidisciplinary clinical operation. *J Am Coll Radiol*. 2014;11:1144–1149.
12. How to use the fishbone tool for root cause analysis. CMS website. https://www.cms.gov/medicare/provider-enrollment-and-certification/qapi/downloads/fishbonerevised.pdf. Accessed November 21, 2018.
13. Patton GA, Gaffney DK, Moeller JH. Facilitation of radiotherapeutic error by computerized record and verify systems. *Int J Radiat Oncol Biol Phys*. 2003;56(1):50–57.
14. Lee K, Tsou I, Wong S, et al. Metastatic spinal cord compression as an oncology emergency—getting our act together. *Int J Qual Health Care*. 2007;19(6):377–381.
15. Gillan C, Davis CA, Moran K, French J, Lisewshi B. The quest for quality: principles to guide medical radiation technology practice. *J Med Imaging Radiat Sci*. 2015;46(4):427–434.
16. Taylor K, Mazur L, Chera B, et al. Application of "A3 thinking" in operational improvements in radiation oncology. In: Guan and Liao, eds., Industrial and Systems Engineering Research Conference Proceedings; Montreal, Canada; 2014. November 22, 2013.
17. Bassuk JA, Washington IM. The A3 problem solving report: a 10-step scientific method to execute performance improvements in an academic research vivarium. *PLoS One*. 2013;8(10):e76833.
18. Varkey P, Kollengode A. Methodologies for quality improvement. In: Pawlicki T, Dunscombe P, Mundt AJ, eds. *Quality and Safety in Radiotherapy*. Boca Raton, FL: CRC Press, Taylor & Francis Group; 2010.
19. Huq SM, Fraass BA, Dunscombe PB, et al. The report of Task Group 100 of the AAPM: application of risk analysis methods to radiation therapy quality management. *Med Phys*. 2016;43(7):4209–4262.
20. About NRC. US Nuclear Regulatory Commission website. www.nrc.gov-/about-nrc.html. Accessed November 14, 2018.
21. Regulations of radioactive materials. U.S. Nuclear Regulatory Commission website. www.nrc.gov/about-nrc/radiation/protects-you/reg-matls.html. Accessed November 14, 2018.
22. EPA's role in radiation protection. U.S. Environmental Protection Agency website. www.epa.gov/radiation/epas-role-radiation-protection. Accessed November 14, 2018.
23. PHMSA. U.S. Department. of Transportation website. https://www.phmsa.dot.gov/about-phmsa/phmsas-mission. Accessed November 14, 2018.
24. Radiation safety. US Food and Drug Administration website. https://www.fda.gov/Radiation-EmittingProducts/RadiationEmittingProductsandProcedures/default.htm. Accessed November 14, 2018.
25. Medical device reporting. US Food and Drug Administration website. https://www.fda.gov/medical-devices/medical-device-safety/medical-device-reporting-mdr-how-report-medical-device-problems. Accessed October 17, 2019.
26. About OSHA. Occupational Safety and Health Administration website. www.osha.gov/about.html. Accessed November 19, 2018.
27. Worker protections against occupational exposure to infectious diseases. Occupational Safety and Health Administration website. https://www.osha.gov/SLTC/bloodbornepathogens/worker_protections.html. Accessed November 19, 2018.
28. Agreement state program. US Nuclear Regulatory Commission website. www.nrc.gov/about-nrc/state-tribal/agreement-states.html. Accessed November 7, 2018.
29. Albert JM, Das P. Quality indicators in radiation oncology. *Int J Radiat Oncol Biol Phys*. 2013;85(4):904–911.
30. About The Joint Commission. The Joint Commission website. www.jointcommission.org/about_us/about_the_joint_commission_main.aspx. Accessed November 7, 2018.
31. Resources: conducting a proactive risk assessment. The Joint Commission website. www.jcrinc.com/assets/1/7/PS17.pdf. Accessed November 5, 2018.
32. ACRO Accreditation. American College of Radiation Oncology website. https://www.acro.org/accreditation. Accessed November 19, 2018.
33. *Manual for ACRO Accreditation*. American College of Radiation Oncology. Seattle, WA. https://www.acro.org/wp-content/uploads/2016/05/Manual-for-ACRO-Accreditation-July-2017.pdf. Accessed October 17, 2019; 2017.
34. Hospital accreditation. DNV-GL Healthcare website. https://www.dnvglhealthcare.com/accreditations/hospital-accreditation. Accessed November 19, 2018.
35. Federal matching shares for Medicaid. *Federal Register*. 2017;82(223):55383–55386. (2017). https://www.gpo.gov/fdsys/pkg/FR-2017-11-21/pdf/2017-24953.pdf. Accessed November 5, 2018.
36. Physician quality reporting system. American College of Radiology website. https://www.acr.org/Practice-Management-Quality-Informatics/Medicare-Value-Based-Programs/PQRS. Accessed November 19, 2018.
37. Fraass B, Doppke K, Hunt M, et al. American Association of Physicists in Medicine Radiation Therapy Committee Task Group 53: quality assurance for clinical radiotherapy treatment planning. *Med Phys*. 1998;25(10):1773–1829.
38. Practice standards. American Society of Radiologic Technologists website. https://www.asrt.org/docs/default-source/practice-standards-published/ps_rt.pdf?sfvrsn=18e076d0_16. Accessed November 19, 2018.
39. APEx standards. American Society for Radiation Oncology website. https://www.astro.org/Daily-Practice/Accreditation/APEx-Process-Overview/APEx-Standards. Accessed November 19, 2018.
40. Merriam-Webster dictionary. Definition of quality. www.merriam-webster.com/dictionary/quality. Accessed November 7, 2018.
41. International Standards Organization. *International Standards Organization Report ISO-8402-1986*. Netherlands: Springer; 1986.
42. Izewska J, Salminen E. Role of quality audits: view from the IAEA. In: Pawlicki T, Dunscombe P, Mundt AJ, eds. *Quality and Safety in Radiotherapy*. Boca Raton, FL: CRC Press, Taylor & Francis Group; 2010.
43. Dunscombe PB, Cooke DL. Perspective on quality and safety in radiotherapy. In: Pawlicki T, Dunscombe P, Mundt AJ, eds. *Quality and Safety in Radiotherapy*. Boca Raton, FL: CRC Press, Taylor & Francis Group; 2010.
44. Specifications manual for Joint Commission national quality measures. Joint Commission website. https://manual.jointcommission.org/releases/TJC2016A/IntroductionTJC.html. Accessed November 19, 2018.
45. Safety is no accident: a framework for quality radiation oncology and care. American Society for Radiation Oncology website. Published 2019. https://www.astro.org/Patient-Care-and-Research/Patient-Safety/Safety-is-no-Accident. Accessed October 18, 2019.
46. ACR-ASTRO practice parameter for radiation oncology. American College of Radiology website; 2018. https://www.acr.org/-/media/ACR/Files/Practice-Parameters/RadOnc.pdf. Accessed November 19, 2018.
47. Surveillance, epidemiology, and end results program. National Cancer Institute website. seer.cancer.gov/data/. Accessed November 19, 2018.
48. Odle TG, Rosier N. *Radiation Therapy Safety: The Critical Role of the Radiation Therapist*. Albuquerque, NM: American Society of Radiologic Technologists Education and Research Foundation, American Society of Radiologic Technologists.

49. American Society of Radiologic Technologists. Radiation therapy staffing and workplace survey 2018.

50. States that regulate by modality. American Society of Radiologic Technologists website. https://www.asrt.org/main/standards-regulations/state-legislative-affairs/states-that-regulate-by-modality. Accessed November 19, 2018.

51. Cheung KY. Role in training. In: Pawlicki T, Dunscombe P, Mundt AJ, eds. *Quality and Safety in Radiotherapy*. Boca Raton, FL: CRC Press, Taylor & Francis Group; 2010.

52. Klein EE, Hanley J, Bayouth J, et al. *Quality Assurance of Medical Accelerators: Report of the American Association of Physicists in Medicine Task Group 142* Published; 2009. www.aapm.org/pubs/reports/RPT_142.pdf. Accessed November 21, 2018.

53. International Atomic Energy Agency. *Comprehensive Audits of Radiotherapy Practices: A Tool for Quality Improvement: Quality Assurance Team for Radiation Oncology (QUATRO)*. Vienna, Austria: International Atomic Energy Agency; 2007.

54. Itri JN, Bakow E, Probyn L, et al. The science of quality improvement. *Acad Radiol*. 2017;24(3):253–262.

55. Donabedian A. The quality of care: how can it be assessed? *JAMA*. 1988;260:1743–1748.

56. Albert JM, Das P. Quality assessment in oncology. *Int J Radiat Oncol Biol Phys*. 2012;83(3):773–781.

57. Viti V. Medical indicators of quality: terminology and examples. In: Pawlicki T, Dunscombe P, Mundt AJ, eds. *Quality and Safety in Radiotherapy*. Boca Raton, FL: CRC Press, Taylor & Francis Group; 2010.

58. Gibata CH, Gossman MS. Role of quality audits: view from North America. In: Pawlicki T, Dunscombe P, Mundt AJ, eds. *Quality and Safety in Radiotherapy*. Boca Raton, FL: CRC Press, Taylor & Francis Group; 2010.

59. Kohn LT, Corrigan J, Donaldson MS. *To Err Is Human: Building a Safer Health System*. Washington, DC: National Academy Press. xxi; 1999.

60. Makary MA, Daniel M. Medical error—the third leading cause of death in the US. *BMJ*. 2016;353(2139):1–5.

61. Deaths: final data for 2019. National vital statistics report. Centers for Disease Control website. https://www.cdc.gov/nchs/data/nvsr/nvsr68/nvsr68_09-508.pdf. Accessed October 18, 2019.

62. Terezakis SA, Pronovost P, Harris K, et al. Safety strategies in an academic radiation oncology department and recommendations for action. *Jt Comm J Qual Patient Saf*. 2011;37(7):291–299.

63. Palta JR, Efstathiou JA, Bekelman JE, et al. Developing a nation radiation oncology registry: from acorns to oaks. *Pract Radiat Oncol*. 2012;2(1):10–17.

64. McIntyre RC. Improving quality improvement. *Am J Surg*. 2012;204:815–825.

65. Hoopes JD, Dicker AP, Eads NL, et al. RO-ILS: radiation oncology incident learning system. A report from the first year of experience. *Pract Radiat Oncol*. 2015;5:312–318.

66. Clarity PSO. *Quarterly Report: Patient Safety Work Produce Q3*. Clarity Group Inc; 2017:1–15.

67. Kalapurakal JA, Zafirovski A, Smith J, et al. A comprehensive quality assurance program for personnel and procedures in radiation oncology: value of voluntary error reporting and checklists. *Int J Radiat Oncol Biol Phys*. 2013;86(2):241–248.

68. Thorton E, Brook OR, Mendiratta-Lala M, Hallett DT, Kruskal JB. Quality initiatives: Application of failure mode and effect analysis in a radiology department. *Radiographics*. 2011;31(1):281–294.

69. Molineu A. Dosimetry equipment and phantoms. In: Pawlicki T, Dunscombe P, Mundt AJ, eds. *Quality and Safety in Radiotherapy*. Boca Raton, FL: CRC Press, Taylor & Francis Group; 2010.

70. Kutcher GJ, Coia L, Gillin M, et al. *Comprehensive Qa for Radiation Oncology: Report of AAPM Radiation Therapy Task Group 40*. Published 1994. www.aapm.org/pubs/reports/RPT_46.PDF. Accessed November 21, 2018.

71. Cadmium. US Department of Labor, Occupational Safety and Health Administration website. www.osha.gov/Publications/3136-08R-2003-English.html. Accessed November 21, 2018.

72. Levy L. Radiation therapy equipment and quality assurance. In: Levy L, ed. *Mosby's Radiation Therapy: Study Guide and Exam Review*. St. Louis, MO: Mosby; 2010.

73. CMS revises meaningful use requirements for 2018. AAP News & Journals website. http://www.aappublications.org/news/2018/05/04/hit050418. Accessed November 20, 2018.

74. International Atomic Energy Agency. *Record and Verify Systems for Radiation Treatment of Cancer: Acceptance Testing, Commissioning and Quality Control*. Vienna, Austria: IAEA; 2013. www-pub.iaea.org/MTCD/Publications/PDF/Pub1607_web.pdf. Accessed November 21, 2018.

75. Song WY. Linear accelerator-based MV and kV imaging systems. In: Pawlicki T, Dunscombe P, Mundt AJ, eds. *Quality and Safety in Radiotherapy*. Boca Raton, FL: CRC Press, Taylor & Francis Group; 2010.

76. Bissonnette JP, Balter PA, Dong F, et al. Quality assurance for image-guided radiation therapy utilizing CT-based technologies: a report of the AAPM TG-179. *Med Phys*. 2012;39(4):1946–1963.

77. Mutic S, Mawlawi OR, Zhu JM. Computed tomography, positron emission tomography, and magnetic resonance imaging. In: Pawlicki T, Dunscombe P, Mundt AJ, eds. *Quality and Safety in Radiotherapy*. Boca Raton, FL: CRC Press, Taylor & Francis Group; 2010.

78. Mutic S, Palta JR, Butker EK, et al. Quality assurance for computed-tomography simulators and the computed-tomography simulation process: report of the AAPM Radiation Therapy Committee Task Group No. 66. *Med Phys*. 2003;30(10):2762 2792.

79. Chen CC, Wan YL, Wai Y, et al. Quality assurance of clinical MRI scanners using ACR MRI phantom: preliminary results. *J Digit Imaging*. 2004;17(4):279–281.

80. Paulson ES, Erickson B, Schultz C, Li A. Comprehensive MRI simulation methodology using a dedicated MRI scanner in radiation oncology for external beam radiation treatment planning. *Med Phys*. 2015;42(1):28–39.

81. Solberg TD, Balter JM, Benedict SH, et al. Quality and safety considerations in stereotactic radiosurgery and stereotactic body radiation therapy. *Pract Radiat Oncol*. 2011;(suppl):1–49.

82. What is a CCD?. Spectral Instruments Inc. website. www.specinst.com/What_Is_A_CCD.html. Accessed November 21, 2018.

83. Hounsell AR, Jordan TJ. Quality control aspects of the Philips multileaf collimator. *Radiother Oncol*. 1997;45:225–233.

84. Fontenot JD, Alkhatib H, Garrett JA, et al. AAPM Medical Physics Practice Guideline 2.a: Commissioning and quality assurance of X-ray-based image-guided radiotherapy systems. *J Appl Clin Med Phys*. 2014;15(1):3–13.

85. Ding X, Zheng Y, Zeidan O, et al. A novel daily QA system for proton therapy. *J Applied Clin Med Physics*. 2013;14(2):4058.

86. Maughan RL. Proton radiotherapy. In: Pawlicki T, Dunscombe P, Mundt AJ, eds. *Quality and Safety in Radiotherapy*. Boca Raton, FL: CRC Press, Taylor & Francis Group; 2010.

87. ACR-AAPM technical standard for the performance of proton beam radiation therapy. American College of Radiology website. https://www.acr.org/-/media/ACR/Files/Practice-Parameters/Proton-Therapy-TS.pdf. Accessed November 21, 2018.

88. Jamema SV. Treatment planning systems. In: Pawlicki T, Dunscombe P, Mundt AJ, eds. *Quality and Safety in Radiotherapy*. Boca Raton, FL: CRC Press, Taylor & Francis Group; 2010.

89. International Commission on Radiation Units and Measurements. *Dose Specifications for Reporting External Beam Therapy With Photons and Electrons*. ICRU Report 29. Bethesda, MD: ICRU; 1978.

90. Nelms BE, Tome WA, Robinson G, et al. Variations in the contouring of organs at risk: test case from a patient with oropharyngeal cancer. *Int J Radiat Oncol Biol Phys*. 2012;82(1):368–378.

91. Breunig J, Hernandez S, Lin J, et al. A system for continual quality improvement of normal tissue delineation for radiation therapy treatment planning. *Int J Radiat Oncol Biol Phys*. 2012;83(5):e703–e708.

20

Surface and Sectional Anatomy

Charles M. Washington

OBJECTIVES

- Relate the importance and use of imaging modalities in radiation therapy.
- Compare and contrast aspects of anatomic positioning, anatomy features, and organ/tissue location used by the radiation oncology team for treatment planning and delivery.
- Discuss the components and function of the lymphatic system and its role in treatment field design.
- Correlate superficial anatomic landmarks and cross-sectional perspectives to deeply seated internal anatomy.

OUTLINE

KEY TERMS

Afferent lymphatic vessels
Anatomic position
Axillary lymphatic pathway
Body cavities
Body habitus
Compensatory vertebral curves
Efferent lymphatic vessels
Immunity
Internal mammary lymphatic pathway

Lymphatic system
Paranasal sinuses
Primary vertebral curves
Right lymphatic duct
Secondary vertebral curves
Spondylolisthesis
Suprasternal notch
Thoracic duct
Transpectoral lymphatic pathway

Radiation therapy practice requires that all team members have keen knowledge of human anatomy and physiology. Radiation therapists learn, early in their education, that they must have a comprehensive understanding of surface and cross-sectional anatomy. Knowledge of human anatomy is essential in simulation, treatment planning, and accurate daily treatment delivery. This chapter focuses on the surface and sectional anatomy used in simulation and treatment delivery performed by the radiation therapist. Surface anatomy is related to deep-seated structures within the human body. An overview of the diagnostic tools used to visualize internal structures is presented, along with a review of lymphatic physiology. This review is included because the lymphatics play a major role in treatment field design and disease management. A brief review of skeletal anatomy is presented to ensure a common basis for understanding important spatial relationships. Surface and sectional, as well as topographic, landmarks are presented in practical radiation therapy applications.

PERSPECTIVE

The primary objective in management of cancer with radiation therapy is to deposit enough dose to a targeted area to result in cancer cell death while minimizing the effect on the surrounding healthy tissues. The challenge is to define a patient-specific therapy plan that localizes the tumor and surrounding dose-limiting tissues, such as the spinal cord, kidney, and eyes. In addition, the radiation therapist must maintain the integrity of the plan throughout its administration. Clinical application is essential in the understanding of a disease process on anatomic grounds, corresponding surface location of internal structures, and the appearance of internal imaged structures.

Visual, palpable, and imaged anatomy forms the basis of clinical examination in radiation therapy.[1] Surface and sectional anatomy provides the foundation that the radiation therapist needs to be effective in simulation, treatment planning, and the daily administration of therapy treatments. Working without this foundation is like traveling from California to Maine for the first time without any planning: we know the general direction of where we want to go, but we do not know the most efficient way to get there. Sectional anatomy emphasizes the physical relationship between internal structures.[2] The radiation therapist must have a complete understanding of imaging modalities that enable tumor visualization, identification of pertinent lymphatic anatomy, and the site-by-site relationship of surface and sectional anatomy. A systematic approach to this information allows the radiation therapist to link vital classroom information to its clinical application.

RELATED IMAGING MODALITIES USED IN SIMULATION AND TUMOR LOCALIZATION

More than any other innovation, the ability to painlessly visualize the interior of the living human body has governed the practice of medicine during the 20th century.[3] In recent years, advancements in medical imaging techniques have allowed for effective ways to diagnose and localize pathologic disorders. The increased ability to image and localize the area of interest allows the treatment team to better target more exact treatment areas. Coupled with advanced immobilization, we can increase the dose delivered to the target while limiting the dose to neighboring areas. The medical imaging modalities used in simulation and tumor localization fit into two categories: ionizing and nonionizing imaging studies. Ionizing imaging studies use ionizing radiation to produce images that primarily show anatomy. Examples of ionizing imaging studies include conventional radiography, computed tomography (CT), and nuclear medicine imaging, particularly positron emission tomography (PET) and the fusion of PET and CT (PET/CT). Nonionizing imaging studies use alternative means of imaging the body, such as magnetic fields in magnetic resonance imaging (MRI) and echoed sound waves in ultrasound scanning.

Conventional Radiography

A radiograph provides a two-dimensional image of the interior of the body. Computerized radiography and digital radiography can also be used to visualize internal anatomy without exposing a physical film. In either case, photostimulable plates or detectors capture the latent images for visualization on computer screens. The latent images produced show the differences in tissue densities of the body; however, x-rays do not always distinguish subtle differences in tissue density. Fig. 20.1 shows a conventional chest radiograph produced with a radiation therapy simulator. The pertinent anatomy can be distinguished and outlined for practical application. Any anomaly, a variation from the standard, is recognizable on the image, as is any structure considered to be dose limiting.

Radiation therapy uses a considerable number of diagnostic imaging tools in its daily practice. Fluoroscopic simulators use specialized diagnostic x-ray equipment to localize the treatment area and reproduce the geometry of the therapeutic beam before treatment. Radiographic localization, once the most commonly used method to localize tumor volumes, is still a viable way to capture treatment planning information.

Computed Tomography

In modern radiation therapy treatment planning and delivery, the use of CT imaging is the most common means of data capture. The translation of three-dimensional information is essential to the complex treatment delivery systems used today, such as intensity-modulated radiation therapy (IMRT), stereotactic radiosurgery, and all image-guided radiation therapies.

CT is an ionizing radiation-based technique in which x-rays interact with detectors after attenuation through body tissues; these

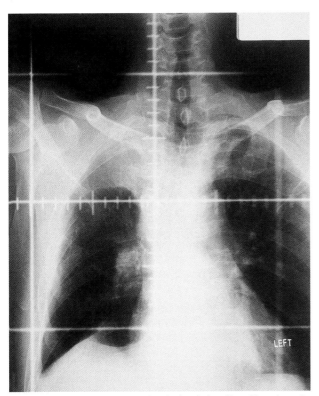

Fig. 20.1 Typical thorax conventional simulation film. Note how bony anatomy is distinguishable from cartilage and soft tissue.

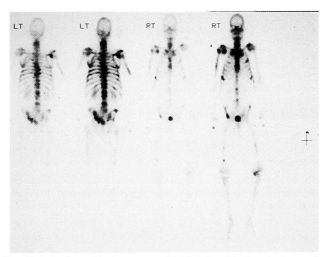

Fig. 20.2 Radionuclide bone scan. Multiple focal lesions in bone of a patient with prostate cancer.

detectors are more sensitive to radiation than x-ray film.[4] CT scanning combines x-ray principles and advanced computer technologies. The x-ray source moves in an arc around the body part being scanned and continually sends out beams of radiation. As the beams pass through the body, the tissues absorb small amounts of radiation, depending on their densities. The beams are converted to signals that are projected onto a computer screen. These images look like radiographs of slices through the body. They are typically perpendicular to the long axis of the patient's body. The CT scan provides important anatomic and spatial relationships at a glance. A series of scans allows the examination of section after section of a patient's anatomy.

The entire CT process takes only seconds for each slice and is completely painless. The detail of the images produced is approximately 10 to 20 times the detail of conventional radiography. Display of CT images reflects the differences among four basic densities: air (black), water (dark/gray), fat/blood (gray/light), and bone/metal (white).[4] CT shows bone detail well. Radiation therapy treatment planning commonly uses CT images, particularly all conformal treatment plans and virtual simulation techniques.

Four-dimensional computed tomography (4D CT): With the implementation of 4D CT, physicists are able to track the movement of a moving tumor (e.g., in the lung) throughout the entire breathing cycle, so physicians can follow exactly where the tumor is located at all points of the cycle. The same technology is used as for gated breathing techniques: a box with indicating markers is placed on the patient's abdomen/chest during the simulation. This enables physicians to determine whether treatment with the gated breathing technique (where radiation is given only during a specific portion of the patient's breathing cycle) allows the planner to minimize the amount of healthy tissue in the field.

Nuclear Medicine Imaging

The branch of medicine that uses radioisotopes in the diagnosis and treatment of disease is known as *nuclear medicine*. Nuclear medicine imaging uses ionizing radiation to provide information about physiology (function) and anatomic structure. This information is typically useful in noted abnormalities from tumor activity, specifically metastatic disease.[5] Sensitive radiation detection devices display images of radioactive drugs taken through the body and their uptake in tissues. Although this imaging technique plays an important role in tumor imaging, it detects disease dissemination more than primary tumors. Bone and liver metastases are localized with nuclear medicine scans. These scans are relatively safe and can provide valuable information. The radionuclide bone scan is the procedure of choice for skeletal scanning. Fig. 20.2 shows a bone scan. Areas of increased uptake, the dark spots, demonstrate high-activity areas that correspond to pathologic changes (uptake in the urinary bladder is normal). The radionuclide liver scan is the initial scan of choice for liver metastasis. Gallium scans localize areas of inflammation and tumor activity in patients with lymphoma. They are useful in monitoring changes in tumor size. Radiation safety procedures are important in nuclear medicine scanning. In both intravenous application and ingestion of radioactive isotopes, care in monitoring patient exposure to ionizing radiation is important. The elimination of isotopes that have run through the body (through urination) also necessitates careful monitoring and precautions.

Positron emission tomographic (PET) scanning uses short-lived radioisotopes such as carbon-11, nitrogen-13, fluorine-18, and oxygen-15 in a solution commonly injected into a patient. The radioisotope circulates through the body and emits positively charged electrons called *positrons*. These positrons collide with conventional electrons in body tissues and cause the release of gamma rays. These rays are detected and recorded. The computer creates a colored PET scan that shows function rather than structure. It can detect blood flow through organs such as the brain and heart, diagnose coronary artery disease, and identify the extent of stroke or heart attack damage. PET is useful in diagnosis of many different cancers. In that way, the physician can prescribe the appropriate treatment regimen early. In addition, PET images are used more and more to outline specific areas of anatomy and then correlated to other imaging studies such as CT and MR in treatment planning. The role of PET/CT is increasing, not only as an oncologic staging tool but also as an effective means of providing additional information for more effective treatment planning; more and more radiation oncology departments rely on PET/CT as an important tool in defining treatment areas. With both anatomic and physiologic information, the potential to visualize extension of disease not always seen on CT scans (because of size) can direct the radiation oncology team to ensure that the treatment field covers all diseased areas. This in itself can translate into better overall treatment results.

Magnetic Resonance Imaging

MRI is becoming increasingly important in radiation oncology. Technical advances in MRI allow departments to not only image-target areas better for more accurate planning but also to aid in the daily delivery of treatment, particularly in adaptive radiation therapies. MRI records data that are based on the magnetic properties of the hydrogen nuclei, which can be thought of as tiny magnets spinning in random directions. These hydrogen nuclei (magnets) interact with neighboring atoms and with all applied magnetic fields.[4] In this imaging modality, a strong uniform magnetic energy is applied to small magnetic fields that lie parallel to the direction of the external magnet. The patient is pulsed with radio waves, which cause the nuclei to send out a weak radio signal that is detected and reworked into a planar image of the body. The images, which indicate cellular activity, look like a CT scan. Fig. 20.3 shows a sagittal MRI scan of the head.

MRI has a diagnostic advantage over CT in that it provides information about chemicals in an organ or tissue. Thus MRI can be used in a noninvasive (one that does not involve puncture or incision of the skin or insertion of a foreign object into the body) biopsy on tumors. The disadvantages of MRI are the expensive magnetic shielding requirements, lower throughput (the number of patients an hour a machine can serve) when compared with CT, and increased cost in comparison with CT. MRI scans are commonly indexed, registered, and fused with CT scans and used in the treatment planning process. In these cases, the best of both imaging modalities is used to outline tumors for better conformal treatment planning.

Although MRI does not require the same precautions as needed with modalities that use ionizing radiation, stringent safety measures are necessary because of the strength of the magnets. The design of the MRI suite requires the identification of zoned safety areas. The team must pay close attention to maintaining an area that is ferrous free (no iron) because the strength of the magnet can cause those items to forcefully fly into the bore of the unit. All items that are used for a patient in this area must be nonmagnetic. Maintaining a safe environment in the MRI suite is critical to providing safe patient care.

Ultrasound

Ultrasound uses high-frequency sound waves that are not heard by the human ear. These waves travel forward and continue to move until they make contact with an object; at that point, a certain amount of the sound bounces back. Submarines use this principle to find other underwater vessels and the depth of the ocean floor. Ultrasound remains a less expensive and less hazardous alternative to the earlier studies.[5] A transducer, a handheld instrument, generates high-frequency sound waves. It moves over the body part that is being examined. The transducer also picks up the returning sound waves. Normal and abnormal tissues exhibit varying densities that reflect sound differently. The resultant image is processed onto a screen and is called a *sonogram.* The images can be a still two-dimensional cross-sectioned image or a moving image, such as the heart of a fetus (real time).

Ultrasound offers no exposure to ionizing radiation, is noninvasive and painless, and requires no contrast media, although a contrast agent has been developed for some applications. However, it does not effectively penetrate bone or air-filled spaces and is therefore not useful in imaging the skull, lungs, or intestines. In radiation therapy, the use of ultrasound continues to increase. It is very helpful in noninvasive determination of internal organ location, as evidenced in the increasing use of

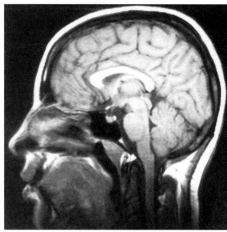

Fig. 20.3 Sagittal magnetic resonance image section through the head. (From Kelley LL, Peterson CM. *Sectional Anatomy for Imaging Professionals.* 4th ed. St. Louis, MO: Mosby; 2018.)

ultrasound to locate and guide brachytherapy implants, to locate tumors within the eye, and to increase positioning efficiency during conformal prostate treatment delivery with IMRT applications. Fig. 20.4 shows a radiation therapist obtaining ultrasound localization information for a patient about to undergo treatment for prostate cancer.

Although all of the mentioned imaging modalities are extremely useful in radiation therapy treatment planning and field design individually, use of multiply image sources in one fused image is extremely important. The use of both computed tomography (CT) and positron emission tomography (PET) and of CT and magnetic resonance imaging (MRI) provides valuable anatomic and physiologic information, which ensures appropriate coverage of tumors that can be "seen" physically and functionally. Image fusion and the process of ensuring that images are registered to each other continue to increase in use in modern treatment planning. PET/CT and MRI simulations are becoming more common in departments each year.

In some instances, images are captured at different points in time on a patient, as is the case with a patient who needs additional treatment after an initial course of radiation therapy. Ensuring that the images are registered accurately requires a process called image deformation. Image deformation is the process of shifting or contorting images to ensure that anatomic features are properly matching or registered. The deformation of the image can help to account for anatomic changes between two time points by altering the anatomy on one image into the exact location of another. The deformation results can help clinicians assess anatomy that may need to be reirradiated and thus better define target areas today as they relate to what was already done earlier.

Modern imaging modalities provide important information to the radiation therapy team for tumor localization and for bladder volume verification. Cross-sectional images are very valuable. They provide views within the patient, and display organs with their normal shape and orientation, typically in treatment position. The direct relationships allow for accurate treatment planning. The patient's surface anatomy can be related to the inner structure. In addition to organs displayed with their normal living shape, normal anatomic relationships can be observed. In particular, the study of sectional images allows the radiation therapy practitioner to develop an excellent three-dimensional concept of anatomy.[2] These modalities provide the basic information necessary for development of critical thinking skills in surface and sectional anatomy that are essential to the role of the radiation therapist.

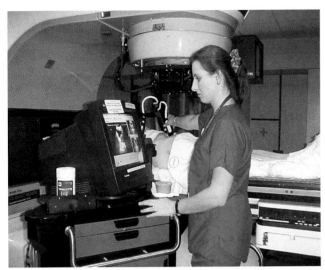

Fig. 20.4 Therapist obtaining ultrasound information for intensity-modulated radiation therapy treatment.

ANATOMIC POSITIONING

Radiation therapy requires daily reproducible positioning for effective treatment delivery. The radiation therapist uses various terms to describe the relationship of anatomic parts, planes, and sections that serve as the foundation in understanding of the body's structural plan.

Definition of Terms

With terms that reference human body position, the body is assumed to be in the anatomic position to allow for clear reference of directional relationships. The anatomic position is one in which the subject stands upright, with feet together flat on the floor, toes pointed forward, arms straight down by the sides of the body with palms facing forward, fingers extended, and thumbs pointing away from the body.[1] Fig. 20.5 shows this position.

Directional terms explain the location of various body structures in relation to each other. These terms are precise and avoid the use of unnecessary words and paint a clear picture for the radiation therapist. *Superior* means toward the head; *inferior*, toward the feet; *medial*, toward the midline of the body; and *lateral*, toward one side or the other. *Anterior* relates to anatomy nearer to the front of the body; *posterior* is nearer to or at the back of the body. *Ipsilateral* refers to a body component on the same side of the body, whereas *contralateral* refers to the opposite side of the body. *Supine* means lying face up; *prone* means lying face down. Table 20.1 outlines the directional terms commonly used by the radiation therapy team.

Planes and Sections

The human body may also be examined with respect to planes, which are imaginary flat surfaces that pass through it. Fig. 20.6 illustrates the standard anatomic planes. The *sagittal plane* divides the body vertically into right or left sides. The *median sagittal plane*, also called the *midsagittal plane*, divides the body into two symmetric right and left sides. There is only one median sagittal plane. A *parasagittal plane* is a vertical plane that is parallel to the median sagittal plane and divides the body into unequal components, both right and left. A *coronal* or *frontal plane* is perpendicular (at right angles) to the sagittal plane and vertically divides the body into anterior and posterior sections. A *horizontal* or *transverse plane* is perpendicular to the midsagittal, parasagittal, and coronal planes and divides the human body into superior and

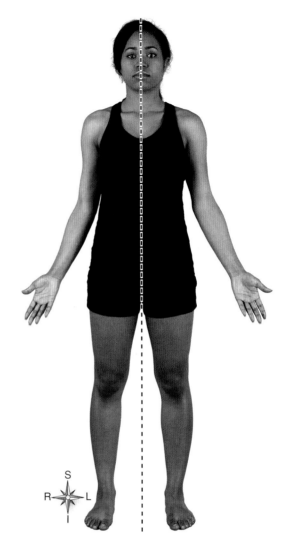

Fig. 20.5 Anatomic position and bilateral symmetry. In the anatomic position, the body is in an erect, or standing, posture with the arms at the sides and palms forward. The head and feet also point forward. The dotted line shows the body's bilateral symmetry. As a result of this organizational feature, the right and left sides of the body are near mirror images of each other. (From Thibodeau GA, Patton KT. *The Human Body in Health & Disease*. 7th ed. St. Louis, MO: Mosby; 2018.)

inferior parts. When a healthcare professional views a body structure, that structure is often seen in a sectional view. A sectional view looks at a flat surface that results from a cut made through the three-dimensional structure.

Surface and cross-sectional anatomies in radiation therapy are not solely a set of definitions or a listing of body parts. The practitioner must relate the body's physical perspective to its overall function. The standardized anatomic terms presented assist in accurate realization of those relationships.

BODY CAVITIES

The spaces within the body that contain internal organs are called body cavities (Fig. 20.7). The two main cavities are the posterior, or dorsal, and the anterior, or ventral, cavities. The dorsal cavity can be further divided into: (1) the spinal or vertebral cavity, protected by the vertebrae, which contains the spinal cord; and (2) the cranial cavity, which contains the brain.

TABLE 20.1	**Anatomic and Directional Terms**	
Term	**Definition**	**Example**
Superior	Toward the top of the body	The manubrium is superior to the body of the sternum.
Inferior	Toward the bottom of the body	The stomach is inferior to the lung.
Anterior	Toward the front of the body	The trachea is anterior to the esophagus, which is anterior to the spinal cord.
Posterior	Nearer to the back (rear)	The esophagus is posterior to the trachea.
Medial	Nearer to the midline; away from the side	The ulna is on the medial side of the forearm.
Lateral	Farther from the midline or to the side	The pleural cavities are lateral to the pericardial cavity.
Ipsilateral	On the same side (of the body)	The ascending colon and appendix are ipsilateral.
Contralateral	On the opposite side (of the body)	The ascending colon and descending colon are contralateral.
Proximal	Nearer to the point of origin or attachment	The humerus is proximal to the radius.
Distal	Away from the point of origin or attachment	The phalanges are distal to the carpals.
Superficial	On or near the body surface	The skin is superficial to the thoracic viscera.
Deep	Away from the body surface	The ribs are deep to the skin of the chest.

Modified from Thibodeau GA, Patton KT. *Anatomy & Physiology*. 6th ed. St. Louis, MO: Mosby; 2007.

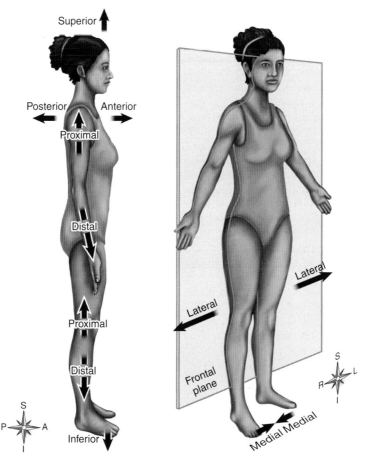

Fig. 20.6 Directions and planes of the body. These planes provide a standardized reference for the radiation therapist. (From Thibodeau GA, Patton KT. *The Human Body in Health & Disease*. 7th ed. St. Louis, MO: Mosby; 2018.)

The anterior cavity is subdivided by a horizontal muscle, called the *diaphragm*, into the thoracic cavity and the abdominopelvic cavity. The thoracic cavity is further divided into a pericardial cavity, which contains the heart and two pleural cavities, including the right and left lungs.

The abdominopelvic cavity has two sections: the upper abdominal cavity and the lower pelvic cavity. No intervening partition exists between the two. The principal structures located in the abdominal cavity are the peritoneum, liver, gallbladder, pancreas, spleen, stomach, and most of the large and small intestines. The pelvic section contains the rest of the large intestine and the rectum, urinary bladder, and internal reproductive system.

The abdominopelvic cavity is large and is divided into four quadrants with a transverse plane placed across the midsagittal plane at the

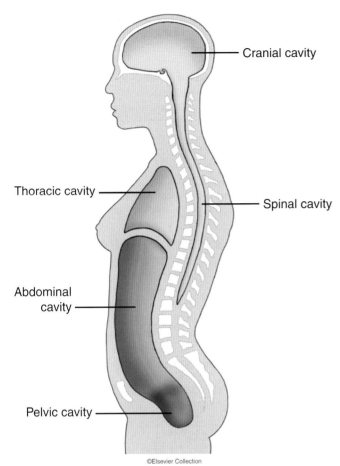

Fig. 20.7 Major body cavities. (Copyright Elsevier Collections.

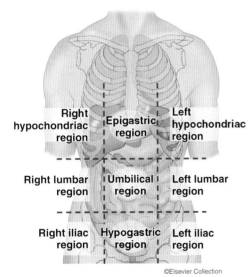

Fig. 20.8 Abdomen broken down into nine regions, showing abdominal structures. (Copyright (C) Elsevier Collections.)

point of the umbilicus (navel). The four quadrants are the right upper, left upper, right lower, and left lower. The abdominal cavity can also be sectioned into several regions. Fig. 20.8 shows the quadrants and regions of the abdomen and pelvis. Table 20.2 outlines the regions of the abdominal cavity.

The surface markings and locations of all structures are approximations and generalizations.[2] However, knowledge of the varying body

types provides the radiation therapist with practical information. If therapists have an idea of where the internal structures are, especially during a simulation, they can locate the placement of the treatment reference points sooner and more accurately. This equates to less time on the simulation table and faster capture of CT scout images for the patient.

BODY HABITUS

Roentgen's discovery of the x-ray allowed scientists at the turn of the 19th century to revolutionize the medical field, both diagnostically and therapeutically.[3] These early radiographs showed differences in the location of internal anatomy from one person to the next. Although everyone had the same organs, the organs were not necessarily in the exact same place. It was agreed that humans are a variable species with regard to structural characteristics, and it is evident that variety in general physique corresponds to great variation in visceral form, position, and motility. Consistency exists between certain physiques and certain types of visceral forms and arrangements. A thorax of certain dimensions obviously can house lungs of only a certain form. The same is true for the abdomen. Knowledge of this can greatly assist the radiation therapist in relating internal anatomy to varying body types.

The physique, or body habitus, of an individual can be classified into four groups. The *hypersthenic habitus* represents about 5% of the population. This body type exhibits a short, wide trunk, great body weight, and a heavy skeletal framework. The abdomen is long with great capacity, the alimentary tract is high, and the stomach is almost thoracic. The pelvic cavity is small. When a chest film of this body type is taken, the cassette may need to be turned crosswise to image the entire chest.

The *sthenic habitus* is similar to the hypersthenic habitus and represents most well-built individuals. Sthenic habitus has the highest rate of occurrence and accounts for about half of the population. These persons are of considerable weight with a heavy skeletal framework when compared with hypersthenic individuals. Like the hypersthenic, the alimentary tract is high but with the stomach located slightly lower in the trunk.

The *hyposthenic habitus,* which represents approximately 35% of the population, has an average physique. This habitus has many of the sthenic characteristics and may be difficult to identify. The abdominal cavity falls between the sthenic and the asthenic.

The *asthenic habitus* has a slenderer physique, light body weight, and a lighter skeletal framework. It is found in 10% of the population. The thorax has long narrow lung fields, with its widest portion in the upper zones. The heart seems to "hang" in the thoracic cavity, almost like a pendant. The asthenic body has an abdomen longer than the hypersthenic and is typically accompanied by a pelvis with great capacity. The alimentary tract is lowest of all types mentioned. Fig. 20.9 compares the various body habitus. Although the internal components are the same in all body types, the locations do vary. These categories can help standardize the variances seen from person to person.

LYMPHATIC SYSTEM

Knowledge of the lymphatic system is important in radiation therapy. For local and regional control of malignant disease processes to be achieved, the anatomy of the lymphatic system must be considered. Many tumors spread through this system; often, areas of tumor spread are predicted based solely on that knowledge. For example, in a head and neck treatment plan, the supraclavicular fossa (SCF) is commonly treated even without clinical evidence of tumor present (prophylactic treatment). This treatment is important because the lymphatic drainage of the head and neck eventually drains to that area, which is the location of the right and left lymphatic ducts. This increases the

TABLE 20.2	**Regions of the Abdominal Cavity**
Region	**Description**
Umbilical	Centrally located around the navel
Lumbar	Regions to the right and left of the navel; lumbar refers to the lower back, which is located here
Epigastric	Central region superior to the umbilical region
Hypochondriac	Regions to the right and left of the epigastric region and inferior to the cartilage of the rib cage
Hypogastric	Central region inferior to the umbilical region
Iliac	Regions to the right and left of the hypogastric region; iliac refers to the hip bones, which are located here

potential for dissemination of disease to other parts of the body. In any examination of surface and cross-sectional anatomy specific to radiation therapy, the lymphatic system is important.

The lymphatic system consists of lymphatic vessels, lymphatic organs, and the fluid that circulates through it, called *lymph.* The system is closely associated with the cardiovascular system and is composed of specialized connective tissue that contains a large quantity of lymphocytes. Lymphatic tissue is found throughout the body.

The lymphatic system has three main functions. First, lymphatic vessels drain tissue spaces of interstitial fluid that escapes from blood capillaries and loose connective tissues, filters it, and returns it to the bloodstream, an essential part of maintaining the overall fluid levels in the body. This function of draining and transporting interstitial fluid is the most important system role.[6] Second, the lymphatic system absorbs fats and transports them to the bloodstream. Third, this intricate system

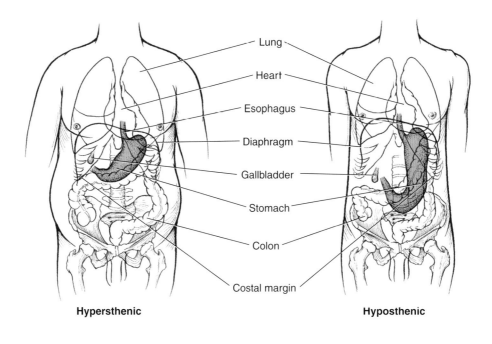

Hypersthenic

Hyposthenic

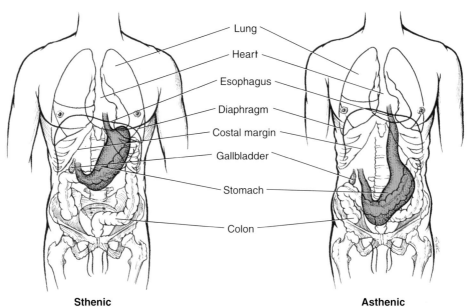

Sthenic

Asthenic

Fig. 20.9 Comparison of the four body habitus. Note that all feature the same structures. However, the internal viscera vary in position from one physique to another.

plays a major role in the body's defense and immunity. Immunity is the ability of the body to defend itself against infectious organisms and foreign bodies. Specifically, lymphocytes and macrophages protect the body by recognizing and responding to the foreign matter.

Lymphatic Vessels

Lymphatic vessels contain lymph. Lymph is excessive tissue fluid that consists mostly of water and plasma proteins from capillaries. It differs from blood by the absence of formed elements. Lymphatic vessels start in spaces between cells; at that point, they are referred to as *lymphatic capillaries*. These lymphatic vessels are extensive. Virtually every region of the body that has a blood supply is richly supplied with these capillaries. It stands to reason that those areas that are avascular do not have the same number of vessels. Examples of these avascular areas are the central nervous system and bone marrow. These lymphatic capillaries are more permeable for substances to enter than are associated blood capillaries. Cellular debris, sloughed off cells, and foreign substances that occur in the intercellular spaces are more readily collected through these lymphatic pathways and transported away for filtration. They start blindly in the interstitial spaces and flow in only one direction.

> Lymphedema, also known as lymphatic obstruction, is a condition of localized fluid retention caused by a compromised lymphatic system. This often becomes a problem in the field of radiation therapy with patients with breast cancer. In surgery to remove and stage breast cancer, surgeons often remove many axillary lymph nodes to see whether the cancer has begun to spread. With this, the natural flow of lymph through the arm is disrupted, and without rehabilitation, lymphedema can occur. In these patients, the arm swells, often reducing circulation; an infection of that limb can develop. Lymphedema can usually be controlled with compression bandages and therapeutic exercises. Surgeons have also begun using a technique known as the sentinel node biopsy in hopes of reducing the risk of lymphedema development by reducing the number of lymph nodes removed during surgery.

The lymphatic capillaries join to form larger lymphatic vessels. Lymphatic vessels resemble veins in structure but have thinner walls and more valves that promote the one-way flow. These larger vessels follow veins and arteries and eventually empty into one of two ducts in the upper thorax—the thoracic duct or the right lymphatic duct—which then flow into the subclavian veins.

Fluid movement in the lymphatic system depends on hydrostatic and osmotic pressures that increase through skeletal muscle contraction. As the muscles around the vessels contract, the lymph is moved past a one-way valve that closes, which prevents the lymph from flowing backward. Respiratory movements create a pressure gradient between two ends of the lymphatic system. Fluid flows from high-pressure areas, such as the abdomen, to low-pressure areas, such as the thorax, where pressure falls as each inhalation occurs.

Lymph Nodes

Along the paths of the lymph vessels are lymph nodes. These nodes vary in size from 2 to 30 mm in length, and they often occur in groups.[6] A lymph node contains both afferent and efferent lymphatic vessels. Afferent lymphatic vessels enter the lymph node at several points along the convex surface. They contain one-way valves that open into the node, bringing the lymph into it. On the other side of the node are efferent vessels. The efferent lymphatic vessels are, overall, smaller in diameter than the afferent vessels; their valves open away from the node, again facilitating one-way flow.[6] More afferent vessels come into a node than efferent vessels come out of it, which slows the flow through

the nodes. This is similar to driving along a four-lane highway during rush hour and getting to a point of road construction that restricts traffic flow to one lane. You can go in only one direction and must wait your turn to move through the area. This slowing of the lymph through the node permits the nodes to effectively filter the lymph, and, through phagocytosis, the endothelial cells of the node engulf, devitalize, and remove contaminants. Fig. 20.10 shows the components of a typical lymph node. The substances can be trapped inside the reticular fibers and pathways throughout the node, which causes edema. Edema is an excessive accumulation of fluid in a tissue that produces swelling. Edema can occur when excessive foreign bodies, lymph, and debris are engulfed in the node. This condition is evident when a person has a cold or the flu. The subdigastric nodes, located in the neck just below the angle of the mandible, become swollen and tender because of the heightened phagocytic activity in that area to rid the body of the trapped contaminants. The swelling goes down as the pathogen is devitalized. Edema also occurs when altered lymphatic pathways cause more than normal amounts of lymph filtration. This condition is commonly seen after mastectomy. The arm on the side of the surgery is often swollen because of the altered natural lymphatic pathways after the operation. The same amount of lymph is redirected through alternate routes, which causes the slowdown of lymphatic flow.

Lymphatic Organs

The spleen is the largest mass of lymphatic tissue in the body at roughly 12 cm in length. It is located posterior to and to the left of the stomach in the abdominal cavity, between the fundus of the stomach and the diaphragm. The spleen actively filters blood, removes old red blood cells, manufactures lymphocytes (particularly B cells, which develop into antibody-producing plasma cells) for immunity surveillance, and stores blood. Because the spleen has no afferent lymphatic vessels, it does not filter lymph. However, the spleen is often thought of as a large lymph node for the blood. During a laparotomy, which is surgical inspection of the abdominal cavity, in patients with lymphoma, this organ is often removed for biopsy and staging purposes. In this case, the bone marrow and liver then assume the functions of the spleen.

The thymus is located along the trachea superior to the heart and posterior to the sternum in the upper thorax. This gland is larger in children than in adults and is more active in pediatric immunity. It generally becomes smaller as we enter adulthood. In adults, if this gland is enlarged, it often is the result of a problem with the immune system, such as in acquired immunodeficiency syndrome. The gland serves as a site where T lymphocytes can mature.

The tonsils are a series of lymphatic nodules embedded in a mucous membrane. They are located at the junction of the oral cavity and pharynx. These collections of lymphoid tissue protect against foreign body infiltration by producing lymphocytes. The pharyngeal tonsils, or adenoids, are in the nasopharynx; the palatine tonsils are in the posterior lateral wall of the oropharynx; and the lingual tonsils are at the base of the tongue in the oropharynx, forming a ring of lymphatic tissue around the posterior oral cavity.

The thoracic duct is on the left side of the body and is typically larger than the right lymphatic duct. It serves the lower extremities, abdomen, left arm, and left side of the head and neck and drains into the left subclavian vein. This duct is approximately 35 to 45 cm in length and begins in front of the second lumbar vertebra (L2), where it is called the *cisterna chyli*. As lymph travels through the lower extremities to the cisterna chyli, it continues its upward trek to the thoracic duct. As it passes through the mediastinum, it bypasses many of the mediastinal node stations. The *right lymphatic duct* serves only the right arm and right side of the head and neck and drains into the right subclavian vein. This duct is approximately 1 to 2 cm in length. These ducts drain into the right and left subclavian veins, which in turn drain to the heart

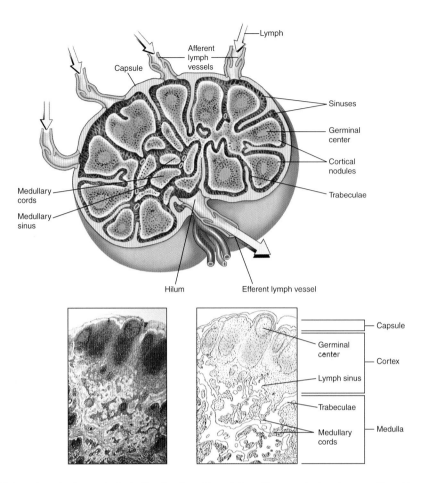

Fig. 20.10 Lymph node. Arrows indicate the direction of lymph flow. The germinal centers are sites of lymphocyte production. As lymph moves through the lymph sinuses, macrophages remove foreign substances. (From Lymphatic system. In: Thibodeau GA, Patton KT, eds. *Anatomy & Physiology*. 6th ed. St. Louis, MO: Mosby; 2007.)

BOX 20.1 Lymphatic Flow Overview

Tissue fluid leaves the cellular interstitial spaces and becomes **lymph**; as it enters a **lymphatic capillary**, it merges with other capillaries to form an **afferent lymphatic vessel**, which enters a **lymph node,** where lymph is filtered. It then leaves the node via an **efferent lymphatic vessel**, which travels to other nodes and then merges with other vessels to form a **lymphatic trunk**, which merges with other trunks and joins a **collecting duct**, either the right lymphatic or the thoracic, which empties into a **subclavian vein**, where lymph is returned to the bloodstream.

---

by way of the superior vena cava. Box 20.1 reviews the flow of lymph through the lymphatic system.

Knowledge of the location of the lymph nodes and direction of lymph flow is important in the diagnosis and prognosis of the spread of metastatic disease. Cancer cells, especially carcinomas from epithelial tissues, often spread through the lymphatic system. Metastatic disease sites are predictable by their lymphatic flow from the primary site.[7] Inadequate knowledge of the lymphatic system may translate into ineffective treatment delivery.

AXIAL SKELETON: SKULL, VERTEBRAL COLUMN, AND THORAX

Most imaging modalities provide valuable information through visualization of differences in anatomic densities. The denser a component, the whiter it appears on a radiographic image. The axial skeleton provides the radiation therapist with a wealth of information used to reference the location of internal anatomy. The following sections briefly review axial skeleton anatomy and provide the reader with a reference necessary in relating internal structures to surface anatomy.

Skull

The skull has approximately 22 bones: 8 true cranial bones and 14 considered facial bones. The cranial bones are mostly joined by sutures, joints held together by connective tissue, which limit movement. The mandible and ossicles, which are bones in the middle ear, are the only bones in the skull not joined by sutures.

The frontal, parietal, temporal, sphenoid, and occipital bones all form the lateral aspect of the skull vault. The first two meet in the midline at the bregma, the roof of the skull, often referred to as the "soft spot," and the last two meet at the lambda. The facial skeleton, or visceral cranium, includes the 14 bones of the face. It consists of two maxillary bones, two zygomatic bones, two nasal bones, two lacrimal bones, two palatine bones, two inferior conchae, one vomer, and one mandible.

Sutures

The four prominent sutures in the skull, or fibrous joints, allow little or no movement between them, which makes the transitions between bones of the skull smooth and stable. The *coronal suture* lies between the frontal bone and the two parietal bones. On either side of the skull, it begins at the bregma and ends at the temporal bone. The sagittal suture lies between the two parietal bones and runs from the bregma to the lambda. The lambdoidal suture is in the posterior portion of the skull and lies between the parietal and occipital bones. Finally, the squamosal sutures,

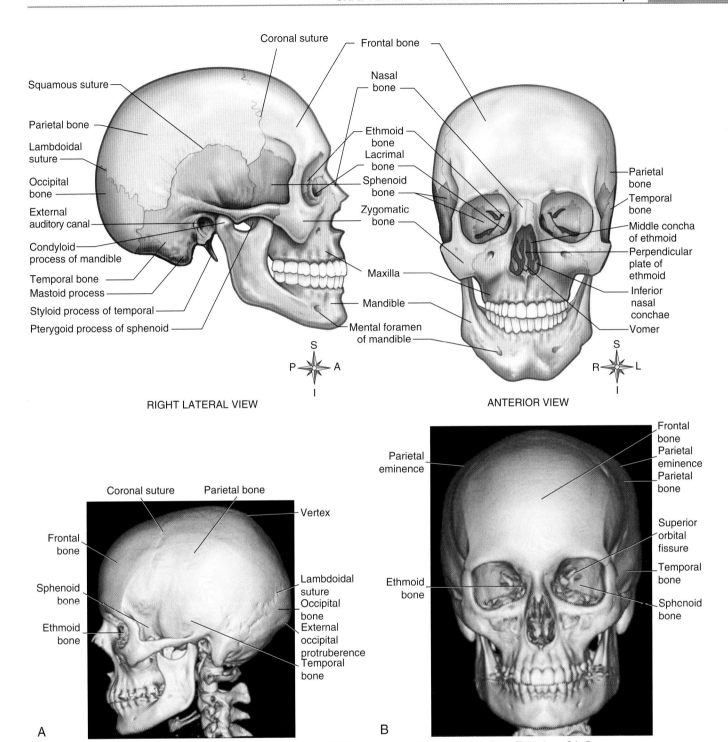

Fig. 20.11 Skull. (A) Lateral view of the skull. (B) Anterior view of the skull. (Top, From Thibodeau GA, Patton KT. *The Human Body in Health & Disease.* 7th ed. St. Louis, MO: Mosby; 2018; Bottom, From Kelley LL, Peterson CM. *Sectional Anatomy for Imaging Professionals.* 4th ed. St. Louis, MO: Mosby; 2018.)

one on each side of the skull, are located near the ears and lie between the parietal and temporal bones. Identification of these sutures radiographically can assist the radiation therapist in locating corresponding underlying structures. Fig. 20.11 shows the bones of the skull and sutures.

Paranasal Sinuses

The bones of the skull and face contain the paranasal sinuses, which are air spaces lined by mucous membranes that reduce the weight of the skull and give a resonant sound to the voice. When a person has sinusitis, an inflammation and blockage of the sinus cavities, the

voice often has a "stuffed-up" tone (loss of resonance). The sinuses are air-filled spaces within the frontal, maxillary, sphenoid, and ethmoid bones. They are lined with mucous membranes and are relatively small at birth. They enlarge during development of the permanent teeth and reach adult size shortly after puberty.[2] The paranasal sinuses are easily seen on plain x-ray, CT, and MRI. Cross sections are an excellent tool to study the surface relations in these areas.[7] Fig. 20.12 shows the paranasal sinuses in two different sections.

The maxillary sinus is a pyramid-shaped cavity that is enclosed in the maxilla. It is the largest of the paranasal sinuses. The roof of the

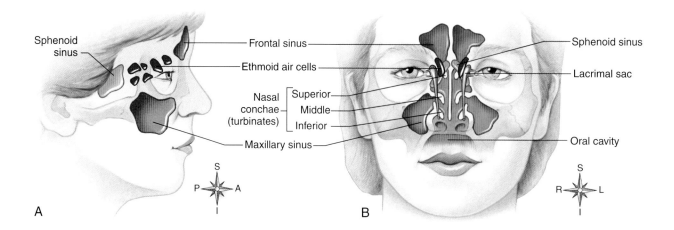

Fig. 20.12 The paranasal sinuses. (A) Lateral view. (B) Frontal view. (From Thibodeau GA, Patton KT. *The Human Body in Health & Disease.* 7th ed. St. Louis, MO: Mosby; 2018.)

sinus forms the floor of the orbit. The frontal sinus lies in the frontal bone above the orbit. It may be located on the surface with a triangle between the following three points: the nasion, a point 3 cm above the nasion, and the junction of the medial and middle thirds of the superior orbital margin (SOM). The sphenoid sinus lies posterior and superior to the nasopharynx, enclosed in the body of the sphenoid bone at the level of the zygomatic arch. Superiorly the sinus is related to the sella turcica (which is approximately 2 cm [3/4 inches] anterior and 2 cm [3/4 inches] superior to the external auditory meatus [EAM]) and the pituitary. The pituitary may be surgically removed through a transsphenoidal approach, one that goes through the nasal cavity; in diseases in which the transsphenoidal approach is not a viable option, a transcranial methodology may be used. The ethmoid sinus is bilateral but consists of a honeycomb of air cells that lie between the middle wall of the orbit and the upper lateral wall of the nose.

Vertebral Column

The vertebral column, located in the midsagittal plane of the posterior cavity, extends from the skull to the pelvis. It consists of separate bones, the vertebrae, which appear as rectangular densities on radiographs.[2] The 33 bones in the adult vertebral column are shown in Fig. 20.13, which also indicates the number of bones in each section. There are 7 cervical, 12 thoracic, 5 lumbar, 5 sacral, and 4 coccygeal vertebrae. At the inferior aspect of the column, the sacrum has five fused bones, whereas the coccyx is composed of four fused bones. Coccygeal segments can vary in number, and some individuals also have six lumbar vertebrae.

The sacrum supports the rest of the vertebral column and thus provides the support necessary for the human body's erectness. The vertebrae are separated by radiolucent fibrocartilage called *intervertebral disks.* In the cervical and thoracic spine, the disks are of similar thickness. In the lumbar spine, the height increases progressively down the column.[2]

The vertebral column is also very flexible. Although limited motion exists between any two neighboring vertebrae, the vertebral column is capable of substantial motion. The column also protects the spinal cord and provides points of attachment for the skull, thorax, and extremities.

Vertebral Characteristics. Most vertebrae share several common characteristics. They have a body that is attached to a posterior vertebral arch. These two components border the vertebral foramen, the passage through which the spinal cord passes. The spinous and transverse processes allow for muscle attachments. The spinous process is posterior

and forms where two laminae meet. These laminae are often palpated in aligning spinal treatment fields. The transverse processes are lateral projections where a pedicle joins a lamina. Fig. 20.14 shows a typical vertebra with its prominent features labeled. It is also important to remember that there are 31 pairs of spinal nerves that run along the spinal cord. These nerves run through the intervertebral and sacral foramina. The nerves terminate at an area termed the *cauda equina* (horse's tail).

The first two vertebrae, C1 and C2, are atypical from all others. C1, the atlas, serves the specialized function of supporting the skull and allowing the head to tilt in the "yes" motion. It has no vertebral body. C2, the axis, has an odontoid process that extends into the ring of the atlas. When the head turns from side to side, it pivots on this process. These two vertebrae are shown in Fig. 20.15. Cervical vertebra number 7 is also somewhat atypical. It has a prominent spinous process that can be palpated at the base of the neck. Anteriorly, the sternal notch is located slightly inferior to this process.

Vertebral Column Curvatures. The vertebral column demonstrates several curvatures that develop at different levels.[2] These curvatures can be classified as either primary or compensatory (secondary) curvatures. Primary vertebral curves are developed in utero as the fetus develops in the C-shaped fetal position, and they are present at birth. Compensatory vertebral curves or secondary vertebral curves develop after birth as the child learns to sit up and walk. Muscular development and coordination influence the rate of secondary curvature development.

The cervical curve extends from the first cervical to the second thoracic vertebrae (C1 to T2). It is convex anteriorly and develops as children learn to hold their head up and sit alone at approximately 4 months of age. This curve is a secondary curvature. The thoracic curve extends from T2 to T12 and is concave anteriorly. This is one of the primary curves of the vertebral column. The lumbar curve runs from T12 to the anterior surface of L5. This convex forward curve develops when a child learns to walk at approximately 1 year of age. The pelvic curve is concave anteriorly and inferiorly and extends from the anterior surfaces of the sacrum and coccyx. This is the other primary curve. The thorax can also have a slightly right or left lateral curve that is influenced by a child's predominate use of the right or left hand during childhood and adolescence.

The cervical, thoracic, lumbar, and pelvic curves are found in the normal human vertebral column. Three abnormal curvatures also are present both clinically and radiographically. *Kyphosis* is an excessive curvature of the vertebral column that is convex posteriorly. This curve

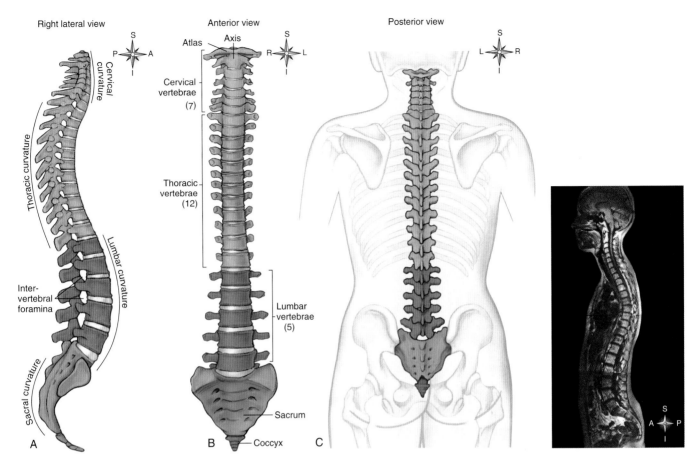

Fig. 20.13 Right lateral view, anterior view, and posterior view of the vertebral column. The image inset shows a midsagittal magnetic resonance image of the vertebral column from the left side. (From Thibodeau GA, Patton KT. *The Human Body in Health & Disease.* 7th ed. St. Louis, MO: Mosby; 2018.)

can develop with degenerative vertebral changes. Scoliosis is an abnormal lateral curvature of the vertebral column with excessive right or left curvature in the thoracic region. This abnormal curvature can develop if only one side (half) of the vertebral bodies are irradiated in pediatric patients, as in the case of patients treated for Wilms' tumor. The radiation slows vertebral body growth on one side and the contralateral side grows at a normal rate, thus creating scoliotic changes. Lordosis is an excessive convexity of the lumbar curve of the spine. Spondylolisthesis occurs when one of the spine's vertebrae (bones) slips forward over the vertebra beneath it. Spondylolisthesis occurs most often in the lumbar spine (low back). Fig. 20.16 shows these abnormal spine curvatures.

Thorax

The illustration in Fig. 20.17 shows the full thorax made up of the bony cage formed by the sternum, costal cartilage, ribs, and thoracic vertebrae to which they are attached.[1,8] The thorax encloses and protects the organs in the thoracic cavity and upper abdomen. It also provides support for the pectoral girdle and upper extremities.

Sternum and Ribs. The sternum, or breastbone, comprises three parts: the manubrium, which is the superior portion; the body, the middle and largest portion; and the xiphoid process, which is the inferior projection that serves as ligament and muscle attachments. The manubrium has a depression called the suprasternal notch (SSN), which occurs at the level of T2 and articulates with the medial ends of the clavicles. This point may be used in measuring the angle of chin tilt in patients with head and neck cancer when thermoplastic immobilization masks are not used. It also serves as

a palpable landmark when setting up an SCF field. The manubrium also articulates with the first two ribs. The junction of the manubrium and the body form the sternal angle, also called the *angle of Louis;* it occurs at the level of T4.

The body of the sternum articulates with the 2nd through 10th ribs. Of the 12 pairs of ribs, the superior 7 pairs are considered true ribs. They are easily seen in the asthenic body habitus and are palpable in most others.[9] They articulate posteriorly with the vertebrae and anteriorly with the sternum directly through a cartilaginous joint. These are known as the *vertebrosternal ribs.* The next three pairs join with the vertebrae posteriorly and anteriorly with the cartilage of the immediately anterior rib. These ribs are classified as *vertebrochondral ribs.* The next (last) pairs articulate only with the vertebrae and do not connect with the sternum in any way; they are called *floating ribs.*

The axial skeleton is easily seen with most imaging techniques used in radiation therapy. A thorough working knowledge of these components serves the radiation therapist in overall daily operations. This information is used in relating the surface and cross-sectional anatomy and the palpable bony landmarks that are used in field placement and treatment planning.

SURFACE AND SECTIONAL ANATOMY AND LANDMARKS OF THE HEAD AND NECK

The human head has various anatomic features that are both interesting and useful to the radiation therapist. These structures are rich in bony moveable soft tissue landmarks and lymphatics commonly used

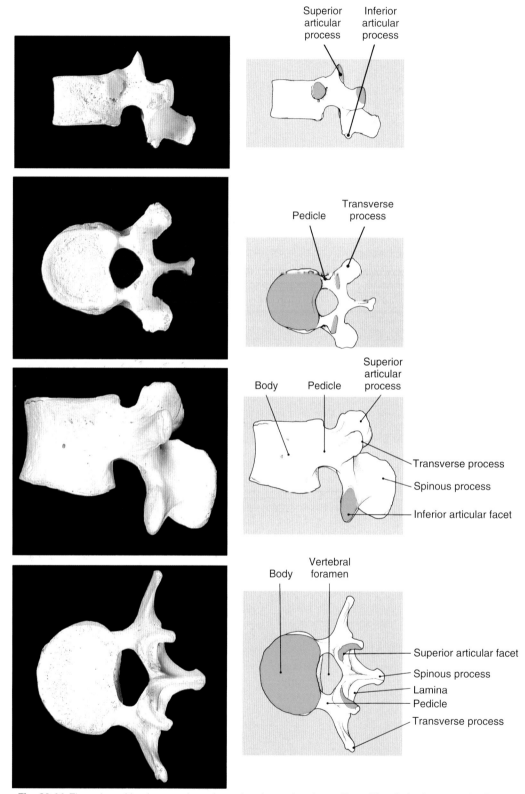

Fig. 20.14 Thoracic and lumbar vertebrae. Lateral and superior views. (From The skeletal system. In: Thibodeau GA, Patton KT. *Anatomy & Physiology.* 6th ed. St. Louis, MO: Mosby; 2007.)

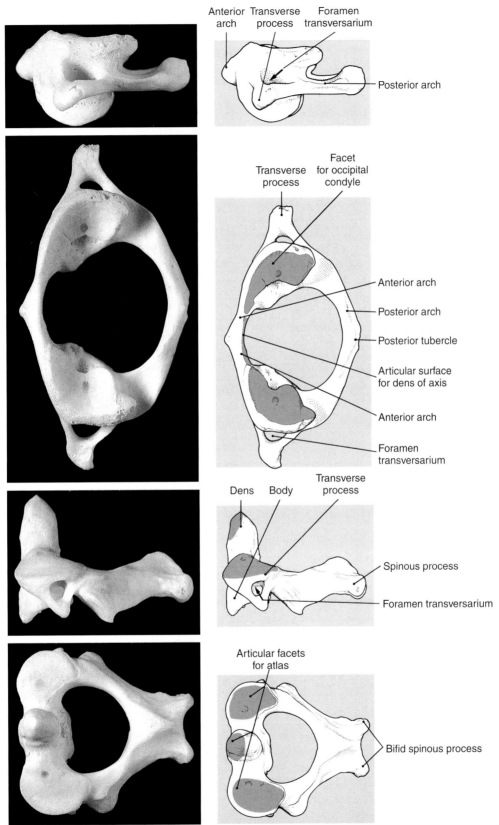

Fig. 20.15 Cervical vertebra. (A) Inferior and superior views of C1, the atlas. (B) Inferior and superior views of C2, the axis. (From Thibodeau GA, Patton KT, editors: Anatomy and physiology, ed 6, St. Louis, 2007, Mosby.)

in field placement, position locations, and so forth. The bony landmarks are stable and are typically used as reference points, as in locating a positioning or central axis tattoo. Soft tissue landmarks can also be extremely useful. However, they tend to be more mobile and provide a less reliable reference than the bony landmarks.

Bony Landmarks: Anterior and Lateral Skull

Figs. 20.18 and 20.19 outline the locations of the following anterior and lateral bony structures.

The frontal bone is the area of maximal convexity on the forehead and articulates with the frontal process of the maxillary bone on the medial side of the orbit.[1,2] Together with the lacrimal bones, it protects the lacrimal duct and glands.

The glabella is the slight elevation directly between the two orbits in the frontal bone. It is just above the base of the nose. This

palpable landmark is more prominent in some individuals than in others.

The nasion is the central depression at the base of the nose. It is formed by the point at which the frontal and nasal bones join.

The superciliary arch starts at the glabella and moves superiorly and laterally above the central portion of the eyebrow. The central part lies superficially to the frontal sinuses on either side and forms the brow of the skull.

The SOM rests just inferior to the eyebrow and is more pronounced on its lateral aspect. The SOM forms the roof of the orbit and serves as one of the points used to delineate the inferior border of whole brain fields (along with the tragus and mastoid tip). When that part of the SOM is in the treatment field, the frontal part of the brain is also in the field.

The maxilla is the bone between the ala (lateral soft tissue prominence) of the nose and the prominence of the cheek. This bone houses the largest of the paranasal sinuses. The inferior alveolar ridge of the maxilla houses the teeth sockets.

The zygomatic bone forms part of the lateral aspect of the orbit and the prominence of the cheek. The articulation between the frontal process of the zygomatic bone and the zygomatic process of the frontal bone can be palpated in the lateral orbital margin (LOM). The mid-zygoma point, a point midway between the EAM and the lateral canthus, lies roughly at the floor of the sphenoid sinus and the roof of the nasopharynx. One centimeter superior to that point corresponds to the floor of the sella turcica, and 1.5 cm superior to the point corresponds to the pituitary gland.

The mastoid process is an extension of the mastoid portion of the temporal bone at the level of the earlobe. It is commonly used to delineate the posterior point of the inferior whole brain border (imaginary line that extends from the SOM to the mastoid tip, commonly through the tragus of the ear).

The external occipital protuberance (EOP; or inion) is the prominence in the posterolateral aspect of the occipital bone of the skull.

The angle of the mandible is the point at which the muscles used for chewing are attached. In addition, several lymph node groups are located inferior and medial to that point. It is also a classic landmark for the tonsils.

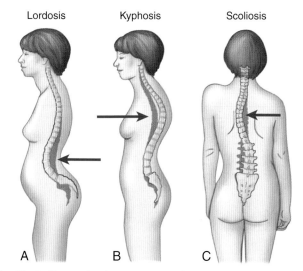

Fig. 20.16 Abnormal spine curvatures. (A) Lordosis. (B) Kyphosis. (C) Scoliosis. (From Thibodeau GA, Patton KT. *The Human Body in Health & Disease*. 7th ed. St. Louis, MO: Mosby; 2018.)

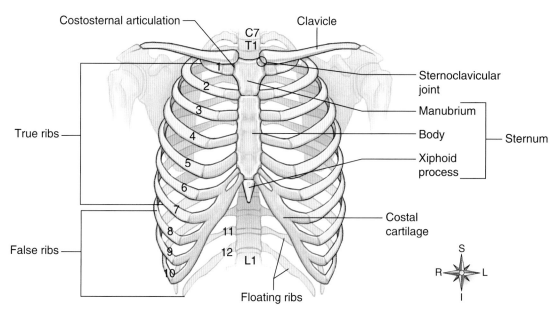

Fig. 20.17 The bony framework of the thorax provides many useful landmarks. (From Thibodeau GA, Patton KT. *The Human Body in Health & Disease*. 7th ed. St. Louis, MO: Mosby; 2018.)

Landmarks Around the Eye

Whenever practical, the landmarks used around the eye should be the bony landmarks. They are radiographically visible and are easily checked if a second course of treatment is necessary in the same or neighboring area. The soft tissue landmarks often vary with age, weight, and surgical changes. They are open to variable interpretation and misinterpretation because of the extreme flexibility of the skin. Fig. 20.20 illustrates these landmarks. The following outlines the important landmarks around the eye.

The SOM forms the upper border of the orbit.

The inferior orbital margin forms the lower border of the bony orbit.

The LOM is a bony landmark that forms the lateral border of the bony orbit.

The medial orbital margin is extremely difficult to palpate and therefore is not clinically useful as an anatomic landmark. It does have some usefulness radiographically.

The inner canthus (IC) is a soft tissue landmark that is formed at the junction of the upper and lower eyelids at the medial aspect of the eye.

The outer canthus (OC) is a soft tissue landmark that is formed at the junction of the upper and lower eyelid at the lateral aspect of the eye.

The punctum lacrimae is a soft tissue landmark that can be used as a point of reference in the surface anatomy of the eye. This white-appearing section of the eye lies just next to the IC on the lower eyelid. Tears are drained through this duct into the lacrimal duct. This opening can become blocked by fibrotic changes from ionizing radiation administered to the area, which cause constant tearing. Extreme caution should be exercised to avoid this occurrence, particularly with treatment of the anterior maxillary sinus field arrangement.

Landmarks Around the Nose

As in the case of the eye, the landmarks used around the nose should be the bony landmarks. Soft tissue landmarks often vary with age, weight, and surgical changes and are open to variable interpretation and misinterpretation because of the extreme flexibility of the skin. Fig. 20.21 illustrates these landmarks. The following outlines the landmarks around the nose; some are reiterated from previous sections.

The lateral ala nasi is a soft tissue landmark formed by the lateral attachment of the ala nasi with the cheek. The inferior ala nasi is a soft tissue landmark formed by the inferior attachment of the ala nasi with the cheek. Both are prominent in most people and can be useful landmarks with measurements in any direction, such as superior to inferior, medial to lateral, and anterior to posterior.

The nasion is the depression of the nose where it joins the forehead at the level of the SOM. It is a useful landmark if it is deep and pronounced and coincides with the crease of the nose. If it is shallow, it is more open to variable interpretation.

The glabella is the bony prominence in the forehead at the level just superior to the SOM. As with the nasion, it is useful if it is prominent and sharp. It is not useful if it is flat or extremely curved, where it, too, is open to misinterpretation.

The ala nasi, dorsum of the nose, and external nares are useful as checkpoints in the surface anatomy of the nose and useful in the positioning of radiation treatment portals.

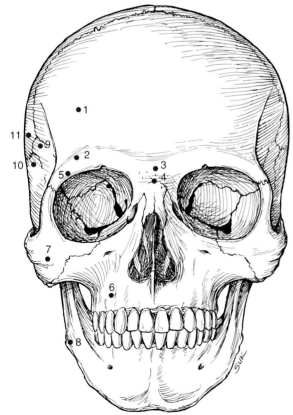

Fig. 20.18 Bony landmarks of the anterior skull: *1*, Frontal bone; *2*, superciliary arch; *3*, glabella; *4*, nasion; *5*, superior orbital margin; *6*, maxilla; *7*, zygomatic bone; *8*, angle of mandible; *9*, sphenoid bone (greater wing); *10*, temporal bone; *11*, parietal bone.

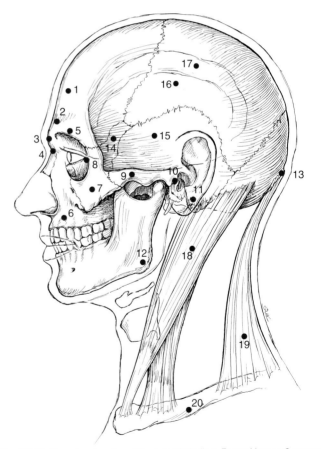

Fig. 20.19 Bony landmarks of the lateral skull: *1*, Frontal bone; *2*, superciliary arch; *3*, glabella; *4*, nasion; *5*, superior orbital margin; *6*, maxilla; *7*, zygomatic bone; *8*, lateral canthus; *9*, midzygoma point; *10*, external acoustic meatus; *11*, mastoid process; *12*, angle of mandible; *13*, external occipital protuberance or inion; *14*, greater wing of sphenoid; *15*, temporal bone; *16*, parietal bone; *17*, parietal eminence; *18*, sternocleidomastoid muscle; *19*, trapezius muscle; *20*, clavicle.

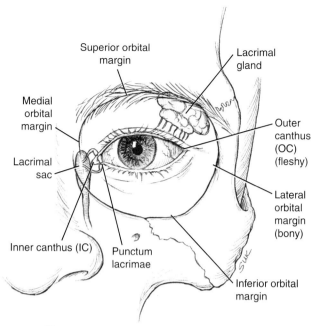

Fig. 20.20 Landmarks around the eye and orbit.

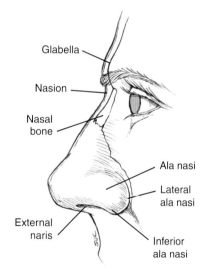

Fig. 20.21 Landmarks around the nose.

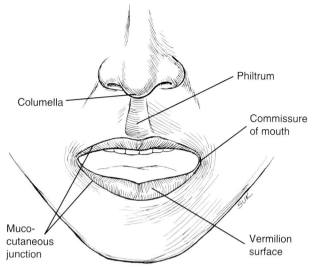

Fig. 20.22 Landmarks around the mouth.

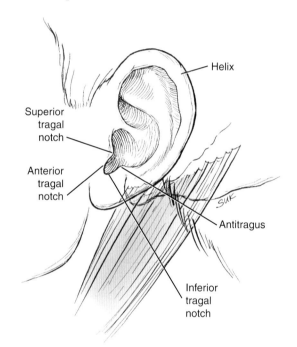

Fig. 20.23 Landmarks around the ear.

Landmarks Around the Mouth

Landmarks around the mouth are generally not very accurate because of the extreme flexibility in the area. Every effort should be made to document these landmarks with reference to more stable anatomic points, if possible. If these landmarks are used, the position of the mouth is important to note, as well as any positioning or immobilization devices used, such as a cork, oral stent, or similar devices. Fig. 20.22 illustrates the landmarks around the mouth.

The commissure of the mouth is formed at the junction of the upper and lower lip. This landmark is extremely mobile.

The mucocutaneous junction is located at the junction of the vermilion border of the lip with the skin of the face.

The columella is located at the junction of the skin of the nose with the skin of the face at the superior end of the philtrum.

Landmarks Around the Ear

The external ear consists of the auricle or pinna, which is formed from a number of irregularly shaped pieces of fibrocartilage covered by skin.

It has a dependent lobule, or earlobe, and an anterior tragus, commonly used as anatomic references.[1,5,10] Parts of the ear are labeled in Fig. 20.23.

The tragus is made up of a stable cartilage that partially covers the EAM in the external ear and is often used in radiation therapy during initial positioning. A pair of optical lasers, coincident with each other, can be focused on the tragus on both sides of the patient. This places the patient's head in a relatively nontilted position because their locations are typically symmetrical. Just anterior to the tragus corresponds to the posterior wall of the nasopharynx. The posterior limit of many head and neck off-cord fields lies at this point.

The tragal notch is the semicircular notch in the ear immediately inferior to the tragus. The superior tragal notch makes up the superior margin of the tragal notch. The inferior tragal notch defines the inferior margin of the tragal notch. The anterior tragal notch makes up the anterior margin of the tragal notch.

Landmarks and Anatomy Around the Neck

The boundaries of the anterior aspect of the neck are the body and angles of the mandible superiorly and the superior border and SSN of

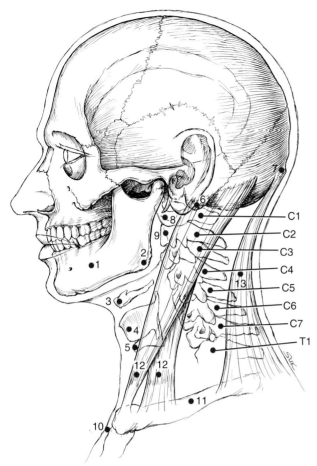

Fig. 20.24 The neck has many useful anatomic landmarks that can assist the radiation therapist. Relating surface structures to deeper anatomy is essential in the practice of radiation therapy. *1,* Body of mandible; *2,* angle of mandible; *3,* hyoid bone; *4,* thyroid cartilage; *5,* cricoid cartilage; *6,* mastoid process; *7,* external occipital protuberance; *8,* atlas; *9,* axis; *10,* suprasternal notch; *11,* clavicle; *12,* sternocleidomastoid muscle; *13,* trapezius muscle.

TABLE 20.3 Cervical Neck Landmarks and Associated Anatomy

Cervical Spine	Associated Anatomy
C1	Transverse process lies just inferior to the mastoid process; may be palpated in the hollow inferior to the ear
C2–C3	Level with the angle of the mandible; lies 5–7 cm below the external occipital protuberance
C4	Located just superior to the hyoid bone of the neck; serves as a point of muscle attachment
C4	Level with the superior portion of the thyroid cartilage and marks the beginning of the larynx
C6	Level with the cricoid cartilage; location of the junction of the larynx to trachea and pharynx to esophagus
C7	First prominent spinous process in the posterior neck

the sternum and the clavicles. The posterior aspect of the neck is bound superiorly by the EOP and laterally by the mastoid processes. The posterior inferior border ends at approximately the level of the seventh cervical vertebra to the first thoracic vertebra (C7 to T1).[2] Fig. 20.24 illustrates the features of the neck anatomy.

The upper cervical vertebrae are not easily palpated; the last cervical and first thoracic vertebrae are the most obvious. The hyoid bone lies opposite the superior border of C4. When the head is in the anatomic position, the hyoid bone may be moved from side to side between the thumb and middle finger, approximately 1 cm below the level of the angle of the mandible, C2 to C3. Table 20.3 relates the location of the cervical bony landmarks to other associated anatomic features.

Pharynx

The pharynx is a membranous tube that extends from the base of the skull to the esophagus. It connects the nasal and oral cavities with the larynx and esophagus. It is divided into the nasopharynx, oropharynx, and laryngopharynx, shown in Fig. 20.25. Note that in a sectional view of the low neck, the therapist can easily remember how to distinguish the order of the spinal cord, esophagus, and trachea. From a posterior to anterior perspective, the order is always SET up: *S,* spinal cord; *E,* esophagus; and *T,* trachea.

1. The nasopharynx, or epipharynx, communicates with the nasal cavity and provides a passageway for air during breathing.

2. The oropharynx, or mesopharynx, opens behind the soft palate into the nasopharynx and functions as a passageway for food moving down from the mouth and for air moving in and out of the nasal cavity.
3. The laryngopharynx, or hypopharynx, is located inferior to the oropharynx and opens into the larynx and esophagus. This structure continues throughout the thorax as the esophagus.

Larynx

The larynx connects to the lower portion of the pharynx above it and to the trachea below it. It extends from the tip of the epiglottis at the level of the junction of C3 and C4 to the lower portion of the cricoid cartilage at the level of the C6 vertebra.[10] The larynx is subdivided into three anatomic regions: the supraglottis, glottis, and subglottis. Fig. 20.26 illustrates sectional views of the larynx. The larynx is actually an enlargement in the airway at the top of the trachea and below the pharynx. It serves as a passageway for air moving in and out of the trachea and functions to prevent foreign objects from entering the trachea. At the level of the inferior margin of the sixth cervical vertebra, the larynx continues as the trachea.

The thyroid cartilage forms a midline prominence, the laryngeal prominence or Adam's apple, which is more obvious in the adult male. The vocal cords are attached to the posterior part of this prominence. The cricoid cartilage serves as the lower border of the larynx and is the only complete ring of cartilage in the respiratory passage; the others are open posteriorly. It is palpable as a narrow horizontal bar inferior to the thyroid cartilage and is at the level of the C6 vertebra.

Nasal and Oral Cavities

The nasal cavity opens to the external environment through the nostrils. Posteriorly, the nostrils are continuous with the nasopharynx and are lined with a ciliated mucous membrane. The oral cavity has a vestibule, which is the space between the cheeks and teeth and the oral cavity proper that opens posteriorly into the oropharynx and houses the soft palate, hard palate, uvula, anterior tongue, and floor of the mouth.

Surface Anatomy of the Neck

Anatomic landmarks around the neck are mainly used as checkpoints and reference points that can establish the patient's position or the anatomic position of the treatment field. The most commonly used landmarks of the neck are as follows:
1. Skin profile
2. Sternocleidomastoid muscle, which is attached to the mastoid and occipital bones superiorly and sternal and clavicular heads

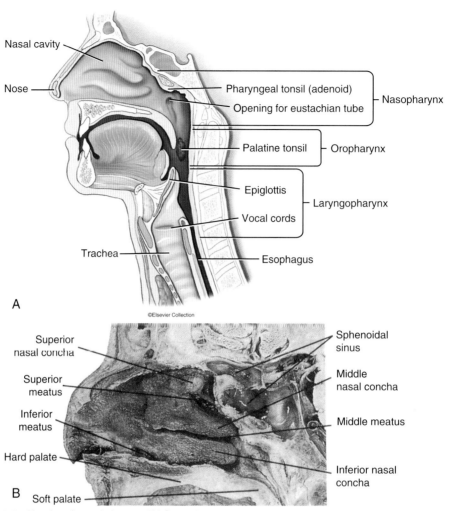

Fig. 20.25 Nasal cavity and pharynx. (A) Sagittal section through the nasal cavity and pharynx viewed from the medial side. (B) Photograph of a sagittal section of the nasal cavity. (A, Copyright Elsevier collection. B, From The lymphatic system and immunity. In: Seeley RR, Stephens TD, Tate P, eds. *Essentials of Anatomy and Physiology.* St. Louis, MO: Mosby; 1991.)

inferiorly. These muscles form the V shape in the neck and are associated with a great number of lymph nodes.

3. Clavicle
4. Thyroid notch
5. Mastoid tip
6. EOP
7. Spinous processes

These surface neck landmarks assist the radiation therapist in referencing locations of treatment fields and dose-limiting structures. They are illustrated in Fig. 20.27.

Lymphatic Drainage of the Head and Neck

The lymphatic drainage of the head and neck is through deep and superficial lymphatic channels, around the base of the skull, and deep and superficial lymph chains. The head and neck area is rich in lymphatics. Enlarged cervical lymph nodes are the most common adenopathy seen in clinical practice.[1] They are typically associated with upper respiratory tract infections but may also be the site of metastatic disease from the head and neck, lungs, breast, or of primary lymphoreticular disease such as Hodgkin disease. The lymph nodes of the head and neck are outlined in the following section. Figs. 20.28 and 20.29 show the lymphatic chains and nodes in the head and neck.

The occipital lymph nodes, typically one to three in number, are located on the back of the head, close to the margin of the trapezius muscle attachment on the occipital bone. These nodes provide efferent flow to the superior deep cervical nodes.

The retroauricular lymph nodes, usually two in number, are situated on the mastoid insertion of the sternocleidomastoid muscle deep to the posterior auricular muscle. They drain the posterior temporo-occipital region of the scalp, auricle, and EAM. They provide efferent drainage to the superior deep cervical nodes.

The deep parotid lymph nodes are arranged into two groups. The first group is embedded in the parotid gland, whose superior border is the temporomandibular joint; posterior border, the mastoid process; inferior border, the angle of the mandible; and anterior border, and the anterior ramus. The second group—the subparotid nodes—are located deep to the gland and lie on the lateral wall of the pharynx. Both drain the nose, eyelid, frontotemporal scalp, EAM, and palate. They provide efferent flow to the superior deep cervical nodes.

The submaxillary lymph nodes are facial nodes that are scattered over the infraorbital region. They span from the groove between the nose and cheek to the zygomatic arch. The buccal lymph nodes are scattered over the buccinator muscle. These nodes drain the eyelids, nose, and cheek and supply efferent flow to the submandibular nodes. The *submandibular lymph nodes* lie on the outer surface of the

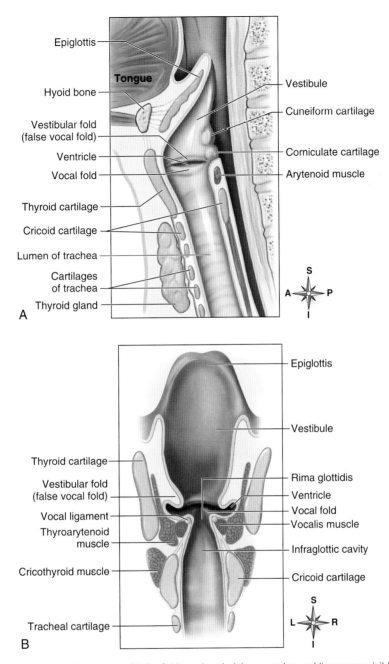

Fig. 20.26 Landmarks of the larynx, with its folds and underlying muscles and ligaments visible. A, Sagittal section. B, Coronal (frontal) section, viewed from behind. (From Patton KT: *Anatomy and physiology*, ed 10, St. Louis, 2019, Elsevier.)

mandible. They drain the scalp, nose, cheek, floor of the mouth, anterior two-thirds of the tongue, gums, teeth, lips, and frontal, ethmoid, and maxillary sinuses. They provide efferent drainage to the superior deep cervical nodes.

The retropharyngeal lymph nodes, one to three in number, lie in the buccopharyngeal fossa, behind the upper part of the pharynx and anterior to the arch of the atlas. These nodes are commonly involved in nasopharyngeal tumors and, subsequently, are included in the treatment fields.

The submental lymph nodes are found in the submental triangle of the digastric muscles, lower gums and lips, tongue, central floor of the

mouth, and skin of the chin. These nodes provide efferent drainage to the submandibular nodes.

The superficial cervical lymph nodes form a group of nodes located below the hyoid bone and in front of the larynx, trachea, and thyroid gland.

The deep cervical lymph nodes form a chain of 20 to 30 nodes along the carotid sheath and around the internal jugular chain along the sternocleidomastoid muscle. The jugulodigastric lymph node, at times called the subdigastric node, is typically located superior to the angle of the mandible and drains the tonsils and the tongue. Inferiorly, the chain spreads out into the subclavian triangle. One of the nodes in this

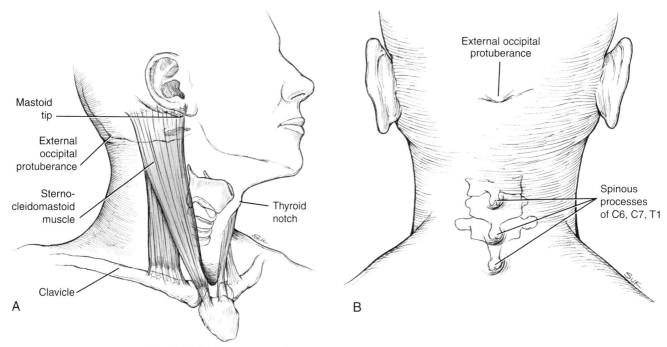

Fig. 20.27 Surface anatomy of the neck: (A) Anterolateral view; (B) posterior view.

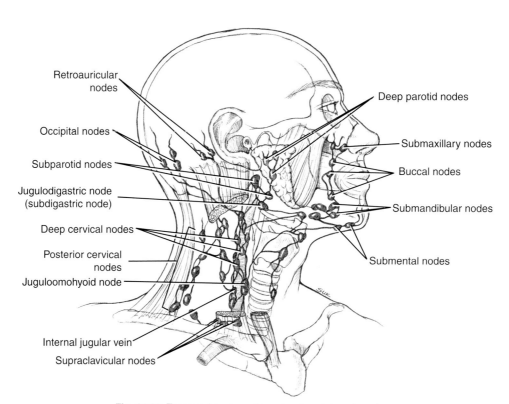

Fig. 20.28 Topographic view of head and neck lymph nodes.

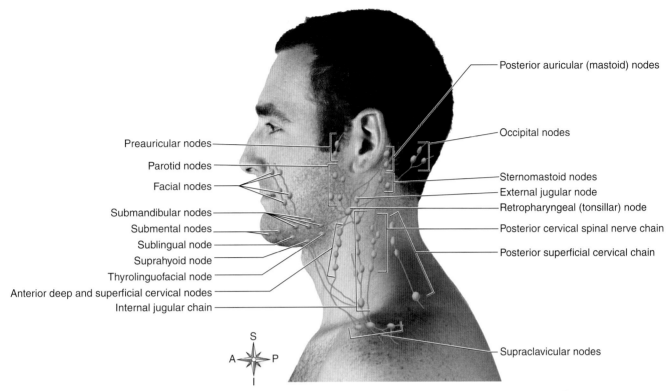

Fig. 20.29 Sagittal view of deep lymph nodes in the head and neck in relation to underlying structures. (From Patton KT: *Anatomy and physiology,* ed 10, St. Louis, 2019, Elsevier.)

group lies in the omohyoid tendon and is known as the juguloomohyoid lymph node.[1,2] When these two nodes are enlarged, carcinoma of the tongue may be indicated, because enlarged neck nodes may be the only sign of the disease. These vessels supply efferent flow to form the jugular trunk, which drains to the thoracic or right lymphatic duct, both in the SCF. The cervical lymph nodes are typically included in the treatment fields of most head and neck cancers that spread through the lymphatics, which include most of these cancers. The fields that encompass the group are commonly called posterior cervical strips.

SURFACE AND SECTIONAL ANATOMY AND LANDMARKS OF THE THORAX AND BREAST

Various malignant diseases manifest themselves in the human thorax. Cancers of the lung, breast, and mediastinal lymphatics require the radiation therapist to have a working knowledge of the surface and sectional anatomy of the thorax. The human thorax has various anatomic features that are commonly used in field placement, position locations, and so forth. The thorax extends from the clavicles superiorly to the costal margin inferiorly.

Anterior Thoracic Landmarks

The clavicles are visible throughout their entire length in the anterior thorax, especially in the asthenic body habitus. The clavicles are easily palpable. The radiation therapist uses the clavicles when outlining a field to treat the lower neck and upper chest lymphatics. The supraclavicular lymph nodes are located superior to the clavicles; they are often treated prophylactically in head and neck and lung cancers. In addition, the brachial plexus, a network of nerves located at the medial section of the clavicle and often involved in superior sulcus (Pancoast) tumors of the lung, can be referenced to this point.

The musculature of the anterior chest wall includes the pectoralis major, pectoralis minor, and deltoid. The pectoralis major is medially attached to the clavicle and superior five costal cartilages. It passes laterally to the axilla. The inferior border of the muscle is not as visible in the female adult because it is covered by the breast.[1,2] The pectoralis minor is overlapped by the pectoralis major. The deltoid muscle forms the rounded portion of the shoulder.

The Breast and Its Landmarks

The male breast remains poorly developed throughout life, whereas the female breast develops to a variable degree during puberty. Although the sizes of the female breasts vary, they typically lie between the second rib superiorly and the sixth rib inferiorly. The female breast is shown in Fig. 20.30. The medial border is the lateral aspect of the sternum, and the lateral border corresponds to the midaxilla. The breast tissue is teardrop shaped; the round, drop portion is situated medially, and the upper outer portion, called the *tail of Spence,* extends into the axilla. The upper limits of tangential treatment fields are typically high near the SSN to include the entire breast and tail of Spence when the SCF is not treated.

The breast can be divided into quadrants: upper outer, upper inner, lower outer, and lower inner. Most tumors are located in the upper outer quadrant of the breast. Tumor location is important in associating the tumor spread patterns. If the breast tumor is located in an inner quadrant, the medially located nodes, such as the internal mammary nodes, may be involved. If the tumor is located in an outer quadrant, the axillary nodes need to be examined for possible involvement. This information is particularly important to the therapist because tumor location and extension dictate field parameters.

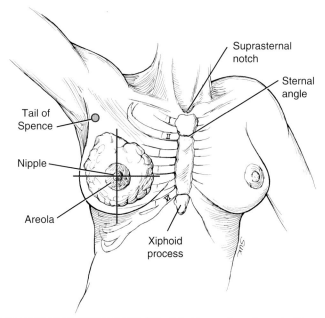

Fig. 20.30 Surface anatomy of the female breast. This gland is teardrop shaped with a portion that extends from the anterior chest wall into the axilla.

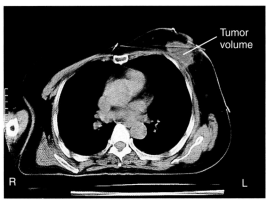

Fig. 20.31 Computed tomographic scan view of the female breast and thorax. The contours of the breast and chest wall from images like this greatly enhance accuracy of treatment planning. Note how tumor volume can easily be related to other internal anatomy.

Other surface anatomy of the breast includes the nipple, areola, and inframammary sulcus. The nipple projects just below the center of the breast. In the male, the nipple lies over the fourth intercostal space; the location varies in the female. The areola is the area that surrounds the nipple. Its coloration changes with varying hormonal levels, as seen in pregnancy. The inframammary sulcus, the inferior point of breast attachment, varies from person to person. In females with large breasts, the breast overhangs this point of attachment and causes considerable concern during its external beam treatment because the breast can bolus itself in these cases.

Radiographically, the breast produces shadows that are easily seen on conventional radiographs. Fig. 20.31 shows a CT scan slice through a section of the thorax and breast. Note how the patient's internal anatomy can be related to the contour of the breast. This information is useful in treatment planning.

Posterior Thoracic Landmarks

The posterior thorax is formed by the structures commonly referred to as the *back*. On initial inspection, the back is made up of various muscles and bony landmarks. The major musculature includes the trapezius, teres major, and latissimus dorsi. The trapezius muscle is a flat triangular muscle that produces a trapezoid shape with the lateral angles at the shoulders and the superior angle at the EOP. The inferior angle is at the level of T12. The teres major is a band of muscle between the inferior angle of the scapula and the humerus; it forms the posterior wall of the axilla. The latissimus dorsi is the broad muscle on either side of the back that spans from the iliac crest of the pelvic bones to the posterior axilla.[1,2,11,12] Fig. 20.32 shows the surface anatomy of the posterior thorax.

The spines of the thoracic vertebrae slope inferiorly; the tips lie more inferior than the corresponding vertebral bodies and are easily palpable. The scapula, the large posterior bone associated with the pectoral girdle, is easily palpated on the back. The spine of the scapula is located at the level of T3. The inferior angle of the scapula is located at the level of T7.

The lower back has a few bony landmarks that serve the radiation therapist well. The crest of the ilium is located at the level of L4. This point is important in locating the subarachnoid space, the point at which lumbar punctures are commonly made. The posterosuperior iliac spine (PSIS) is approximately 5 cm from midline, is easily palpable, and lies at the level of S2.

Internal and Sectional Anatomy of the Thorax

Bone detail can easily be visualized with CT scan sections. MRI shows soft tissue anatomy not clearly seen with conventional x-ray equipment. Fascial planes are identified, which allows separation of organ systems, vascular supply, muscles, bone, and lymphatic system.[4,13,14] The thorax provides much anatomic information that the radiation therapist uses in the daily administration of ionizing radiation.

The trachea is the part of the airway that begins at the inferior cricoid cartilage at the level of C6. It is approximately 10 cm long and

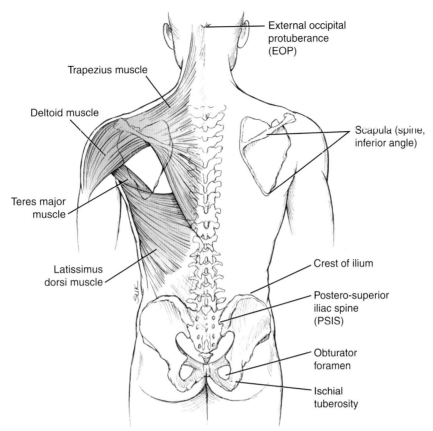

Fig. 20.32 Surface anatomy of the posterior thorax.

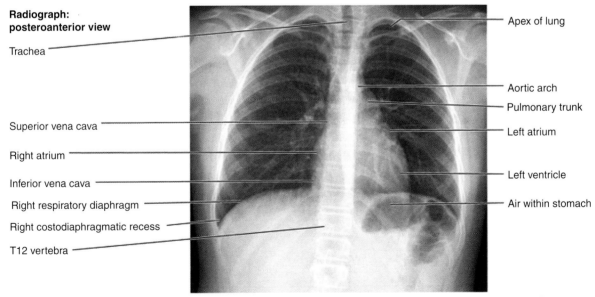

Fig. 20.33 This x-ray image shows the trachea and its distal bifurcation, the carina. The branching typically occurs at T3 to T4.

extends to a point of bifurcation, called the carina, at the level of T4 to T5. Topically, it corresponds to the angle of Louis (Fig. 20.33). The bifurcation forms the beginning of the right and left main bronchi, which can assist the therapist in locating the initial location of treatment field borders, especially lung cancer fields whose inferior border commonly lies a few centimeters below this anatomic reference point.

The diaphragm is the dome-shaped muscle that separates the thorax and abdomen. It is important in respiration and lies between T10 and T11. The esophagus and inferior vena cava pass through the diaphragm at the level of T8 to T9, whereas the descending aorta goes through at the level of T11 to T12. These features are shown in cross section in Fig. 20.34.

The pleural cavity extends superiorly 3 cm above the middle third of the clavicle. The anterior border of the pleural cavity reaches the midline of the sternal angle. The pleura are more extensive in the peripheral regions around the outer chest wall. The diaphragm bulges up into each pleural cavity from below. The pleura mark the limit of expansion of the lungs.[1,2]

The lungs correspond closely with the pleura, except in the inferior aspect, where they do not extend down into the lateral recesses. The anterior border of the right lung corresponds to the right junction of the costal and mediastinal pleura down to the level of the sixth chondrosternal joint. The anterior border of the left lung curves away laterally from the line of pleural reflection. The surface projection of the lung and pleura is noted in Fig. 20.35.

The heart rests directly on the diaphragm in the pericardial cavity and is covered anteriorly by the body of the sternum. The base of the heart lies at the level of T4. A cardiac shadow can clearly be seen in a radiograph of the chest.

Associated with the thorax and heart are an abundance of arteries and veins—the great vessels. The aorta has ascending and descending components. The ascending aorta runs from the aortic orifice at the medial end of the third left intercostal space up to the second right chondrosternal joint. This arch continues above the right side of the sternal angle and then turns down behind the second left costal cartilage. The descending aorta runs down behind this cartilage, gradually moving across to reach a point just to the left of midline, approximately 9 cm below the xiphisternal joint, where it enters the abdomen. The innominate left common carotid and left subclavian arteries extend from this aortic arch. The superior vena cava is located at the level of T4. It runs down through the pericardium, where it enters the heart. The inferior vena cava does not extend a great distance in the thorax; it lies in the right cardiodiaphragmatic angle and enters the heart behind the sixth right costal cartilage.

Lymphatics of the Breast and Thorax

The lymphatic drainage of the thorax and breast is important to the radiation therapist. The thorax is rich in lymphatic vessels. The lymphatics of the axilla, SCF, and mediastinum play a major role in radiation therapy field arrangement of breast, head and neck, lung, and

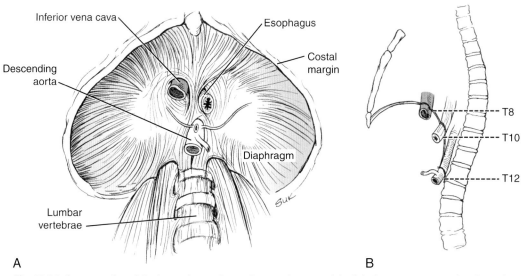

Fig. 20.34 Cross section of the lower thorax shows the esophagus and the inferior vena cava passing through the diaphragm. (A) Inferior surface of the diaphragm. (B) Sagittal view of the diaphragm.

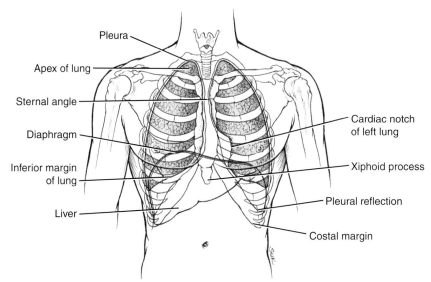

Fig. 20.35 Surface projection of the lung and pleura.

lymphatic cancers. The lymph nodes of the thorax are divided into nodes that drain the thoracic wall and breast and those that drain the thoracic viscera.

Breast Lymphatics. Three lymphatic pathways are associated with the breast: the axillary, transpectoral, and internal mammary pathways. These pathways are the major routes of lymphatic drainage for

the breast. Specific lymph node groups are associated with each pathway and are shown in Fig. 20.36.

The axillary lymphatic pathway comes from trunks of the upper and lower half of the breast. Lymph is collected in lobules that follow ducts, which anastomose behind the areola of the breast; from that point, they drain to the axilla. This pathway is also referred to as the *principal pathway*. The nodes of this pathway drain the lateral half of the breast. These nodes are important to note in invasive breast cancers: axillary nodes are commonly biopsied for assessment of disease spread. The axillary lymph nodes are commonly at the level of the second to third intercostal spaces and can be divided into low, mid-, and apical axillary nodes.

The transpectoral lymphatic pathway passes through the pectoralis major muscle and provides efferent drainage to the supraclavicular and infraclavicular fossa nodes. One of the intermediate nodes in the infraclavicular fossa worth noting is Rotter's node. Nodes of the SCF and low neck, generally 1 to 3 cm deep, are often treated when there is involvement of the transpectoral pathway. The scalene node, found in the low neck/SCF, is often biopsied to note disease spread.

The internal mammary lymphatic pathway runs toward the midline and passes through the pectoralis major and intercostal muscles close to the body of the sternum (T4 to T9). Associated with this pathway are the internal mammary nodes. These nodes are more commonly involved with primary breast cancers that are located in the inner breast quadrants and with positive axillary nodes. These nodes are generally 2.5 cm from midline (with variations from 0 to 5 cm) and are approximately 2.5 cm deep (with variations from 1 to 5 cm). CT scans are extremely helpful to the radiation oncology team in assessment of the location of these nodes. The lateral location and depth assist in determination of the field width and treatment energy, respectively.

Breast lymphatic flow is also important from a surgical standpoint. With radical breast surgery, lymphatic flow is often compromised. Because the channels of flow are altered with surgical intervention, the

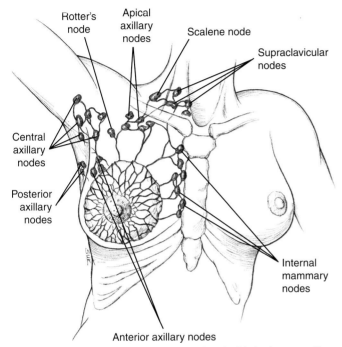

Fig. 20.36 The lymphatic pathways associated with the breast: axillary, transpectoral, and internal mammary.

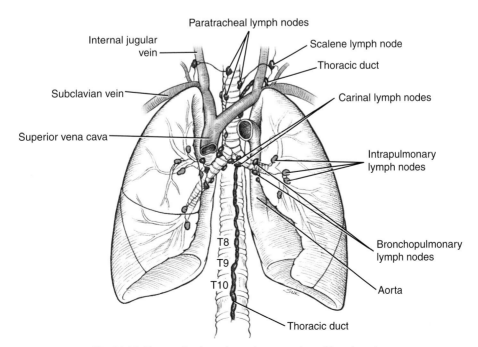

Fig. 20.37 The mediastinum has a large number of lymph nodes.

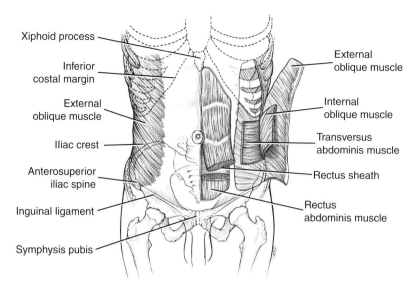

Xiphoid process

Inferior
costal margin

External
oblique muscle

Iliac crest

Anterosuperior
iliac spine

Inguinal ligament

Symphysis pubis

External
oblique muscle

Internal
oblique muscle

Transversus
abdominis muscle

Rectus sheath

Rectus
abdominis muscle

Fig. 20.38 The muscles of the anterior and lateral abdominal wall work in unison to provide structure and stability to the torso.

lymph has fewer drainage paths back to the cardiovascular system. This slowed drainage causes edema that is sometimes seen in the arms of patients who have received radical breast surgery. Exercise and elevation of the limb help drain stagnant lymph. This complication has led the cancer management team to use less radical surgery when possible, along with other modalities.

Thoracic Lymphatics. The mediastinum has a rich intercommunicating network of lymphatics. The most important nodes to note are the lymphatics of the thoracic viscera and pulmonary veins. They are commonly involved in Hodgkin disease and in lung cancers, in which they can be radiographically seen as a widened mediastinum. The lymphatics of the lung and mediastinum are shown in Fig. 20.37.

The superior mediastinal nodes are located in the superior mediastinum. They lie anterior to the brachiocephalic veins, the aortic arch, and the large arterial trunks that arise from the aorta. They receive lymphatic vessels from the thymus, heart, pericardium, mediastinal pleura, and anterior hilum. The tracheal nodes extend along both sides of the thoracic trachea and are also called the paratracheal nodes. The superior tracheobronchial nodes are located on each side of the trachea. They are superior and lateral to the angle at which the trachea bifurcates into the two primary bronchi.

The inferior mediastinal nodes are located in the inferior mediastinum. The inferior tracheobronchial nodes lie in the angle below the bifurcation of the trachea. They are also called the carinal nodes. The bronchopulmonary nodes, often called the hilar nodes, are found at the hilus of each lung at the site of the division of the main bronchi and pulmonary vessels into the lobular bronchi and vessels. These nodes are involved in most lung cancer cases. The pulmonary nodes, also known as the intrapulmonary nodes, are found in the lung parenchyma along the secondary and tertiary bronchi.

In the right lung, all three lobes drain to the intrapulmonary and hilar nodes. They then flow to the carinal nodes and then to the paratracheal nodes before they reach the brachiocephalic vein through the scalene node and right lymphatic duct. In the left lung, the upper lobe drains to the pulmonary and hilar nodes, carinal nodes, left superior paratracheal nodes, and then the brachiocephalic vein through the thoracic duct. The

left lower lobe drains to the pulmonary and hilar nodes, then to the right paratracheal nodes, where it follows the path outlined for the right lung. This is important when designing the treatment field of a patient with lung cancer.

SURFACE AND SECTIONAL ANATOMY AND LANDMARKS OF THE ABDOMEN AND PELVIS

The abdomen and pelvis house many organs that are treated for malignant disease. Management presents treatment planning challenges for the radiation therapist and medical dosimetrist because of the abundance of radiosensitive structures within the abdominal and pelvic cavities. Treatment of a colorectal cancer to a dose of 60 Gy or more can be difficult when the neighboring anatomy tolerates much less. Knowledge of surface and cross-sectional anatomy of the abdomen and pelvis is essential in radiation therapy. The radiation therapist must be able to bridge knowledge of surface and sectional anatomy with various body habitus to visualize internal anatomy. However, relating internal structures to the topography of the area is not without certain challenges, particularly in the anterior abdomen. When compared with the head, neck, and thorax, the anterior abdomen does not have as many bony landmarks to reference. However, some stable bony landmarks in the pelvis are commonly referenced.

Anterior Abdominal Wall

The anterior abdominal wall is bordered superiorly by the inferior costal margin and inferiorly by the symphysis pubis, inguinal ligament, anterosuperior iliac spine (ASIS), and iliac crest. The anterior aspect of the wall is formed by sheets of interlacing muscles that provide stability and form to the abdomen. The major muscles that help form the anterior abdominal wall include the rectus abdominis, transverse abdominis, internal oblique, and external oblique.

The external oblique muscle extends from the lower eight ribs to an insertion point that spans from the iliac crest to the midline aponeurosis, a sheetlike tendon that joins one muscle to another. It extends from the outer lateral body to the midline.

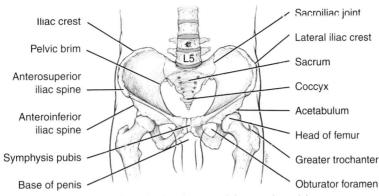

Fig. 20.39 Bony landmarks around the anterior pelvis.

The internal oblique muscle spans from the iliac crest and inguinal ligament to the cartilage of the last four ribs. It runs in a midline to an outer lateral perspective.

The transverse abdominis muscle runs from the iliac crest, inguinal ligament, and last six rib cartilages to the xiphoid process, linea alba (a tough fibrous band that extends from the xiphoid process to the symphysis pubis), and pubis on both sides. Thus this muscle runs from side to side.

The rectus abdominis muscle is commonly called the "six pack" by sports buffs. This muscle runs from the symphysis pubis to the xiphoid process and has three transverse fibrous bands that separate the muscle into six sections that are prominent in individuals with pronounced muscular tone.

These muscles work together in providing structure to the anterior abdominal wall. Fig. 20.38 shows the interrelated nature of these muscles.

Several structures can be palpated in the abdomen. The xiphoid process lies in the epigastric region at the level of T9. This bony landmark is very stable. The radiation therapist typically uses this structure and the SSN to ensure that a patient is lying straight on the treatment couch. If both landmarks are in line with the projection of a sagittal laser, the thorax is usually straight. The xiphoid can also be used in conjunction with the symphysis pubis or associated soft tissue landmarks to ensure that the lower body is straight. The cartilages of the 7th to 10th ribs form the costal margin, which forms the inferior border of the rib cage. The umbilicus, also known as the *navel* or *belly button,* is an inconsistent, mobile landmark on the anterior abdomen. It is typically at the level of L4 when an individual is in a recumbent position. When standing, in the infant, and in the pendulous abdomen, it lies at a lower level.

Posterior Abdominal Wall (Trunk)

In the posterior wall, the lower ribs, lumbar spines, PSIS, and iliac crest are palpable. A line, called the *intercristal line,* can be drawn between the iliac crests.[1] This line typically passes between the spines of the third and fourth lumbar vertebrae, a location important in lumbar punctures.

Landmarks of the Anterior Pelvis

The anterior pelvis has several bony and soft tissue landmarks that are useful to the radiation therapist. They are outlined in the following section and shown in Fig. 20.39.

The iliac crest extends from the ASIS to the PSIS. The ASIS is palpable, and measurements may be taken from it in the superoinferior or mediolateral direction. It is often used in referencing the

location of the femur. The lateral iliac crest is also easily palpable and, being on the lateral pelvic wall, may be used as a transverse level on either the anterior or the posterior pelvis. The lateral iliac crest level is the line that joins the right and left lateral iliac crests. These crests are the most superior margin of the ilium on the lateral pelvic wall. Measurements may be taken from this level in the superoinferior direction.

The head of the femur and greater trochanter, although not direct components of the true pelvis, are important to note when considering the lateral pelvic anatomy. The head of the femur articulates with the hip at the acetabulum. If this is irradiated beyond tolerance, fibrotic changes can occur and cause painful or limited motion of the joint. Usually, this joint is shielded in moderate to large pelvic portals to limit this occurrence. The greater trochanter is the only part of the proximal femur that can be palpated; therefore its relationship to bony points of the hip bone is important.[6] The radiation therapist uses the greater trochanter when aligning patients during simulation to alleviate pelvis rotation. The patient should be horizontally level when the greater trochanters are at the same height from the tabletop. The radiation therapist can measure this with a ruler and optical lasers.

The symphysis pubis appears as the 5-mm midline gap between the inferior parts of the pelvic bones.[2] The upper border pubis is the palpable upper border of the midline pubic bone. It is fairly easy to palpate except in extremely obese patients. When it is palpated, care should be taken to allow for overlying tissue. The lower border pubis is the palpable lower border of the pubic bone in midline. It is not as easily palpable as the upper border pubis because it lies more inferiorly and posteriorly. All of these can be accurately located radiographically. The radiation therapist uses these components when setting the anterior border of lateral prostate fields (the prostate lies immediately posterior to the symphysis pubis).

The ischial tuberosities are located in the inferior portion of the pelvis. This corresponds to the lower region of the buttock. When a person sits down, the ischial tuberosities bear the weight of the body. Many radiation oncologists use the ischial tuberosities as the inferior border of the anterior and posterior prostate treatment portals.

When pelvic irradiation is indicated, the radiation therapist can use the anatomy of the perineum, the diamond-shaped area bounded laterally by the ischial tuberosities, anteriorly by the symphysis pubis, and posteriorly by the coccyx, to assist in portal location. Treatment lines in these areas commonly fade because of perspiration and garment rubbing.[6] Knowledge of the area can thus provide a practical means of field verification. Both male and female anatomies have useful landmarks.

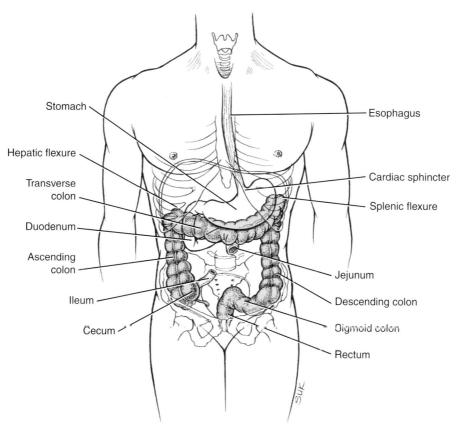

Fig. 20.40 Surface projection of the alimentary organs.

The anterior commissure of the labia majora is easily distinguishable in the female. It is an important soft tissue landmark because it is used as a reference point from which the upper or lower border pubis is measured. Thus checking back to this soft tissue landmark may eliminate variations in the palpation of the pubic bone.

The base of the penis is taken as the line that joins the anterior skin of the penis with the skin of the anterior pelvic wall. This level is used as a reference point from which the upper or lower border pubis is measured in the male. A therapist may measure changes in the lateral position of prostate fields by referencing appropriate measurements from the base of the penis.

Landmarks of the Posterior Pelvis

The most commonly used bony surface landmarks of the posterior pelvis are the PSISs, the coccyx, the iliac crests, and the lateral iliac crests. Because the latter two were also mentioned in the previous section, only the PSIS and coccyx are discussed here. The PSISs are indicated by dimples above and medial to the buttock, approximately 5 to 6 cm from the midline. They are palpable, and measurements may be taken in the superoinferior or mediolateral directions. The coccyx lies deep to the natal cleft, with its inferior end approximately 1 cm from the anus.

Abdominopelvic Viscera

The organs of the abdomen and pelvis can be visualized with various means. Radiographs, CT, MRI, and ultrasound are commonly used to provide information concerning organ location. Note that the location of any organ in the abdomen and pelvis can vary with respiration, anatomic position, and level of fullness, which is why placement of radiation therapy patients in a reproducible position that limits movement daily is extremely important. As observed previously, body habitus

affects the location of internal organs. This holds true for the abdomen and pelvis as well. This section examines the location of the abdominal and pelvic viscera.

Location of the Alimentary Organs

The esophagus begins at the lower border of the cricoid cartilage in the neck and travels through the diaphragm to the cardiac sphincter, the entrance to the stomach, at the level of T10 approximately 2 to 3 cm to the left of midline. For radiographic visualization of the esophagus, the patient commonly is instructed to swallow a radiopaque substance such as barium before examination.

The duodenum, a C-shaped section of the small bowel approximately 25 cm in length, starts to the right of midline at the edge of the epigastric region. The stomach lies between the duodenum and the distal esophagus and is of variable size and location, partly covered by the left rib cage and filling the epigastric region. The root of the small gut mesentery, made up of sections called the *jejunum* and *ileum,* extends from the duodenum to the inlet to the large bowel.[1,2]

The start of the large bowel is the cecum. It lies in the right iliac region at the level of L4. The ascending colon (15 cm in length) and hepatic flexure of the colon on the right side and the splenic flexure and descending colon (25 cm in length) on the left side are largely retroperitoneal structures, whereas the transverse and sigmoid colon have a mesentery and vary in their position from one person to the next.[1,2] However, similarities are found within common body habitus. The rectum starts at the level of S3 and ends approximately 4 cm from the anus. It is one of the dose-limiting structures when prostate treatment fields are outlined. Rectal visualization is thus important during the simulation process.

Fig. 20.40 delineates the surface projections of the alimentary tract in the abdomen and pelvis.

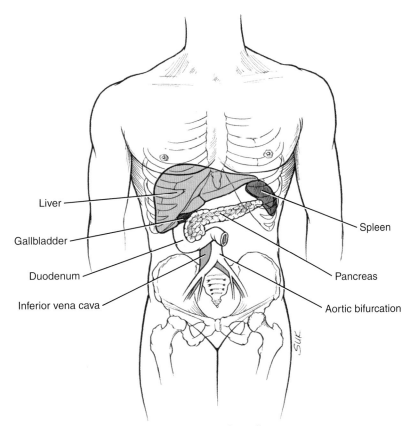

Fig. 20.41 Surface projection of nonalimentary organs.

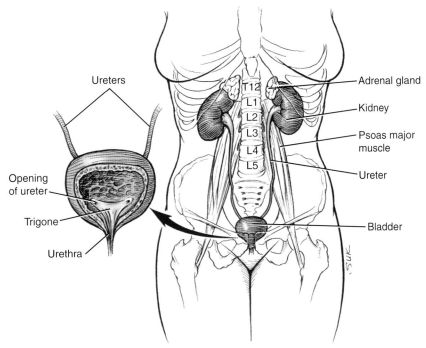

Fig. 20.42 Surface projection of the urinary tract and adrenal glands.

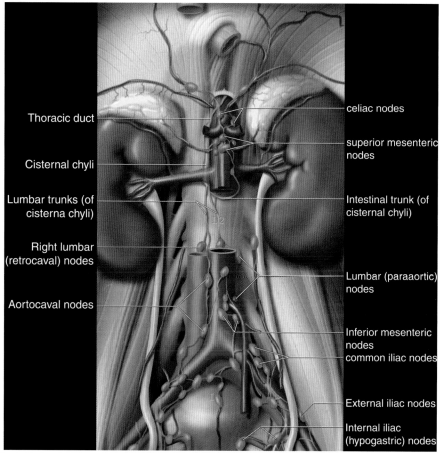

Fig. 20.43 Abdominal lymph nodes. (From Woodward PJ, et al.: Imaging Anatomy: Ultrasound, ed 2, Philadelphia, 2018, Elsevier.)

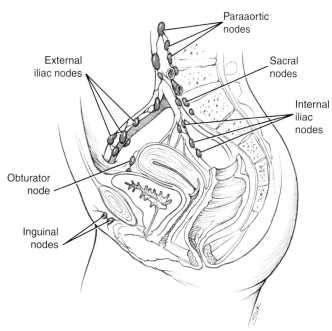

Fig. 20.44 Lymphatics of the pelvis.

Location of Nonalimentary Organs

The radiation therapist benefits from a working knowledge of the nonalimentary organs of the abdomen and pelvis. Many times these organs are involved in malignant processes and must be included in the patient's treatment scheme. Fig. 20.41 shows the surface projections of the organs outlined here.

The liver is an irregularly shaped organ located in the right hypochondriac region of the abdomen above the costal margin. The superior margin of the liver, which bulges into the diaphragm, is at the level of T7 to T8. The liver is commonly imaged with CT scan, ultrasound, and nuclear medicine studies.

The gallbladder is located below the lower border of the liver and contacts the anterior abdominal wall where the right lateral border of the rectus abdominis crosses the ninth costal cartilage. This location is called the *transpyloric plane.* Again, ultrasound is useful in distinguishing biliary obstructions and gallstones.

The spleen, mentioned previously as a lymph node for the blood, is located posteriorly approximately 5 cm to the left of midline at the level of T10 to T11. The healthy organ lies beneath the 9th through 11th ribs on the left side of the body. This organ is often examined surgically in patients with lymphoma to determine disease extension. If the organ is removed for biopsy, the splenic pedicle, the point of attachment of the organ to its vascular and lymphatic connections, is included in the abdominal treatment field for Hodgkin disease.

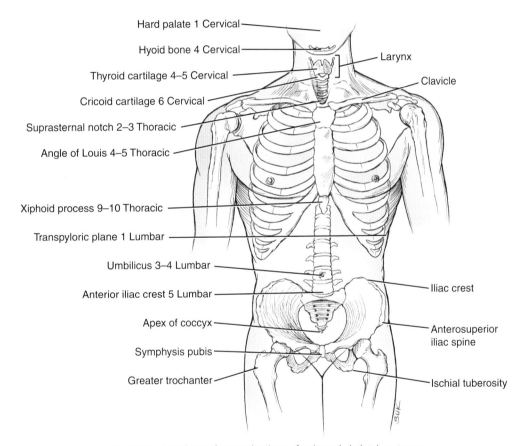

Hard palate 1 Cervical

Hyoid bone 4 Cervical

Thyroid cartilage 4–5 Cervical

Cricoid cartilage 6 Cervical

Suprasternal notch 2–3 Thoracic

Angle of Louis 4–5 Thoracic

Xiphoid process 9–10 Thoracic

Transpyloric plane 1 Lumbar

Umbilicus 3–4 Lumbar

Anterior iliac crest 5 Lumbar

Apex of coccyx

Symphysis pubis

Greater trochanter

Larynx

Clavicle

Iliac crest

Anterosuperior iliac spine

Ischial tuberosity

Fig. 20.45 Anterior surface projections of selected skeletal anatomy.

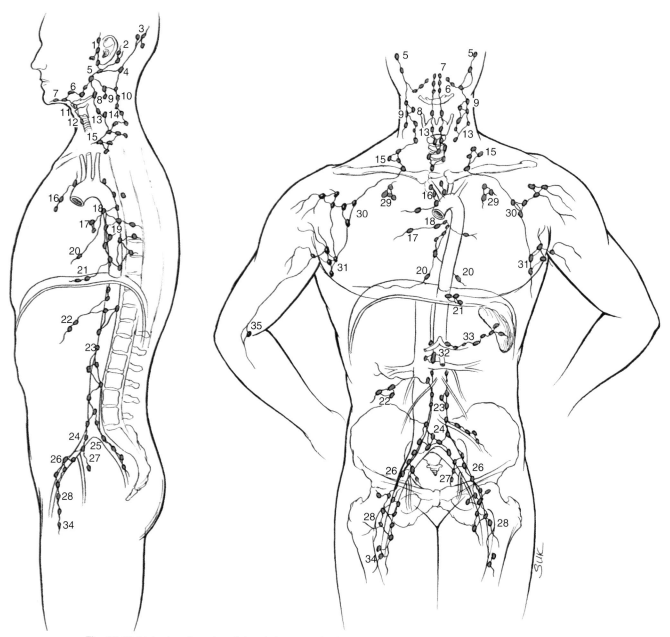

Fig. 20.46 Major lymph nodes of the abdomen and pelvis: *1,* Preauricular; *2,* mastoid; *3,* occipital; *4,* upper cervical; *5,* parotid; *6,* submaxillary; *7,* submental; *8,* jugulodigastric; *9,* upper deep cervical; *10,* spinal accessory chain; *11,* infrahyoid; *12,* pretracheal; *13,* juguloomohyoid; *14,* lower deep cervical; *15,* supraclavicular; *16,* mediastinal; *17,* interlobar; *18,* intertracheal; *19,* posterior mediastinal; *20,* lateral pericardial; *21,* diaphragmatic; *22,* mesenteric; *23,* para-aortic; *24,* common iliac; *25,* lateral sacral; *26,* external iliac; *27,* hypogastric; *28,* inguinal; *29,* interpectoral; *30,* axillary apex; *31,* axillary; *32,* cisterna chyli; *33,* splenic; *34,* femoral; *35,* epitrochlear.

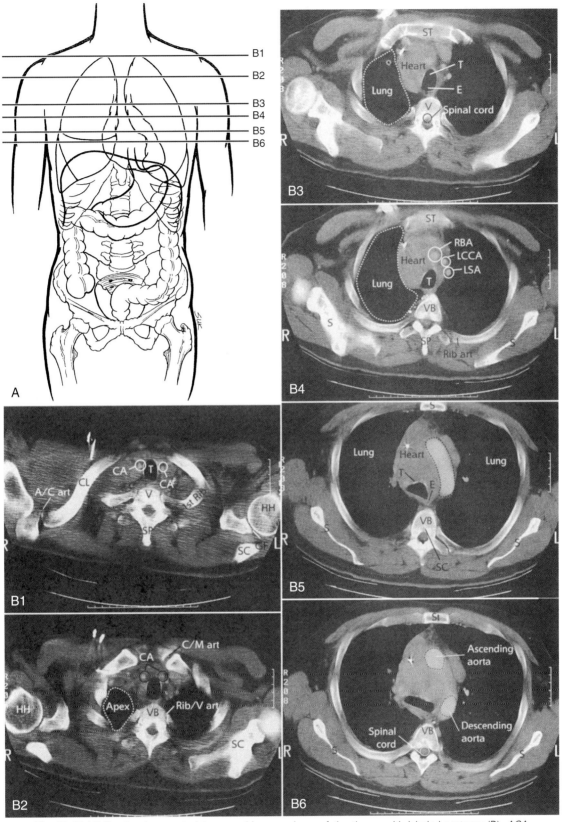

Fig. 20.47 (A) Sectional computed tomographic scan views of the thorax with labeled anatomy (B). *ACA,* Ascending aorta; *A/C art,* acromial clavicular articulation; *CA,* carotid artery; *CL,* clavicle; *C/M art,* clavicular macrobial articular; *DCA,* descending aorta; *E,* esophagus; *GF,* glenoid fossa; *HH,* humeral head; *LCCA,* left common carotid artery; *LSA,* left subclavian artery; *RBA,* right bronchocephalic artery; *Rib/V art,* rib/vertebral artery; *SC,* scapula; *SP,* spinous; *ST,* sternum; *T,* trachea; *V,* vein; *VB,* vertebral body.

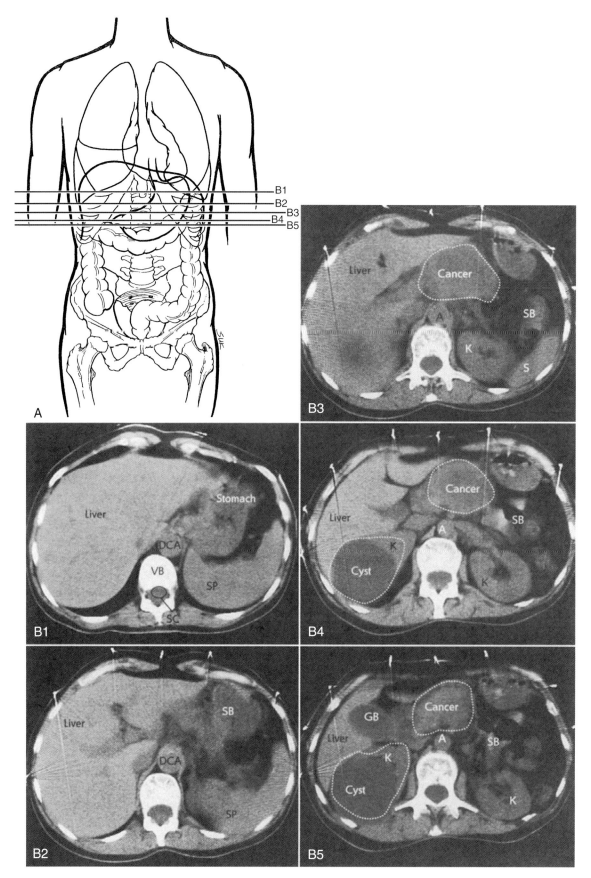

Fig. 20.48 (A) Sectional computed tomographic scan views of the abdomen with labeled anatomy (B). *A,* Aorta; *DCA,* descending aorta; *GB,* gallbladder; *K,* kidney; *L,* liver; *S,* spleen; *SB,* small bowel; *SC,* spinal cord; *SP,* spinous process; *VB,* vertebral body.

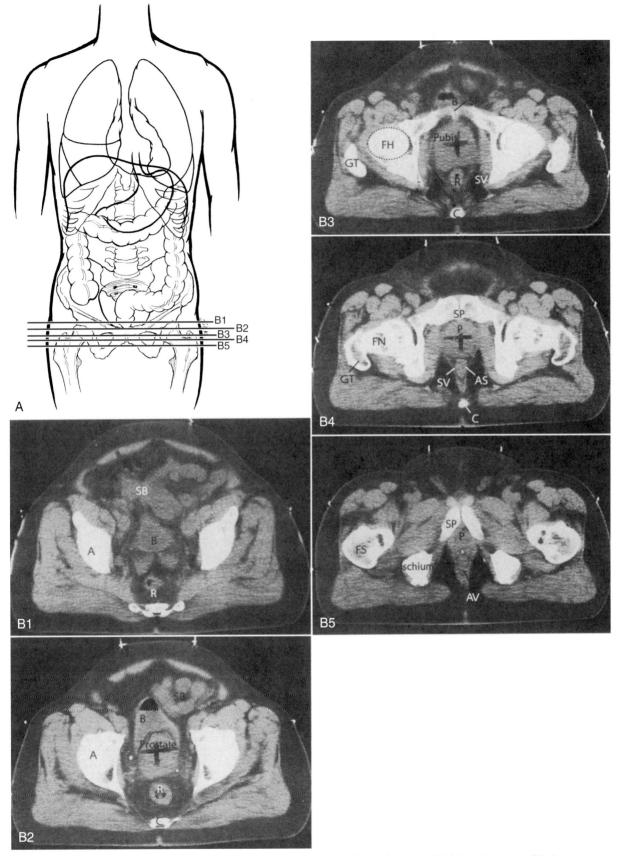

Fig. 20.49 (A) Sectional computed tomographic scan view of the male pelvis with labeled anatomy (B). *A,* Acetabulum; *AS,* axial sphincter; *AV,* anal verge; *B,* bladder; *C,* coccyx; *FH,* femoral head; *FN,* femoral neck; *FS,* femoral shaft; *GT,* greater tuberosity; *I,* ischium; *P,* prostate; *R,* rectum; *S,* sacrum; *SB,* small bowel; *SP,* symphysis pubis; *SV,* seminal vesicles.

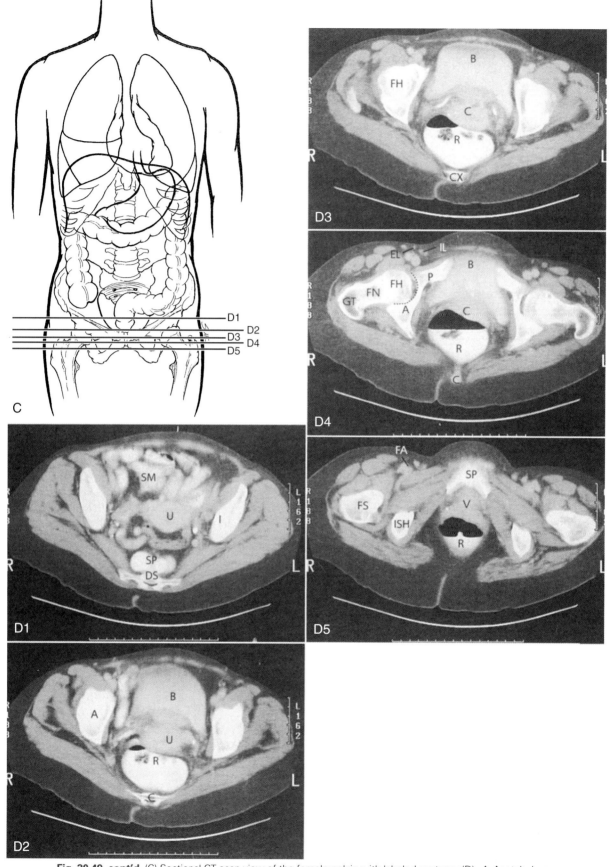

Fig. 20.49, cont'd (C) Sectional CT scan view of the female pelvis with labeled anatomy (D). *A,* Acetabulum; *B,* bladder; *C,* cervix; *CX,* coccyx; *DS,* descending sigmoid; *EL,* external iliac; *FA,* femoral artery; *FH,* femoral head; *FN,* femoral neck; *FS,* femoral shaft; *GT,* greater tuberosity; *I,* ilium; *IL,* internal iliac; *ISH,* ischium; *P,* pubis; *R,* rectum; *SM,* small intestine; *SP,* symphysis pubis; *U,* uterus; *V,* vagina.

Three components, the head, body, and tail, compose the pancreas. The head of the pancreas is located in the C section of the duodenum. The body extends slightly superiorly to the left across midline, at the level of L1. The tail of the pancreas passes into the hilum, a concave point of an organ that has vascular inlets and outlets, of the spleen.

Location of the Urinary Tract Organs

The kidneys lie on the posterior abdominal wall in the retroperitoneal space. The hilum of the right kidney is at the level of L2, whereas the hilum of the left is at the level of L1. The right kidney lies lower than the left because of the presence of the adjacent liver. Superior and medial to each kidney are the adrenal glands. The kidneys are generally not fixed to the abdominal wall; they can move as much as 2 cm with respiration. When the radiation therapist outlines the location of these radiation-sensitive structures, this movement is important to take into account.

The ureters are tubular structures that transport urine from the kidneys to the urinary bladder. They run anterior to the psoas muscles and enter the pelvis lateral to the sacroiliac (SI) joint. The ureters, as well as the kidneys, are commonly imaged with CT scan, ultrasound, and intravenous and retrograde studies.

The urinary bladder is located in the pelvis. The neck of the bladder lies posterior to the symphysis pubis and anterior to the rectum. This organ also lies immediately superior to the prostate in the male. The urinary bladder is a dose-limiting structure in the treatment of prostatic cancer. It is commonly visualized with contrast agents during the simulation process.

The topographic relations of the urinary tract organs are shown in Fig. 20.42.

Lymphatics of the Abdomen and Pelvis

The lymphatic drainage routes for the abdomen and pelvis are important to the radiation therapist. An abundance of lymphatic vessels is found in this section of the body. Those of the retroperitoneum and pelvis play a major role in radiation therapy field arrangement of gynecologic, genitourinary, and lymphatic cancers. Figs. 20.43 and 20.44 show the nodes and nodal groups outlined here.

The lymphatic pathways and nodes of the abdomen are often referred to as the *visceral nodes* because they are closely associated with the abdominal organs. The three principal groups of nodes of the abdomen that drain the corresponding viscera before entering the cisterna chyli or the thoracic duct are the celiac, superior mesenteric, and inferior mesenteric groups, also called the *preaortic nodes.*

The celiac nodes include the nodes that drain the stomach, greater omentum, liver, gallbladder, and spleen and most of the lymph from the pancreas and duodenum. The superior mesenteric nodes drain part of the head of the pancreas; a portion of the duodenum; the entire jejunum, ileum, appendix, cecum, and ascending colon; and most of the transverse colon. The inferior mesenteric nodes drain the descending colon, the left side of the mesentery, the sigmoid colon, and the rectum.

The posterior abdominal wall has a rich network of lymphatic vessels. The paraaortic nodes provide efferent drainage to the cisterna chyli, which is the beginning of the thoracic duct. These nodes run adjacent to the abdominal aorta from T12 to L4. This major section of the lymphatic system eventually receives lymph from most of the lower regions of the body. The paraaortics directly drain the uterus, ovary, kidneys, and testicles. An interesting note is that embryonically the testes develop near the kidneys and descend into the scrotum after birth. As they descend, they take the vascular and lymphatic vessels with them as direct means for blood and lymph flow.

The common iliac nodes lie at the bifurcation of the abdominal aorta at the level of L4. These nodes directly drain the urinary bladder, prostate, cervix, and vagina. This chain moves laterally and breaks up into the external and internal iliac nodes. The external iliac nodes drain the urinary bladder, prostate, cervix, testes, vagina, and ovaries. The internal iliac nodes, also known as the hypogastric nodes, drain the vagina, cervix, prostate, and urinary bladder. These nodes are more medial and posterior to the external iliac nodes previously mentioned.

The inguinal nodes are more superficial than the previously mentioned nodes. These nodes directly drain the vulva, uterus, ovaries, and vagina. These nodes are commonly treated with electrons because of their superficial location.

APPLIED TECHNOLOGY

Practical application of the material presented in this chapter is important. To enhance the comprehensive understanding of the relationships presented, the last section of this chapter presents diagrams that relate structures to vertebral body levels and CT scans through the head, neck, thorax, abdomen, and pelvis. The appropriate structures pertinent to the radiation oncology practitioner are shown. Figs. 20.45 through 20.49 show these diagrams and scans.

■ SUMMARY

- Radiation therapy requires its practitioners to have a keen knowledge and understanding of surface and sectional anatomy.
- The complex simulation procedures and planning used in patient treatment mandate strict attention to detail.
- The radiation therapist must use information provided by several imaging modalities to achieve the ultimate goal: administration of a tumoricidal dose of radiation to the tumor and tumor bed with as much normal tissue spared as possible.
- The lymphatic vessels play a major role in treatment field delineation and disease management.
- The complexity of radiation therapy requires the radiation therapist to use all available means to function effectively. All therapists should review their practical skills in surface and sectional anatomy because they are crucial for accurate treatment planning and delivery.
- For patients to completely benefit from the new technology in radiation therapy, the radiation therapist must have a strong anatomic base that allows effective treatment delivery.

- Medical imaging greatly assists not only in targeting but also in promoting greater treatment delivery options through more precise and exacting means.
- Body habitus knowledge helps the radiation therapist quickly locate treatment areas and relate internal structure location as related to body type. Knowledge of how the human body varies is essential to effective practice.
- The lymphatic system and its related components depict possible routes of tumor spread. The system's one-way flow makes the spread patterns predictable. Closely associated with neighboring structures and the cardiovascular system, the lymphatic channels and extent of their involvement in a cancer diagnosis are essential in the radiation treatment field design and delivery.
- Anatomic landmarks are important tools in locating and recalling treatment areas. Two types of landmarks should be considered: bony and soft tissue. Although all provide useful information, the bony landmarks are more stable and more predictably referenced. Soft tissue landmarks are useful in locating general areas but may not be as exact in comparison.

REVIEW QUESTIONS

The answers to the Review Questions can be found by logging on to our website at: http://evolve.elsevier.com/Washington/principles

1. Which plane goes through the middle of the body from the front to back through the sagittal suture of the skull that divides the body into two equal parts?
   a. Midsagittal.
   b. Coronal.
   c. Horizontal.
   d. Superior.

2. Which muscle partitions the anterior cavity into the thoracic and abdominal portions?
   a. Diaphragm.
   b. Rectus abdominus.
   c. Trapezius.
   d. Pectoralis major.

3. Which vessel returns lymph from the entire body back into the bloodstream, except for the upper right limb and the right side of the thorax, head, and neck?
   a. Cisterna chyli.
   b. Thoracic duct.
   c. Right lymphatic duct.
   d. Superior vena cava.

4. The angle of the mandible is generally located at which vertebra number level?
   a. C1.
   b. C4.
   c. T1.
   d. T4.

5. Which structures run anterior to the psoas stripes (muscles) and enter the pelvis lateral to the SI joint? (Tumors in these structures are very rare.)
   a. Kidneys.
   b. Urethra.
   c. Ureters.
   d. Adrenal glands.

6. If the punctum lacrimae of the eye is overirradiated, fibrotic changes can occur. If this happens, what is a clinical sign?
   a. Dry eye.
   b. Constantly tearing eye.
   c. Cataracts.
   d. Ocular muscle atrophy.

7. In the lower neck, the esophagus lies:
   a. Anterior to the trachea and posterior to the spinal cord.
   b. Anterior to the spinal cord and posterior to the trachea.
   c. Anterior to the trachea and inferior to the spinal cord.
   d. Inferior to the spinal cord and posterior to the trachea.

8. Which of the following are examples of primary curves?
   I. Thoracic.
   II. Lateral.
   III. Pelvic.
      a. I and II.
      b. I and III.
      c. II and III.
      d. I, II, and III.

9. The trachea is a hollow tube approximately 10 cm in length that extends from the larynx to a bifurcation called the:
   a. Bronchus.
   b. Carina.
   c. Bronchiole.
   d. Lung.

10. Which of the following is a commonly used soft tissue landmark of the anterior pelvis?
    a. Umbilicus.
    b. Base of the penis.
    c. Both a and b.
    d. Neither a nor b.

QUESTIONS TO PONDER

1. Examine the process of how lymph is transported through the lymphatic system.
2. Describe how the directional flow of lymph is facilitated through the lymphatic system.
3. Describe events that can occur if lymphatic channels are compromised through either surgical or radiation damage.
4. Why are landmarks around the mouth, and other soft tissue landmarks, not very accurate? What do we have to do to use them accurately?
5. How could a therapist locate the pituitary gland using only topographic landmarks?
6. Describe how the radiation therapist uses body habitus in localizing a patient's internal organs.
7. What is the significance of including a portion of lung tissue in the tangential fields of the patient undergoing treatment for breast cancer?
8. Analyze the relationship of surface anatomy knowledge with performance of effective simulation procedures. How can this knowledge also affect daily treatment administrations?

REFERENCES

1. Lumley JSP. *Surface Anatomy: The Anatomical Basis of Clinical Examination.* 4th ed. London, UK: Churchill Livingstone; 2008.
2. Keogh B, Ebbs S. *Normal Surface Anatomy.* Philadelphia, PA: Lippincott; 1984.
3. Khan FM, Gerbi BJ. *Treatment Planning in Radiation Oncology.* 3rd ed. Philadelphia, PA: Lippincott Williams & Wilkins; 2012.
4. El-Khoury GY, Montgomery WJ, Bergman RA. *Sectional Anatomy by MRI and CT.* Churchill Livingstone; 2007.
5. Christianson PE, Waterstram-Rich KM. *Nuclear Medicine and PET/CT: Technology and Techniques.* 7th ed. St. Louis, MO: Mosby; 2012.
6. Foldi M, Strosenreuther R. *Foundations of Manual Lymph Drainage.* 3rd ed. St. Louis, MO: Mosby; 2005.
7. Philippou M, et al. Cross-sectional anatomy of the nose and paranasal sinuses. *Rhinology.* 1990;28:221–230.
8. Tortora GJ, Grabowski SR. *Principles of Human Anatomy.* 13th ed. NJ Hoboken: John Wiley & Sons; 1999.
9. Kelley LL, Peterson CM. *Sectional Anatomy for Imaging Professionals.* 3rd ed. St. Louis, MO: Mosby; 2012.
10. Shaver ML , Batra P. In: Cox JD, Ang KK, eds. *Radiation Oncology: Rationale, Techniques, Results.* 9th ed. St. Louis, MO: Mosby; 2010.

11. Collins JD, et al. Anatomy of the abdomen, back, and pelvis as displayed by magnetic resonance imaging: part two. *J Natl Med Assoc.* 1989;81: 809–813.
12. Collins JD, et al. Anatomy of the abdomen, back, and pelvis as displayed by magnetic resonance imaging: part three. *J Natl Med Assoc.* 1989;81:857–861.
13. Collins JD, et al. Anatomy of the abdomen, back, and pelvis as displayed by magnetic resonance imaging: part one. *J Natl Med Assoc.* 1989;81: 680–684.
14. Collins JD, et al. Magnetic resonance imaging of chest wall lesions. *J Natl Med Assoc.* 1991;83:352–360.

BIBLIOGRAPHY

Hoppe RT, Phillips TL, Roach M. *Leibel and Phillips Textbook of Radiation Oncology.* St. Louis, MO: Elsevier; 2010.

Stewart GS. Trends in radiation therapy for the treatment of lung cancer. *Nurs Clin North Am.* 1992;27:643–651.

Thibodeau GA, Patton KT. *Anatomy & Physiology.* 6th ed. St. Louis, MO: Mosby; 2007.

Vann AM, Dasher BG, Wiggers NH, Chestnut SK, Markwalter PS. *Portal Design in Radiation Therapy.* Phoenix Printing, Augusta, GA

Wechsler RJ, Steiner RM. Cross-sectional imaging of the chest wall. *J Thorac Imag.* 1989;4:29–40.

21

Computed Tomography Simulation Procedures

Nora Uricchio, Ronnie G. Lozano

OBJECTIVES

- Describe the evolution of the radiation therapy simulation process from a historic perspective.
- Define common acronyms and nomenclature used during the simulation process.
- Define the target volumes as described in the International Commission on Radiation Units and Measurements Report 62.
- Describe the benefits and considerations of computed tomography simulation.
- Identify commonly used positioning and immobilization devices for various parts of the body and special procedures.
- State considerations to create and achieve reproducible patient setups.
- Compare and contrast the benefits and contraindications of contrast agents used with computed tomography simulation.
- Discuss common uses of contrast media for various body parts.
- Provide a general description of the following steps in the simulation process: presimulation planning, patient positioning, patient immobilization, preparation of the room, explanation of the simulation procedure, setting of field parameters, and documentation of pertinent data.

- State the importance of topograms (scout image) in the computed tomography simulation process.
- State scan parameters that are commonly adjusted based on the patient or area that is simulated.
- Describe shift and no-shift methods for simulation.
- Describe techniques for isocenter localization.
- State the benefits of the use of movable patient marking systems.
- Compare different methods of motion management including four-dimensional computed tomography.
- Describe surface imaging and state the benefits of use.
- Summarize the benefits, challenges, and uses of magnetic resonance imaging. Describe safety requirements. State the benefits and challenges of magnetic resonance imaging simulation only.
- Describe the simulation process that includes positron emission tomography and computed tomography.
- State quality assurance procedures for the computed tomography simulator.

OUTLINE

KEY TERMS

Clinical target volume
Contrast media
Digitally reconstructed radiograph
Field of view
Field size
Four-dimensional computed tomography
International Commission on Radiation Units and Measurements
Image fusion
Image-guided radiation therapy
Immobilization devices
Interfraction motion
Internal target volume
Intrafraction motion
Localization
Maximum intensity projection
Magnetic resonance imaging

Organ at risk
Osmolality
Planning target volume
Port film
Positioning aids
Positron emission tomography
Prospective axial
Radiopaque marker
Scan field of view
Separation
Simulation
Single-photon emission computed tomography
Stereotactic radiosurgery
Stereotactic body radiation therapy
Surface guided radiation therapy
Verification
Virtual simulation

INTRODUCTION

The goal of radiation therapy is to deliver a dose of radiation to the target volume and simultaneously reduce the dose to the normal surrounding tissue. This requires a high degree of precision and accuracy. The right combination of high-technology equipment, such as the computed tomography (CT) simulator, and the involvement of dedicated professionals can sometimes make the difference between a geographic miss and curing the patient of cancer (Box 21.1).[1]

Patients treated with radiation therapy, either for cure or for palliation, will undergo numerous processes, ranging from diagnosis to ongoing patient follow-up. There are various steps (Fig. 21.1) that a patient will experience as part of the entire process of external beam radiation therapy. Before treatment planning can begin, a simulation procedure is necessary. In many cases, the ultimate success of treatment is directly related to the effectiveness of the simulation procedure. This procedure determines and documents patient immobilization and positioning for their course of treatment. During simulation,

the physician and other members of the radiation therapy team use acquired images and CT simulation software to localize the treatment isocenter, define the size and shape of the treatment volume relative to important normal tissues, and translate this information back on the patient with a laser-based patient marking system. The patient is marked and documented for daily setup and treatment. This information is used to initiate the treatment planning process.

Advancements in medical imaging have revolutionized how we simulate and plan radiation therapy treatments. Other medical imaging modalities and techniques, such as magnetic resonance imaging (MRI), positron emission tomography (PET), and single-photon emission computed tomography (SPECT), have provided valuable information that is often incorporated into the simulation planning process by a complex process of image fusion.[2] This multidisciplinary approach has allowed for more accurate treatment simulation, treatment planning, and treatment delivery. CT technology continues to evolve, and methods such as four-dimensional (4D) CT are available to evaluate tumor and critical structure motion. This technology also led to an increased

---

BOX 21.1 ACR–ASTRO Practice Parameter for Radiation Oncology

Equipment Requirements

A. Core Radiation Oncology Capabilities: At a minimum, the radiation oncology facility must have these core capabilities: a megavoltage radiation therapy delivery system, a computer-based treatment planning system, a treatment management system, access to simulation equipment, and the ability to fabricate or obtain customized treatment aids. The following specific equipment must be available to patients in all facilities:

1. Megavoltage radiation therapy equipment such as high-energy photon equipment capable of delivering three-dimensional (3D) conformal therapy and intensity-modulated radiation therapy (IMRT). Computed tomography (CT) simulator capable of duplicating the setups of the facility's megavoltage units and producing either standard images or digitally reconstructed radiographs of the fields to be treated. A dedicated CT simulator is preferred but could be substituted with a diagnostic CT scanner modified to obtain imaging data replicating patient treatment position and suitable for radiation therapy treatment planning. Satellite facilities must have access to simulator equipment. The CT scanner should have a gantry diameter sufficient to accommodate the patient in normal treatment positions as encountered in the clinic.

2. Computerized dosimetry equipment capable of providing external beam isodose curves as well as Practice Parameter 9 Radiation Oncology brachytherapy isodose curves, 3D IMRT treatment planning, and dose-volume histograms.

3. Physics calibration devices for all equipment, including a field dosimetry system (electrometer and ion chamber) and an Accredited Dosimetry Calibration Laboratory (ADCL) calibrated local standard dosimetry system.

4. Physics equipment and/or software for IMRT quality assurance (QA) measurement and analysis.

5. Beam-shaping devices.

6. Immobilization devices

7. An in vivo dosimetry system or capability.

B. Specialized Radiation Oncology Capabilities: The facility should have available equipment to provide specialized treatments such as low-dose-rate brachytherapy and high-dose-rate brachytherapy, stereotactic body radiation therapy (SBRT), stereotactic radiosurgery (SRS), radionuclide therapy, electron beam, or other capabilities for treating skin or superficial lesions, or the ability to refer for these services.

From the American College of Radiology ACR practice guideline for radiation oncology, Revised 2018.

DIAGNOSIS

- screening
- cancer imaging
- pathology
- staging

THERAPEUTIC DECISIONS

- cure
- palliation
- benign
- surgery/radiation/chemotherapy
- patient interview

SIMULATION

- fluoroscopy-based
- CT simulation
- patient positioning
- immobilization devices
- digitally reconstructed radiographs (DRRs)

TREATMENT PLANNING

- identifying planning target volume
- identifying critical structures
- selection of treatment technique
- isodose distribution
- calculation of treatment beams
- optimization

TREATMENT

- treatment verification and imaging
- dosimetry checks
- treatment delivery and monitoring
- patient assessment
- record keeping

PATIENT FOLLOW-UP

- patient assessment
- normal tissue response
- tumor control

Fig. 21.1 The various steps involved in the process of external beam treatment. The process may vary somewhat depending on the treatment goal. It is the team approach, involving each member, that usually provides effective planning. *CT,* Computed tomography. (Modified from Van Dyk J, Mah K. Simulators and CT scanners. In: Williams JR, Thwaites DI, eds. *Radiotherapy Physics in Practice.* Oxford, UK: Oxford University Press; 2000.)

interest in treating moving targets. Research is aimed at delivering higher doses to tumors with the hope of achieving greater control of the disease.

Radiation oncologists define the target volume not just in two dimensions, but also in three and sometimes four dimensions (the fourth dimension includes motion). With intensity-modulated radiation therapy (IMRT) and image-guided radiation therapy (IGRT), it is possible, and in many situations advantageous, to escalate the dose to the tumor volume. CT imaging and simulation, along with other imaging modalities, allow the visualization of anatomy in three dimensions and, with 4D CT, also account for any tumor motion. This enables the physician and treatment planner to conform the dose around the target volume more closely and irradiate the tumor with the highest possible dose while sparing healthy tissues.[3]

In this chapter, the complexities of CT-based simulation are introduced and discussed. This includes nomenclature (definitions) and the importance of patient assessment and education before the simulation procedure. Patient immobilization, patient positioning, and the other steps involved to acquire a CT scan in the simulation process are outlined and detailed. Techniques for isocenter localization and patient marking by using an external patient marking laser system are

introduced. The use of additional imaging techniques such as 4D CT, PET, and MRI are also described as they relate to CT simulation.

HISTORIC PERSPECTIVE

In the early days of radiation therapy treatment, simulation was performed on the treatment unit.[4] This simulation took time from the treatment room. The treatment accuracy was evaluated by a poor-quality port film. The poor quality was as a result of the predominate Compton scatter interaction in the MV range (Fig. 21.2).

While technology advanced and the demand for more accurate treatments increased, conventional simulation was developed. Conventional simulation, also referred to as *fluoroscopy-based simulation*, implies the use of a piece of x-ray equipment capable of the same mechanical movements as a linear accelerator. Conventional simulators mimic the mechanical, geometric, and optical conditions of the treatment units and display a representation of the treatment field on the patient's skin.[5] These simulators used fluoroscopy and kV x-rays to establish treatment fields, and the patient could be marked for daily setup to deliver the planned treatment. (Fig. 21.3)

During a conventional simulation procedure, time could be scheduled to position, immobilize, and align the patient and target volume with the simulator's isocenter, providing more accurate data and lessening the burden on the treatment unit. Images created on the conventional simulator, with the aid of fluoroscopy and diagnostic-quality images, greatly improved the simulation process.

During the conventional simulation process, patients were contoured only at the central axis (CA) and, at times, certain levels above and below CA by using solder or plaster contouring methods. These patient contours had to be manually digitized into the planning system by using a digitizer interface. All treatment beam and field size information were manually entered into the planning system. If beam modifiers such as Cerrobend blocks were used to block portions of the field, then they too had to be digitized into the planning system. Treatments were often simple anteroposterior (AP)/posteroanterior (PA) four-field techniques delivered to a large area.

Conventional simulators evolved during the years, and improvements were made to two-dimensional (2D) imaging and the display of these images. Film-based x-rays were soon replaced by digital images. Simulation software greatly improved, and systems soon had the ability to electronically export beam and field information from the simulator to treatment planning computers or record-and-verify systems. This eliminated the need for manually entering and digitizing this information into the treatment planning system. These systems could also import beam and treatment field information from the treatment planning computers. This allowed for treatment plan information and patient positioning to be verified by fluoroscopy and static digital x-rays on the simulator before the first treatment delivery. Another improvement to the conventional simulator was the addition of volumetric cone-beam CT (CBCT) technology. This replaced the need for manual solder or plaster patient contour methods and expanded the ability to verify the accuracy of generated treatment plans and patient positioning before treatment.

Although CT proved to be beneficial, the technology was lacking in regard to facilitating the transfer of the CT information to the treatment planning system. In the late 1970s and early 1980s, attempts were made to market a type of CT scanner specifically for radiation therapy simulation. This failed for two reasons: the lack of high-quality digitally reconstructed radiographs (DRRs) and a limited treatment planning system that did not allow for interactive definition of target volumes and dose calculations. It took several years to realize the full potential that CT can have on the radiation therapy simulation and treatment planning process.

Until the 1990s, most simulation procedures were performed on the conventional fluoroscopy-based simulator. Several developments

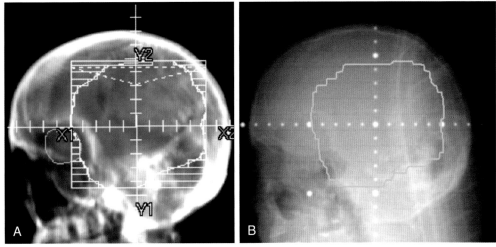

Fig. 21.2 Imaging with diagnostic and high-energy photons. (A) Simulator image of a brain tumor patient, with a block indicated by the outline. (B) Portal image of the patient in A shows the blocked area and context around the treatment region. Contrast is much higher in A because of increased amount of photoelectric effect. Contrast is poorer and of more limited range in B because of dominance of the Compton effect. (From Gunderson LL, Tepper JE. *Clinical Radiation Oncology.* 4th ed. Philadelphia, PA: Elsevier; 2016.)

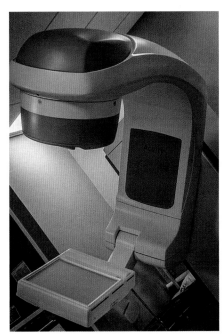

Fig. 21.3 A conventional simulator with a digital imager. (Courtesy of Shahzeb Ahmad, Hartford Hospital, Hartford, CT.)

occurred in the early 1990s that greatly affected radiation treatment planning and led to the widespread use of CT simulation.[6]

1. Virtual simulation was introduced, which provided the ability to design the fields without a conventional simulator and with better visualization of internal structures by using three-dimensional (3D) images on the computer.
2. Treatment planning computers were developed with more sophisticated algorithms and faster computer speeds that could carry out 3D treatment planning by using CT images.
3. A true virtual simulator allowed for a CT scan to be acquired, and a virtual patient could be reconstructed from the CT images. Procedures usually performed on a conventional simulator could now be performed by using the simulation software, and kV x-rays were replaced by high-resolution DRRs that could be compared with port films generated on the linear accelerator.

One of the first commercially available CT virtual simulation systems was developed by Picker X-ray. This system was a diagnostic CT scanner with a virtual simulation workstation.

CT scanning has been used, in some fashion, in radiation therapy almost as long as the CT scanner has been in existence, providing information necessary to plan the patient's treatment.

Since the introduction of virtual simulation, there have been many advances in treatment delivery techniques that necessitate the need for more precise simulation and treatment planning.

Simulation has become much more demanding and requires increased accuracy and precision in identifying the tumor and surrounding critical structures compared with the technology of 25 years ago.

Regardless of the method of simulation that is used, the outcome is the same. Simulation should define the anatomic area to be treated so that it is reproducible for daily treatment. An elaborate and complicated simulation is of no value unless it is reproducible on the treatment unit.

Nomenclature

Before a discussion of exactly what simulation is, a review of several key definitions and acronyms, designed to provide a foundation in simulation procedures, is helpful.

Simulation is the process of determining the patient treatment position, the volume to be treated, and the normal structures in or surrounding that volume.[1] The standard simulation equipment includes a CT scanner, software to perform target volume definition and treatment planning dose calculation, and the production of DRRs. Other imaging modalities such as MRI and PET/CT can be used. Images can be fused together to gain complete anatomical and physiological information to create the best treatment plan.

Immobilization devices: An essential component of simulation is making devices that assist in reproducing the treatment position while restricting movement, ensuring comfort and reproducibility of the patient position.

Localization refers to geometric definition of the position and extent of the tumor or anatomic structures by reference of surface marks that can be used for treatment setup purposes.[7] The radiation oncologist and radiation therapist, along with other team members, localize the tumor volume and critical normal structures by using clinical, radiographic, and/or CT, MRI, and PET image information.

Verification is a final check to ensure that each of the planned treatment beams covers the tumor or target volume and does not irradiate critical normal structures.[7] This is usually done on a treatment unit. Verification involves taking radiographic images or portal images of each of the treatment beams with the patient in the simulated position. It is an essential process that provides verification of the treatment plan.

Radiopaque marker refers to a material with a high atomic number. It is usually made of lead, copper, or solder wire. Frequently, it is used on the surface of a patient or appropriately placed in a body cavity. This is done to delineate special points of interest for calculation purposes or to mark critical structures requiring visualization during treatment planning. Small radiopaque markers are often used to mark specific points on a patient during the CT acquisition phase of the simulation procedure.

Contrast media is a compound or agent used as an aid in visualizing internal structures, because it has the ability to enhance the differences in adjacent anatomic structures. Barium (atomic number of 56) and iodine (atomic number of 53) are compounds commonly used to visualize anatomic structures with x-rays.

Separation refers to the measurement of the thickness of a patient along the CA or at any other specified point within the irradiated volume. Separations are helpful in calculating the amount of tissue in front of, behind, or around a tumor. A caliper, which is a graduated ruled instrument with one sliding leg and one that is stationary, is used to determine the patient's thickness. A patient's separation is also referred to as the *intrafield distance*, or sometimes the *innerfield distance*. Separations are easily acquired in virtual simulation and treatment planning by line measurements in the software.

Field size involves the dimensions of a treatment field at the isocenter, which are represented by width × length. This measurement, determined by the collimator opening in the simulation software, treatment planning system, and on the treatment unit, defines the dimensions of the treatment portal at the isocenter.

A DRR is a two-dimensional image reconstructed from CT data that shows a beam's-eye view (BEV) of the treatment field. The DRR is created at the given isocenter determined by the treatment plan.

Interfraction motion is the change in target position from one fraction to another.

Intrafraction motion is the change in target position during treatment delivery as might occur in the thorax with respirations.

There are several definitions related to the patient planning process provided by the International Commission on Radiation Units and Measurements (ICRU) in an effort to standardize radiation therapy terminology.[7] Fig. 21.4 illustrates several target volumes described by ICRU Report 50.[7] Uniform application of these terms when radiation treatments are prescribed, recorded, and reported helps with the comparison of treatment results from different centers. Four specific target volumes are further defined (see Fig. 21.4): gross tumor volume (GTV), clinical target volume (CTV), planning target volume (PTV), and internal target volume (ITV).[7] ICRU Report 62[7] updates ICRU Report 50 regarding a further defining of organs at risk (OAR), which are critical structures that may limit the amount of radiation delivered to the tumor volume.

Gross tumor volume indicates the gross palpable or visible tumor.

Clinical target volume indicates the gross palpable or visible tumor (GTV) and a surrounding volume of tissue that may contain subclinical or microscopic disease.

Planning target volume indicates the CTV plus margins for geometric uncertainties, such as patient motion, beam penumbra, and treatment setup differences.

Internal target volume indicates the CTV plus an internal margin that accounts for tumor motion.

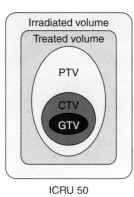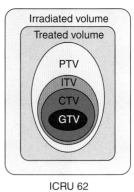

Fig. 21.4 Definition of target volumes used in radiation therapy from International Commission on Radiation Units and Measurements Reports 50 and 62. *CTV,* Clinical target volume; *GTV,* gross tumor volume; *ITV,* internal target volume; *PTV,* planning target volume.

INTERNATIONAL COMMISSION ON RADIATION UNITS AND MEASUREMENTS REPORT 62[7]

One of the important factors in the success of the current three-dimensional (3D) treatment planning process is the standardization of nomenclature achieved by the International Commission on Radiation Units and Measurements (ICRU)'s Report 50, published in 1993.[7] This report provided the radiation oncology community a language and methodology for image-based 3D planning to define the volumes of known tumor, suspected microscopic spread, and marginal volumes necessary to account for setup variations and organ and patient motion. ICRU Report 62[7] was published in 1999 as a supplement to Report 50 to more accurately formulate some of the definitions, take into account the consequences of the advances made in recent years, and address perceived limitations of Report 50. Report 50 was perhaps criticized mostly for the fact that it did not account for organs at risk (OAR) positional uncertainties. (See www.icru.org for additional information.)

Acronyms

A common language evolves in communicating thoughts and ideas between team members. An introduction to several more important acronyms used in the radiation therapy department will be helpful. Many of the useful acronyms are illustrated in Fig. 21.5 and defined in Table 21.1.

SIMULATION PROCEDURES

The simulation process, patient positioning and imaging, involves the participation of several team members, each with a variety of unique skills. A solid foundation in the theory and application of radiation oncology techniques and effective patient care skills are essential to provide comfort and care for the patient throughout the simulation process. The team approach, involving each member, provides effective planning as well as localization and documentation of the patient's disease in relationship to normal tissue structures. Table 21.2 identifies key staff functions in the radiation therapy process from diagnosis to patient follow-up.

Equipment requirements for a radiation therapy CT simulator include a CT scanner with fast CT acquisition time, multislice technology, axial and helical scanning capabilities, and a wide bore larger than 75 cm to accommodate immobilization devices.[9] Additional technology includes an external laser marking system and virtual simulation software.[5] Other options include gating technology to perform motion-correlated scans, which is also called 4D CT and surface-guided radiation therapy technology.[11]

The localization and verification of a treatment field during CT simulation must reflect precisely what will happen in the treatment room when a prescribed dose of radiation therapy is delivered. CT simulation

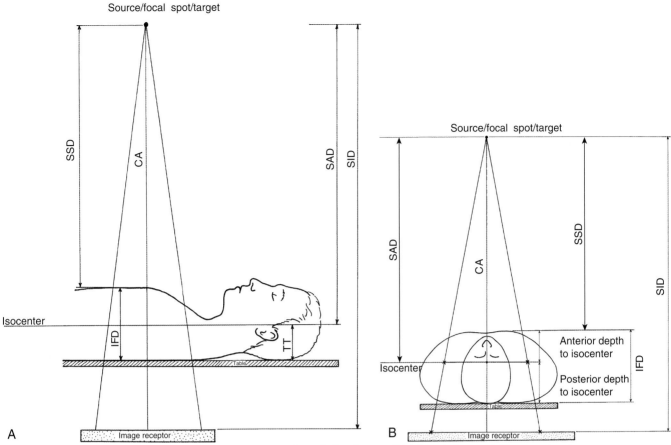

Fig. 21.5 A list of common acronyms used in radiation therapy. (A) A lateral view, and (B) a superior view illustrating terms in a transverse plane. *CA,* Central axis; *IFD,* intrafield distance; *SAD,* source-axis distance; *SID,* source-image distance; *SSD,* source-skin distance.

TABLE 21.1	**Acronyms and Terminology Used During Radiation Therapy Treatment and Fluoroscopy-Based Simulation Procedures**
Acronym/Term	**Definition**
CA (CAX)	Central axis is a line perpendicular to the cross section of the simulation or treatment field. It is the only imaginary line emanating from the source (focal spot) of radiation that is not divergent.
IFD	Intrafield distance (also called *separation*) is a measurement used for treatment planning purposes to determine the thickness of a body part from entrance point to exit point, often measured along the CA.
Image	Any process used to capture the x-ray, magnetic resonance image (MRI), or sonographic information, including film, electronic, or digitally reconstructed radiograph (DRR).
Isocenter	Point in space where radiation beams intersect from any of the 360-degree gantry angles. It is similar to the spokes of a bicycle wheel intersecting at the axle.
SAD	Source-axis distance is the distance from the source of radiation to the axis of the radiation beam or isocenter (also referred to as *TAD [target-axis distance]*).
TID	Target-image receptor distance is the distance from the target of radiation to the imager.
SSD	Source-skin distance is the distance from the source of radiation to the skin surface of the patient (also referred to as *TSD [target-source distance]*).
Source/focal spot	Geometric point or area where the radiation beam emerges and fans out or diverges as it moves farther from the source, target, or focal spot.

Other acronyms are used by the radiation therapy team during the simulation and treatment process. The more common ones are listed as a reference.

TABLE 21.2 **Key Staff Functions in the Radiation Therapy Process**	
Function	**Team Member(s)**
Diagnosis	Pathologist Referring physician Radiation oncologist
Therapeutic decisions	Radiation oncologist Referring physician
Target volume localization	Radiation oncologist Radiation therapist Dosimetrist Physicist
Simulation and treatment planning	Radiation oncologist Radiation therapist Physicist Dosimetrist
Fabrication of treatment aids	Radiation therapist Dosimetrist
Treatment	Radiation therapist Radiation oncologist Dosimetrist Physicist
Patient evaluation during treatment	Radiation oncologist Radiation therapist Oncology nurse
Patient follow-up	Radiation oncologist Oncology nurse

is part of the treatment planning process and includes both the actual CT scanner and the virtual simulation software, which may reside on the CT simulator or in the treatment planning software (Fig. 21.6).

CT scanners manufactured for oncology have flat couch tops often indexed that mimic the flat therapy couch tops available on the linear accelerator. This allows for the universal use of many immobilization devices between CT and treatment. Some CT units that are also used for diagnostic imaging have couch tops that may have a concave curve. If so, then a flat couch table insert must be placed on the curved couch to simulate the treatment table (Fig. 21.7). The CT scanner may have limitations on the number and type of immobilization devices it can accommodate, depending on the size of the aperture. Scanners designed for CT simulation usually have large or wide bores.

Optimizing the patient position and immobilization device depends on several factors, including the patient's medical condition and treatment technique. Immobilization devices are commercially available and commonly used to aid in patient positioning. Custom devices can also be fabricated by the radiation therapist. Patient position, beam alignment, and the planning volume must be the same at the end of treatment planning as at the beginning of treatment. Policies and procedures should be developed within the radiation therapy department related to the unique issues involved in CT and virtual simulation procedures. Before introducing the many steps involved in the CT simulation process (Box 21.2), some of the benefits and considerations are listed.[10]

Benefits of Computed Tomography Simulation

Once the CT scan is acquired and reconstructed, all anatomic data needed to plan the treatment are readily available. The benefits of CT simulation are as follows[3,7]:
1. Accurate delineation of 3D volumes in the patient's treatment position with the ability to outline tumor volume and critical structures, also known as OAR, and view these structures in three dimensions.
2. The isocenter can be placed quickly and accurately in any location.
3. A virtual patient provides flexibility to create or change any factor of the treatment plan.
4. More information/data for measurements postsimulation.
5. Cone down or boost fields can be accomplished without the patient present (virtual simulation).
6. A BEV display allows anatomy to be viewed from the perspective of the radiation beam.
7. CT simulation allows field shaping electronically at the graphic display station.
8. Virtual simulation allows comparison of beams and construction of DRRs without the patient present.
9. CT simulation allows for downstream calculation and viewing of dose distribution based on patient anatomy.
10. Virtual simulation confers the ability to mitigate intrafraction motion with 4D CT.
11. Simulation results in an easier procedure for the patient because of reduction in procedure time.
12. All information is archived digitally, which facilitates data recovery and streamlines storage.
13. CT exposure can be quantified and recorded.

Considerations of Computed Tomography Simulation
1. The size of the aperture of the CT scanner must be large enough to accommodate patients in the treatment position with complex immobilization devices.
2. Scanning and display fields of view must be large enough so that the patient's entire external contour can be visualized.
3. The patient couch must be flat and level so that the patient position can be replicated in the treatment room, and the couch must travel perpendicular to the bore to ensure that the patient position is accurately reproduced by the CT set in the longitudinal direction.
4. An external marking laser system to localize the isocenter must be present.
5. The time between the start of CT acquisition and patient marking must be minimized to avoid potential patient movement and localization errors.
6. Careful consideration must be taken when CT numbers are used for dose inhomogeneity corrections during dosage calculations.
7. Treatment machine parameters, beam-shaping devices, and treatment accessories such as multileaf collimator (MLC) verification cannot be verified on the CT scanner.
8. Interfraction variability should be reduced by ensuring the patient is comfortable and in a reproducible position.
9. Monitor CT dose.

COMPUTED TOMOGRAPHY SIMULATION PROCEDURES

Virtual simulation is defined as a CT image-based simulation process that uses 2D and 3D reconstructions of the patient. This includes transverse, sagittal, and coronal 2D images, DRRs, and 3D renderings of the patient. Once scans are completed through the area of interest, the information is loaded into the virtual simulation software on the CT scanner, exported to a virtual simulation workstation, or exported to a treatment planning computer via a local area network. Then physicians working with radiation therapists and medical dosimetrists can delineate tumor volume and other critical structures. Isocenter, treatment beams, and beam modifiers can also be established. A boost field can also be

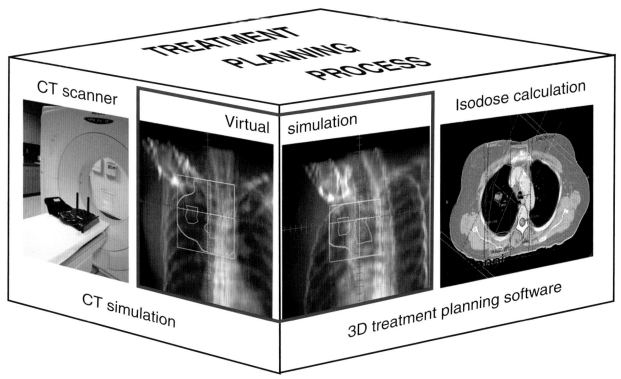

Fig. 21.6 Computed tomography *(CT)* simulation is part of the treatment planning process and includes both the actual CT scanner and the virtual simulation workstation. The treatment planning system includes the virtual simulation workstation and dosage calculation computer. Virtual simulation is defined as the simulation process without the patient actually present. Data are collected from the CT scanning process and then manipulated with the help of the treatment planning software. *3D,* Three-dimensional.

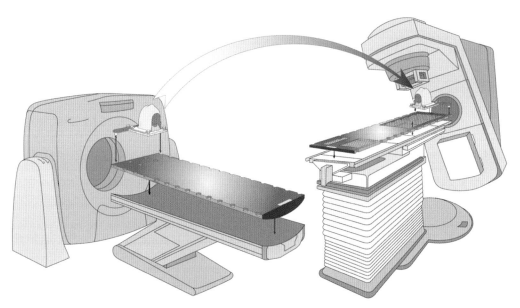

Fig. 21.7 A computed tomography simulator and linear accelerator both demonstrate a thermoplastic mask used primarily to immobilize the head and neck area, indexed to the simulator and treatment couch. Note the small notches along the lateral edge of each tabletop used for indexing the immobilization device. (Courtesy of MED-TEC, Orange City, IA.)

developed and prescribed, based on the patient's reference marks, without the patient present; thus the term virtual simulation is used.

In the following section, specific CT simulation procedures are discussed in detail. The CT simulation process consists of explanation of the procedure to the patient, fabrication and indexing of immobilization devices, CT data acquisition, target and healthy tissue localization, virtual simulation of treatment fields, and marking of the patient.

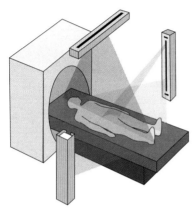

Fig. 21.8 External lasers are used to mark the patient to delineate the treatment area.

Presimulation Planning

The importance of the therapist and physician consultation before the actual simulation cannot be overemphasized. Radiation oncologists, even within the same institution, vary in their approach to simulation and treatment. The physician and therapist should be aware of the limitations of the CT scanner, especially regarding immobilization and patient positioning. Discussion with the patient should also include the time involved for the procedure, patient positioning, and the use of contrast (if applicable). Ideally, an assessment of all relevant patient information and an evaluation of possible treatment approaches is completed before the patient arrives. This is especially true for difficult cases involving patients who have had previous treatment or extensive disease.[12] Minimally, the patient's history and physical examination notes should be reviewed by the radiation oncologist and radiation therapist, along with all other available pertinent information, such as radiographs, PET, CT, and MRI scans, pathology reports, and operative reports.

Patient Positioning

One of the weakest links in treatment planning and treatment delivery is patient positioning.[3] If the patient is not comfortable and does not remain still during treatment administration, then sophisticated treatment plans and elaborate immobilization devices are not as effective.[1] If a stable position cannot be maintained and reproduced daily, the result is a geometric miss of the target volume and irradiation of greater amounts of uninvolved normal tissue.[13] Thus daily reproduction of the prescribed, simulated, and planned treatment is essential to its outcome. A patient's age, weight, and general health, as well as the anatomic area to be simulated, should be taken into consideration to determine the optimal patient position. The positioning of the patient for treatment is usually depicted by a patient alignment system (Fig. 21.8). Three directional lasers, which are projected onto the patient,

accomplish this through the transverse, coronal, and sagittal planes. Usually, India ink tattoos, visual skin marks, or references to topographic anatomy are used to delineate the treatment area on the patient during the simulation procedure.

For most simulation procedures, the patient is positioned supine or prone, usually utilizing an immobilization device that minimizes or prohibits patient movement. Immobilization devices improve the accuracy and reproducibility of treatment setup and delivery, enabling the integrity of a patient's position throughout their course of treatment.

Patient Immobilization

Accuracy and reproducibility of daily setup are essential to reduce possible treatment complications. Small decreases in the absorbed dose of the tumor may make large differences in tumor control. In a similar manner, once the threshold for normal tissue injury has been reached, small increases in dose may greatly increase the risk of complications.[13] Thus the need for accurate patient positioning and the maintenance of that position by immobilization is critical.

Although the need for immobilization is apparent, achieving it is not always simple or easy. Effective immobilization devices constrain the patient from moving during treatment and perform the following functions:

- Aid in daily treatment setup and reproducibility.
- Provide immobilization of the patient or treatment area with minimal discomfort to the patient.
- Support the conditions prescribed in the treatment plan.
- Increase precision and accuracy of treatment.
- May be indexed to the simulation and treatment tabletops.
- Are rigid and durable enough to withstand an entire course of treatment, often as long as 6 to 8 weeks.
- Facilitate the patient's condition and treatment unit limitations.

Immobilization and positioning aids that can be adapted for many patients with minimal modification and that are cost-effective are desirable. The aids need to be made of materials that do not cause CT artifacts.[1] Many newer devices are also MRI compatible with no metal parts.

Devices can usually be broadly divided into three categories: positioning aids, simple immobilization, and complex immobilization.[14] Patient positioning aids are devices designed to place the patient in a particular position for treatment. There is usually very little structure in these devices to ensure that the patient does not move. **Simple immobilization devices** restrict some movement but usually require the patient's voluntary cooperation. **Complex immobilization devices** are individualized immobilizers that are usually constructed for a single patient and that restrict patient movement and ensure reproducibility in positioning.

Positioning aids may be the most commonly used devices in patient setup. In general, they are widely available and easy to use and may be used for more than one patient, thus making them convenient and inexpensive. Most are designed to be comfortable for the patient, which encourages him or her to maintain proper treatment position. These devices will not, however, prevent patient movement during treatment. The patient must be cooperative and fully understand the importance of not moving during setup or treatment for the devices to be effective.

Head holders are probably the most commonly used positioning aid. They are usually made of formed plastic (attenuate less radiation) or molded polyurethane foam. They come in a variety of heights and neck contours. The different heights and contours allow for the desired head and neck angulation (flexion or extension) to achieve the desired treatment position. Couch tops and overlays are available to help facilitate positioning and immobilization devices.

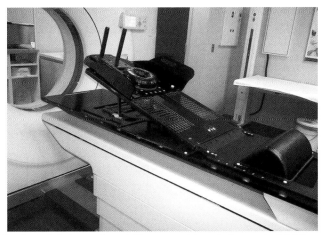

Fig. 21.9 Q-fix breast board. (Courtesy of Angela Darmanin, Middlesex Hospital, Middlesex, CT.)

Patients who must be treated in a prone position may use different versions of a support device such as a prone pillow. A variety of sponge pillows and foam cushions are available. Various sizes and shapes are useful in different treatment positions. Foam cushions and pillows also tend to make patients more comfortable on hard treatment and simulation tables. Comfortable patients are more likely to be cooperative and are better able to maintain treatment position, both of which contribute to setup reproducibility and treatment accuracy.

In addition, other devices used to set up and position specific treatment areas, such as for breast and pelvic treatments, are available. A traditional breast board (Fig. 21.9) may be used to abduct the affected arm and shoulder away from the chest wall and, at the same time, elevate the patient on an adjustable angle board for patient positioning and daily reproducibility. A "wingboard" (Fig. 21.10) is more commonly used to abduct both arms above the patient's head and may be preferred for CT simulation. A "belly board" (Fig. 21.11) is commonly used to treat pelvic malignancies with the patient in the prone position. It has adjustable inserts to accommodate a variety of patients and provides a means of reducing the amount of small bowel in the treatment field.

Simple immobilization devices are commonly used in addition to positioning aids. They typically provide some restriction of movement and stability of treatment position in cooperative patients. However, patients who insist on moving or are unable to remain still because of their disease condition will not be entirely immobilized by these devices.

A very simple and accessible immobilization device is the rubber band. Large rubber bands, approximately 1 to 2 cm in width, can be used to bind the patient's feet together when he or she is in supine position. The bands help to ensure that the legs and feet are consistently in a reproducible position by limiting hip motion or rotation. In choosing to use any simple immobilization device, the radiation therapist must keep the patient in mind. Patients must understand the importance of holding still during treatment and must cooperate with the radiation therapist; otherwise, any simple immobilization device will be ineffective.

Complex immobilization devices are popular because of the increased use of IMRT and stereotactic treatment planning techniques, which demand rigid immobilization. Because each device is individualized, they tend to be more costly. However, the advantages are that unusual patient positions can be achieved, and, in many cases, portal markings can be made on the device, thus limiting the need for patients to keep skin markings or tattoos. Complex immobilization devices can

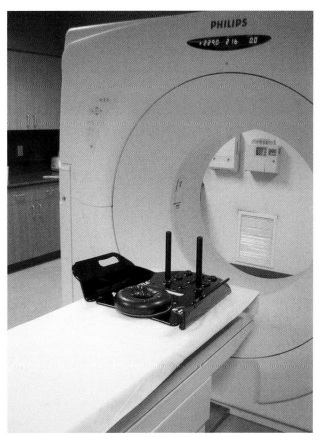

Fig. 21.10 A "wingboard" is used to abduct both arms above the patient's head and may be preferred for computed tomography simulation. (Courtesy of Paula Keogh, Maine Medical Center, Portland, ME.)

be made of a number of different products, such as plaster, carbon fiber, plastic, and polystyrene foam (Styrofoam; Dow Chemical Company). The materials used will depend on the treatment area, the availability of materials, and the individual practitioner's preference.

Use of a foaming agent, such as Alpha Cradle (Smithers Medical Products, Inc, North Danton, OH) (Fig. 21.12) is one method of immobilizing patients. It can be used to immobilize most anatomic areas, such as the head and neck area, thorax, pelvis, and extremities. Before construction for the individualized patient, a shell with a plastic bag or other protective sheeting and a set of foaming agents are set aside. When the foaming agents are combined and placed in the plastic-covered shell, they react chemically and begin to expand. When a patient is positioned in the shell, the foam automatically contours or molds around the patient and hardens. The chemical reaction of the foaming agents produces a small amount of heat, which most patients do not find uncomfortable. One concern with this type of immobilization device is the safe use of the foaming agents. Inappropriate use of the agents and inaccurate disposal of their containers after use could lead to environmental problems, hazardous situations, or both.[15]

Another immobilization device that is currently available is the vacuum cushion (Fig. 21.13). This device consists of a cushion and a vacuum compression pump. The patient is placed into treatment position on a partially inflated cushion. Air in the cushion is partially evacuated until it is semirigid, and the therapist molds it around the area to be immobilized. Once the shape is established, the vacuum procedure is completed until the cushion is completely rigid. Cushions are available in several shapes and sizes to accommodate most anatomic sites. The advantage to using this system is that the cushions can be inflated, cleaned, and reused after a patient has completed his or her treatment

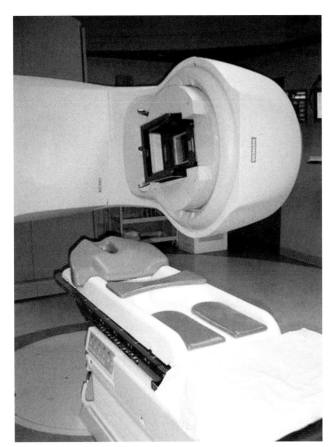

Fig. 21.11 A "belly board" is commonly used to treat patients in the prone position. (Courtesy of Paula Keogh, Maine Medical Center, Portland, ME.)

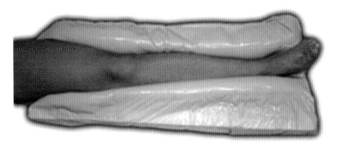

Fig. 21.12 Alpha Cradle. (Reproduced from "Alpha Cradle brand Lower Extremity Form" manufactured and distributed by Smithers Medical Products.)

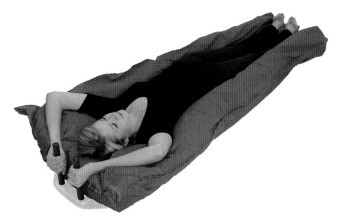

Fig. 21.13 Vacuum mold. (Courtesy Qfix, Avondale, PA.)

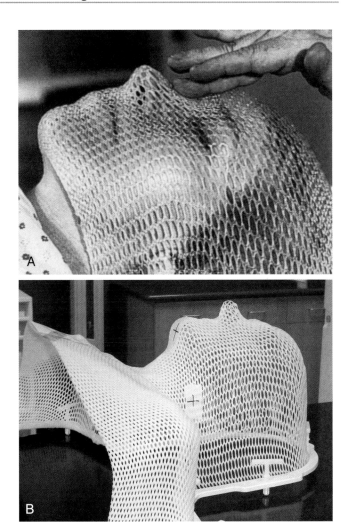

Fig. 21.14 (A) Aquaplast mask. (B) Thermoplastic immobilization device for head and shoulders. (A, Courtesy of WFR/Aquaplast Corporation, Wyckoff, NJ. B, Courtesy of Paula Keogh, Maine Medical Center, Portland, ME.)

course. Vacuum cushions form a custom mold of a patient's anatomic contours, allowing for proper positioning and reproducibility between treatments.

Thermoplastic molds are another commonly used immobilization device (Fig. 21.14). The thermoplastic mold becomes pliable when warmed in a hot water bath. When pliable, it can be shaped around the patient. It is lightweight and easy to use in making immobilization devices, and is very popular for immobilization for head and neck treatment. Use of a thermoplastic mold requires the addition of a headrest and some type of frame to secure the mask on the patient and to the table during setup and treatment. Bite blocks may also be used with a mask to position the chin and move the tongue out of the treatment area. In addition to the headrest, a custom made vacuum bag or moldable cushions for increased immobilization of the head can be used. The customizable cushion contains polystyrene beads in a soft fabric bag which, when activated with water, becomes rigid. Although thermoplastic molds have traditionally been used for immobilization of the head, other uses include the head and shoulders (see Fig. 21.14B), pelvic immobilization, extremities, full body molds, and supports for large breasts and in brachytherapy procedures.

In addition to the immobilization the thermoplastic device provides, patient markings can be made directly on the mask or on tape placed on the mask. The casts may be cut to further increase patient comfort, especially if the mask is tight around the eyes and forehead or if a patient feels claustrophobic. It should be noted, however, that excessive cutting reduces the integrity of this immobilizer. There are currently thermoplastic molds that have an open face area, which avoids the need for cutting. To further position the mouth, a custom bite block can be used when you want to displace the hard palate, mandible, or tongue away from the treatment volume. It can also be used to help maintain the position of the chin. Bite blocks can be made of cork, Aquaplast (Qfix, Avondale, PA) pellets, or dental putty.

Modifications in the mask to accommodate weight loss or reduction in swelling can be made on a completed mask at any time during the course of treatment. A heat gun may be used to heat the problem area until it is pliable, and then changes may be made. Any changes to the mask may require a new CT simulation scan. The devices should be modified only after a discussion with the physician and medical dosimetrist.

Although complex immobilization devices are somewhat time consuming and costly to make, they allow for customized patient positioning options. They typically provide more stability, prevent patient movement, and usually save time in daily treatment procedures, thus justifying the cost for many practitioners.

With the use of record-and-verify systems, tolerances may be set on many of the treatment unit's positions, such as couch height and couch positions in the left/right and inferior/superior directions. Indexing complex immobilization devices, such as thermoplastic immobilization devices and foaming agent devices to the treatment couch, may provide for "tighter" tolerance settings. Specific points may be marked during the simulation process on the immobilization device and will correspond to the relative position of the device located on the treatment couch. In some situations, the immobilization device is secured to the same spot, perhaps through predrilled holes along the lateral length of the tabletop, on both the simulator and treatment couch. During the treatment setup process, the immobilization device is indexed or positioned on the treatment couch in the same position it was in during simulation.

Some of the devices are simple, yet effective, in immobilizing patients. Others are more complex and are made individually for the particular patient. The choice of immobilization devices depends on many considerations, including the condition of the patient, the area to be treated, and the availability and cost of materials. Radiation therapists must be prepared to recommend and use the appropriate device for a particular patient to ensure the best possible treatment outcome for that patient.

Certain accommodations for unique cases and an assessment of the complexity of the simulation procedure are required. It is important to consider the patient's fears and anxieties, especially when performing simulations on small children and others with special needs. For all cases, if a clear treatment approach is known at the beginning of the simulation, the procedure will go more efficiently and accurately, enhancing the patient's confidence in the entire process and reducing the time needed to complete it.[15] The patient should be positioned per direction of the radiation oncologist. All positioning information should be recorded for daily patient setup.

Tips to ensure patient setup reproducibility and quality imaging:
1. The patient must be cooperative and relaxed. This can only occur with good communication. Clearly explain the procedure to the patient.
2. Take extra care to construct an immobilization device to ensure accuracy. Follow manufacturer recommendations for making the immobilization device.
3. Straighten the patient, restraighten, and repeat the topogram (scout) if necessary.

Special Procedure Immobilization

Leksell introduced radiosurgery in 1951. Stereotactic radiosurgery (SRS) consists of narrow beams of radiation that are targeted within the brain to the submillimeter tolerance. The immobilization consisted of a frame that is affixed to the head of the patient's skull, a procedure that is invasive and painful.[11] Currently, there are commercially available frameless immobilization systems for patients who receive SRS (Fig. 21.15).

Another special procedure, stereotactic body radiation therapy (SBRT) immobilization consists of an extended vacuum bag molded specifically for each patient. There is also an abdominal compression device that places pressure on the abdomen to restrict breathing motion, resulting in decreased tumor movement.

Pediatric patient immobilization can be very challenging. Often the pediatric patient will need anesthesia. Immobilization and positioning may need to be altered to accommodate the needs of the anesthesia equipment. Also, there are not many commercially available immobilization devices for the pediatric population. Adult devices that are used with children often lack immobilization, which makes it difficult to reproduce the setup daily.

Room Preparation

Effective use of time on the simulator is essential. Proper room preparation can aid in the effective use of that time. Having all materials readily available, such as a camera to photograph the setup area, markers, small, metal pellet that can be seen in radiographic images, and tape, will ensure efficient use of time. A review of all the pertinent information needed for the simulation procedure allows the therapist to prepare the simulation room in advance. The time demands on the simulator can be pressing; one simulator can serve two or three treatment units. Special attention should be given to the fabrication and registration of immobilization devices because of the aperture (bore) size of the scanner. A large-diameter CT aperture is desired to allow patient positioning that exactly matches the treatment position. Patient immobilization devices should be used that will minimize image artifacts. Each institution has a preferred method to position and immobilize the patient for various setups. Here are some examples.

Head and Neck
- Ensure the patient has removed jewelry.
- Dentures may be removed or kept in, depending on the department protocol.
- A headrest (which can range from A to F) and/or a fabricated custom cushion to position the head should be used. If needed, construct and position a bite block.

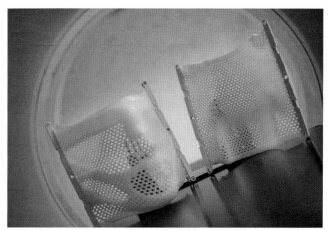

Fig. 21.15 Stereotactic aquaplast mask. (Courtesy of Shahzeb Ahmad, Hartford Hospital, Hartford, CT.)

- Straighten the patient's head by using outer canthus or external auditory meatus. Mark the patient on the head and chest for positioning reference. Place reference marks on the head and neck to ensure the patient maintains position during immobilization fabrication. CT topograms can be used to confirm patient positioning before creating immobilization devices.
- Create a thermoplastic mask, taking great care to ensure the patient's head remains straight. Mold the mask around the patient's nose, chin, and head. Follow the manufacturer's instructions. Allow the mask to cool, following the provided instructions. Some institutions briefly remove the mask before the scan in order for it to cool completely. Use of moist towels applied to the mask will reduce the cooling time. Place CT radiopaque skin markers, designed for CT, as reference marks and additional marks if needed to visualize a surgical scar or area of interest. These will be seen on the CT scan without causing major artifacts.
- Pull straps or some other mechanism can be used to pull or push the top of the patient's shoulders down inferiorly and out of the treatment field. The primary purpose is to move the patient's shoulders out of lateral head and neck fields.

Thorax

- Position the patient with his or her arms overhead on a wing board with a headrest. Often used is the B headrest, which positions the head in a neutral position, or a C headrest may be used to elevate the chin.
- An Alpha Cradle or vacuum bag may be used to provide additional support/positioning of the patient's arms.
- A knee sponge is usually used for patient comfort.
- Straighten the patient by using the suprasternal notch and xiphoid tip. Perform a topogram to ensure straightness. Repeat if necessary.
- Because the patient generally receives part of the treatment through the treatment couch from a direct posterior field or posterior oblique portals, a table pad is not recommended. A cushion on the table may interfere with reproducibility and beam attenuation. If the patient is in severe pain, accommodations requiring a pad or cushion during treatment and simulation can be calculated.

Supine Pelvis

- Ensure patients have followed the instructions before the sim.
- Patients may have been instructed to have a full bladder to help move the small bowel out of the irradiated volume or an empty bladder to reduce the treatment volume.
- Position the patient with a comfortable support under his or her head and with the hands on chest folded or holding a foam ring.
- Immobilize the patient's legs with an Alpha Cradle, vacuum bag, or a rubber band around the feet to immobilize the lower extremities.
- Patients with tumors in the lower pelvis such as anus, vagina, vulva, or inguinal node involvement should be positioned with frog legs. This will eliminate skin folds and allow for better visualization of the target area.
- Straighten the patient. Perform a topogram to ensure straightness. Repeat if necessary.
- Contrast agents can be used to visualize the small bowel, large intestine, bladder, or rectum. Oral contrast to enhance the small bowel would be given several hours before the exam.
- Radiopaque markers may be placed on the inferior-most extension of the target area or on lymph nodes.

Prone Pelvis

- Position the patient on a belly board with a prone pillow. This will help displace the small bowel and minimize treatment side effects.

- Record the indexed position of the patient on the belly board. If this does not occur, the small bowel may be pushed into the field, or dosimetric variations can occur because of a change in patient positioning.
- Straighten the patient. Perform a topogram to ensure straightness. Repeat if necessary.

Breast

- Position the patient with one or both arms up. Use a breast board, wing board, or other device for arm immobilization and reproducibility. If using a breast board, the angle should be selected to prevent the breast from falling superiorly. The head is turned toward the unaffected side.
- The physician or therapist may outline breast tissue and mark the scar with radiopaque markers.
- Straighten the patient by using the suprasternal notch and xiphoid tip. Perform a topogram to ensure straightness. Repeat if necessary.
- A knee sponge is usually used for patient comfort.
- Women with large pendulous breasts pose a challenge. Eliminate the skin folds in the inframammary area by using a breast cup or ring. Another option is using the prone position.

Establishing a definite treatment approach at the beginning of the simulation procedure allows the process to proceed more efficiently and accurately. The patient gains confidence in the radiation therapy staff when the first impression of the department is positive. This can be enhanced if the simulation procedure is professional, accurate, organized, and not rushed. It also provides an opportunity to educate the patient and answer questions concerning the treatment process, side effects, and skin care.

Explanation of Simulation Procedure

Patients should be instructed on how to change and to remove all metallic objects, including jewelry, dentures, eyeglasses, and hair accessories, from the area of interest. Simulation time may also vary depending on the institution and the needs of the patient. It is possible to complete the patient portion of the simulation (data acquisition and marking) in 20 to 60 minutes. Patients should be told the purpose of the procedure and to remain still and breathe normally. Depending on the area that is treated and the treatment type, patients may be asked to hold their breath during a scan. Scans may be done at full inhalation and at full exhalation. This is a simple version of creating a 4D CT. They should be assured that visible and audible monitoring will take place during the scanning process even though the therapist is not in the room. They should also be told that the table will move during the procedure and, if contrast is administered, that they may experience a metallic taste in their mouth and/or a warm, flushing sensation throughout their body.

Assessment. The therapist must assess the patient's needs, recognize cultural differences, respond to nonverbal communication, and then attempt to communicate therapeutically and effectively with the patient.

The radiation therapist should assess the patient's physical condition and emotional state to determine whether the patient is nervous, fearful, or withdrawn. If a patient requires oxygen or medications, or has difficulty standing, sitting, or walking, the therapist can try to make the patient more comfortable. If a patient has difficulty hearing or speaking, provisions can also be made. Good observation and listening skills are essential to proper patient assessment.

Communication. Our entire healthcare system is based on effective communication. Miscommunication can have a major effect on the patient's care. If there are distractions in the area, such as unwanted noises or the usual distractions of a radiation oncology department, it may be preferable to retreat to a private area to communicate with the patient (the simulator room is much better for this than a busy waiting room). Radiation therapists must establish an environment where they can facilitate communication clearly, effectively, and therapeutically. Before the simulation procedure, the therapist should explain the procedure in a manner appropriate to the patient's level of understanding and inform the patient what will be required of him or her during the procedure. This should be done in a professionally responsible and compassionate manner.

Educating the Patient and Family. Professionally, the radiation therapist is obligated to educate the patient not only about the physical aspects of radiation therapy that the patient can see and feel but also about the emotional aspects of radiation therapy. The simulation treatment procedure should be explained in detail. This explanation should be done slowly and clearly, with use of all therapeutic communication techniques. The equipment must be explained to the patient. It is helpful to mention that the simulation is not an actual treatment and that the simulator is a CT scanner, not a therapeutic treatment machine. The patient should be shown where he or she will lie on the table, which way the head should be placed, whether the patient will be supine or prone, and the positioning/immobilization devices chosen for the procedure. Basic patient positioning should be communicated along with an explanation of why that position is needed. This explanation facilitates patient cooperation.

The patient should also be given an explanation of what procedures will follow after the simulation. This might include instructions on how to take care of the skin marks, as well as the skin itself, before the treatments begin and throughout the course of treatment. Any special instructions that the patient must follow before he or she receives treatment, such as arriving for treatment with a full or empty bladder, should be communicated at this time. When barium (oral or rectal) is used during the simulation, follow-up instructions are needed. An appointment time for the first treatment should be discussed and established. The therapist's name and department number should be provided in case communication is necessary before the next appointment.

CONTRAST AGENTS

When performing CT, contrast media may be used to help differentiate anatomic structures or highlight an abnormality. Contrast can be administered into the body via four methods: intravascularly (intravenously [IV]), orally, intrathecally, or intraarteriorly. The most common methods of administration contrast during CT simulation are oral, IV, and intracavitary.[16]

Medical History

Before any contrast media is injected into the patient, a thorough medical history must be obtained to evaluate the possibility of an adverse reaction to contrast media.[16] Patients receiving contrast media usually complete a questionnaire or are asked several questions to determine whether they have a rare allergy to the contrast agent and are at risk for any side effects, some of which may be minor and some of which may be life-threatening (Box 21.3).

A common agent used to localize the gastrointestinal tract is barium sulfate. Barium is not water soluble. Therefore patients with a high risk of gastrointestinal perforation would not receive barium sulfate and instead would receive an aqueous iodinated agent such as diatrizoate meglumine and diatrizoate sodium (Gastrograffin, Bracco Diagnostic Inc.). Both can be administered orally or rectally. Table 21.3 lists the factors that increase the risk for an adverse reaction to contrast agents.[1]

BOX 21.3 Administration of Intravenous Contrast Sample Questionnaire

1. Have you ever received iodinated contrast media before?
2. Have you ever had a reaction to iodinated contrast media?
3. Do you have any allergies to food or medications?
4. Do you have any of the following conditions?
   - Allergies (Have you had an allergic reaction to contrast in the past?)
   - Asthma
   - Kidney problems
   - Cardiac disease
   - Diabetes
   - High blood pressure
   - Sickle cell anemia
   - Multiple myeloma
   - Pheochromocytoma
5. Is there any chance that you are pregnant?
6. Have you had anything to eat or drink within the last 4 hours?

TABLE 21.3 Patient History Factors in Barium Sulfate Examinations

Factor	Importance
Age	Ability to communicate, hear, and follow directions ↑ Risk of colon perforation caused by loss of tissue tone
Diverticulitis or ulcerative colitis	↑ Difficulty in holding an enema ↑ Risk of colon perforation
Long-term steroid therapy	↑ Risk of colon perforation
Colon biopsy within previous 2 weeks	Lower gastrointestinal series contraindicated
Mental retardation, confusion, or dizziness	↑ Risk of aspiration during upper gastrointestinal series
Recent onset of constipation or diarrhea	↑ Risk of colon perforation or tumor rupture
Nausea and vomiting	↑ Risk of aspiration during upper gastrointestinal series

↑, Increased.
From Adler AM, Carlton RR. *Introduction to Radiologic Sciences and Patient Care.* 6th ed. St. Louis, MO: Saunders; 2016.

Patients with risk factors for receiving IV contrast are patients who are older than 60 years, are diabetic, have impaired kidney function, have a history of hypertension, or have had a reaction to contrast in the past.[17] Patients at high risk may need to receive bloodwork to evaluate kidney function before their simulation session. Creatinine levels and/or estimated glomerular filtration rate (EGFR) are obtained to assess the patient's kidney function. If the patient's creatinine is near an unsafe level or the EGFR is less than 60, the amount of contrast that is necessary would be decreased or not given to the patient. In some patients, the administration of iodinated contrast media can cause kidney damage and require temporary or permanent dialysis. This may be more likely in patients with an elevated creatinine level. The risk may be reduced in some patients by using a low-osmolality contrast medium.

TABLE 21.4 Patient History Factors in Water-Soluble Iodine Contrast Examinations

Factors	Importance
Age	↑ Risk with increased age
Allergies or asthma	↑ Risk of allergic-like reactions
Diabetes	Insulin usually given before procedure; these patients should be scheduled before others
Coronary artery disease	↑ Risk of tachycardia, bradycardia, hypertension, myocardial infarction (heart attack)
Hypertension	Hypertension with tachycardia
Renal disease	Inform physician if creatinine level is higher than 1.4 mg/dL
Multiple myeloma	Abnormal protein binds with contrast and can cause renal failure Patients must be hydrated
Confusion or dizziness	Blood-brain barrier effects
Sickle cell anemia or family history of chronic obstructive pulmonary disease	↑ Risk of blood clots ↑ Risk of dyspnea (difficulty in breathing)
Previous iodine contrast examinations	Did the patient have difficulties with procedure?
History of blood clots	↑ Risk of blood clots
Use of beta-blockers	↑ Risk of anaphylactoid reactions
Use of calcium channel blockers	↑ Risk of heart block
Use of metformin (Glucophage)	↑ Risk of lactic acidosis if renal failure occurs

↑, Increased.
From Adler AM, Carlton RR. *Introduction to Radiologic Sciences and Patient Care.* 6th ed. St. Louis, MO: Saunders; 2016.

IV contrast can be ionic iodine or nonionic iodine. Ionic iodine contrast media have a high osmolality, which is a measure of the total number of particles in solution per kilogram of water.[16] When contrast media is injected into the blood vessel, the ionic contrast media has an effect of displacing water in the body. Through osmosis, water moves from the body cells into the vascular system, causing hypervolemia and vessel dilation. The high osmolality of contrast media attracts water to move into blood vessels. This produces pain and discomfort and may cause a decrease in blood pressure because of vessel dilation or may increase blood pressure because of hypervolemia.[16] If a patient is dehydrated, the decreased body cell volume can result in shock. Use of a lower-osmolality substance such as nonionic iodine decreases the risk of these side effects. Adverse reactions have rarely been seen when nonionic substances are used. However, a careful medical history needs to be taken. A list of patient history factors is given in Table 21.4.[16]

IV contrast is usually an iodine-based solution injected into the vein by using a power-assisted injector, or it may simply be hand injected by using a syringe. A power injector allows the contrast to be delivered at a rapid, consistent rate during the CT scan. The nonionic contrast often comes in prefilled vials specifically made for the power injector. Injection of contrast media at a rapid rate can be painful for the patient because of the viscosity (thickness of substance) of the contrast media concentration and the size of the molecule. Heating the contrast media

BOX 21.4 Steps for Using a Power Injector

1. Check to be sure the patient questionnaire was completed. Note any precautions as stated by the therapist, nurse or physician.
2. Have an anaphylactic kit on hand.
3. Retrieve appropriate contrast media from warmer.
4. Check expiration date of contrast to be injected. Do not use if expired.
5. Place syringe in power injector according to manufacturer specifications.
   a. Remove covering of syringe. The tip of the syringe is sterile. Connect tubing to syringe by using sterile technique.
   b. Remove air in syringe and intravenous line.
   c. Connect to patient's intravenous site.
6. Position and immobilize patient.
   a. Select protocol for rate and amount of contrast to be injected. These are often predetermined based on the protocol for the department.
   b. If a smaller needle was used in the patient, the rate of administration is decreased.
7. Prepare scanner. Do not begin scan yet.
8. Begin power injection.
   a. Depending on what needs to be visualized, the scan will begin as dictated by the physician.
   b. Some departments will not inject the contrast unless a physician or nurse is present.

to body temperature in a warmer reduces viscosity and facilitates rapid injection.[2] Many departments will discard the contrast media if it has been in the warmer for as long as 30 days and has not been used. Box 21.4 lists the steps necessary to connect the power injector.

Once the iodine-based liquid is injected, it causes many organs and structures, such as the kidneys and blood vessels, to become much more visible on the CT scan. While CT images are acquired, the beam of radiation is attenuated or absorbed while it passes through the blood vessels and organs filled with the high-density contrast agent. This causes the blood vessels and organs containing the contrast to "enhance" and show up as white areas on the CT images.

Contrast media are often manufactured specifically for CT. High-atomic number contrast media can create star artifacts on the CT scans (artifacts are discussed in Chapter 6). Usually between 30 and 100 mL of contrast is used for a CT simulation examination, depending mostly on the patient's age and weight. Some centers may use a chart based on the patient's weight to determine a more specific dose. For example, smaller patients may receive 75 mL, and larger patients may receive 150 mL of the iodinated contrast for their examination. Once the contrast media is administered, patients should be monitored for side effects. Some 70% of adverse reactions occur within 5 minutes; most others occur within 30 minutes.[16] High-risk patients should be monitored for longer than 30 minutes. The most common reaction is a feeling of warmth and discomfort at the injection site. Box 21.5 lists categories of reactions, and Box 21.6 states how to manage the acute reactions to contrast media.

Contrast is often used to enhance structures in patients with a specific pathology, such as head and neck, lung, brain, abdominal, and pelvic tumors.[15] Timing of the contrast injection is critical. It may be injected before the scan or during the scan, depending on what area of the body must be visualized. The following section discusses sites where contrast is most commonly administered during CT simulation, the contrast used, and how and when it is administered.

Head and Neck and Lung. In patients with head and neck cancer and lung tumors, contrast may be administered with a power injector, often just seconds before the scan. The purpose of the contrast is to highlight

BOX 21.5 Categories of Reactions to Contrast Media

Mild

Signs and symptoms are self-limited without evidence of progression. Mild reactions include:

Allergic-Like

Limited urticaria/pruritis
Limited cutaneous edema
Limited "itchy"/"scratchy" throat
Nasal congestion
Sneezing/conjunctivitis/rhinorrhea

Physiologic

Limited nausea/vomiting
Transient flushing/warmth/chills
Headache/dizziness/anxiety/altered taste
Mild hypertension
Vasovagal reaction that resolves spontaneously
Treatment: Requires observation to confirm resolution and/or lack of progression but usually no treatment. Patient reassurance is usually helpful.

Moderate

Signs and symptoms are more pronounced and commonly require medical management. Some of these reactions have the potential to become severe if not treated. Moderate reactions include:

Allergic-Like

Diffuse urticaria/pruritis
Diffuse erythema, stable vital signs
Facial edema without dyspnea
Throat tightness or hoarseness without dyspnea
  Wheezing/bronchospasm, mild or no hypoxia

Physiologic

Protracted nausea/vomiting
Hypertensive urgency

Isolated chest pain
Vasovagal reaction that requires and is responsive to treatment
  Treatment: Clinical findings should be considered as indications for immediate treatment. These situations require close, careful observation for possible progression to a life-threatening event.

Severe

Signs and symptoms are often life-threatening and can result in permanent morbidity or death if not managed appropriately.
Cardiopulmonary arrest is a nonspecific end-stage result that can be caused by a variety of the following severe reactions, both allergic-like and physiologic. If it is unclear what etiology caused the cardiopulmonary arrest, it may be judicious to assume that the reaction is/was an allergic-like one.
Pulmonary edema is a rare severe reaction that can occur in patients with tenuous cardiac reserve (cardiogenic pulmonary edema) or in patients with normal cardiac function (noncardiogenic pulmonary edema). Noncardiogenic pulmonary edema can be allergic-like or physiologic; if the etiology is unclear, it may be judicious to assume that the reaction is/was an allergic-like one.
Severe reactions include:

Allergic-Like

Diffuse edema, or facial edema with dyspnea
Diffuse erythema with hypotension
Laryngeal edema with stridor and/or hypoxia
Wheezing/bronchospasm, significant hypoxia
Anaphylactic shock (hypotension + tachycardia)

Physiologic

Vasovagal reaction resistant to treatment
Arrhythmia
Convulsions, seizures
Hypertensive emergency
  Treatment: Requires *prompt* recognition and treatment; almost always requires hospitalization.

From American College of Radiology. *Manual on Contrast Media*, version 10.3, 2018. https://www.acr.org/Clinical-Resources/Contrast-Manual. Accessed October 29, 2019.

---

the vessels and distinguish them from lymph nodes or a mass.[5] Injection of contrast immediately before the scan allows the images to be captured when the contrast is in the vessels.

Brain. IV contrast is administered 10 to 30 minutes before the scan through an IV push. Because tumors are usually more vascular than normal anatomy, contrast media will highlight the tumor more than the normal structures.

Abdomen: Liver. The power injector may also be used if the physician would like to enhance some of the blood vessels in and around the liver, which has dual blood supply from both the portal vein and the hepatic artery. Scanning that occurs approximately 20 to 40 seconds after the initiation of the injection will visualize the hepatic arterial phase. The venous phase occurs from 60 to 90 seconds after the start of the injection. If scanning occurs after the portal venous phase, then many hepatic tumors may not be visualized on the images.[16] A higher flow rate (rate of contrast injection) may be used to administer the contrast more quickly.

Pelvis. In some patients with prostate tumors, a delayed scan may be required. IV contrast would be administered before the scan through

an IV push. Allowing a minimum of 15 minutes after the injection will allow the contrast to filter through the heart and blood vessels to the bladder to allow better visualization of the pelvic anatomy.[16,18] To visualize the rectum, a radiopaque marker can be placed in or near these structures. Sometimes barium is given several hours before the examination to allow visualization of the small bowel.

Gastrointestinal Tumors. A barium paste can be used to coat the esophagus. Dilute barium sulfate solution, if there is no concern of perforation, will highlight the stomach or small bowel during an abdominal CT scan. If the physician would like to see the small bowel, the patient is given the barium a minimum of 30 to 60 minutes before the simulation.

When scanning a patient for treatment planning, some radiation oncologists prefer to minimize the use of contrast agents because the image of the contrast on the scan may alter dose calculations and cause certain structures to appear more dense than they really are. Inaccurate dose calculations could occur because some treatment planning systems may interpret the area of contrast, registering a high Hounsfield unit (HU) similar to bone, that would attenuate the beam more than it would the actual soft tissue that is highlighted by the contrast. If contrast is used, then a CT scan can be performed without contrast and

---

BOX 21.6   Management of Acute Reactions to Contrast Media in Adults

Urticaria (Hives)

1. Discontinue injection if not completed
2. No treatment needed in most cases
3. Give histamine (H_1)-receptor blocker, diphenhydramine (Benadryl) PO/IM/IV, 25–50 mg
4. If severe or widely disseminated, α-agonist (arteriolar and venous constriction)
5. Epinephrine SC (1:1000), 0.1–0.3 mL (0.1–0.3 mg) (if no cardiac contraindications)

Facial or Laryngeal Edema

1. Give α-agonist (arteriolar and venous constriction), epinephrine IM (1:1,000) 0.1–0.3 mL (0.1–0.3 mg) or, if hypotension is evident, epinephrine (1:10,000) slowly by IV, 1 mL (0.1 mg)
2. Repeat as needed to a maximum of 1 mg
3. Give O_2, 6–10 L/min (via mask)

   If patient is not responsive to therapy or if there is obvious acute laryngeal edema, seek appropriate assistance (e.g., a cardiopulmonary arrest response team)

Bronchospasm

1. Give O_2, 6–10 L/min (via mask)
2. Monitor electrocardiogram, O_2 saturation (pulse oximeter), and blood pressure
3. Give β-agonist inhalers (bronchiolar dilators, such as metaproterenol [Alupent], terbutaline [Brethaire], or albuterol [Proventil, Ventolin]) 2–3 puffs; repeat prn. If patient is unresponsive to inhalers, use subcutaneous (SC), IM, or IV epinephrine
4. Give epinephrine SC or IM (1:1000), 0.1–0.3 mL (0.1–0.3 mg) or, if hypotension is evident, administer epinephrine (1:10,000), slowly via IV, 1 mL (0.1 mg)
5. Repeat as needed to a maximum of 1 mg

   Call for assistance (e.g., cardiopulmonary arrest response team) for severe bronchospasm or if O_2 saturation <88% persists

Hypotension With Tachycardia

1. Ensure patient's legs are elevated 60 degrees or more (preferred) or in the Trendelenburg position
2. Monitor electrocardiogram, pulse oximeter, and blood pressure
3. Give O_2, 6–10 L/min (via mask)
4. Rapid IV administration of large volumes of isotonic lactated Ringer or normal saline

If patient is poorly responsive: administer epinephrine (1:10,000), slowly by IV, 1 mL (0.1 mg)

   Repeat as needed to a maximum of 1 mg

   If patient is still poorly responsive, seek appropriate assistance (e.g., cardiopulmonary arrest response team)

Hypotension With Bradycardia (Vagal Reaction)

1. Monitor vital signs
2. Ensure patient's legs are elevated 60 degrees or more (preferred) or in the Trendelenburg position
3. Secure airway, give O_2, 6–10 L/min (via mask)
4. Secure IV access, rapid administration of lactated Ringer or normal saline
5. Give atropine, 0.6–1 mg, by IV slowly if patient does not respond quickly to steps 2 through 4
6. Repeat atropine to a total dose of 0.04 mg/kg (2–3 mg) in adults
7. Ensure complete resolution of hypotension and bradycardia before discharge

Hypertension, Severe

1. Give O_2, 6–10 L/min (via mask)
2. Monitor electrocardiogram, pulse oximeter, and blood pressure
3. Give nitroglycerin, 0.4-mg tablet, sublingual (may repeat 3×), or topical 2% ointment, apply 1-inch strip
4. If no response, consider labetalol 20 mg IV, then 20–80 mg IV, q10 min to 300 mg
5. Transfer to intensive care unit or emergency department

Seizures or Convulsions

1. Give O_2, 6–10 L/min (via mask)
2. Consider diazepam (Valium), 5 mg IV (or more, as appropriate), or midazolam (Versed), 0.5–1 mg IV
3. If longer effect needed, obtain consultation; consider Lorazepam infusion, IV 2–4 mg; administer slowly, to maximum dose of 4 mg
4. Careful monitoring of vital signs required, particularly of PO_2 because of risk of respiratory depression with benzodiazepine administration
5. Consider use of cardiopulmonary arrest response team for intubation if needed

Pulmonary Edema

1. Elevate patient's torso
2. Give O_2, 6–10 L/min (via mask)
3. Give diuretics: furosemide (Lasix), 20–40 mg IV, slow push
4. Transfer to intensive care unit or emergency department

IM, Intramuscular; *IV,* intravenous; *PO,* orally; *PO_2,* partial pressure of oxygen; *prn,* as needed; *q10min,* every 10 minutes; *SC,* subcutaneous. From American College of Radiology. *Manual on Contrast Media,* version 10.3, 2018. https://www.acr.org/Clinical-Resources/Contrast-Manual.

---

then repeated with contrast. Another option is for the dosimetrist, at the direction of the physician, to contour the structures outlined by the contrast and change the HU to one for that structure. Contrast media and markers must have a low atomic number to reduce the effects of unwanted artifacts on the image. There are many commercially available contrast media and markers developed specifically for CT scanning. A summary of contrast materials used is listed in Table 21.5.

Important points to remember:
- Have patients complete a questionnaire to identify any risk of a reaction to contrast.
- Ensure patients have fasted if necessary.
- Perform a CT scan without contrast and complete again with contrast for treatment planning purposes.

PATIENT POSITIONING IN THE COMPUTED TOMOGRAPHY SCANNER

The transfer of information, such as the exact location of immobilization devices from simulation to the treatment machine, is improved when devices are referenced or indexed to the treatment table. The patient and immobilization device are then "locked" into place on the treatment table to recreate the patient position on the CT simulator.

The patient should be positioned carefully so that the area of interest/treatment is in the center of the CT bore and scan field of view, which is the area for which projection data are collected for a CT scan. This will help to eliminate image artifacts, provide the best image quality, and ensure the field of view (FOV) encompasses the entire external patient contour. Positioning the patient in the center of the bore also yields lower radiation dose delivery to the patient.

TABLE 21.5	**Summary of Use of Contrast Media**			
Area	Contrast	Method of Administration	Patient Preparation	Timing of Administration
Lung, head, and neck	Ionic or nonionic	IV	NPO 4 hours before exam	Seconds before scan
Pelvis	Markers Barium	Placed in rectum/vagina Oral	None	Placed in orifice before scan
Brain	Ionic or nonionic	IV	NPO 4 hours before exam	10–30 minutes before scan
Prostate	Ionic or nonionic	IV	NPO 4 hours before exam	
GI visualization	Diluted barium	Oral	Drink 30 minutes before scan	

GI, Gastrointestinal; *IV,* intravenous; *NPO,* nothing by mouth.

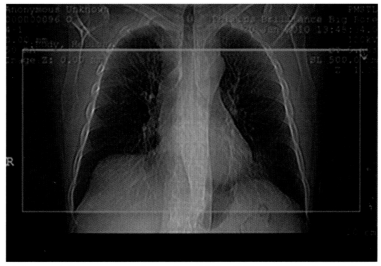

Fig. 21.16 Anteroposterior topograms. (Image from Philips Brilliance CT Big Bore, Philips Healthcare.)

For diagnostic CT imaging, it is common practice to offset the FOV during CT planning to include the area of interest when the patient is not well centered within the CT bore. FOV offsets can be incompatible with some of the commercially available external laser marking systems and are not suggested during CT planning for radiation therapy.

Initially, the patient should be clinically straightened by using the external laser system and any useful topographic anatomy. With use of the lasers, temporary reference marks can be drawn on the patient. These marks may be used later in the simulation process as a reference to check patient positioning or help place fiducials after topograms are acquired (if fiducial marks are required by the virtual simulation software).

Before beginning the scan, the radiation therapist should check that any immobilization or positioning devices and the patient will travel through the aperture (bore) of the CT scanner with sufficient clearance. For example, a patient treated for breast cancer with a steep slope may need an angle board for treatment. Depending on the type and angle of the breast board, the patient position, and the immobilization device used, the patient may not fit into the scanner without collision.

COMPUTED TOMOGRAPHY TOPOGRAMS

Topogram scans (e.g., surviews, pilots, scouts, scanogram images) are typically the first images acquired during the CT simulation procedure. Commonly an AP scan, lateral scan, or both, are taken.[1] The radiation therapist collaborates with the radiation oncologist to define the area to be imaged and the length of the topogram. Topograms are used to assess alignment of the patient in the CT bore (Fig. 21.16). Geometric tools such as image

length crosshairs or grids are usually available in the scanner software to aid in patient adjustment and alignment, to ensure the patient is straight and centered into the bore properly. The topogram scans are also the images that will be used to plan the actual helical or axial CT scan start and end positions superiorly and inferiorly. Modern CT scanners designed for radiation therapy allow multiple topograms to be taken, so, if desired, the patient can be repositioned between images. During the acquisition of these images, the x-ray tube is stationary, and the table moves through the gantry. After topogram images are taken and the patient is aligned properly, the radiation therapist can use the external laser system to place fiducial marks (reference BBs) on the patient in a stable location (if required by the virtual simulation software/treatment planning system) and plan the CT scan that will be used for the virtual simulation.

COMPUTED TOMOGRAPHY DATA ACQUISITION

Almost all CT scanners designed today for CT simulation are multislice units, all of which are capable of helical (or spiral) and axial scanning. Helical, or volume, scanning greatly reduces scan time, and today's reconstructed helical images are comparable in image quality to those acquired in axial mode. Most CT simulation scanning protocols use a helical acquisition to reduce the amount of time the patient is on the table during the simulation procedure. Actual scan time for a routine helical CT is just a few seconds, and the images reconstruct almost instantly, allowing for quick image launch into CT simulation software and export to a CT simulation workstation or treatment planning system with simulation capabilities. Today's gold standard, multislice helical scanning, will be discussed in the following paragraphs.

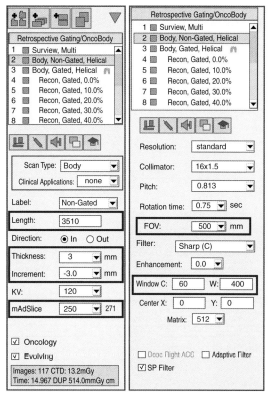

Fig. 21.17 Brilliance CT Big Bore (Phillips) protocol parameters. Commonly adjusted parameters may include mAs, slice thickness, slice increment, window level, window width, and scan length.

The first step of the multislice helical scanning process is to manually enter or load patient demographics. Next, position and immobilize the patient as described above and give ample time for the patient to relax on the CT couch. This will ensure daily treatment setup will better match the simulated position.

A scan protocol that contains topograms, helical scans, and their associated scan parameters should be selected. Protocols are typically site specific and may be modified as needed. Common protocol parameters include kilovolt peak (kVp), mAs, display FOV (DFOV), pitch, resolution, slice thickness, slice increment, rotation speed, scan length, filters, window level (represents the central HU of all the CT numbers), window width (range of numbers displayed or the contrast on a CT image), dose savings techniques, collimation, and image matrix (see Chapter 6 for a detailed descriptions of these parameters). Parameters may be adjusted based on patient size and area of interest. Commonly adjusted parameters may include mAs, slice thickness, slice increment, DFOV, window level, window width, and scan length. For example, the mAs may be preset by the selected protocol but may be modified to accommodate the size of the patient.

Slice thickness is important, especially as it relates to treatment planning. Three-dimensional conformal and IMRT treatment planning may require a slice thickness of 2 to 3 mm, although more complex cases such as SBRT or SRS may require 2 mm or less. Slice increment also tends to match slice thickness, yielding a contiguous scan as opposed to a diagnostic CT scan, which may have slices that overlap. Default scanning protocols may also contain preset DFOV settings. The DFOV should be closely evaluated and optimized to ensure that the patient surface is not clipped in the scan while keeping the DFOV as small as possible to ensure optimal image quality (Fig. 21.17).

When planning the helical CT scan on the acquired topograms, the radiation therapist works with the radiation oncologist and medical dosimetrist to ensure the scan will cover the area of interest and include enough additional anatomy to ensure proper coverage for the treatment plan. The treatment planning system typically requires data (patient anatomy) 5 to 10 cm beyond treatment beam borders for scatter calculation. Care must also be taken to ensure that the entire head is scanned if included in the treatment area. This is best done by acquiring at least one or more slices in air superior to the patient's vertex. These techniques also allow the treatment planner to use noncoplanar beams, if necessary, to satisfy treatment planning protocol criteria.

For treatment planning, a primary CT data set is acquired for dose calculation. As previously mentioned, the initial scan is free of contrast media for dosimetric reasons. After this, contrast may be administered if requested by the physician for additional image acquisitions. Secondary image data sets such as contrast CT, MRI, PET, and SPECT images are used to assist in target delineation once registered and fused to the primary image set in the simulation software or treatment planning system.

> Note: If a contrast computed tomography (CT) is to be used as the primary data set for dose computation, care must be taken by the dosimetrist to apply appropriate tissue corrections in the treatment planning system.

Once the CT images have been acquired and reconstructed, they are then exported via digital imaging and communications in medicine (DICOM) and imported into a virtual simulation workstation, treatment planning system, or simulation software that may reside on the CT console.

METHODS OF SIMULATION WITH COMPUTED TOMOGRAPHY IMAGES

During CT imaging for radiation therapy treatment planning, a set of reference or setup marks should be placed on the patient so the treatment position can be later reproduced at the treatment machine. The workflow to establish the location of these patient setup marks can be described as "shift" and "no-shift" methods.[18] Both methods will be discussed in the following section. Department resources and physician preference typically determine which method is used. These methods are outlined in Box 21.7. For the shift and no-shift simulation methods, a set of reference marks should be placed on the patient so the treatment position can be reproduced later at the treatment machine.[19]

Shift method: This method is based on a procedure in which the reference marks are placed on the patient before the CT scan in a somewhat arbitrary location that is close to the desired anatomic treatment isocenter. The reference point placement can be based on the therapist's understanding of the diagnostic workup (e.g., CT, MRI, PET, palpation) or the physician's instructions. After the CT scan, the patient can go home, and the images are transferred to the treatment planning workstation. Later, the physician contours the target volumes and determines the treatment isocenter coordinates. Shifts (distances in three directions) between the reference marks placed on the patient while he or she was on the CT scanner and the treatment isocenter are then calculated. On the first day of treatment, the patient is positioned to the initial reference marks and then *shifted* to the new treatment isocenter by using the calculated shifts from the treatment plan. Initial reference marks are then removed, and the new treatment isocenter is marked on the patient.[19,20] This process is illustrated in Fig. 21.18. These shifts can introduce uncertainties in patient treatment because of inexact shifting and patient remarking, or occasionally because of incorrect shifts. Once there are incorrect shifts, exact corrections are very difficult to determine, and some residual error inevitably remains. Additionally, this process can be inefficient, as the patient has to be

BOX 21.7 Summary of Computed Tomography Simulation Major Steps

No-Shift Method	Shift Method
During Simulation Planning	**During Simulation Planning**
• Explanation of procedure	• Explanation of procedure
• Straighten patient	• Straighten patient
• Immobilization and positioning	• Immobilization and positioning
• Administration of contrast media (if applicable)	• Administration of contrast media (if applicable)
• Mark reference points on patient by using laser system	• Mark reference points on patient by using laser system
• Take topograms (preliminary image)	• Take topogram (preliminary image)
• Physician selects area to scan	• Physician selects area to scan
	• Place fiducial markers at reference points before scan
CT Scan Is Performed	
• CT scan completed by using specific department protocol	**CT Scan Is Performed**
• Transfer reconstructed images to virtual simulation station	• CT scan completed by using specific department protocol
	• Transfer reconstructed image to treatment planning system
Virtual Simulation Software	
• Contouring	**Treatment Planning**
• Localize tumor and target volumes and normal structures	• Treatment isocenter is determined
• Determination of target isocenter and transfer to patient by using laser system	• Treatment plan is completed
	• Shifts from reference marks to treatment isocenter are established
• Patient is marked during procedure and patient leaves	
• Transfer CT data to treatment planning system	**Treatment Machine**
	• First day of treatment, shifts are made from reference marks to treatment isocenter
	• Verification with onboard imaging
	• Patient is re-marked at isocenter location for daily setup

CT, Computed tomography.

remarked before treatment, occupying the treatment machine or requiring separate treatment setup verification.[19]

No-shift method: For this method, the patient is scanned and, while the patient is still on the CT couch, the images are reviewed by the physician and the treatment isocenter is determined based on the areas contoured on the CT images. The isocenter coordinates are then programmed into the movable lasers in the scanner room, and the patient is marked accordingly. The patient then goes home with marks that will actually be used for treatment delivery. This process is illustrated in Fig. 21.19. Determination of the isocenter can be performed by CT simulator staff, a physician, or a dosimetrist.[19]

To determine the isocenter that is marked on the patient, the no-shift method requires a review of CT images by using virtual simulation software. Workstations are commercially available from several imaging and treatment planning software vendors.[19] Today, virtual simulation software resides not only on remote workstations; it can reside directly on the CT scanner console as an application. To transfer the isocenter coordinates from virtual simulation software to the patient's skin accurately, the patient needs to remain still in the scanning position while images are processed.[19] This no-shift method of virtual simulation software allows treatment isocenters to be established and the marking of the patient at the time of the CT simulation. Establishing treatment isocenters and marking the patient at the time of the CT scan allows for the patient to be positioned more efficiently, increases throughput in the department, and helps to avoid potential patient shift errors (or fail to shift errors) on the treatment machine. This method of CT simulation has become increasingly popular and is typically the preferred method.

Techniques for Isocenter Localization

Isocenter localization procedures are divided into three methods: (1) external skin fiducials, (2) computing the isocenter based on field border placement, and (3) placement of the isocenter based on treatment volume or contour information. Each method is described in the following paragraphs.

The first method is placement of the isocenter anatomically based on external skin fiducials, anatomy of interest, or physician direction. Manual (visual) placement of the isocenter on the CT image in the proper location by using virtual simulation tools yields a fast, effective, and simple placement.

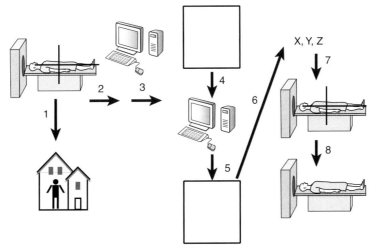

Fig. 21.18 Shift method. In this simulation method, initial marks are placed on the patient before the scan. During treatment planning, shifts (*X, Y, Z*) from the initial marks to the treatment isocenter are then determined. These shifts are applied before patient treatment, and the patient is then re-marked.

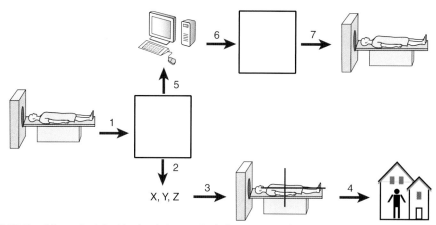

Fig. 21.19 No-shift method. In this simulation method, the treatment isocenter is marked while the patient is still in the computed tomography simulator (step 3). The patient goes home with marks that will be used for treatment. On the first treatment day, there are no adjustments in patient setup, shifts, or re-marking. This is exactly the same process that would be performed with a conventional simulator.

The second method is to compute the isocenter based on field border placement. For example, during a whole-brain simulation, the physician may define the treatment borders of the beam (field edges), and then the simulation software can compute the isocenter midfield. The software can also then place the isocenter at midplane if desired. This simulation technique is very common in emergency treatments or "sim and treat" situations and very similar to conventional fluoroscopy simulation techniques.

The third method of isocenter placement is treatment volume or contour based. Here, the physician would be required to delineate or segment a target volume. Virtual simulation software can then place the isocenter automatically to the geometric center of the defined structure. This simulation technique can greatly streamline workflow, as the data can be exported to the treatment planning computer with contours predefined. Complex treatment plans require contoured volumes before any treatment planning can be accomplished.

Advanced cases may use a combination of the three techniques. Breast simulations may use a combination of volume-based and field-based approaches. These techniques are typically department or physician defined.

Integration With Treatment Planning

Once the CT simulation has been completed, the digital data must be transferred to the treatment planning system. This typically includes the CT images, any contoured structures, established isocenters, and treatment beams along with any beam modifiers. This can be accomplished via specific DICOM protocols (which is the standard format used to transfer information between the imaging devices, virtual simulation systems, and the treatment planning system). When beam arrangements are created using CT simulation, gantry limits, collimator limits, and table angle limits must be kept in mind. It is possible to create a treatment plan that cannot be executed in the treatment room, especially if the gantry and couch are oriented so that they cause a collision.

Multiple imaging studies of the same patient are often used to produce all the information needed for the accurate identification of target volume and critical organs.[9,21] Image registration and correlation or image fusion are used to identify preoperative volume and transfer to postoperative scans. The CT can be fused with MRI and PET scans,

which allow better soft tissue contrast and display information about the metabolic behavior of a tumor, respectively.[9]

For example, a patient with a nasopharyngeal tumor may have had both MRI and CT diagnostic scans that showed bony invasion on the CT, whereas the high-intensity areas on MRI showed the extent of soft tissue tumor involvement. This information is important in the design of tumor volumes.[1] Maurer and Fitzpatrick[22] define registration as the determination of a one-to-one mapping between two coordinates in one space and those in another, such that points in the two spaces that correspond to the same anatomic point are mapped to each other. The fusion process of image registration begins with two sets of images. The treatment planner locates image features on both sets that are the same. These features can include a bony prominence or a soft tissue structure. A manual match mode allows the treatment planner to select three points on both scans. In addition to the points selected, scans can be overlaid and the dosimetrist is able to rotate the scans to get the best match. One of the challenges with image registration is that often the patients are not in the same position or the modalities are different, making it difficult to fuse the two images. Automatic fusion algorithms have also been developed that look for spatial relationships within the data sets. Although some discrepancies between data sets may yield undesirable results, deformable image registration techniques have been developed for these situations. Once the physician has approved the fused images, outlines of treatment volumes and critical structures can take into account all the information of the fused images (Fig. 21.20).

PATIENT MARKING SYSTEM

Either isocenter or field edge marking systems are available for CT simulation. The patient is temporarily marked with reference points before scanning: usually an anterior/posterior mark and two lateral points. After the target volume has been determined, the computer calculates the isocenter with reference to the temporary marks. The lasers and/or couch are then adjusted automatically so the patient can be marked. Some simulation software does not require the use of these reference marks, and they may not be necessary to compute the marked isocenter. Movable lasers display the triangulation, or treatment setup point on the skin representing the three major planes: transverse, sagittal, and coronal.[2] Field edge marking systems are available with some CT

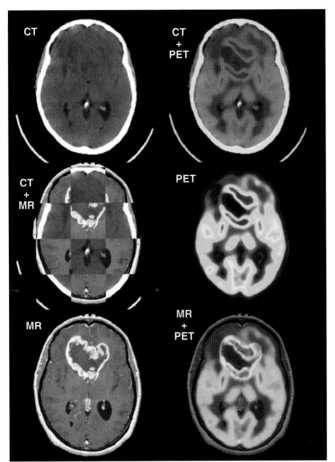

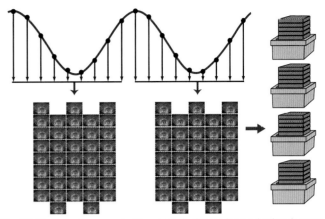

Fig. 21.21 A single computed tomography image is acquired and reconstructed into multiple phases (data sets) of respiration.

Fig. 21.20 Multimodality visualization of a brain tumor fusing a computed tomography *(CT)* scan, magnetic resonance image *(MRI)*, and positron emission tomography *(PET)* scan of the same patient. (From Leibel SA, Phillips TL. *Textbook of Radiation Oncology*. 3rd ed. Philadelphia, PA: Saunders; 2010.)

scanner laser systems and are used to control the position of lasers that identify the superior, inferior, and lateral field borders and/or isocenter on the patient's skin.

The LAP laser company has developed a CT positional laser system that consists of a laser tracking system, which has two sidewall cross lasers (with a movable horizontal line) and one overhead laser with a movable sagittal line. These lasers provide movement in two dimensions, and the CT tabletop (couch) movement (in and out) provides the third dimension. The lasers can be controlled through most treatment planning systems, with the CT simulation software or with the remote handheld pendant. Lasers can accept exported coordinates from treatment planning systems, and virtual simulation software allowing easy and accurate movement to the marking location. Diode lasers are typically available in green or red. Not only does the integrated green laser enhance contrast on various skin tones, especially dark skin tones; its unique design incorporates power-stabilizing circuitry that extends diode life.[13]

> A computed tomography (CT) simulation laser system can consist of a single overhead laser line that moves to project the sagittal plane, two vertical moving lateral lasers to project the coronal plane, and fixed lasers to project the transverse plane. Do not stare at the laser lights, although they are low in power. They can cause retinal damage.

DOCUMENTING DATA

Information documented in the treatment chart to aid in the daily setup of the patient may be organized in several ways and is usually institutionally dependent. Patient position and immobilization devices must be documented. A digital camera can capture the patient's position and immobilization devices as they appeared during the simulation process. This information can then be transferred to the electronic medical record for use during treatment. With CT simulation, the exact field size, gantry position, shielding, and isocenter are often determined during the simulation and transferred to the treatment planning system. Once the treatment plan is completed, it is exported and recorded in the record-and-verify system for archival and treatment delivery on the linear accelerator.

USE OF FOUR-DIMENSIONAL COMPUTED TOMOGRAPHY IN VIRTUAL SIMULATION

For many years, motion artifacts have been recognized with CT scanning. With the advancements in tumor localization in radiation therapy, breathing motion remains a challenge in localizing lung, thorax, and upper abdomen tumors.[20] Organs can move several centimeters during a few seconds.[9] One method to overcome breathing motion artifacts is for the patient hold his or her breath during the scan, often at full inhalation, which is called "deep inspiration breath hold" (DIBH) or "full exhalation."[1] Scans may also be taken at a full expiration breath hold. However, many patients cannot hold their breath for long periods of time, and the amount of inspiration or expiration is not very reproducible. Scan modes such as prospective axial and prospective helical were created to help mitigate these issues. Prospective axial is a scanning method in which the scanner is triggered to acquire an image set at a specific point of respiration while letting the patient breathe freely during the scan. The reconstructed data set is a predetermined point of respiration. Prospective helical scanning is very similar to a standard helical scan; however, it is acquired during a breath hold. A newer and more sophisticated approach, 4D CT, correlates very low pitch (slow) scan data with patient respiration via a recorded respiratory waveform. Many phases of respiration are reconstructed, yielding multiple CT scans at different points of the breathing cycle (Fig. 21.21).

Prospective methods do not represent the entire breathing cycle in the way that a 4D CT can. Retrospective 4D CT techniques are currently used to account for the moving tumor volumes. 4D CT phases may be binned either linearly or based on amplitude of the respiratory waveform. Linear phase reconstruction will use all of the raw data for image reconstruction. This can cause image artifacts when patients

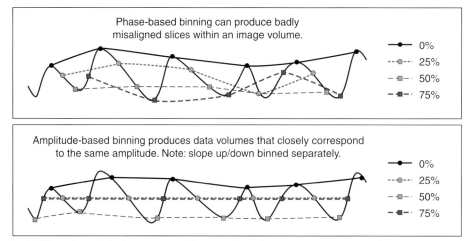

Fig. 21.22 Phase-based binning can create image artifacts because the amplitude of each breath may vary throughout the scan (upper waveform). The patient anatomy may be in a different location during breaths that vary in amplitude, creating an artifact on the reconstructed phases of data. One amplitude-based binning method calculates an amplitude threshold and produces data volumes that closely correspond to the same amplitude, thus minimizing artifacts from irregular breathing (lower waveform).

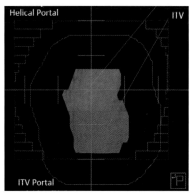

Fig. 21.23 Internal target volume portals *(ITVs)*, created by using four-dimensional computed tomography (4D CT), are optimal in conforming to target motion. Note that the inferior margin of the helical portal does not provide an adequate margin around the true target motion.

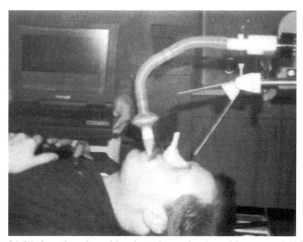

Fig 21.24 A patient breathing into the active breathing control (ABC) apparatus. A nose clip is used to make sure that the breathing is through the ABC unit. (From Bragg DG, Rubin P, Hricak H, eds. *Oncologic Imaging.* 2nd ed. Philadelphia, PA: Saunders; 2002:116.)

with irregular breathing are scanned. Amplitude-based binning eliminates data from irregular breathing cycles that may cause these artifacts, and produces data volumes that closely correspond to the same amplitude (Fig. 21.22).

After scanning, 4D CT reconstructed data sets can be loaded into simulation or treatment planning software and played in as a "movie" loop to demonstrate respiration and assess tumor motion. Another application of 4D CT is to generate treatment margins that include the extent of tumor motion or excursion. This could traditionally be achieved on single-slice CT scanners with a "free breathing" scan. The patient was instructed to breathe normally during a standard CT acquisition. The slow scan during multiple breaths caused a blurring of the target that was used to create contours that encompassed the full motion.

Modern-day multislice scanners have evolved and have far faster scan times as compared with single-slice scanners. Even though the patient is breathing freely during this scan, there will be very little target blur or representation of target excursion. The use of 4D CT mitigates this limitation of data and allows tumor volume contours to be more representative of traditional "free breathing" scans. The contouring of moving targets on a modern multislice helical standard image acquisition may lead to geometric misses of the target (Fig. 21.23).

To perform 4D CT scanning, a method to measure the respiratory phase is needed. This can be accomplished by using a spirometer (a respiratory therapy machine that measures various lung volumes; Fig. 21.24) or a measurement of the motion of the abdomen, which usually consists of a device strapped to the abdomen that records the breathing cycle.[1] Also, an infrared camera (Fig. 21.25) can be used to track the motion of an infrared marker block placed on the patient's chest or abdomen.

The patient's breathing waveform will be recorded, and the pitch is set according to the breath rate. A very slow pitch such as 0.06 may be used for helical scanning, which allows for multiple samples per couch position, recording the patient's anatomy at the various phases of the breathing cycle.[23] Some vendors use axial step and shoot to achieve this instead of low-pitch helical scanning. This scan will then be placed into tidal volume bins according to which phase of the breathing cycle each projection or slice was acquired.

If respiratory gating will be used on the treatment machine, the physician may select only a few phases to create a treatment plan. This will allow a plan to be created with a smaller tumor volume and will be treated only at the planning phases of the respiratory cycle. The advantage to this method is the ability to spare normal lung and heart tissue and ensure maximum dose coverage to the tumor. A maximum intensity projection (MIP) can be created to assist with planning (Fig. 21.26). This takes multiple phases of respiration and adds the brightest voxels (volume elements) from each to create a new data set.[1]

For lung cases, the MIP may represent the maximum amount of tumor movement during the respiratory cycle. A MIP may be generated by using the full range of phases if a nongated treatment is delivered. Treatment planning can then include the entire motion of the tumor volume. A subset MIP may also be created by using only treatment phases for gated treatments. MinIP (minimum intensity projection) and Avg (average) projections are also available. MinIPs use multiple phases of respiration and add the darkest voxels from each to create a new data set. MinIPs may be useful for hypodense targets such as liver tumors. Avg IPs use multiple phases of respiration and average them with equal weight to create a new data set. Avg IPs may be used for dose calculation and normal structure delineation (Fig. 21.27).

Surface Imaging in Radiation Therapy

Surface-guided radiation therapy (SGRT) is the use of an optical-based video system or laser scanning that allows the patient's surface to be monitored during radiation therapy treatments.[24] Surface imaging provides 3D imaging of the patient representing six directions of movement: vertical, longitudinal, lateral, pitch, roll, and yaw. Pitch is a horizontal axis rotation, roll is a longitudinal axis, and yaw is a vertical axis rotation (Fig. 21.28). These nonradiographic,

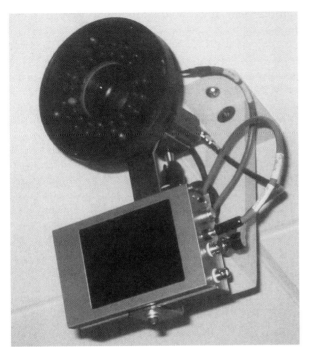

Fig. 21.25 Charged-coupled device video camera attached to infrared illuminator for tracking the respiratory motion. (From Hoppe R, Phillips T, Roach M. *Leibel and Phillips Textbook of Radiation Oncology.* Philadelphia, PA: Saunders; 2010.)

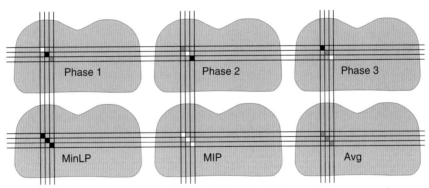

Phase 1 Phase 2 Phase 3

MinLP MIP Avg

Fig. 21.26 Intensity projections are created by combining the minimum, average, or maximum computed tomography (CT) numbers from all selected four-dimensional (4D) CT phases.

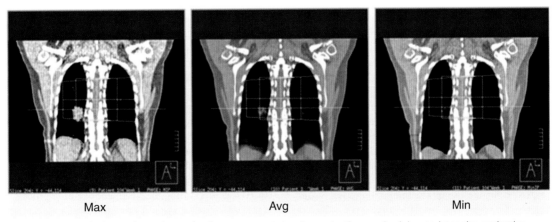

Max Avg Min

Fig 21.27 Maximum intensity projection, average intensity projection. and minimum intensity projection (Philips Healthcare).

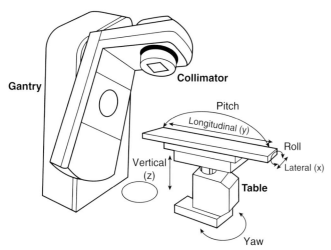

Fig. 21.28 The surface imaging system detects three translational and three rotational references for patient alignment. Directional variations that affect treatment alignment are measured in the *X* (lateral), *Y* (longitudinal), and *Z* (vertical) directions. Rotational variations include pitch, roll, and yaw. (Reprinted with permission from the American Society of Radiologic Technologists for educational purposes. ©2013. All rights reserved.)

noninvasive systems provide intrafaction monitoring during treatments.[25] Intrafraction motion, motion occurring during the treatment, can arise from patient movement or organ motion that occurs from breathing.[25] Monitoring the patient continuously can reduce setup variability, improve target localization, and reduce positioning uncertainty. This can lead to a reduction in PTV size, thereby lowering the dose to normal tissues and associated side effects.[25] Good examples are respiratory gating and DIBH techniques that are used to reduce the irradiated lung volume and limit doses to other critical structures such as the heart.[25]

Other benefits of the daily surface imaging include no radiation exposure, reduction of imaging dose, greater comfort for the patients with decreased amount of immobilization, and improved setup efficiency.[24,25] Surface imaging can be used for sites including intracranial, breast, head and neck, and extremities.[25]

For surface imaging to be successful, the patient's skin surface needs to be visible and not obscured by the gantry, imaging arms, or other components of the equipment. Clothing and sheets must also be removed, thus leaving patients exposed in the treatment room.[25] Additional training, quality assurance (QA), and time are needed develop the protocols to include surface imaging in the workflow.[26]

Surface imaging begins with CT simulation. The external contour of the patient is necessary for the surface tracking to occur. The reference contour is obtained in one of two methods. The reference surface image can be taken from the external surface of the CT scan from the treatment planning system.[25] If the CT simulator has a video surface tracking system, the surface contour can be captured at the time of simulation.[26] The first day of treatment, when Cone Beam CT 2-dimensional/2-dimensional images (CBCT/2D/2D) images are taken, a new reference image may be taken to be used during treatment.

Intrafraction patient monitoring has distinct advantages including easy and quick shifts; use with DIBH to enable fast, reliable treatment; six-dimensional isocenter correction; and SRS for noncoplanar treatment fields. The use of surface tracking with intracranial lesions require a high-resolution image to detect submillimeter motions verses a larger surface needed for the use of breathing monitoring.[25] Studies show the use of SGRT with breast cancer treatment can reduce the setup time, decrease the number of weekly portal images, and produce more accurate results than the use of tattoos.[27–29]

Magnetic Resonance Imaging in Simulation

MRI is becoming more important in radiation therapy. MRI has been used successfully in SRS procedures for more than a decade. The superior contrast resolution of the MRI image compared with CT allows better visualization of soft tissue and can also provide functional information.[30] The better soft tissue contrast and resolution than CT allows the tumor volume to be better defined, especially in the brain, head and neck, liver, pelvis, prostate, and sarcomas.[2]

Human tissues are made up of mostly water, which contains hydrogen protons. MRI uses magnetic and radio waves to align the plentiful hydrogen protons. Hydrogen protons are randomly aligned and spin on their axes. When a strong magnetic field of the MRI unit is applied, hydrogen protons align with the magnetic field. They are still pointed in different directions. A radiofrequency (RF) wave is sent into the body, which aligns the hydrogen protons to line up perpendicularly to the main magnet. The RF wave is then turned off. The protons realign with the magnetic field (called T1 relaxation) and fan out (called T2 relaxation). While the protons are manipulated by the RF waves and realign with the magnetic field, electric signals are created and recorded by a receiver coil. The image is formed from those signals. (Detailed information about how MRI images are created can be read in "Medical Imaging," Chapter 6)

The relaxation rate depends on the type of tissue, and image contrast comes from the tissue relaxation properties. Because the signal produced by the protons is fairly small, it is best if the receiving coils are close to the area being imaged. There are different types of coils for various body parts, such as head coils for brain imaging, spine coils, and surface coils for various extremities. This can pose challenges in the use of MRI units for radiation therapy imaging because of positioning and immobilization devices for radiation therapy treatment. Coils avoid compression of patient contours and avoid the laser system. For example, an article published on MRI simulation and planning of pediatric radiation therapy provided coils beneath the tabletop and included flexible anterior coils as the receiver coils when imaging the thorax, abdomen, and pelvis.[31]

The use of MRI poses some risks different than the risks from radiation exposure. The most serious risks have been termed missile effect or projectile injuries when ferromagnetic objects are pulled into the scanner at high speed.[30] Because of this risk to both patients and healthcare workers, the American College of Radiology (ACR) developed practice guidelines. All MRI sites need to establish and maintain safety policies (https://www.acr.org/Clinical-Resources/Radiology-Safety/MR-Safety). The ACR identifies four zones:

Zone 1: Area accessible to the general public. No magnetic hazards in this area. Uncontrolled area

Zone 2: Patients are under general supervision of MR
- Screening questions asked about MR, patient histories obtained

Zone 3: Restrict access to MR personnel
- Imaging control and computer rooms

Zone 4: MR scanner room.
- Marked clearly as potentially hazardous area
- Extremely strong magnetic fields

All equipment, including positioning and immobilization devices, must be MRI compatible. All employees must complete a screening survey and have proper training to access Zone 3. Patients complete screening questions in Zone 2. For a sample questionnaire, visit https://www.acr.org/Clinical-Resources/Radiology-Safety/MR-Safety.

In most clinical settings, MRI and CT are completed. Images are fused together during the treatment planning process.[32] CT has been necessary for dose calculation and is used to create reference images for CBCT during treatment. MRI simulators in the radiation oncology department should have a wide bore (70 cm), flat tabletop, and external

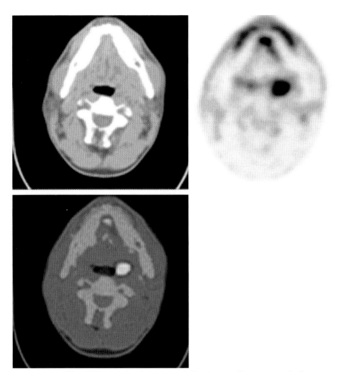

Fig. 21.29 The CT scan in the upper left shows the anatomic features; the PET scan on the upper right demonstrates elevated FDG activity; the fused PET-CT scan is on the bottom left and shows both anatomic form and tissue function. (From Paulino AC. *PET-CT in Radiotherapy Treatment Planning.* Philadelphia, PA: Saunders; 2008.)

positioning lasers similar to those used in the CT simulator. Patients who have multiple scans may receive temporary skin marks from CT and then get permanent marks in the MRI scanner. The room must be designed to keep out unwanted RF waves to keep electromagnetic noise outside. This can be accomplished by having a faraday shield (Faraday cage) such as a copper-lined room.[30]

Magnetic Resonance Imaging–Only Simulation

There is growing interest to substitute CT simulation for MRI-only simulation. This is a result of the superior quality of MR images to delineate target and normal tissues. MRI-only simulation would improve workflow by eliminating the need for a CT scan. It would also reduce ambiguities by eliminating MR-CT registration errors and ease planning logistics for patients.[32] The major challenge is in performing dose calculations. Unlike CT, there is a lack of correspondence between the attenuation of the tissue and the voxel intensity. MRI relates to the proton density and magnetic relaxation rates. Bone and air/lung tissue both appear dark on an MRI. There are some algorithms developed to generate a synthetic or substitute CT image.[30] The use of these algorithms allows planning to be completed on the MRI/synthetic CT image.[32] Philips has commercially available software, MRCAT, that creates a CT dose-equivalent plan from MRI only.

Positron Emission Tomography-Computed Tomography Imaging

PET uses functional molecular imaging that enables the visualization of biological processes in the body; however, it has poor anatomic precision. PET can be performed along with a CT scan (PET-CT), which provides anatomic detail. Images can be "registered," which allows the CT and PET to be fused and viewed together. PET-CT is used to diagnose, stage, and follow up cancers and aids in identifying the tumor volume and surrounding patient anatomy during simulation.[33]

When patients are scheduled for a PET-CT scan, they are injected with a beta decay radiotracer called *Fludeoxyglucose* (FDG), which has a 110-minute half-life.[20] The FDG actively accumulates in organs with high glucose utilization, which occurs in areas of more metabolic activity, such as disease sites. PET imaging is helpful in showing increased areas of nodal activity and metastatic disease[3,20] (Fig. 21.29). Once injected, the patient will be asked to sit quietly, avoiding movement and talking for approximately 60 minutes because motion can increase metabolic activity and be displayed as disease in the body.

If the PET-CT scanner is in the radiation oncology department, the patient will be immobilized in the treatment position on a flat tabletop surface (just as in the CT scanner). Immobilization devices need to be constructed to enable the patient to travel through the bore of the scanner. Many facilities will fabricate the immobilization devices before the injection and exam, or on a previous date.

There are some challenges associated with use of the PET-CT scanner in radiation oncology. At the time of CT simulation, patients are radioactive from the injected radioisotope, which increases exposure for the therapists. If the PET-CT resides in the radiation therapy department, the facility must staff nuclear medicine technologists or share staff with the nuclear medicine department. The radiation therapists are able to perform the CT scans but are not able to perform the PET portion because of the use of the radioactive isotope. If the scanner is located in the nuclear medicine department, the radiation therapists must be present to assist with patient positioning, immobilization, the simulation procedure (if applicable), and any patient marking. Lastly, it can be very taxing and challenging for the patient to be immobile and positioned for than extended amount of time. Patients who are claustrophobic may have difficulty with the scan.

A PET-CT completed for diagnostic purposes can be fused with the CT acquired during the simulation process and used for treatment planning. This assists the radiation oncologist and medical dosimetrist with target volume definition and treatment planning. The patient is often not in the same position for both scans (CT simulation and PET-CT). This can result in a poor or unusable image fusion. Diagnostic PET-CT scanners have curved tabletops, which cause difficulty in fusing the images to the treatment planning CT acquired with a flat tabletop. It is preferable to have the patient in the treatment position in the appropriate immobilization devices for both procedures to ensure accurate fusion. Flat tabletops are available for most diagnostic PET-CT scanners. PET-CT simulators designed for radiation therapy use, have large bores and a flat couch very similar to CT simulators.

ROOM DESIGN

The design of a simulator room is a process that must involve the expertise of numerous professionals, including an architect, an engineer, and a radiologic physicist. Input should also be encouraged from the therapists and the radiation oncologists in the department. Before designing the room, the site must be chosen. The ideal location is close to the treatment machines. This location facilitates communication among all parties involved in the patient's treatment.

Space Allocations

The simulator room should be of sufficient size to accommodate not only the machine and all of its components but also its full range of motions. The equipment will have a longer life if sufficient space is provided. It will also be a more pleasant work area if personnel have room to comfortably perform their duties, such as preparing the patient for simulation, constructing immobilization devices, and preparing contrast media.

Space must also be allocated for a good-sized counter that should include a sink, workspace, and writing area. The workspace should be of sufficient size to allow for the manufacture of various immobilization devices used in radiation therapy. Cabinets and drawer space for the storage of simulation equipment and spare simulator parts are necessary in any simulator room. In addition, storage space should be available for routine immobilization devices and other related equipment such as a breast board, belly board, wing board, and, especially, a hot water tank used in the construction of thermoplastic immobilization devices.

The control area is normally set in one corner of the room, usually near the entrance. This area is designed to protect the operators from radiation and to house the simulator's controls, treatment planning equipment if a CT simulator is used, and x-ray generator. It must be large enough for several pieces of equipment, which might include a record-and-verify system and one or more liquid-crystal display monitors, a work area, and numerous personnel. It is always important that the operator have full visual and aural contact with the patient. A lead glass window may be installed for patient visualization. As with all radiation equipment, room shielding is an important consideration. Radiation rooms are most commonly shielded with lead or concrete or a combination of the two. The specifics of room shielding can be found in Chapter 17.

Other Considerations

There are several other considerations worth mentioning concerning the simulator. Simulator manufacturers have very specific requirements for ventilation of the room. They reserve the right to negate the warranty if these requirements are not met. The lighting system is also important. The intensity must be adjustable, with independent control of the room and the control area. For conventional simulation, visualization of the light field is easier in low light, as is the fluoroscopy image. On the other hand, certain simulation duties need maximum light, such as recording pertinent information, preparing contrast materials, or constructing an immobilization device. Task lighting in certain areas, such as under cabinets, is very beneficial.

CT simulator external positioning and patient marking lasers, which project a small red, green, or blue beam of light toward the patient during the simulation process, must be installed and be highly accurate. There are several systems available, and the department personnel must choose the style they believe best suits their needs. Side lasers are more stable if they are recessed in the wall to prevent inadvertent collisions. A third overhead laser is installed and represents the anterior CA. These lasers systems assist in patient positioning and patient marking during the CT simulation procedure. Today's systems can be controlled by a computer and have movable lasers that typically move left/right and up/down. The computer can be networked to virtual simulation and treatment planning systems and receive image and treatment plan information to translate on the patient. Some systems include movable lasers that will cast an established field size, block, or MLC pattern on the patient. These lasers can also

provide the therapist several external reference points in relationship to the position of the isocenter and assist with marking various setup points.[35] Daily checks, which provide strict quality control of the positional lasers, are a must.

Many of the factors used in consideration of the simulator room design, such as space allocations, equipment motions, and shielding design, allow for more efficient use of this essential piece of equipment. Because the time invested during the simulation process can seriously affect the outcome of a patient's treatment plan, a thorough knowledge of the simulator, its use, and its limitations is necessary if the simulator's maximum potential is to be achieved.

QUALITY ASSURANCE

CT scanners used for radiation therapy simulation should have similar mechanical checks as linear accelerators because they are meant to simulate the geometry of the treatment beam.[16] Both mechanical checks and image quality performance checks should be evaluated according to the guidelines in the 2003 report of the American Association of Physicists in Medicine Radiation Therapy Committee Task Group No. 66,[35] which outlines QA for CT simulators and the CT simulation process. These guidelines (Tables 19.8 and 19.9) can be used to establish a department-specific QA program based on the amount of CT simulation experience and departmental goals.

Daily warmup procedures for the CT simulator include warming up the x-ray tube according to the manufacturer's specifications, checking the laser systems, and scanning a water phantom. The water phantom scan checks noise levels by comparing the Hounsfield number of water at various areas of the phantom. These levels should be within plus or minus 3 from zero. The scan should have a large enough region of interest. If scanning air, the Hounsfield number should read −1000 with ±1 variance allowed.[19,20] The quality of the beam must be checked yearly, including spatial resolution, contrast resolution, and correlation of Hounsfield numbers with electron density.[19,20] Monthly tests include CT (Hounsfield) number/electron density verification, reconstruction slice location, image transfer protocols, left/right registration, and distance between known points in the image.[23]

For more information regarding quality assurance for radiation therapy computed tomography (CT) simulators, see the American Association of Physicists in Medicine (AAPM) website at http://www.aapm.org/pubs/reports/.

The publication by the AAPM, "Quality Assurance for Computed-Tomography Simulators and the Computed-Tomography-Simulation Process: Report of the AAPM Radiation Therapy Committee, Task Group No. 66, Report No. 83," is available for review on the website.

SUMMARY

- The use of CT simulation is the primary method of simulation. CT simulation provides more complete anatomic patient data, which allow for better treatment planning.
- Benefits of CT simulation include the ability to view all critical structures, which allows for more accurate treatment planning.
- CT image data can be used for radiation therapy dose calculations.
- Because the CT scanner does not reflect the geometry of the linear accelerator, careful simulation must occur to ensure the ability to treat the patient as planned.
- Contrast media are most commonly used to enhance structures in patients with a specific pathology, such as head and neck, lung, brain, abdominal, and pelvic tumors.

- The most common contrast agents are barium, given orally or rectally, and ionic or nonionic iodinated contrast, which is given through an IV line. A patient questionnaire must be completed before contrast media is administered.
- Communicating with and reassuring the patient are key to performing a successful simulation.
- The patient needs to be in the center of the FOV so that the patient's contour is not cut off. This also helps minimize dose to the patient and ensure a good-quality image.
- CT scan protocols need to be selected for the appropriate area being scanned. Protocols can be altered to optimize the images and minimize patient dose.

- There are several methods for isocenter localization:
- Respiratory gating can be used during simulation. These benefits result in better treatment planning, resulting in better patient care.
- Intrafraction motion surface imaging tracking enables reduced dose to critical structures.

- PET-CT, MRI, and other imaging modalities are essential in radiation therapy treatment planning.
- MRI-only simulation is being used because of the commercially available algorithms to generate a substitute CT for treatment planning purposes.

REVIEW QUESTIONS

The answers to the Review Questions can be found by logging on to our website at: http://evolve.elsevier.com/Washington/principles

1. Presimulation planning is important because it:
   a. Will involve determining patient positioning and the selection or preparation of immobilization devices.
   b. Will help determine the patient's separation.
   c. Will be helpful in determining any radiographic exposure techniques used during simulation.
   d. Will involve the patient and his or her family in the treatment process.
2. The GTV treatment volume will contain:
   a. Tumor.
   b. Involved lymphatics.
   c. Normal tissue.
   d. All of the above.
3. _____ is the initial phase of treatment planning in which actual visualization of the treatment volume is documented before treatment.
   a. Initial consultation.
   b. Simulation.
   c. Brachytherapy.
   d. Radiation treatment.
4. With PET scanning, _____is injected into the patient used to create the image.
   a. 18F fluorothymidine.
   b. FDG.
   c. Gallium.
   d. Iodine 131.
5. Which of the following is not a desirable quality of an effective and useful immobilization device?
   a. Ensures immobilization with minimal patient discomfort.
   b. Requires additional setup time.
   c. Is durable enough to withstand the entire treatment plan.
   d. Achieves conditions prescribed in the treatment plan.
6. Patient immobilization is important because:
   a. Sophisticated treatment planning techniques allow more accurate delivery of treatment.
   b. Missing the tumor once or twice in a treatment course can reduce the planned dose by 10% or more.

   c. Daily reproduction of the planned treatment is essential to treatment outcomes.
   d. All of the above.
7. Contrast media may be given to patients with a brain tumor:
   a. 10 minutes before scan.
   b. Immediately before the scan.
   c. The day before the scan.
   d. Time does not matter.
8. The no-shift method of simulation include all of the following except:
   a. The physician determines the isocenter location after the patient has completed the simulation process.
   b. The patient is tattooed at the isocenter.
   c. Moveable lasers are used to mark the isocenter.
   d. The virtual simulation workstation is used.
9. Respiratory gating used during CT simulation consists of recording the patient's breathing pattern and scanning:
   a. At full exhalation.
   b. With a fast pitch during the entire breathing pattern.
   c. At full inhalation.
   d. With a slow pitch during the entire breathing pattern.
10. In 4D CT, the fourth dimension is:
    a. Motion.
    b. Left/right.
    c. Up/down.
    d. In/out.
11. _____ provides a 3D imaging of the patient of the patient representing six directions of movement: vertical, longitudinal, lateral, pitch, roll, and yaw in six directions.
    a. Four-dimensional-CT.
    b. Respiratory gating.
    c. Surface imaging.
    d. CBCT.
12. The benefit of MRI-only simulation includes all but:
    a. Superior quality of MR images versus CT.
    b. No radiation exposure.
    c. Improved workflow.
    d. Increased MR-CT registration errors.

QUESTIONS TO PONDER

1. Discuss the importance of contrast agents used in CT simulation.
2. Describe, as though you were educating an interested patient, the purpose of the CT simulation procedure.
3. Explain the purpose of each of the components of the CT simulator.

4. Discuss the process of tumor localization and treatment planning used in CT simulation.
5. What are the advantages and disadvantages of CT simulation versus conventional simulation?
6. Compare PET and MRI imaging as it relates to CT simulation.

REFERENCES

1. American College of Radiology. *ACR Practice Guidelines for Radiation Oncology.* Reston, VA: American College of Radiology; 2004.
2. Hoppe R, Phillips T, Roach M. *Leibel and Phillips Textbook of Radiation Oncology.* Philadelphia, PA: Saunders; 2010.
3. Cox J, Ang K. *Radiation Oncology.* 9th ed. St. Louis, MO: Elsevier; 2010.
4. Bomford CK, Craig LM, Hanna FA, Innes GS, Lillicrap SC, Morgan RL. Treatment simulators. *Br J Radiol Suppl.* 1981;16:1–31.
5. Purdy JA. Principles of radiologic physics, dosimetry and treatment planning. In: Halperin EC, Perez CA, Brady LW, eds. *Principles and Practice of Radiation Oncology.* Philadelphia, PA: Lippincott Williams & Wilkins; 2013.
6. Sherouse GW, Novins KL, Chaney EL. Computation of digitally reconstructed radiographs for use in radiotherapy treatment design. *Int J Radiat Oncol Biol Phys.* 1990;18:651–658.
7. International Commission on Radiation Units and Measurements. *Prescribing, Recording, and Reporting Photon Beam Therapy* (Report 50). Bethesda, MD: International Commission on Radiation Units and Measurements; 1993.
8. International Commission on Radiation Units and Measurements. *Prescribing, Recording and Reporting Photon Beam Therapy* (Report 62). Bethesda, MD: International Commission on Radiation Units and Measurements; 1999.
9. Khan F, Gibbons J, Sperduto P. *Treatment Planning in Radiation Oncology.* 4th ed. Philadelphia, PA: Wolters Kluwer; 2016.
10. Pereira G, Traughber M, Muzic R. The role of imaging in radiation therapy planning: past present, and future. *Biomed Res Int.* 2014;2014:231090.
11. Small WJr. *Clinical Radiation Oncology.* 3rd ed. Hoboken, NJ: John Wiley & Sons, Inc; 2017.
12. Hunt M, Hoboken, NJ, Coia L. The treatment planning process. In: Purdy JA, Starkschall G, eds. *3D Planning and Conformal Radiation Therapy.* Madison, WI: Advanced Medical Publishers; 1999.
13. Khan FM, Gibbons J. *The Physics of Radiation Therapy.* 5th ed. Baltimore, MD: Lippincott Williams & Wilkins; 2014.
14. Symonds P, Deehan C, Meredith C, et al. *Walter and Miller's Textbook of Radiotherapy: Radiation Physics, Therapy and Oncology.* 7th ed. Philadelphia, PA: Elsevier; 2012.
15. Bentel GC. Patient positioning and immobilization in radiation oncology. McGraw-Hill.
16. Adler A, Carlton R. *Introduction to Radiographic Sciences and Patient Care.* 6th ed. Philadelphia, PA: Saunders; 2015.
17. Contrast manual. American College of Radiology website. https://www.acr.org/Clinical-Resources/Contrast-Manual. Accessed January 7, 2019.
18. Pereira G, Traughber M, Muzic R. The role of imaging in radiation therapy planning: past present, and future. *Biomed Res Int.* 2014;2014:231090.
19. Mutic S. Tumor LOC software: intent and clinical use. http://www.healthcare.philips.com/me_en/about/events/arabhealth/pdfs/Imaging_Systems/Tumor_LOC_White_Paper.pdf. Accessed January 9, 2019.
20. Seeram E. *Computed Tomography: Physical Principles, Clinical Applications, and Quality Control.* 4th ed. St. Louis, MO: Saunders Elsevier; 2015.
21. O'Connor-Hartsell S, Hartsell W. Minimizing errors in patient positioning. *Radiat Ther.* 1994;3:15–19.
22. Maurer C, Fitzpatrick J. A review of medical image registration. In: Maciunas R, ed. *Interactive Image Guided Neurosurgery.* Park Ridge, IL: American Association of Neurological Surgeons; 1993.
23. Hunt M, Coia L. The treatment planning process. In: Purdy JA, Starkschall G, eds. *3D Planning and Conformal Radiation Therapy.* Madison, WI: Advanced Medical Publishers; 1995.
24. Chelbik A. Surface imaging in radiation therapy. *Radiol Technol.* 2017;26(1):23–41.
25. Hoisak JDP, Pawlicki T. The role of optical surface imaging systems in radiation therapy. *Semin Radiat Oncol.* 2018;28(3):185–193.
26. Freislederer P. SP-0245: surface guided radiation therapy: a new reality, pros and cons. *Radiother Oncol.* 2018;127:S126.
27. Liszeski B. *Image-Guided Radiation Therapy: Surface Tracking.* Albuquerque, NM: ASRT; 2013.
28. Herron E, Murray M, Hilton L, Goldstein T, Ogunleye TB, Bailey D. Surface guided radiation therapy as a replacement for patient marks in treatment of breast cancer. *Int J Radiat Oncol Biol Phys.* 2018;102:e492–e493.
29. Kost S, Shah CS, Xia P, Guo B. Setup time and positioning accuracy in breast radiation therapy using surface guided radiation therapy. *Int J Radiat Oncol Biol Phys.* 2018;102:e481–e482.
30. Keller R. Magnetic resonance imaging in radiation therapy. *Radiol Technol.* 2018;27(1):21–41.
31. Hua C-H, Uh J, Krasin MJ, et al. Clinical implementation of magnetic resonance imaging systems for simulation and planning of pediatric radiation therapy. *J Med Radiat Sci.* 2018;49(2):153–163.
32. Kerkmeijer LGW, Maspero M, Meijer GJ, van der Voort van Zyp JRN, de Boer HCJ, van den Berg CAT. Magnetic resonance imaging only workflow for radiotherapy simulation and planning in prostate cancer. *Clin Oncol.* 2018;30(11):692–701.
33. Furlow B. PET-CT cancer imaging. *Radiol Technol.* 2018;90(2):149CT–168CT.
34. LAP Laser systems for measurement and projection LAP Laser website. https://www.lap-laser.com/. Accessed January 8, 2019.
35. Mutic S, Palta JR, Butker EK, et al. Quality assurance for computed-tomography simulators and the computed-tomography-simulation process: report of the AAPM Radiation Therapy Committee Task Group No. 66. *Med Phys.* 2003;30(10):2762–2792.

Photon Dosimetry Concepts and Calculations

Charles M. Washington

OUTLINE

OBJECTIVES

- Identify and accurately apply the information in a radiation therapy prescription to calculate the treatment time (i.e., monitor unit or minute setting).
- Define the terms used in radiation therapy to calculate the monitor unit setting and minute setting and the dose to selected points of interest.
- Define machine output in terms of dose rate.
- Identify the major data tables necessary to perform a radiation treatment time calculation.
- Calculate an equivalent square of a rectangular field with Sterling formula.
- Analyze the need for percentage depth dose, tissue-air ratio, tissue-phantom ratio, and tissue-maximum ratio tables.
- Identify the differences in calculation models used for nonisocentric versus isocentric calculations.
- Apply the correct calculation model to determine the monitor unit setting and doses to points of interest.
- Explain the effect on the treatment time calculation with use of wedge filters, compensating filters, and a block tray.
- Calculate changes in dose rate as a function of distance from the target with the inverse square law.
- Describe the effect of the inverse square law on the monitor unit setting.
- Calculate the monitor unit setting for a given patient treatment.
- Calculate the dose to points of interest such as the dose to the cord and the dose to the depth of maximum equilibrium.

KEY TERMS

Absorbed dose

Backscatter factor

Dose rate

Effective field size

Equivalent square

Equivalent square of rectangular fields

Field size

Isocenter

Monitor units

Output

Output factor

Peak scatter factor

Percentage depth dose

Radiation therapy prescription

Source-axis distance

Source-skin distance

Tissue absorption factors

Tissue-air ratio

Tissue-maximum ratio

Tissue-phantom ratio

Treatment time

Effectively delivering ionizing radiation for cancer treatment requires intricate knowledge of anatomy, physics, and biologic responses. The success or failure of a radiation therapy treatment course depends on both precise and accurate administration of radiation to a localized site that has been prescribed by a radiation oncologist. The treatment planning team must quantify the overall prescribed dose of radiation and determine how much dose will be delivered over the outlined time frame. Many parameters of photon beam dose calculation must be addressed; the radiation therapist, medical dosimetrist, and physicist must be able to determine treatment machine settings to deliver the prescribed dose through manual and computerized methods.

Today, there is greater emphasis on computer-based calculation models, and many oncology departments use sophisticated treatment planning and calculation software to verify the monitor units (MUs) derived by the computer. In addition, with three-dimensional and adaptive treatment planning, more importance is placed on determination of the dose delivery to volumes of tissues, such as the clinical target volume.

With computerized planning as the standard of treatment planning today, it is increasingly important to ensure understanding of the relationships between prescribed dose, individualized patient body profiles, and delivery equipment to fully appreciate the modern treatment planning process. In this chapter, the emphasis is placed on manual calculation of the MU setting for a dose prescribed to a single point and on calculation of the dose to other points, such as spinal cord and doses to the depth of maximum equilibrium (D_{max}). The effective use of new treatment planning technology requires a fundamental understanding of the factors that affect dose delivery and a comfort level with MU and point-dose calculations. Coverage of every established method of performing dose calculations is not possible because most clinical settings have site-specific methods for calculation of dose, normally determined by a medical physicist. This chapter provides clinical examples of dose calculations, both MU and time, and examples that encompass the components used in treatment planning. This allows the treatment planning and delivery team to use the principles presented with the calculation methods used in any radiation therapy center.

Written with the beginning practitioner in mind, a brief review of terminology and concepts provides a basic overview, beginning with basic calculations and then moving toward the more advanced calculations.

RADIATION THERAPY PRESCRIPTION

The radiation therapy prescription is a communication tool between the radiation oncologist and the treatment planning and delivery team, particularly the radiation therapist, medical dosimetrist, and medical physicist. The prescription, whether in a handwritten or electronic format, provides the information necessary to administer the appropriate radiation treatment. This legal document defines the treatment volume, intended tumor dose (TD), number of treatments, dose per treatment, and frequency of treatment.[3] The prescription also states the type and energy of radiation, beam-shaping devices such as wedges and compensators, and any other appropriate factors. The radiation therapist must be able to discuss with the patient the treatment procedure, the function of the devices, and the treatment side effects. In practice, there is no standard radiation therapy prescription. The organization and detail of prescriptions vary from one radiation oncology center to another. The radiation prescription must be clear, precise, and complete. For example, if a thorax is to be treated with anterior and posterior (AP/PA) opposed fields, the prescription commonly sets a spinal cord limit not to exceed 4500 cGy. This instruction should be clear and without need for interpretation. Every parameter and phase of the treatment must be clearly defined within the radiation therapy prescription.

The radiation oncologist commonly defines the region to be treated, technique, treatment machine, energy, fractionation, and daily and total doses within a radiation prescription form. All of the necessary parameters may be located in one or more areas of the treatment record. Most oncology centers use some type of computerized patient management systems. The patient treatment instructions may be found on one screen, whereas the field sizes and gantry, collimator, and couch angles may be found on another. Virtually all patients have a computerized isodose, 3D treatment, intensity-modulated radiation therapy (IMRT), volumetric modulated arc therapy, or stereotactic body radiation therapy treatment plan that is also part of the patient record. The computerized plans (e.g., isodose plan) should document required treatment parameters set for the patient: field sizes, treatment machine angles, doses, beam weighting, modifiers (wedges or compensators), multileaf collimator (MLC) setting, or customized Cerrobend blocks. Again, these plans are considered part of the radiation therapy prescription and should always be dated and signed by the radiation oncologist.

The radiation therapist, medical dosimetrist, and medical physicist must ensure that all parts of the prescription match before treatment delivery. For example, the doses, beam energy, treatment machines, and so forth, should be the same on the prescription form and the computerized plan.

CONCEPTS USED IN PHOTON BEAM DOSE CALCULATIONS

When ionizing radiation is administered to a patient, many factors must be considered and formally identified. As noted previously, beam energy, distance from the source of radiation, and field size, are just a few of the variables that must be addressed for accurate calculation of treatment time (length of time a unit is physically activated to deliver a prescribed, measured dose) or MU setting. Note that the MU can be thought of as the

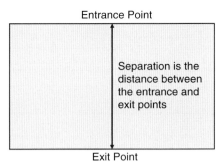

Fig. 22.1 Diagram shows patient separation as the distance between the beam entrance and exit points.

treatment "time" for a linear accelerator. Other technologies for which the treatment time is set in minutes include Gamma Knife, cobalt-60, orthovoltage, and high-dose-rate brachytherapy. The radiation physicist uses mathematics, computers, and specialized treatment planning equipment to develop dose calculation data used by the treatment team. Many of the data are organized in tables to provide quick reference for manual calculations. Before any attempt at dose calculation is made, a number of terms must be defined. The nomenclature outlines the parameters necessary for accurate treatment delivery. Remember that different approaches, methods, and terms are used for dose and MU calculations. The radiation therapist, medical dosimetrist, and medical physicist must ensure that the appropriate information for each individual application is used.

Dose

Everyone involved with treatment planning and delivery must have a clear idea of what is meant by dose. The *dose,* or absorbed dose, is measured at a specific point in a medium (typically a patient or phantom) and refers to the energy deposited at that point. Dose is commonly measured in gray (Gy), which is defined so that 1 Gy equals 1 J/kg.[2,3] Note that before the gray, the rad was the unit of absorbed dose: 100 rad equals 1 Gy, and 1 rad equals 1 cGy.

Depth

Depth is the distance beneath the skin surface where the prescribed dose is to be delivered. Sometimes the radiation oncologist specifies the depth of calculation. For example, when an area is treated with a single treatment field, the radiation oncologist states the exact point, or depth, for the calculation. With use of a posterior field for treatment of vertebral body metastasis, the radiation therapy prescription may state that a dose of 3 Gy to a depth of 5.0 cm is to be delivered. For opposed fields, the patient's midplane is often used for the depth of calculation. Most multiple field arrangements use the isocenter, or intersection of the beams, for the calculation depth. Treatment techniques, such as stereotactic, also require that the dose is prescribed to a volume, whereas IMRT techniques require that doses are specified to a number of volumes. Computed tomographic (CT) scans, which provide visual information on the patient's shape (contour) and location of organs and other anatomic structures, are useful in determination of the point of calculation. CT scan is the basis for most treatment planning systems. Often information from other scans, such as magnetic resonance imaging and positron emission tomography, can be fused onto the CT scan to provide more in-depth information. The depth of the calculation affects measurements of dose attenuation.

Separation

Separation is a measurement of the patient's thickness from the point of beam entry to the point of beam exit (Fig. 22.1). With calculation of a treatment time or MU setting, the separation is normally measured along

the beam's central axis. The separation can be measured directly with calipers, measured indirectly with the source-skin distance (SSD) readings supplied by optical distance indicators (ODIs) located on the treatment units or measured from the treatment plan. Often, for parallel opposed treatment fields (two fields focused at a point of specification directed 180 degrees apart), the calculation is done to deliver the prescribed dose at the patient's midplane or midseparation. To find the midseparation, the total separation is divided by 2. For example, if the treatment prescription requires delivery of 2 Gy per fraction at midseparation with use of opposed fields, the patient's separation at the central axis is measured. If the separation is measured as 20 cm, the midseparation (midplane) is 10 cm. In that case, a depth of 10 cm is used for the MU calculation.

Source-Skin Distance or Target-Skin Distance

Source-skin distance or target-skin distance (TSD) is the distance from the source or target of the treatment machine to the surface of the patient or phantom (a volume of tissue equivalent material). The SSD/TSD is normally measured with an ODI. This device projects a distance scale onto the patient's skin (Fig. 22.2A). The number read is the distance from the source of photons to the patient's skin surface.

> Setting and verification of the appropriate SSD on a daily basis is crucial to the accurate delivery of the radiation treatment plan. Many radiation treatment centers ensure that the radiation therapist does so by requiring weekly documentation of the SSD of all fields. The nature of the disease and the side effects of various treatments cause a high tendency for weight loss, specifically in the head and neck region and in the lung and abdomen. There is discussion on the value of the radiation therapist verifying SSDs. Some believe that a weekly check of the isocenter with an anteroposterior and lateral view or with cone beam technology is adequate. However, others believe that this simple check is still a valuable component of quality assurance. With verification and documentation of weekly SSDs, dosimetrists can note any change and account for it by changing MUs or altering the plan. If the SSD changes significantly, the patient may need resimulation and/or modifications to any immobilization devices used.

Source-Axis Distance, Target-Axis Distance, and Isocenter

The source-axis distance (SAD) or target-axis distance is the distance from the source of photons to the isocenter of the treatment machine (Fig. 22.2B). Although these terms have been used interchangeably, the term *SAD or SSD* is used for simplicity. The isocenter is the intersection of the axis of rotation of the gantry and the axis of rotation of the collimator for the treatment unit. This is usually a point in space at a specified distance from the source or target that the gantry rotates around. Cobalt-60 treatment machines typically have a SAD of 80 cm, whereas the SAD for modern linear accelerators is 100 cm. When the gantry rotates around the patient, the SSD continually changes; however, the SAD and isocenter are at a fixed distance and therefore do not change. In an isocentric treatment, the isocenter is established inside the patient. The treatment machines are designed so that the gantry rotates around this reference point.

Field Size

Field size refers to the physical dimensions set on the collimators of the therapy unit that determine the size of the treatment field at a reference distance. Depending on the type of machine, this is the setting for the *x* and *y* jaws or the upper and lower jaws. Older technologies could only produce symmetric fields (both collimators being equidistant from the central axis). Modern technology allows for independent or asymmetric setting of the jaws. For example, a "10-cm"-wide field could have the jaws set at −4 cm and +6 cm, which has one jaw 4 cm from the

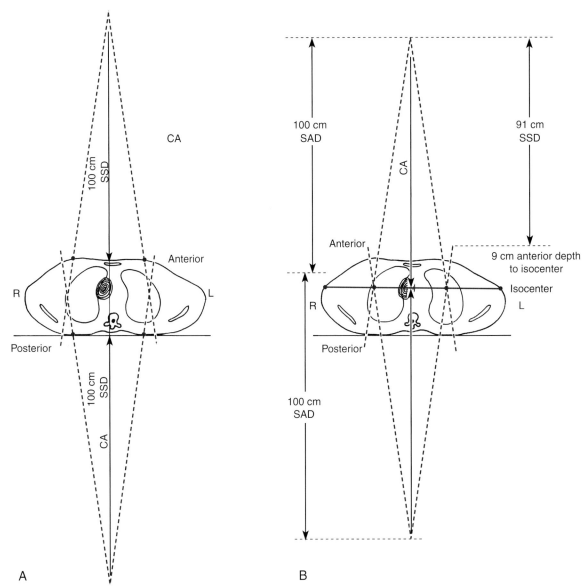

Fig. 22.2 Differences are shown between (A) a source-skin distance *(SSD)* approach, where the field size is defined on the surface, and (B) a source-axis distance *(SAD)* approach, where the field size is defined at a depth calculated within the patient. Both methods used in the planning and delivery of a prescribed course of radiation therapy require careful documentation.

central axis and the other jaw 6 cm from the central axis. Asymmetric jaws and MLC settings require more complicated dosimetry than the historic-type symmetric jaws. The field size is normally defined at the machine's isocenter. For example, when a field size of 10 × 10 cm is set on the treatment unit (*x* and *y* digital readouts), the square treatment field measures 10 × 10 cm at the isocentric distance for that particular machine. On most linear accelerators, the isocenter distance is at 100 cm. On a cobalt-60 machine, the distance is at 80 cm.

Field size changes with distance from the source of radiation because of divergence. The 10 × 10 cm field size measures smaller at distances shorter than the isocentric distance and larger at distances greater than the isocentric distance. In an isocentric patient treatment, the field size set is inside the patient at the isocenter distance. This is called an *SAD treatment.* The physical size measured on the patient's surface at that point is smaller because it is at a distance shorter than the isocenter. In the nonisocentric (SSD) patient treatment, the field size set on the collimator is the same as measured on the skin surface because the isocentric distance is set at the skin surface in this instance.

For an extended distance treatment (>100 cm to the skin), the field size on the skin is greater than the field size at the isocenter because of the increased distance.

Scatter

The radiation treatment beam is composed of both primary and scatter radiation. Any interaction of the primary radiation may result in scatter. When the primary beam interacts with matter, the result is scatter radiation made up of photons or electrons. A change of direction is associated with scatter radiation. When an electron interacts with the target in the linear accelerator, photons are produced. These photons are the primary beam. As the primary photons travel to the patient, they interact with the flattening filter; then, some of them interact with the collimator. When the primary photon interacts with the collimator, the photon beam may also be deflected back toward the patient. The deflected photons are considered scatter radiation. When the photons reach the patient and travel through the patient, they interact mostly with the electrons. Many of these photons change direction with each

TABLE 22.1	Approximate Depths of Maximum Equilibrium
Beam Energy	**Depth of D_{max} (cm)**
200 kV	0.0
1.25 MV	0.5
4 MV	1.0
6 MV	1.5
10 MV	2.5
20 MV	3.5
25 MV	5.0

D_{max}, Depth of maximum equilibrium.

electron interaction and thus create scatter radiation within the patient. Radiation that is scattered back toward the surface of the patient is called *backscatter* (this is covered in more detail later in this chapter). The absorbed dose received by the patient results from secondary radiation caused by interactions in which the primary and scattered photons impart energy to the electrons. Then, the electron undergoes tens of thousands of collisions while giving up some energy at each collision. Most of the absorbed dose that is received by the patient results from the collisions of the scattered electrons with other electrons.

Depth of Maximum Equilibrium

The *depth of maximum equilibrium* (D_{max}) is the depth at which electronic equilibrium occurs for photon beams. D_{max} is the point at which the maximum absorbed dose occurs for single-field photon beams and mainly depends on the energy of the beam. The depth of maximum ionization increases as the energy of the photon beam increases. D_{max} occurs at the surface (or within a few millimeters of the surface) for low-energy photon beams (KV) and beneath the surface for megavoltage photon beams (MV). Other factors such as field size and distance may influence the depth at which maximum ionization occurs. Table 22.1 lists the approximate depth of D_{max} for various photon beam energies. When the depth of D_{max} occurs at a significant depth (1.0 to 4.0 cm) below the skin, the dose to the skin is reduced. This principle is an important concept that is known as *skin sparing*.

Knowledge of the dose at D_{max} is important at times. When a patient is treated with a single field, the dose at D_{max} should be calculated and recorded because the dose at D_{max} is higher than the prescribed dose. The dose at D_{max} is also greater than the prescribed dose when opposed treatment fields are used to treat the patient and are greater than the dose delivered to the patient's midplane. The dose at D_{max} is slightly greater than the midplane dose for high-energy treatment beams and for patients with a small separation. When low-energy treatment beams (cobalt-60 and 6 MV) are used, the dose at D_{max} can be significantly higher than the midplane dose. This is especially true for large patient separations. When megavoltage photon beams are used, calculation of the dose at D_{max} may not be necessary with use of multiple field arrangements to treat the patient. With use of many fields, the dose at D_{max} is normally less than the prescribed dose.

Output

The output can be referred to as the dose rate (cGy/MU) of the machine; in the past, it has been measured in the absence of a scattering phantom and in tissue equivalent material.[2] Referencing the Task Group-51 (TG51) protocol and the TG51 addendum, the dose rate is measured in a phantom.[1,5] It is the amount of radiation "exposure" produced by a treatment machine or source as specified at a reference field size and at a specified reference distance. The reference field size and distance are used so that standardized measurements may be related to those that vary from the standards. The reference field size is often a 10×10 cm field measured at the isocenter. Changing the field size, distance, or attenuating medium changes the dose rate. Dose rate increases with increased field size. Remember that a therapeutic beam of radiation is made up of primary and scatter radiation and measured at a point of reference. If the field size is increased on a treatment machine, the primary component remains the same. However, the increased area causes increased scatter, which adds to the output (all other parameters remaining constant). If the distance from the source of radiation to the point of measurement increases, then the dose rate decreases because of the inverse square law. An example of output on a cobalt-60 unit may be 100 cGy/min, whereas a linear accelerator reference output may be 1.0 cGy/MU at the reference field size and distance.

Output Factor

The output factor is the ratio of the dose rate of a given field size to the dose rate of the reference field size. The output factor allows for the change in scatter as the collimator setting changes. The output factor is usually normalized or referenced to a 10×10 cm field size, which means that the output factor for a 10×10 cm field size is 1.00 for the linear accelerator or cobalt-60 unit. The output factor is greater than 1.00 for field sizes larger than 10×10 cm because of an increase in scatter as the collimator setting is increased. The output factor is less than 1.00 for field sizes smaller than 10×10 cm because of a decrease in scatter as the collimator setting is decreased.

The term *output factor* may be a generic term. Many institutions use other terminology, such as *relative output factor, collimator scatter factor, field size correction factor,* and *phantom scatter factor*. Khan[4] defines measured values for collimator scatter factor and total scatter factors and a derived value for phantom scatter factor. The authors use the conventions defined by Kahn in this chapter (collimator scatter factor [Sc], phantom or patient scatter factor [Sp], and combined collimator and phantom scatter [Sc, p]).

Output factors relate the dose rate of a given collimator setting to the dose rate of the reference field size and are useful and practical for calculations that involve linear accelerators and cobalt-60 treatment machines. The reference dose rate (RDR) for the cobalt-60 treatment machine constantly changes because of the decaying of the cobalt-60 radioisotope used as the source of gamma ray emissions in these machines. Usually, the RDR is updated monthly. Although the RDR is changed every month, the output factors do not change; therefore with use of output factors, only the RDR must be changed. Normally, the RDR is 1.0 cGy/MU for linear accelerators. The RDR does not normally change for linear accelerators, which means that in some centers, the output factor is the dose rate for that field size (any number multiplied by 1 does not change). For example, say that the RDR is 1.0 cGy/MU for a 10×10 cm field size measured at 100 cm from the target in free space. Also say that the output factor for the 15×15 cm collimator setting is 1.02 (larger than 1.00 because the field size is greater than the reference). The dose rate for the 15×15 cm collimator setting can be calculated as follows:

$$\text{Dose Rate}_{(\text{Given Field Size})} = \text{Dose Rate}_{(\text{Reference Field Size})} \times \text{Output Factor}_{(\text{Given Field Size})}$$

$$\text{Dose Rate}_{(\text{Field Size } 15 \times 15)} = 1.0 \text{ cGy/MU} \times 1.02$$

$$\text{Dose Rate}_{(\text{Field Size } 15 \times 15)} = 1.02 \text{ cGy/MU}$$

Today, some treatment centers use more than one output factor. For example, some calculation models require the use of a collimator scatter factor (Sc) and a phantom scatter factor (Sp). Sc is used to determine the scatter, usually measured in air, from the collimators (or head scatter, which is defined subsequently), and Sp is used to determine the scatter from the patient. Later in the chapter, it is shown that both Sc and Sp can simplify the MU calculation.

Historically, the scatter that is generated in the treatment head is called *collimator scatter*. However, scatter is generated in both the collimator and the flattening filter. The combination of scatter generated in the flattening filter and collimator is known as *head scatter*. When the primary beam passes through the flattening filter, some photons are absorbed, some pass through, and some are scattered. These scattered photons are spread out spatially across the flattening filter. In essence, the flattening filter acts as a second source of photons that is broader than the primary source. Imagine looking from the patient back to the x-ray target; you can see the entire flattening filter if the collimators are open wide enough. If the collimators are then partially closed, part of the filter is blocked from your view. Thus as the field size changes, the amount of scatter from the flattening filter that reaches the patient changes.

Note that modern linear accelerators may offer flattening filter free applications. Although IMRT offers improved dose conformity to the target, it tends to have higher MUs compared with three-dimensional techniques, contributing to higher leakage from the gantry head and consequently increased dose to normal tissues and whole body.[10] To reduce the unnecessary scatter from the gantry head and shorten the treatment time for IMRT delivery, removal of the flattening filter has been a logical choice to reduce the scatter. This is an example of how technological advances address fundamental operational challenges.

Inverse Square Law

The inverse square law is a mathematic relationship that describes the change in beam intensity caused by the divergence of the beam. As the beam of radiation diverges or spreads out, a decrease in the intensity is seen. Therefore as the distance from the source of radiation increases, the intensity decreases. For example, a photon beam that is made up of 400 photons is administered in a field size of 10×10 cm at a distance of 100 cm. The area of the beam is 100 cm^2 (with the formula width $\times$ length). If the photon coverage is uniform, intensity is 4 photons/cm^2. At a distance of 200 cm, the field size doubles to dimensions of 20×20 cm. The area of this field is then 400 cm^2. Still only 400 photons cover this larger area. Now if the photon coverage is uniform, there is 1 photon/cm^2. With doubling of the distance, the intensity or number of photons per square centimeter has decreased to one-fourth of the original intensity.

One practical application of the inverse square law is its effect on the output or dose rate of the treatment machine. The dose rate is commonly measured at the isocenter of the treatment machine. For linear accelerators, the dose rate at the isocenter for a 10×10 cm field is often 1.0 cGy/MU. When the MUs are calculated for treatment at distances greater than the standard, the inverse square law is used to account for the decrease in dose rate at distances beyond the isocenter. The dose rate of the beam is inversely proportional to the square of the distance, which means that even a small change in distance can have a large effect on the dose rate. For example, if the dose rate is 1.0 cGy/MU at 100 cm, then the dose rate is 0.64 cGy/MU at 125 cm (see the following method used to calculate the change in dose rate).

The equation commonly used for the inverse square law is as follows:

$$I_1/I_2 = (d_2)^2/(d_1)^2$$

with *I* for intensity and *d* for distance. This equation may be used to find the change in dose rate with a change in distance (note that the general term *I*, intensity, is replaced with a more specific term, dose rate

at distance). The following equation is used to calculate the dose rate at distances other than the reference (isocenter) distance:

$$\text{Dose Rate at Distance}_1/\text{Dose Rate at Distance}_2 = (\text{Distance}_2)^2/(\text{Distance}_1)^2$$

Example: The dose rate at 100 cm is 1.0 cGy/MU. Calculate the dose rate at 125 cm. For this example, distance 1 is defined as 125 cm and distance 2 as 100 cm. Rearranging the previous equation, we get the following:

$$\text{Dose Rate at Distance}_1 = \text{Dose Rate at Distance}_2 \times (\text{Distance}_2)^2/(\text{Distance}_1)^2$$

Substituting the values in our example, we have the following:

$$\text{Dose Rate at 125 cm} = \text{Dose Rate at 100 cm} \times (100 \text{ cm})^2/(125 \text{ cm})^2$$

$$\text{Dose Rate at 125 cm} = 1.0 \text{ cGy/MU} \times (100 \text{ cm})^2/(125 \text{ cm})^2$$

$$\text{Dose Rate at 125 cm} = 0.64 \text{ cGy/MU}$$

The following is a second example for calculating the dose rate at a different distance with the inverse square law.

Example: The dose rate of a linear accelerator is 1.0 cGy/MU at a distance of 100 cm. Calculate the dose rate at 90 cm. Distance$_1$ is defined as 90 cm for this example. Rearranging the previous equation, we get the following:

$$\text{Dose Rate at Distance}_1 = \text{Dose Rate at Distance}_2 \times (\text{Distance}_2)^2/(\text{Distance}_1)^2$$

Substituting the values in our example, we have the following:

$$\text{Dose Rate at 90 cm} = \text{Dose Rate at 100 cm} \times (100 \text{ cm})^2/(90 \text{ cm})^2$$

$$\text{Dose Rate at 90 cm} = 1.0 \text{ cGy/MU} \times (100 \text{ cm})^2/(90 \text{ cm})^2$$

$$\text{Dose Rate at 90 cm} = 1.235 \text{ cGy/MU}$$

Note that in this chapter, the correction for distance in the MU and dose calculations is referred to as the *inverse square correction factor* (ISCF). Some clinics may refer to this correction as the *distance correction factor*.

Equivalent Squares of Rectangular Fields

A square field is a field that has equal dimensions for the field width and length, such as a 10×10 cm field. A rectangular field has a field width and length that are different, as is the case with a 10×15 cm field; in a clinical setting, most patients are treated with rectangular fields of different sizes. Treatment calculation tables use field size as a qualifying parameter. Use of different rectangular field sizes requires extensive tables with thousands of number combinations. Thus a method is needed to make the amount of data and number of tables manageable.

Equivalent square of rectangular fields (ESRF) postulates that, for an arbitrary rectangular field, there exists an equivalent square (ES) field sharing certain dosimetric characteristics.[11] That concept provides a pathway for estimating a rectangular field's properties (e.g., central axis percentage depth dose [PDD], scatter factor) from measurements performed on square fields. For a rectangular field with width (a) and length (b), Sterling's approximation formula of 4 times

TABLE 22.2 Sample Equivalent Squares of Rectangular Fields Chart

Long Axis (cm)	0.5	1.0	2.0	3.0	4.0	5.0	6.0	7.0	8.0	9.0	10.0	11.0	12.0
0.5	0.5												
1	0.7	1.0											
2	0.9	1.4	2.0										
3	1.0	1.6	2.4	3.0									
4	1.1	1.7	2.7	3.4	4.0								
5	1.2	1.8	2.9	3.8	4.5	5.0							
6	1.2	1.9	3.1	4.1	4.8	5.5	6.0						
7	1.2	2.0	3.3	4.3	5.1	5.8	6.5	7.0					
8	1.2	2.1	3.4	4.5	5.4	6.2	6.9	7.5	8.0				
9	1.2	2.1	3.5	4.6	5.6	6.5	7.2	7.9	8.5	9.0			
10	1.3	2.2	3.6	4.8	5.8	6.7	7.5	8.2	8.9	9.5	10.0		
11	1.3	2.2	3.7	4.9	6.0	6.9	7.8	8.5	9.3	9.9	10.5	11.0	
12	1.3	2.2	3.7	5.0	6.1	7.1	8.0	8.8	9.6	10.3	10.9	11.5	12.0
13	1.3	2.2	3.8	5.1	6.2	7.2	8.2	9.1	9.9	10.6	11.3	11.9	12.5
14	1.3	2.3	3.8	5.1	6.3	7.4	8.4	9.3	10.1	10.9	11.6	12.3	12.9
15	1.3	2.3	3.9	5.2	6.4	7.5	8.5	9.5	10.3	11.2	11.9	12.6	13.3
16	1.3	2.3	3.9	5.3	6.5	7.6	8.6	9.6	10.5	11.4	12.2	12.9	13.7
17	1.3	2.3	3.9	5.3	6.5	7.7	8.8	9.8	10.7	11.6	12.4	13.2	14.0
18	1.3	2.3	3.9	5.3	6.6	7.8	8.9	9.9	10.9	11.8	12.6	13.5	14.3
19	1.4	2.3	4.0	5.4	6.6	7.8	8.9	10.0	11.0	11.9	12.8	13.7	14.5
20	1.4	2.3	4.0	5.4	6.7	7.9	9.0	10.1	11.1	12.1	13.0	13.9	14.7
40	1.4	2.4	4.1	5.6	7.0	8.3	9.5	10.7	11.9	13.0	14.1	15.2	16.3

the area divided by the perimeter was historically the first widely used and remains the primary choice in current medical physics practice and is almost a synonym for ES calculations because of its simple mathematical structure and good prediction power for conventionally shaped and sized fields.[11] In the application of the Sterling formula, the number derived from the calculation is one side of the square field that has approximately the same measurable scattering and attenuation characteristics as the original rectangular field, essentially taking field shape into account. This formula is an approximation and should be used when an ESRF table is not available. In general, if the ratio of width or length exceeds 2 (e.g., a 16 × 4 cm field), the use of standardized tables of ESs is recommended. Table 22.2 is an example of a chart that shows ESRF.

Although a formula or equation may appear to be an exact calculation, the Sterling formula does not always account for the loss of scatter back to the central point (e.g., central axis, isocenter), so its accuracy, especially for extremely elongated fields, still leaves room for improvement.[11] For example, with the formula, the following results are obtained for a 12.0 × 16.0 cm field size and a 7.0 × 40.0 cm field size: 13.7 cm and 11.9 cm, respectively. However, with reference to the ES table, the ESs of the fields are 13.7 and 10.7. Thus for the field where both the width and the length are similar, the formula and the table produce the same or similar results. However, when one dimension of the field is much greater than the other dimension, the formula and table produce two very different results. The table "based on measurements" provides a more accurate result than Sterling formula.

Another calculation method for ES estimation, weighted power mean (WPM), outperformed the Sterling formula on three tests, and with increasing utilization of very elongated, small rectangular fields in modern radiation therapy, improved photon output factor estimation is expected by considering the WPM formula in treatment planning and secondary MU check.[11]

Example: Use the Sterling formula to calculate the ES for a field of dimensions 10 cm × 20 cm:

$$ES = 4 \ (Area/Perimeter)$$

$$ES = 4 \ (10 \times 20) / ([10 \times 2] + [20 \times 2])$$

$$ES = 4 \ (200)/60$$

$$ES = 13.3$$

The ESRF tables are commonly used to find the output, output factor, and tissue absorption factors. Most radiation beam data tables are constructed so that the ESRF must be known to use the table. For example, for the output factor for a square field, the ES is found to be 10 × 10 cm.[9] The output factor for a 10 × 10 cm field is used because it is effectively the same as that of a 7 × 19 cm field, all other parameters remaining unchanged. The output factor for a 10 × 10 cm field is 1.000. Therefore the output factor for a 7 × 19 cm field is also 1.000.

When MLCs or blocks are used to customize the shape of the treatment area, two portions of the field are created. The first is the area being shielded, and the second is the area being treated. When looking at the area being treated, its dimensions must be determined. This derived field size is called the effective field size (EFS) or *blocked field size*, which is the equivalent rectangular field dimension of the open or treated area within the collimator field dimensions. Usually some method of approximation is used to determine the EFS (a square or rectangular field that approximates the same physical volume as the blocked shape). The EFS is normally smaller than the collimator field size, although it may be larger for some extended distance treatments. The general rules for measurement of EFS are as follows:

1. Basic field shape should be maintained for the effective field (a field that looks like an elongated rectangle should retain a rectangular shape after measurement).
2. One should visualize the closest rectangular area that can be adapted to the irregular field.
3. The rectangular field is converted to an ES.

The actual collimator setting ES may be used to determine the Sc. The EFS ES is normally used to determine the Sp and tissue absorption factors, such as the PDD, tissue-air ratio (TAR), tissue-phantom ratio (TPR), or tissue-maximum ratio (TMR), which are discussed in the following section. (Special note: Whether to use the actual ES or EFS may be based on the construction of the linear accelerator and manufacturer's placement of the MLCs within the treatment unit head. Some manufacturers construct the treatment head so that the MLC is on the proximal side of the x and y jaws. Other manufacturers have the MLC on the distal side of the jaws.)

TISSUE ABSORPTION FACTORS

As the beam of radiation travels through the body, it gives up energy. The more tissue the beam traverses, the more it is attenuated (the more energy it gives up). A number of different methods have been used for measurement of the attenuation of the beam as it travels through tissue. In historic order, they are PDD, TAR, TMR, and TPR. The first of these methods used in a treatment setting was PDD. Remember that in the early days of radiation therapy, patients were treated with an SSD technique, which is referred to as a *nonisocentric treatment* in this chapter. PDD was primarily developed for SSD treatments. With appropriate corrections, any of the four methods (PDD, TAR, TPR, and TMR) may be used for SSD or SAD treatments. However, PDD works best with SSD (nonisocentric) treatments, whereas TAR, TMR, and TPR work very well with SAD (isocentric) treatments.

> As previously stated, when a photon beam is directed, it immediately begins to release its energy. Because of this, a dose is released from the point of beam entry into the body and continues on, also depositing some exit dose as it leaves the body; therefore the dose must be modified to ensure that the tolerance dose of any surrounding structures is not exceeded.
>
> The characteristics of a proton beam are dramatically different. With proton therapy, the physician can predict and control the exact depth at which the beam is deposited in the patient. The position that the physician picks to deposit the dose is called the Bragg peak. After the beam reaches the Bragg peak, the dose is deposited, and then there is quick falloff of the beam to eliminate exit dose. This allows the physician to increase the tumoricidal dose (tumor lethal dose) delivered to the patient because the effect on surrounding critical structures is minimal, which reduces toxicity and increases chances of tumor control.[6]

Percentage Depth Dose

The PDD is the ratio, expressed as a percentage, of the absorbed dose at a given depth to the absorbed dose at a fixed reference depth, usually D_{max},[9] (Fig. 22.3) as follows:

$$PDD = \text{Absorbed Dose at Depth} / \text{Absorbed Dose at } D_{maxa} \times 100\%$$

Normally, the depth of D_{max} is used for the fixed reference depth. PDD is dependent on four factors: energy, depth, field size, and SSD. PDD increases as the energy, field size, and SSD increase. This is a direct relationship. Higher energies are more penetrating, so a greater percentage of dose is available at a specific depth compared with a lower energy. As field size increases, more scatter is added to the deposited beam, thus increasing PDD. As the distance from the

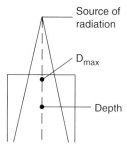

Fig. 22.3 Diagram of percentage depth dose (PDD). PDD measures the dose along the central ray at depth as it compares with the dose at depth of maximum equilibrium *(D$_{max}$)*.

source of radiation to the patient (phantom) surface increases, the PDD increases. The increase in PDD is based on a mathematic relationship and is discussed in the section for the Mayneord "F" factor. PDD decreases as the depth in tissue increases (inverse relationship) because dose is deposited in tissue as it traverses it; thus a smaller percentage is available at greater depths.

Tissue-Air Ratio

The TAR is the ratio of the absorbed dose at a given depth in phantom to the absorbed dose at the same point in free space (Fig. 22.4):

$$TAR = \text{Dose in Tissue} / \text{Dose in Air}$$

Free space (in air) is a term used for measurements that use a buildup cap or mini-phantom (a small volume of tissue equivalent material that does not include full scatter). A maxi-phantom (phantom) is a large volume of tissue equivalent material that produces "full scatter." A true air measurement may not be possible. A buildup cap is a device made of acrylic or other phantom material that is placed over an ionization chamber to produce conditions of electronic equilibrium, which allows for a more accurate measurement. The mini-phantom is a sphere of tissue-equivalent material that surrounds a point of interest. There is just enough material to produce buildup at the center (depth of D_{max}).[4] The ionization chamber then measures the flow of electrons and eventually the dose rate of the treatment machine (Fig. 22.5).

In determination of the TAR, the dose is measured at a reference distance from the target but within two sets of conditions. The first measurement is in free space (buildup cap or mini-phantom), and the second measurement is in phantom (the point of measurement does not change between the two measurements). The amount of phantom material used for the second measurement corresponds to the depth of interest.

The TAR depends on energy, field size, and depth.[4] TAR increases as the energy and field size increase and decreases as the depth increases. These characteristics are consistent with PDD. However, TAR is independent of SSD (distance) because both of the measurements for the "ratio" are measured at the same distance from the source of radiation. TAR is normally used to perform calculations for SAD treatments that involve low-energy treatment units such as a cobalt-60 or a 4-MV linear accelerator. Few treatment centers use TAR for energies greater than 4 MV.

Scatter-Air Ratio

The absorbed dose of radiation used to treat cancer is made up of two distinct components as it is measured along the central ray of the beam at the point of calculation: primary radiation that is emitted from the treatment unit and scatter radiation from the surrounding irradiated tissue. The primary part of total absorbed dose is represented by the zero-area (zero field size) TAR. This zero-area TAR cannot be measured directly. The difference between the TAR for a field of definite area and

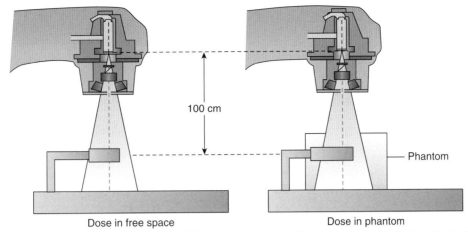

Fig. 22.4 Diagram of tissue-air ratio (TAR). TAR compares the dose in tissue at a specific depth with the dose in air at the same distance from the source (at the isocenter). When the depth in tissue corresponds to the level of dose at depth of maximum equilibrium (D_{max}), the TAR is known as the backscatter or peak/phantom scatter factor.

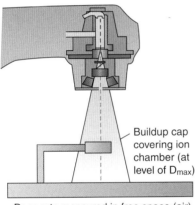

Fig. 22.5 Dose rate measured in air. A buildup cap over the ionization measuring chamber allows for maximum scatter component to be accounted for. D_{max}, Depth of maximum equilibrium.

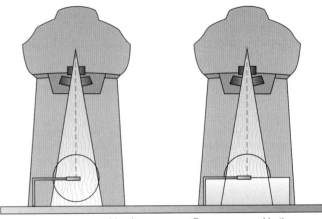

Fig. 22.6 Backscatter or peak/phantom scatter factor relates dose in tissue to dose in air at the level of maximum equilibrium. D_{max}, Depth of maximum equilibrium.

that for a zero area is a measure of the contribution from scattered radiation. The contribution of scatter to points of calculation in the irradiated tissue, along the central ray, and points off axis is particularly important as the irregular shapes of the treatment fields are considered. The intensity of the beam can vary across the field. The variation is mainly dependent on depth and distance from the central axis. With calculation of doses to points that are off axis (i.e., do not lie on the central axis), off-axis ratios, off-axis factors, or off-center ratios are used.

Off-axis point doses can also be calculated to good approximation by entering the appropriate SSD and depth, with allowance for off-axis output profile in determining the primary dose contribution. In their use, they are added back to adjusted SAR values to calculate an effective TAR for a specific field geometry, so the result is not sensitive to what model was used, provided the same one is used to derive the SAR. Virtually all modern treatment planning computer systems include irregular field algorithms to accurately calculate treatment doses for shaped fields.[3]

Backscatter Factor and Peak Scatter Factor

The backscatter factor (BSF) or peak scatter factor (PSF) is the ratio of the dose rate with a scattering medium (water or phantom) to the dose rate at the same point without a scattering medium (air) at the depth (level) of maximum equilibrium.[2–4,7] Backscatter is then a TAR at the depth (level) of D_{max}. The BSF

is measured at the surface for orthovoltage and other low-energy x-ray treatment machines (energies <400 kV; Fig. 22.6). The BSF is measured at the depth of D_{max} for megavoltage photon beams. The preferred terminology is to use BSF for low-energy beams and PSF for high-energy beams (>4 MV). The PSF is sometimes normalized to a reference field size, usually 10×10 cm, for energies of 4 MV and higher.[2]

Tissue-Phantom Ratio and Tissue-Maximum Ratio

The TPR is the ratio of the absorbed dose at a given depth in phantom to the absorbed dose at the same point at a reference depth in phantom as follows:

$$TPR = \text{Dose in Tissue/Dose in Phantom}$$

The reference depth may be any depth (e.g., 5.0 cm). If the reference depth is chosen to be the depth of D_{max}, then the TPR is referred to as the TMR, as seen in Fig. 22.7:

$$TMR = \text{Dose in Tissue/Dose in Phantom } (D_{max})$$

The TMR is related to the TAR by the formula TAR = TMR × BSF for low-energy beams or TAR = TMR × PSF for high-energy beams.

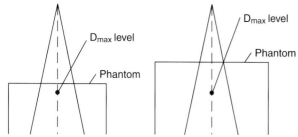

Fig. 22.7 Tissue-maximum ratio compares dose at the depth of maximum equilibrium *(D_max)* with dose at the depth where the distance from the source to each point is the same. If another point of reference is used instead of D_{max}, the relationship is known as tissue-phantom ratio.

The TMR and TPR were developed because of difficulties in measurement of the TAR for high-energy beams. TAR is measured with some form of a buildup cap (small-volume tissue-equivalent material). With high-energy beams, a large buildup cap is needed for accurate measurement. As the buildup cap becomes increasingly larger, phantom scatter is introduced into the "free space" of the TAR. A buildup cap is not needed for measurement of TPR or TMR because both measurements are done in phantom. Thus TMR overcame the problem of getting a true free space measurement.

Because the depth of D_{max} depends on field size, the reference depths for TMR change with field size accordingly. One advantage of a TPR over a TMR is that the reference depth does not change with field size. With use of a reference depth of D_{max} for the 10 × 10 cm field size, the dependence of the depth of D_{max} with field size has been eliminated with the use of TPR.

In determination of the TMR and TPR, the dose is measured at one distance from the target but at two different depths in phantom-specific conditions. The first measurement is at the depth of D_{max} or another established standard, and the second measurement is at the desired depth. The point of measurement does not change between the two measurements. The amount of phantom material used for the second measurement is determined by the depth of interest. The value of TMR is never greater than 1.00, and the value of TPR has no upper limit. The deeper the reference depth, the greater the TPR.[8] See Box 22.1 for a summary of tissue absorption factors.

Dose Rate Modification Factors

Any device placed in the path of the radiation beam attenuates some of it. The transmission factor is the ratio of the radiation dose with the device to the radiation dose without the device and accounts for the material in the beam's path. Examples of such factors include tray transmission, wedge, and compensating filter factors.

Tray Transmission Factor

Most modern linear accelerators have MLCs and, for most situations, have eliminated the need for Cerrobend blocks that are mounted onto or placed on a block tray. Most block trays are made of a plastic derivative. When a tray is used, some of the beam is absorbed by the tray, and the MU setting must be increased to ensure that the prescribed dose is delivered. The *tray transmission factor* (tray factor) defines how much of the radiation is transmitted through a block tray. The medical physicist takes two measurements: the first measurement is with the tray in the path of the beam, and the second measurement is without the tray in the path of the beam. The ratio of these two measurements is known as the tray transmission factor. For example, if a dose with the tray in place is measured as 97 cGy and the dose without the tray is 100 cGy, the

---

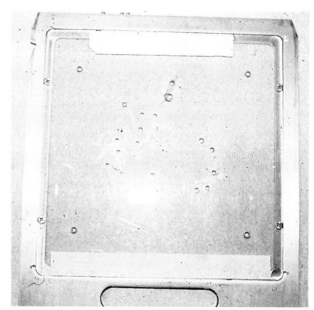

Fig. 22.8 Typical blocking tray used to support standardized or custom shielding blocks.

ratio of the two doses, 97/100, yields a tray transmission factor of 0.97. This means that 97% of the radiation is transmitted through the tray and 3% of the radiation is attenuated. Tray factors vary with beam energy. As energy increases, the effect of the material in the beam's path is lessened because of the increased penetrating power of the higher energy. Thus departments may use the same trays on different treatment units (Fig. 22.8) and simply use an appropriate tray factor for the energy with which it is used.

For delivery of an accurate dose to the patient, the radiation attenuated by the tray must be taken into consideration. This is normally done with the tray transmission factor as a dose rate modifier. When the tray transmission factor is handled in this manner, it should always be represented by a number less than 1.00. Although this is the method used in this chapter, some therapy departments may multiply the MU or time setting by a tray factor that is greater than 1.00. For example, if the calculated MU setting before the tray is taken into account is 100 MU and the tray factor is 1.03 (denoting 3% attenuation), with the 100 MU multiplied by 1.03, a corrected MU setting of 103 is obtained. When the tray factor is greater than 1.00, it is not a tray transmission factor and cannot be multiplied by the dose rate to account for the attenuation. In these cases, the machine setting must be increased by this factor.

Wedge and Compensator Filter Transmission Factors

The wedge transmission factor (wedge factor) depicts the amount of the radiation transmitted through a physical or virtual wedge placed

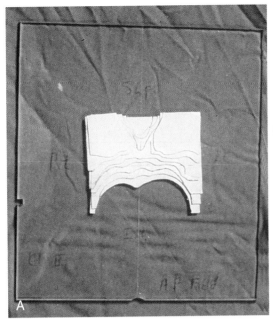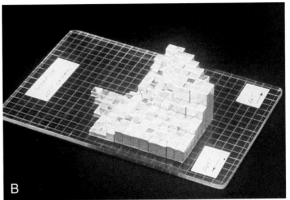

Fig. 22.9 Compensator filters. (A) Lead sheet compensator filter. (B) Aluminum cube compensator filter. These filters attenuate the beam so that topographic variances are accounted for. Through this process, the distribution of dose at depths below the surface is even.

in the beam to shape the beam delivery. A physical wedge is made of a dense material, usually lead or steel, that attenuates the radiation beam progressively across a field. The thinner side of the wedge attenuates less of the beam than does the thicker side, which results in an alteration of the beam isodose patterns.[2,3] The physicist takes several measurements and defines the wedge transmission factor, which is specific for each beam energy with which it is used. If a wedge has a wedge transmission factor of 0.67, 67% of the radiation is transmitted through the wedge, and 33% of the radiation is attenuated. To deliver the correct dose to the patient, a correction must be made for this amount of beam attenuation. In addition to physical wedges, some methods can be used to simulate the effects of a physical wedge. Dynamic wedge, enhanced dynamic wedge, virtual wedge, and omni wedge are names used by various manufacturers for systems with no physical wedge. A physical wedge when placed in the path of the beam changes the intensity across the field and creates a "tilting" of the isodose curves. The angle of "tilt" is the wedge angle. For example, a 45-degree physical wedge produces a 45-degree tilt in the isodose curves. Dynamic, virtual, and other systems use no physical wedge. Instead, the change in intensity across the field is created by computer-controlled movement of one of the independent jaws across the field while the beam is on.

The compensator filter transmission factor is measured in the same manner as the wedge transmission factor. A compensator filter alters the isodose patterns, just as in the wedge (Fig. 22.9). However, the compensator filter is individually produced for each patient and alters the patterns so that they are at maximum efficiency for that patient. Both factors are normally multiplied into the dose rate with a treatment unit calculation. Examples of treatment unit calculations that involve physical wedges and compensators can be found in the section on applications. Remember that anytime a tray, wedge, or compensating filter is used, the MU setting must be adjusted upward to account for the radiation that is absorbed by one of these accessory devices.

PRACTICAL APPLICATIONS OF PHOTON BEAM DOSE CALCULATIONS

A comprehensive understanding of the factors that affect radiation treatment delivery is extremely important to the radiation oncology team. Small changes in parameters can change the dose administered to the patient. A field size set incorrectly changes the machine output in reference to the patient. A sagging tabletop that inaccurately sets the patient at a wrong distance can have the same effect. With all this in mind and with a continued focus on the relationships presented, this section presents practical applications of treatment unit calculations. Tables needed for the calculations are located within the chapter.

Treatment Unit Calculations: General Equation

With attempts to perform treatment unit calculations, a number of variables must be accounted for. Field size variations, energy changes, and modifiers in the beam's path can alter the amount of radiation received by a patient, as either an underdose or an overdose. Although the complexity of each calculation varies within these parameters, one basic equation addresses virtually every scenario. The general equation for performing MU or treatment time calculation can be represented as follows:
Linear accelerator:

$$\text{MU} = \text{Dose at a Point/Dose Rate at That Point}$$

Cobalt-60:

$$\text{Minute Setting} = \text{Dose at a Point / Dose Rate at That Point}$$

The MU setting represents the setting to be used on a linear accelerator, and the time setting represents the minutes for a cobalt-60 treatment unit. The dose at a point represents the prescribed dose as determined by the radiation oncologist. The dose rate at that point represents the dose rate of the treatment unit at the point of calculation (depth or point as identified in the prescription). Three general points are necessary with a treatment calculation: (1) one must know the dose

BOX 22.2   Six-Step Process

1. Determine the equivalent square for the collimator setting
   Used to determine collimator scatter factor (Sc)
2. Determine the effective field size
   Used to determine both phantom or patient scatter factor (Sp) and the tissue absorption factor
3. Determine the appropriate tissue absorption table
   Percentage depth dose (PDD), tissue-air ratio (TAR), tissue-maximum ratio (TMR), or tissue-phantom ratio (TPR)
4. Determine the prescribed dose
   Usually from the radiation therapy prescription
5. Look up the factors with use of the appropriate data tables
   Reference dose rate, Sc, Sp, other factors (tray factor, wedge factor, etc.)
6. Use the appropriate equation to calculate the minute or monitor unit setting

BOX 22.3   PDD Inverse Square Correction Factor

The reference distance for cobalt-60 is 80 cm, and the depth of maximum equilibrium (D_{max}) is 0.5 cm. Therefore 80.5 cm is used for cobalt-60 calculations with use of percentage depth dose (PDD).

The reference distance for a 6-MV linear accelerator is 100 cm, and the depth of D_{max} is 1.5 cm. Therefore 101.5 cm is used for 6-MV linear accelerator calculations with use of PDD.

BOX 22.4   Equations Used for SSD Calculations

Calculation of the minute setting for cobalt-60 treatments with use of percentage depth dose (PDD):

   Minute Setting = Prescribed Dose/ reference dose rate (RDR) × inverse square correction factor inverse square correction factor (ISCF) × collimator scatter factor (Sc) × phantom or patient scatter factor (Sp) × (percentage depth dose [PDD]/100) × Other Factors

Calculation of the monitor unit setting with use of percentage depth dose (PDD):

   Monitor unit (MU) Setting = Prescribed Dose/ reference dose rate (RDR) × inverse square correction factor (ISCF) × collimator scatter factor (Sc) × phantom or patient scatter factor (Sp) × (percentage depth dose [PDD]/100) × Other Factors

Calculation of the dose to a point with use of percentage depth dose (PDD): ratio method:

   $Dose_A$/percentage depth dose $(PDD)_A = Dose_B$/percentage depth dose $(PDD)_B$

Calculation of the dose to a point with use of percentage depth dose (PDD): special equations:

   Given Dose = tumor dose (TD)/percentage depth dose $(PDD)_{tumor\ dose\ (TD)}$ × 100
   Tumor Dose = Given Dose × percentage depth dose $(PDD)_{tumor\ dose\ (TD)}$/100

at a point, (2) one must know the dose rate at that point, and (3) the dose and dose rate must be in the same medium (usually tissue).

Normally the dose and dose rate are expressed in tissue with use of PPD or TPR/TMR. When TAR is used, the dose rate is expressed in air.

SOURCE-SKIN DISTANCE (NONISOCENTRIC) TREATMENT CALCULATIONS

An SSD treatment occurs when the patient's skin surface is set up at the reference distance (or isocenter distance). Therefore in an SSD treatment, the field size is defined on the patient's skin. Knowledge of the reference (isocenter) distance is important because the distance can vary for treatment unit type: cobalt-60 is typically 80 cm, and linear accelerators are 100 cm. These are the respective distances used in this chapter. The output or dose rate of the machine for SSD treatments should be expressed at the depth of D_{max}; the field size is defined at the skin surface, and the dose rate is measured in tissue at the depth of D_{max}.

For nonisocentric SSD treatment calculations, a six-step process can be used:

Step 1. Determine the ES of the collimator setting (used for the Sc).

Step 2. Determine the EFS ES of the treated area used for phantom or patient scatter Sp and the PDD, if applicable.

Step 3. Determine the appropriate table.

Step 4. Determine the prescribed dose.

Step 5. Look up the factors with use of the appropriate data tables (located within the chapter).

Step 6. Use the appropriate equation to determine the treatment unit setting.

These six steps are used in all the examples for calculating the minute setting for a cobalt-60 treatment machine or the MU setting for a linear accelerator treatment machine (Box 22.2).

The advantages of using PDD for calculations are as follows:

- The PDD is normalized to the depth of D_{max}; the PDD at D_{max} is 100%. Therefore, calculation of doses at various depths is easy because the PDD at each depth is the percentage of the D_{max} dose or percentage. For example, the PDD at a depth of 5 cm is 85.0. So, the dose delivered to a depth of 5 cm is 85% of the dose at D_{max}. Thus, if the D_{max} dose is 200 cGy, then the dose at a depth of 5 cm is equal to 85% of 200, or 170 cGy.
- The field size on the surface (skin) is used to look up the PDD at each depth. (Note: Later we see that for TAR, TMR, and TPR, the field size changes at each depth and a field size correction must be calculated.)
- As long as the patient is treated at the reference distance, the ISCF is 1.000.

The disadvantage to use of PDD for calculations is that if the patient is treated at any distance other than the reference distance, the PDD

must be recalculated for the new distance with Mayneord factor, and an ISCF must be applied to the RDR.

With use of PDD, the ISCF equation is (reference SSD + depth of D_{max})^2/(treatment SSD + depth of D_{max})^2 (Boxes 22.3 and 22.4).

Although most radiation oncology departments no longer have cobalt-60 treatment units, one example of a treatment time calculation is provided. Cobalt-60 calculations, for the most part, are identical to those for linear accelerator calculations.

Example 1: A patient is treated on the cobalt-60 treatment machine at 80 cm SSD to his thoracic lumbar/sacral spine. The patient is prone and is treated through a single treatment field. The collimator setting is 7 × 15 cm. Some blocking is used to shape the field. The blocks are mounted to a 5-mm-thick solid Lucite tray. The prescription states that a dose of 3000 cGy is to be delivered to a depth of 5 cm in 10 fractions. Calculate the treatment time.

This is the most basic calculation and involves only the RDR, scatter factors (Sc and Sp), and PDD. Because no blocking is used, the ES for the collimator setting or actual field size is used to look up Sc, Sp, and PDD.

Step 1. Determine the ES of the collimator setting.

   The ES, from a table of ESRFs of a 7 × 15 cm field, is 9.5 cm^2 (see Table 22.2).

Step 2. Determine the EFS ES.

   This step is because of the blocking, and the EFS is determined to be 8.0.

Step 3. Determine the appropriate tissue absorption factor table.

   The patient is treated with nonisocentric treatment. Therefore, PDD is used for the calculation.

Step 4. Determine the prescribed dose.

   From the prescription, the total prescribed dose to a depth of 5 cm is 3000 cGy. This dose is to be delivered in 10 fractions. Therefore, the

TABLE 22.3 Reference Dose Rate

Treatment Machine	Dose Rate Specified	Reference Dose Rate for a 10 × 10 cm Collimator Setting
Cobalt 60	SSD/PDD	51.7 cGy/min at depth of D_{max}
Cobalt 60	SAD/TAR	50.6 cGy/min in air at 80 cm
6 MV	SSD/PDD	0.993 cGy/MU at depth of D_{max}
6 MV	SAD/TAR	1.000 cGy/MU in air at 100 cm
6 MV	SAD/TMR/TPR	1.000 cGy/MU in tissue at 100 cm

D_{max}, Dose at maximum equilibrium; *PDD*, percentage depth dose; *SAD*, source-axis distance; *SSD*, source-skin distance; *TAR*, tissue-air ratio; *TMR*, tissue-maximum ratio; *TPR*, tissue-phantom ratio.

dose per fraction is 300 cGy. To obtain the dose per fraction, divide the total dose by the number of fractions as follows:

$$\text{Dose per Fraction} = \text{Total Prescribed Dose/Number of Fractions}$$

$$\text{Dose per Fraction} = 3000 \text{ cGy/10 Fractions}$$

$$\text{Dose per Fraction} = 300 \text{ cGy}$$

$$\text{Dose per Treatment Field} = \text{Dose per Fraction/Number of Fields}$$

$$\text{Dose per Treatment Field} = 300 \text{ cGy/1}$$

$$\text{Dose per Treatment Field} = 300 \text{ cGy}$$

Step 5. Look up the factors with use of the appropriate data tables.

The factors for the dose rate at a point are (1) reference dose rate, (2) collimator scatter, (3) phantom scatter factor, and (4) tissue absorption factor, in this case, PDD and the tray factor. The following information can be obtained in the data tables located within the chapter (Tables 22.3 through 22.10):

$$\text{Reference Dose Rate} = 51.7 \text{ cGy/min (see Table 22.3)}$$

$$\text{Sc for } (7 \times 15 \text{ cm}) \left[9.5^2\right] = 0.9965 \text{ (see Table 22.4, Sc)}$$

$$\text{Sp for } (8.0 \text{ cm}) = 0.993 \text{ (see Table 22.4, Sp)}$$

$$\text{PDD } (5,8,80) = 76.9 \text{ (see Table 22.5)}$$

$$\text{Tray Factor} = 0.96$$

Step 6. Use the appropriate equation for determining the treatment setting.

$$\text{Time Setting} = \text{Dose at Point/Dose Rate at That Point}$$

therefore

$$\text{Time Setting} = \text{Prescribed Dose/RDR} \times \text{ISCF} \times \text{Sc} \times \text{Sp} \times \text{PDD/100}$$

$$\text{Time Setting} = 300 \text{ cGy/51.7 cGy/min} \times (80.5/80.5)^2 \times 0.9965 \times 0.993 \times (76.9/100) \times 0.96$$

$$\text{Time Setting} = 300 \text{ cGy/37.77 cGy/min}$$

$$\text{Time Setting} = 7.94 \text{ minutes}$$

The treatment unit has to be set for 7.94 minutes to treat a 7 × 15 cm field size at 80 cm SSD to deliver 300 cGy to a depth of 5 cm.

Again, the previous six-step process is used throughout this chapter for linear accelerator MU setting calculations.

The treatment time for the cobalt-60 machine is given in real time (i.e., minutes). The dose rate for the cobalt-60 machine is defined in centigray per minute. Real time is used with the cobalt-60 machine because the dose rate is caused by the radioactive decay of the isotope source. The half-life of cobalt-60 is approximately 5.3 years, which means that after 5.3 years, the dose rate of the unit is half of its original dose rate. For example, if the dose rate is 50 cGy/min today, then the dose rate will be 25 cGy/min 5.3 years from today. As the dose rate decreases, the time it takes to deliver the prescribed dose increases.

Because the rate of decay for the cobalt-60 machine is relatively slow, the dose rate can be assumed to be constant over a short period of time. The time frame for this constant dose rate is 1 month. Thus, every month, the minute settings used to treat the patient with the cobalt-60 machine must be adjusted. The rate of adjustment is approximately 1.1% each month. The following equation can be used to make the monthly adjustment in the minute setting for patients who are already on treatment:

$$\text{New Minute Setting} = \text{Old Minute Setting} \times 1.01$$

If 2.00 minutes are needed to deliver 100 cGy on January 1, then 2.02 minutes are needed to deliver 100 cGy on February 1. Also, because of the slow decay or long half-life, the dose rate of the cobalt-60 machine is considered constant for a given treatment. In Example 1, the treatment time is 7.94 minutes. If the treatment continued into the following month, the therapist would need to set 8.02 minutes to deliver the 300 cGy (7.94 × 1.01).

LINEAR ACCELERATOR NONISOCENTRIC MONITOR UNIT SETTING CALCULATIONS

The major difference in the time setting calculation for the cobalt-60 machine and the MU setting calculation for the linear accelerator is in the measurement of the reference dose rate. The reference dose rate for the cobalt-60 treatment machine is measured in centigray per minute, whereas the reference dose rate for the linear accelerator is measured in centigray per MU.

With the dose rate for the linear accelerator, a look at a simple time, distance, and speed calculation might be helpful. The following formula can be used to calculate the time necessary to drive a given distance:

$$\text{Time} = \text{Distance/Speed}$$

If a driver makes a 450-mile trip, driving the entire distance at exactly 50 miles per hour, exactly 9 hours are necessary to complete the trip:

$$\text{Time} = 450 \text{ miles/50 miles/hour}$$

$$\text{Time} = 9 \text{ hours}$$

TABLE 22.4   Scatter Factors

Scatter Factor for Collimator Scatter (SC; Used with PDD, TAR, TMR/TPR)

Mach/Eq Sq	4.0	5.0	6.0	7.0	8.0	9.0	10.0	11.0	12.0	13.0	14.0	15.0	16.0	17.0	18.0	19.0	20.0	22.0	24.0	26.0	28.0	30.0	32.0	35.0
Cobalt 60	0.946	0.961	0.975	0.981	0.987	0.993	1.000	1.006	1.012	1.018	1.024	1.030	1.035	1.039	1.044	1.048	1.053	1.057	1.061	1.063	1.063	1.063		
6 MV	0.948	0.961	0.970	0.979	0.987	0.994	1.000	1.004	1.008	1.013	1.017	1.021	1.024	1.028	1.031	1.035	1.038	1.041	1.045	1.048	1.051	1.052	1.053	1.055
10 MV	0.938	0.951	0.962	0.973	0.982	0.991	1.000	1.005	1.009	1.014	1.018	1.023	1.026	1.030	1.033	1.037	1.040	1.044	1.048	1.051	1.052	1.054	1.057	1.061
18 MV	0.914	0.931	0.948	0.965	0.978	0.989	1.000	1.006	1.012	1.017	1.023	1.029	1.032	1.036	1.039	1.043	1.046	1.052	1.057	1.063	1.066	1.067	1.069	1.070

Scatter Factor/Combined Scatter (SC, SP)

Mach/Eq Sq	4.0	5.0	6.0	7.0	8.0	9.0	10.0	11.0	12.0	13.0	14.0	15.0	16.0	17.0	18.0	19.0	20.0	22.0	24.0	26.0	28.0	30.0	32.0	35.0
Cobalt 60	0.928	0.945	0.962	0.971	0.980	0.990	1.000	1.009	1.019	1.028	1.037	1.046	1.053	1.060	1.067	1.074	1.081	1.089	1.096	1.102	1.105	1.109		
6 MV	0.927	0.940	0.954	0.967	0.979	0.990	1.000	1.007	1.014	1.021	1.028	1.035	1.039	1.044	1.049	1.053	1.058	1.065	1.072	1.079	1.084	1.088	1.092	1.098
10 MV	0.925	0.938	0.953	0.967	0.979	0.990	1.000	1.005	1.011	1.016	1.022	1.027	1.032	1.037	1.041	1.046	1.051	1.058	1.065	1.069	1.071	1.073	1.077	1.081
18 MV	0.904	0.922	0.941	0.961	0.976	0.988	1.000	1.007	1.014	1.021	1.028	1.036	1.041	1.046	1.051	1.056	1.060	1.067	1.073	1.079	1.084	1.087	1.090	1.093

Scatter Factor For Phantom Scatter (SP; Used With PDD, TMR/TPR)

Mach/Eq Sq	4.0	5.0	6.0	7.0	8.0	9.0	10.0	11.0	12.0	13.0	14.0	15.0	16.0	17.0	18.0	19.0	20.0	22.0	24.0	26.0	28.0	30.0	32.0	35.0
Cobalt 60	0.981	0.983	0.987	0.990	0.993	0.997	1.000	1.003	1.007	1.010	1.013	1.016	1.017	1.020	1.022	1.025	1.327	1.030	1.033	1.037	1.040	1.043		
6 MV	0.978	0.978	0.984	0.988	0.992	0.996	1.000	1.003	1.006	1.008	1.011	1.014	1.015	1.016	1.017	1.017	1.319	1.023	1.026	1.030	1.031	1.034	1.037	1.041
10 MV	0.986	0.986	0.991	0.994	0.997	0.999	1.000	1.000	1.002	1.002	1.004	1.004	1.006	1.007	1.008	1.009	1.311	1.013	1.016	1.017	1.018	1.018	1.019	1.019
18 MV	0.989	0.990	0.993	0.996	0.998	0.999	1.000	1.001	1.002	1.004	1.005	1.007	1.009	1.010	1.012	1.012	1.313	1.014	1.015	1.015	1.017	1.019	1.020	1.021

EQ SQ, Equivalent square; Mach, Machine; PDD, percent depth dose; TAR, tissue-air ratio; TMR, tissue-maximum ratio; TPR, tissue-phantom ratio.

TABLE 22.5 Percentage Depth Dose For Cobalt-60 at 80-cm Source-Skin Distance

Depth (cm)	EQ SQ 0.0	4.0	5.0	6.0	7.0	8.0	9.0	10.0	11.0	12.0	13.0	14.0	15.0	16.0	17.0	18.0	19.0	20.0	22.0	24.0	26.0	28.0	30.0
0.0	14.9	15.0	17.4	19.8	21.7	23.6	25.5	27.4	28.1	28.8	29.5	30.1	30.8	32.3	33.7	35.2	36.7	38.1	41.2	44.3	47.4	50.4	53.4
0.5	100.0	100.0	100.0	100.0	100.0	100.0	100.0	100.0	100.0	100.0	100.0	100.0	100.0	100.0	100.0	100.0	100.0	100.0	100.0	100.0	100.0	100.0	100.0
1.0	95.6	96.4	96.6	96.8	96.9	97.0	97.0	97.1	97.1	97.1	97.2	97.2	97.2	97.3	97.3	97.4	97.4	97.5	97.7	97.8	98.0	98.1	98.2
2.0	87.4	90.2	90.7	91.3	91.6	92.0	92.3	92.6	92.8	92.9	93.1	93.3	93.5	93.6	93.7	93.8	93.9	94.0	94.1	94.2	94.3	94.4	94.4
3.0	80.1	84.2	85.1	85.8	86.4	87.0	87.4	87.8	88.1	88.5	88.8	89.1	89.3	89.5	89.7	89.9	90.1	90.1	90.2	90.3	90.4	90.5	90.4
4.0	73.2	78.4	79.4	80.4	81.2	81.9	82.6	83.1	83.5	84.0	84.4	84.8	85.1	85.3	85.5	85.8	86.0	86.0	86.1	86.2	86.4	86.5	86.3
5.0	67.1	72.9	74.0	75.1	76.0	76.9	77.7	78.3	78.8	79.4	79.9	80.4	80.7	81.0	81.3	81.6	81.9	81.9	82.0	82.1	82.2	82.3	82.1
6.0	61.4	67.7	68.9	70.1	71.1	72.0	72.9	73.6	74.2	74.8	75.4	76.0	76.3	76.7	77.0	77.3	77.5	77.6	77.7	77.9	78.1	78.2	78.0
7.0	56.2	62.7	64.0	65.3	66.4	67.4	68.3	69.0	69.7	70.3	71.0	71.6	71.9	72.3	72.7	73.1	73.3	73.4	73.6	73.7	73.9	74.0	73.8
8.0	51.5	58.0	59.4	60.7	61.9	62.9	63.9	64.6	65.3	66.1	66.8	67.4	67.8	68.2	68.6	69.1	69.2	69.3	69.5	69.7	69.9	69.9	69.7
9.0	47.3	53.7	55.1	56.4	57.5	58.6	59.6	60.4	61.1	61.9	62.6	63.2	63.6	64.1	64.5	65.0	65.1	65.2	65.4	65.7	65.9	65.9	65.8
10.0	43.3	49.7	51.0	52.3	53.5	54.5	55.6	56.3	57.1	57.9	58.6	59.2	59.7	60.2	60.6	61.1	61.2	61.3	61.6	61.9	62.1	62.1	61.9
11.0	39.8	45.9	47.2	48.5	49.7	50.7	51.7	52.5	53.3	54.1	54.9	55.4	55.9	56.4	56.9	57.3	57.4	57.5	57.8	58.1	58.4	58.4	58.2
12.0	36.4	42.4	43.7	45.0	46.2	47.2	48.1	48.9	49.7	50.5	51.3	51.8	52.3	52.8	53.3	53.6	53.8	53.9	54.3	54.6	55.0	54.8	54.7
13.0	33.4	39.2	40.5	41.6	42.8	43.8	44.7	45.5	46.3	47.1	47.8	48.3	48.8	49.4	49.9	50.1	50.3	50.5	50.9	51.2	51.6	51.4	51.3
14.0	30.7	36.1	37.4	38.6	39.6	40.6	41.5	42.3	43.1	43.9	44.6	45.1	45.6	46.1	46.7	46.8	47.0	47.2	47.6	48.0	48.3	48.1	48.0
15.0	28.1	33.4	34.6	35.7	36.7	37.7	38.5	39.3	40.0	40.8	41.5	42.0	42.5	43.1	43.6	43.8	43.9	44.1	44.6	45.0	45.2	45.1	44.9
16.0	25.9	30.8	31.9	33.0	34.0	34.9	35.7	36.4	37.2	38.0	38.6	39.1	39.6	40.2	40.6	40.8	41.0	41.2	41.6	42.1	42.2	42.1	42.0
17.0	23.8	28.4	29.5	30.5	31.4	32.3	33.1	33.8	34.6	35.3	35.9	36.4	36.9	37.5	37.8	38.0	38.3	38.5	38.9	39.4	39.5	39.3	39.2
18.0	21.8	26.2	27.2	28.2	29.1	30.0	30.7	31.4	32.1	32.8	33.4	33.9	34.4	34.9	35.2	35.4	35.6	35.9	36.3	36.8	36.8	36.7	36.6
19.0	20.0	24.2	25.1	26.0	26.9	27.7	28.4	29.1	29.8	30.5	31.0	31.5	32.0	32.5	32.8	33.0	33.2	33.5	33.9	34.4	34.4	34.3	34.2
20.0	18.4	22.3	23.2	24.1	24.9	25.7	26.3	27.0	27.6	28.3	28.8	29.3	29.8	30.3	30.5	30.7	30.9	31.2	31.7	32.2	32.1	32.0	31.9
21.0	17.0	20.6	21.5	22.3	23.1	23.8	24.4	25.0	25.7	26.3	26.8	27.2	27.7	28.1	28.4	28.6	28.8	29.1	29.6	30.0	29.9	29.8	29.7
22.0	15.6	19.0	19.8	20.6	21.3	22.0	22.6	23.2	23.8	24.3	24.8	25.3	25.7	26.1	26.3	26.6	26.8	27.0	27.5	27.9	27.8	27.7	27.6
23.0	14.3	17.5	18.3	19.0	19.7	20.4	20.9	21.5	22.1	22.6	23.1	23.5	23.9	24.3	24.5	24.7	25.0	25.2	25.7	26.0	25.9	25.8	25.7
24.0	13.1	16.1	16.8	17.5	18.2	18.8	19.3	19.9	20.4	20.9	21.4	21.8	22.2	22.5	22.7	23.0	23.2	23.4	23.9	24.1	24.1	24.0	23.9
25.0	12.1	14.9	15.6	16.2	16.8	17.4	17.9	18.5	19.0	19.5	19.9	20.3	20.7	20.9	21.2	21.4	21.6	21.8	22.3	22.5	22.4	22.3	22.3
26.0	11.1	13.7	14.3	14.9	15.5	16.1	16.6	17.1	17.6	18.0	18.4	18.8	19.2	19.4	19.6	19.8	20.1	20.3	20.8	20.9	20.8	20.7	20.7
27.0	10.2	12.7	13.3	13.8	14.4	14.9	15.4	15.8	16.3	16.7	17.1	17.5	17.8	18.1	18.3	18.5	18.7	18.9	19.4	19.4	19.4	19.3	19.2
28.0	9.4	11.7	12.2	12.8	13.3	13.7	14.2	14.6	15.1	15.5	15.8	16.2	16.5	16.7	17.0	17.2	17.4	17.6	18.0	18.0	18.0	17.9	17.9
29.0	8.7	10.8	11.3	11.8	12.3	12.7	13.1	13.6	14.0	14.4	14.7	15.1	15.4	15.6	15.8	16.0	16.2	16.4	16.8	16.7	16.7	16.6	16.6
30.0	8.0	9.9	10.4	10.9	11.3	11.7	12.1	12.5	12.9	13.3	13.6	13.9	14.2	14.4	14.6	14.8	15.0	15.2	15.6	15.5	15.5	15.4	15.4
BSF/PSF	1.000	1.015	1.018	1.021	1.025	1.028	1.032	1.035	1.038	1.041	1.045	1.048	1.051	1.053	1.056	1.058	1.061	1.063	1.066	1.070	1.073	1.077	1.080

BSF, Backscatter factor; EQ SQ, equivalent square; PSF, peak scatter factor.

TABLE 22.6 Percentage Depth Dose For 6 MV at 100-cm Source-Skin Distance

EQ SQ Depth (cm)	0.0	4.0	5.0	6.0	7.0	8.0	9.0	10.0	11.0	12.0	13.0	14.0	15.0	16.0	17.0	18.0	19.0	20.0	22.0	24.0	26.0	28.0	30.0	32.0	35.0
0.0	19.2	19.2	19.2	20.5	21.8	23.0	24.3	25.6	26.7	27.9	29.1	30.2	31.4	32.6	33.8	35.1	36.3	37.5	39.0	40.4	41.9	43.2	44.5	45.7	47.6
1.0	96.8	96.9	96.9	97.0	97.0	97.0	97.1	97.1	97.2	97.2	97.3	97.3	97.4	97.4	97.5	97.5	97.6	97.6	97.7	97.8	98.0	98.1	98.1	98.2	98.3
1.5	100.0	100.0	100.0	100.0	100.0	100.0	100.0	100.0	100.0	100.0	100.0	100.0	100.0	100.0	100.0	100.0	100.0	100.0	100.0	100.0	100.0	100.0	100.0	100.0	100.0
2.0	97.4	98.2	98.4	98.4	98.5	98.5	98.6	98.6	98.6	98.6	98.6	98.6	98.6	98.6	98.6	98.7	98.7	98.7	98.7	98.7	98.7	98.7	98.7	98.7	98.7
3.0	91.1	93.8	94.4	94.7	94.9	95.0	95.0	95.1	95.1	95.1	95.2	95.2	95.2	95.3	95.3	95.4	95.4	95.5	95.5	95.6	95.6	95.6	95.6	95.6	95.5
4.0	85.3	89.6	90.6	90.9	91.3	91.4	91.5	91.5	91.5	91.6	91.6	91.7	91.7	91.8	91.9	92.0	92.1	92.2	92.2	92.3	92.4	92.3	92.3	92.3	92.2
5.0	79.9	84.5	85.6	86.1	86.6	86.8	87.0	87.1	87.3	87.5	87.7	87.8	87.9	88.1	88.2	88.3	88.5	88.6	88.7	88.8	89.0	89.0	89.0	89.0	88.9
6.0	74.8	79.7	80.9	81.5	82.1	82.4	82.7	83.0	83.2	83.5	83.8	84.0	84.1	84.3	84.5	84.7	84.8	85.0	85.2	85.4	85.6	85.6	85.7	85.8	85.7
7.0	70.1	75.1	76.3	77.1	77.8	78.3	78.7	79.0	79.3	79.6	79.9	80.3	80.4	80.6	80.8	81.0	81.2	81.4	81.7	82.0	82.2	82.3	82.4	82.5	82.3
8.0	65.7	70.8	72.1	72.9	73.7	74.2	74.7	75.1	75.5	75.9	76.2	76.6	76.8	77.0	77.3	77.5	77.8	77.9	78.3	78.6	78.8	78.9	79.0	79.1	79.0
9.0	61.5	66.7	68.0	68.9	69.8	70.4	71.0	71.4	71.8	72.2	72.6	73.0	73.2	73.5	73.8	74.1	74.3	74.5	74.9	75.3	75.5	75.6	75.8	76.0	75.7
10.0	57.7	62.8	64.1	65.1	66.1	66.7	67.4	67.8	68.3	68.8	69.2	69.6	69.8	70.1	70.5	70.8	71.0	71.2	71.6	72.0	72.3	72.5	72.7	72.8	72.6
11.0	54.0	59.2	60.4	61.5	62.4	63.1	63.8	64.2	64.8	65.3	65.8	66.1	66.4	66.8	67.1	67.5	67.7	67.9	68.4	68.8	69.0	69.2	69.4	69.6	69.3
12.0	50.7	55.7	57.0	58.0	58.9	59.7	60.4	60.9	61.4	61.9	62.4	62.8	63.1	63.5	63.9	64.3	64.5	64.8	65.3	65.8	66.0	66.2	66.4	66.5	66.2
13.0	47.5	52.4	53.6	54.6	55.6	56.4	57.2	57.7	58.2	58.8	59.3	59.7	60.0	60.4	60.8	61.2	61.5	61.7	62.2	62.7	63.0	63.2	63.4	63.5	63.3
14.0	44.6	49.4	50.6	51.6	52.5	53.3	54.1	54.6	55.1	55.7	56.3	56.6	57.0	57.4	57.8	58.2	58.5	58.8	59.4	59.9	60.1	60.3	60.6	60.6	60.4
15.0	41.8	46.6	47.8	48.7	49.6	50.5	51.2	51.7	52.3	52.9	53.5	53.9	54.2	54.7	55.1	55.5	55.8	56.1	56.6	57.1	57.4	57.6	57.9	57.8	57.6
16.0	39.2	43.9	45.1	46.0	46.9	47.8	48.5	49.1	49.7	50.3	50.9	51.2	51.6	52.0	52.5	52.8	53.1	53.4	54.0	54.5	54.8	55.1	55.4	55.2	55.1
17.0	36.8	41.4	42.5	43.5	44.3	45.2	45.9	46.4	47.1	47.7	48.2	48.6	49.0	49.4	49.9	50.2	50.6	50.9	51.5	52.0	52.3	52.6	52.9	52.7	52.6
18.0	34.5	39.0	40.1	41.0	41.9	42.7	43.4	44.0	44.6	45.3	45.8	46.2	46.6	47.0	47.5	47.8	48.2	48.5	49.1	49.6	49.9	50.2	50.5	50.3	50.2
19.0	32.4	36.8	37.8	38.7	39.6	40.5	41.1	41.7	42.3	43.0	43.5	43.9	44.3	44.7	45.1	45.5	45.8	46.1	46.8	47.2	47.6	48.0	48.2	48.0	47.9
20.0	30.4	34.6	35.7	36.6	37.4	38.2	38.9	39.5	40.1	40.7	41.2	41.6	42.0	42.5	42.9	43.2	43.6	43.9	44.6	45.0	45.4	45.7	45.9	45.8	45.6
21.0	28.6	32.7	33.7	34.5	35.3	36.1	36.8	37.4	38.0	38.6	39.1	39.5	39.9	40.3	40.7	41.1	41.4	41.8	42.4	42.9	43.2	43.6	43.7	43.6	43.5
22.0	26.8	30.8	31.8	32.6	33.4	34.2	34.8	35.4	36.0	36.9	37.1	37.5	37.9	38.3	38.7	39.1	39.4	39.8	40.4	40.8	41.2	41.6	41.7	41.6	41.5
23.0	25.2	29.1	30.0	30.8	31.6	32.4	33.0	33.6	34.2	34.8	35.2	35.6	36.0	36.4	36.8	37.2	37.5	37.9	38.5	38.9	39.3	39.7	39.8	39.6	39.5
24.0	23.6	27.5	28.4	29.1	29.9	30.6	31.2	31.8	32.4	32.9	33.4	33.7	34.1	34.6	35.0	35.3	35.7	36.0	36.7	37.1	37.5	37.9	37.8	37.7	37.6
25.0	22.2	26.0	26.8	27.6	28.3	29.0	29.6	30.1	30.7	31.3	31.7	32.0	32.4	32.9	33.2	33.6	33.9	34.3	34.9	35.3	35.7	36.1	36.0	35.9	35.8
26.0	20.9	24.5	25.3	26.0	26.7	27.4	27.9	28.5	29.1	29.6	30.0	30.4	30.8	31.2	31.5	31.9	32.2	32.6	33.2	33.6	34.0	34.4	34.3	34.2	34.1
27.0	19.6	23.2	24.0	24.7	25.3	26.0	26.5	27.0	27.6	28.1	28.4	28.8	29.2	29.6	30.0	30.3	30.7	31.0	31.6	32.0	32.4	32.7	32.6	32.6	32.4
28.0	18.4	21.9	22.6	23.3	24.0	24.6	25.1	25.6	26.1	26.6	26.9	27.3	27.7	28.1	28.4	28.8	29.2	29.5	30.1	30.5	30.9	31.1	31.1	31.0	30.9
29.0	17.3	20.7	21.4	22.0	22.7	23.3	23.7	24.2	24.7	25.2	25.6	25.9	26.3	26.7	27.0	27.4	27.7	28.1	28.6	29.0	29.4	29.6	29.5	29.5	29.4
30.0	16.2	19.5	20.2	20.8	21.4	22.0	22.4	22.9	23.4	23.8	24.2	24.6	24.9	25.3	25.7	26.0	26.4	26.7	27.2	27.6	28.0	28.1	28.0	28.0	27.9
PSF	1.000	1.002	1.003	1.007	1.012	1.016	1.021	1.025	1.028	1.031	1.033	1.036	1.039	1.040	1.041	1.043	1.044	1.045	1.048	1.051	1.054	1.057	1.060	1.063	1.067

EQ SQ, Equivalent square; PSF, peak scatter factor.

TABLE 22.7 Percentage Depth Dose For 18 MV at 100-cm Source-Skin Distance

EQ SQ Depth (cm)	0.0	4.0	5.0	6.0	7.0	8.0	9.0	10.0	11.0	12.0	13.0	14.0	15.0	16.0	17.0	18.0	19.0	20.0	22.0	24.0	26.0	28.0	30.0	32.0
0.0	10.0	10.0	10.1	11.7	13.4	15.4	17.6	19.8	21.3	22.8	24.3	25.8	27.3	28.7	30.1	31.5	32.9	34.4	36.2	38.0	35.3	41.2	42.0	42.9
1.0	77.8	77.8	77.8	78.3	78.7	79.3	80.0	80.6	80.9	81.2	81.6	81.9	82.2	82.7	83.2	83.7	84.2	84.7	85.2	85.7	86.2	86.5	86.8	87.0
2.0	95.4	95.5	95.5	95.6	95.7	95.8	96.0	96.2	96.2	96.2	96.2	96.2	96.3	96.5	96.7	96.9	97.2	97.4	97.5	97.7	97.8	97.9	98.0	98.0
3.0	98.3	98.4	98.4	98.4	98.4	98.5	98.6	98.6	98.6	98.6	98.6	98.6	98.7	98.7	98.8	98.9	99.0	99.0	99.1	99.1	99.2	99.2	99.3	99.3
3.5	100.0	100.0	100.0	100.0	100.0	100.0	100.0	100.0	100.0	100.0	100.0	100.0	100.0	100.0	100.0	100.0	100.0	100.0	100.0	100.0	100.0	100.0	100.0	100.0
4.0	98.1	98.8	98.9	98.9	98.9	98.9	98.9	98.9	98.9	98.8	98.8	98.8	98.8	98.8	98.8	98.8	98.8	98.8	98.8	98.7	98.7	98.8	98.8	98.8
5.0	93.5	95.8	96.3	96.3	96.2	96.2	96.1	96.1	96.1	96.0	96.0	96.0	95.9	95.9	95.9	95.8	95.8	95.7	95.7	95.7	95.7	95.7	95.7	95.8
6.0	89.0	92.8	93.4	93.4	93.4	93.3	93.3	93.3	93.2	93.2	93.2	93.1	93.1	93.0	93.0	92.9	92.9	92.8	92.8	92.8	92.8	92.9	92.9	93.0
7.0	84.9	89.0	89.8	89.8	89.9	89.8	89.8	89.8	89.8	89.8	89.8	89.8	89.8	89.8	89.7	89.7	89.6	89.6	89.6	89.6	89.6	89.7	89.8	89.8
8.0	81.0	85.4	86.2	86.3	86.4	86.4	86.4	86.5	86.5	86.6	86.6	86.7	86.6	86.6	86.5	86.5	86.4	86.4	86.4	86.4	86.5	86.6	86.7	86.8
9.0	77.2	81.8	82.6	82.9	83.1	83.0	83.0	83.1	83.2	83.2	83.3	83.4	83.4	83.4	83.4	83.3	83.3	83.3	83.3	83.4	83.6	83.7	83.8	83.9
10.0	73.6	78.3	79.1	79.5	79.7	79.9	79.7	79.9	80.0	80.1	80.3	80.3	80.3	80.3	80.3	80.3	80.2	80.3	80.3	80.4	80.6	80.8	81.0	81.1
11.0	70.2	74.9	75.7	76.1	76.4	76.5	76.6	76.7	76.9	77.0	77.1	77.2	77.3	77.3	77.3	77.3	77.3	77.3	77.4	77.5	77.7	77.9	78.0	78.1
12.0	67.0	71.7	72.5	72.9	73.2	73.3	73.5	73.6	73.8	73.9	74.1	74.2	74.3	74.3	74.4	74.4	74.4	74.4	74.5	74.6	74.9	75.0	75.2	75.2
13.0	64.0	68.7	69.4	69.8	70.1	70.3	70.5	70.7	70.9	71.0	71.2	71.3	71.4	71.5	71.6	71.6	71.6	71.6	71.7	71.9	72.1	72.3	72.4	72.5
14.0	61.0	65.7	66.4	66.8	67.1	67.4	67.7	67.9	68.0	68.2	68.3	68.5	68.6	68.8	68.9	68.9	68.9	69.0	69.1	69.3	69.5	69.7	69.8	69.8
15.0	58.3	62.8	63.6	64.0	64.4	64.7	64.9	65.1	65.3	65.5	65.7	65.9	66.0	66.2	66.3	66.3	66.3	66.4	66.6	66.8	67.0	67.2	67.4	67.4
16.0	55.6	60.2	60.9	61.4	61.7	62.1	62.4	62.6	62.8	63.0	63.2	63.4	63.5	63.7	63.8	63.8	63.9	64.0	64.2	64.4	64.7	64.9	65.0	65.0
17.0	53.1	57.6	58.3	58.8	59.1	59.5	59.8	60.0	60.3	60.5	60.8	61.0	61.1	61.3	61.4	61.5	61.5	61.6	61.8	62.1	62.3	62.5	62.8	62.7
18.0	50.7	55.1	55.8	56.4	56.7	57.1	57.4	57.7	58.0	58.2	58.5	58.7	58.8	58.9	59.1	59.1	59.2	59.3	59.6	59.8	60.1	60.3	60.5	60.4
19.0	48.4	52.8	53.5	54.0	54.4	54.7	55.0	55.3	55.6	56.0	56.2	56.4	56.6	56.7	56.8	56.9	57.0	57.1	57.3	57.6	57.9	58.2	58.3	58.2
20.0	46.3	50.5	51.2	51.7	52.1	52.4	52.8	53.1	53.4	53.7	54.0	54.2	54.3	54.5	54.6	54.7	54.8	54.9	55.2	55.5	55.9	56.1	56.2	56.1
21.0	44.2	48.3	49.0	49.6	49.9	50.3	50.6	51.0	51.3	51.7	51.9	52.1	52.2	52.4	52.5	52.6	52.7	52.9	53.2	53.5	53.9	54.1	54.2	54.1
22.0	42.3	46.3	46.9	47.5	47.8	48.2	48.6	48.9	49.3	49.6	49.9	50.0	50.2	50.4	50.5	50.6	50.7	50.9	51.3	51.6	51.9	52.2	52.3	52.2
23.0	40.4	44.3	45.0	45.5	45.9	46.3	46.6	47.0	47.3	47.7	47.9	48.1	48.3	48.4	48.5	48.7	48.8	49.0	49.4	49.7	50.0	50.3	50.3	50.2
24.0	38.6	42.4	43.1	43.7	44.0	44.4	44.7	45.1	45.4	45.8	46.0	46.2	46.4	46.6	46.8	46.9	47.0	47.2	47.5	47.8	48.2	48.5	48.4	48.4
25.0	36.9	40.7	41.3	41.9	42.2	42.6	42.9	43.3	43.6	44.0	44.2	44.4	44.6	44.9	45.0	45.1	45.2	45.4	45.8	46.1	46.4	46.7	46.6	46.6
26.0	35.3	38.9	39.6	40.2	40.5	40.9	41.2	41.6	41.9	42.2	42.5	42.7	42.9	43.1	43.2	43.4	43.5	43.7	44.0	44.4	44.7	44.9	44.9	44.8
27.0	33.7	37.3	38.0	38.5	38.9	39.2	39.6	39.9	40.3	40.6	40.8	41.0	41.3	41.5	41.6	41.7	41.9	42.0	42.4	42.7	43.0	43.3	43.2	43.1
28.0	32.2	35.7	36.4	36.9	37.3	37.7	38.0	38.3	38.7	39.0	39.2	39.5	39.7	39.9	40.0	40.1	40.3	40.4	40.8	41.1	41.5	41.6	41.6	41.5
29.0	30.9	34.3	34.9	35.4	35.8	36.1	36.5	36.8	37.1	37.4	37.7	37.9	38.2	38.4	38.5	38.6	38.7	38.7	39.3	39.6	39.9	40.1	40.0	40.0
30.0	29.5	32.9	33.5	34.0	34.3	34.7	35.0	35.3	35.6	35.9	36.2	36.4	36.7	36.9	37.0	37.1	37.3	37.4	37.8	38.1	38.5	38.6	38.5	38.5
PSF	1.000	1.002	1.003	1.006	1.009	1.011	1.012	1.013	1.014	1.015	1.017	1.018	1.019	1.021	1.022	1.024	1.025	1.027	1.028	1.028	1.029	1.030	1.031	1.033

EQ SQ, Equivalent square; *PSF,* peak scatter factor.

TABLE 22.8   Tissue-air Ratio for 6 MV

EQ SQ Depth (cm)	0.0	4.0	5.0	6.0	7.0	8.0	9.0	10.0	11.0	12.0	13.0	14.0	15.0	16.0	17.0	18.0	19.0	20.0	22.0	24.0	26.0	28.0	30.0	32.0	35.0
0.0	0.186	0.187	0.187	0.200	0.213	0.227	0.240	0.254	0.266	0.279	0.291	0.304	0.316	0.329	0.342	0.354	0.367	0.380	0.396	0.412	0.428	0.443	0.457	0.471	0.492
1.0	0.957	0.960	0.961	0.965	0.970	0.974	0.979	0.984	0.987	0.990	0.994	0.997	1.000	1.002	1.003	1.005	1.006	1.008	1.012	1.017	1.021	1.025	1.028	1.032	1.037
1.5	1.000	1.002	1.003	1.007	1.012	1.016	1.021	1.025	1.028	1.031	1.033	1.036	1.039	1.040	1.041	1.043	1.044	1.045	1.048	1.051	1.054	1.057	1.060	1.063	1.067
2.0	0.982	0.992	0.994	0.999	1.004	1.009	1.014	1.018	1.021	1.024	1.027	1.030	1.032	1.034	1.035	1.037	1.038	1.039	1.043	1.046	1.049	1.052	1.055	1.057	1.061
3.0	0.936	0.966	0.973	0.979	0.986	0.991	0.996	1.001	1.004	1.007	1.010	1.013	1.016	1.018	1.020	1.021	1.023	1.025	1.028	1.032	1.035	1.038	1.041	1.043	1.047
4.0	0.894	0.940	0.951	0.959	0.966	0.972	0.977	0.982	0.985	0.988	0.991	0.994	0.997	0.999	1.001	1.004	1.006	1.008	1.012	1.015	1.019	1.022	1.025	1.027	1.031
5.0	0.853	0.903	0.915	0.924	0.933	0.941	0.946	0.952	0.956	0.961	0.965	0.970	0.974	0.977	0.979	0.982	0.984	0.987	0.991	0.996	1.000	1.003	1.006	1.009	1.013
6.0	0.814	0.867	0.880	0.890	0.900	0.909	0.916	0.923	0.928	0.933	0.939	0.944	0.949	0.952	0.955	0.958	0.961	0.964	0.969	0.974	0.979	0.984	0.987	0.990	0.995
7.0	0.777	0.831	0.845	0.857	0.868	0.878	0.886	0.894	0.900	0.906	0.911	0.917	0.923	0.926	0.930	0.933	0.937	0.940	0.946	0.951	0.957	0.962	0.965	0.969	0.974
8.0	0.742	0.798	0.812	0.824	0.837	0.847	0.856	0.865	0.871	0.878	0.884	0.891	0.897	0.901	0.905	0.908	0.912	0.916	0.922	0.928	0.934	0.939	0.943	0.946	0.952
9.0	0.708	0.765	0.779	0.792	0.805	0.817	0.826	0.836	0.843	0.850	0.856	0.863	0.870	0.874	0.878	0.883	0.887	0.891	0.898	0.904	0.911	0.916	0.920	0.924	0.930
10.0	0.676	0.733	0.747	0.761	0.775	0.787	0.798	0.808	0.815	0.822	0.830	0.837	0.844	0.848	0.853	0.857	0.862	0.866	0.873	0.880	0.887	0.892	0.897	0.901	0.908
11.0	0.645	0.702	0.716	0.730	0.744	0.756	0.767	0.778	0.786	0.793	0.801	0.808	0.816	0.821	0.826	0.830	0.835	0.840	0.847	0.854	0.861	0.867	0.872	0.876	0.883
12.0	0.616	0.672	0.686	0.700	0.714	0.727	0.738	0.749	0.757	0.765	0.772	0.780	0.788	0.793	0.798	0.804	0.809	0.814	0.822	0.829	0.837	0.843	0.848	0.852	0.859
13.0	0.588	0.643	0.657	0.671	0.684	0.697	0.709	0.721	0.729	0.737	0.745	0.753	0.761	0.766	0.772	0.777	0.783	0.788	0.796	0.804	0.812	0.818	0.823	0.828	0.835
14.0	0.561	0.616	0.630	0.643	0.656	0.669	0.681	0.693	0.701	0.709	0.718	0.726	0.734	0.740	0.745	0.751	0.756	0.762	0.771	0.779	0.788	0.794	0.799	0.804	0.811
15.0	0.536	0.590	0.604	0.617	0.630	0.642	0.655	0.667	0.675	0.684	0.692	0.701	0.709	0.715	0.721	0.726	0.732	0.738	0.747	0.755	0.764	0.771	0.776	0.781	0.788
16.0	0.511	0.565	0.579	0.592	0.605	0.617	0.630	0.642	0.651	0.659	0.668	0.676	0.685	0.691	0.697	0.702	0.708	0.714	0.723	0.732	0.741	0.748	0.753	0.758	0.766
17.0	0.488	0.542	0.555	0.568	0.581	0.593	0.605	0.617	0.626	0.634	0.643	0.651	0.660	0.666	0.672	0.678	0.684	0.690	0.699	0.708	0.717	0.725	0.730	0.736	0.744
18.0	0.466	0.518	0.531	0.544	0.557	0.569	0.581	0.593	0.602	0.611	0.619	0.628	0.637	0.643	0.649	0.655	0.661	0.667	0.676	0.686	0.695	0.703	0.708	0.714	0.722
19.0	0.445	0.496	0.509	0.521	0.534	0.546	0.558	0.570	0.579	0.588	0.596	0.605	0.614	0.620	0.626	0.632	0.638	0.644	0.653	0.663	0.672	0.680	0.686	0.692	0.701
20.0	0.424	0.474	0.478	0.499	0.512	0.524	0.535	0.547	0.556	0.565	0.573	0.582	0.591	0.597	0.603	0.609	0.615	0.621	0.631	0.640	0.650	0.658	0.664	0.670	0.679
21.0	0.405	0.455	0.467	0.479	0.490	0.502	0.513	0.525	0.534	0.543	0.551	0.560	0.569	0.575	0.581	0.587	0.593	0.599	0.609	0.618	0.628	0.636	0.642	0.649	0.658
22.0	0.387	0.435	0.447	0.459	0.470	0.482	0.493	0.504	0.513	0.522	0.530	0.539	0.548	0.554	0.560	0.566	0.572	0.578	0.588	0.597	0.607	0.615	0.622	0.628	0.638
23.0	0.370	0.417	0.429	0.440	0.451	0.463	0.474	0.485	0.493	0.502	0.510	0.519	0.528	0.534	0.539	0.546	0.552	0.558	0.567	0.577	0.587	0.595	0.602	0.608	0.618
24.0	0.352	0.399	0.411	0.422	0.433	0.443	0.454	0.465	0.473	0.482	0.490	0.499	0.507	0.513	0.519	0.525	0.531	0.537	0.547	0.557	0.567	0.575	0.582	0.588	0.598
25.0	0.337	0.383	0.394	0.405	0.415	0.426	0.436	0.447	0.455	0.463	0.471	0.480	0.488	0.494	0.500	0.506	0.512	0.518	0.528	0.538	0.548	0.556	0.562	0.569	0.579
26.0	0.321	0.366	0.377	0.387	0.398	0.408	0.418	0.428	0.436	0.444	0.453	0.461	0.469	0.475	0.481	0.486	0.492	0.498	0.508	0.518	0.528	0.536	0.543	0.549	0.559
27.0	0.307	0.351	0.362	0.372	0.382	0.392	0.402	0.412	0.419	0.427	0.435	0.443	0.451	0.457	0.462	0.468	0.474	0.480	0.490	0.500	0.510	0.518	0.525	0.531	0.541
28.0	0.292	0.336	0.347	0.357	0.366	0.376	0.385	0.395	0.403	0.410	0.418	0.425	0.433	0.439	0.444	0.450	0.455	0.461	0.471	0.482	0.492	0.500	0.507	0.513	0.523
29.0	0.279	0.322	0.333	0.342	0.351	0.361	0.370	0.379	0.386	0.394	0.401	0.409	0.416	0.422	0.427	0.433	0.438	0.444	0.454	0.464	0.474	0.483	0.489	0.495	0.505
30.0	0.266	0.308	0.318	0.327	0.336	0.345	0.354	0.363	0.370	0.377	0.385	0.392	0.399	0.405	0.410	0.416	0.421	0.427	0.437	0.447	0.457	0.465	0.471	0.478	0.487

EQ SQ, Equivalent square.

TABLE 22.9 Tissue-maximum Ratio for 6 MV

EQ SQ Depth (cm)	0.0	4.0	5.0	6.0	7.0	8.0	9.0	10.0	11.0	12.0	13.0	14.0	15.0	16.0	17.0	18.0	19.0	20.0	22.0	24.0	26.0	28.0	30.0	32.0	35.0
0.0	0.186	0.187	0.186	0.199	0.210	0.223	0.235	0.248	0.259	0.271	0.282	0.293	0.304	0.316	0.329	0.339	0.352	0.364	0.378	0.392	0.406	0.419	0.431	0.443	0.461
1.0	0.957	0.958	0.958	0.958	0.958	0.959	0.959	0.960	0.960	0.960	0.962	0.962	0.962	0.963	0.963	0.964	0.964	0.965	0.966	0.968	0.969	0.970	0.970	0.971	0.972
1.5	1.000	1.000	1.000	1.000	1.000	1.000	1.000	1.000	1.000	1.000	1.000	1.000	1.000	1.000	1.000	1.000	1.000	1.000	1.000	1.000	1.000	1.000	1.000	1.000	1.000
2.0	0.982	0.990	0.991	0.992	0.992	0.993	0.993	0.993	0.993	0.993	0.994	0.994	0.993	0.994	0.994	0.994	0.994	0.994	0.995	0.995	0.995	0.995	0.995	0.994	0.994
3.0	0.936	0.964	0.970	0.972	0.974	0.975	0.976	0.977	0.977	0.977	0.978	0.978	0.978	0.979	0.980	0.979	0.980	0.981	0.981	0.982	0.982	0.982	0.982	0.981	0.981
4.0	0.894	0.938	0.948	0.952	0.955	0.957	0.957	0.958	0.958	0.958	0.959	0.959	0.960	0.961	0.962	0.963	0.964	0.965	0.966	0.966	0.967	0.967	0.967	0.966	0.966
5.0	0.853	0.901	0.912	0.918	0.922	0.926	0.927	0.929	0.930	0.932	0.934	0.936	0.937	0.939	0.940	0.942	0.943	0.944	0.946	0.948	0.949	0.949	0.949	0.949	0.949
6.0	0.814	0.865	0.877	0.884	0.889	0.895	0.897	0.900	0.903	0.905	0.909	0.911	0.913	0.915	0.917	0.919	0.920	0.922	0.925	0.927	0.929	0.931	0.931	0.931	0.933
7.0	0.777	0.829	0.842	0.851	0.858	0.864	0.868	0.872	0.875	0.879	0.882	0.885	0.888	0.891	0.893	0.895	0.898	0.900	0.903	0.905	0.908	0.910	0.910	0.912	0.913
8.0	0.742	0.796	0.810	0.818	0.827	0.834	0.838	0.844	0.847	0.852	0.856	0.860	0.863	0.866	0.869	0.871	0.874	0.877	0.880	0.883	0.886	0.888	0.890	0.890	0.892
9.0	0.708	0.763	0.777	0.786	0.795	0.804	0.809	0.816	0.820	0.824	0.829	0.833	0.837	0.840	0.843	0.847	0.850	0.853	0.857	0.860	0.864	0.867	0.868	0.869	0.872
10.0	0.676	0.732	0.745	0.756	0.766	0.775	0.782	0.788	0.793	0.797	0.803	0.808	0.812	0.816	0.819	0.822	0.826	0.829	0.833	0.837	0.842	0.844	0.846	0.848	0.851
11.0	0.645	0.701	0.714	0.725	0.735	0.744	0.751	0.759	0.765	0.769	0.775	0.780	0.785	0.789	0.793	0.796	0.800	0.804	0.808	0.813	0.817	0.820	0.823	0.824	0.828
12.0	0.616	0.671	0.684	0.695	0.706	0.716	0.723	0.731	0.736	0.742	0.747	0.753	0.758	0.763	0.767	0.771	0.775	0.779	0.784	0.789	0.794	0.798	0.800	0.802	0.805
13.0	0.588	0.642	0.655	0.666	0.676	0.686	0.694	0.703	0.709	0.715	0.721	0.727	0.732	0.737	0.742	0.745	0.750	0.754	0.760	0.765	0.770	0.774	0.776	0.779	0.783
14.0	0.561	0.615	0.628	0.639	0.648	0.658	0.667	0.676	0.682	0.688	0.695	0.701	0.706	0.711	0.716	0.720	0.724	0.729	0.736	0.741	0.748	0.751	0.754	0.756	0.760
15.0	0.536	0.589	0.602	0.613	0.623	0.630	0.642	0.651	0.657	0.663	0.670	0.677	0.682	0.688	0.693	0.696	0.701	0.706	0.713	0.718	0.725	0.729	0.732	0.735	0.739
16.0	0.511	0.564	0.577	0.588	0.598	0.607	0.617	0.626	0.633	0.639	0.647	0.653	0.659	0.665	0.670	0.673	0.678	0.683	0.690	0.696	0.703	0.708	0.710	0.713	0.718
17.0	0.488	0.541	0.553	0.564	0.574	0.584	0.593	0.602	0.609	0.615	0.622	0.628	0.635	0.641	0.646	0.650	0.655	0.660	0.667	0.674	0.680	0.686	0.689	0.692	0.697
18.0	0.466	0.517	0.529	0.540	0.550	0.560	0.569	0.579	0.586	0.593	0.599	0.606	0.613	0.618	0.623	0.628	0.633	0.638	0.645	0.653	0.659	0.665	0.668	0.672	0.677
19.0	0.445	0.495	0.507	0.517	0.528	0.537	0.547	0.556	0.563	0.570	0.577	0.584	0.591	0.596	0.601	0.606	0.611	0.616	0.623	0.631	0.638	0.643	0.647	0.651	0.657
20.0	0.424	0.473	0.486	0.496	0.506	0.516	0.524	0.534	0.541	0.548	0.555	0.562	0.569	0.574	0.579	0.584	0.589	0.594	0.602	0.609	0.617	0.623	0.626	0.630	0.636
21.0	0.405	0.454	0.466	0.476	0.484	0.494	0.502	0.512	0.519	0.527	0.533	0.541	0.548	0.553	0.558	0.563	0.568	0.573	0.581	0.588	0.596	0.602	0.606	0.611	0.616
22.0	0.387	0.434	0.446	0.456	0.464	0.474	0.483	0.492	0.499	0.506	0.513	0.520	0.527	0.533	0.538	0.543	0.548	0.553	0.561	0.568	0.576	0.582	0.587	0.591	0.598
23.0	0.370	0.416	0.428	0.437	0.446	0.456	0.464	0.473	0.480	0.487	0.494	0.501	0.508	0.513	0.518	0.523	0.529	0.534	0.541	0.549	0.557	0.563	0.568	0.572	0.579
24.0	0.352	0.398	0.410	0.419	0.428	0.436	0.445	0.454	0.460	0.468	0.474	0.482	0.488	0.494	0.499	0.503	0.509	0.514	0.522	0.530	0.538	0.544	0.549	0.553	0.560
25.0	0.337	0.382	0.393	0.402	0.410	0.419	0.427	0.436	0.443	0.449	0.456	0.463	0.470	0.475	0.480	0.485	0.490	0.496	0.504	0.512	0.520	0.526	0.530	0.535	0.543
26.0	0.321	0.365	0.376	0.384	0.393	0.402	0.409	0.418	0.424	0.431	0.439	0.445	0.451	0.457	0.462	0.466	0.471	0.477	0.485	0.493	0.501	0.507	0.512	0.516	0.524
27.0	0.307	0.350	0.361	0.369	0.377	0.386	0.394	0.402	0.408	0.414	0.421	0.428	0.434	0.439	0.444	0.449	0.454	0.459	0.468	0.476	0.484	0.490	0.495	0.500	0.507
28.0	0.292	0.335	0.346	0.355	0.362	0.370	0.377	0.385	0.392	0.398	0.405	0.410	0.417	0.422	0.427	0.431	0.436	0.441	0.449	0.459	0.467	0.473	0.478	0.483	0.490
29.0	0.279	0.321	0.332	0.340	0.344	0.355	0.362	0.370	0.375	0.382	0.388	0.395	0.400	0.405	0.410	0.415	0.420	0.425	0.433	0.441	0.450	0.457	0.461	0.466	0.473
30.0	0.266	0.307	0.317	0.325	0.332	0.340	0.347	0.354	0.360	0.366	0.373	0.378	0.384	0.389	0.394	0.399	0.403	0.409	0.417	0.425	0.434	0.440	0.444	0.450	0.456

EQ SQ, Equivalent square.

TABLE 22.10   Tray, Wedge, and Compensator Factors

	Tray	Factor	Wedge	Factor	Brass Compensator	Factor
Cobalt-60	5 mm solid	0.96	15 degree	0.828	1 mm	0.956
	5 mm slotted	0.97	30 degree	0.744	2 mm	0.914
			45 degree	0.653	3 mm	0.874
			60 degree	0.424	4 mm	0.835
6 MV	5 mm solid	0.97	15 degree	0.828	1 mm	0.965
	5 mm slotted	0.98	30 degree	0.714	2 mm	0.931
			45 degree	0.580	3 mm	0.899
			60 degree	0.424	4 mm	0.867
18 MV	5 mm solid	0.98	15 degree	0.866	1 mm	0.945
	5 mm slotted	0.99	30 degree	0.775	2 mm	0.927
			45 degree	0.656	3 mm	0.918
			60 degree	0.449	4 mm	0.892

No matter how many times this trip is made, the trip is 9 hours as long as a constant speed of 50 miles per hour is maintained. This type of constant speed (dose rate) happens in the cobalt-60 machine and is the principle behind the time setting calculation. In the linear accelerator, the "dose rate" varies slightly from one moment to the next. If the dose from the linear accelerator is measured with real time, the dose can be different each time. Therefore, real time cannot be used to deliver the prescribed dose with a linear accelerator. Instead, a different system of time called *MU* is used. In the example, 450 miles are traveled each trip regardless of the speed. Depending on traffic conditions, the time needed to go 450 miles changes each day. The MU setting ensures that the same dose is delivered at each treatment regardless of the "real-time" conditions. The rate at which the MUs are delivered is the MU per minute rate. The MU/minute setting can be adjusted by the therapist. This rate is usually in the range of 400 to 1000 MU/minute. Assume that the MU/minute has been set to deliver 600 MU/minute. The prescription requires a total of 300 MU to be delivered. In theory, the linear accelerator should deliver the 300 MU in 0.5 minutes. However, because of slight fluctuations in the 600 MU/minute delivery rate, the actual treatment time may be slightly greater than the 0.5 minutes. If the beam is turned on for exactly 0.5 minutes each treatment, the patient may not receive the exact same dose each day. However, with delivery of 300 MU each day, the patient is treated to the same dose each day.

Linear Accelerator Nonisocentric Calculations

Examples 2, 3, and 4 demonstrate MU calculations, starting with the most basic calculation and progressing in complexity.

Example 2: A patient is treated on the 6-MV linear accelerator at 100 cm SSD. The collimator setting is 10×10 cm. No blocking is used for this treatment. The prescription states that a dose of 3000 cGy is to be delivered to a depth of 5 cm in 10 fractions. Calculate the MU setting.

Step 1. Determine the ES for the collimator setting: 10.

Step 2. Determine the EFS: no blocks; therefore the EFS is also 10.

Step 3. Determine the appropriate tissue absorption factor: nonisocentric treatment; therefore, PDD.

Step 4. Determine the prescribed dose: 300 cGy per fraction.

Step 5. Look up the factors: the factors for the dose rate at a point are RDR, Sc, Sp, and PDD.

$$\text{Reference Dose Rate} = 0.993 \text{ cGy/MU} \text{ (see Table 22.3)}$$

$$\text{Sc } (10 \times 10 \text{ cm}) = 1.000 \text{ (see Table 22.4)}$$

$$\text{Sp } (10 \times 10 \text{ cm}) = 1.000 \text{ (see Table 22.4)}$$

$$\text{PDD } (5,10,100) = 87.1 \text{ (see Table 22.6)}$$

$$\text{MU Setting} = \text{Prescribed Dose/RDR} \times \text{SCF} \times \text{Sc} \times \text{Sp} \times \text{PDD}/100$$

$$\text{MU Setting} = 300 \text{ cGy}/0.993 \text{ cGy/MU} \times (101.5/101.5)^2 \times 1.00 \times 1.0 \times 87.1/100$$

$$\text{MU Setting} = 300 \text{ cGy}/0.8649 \text{ cGy/MU}$$

$$\text{MU Setting} = 347 \text{ MU}$$

If the collimator setting is changed from 10×10 cm to 15×15 cm, is the MU setting greater than or less than 347 MU? (See Example 3.)

Both the scatter (Sc and Sp) and PDD increase with the increased collimator setting. Thus, the dose rate at the calculation point should increase, and therefore, the MU setting is less than 347 MU.

Example 3: A patient is treated on the 6-MV linear accelerator at 100 cm SSD. The collimator setting is 15×15 cm. No blocking is used for this treatment. The prescription states that a dose of 3000 cGy is to be delivered to a depth of 5 cm in 10 fractions. Calculate the MU setting.

$$\text{Reference Dose Rate} = 0.993 \text{ cGy/MU} \text{ (see Table 22.3)}$$

$$\text{Sc } (15 \times 15 \text{ cm}) = 1.021 \text{ (see Table 22.4)}$$

$$\text{Sp } (15 \times 15 \text{ cm}) = 1.014 \text{ (see Table 22.4)}$$

$$\text{PDD } (5,15,100) = 87.9 \text{ (see Table 22.6)}$$

$$\text{MU Setting} = \text{Prescribed Dose/RDR} \times \text{ISCF} \times \text{Sc} \times \text{Sp} \times \text{PDD}/100$$

$$\text{MU Setting} = 300 \text{ cGy}/0.993 \times (101.5/101.5)^2 \times 1.021 \times 1.014 \times 87.9/100$$

$$\text{MU Setting} = 300 \text{ cGy}/0.0937$$

MU Setting = 332 MU

Example 4: A patient is treated on the 6-MV linear accelerator at 100 cm SSD. The collimator setting is 15 × 15 cm. With multileaf collimator, the field is blocked to an EFS of an 8 × 8 cm ES. The prescription states that a dose of 3000 cGy is to be delivered to a depth of 5 cm in 10 fractions.

(Note: The six-step process is used; however, it is no longer outlined step by step.)

The prescribed dose is 300 cGy per fraction.

The factors for the dose rate at a point are RDR, Sc, Sp, and PDD.

Reference Dose Rate = 0.993 cGy/MU (see Table 22.3)

Sc (15 × 15 cm) = 1.021 (see Table 22.4)

Sp (8 × 8 cm) = 0.992 (see Table 22.4)

PDD (5,8,100) = 86.8 (see Table 22.6)

MU Setting = Prescribed Dose/RDR × ISCF × Sc × (15 × 15) × Sp × (8 × 8) × PDD/100

$$\text{MU Setting} = 300 \text{ cGy}/0.933 \text{ cGy/MU} \times (101.5/101.5)^2 \times 1.021 \times 0.992 \times 86.8/100$$

MU Setting = 300 cGy 0.8730 cGy/MU

MU Setting = 344 MU

Note that the blocks created a smaller treated volume, and thus there was a reduction in the Sp and PDD compared with Example 3. To compensate for the reductions in Sp and PDD, the MU setting needs to be increased for Example 4. The MU setting for Example 3 was 332 MU, and the setting for Example 4 was 344 MU. Again, note that smaller field sizes require higher MU settings than do larger field sizes. In addition, fields that have any device such as a block tray wedge or compensator also require higher MU settings than fields that do not have these devices.

EXTENDED DISTANCE CALCULATIONS WITH PERCENTAGE DEPTH DOSE AND SOURCE-SKIN DISTANCE TREATMENT

On occasion, anatomical areas of a patient's body must be treated that are larger than the collimator areas achievable with conventional radiation therapy treatment units. This is the case in total body, total skin irradiation techniques, and various other field arrangements. In these cases, larger field areas are possible with extension of the distance of the treatment area. Because of divergence, as the distance from the source increases, the field size increases. In this manner, very large areas can be treated in a single field. The alternative is to split the treatment fields up into areas that can be accommodated at conventional distances with the challenge of accurate matching of divergent fields. To avoid this challenge, extended distances are commonly used. For example, the isocenter on a linear accelerator is 100 cm. In a standard SSD treatment, the patient is treated at 100 cm SSD. However, for a larger field, the patient may be set up at 125 cm SSD. To reiterate, an extended distance treatment is one in which the patient is set up at a distance beyond the isocenter or reference distance.[8]

With this type of calculation, several points must be considered. PDD is used for the calculation because its arrangement is nonisocentric. PDD depends on four factors: energy, field size, depth, and SSD. If any of these factors change, the PDD changes. If the energy is increased from cobalt-60 (1.25 MeV) to 6 MV, the PDD increases because of increased penetrating power. If the field size, at a given energy, changes from 10 × 10 cm to 15 × 15 cm, the PDD increases because of an increase in scatter. If the depth is increased from 6 cm to 10 cm, the PDD decreases because more attenuation and beam absorption occur. As the SSD is increased, the PDD increases because of a change in the inverse square law with a change in distance. As a result of these changes, special considerations must be used to calculate treatment times and MUs at extended distance treatment with use of PDD.

Mayneord Factor

The Mayneord factor is a special application of the inverse square law. Many forms of the Mayneord factor are cited by different authorities. If it is understood where the numbers for the Mayneord factor are derived from, the likelihood of applying the numbers correctly is increased, which results in no real need to memorize what appears to be a complex equation.

Reference or standard-distance PDD values are determined from direct measurement. When patients are treated at an extended distance, the distance from the source of radiation to the depth of D_{max} and the depth of the calculation point also changes. Note that the distances are what change and not the specified depth of treatment. If a patient is treated on a 6-MV linear accelerator with a 10 × 10 cm field size at 100 SSD to a depth of 8 cm and the distance is extended to 125 SSD, the depth of D_{max} and the point of calculation remain the same; the depths are 1.5 cm and 8 cm, respectively. However, the distances to these points for a 125-cm SSD treatment are 126.5 cm (125.0 + 1.5 cm) and 133 cm (125.0 + 8.0 cm), respectively (Fig. 22.10).

Other factors must be considered. The energy of the treatment machine is the same in the standard and extended distance treatment. A 6-MV accelerator has the same energy at 125 cm as it does at 100 cm. If the field size is 10 × 10 cm in both cases and the depth of calculation is 8 cm for both treatments, these factors should have little or no effect on the calculation. Because the 10 × 10 cm field is defined on the skin in both treatments, the field size at the calculation point is slightly different because of divergence. This slightly changes the amount of scatter. The major change results from the change in distance. The original distances from source to D_{max} and depth are 101.5 and 108 cm, respectively. These distances should be removed from the measured PDD by multiplying by the inverse as follows:

$$(108)^2 / (101.5)^2$$

Then, the correct distance is used in the calculation by multiplying by the square of the ratio of the new distances:

$$(126.5)^2 / (133)^2$$

This allows for the correct attenuation of the beam for the new distances. These derived correction factors are then multiplied by the PDD referenced from the table, the result being the new PDD for the extended distances.

The Mayneord factor can be calculated with use of these distances. Note that the depth of D_{max} is 1.5 cm for a 6-MV linear accelerator and is reflected in the numbers. The PDD (8,10,100) is 75.1%.

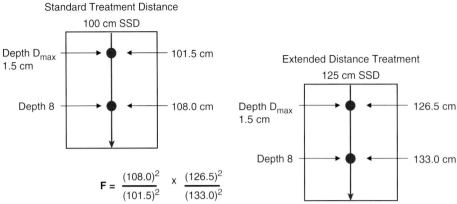

Standard Treatment Distance
100 cm SSD

Depth D_{max} 1.5 cm — 101.5 cm

Depth 8 — 108.0 cm

Extended Distance Treatment
125 cm SSD

Depth D_{max} 1.5 cm — 126.5 cm

Depth 8 — 133.0 cm

$$F = \frac{(108.0)^2}{(101.5)^2} \times \frac{(126.5)^2}{(133.0)^2}$$

Fig. 22.10 Diagram shows the Mayneord factor.

The original distances were 101.5 cm and 108 cm. The new distances are 126.5 cm and 133 cm:

$$\text{New PDD}_{(8,10,125)} = 75.1 \times (108)^2 / (101.5)^2$$
$$\times (126.5)^2 / (133)^2$$

$$\text{New PDD} = 76.9$$

Again, the Mayneord factor is an inverse square correction of the PDD. It can also be used in shortened treatment distances. Note that the Mayneord factor does not account for changes in scatter because of a change in beam divergence. Actually, beam divergence decreases at extended distances; therefore there is a small decrease in scatter. Thus the Mayneord factor gives the approximate value for the new PDD. For the exact value for the new PDD, actual beam measurements with use of an ionization chamber or other appropriate devices are necessary.

Hint: Mayneord factor should always be greater than 1.0 for extended distance treatments. If the treatment distance is decreased, Mayneord factor is less than 1.0.

Try the following: Patient 1 is treated at 100 cm SSD with a 10-cm-wide field on the skin surface. Patient 2 is treated at 200 cm SSD with a 10-cm-wide field on the skin. Now calculate the field size at depth of 10 cm for each patient. Your answers should be 11.0 cm wide for Patient 1 and 10.5 cm wide field for Patient 2. Scatter is less for a 10.5-cm field than for an 11.0-cm field.

The following example uses the Mayneord factor in the calculation of a MU setting for a 6-MV accelerator.

Example 5: A patient is treated on the 6-MV treatment unit at an extended distance of 125 cm. The collimator setting is 20 × 20 cm, and the field size on the patient's skin is 25 × 25 cm. The prescription states that a dose of 3000 cGy is to be delivered to a depth of 5 cm in 10 fractions with a single posterior treatment field arrangement. Calculate the MU setting.

A similar process can be used for extended distance calculations. Use the same five steps discussed previously and add a sixth step for the Mayneord factor.

The collimator setting is 20 × 20 cm, which is conveniently the ES.

The field size at the treatment SSD of 125 cm is 25 × 25 cm; therefore the EFS ES is 25^2 cm.

$$\text{Reference Dose Rate} = 0.993 \text{ cGy/MU}$$

$$\text{Sc} (20 \times 20 \text{ cm}) = 1.038$$

$$\text{Sp} (25 \times 25 \text{ cm}) = 1.028$$

$$\text{PDD} (5,25,100) = 88.9$$

The prescribed dose is 3000 cGy in 10 fractions; therefore the daily prescribed dose is 300 cGy/fraction.

The original distances when the PDD was measured were 101.5 cm to the depth of D_{max} and 105 cm to a depth of 5 cm. Thus the inverses of these distances are 105/101.5. The patient is treated at 125 cm SSD; therefore the distances to the depth of D_{max} and the depth of calculation are 126.5 and 130, respectively (125.0 + 1.5 = 126.5 and 125.0 + 5.0 = 130.0).

Calculate the new PDD with the Mayneord factor. Determine the PDD at a depth of 5 cm.

$$\text{New PDD}_{(5,25,100)} = 88.9 \times (105)^2 / (101.5)^2$$
$$\times (126.5)^2 / (131)^2$$

$$\text{New PDD} = 90.08$$

The equation to be used is, again, a variation of dose divided by dose rate. The dose rate is affected by the factors mentioned in the problem. Because the treatment is at an extended distance, the intensity of the beam is affected by the inverse square law. Although the PDD increased because of the extended distance, the intensity (dose rate) of the beam decreases because of the increased distance. The correction relates the distance from the source to the point of treatment unit calibration (where referenced data were measured) and the treatment SSD plus D_{max}. The inverse square correction is then included as a dose rate correction in the denominator of the equation. It may be written as follows:

$$\text{Inverse Square Correction} = (\text{Reference Source Calibration}$$
$$\text{Distance}^2 / (\text{Treatment SDD}$$
$$+ D_{max}^2 \times \text{PDD}/100$$

The treatment time can now be calculated as follows:

$$\text{MU Setting} = \text{Prescribed Dose}/\text{RDR}$$
$$\times \text{inverse square correction}$$
$$\times \text{Sc} \times \text{Sp} \times \text{PDD}$$

$$\text{MU Setting} = 300 \text{ cGy}/0.993 \text{ cGy/MU} \times (101.5/126.5)^2$$
$$\times 1.038 \times 1.028 \times 90.08/100$$

$$\text{MU Setting} = 300 \text{ cGy}/0.6145 \text{ cGy/MU}$$

$$\text{MU Setting} = 488 \text{ MU}$$

Again, note that as the treatment distance increases, the MU setting increases to offset the loss of intensity from the increased distance.

Calculation of the Given Dose for a Source-Skin Distance Treatment with Percentage Depth Dose

Often, knowledge of the dose to points other than the prescription point is important. Dose-limiting and critical structures are anatomic sites that cannot withstand the same amount of exposure as neighboring tissues without damage. The spinal cord, bowel, and lens of the eye are examples of dose-limiting structures that are commonly monitored. The anatomy to be monitored is determined chiefly by the region of the body being irradiated.

The SSD calculations are often done at D_{max}. When a single field is used to treat a patient, such as a posterior spine field, the dose at D_{max} is known as the *given dose*. Other names for the given dose are *applied dose, entrance dose, peak absorbed dose,* and D_{max} *dose.* This point is where the PDD is equal to 100%. As the depth increases from that point, the PDD decreases. If a prescription calls for the administration of 300 cGy to a certain depth below D_{max} through a single field, the given dose has to be more than the 300 cGy based on these concepts. The dose at depth is also called the *TD.* This is done for cobalt-60 as well as for linear accelerators. Each treatment field has its own given dose. The given dose can be calculated with use of the ratio of the prescribed dose for the field and the PDD at the depth of the prescribed dose as follows:

$$\text{Given Dose} = \text{TD/PDD} \times 100$$

When the PDD is written, the convention used is PDD (d,s,SSD), which indicates that this refers to the PDD at depth (d), for ES (s), at the treatment distance (SSD). If the PDD at a depth of 5 cm for a 10×10 cm field treatment at 100 cm SSD is 78.3%, the convention for writing this information is PDD (5,10,100) = 78.3%.

A direct relationship exists between the dose and the PDD at a point. Thus a ratio or direct proportion can be established as follows:

$$\text{Dose}_A/\text{PDD}_A = \text{Dose}_B/\text{PDD}_B$$

Note that the previous equation can be used to calculate the dose to any point of interest (on the central axis) with use of PDD. In this chapter, this equation is referred to as the *ratio method* for calculating the dose.

The following example calculates the given dose.

Example 6: A patient is treated on the 6-MV linear accelerator at 100 cm SSD. The collimator setting is 15×15 cm. No MLC is used for this treatment. The prescription states that a dose of 300 cGy per fraction is to be delivered at a depth of 5 cm. Calculate the given dose.

From data given in Table 22.6, the PDD (5,15,100) is 87.9.

$$\text{Given Dose} = \text{TD/PDD} \times 100$$

$$\text{Given Dose} = 300 \text{ cGy/87.9}$$

$$\text{Given Dose} = 341.3 \text{ cGy}$$

As expected, the given dose is greater than the TD.

Any other point along the central axis can be found if the depth and PDD are known. If a dose at a depth of 3 cm is sought in the preceding example, it is somewhere between the dose at D_{max} and the dose at 5 cm. With looking up the PDD at the desired depth, the information can be derived.

In earlier years of radiation therapy, the use of lower-energy machines and the resultant higher given doses presented problems. To treat tumors at depth, the superficial tissues needed higher doses. Coupled with the use of lower-energy therapy machines that had a shallower D_{max}, heightened skin reactions were common, and sometimes, the administration of radiation therapy was limited.

On rare occasions, nonisocentric treatments are done for parallel opposed fields. At those times, the radiation oncology team may benefit from noting the total dose at D_{max}. In this case, the given dose is added to the exit dose. The exit dose is the dose absorbed by a point that is located at the depth of D_{max} at the exit of the beam. For example, the depth of D_{max} for a 6-MV photon beam is approximately 1.5 cm. If a patient is treated with parallel opposed AP/PA photon beams and the patient's central axis separation is 20 cm, the total D_{max} dose can be calculated. The given dose is calculated at a depth of 1.5 cm and the exit dose at a depth of 18.5 cm (20 cm – 1.5 cm). The following example calculates the total D_{max} dose and cord dose with a linear accelerator. Each field contributes to the total dose of each.

Example 7: A patient is treated on the 6-MV linear accelerator at 100 cm SSD. The collimator setting is 15×15 cm. The MLC reduces the treated area to an 8×8 cm EFS. The prescription states that a dose of 3600 cGy is to be delivered to a depth of 10 cm in 20 fractions using an AP/PA treatment field arrangement. The patient's central axis separation is 20 cm. The cord lies 3.0 cm beneath the posterior skin surface. Calculate the total D_{max} dose and the cord dose.

We see that, in this arrangement, the cord calculation point lies 3.0 cm from the posterior surface and 17.0 cm from the anterior surface. It is important to note here that all points of calculation are along the central axis. To obtain the anterior depth of the cord, the posterior depth of the cord should be subtracted from the patient's total separation (20.0 cm – 3.0 cm = 17.0 cm). The depth of D_{max} for the 6-MV linear accelerator is 1.5 cm. The depth of the posterior field exit point is 18.5 cm (20.0 cm – 1.5 cm).

The factors required for this calculation are as follows:

$$\text{PDD } (1.5,8,100) = 100.0 \text{ (PDD at the Depth of } D_{max})$$

$$\text{PDD } (3,8,100) = 95.0 \text{ (PDD at the Depth of 3 cm}$$
$$\text{for Posterior Cord Dose)}$$

$$\text{PDD } (10,8,100) = 66.7 \text{ (PDD at the Depth of 10 cm}$$
$$\text{for Midplane Dose)}$$

$$\text{PDD } (17,8,100) = 45.2 \text{ (PDD at the Depth of 17 cm}$$
$$\text{for Anterior Cord Dose)}$$

$$\text{PDD } (18.5,8,100) = 41.6 \text{ (PDD at the Depth of 18.5 cm,}$$
$$\text{which represents the Exit Dose)}$$

Determination of Total D_{max} Dose

A. Calculate the anterior dose contribution to D_{max} (given dose). In this problem, the direct proportion formula is used as follows:

$$\text{Dose at Point A/PDD at Point A} = \text{Dose at Point B/}$$
$$\text{PDD at Point B}$$

$$Dose_{1.5\ cm}/PDD_{1.5\ cm} = Dose_{10\ cm}/PDD_{10\ cm}$$

$$Dose_{1.5\ cm}/100 = 90\ cGy/66.7$$

$$Dose_{1.5\ cm} = 134.9\ cGy$$

A. Calculate the posterior dose contribution to D_{max} (exit dose). With use of the exit point (A) and D_{max} point (B), depths are 18.5 cm and 1.5 cm, respectively:

$$Dose_{1.5\ cm}/PDD_{1.5\ cm} = Dose_{18.5\ cm}/PDD_{18.5\ cm}$$

$$134.9\ cGy/100 = Dose_{18.5\ cm}/41.6$$

$$Dose_{18.5\ cm} = 56.1\ cGy$$

I. Add the AP/PA dose contributions to obtain total D_{max} dose.

$$D_{max}Dose\ (Total) = D_{max}Dose\ (Anterior) \\ + D_{max}Dose\ (Posterior)$$

$$D_{max}Dose\ (Total) = 134.9 + 56.1$$

$$D_{max}Dose\ (Total) = 191.0\ cGy$$

Determination of Cord Dose (Contribution from Both Fields)

A. Calculate the anterior dose contribution to the cord. With use of the cord point (A) and D_{max} (B), depths are 17.0 cm and 1.5 cm, respectively:

$$Dose_{17\ cm}/PDD_{17\ cm} = Dose_{1.5\ cm}/PDD_{1.5\ cm}$$

$$Dose_{17\ cm}/45.2 = 134.9\ cGy/100$$

$$Dose_{17\ cm} = 61.0\ cGy$$

A. Calculate the posterior dose contribution to the cord. With use of the cord point (A) and D_{max} point (B), depths are 3.0 cm and 1.5 cm, respectively:

$$Dose_{3\ cm}/PDD_{3\ cm} = Dose_{1.5\ cm}/PDD_{1.5\ cm}$$

$$Dose_{3\ cm}/95.0 = 134.9\ cGy/100$$

$$Dose_{3\ cm} = 128.2\ cGy$$

I. Add the AP/PA dose contributions to obtain the total cord dose.

$$Cord\ Dose\ (Total) = Cord\ Dose\ (Anterior) + Cord \\ Dose\ (Posterior)$$

$$Cord\ Dose\ (Total) = 61.0\ cGy + 128.2\ cGy$$

$$Cord\ Dose\ (Total) = 189.2\ cGy$$

If this calculation is done on a cobalt-60 treatment machine (1.25 MeV) and compared with the preceding calculation, the following chart is built:

Point of Calculation	Cobalt-60	6-MV	% Difference
Total dose at D_{max}	212.8	191.0	11.4
Total cord dose	197.0	189.2	4.1
Total dose to midplane	180.0	180.0	0.0

Although the midplane dose is constant in both cases, the total doses to D_{max} and the cord are different for the two energies. The data show that the total dose at D_{max} and the cord dose are less for higher treatment energies. Both doses are even less for energies of 10 MV, 18 MV, or greater. One of the advantages of higher energy beams, especially for parallel opposed treatment field arrangements, is that the total dose at D_{max} is significantly less. In this case, the patient receives approximately 4.1% less dose to the cord if a 6-MV beam is used instead of the cobalt 60 beam.

SOURCE-AXIS DISTANCE (ISOCENTRIC) CALCULATIONS

An SAD or isocentric treatment occurs when the treatment machine's isocenter is established at some reference point within the patient. When this is established, it can also be referred to as an *isocentric technique*. Because the field size is defined at the isocenter, the collimated field matches the field size setting inside the patient at the isocenter and not on the skin surface as seen in the nonisocentric SSD treatment.

One advantage that SAD treatment techniques have over SSD techniques is that when the patient has been properly positioned and the isocenter for the treatment has been established, there is usually no movement of the patient or treatment table relative to the treatment isocenter for each of the subsequent treatment fields. For example, a patient is treated with an AP/PA treatment field arrangement on a 6-MV, 100-cm isocentric linear accelerator. The patient's central axis separation is 20 cm, and the dose is calculated at the patient's midplane (equal distance established from both AP/PA skin surfaces). If this arrangement is treated with an SSD technique, the anterior field is established at 100 cm to the anterior skin surface. After treatment of the anterior field, the gantry is rotated 180 degrees for treatment of the posterior field. However, the treatment table has to be raised until the ODI reads 100 cm on the patient's posterior skin surface.

In treatment of the same patient with an SAD (isocentric) technique, the anterior SSD is established at 90 cm. The isocenter is positioned 10 cm beneath the anterior skin surface and 10 cm beneath the posterior skin surface, which makes it midplane as prescribed. (Note that the 10-cm anterior depth and 10-cm posterior depth add up to the 20-cm central axis separation.) The SAD is 100 cm (90 cm SSD + 10 cm depth). After the anterior field is treated, the gantry is rotated 180 degrees for treatment of the posterior field. However, in an isocentric technique, the gantry is rotating about the isocenter, which has been established inside the patient. Therefore the patient is at the correct posterior SSD of 90 cm without the treatment table being raised or lowered. Less movement between treatment fields lowers the chance of treatment errors from positioning variations that occur during patient movement.

For calculation of the MU setting or doses to specific points, TAR, TMR, and TPR work very well for isocentric techniques. PDD can also be used for isocentric treatment techniques. However, two main differences from PDD affect calculations with TAR, TMR, or TPR. Both are caused by the way PDD and TAR, TMR, and TPR are calculated. PDD is calculated from two measurements at two different points in space. TAR, TMR, and TPR are calculated from two measurements at the same point in space. This affects the beam geometry (field divergence) and application of the inverse square law.

First, when TAR is used for calculations, the field size at the point of calculation must be used. In some conditions, the field size at the point of interest must be determined. One example is with determination of a dose delivered to points other than the isocenter along the central axis. In this case, the treatment field size at the alternate point changes because of beam divergence and needs to be calculated. Another effect on the calculation involves the application of the inverse square law. An inverse square correction is needed when the dose to a point other than the isocenter is calculated. These points are covered in greater detail in the example problems (Box 22.5).

The same basic six-step process described previously in the section on nonisocentric calculations with PDD is used with these isocentric technique calculations:

Step 1. Determine the ES of the collimator setting (used for Sc).
Step 2. Determine the ES of the EFS (used for TAR, TMR, or TPR and Sp when appropriate).
Step 3. Determine the appropriate tissue absorption table.
Step 4. Determine the prescribed dose.
Step 5. Look up the factors with use of the appropriate data tables.
Step 6. Use the appropriate equation for determining the MU setting.

Example 8: A patient is treated on the 6-MV linear accelerator treatment machine at 100 cm SAD. The treatment SSD is 95 cm. The collimator setting is 15 × 15 cm. The MLC reduces the treated area to an 8 × 8 cm EFS. The prescription states that a dose of 3000 cGy is to be delivered to a depth of 5 cm in 10 fractions through a single field. Calculate the MU setting with use of TAR.

Step 1. The collimator ES is 15.0.
Step 2. The EFS is 8.0.
Step 3. TAR is used for the calculation. (Reminder: With use of TAR, only Sc is used because Sp is "built into" the TAR table).

BOX 22.5 Isocentric Calculation Process

Equations used for isocentric (SAD) calculations

Calculation of the Monitor Unit Setting

TAR Calculations
Monitor unit (MU) Settings = Prescribed Dose/ reference dose rate (RDR) × inverse square correction factor (ISCF) × collimator scatter factor (Sc) × TAR × Other Factors

TMR Calculations
Monitor unit (MU) Settings = Prescribed Dose/ reference dose rate (RDR) × inverse square correction factor (ISCF) × collimator scatter factor (Sc) × phantom or patient scatter factor (Sp) × TMR × Other Factors

TPR Calculations
Monitor unit (MU) Settings = Prescribed Dose/ reference dose rate (RDR) × inverse square correction factor (ISCF) × collimator scatter factor (Sc) × phantom or patient scatter factor (Sp) × TPR × Other Factors

Calculation of Changes in Field Size with Distance
Field Size$_A$/Distance$_A$ = Field Size$_B$/Distance$_B$

Calculation of Dose to a Point with TAR, TMR, and TPR
Dose$_A$ = Dose$_B$/TAR$_B$ × source calculation point dose (SCPD$_B$)^2/(SCPD$_A$)^2 × TAR$_A$
Dose$_A$ = Dose$_B$/TMR$_B$ × source calculation point dose (SCPD$_B$)^2/(SCPD$_A$)^2 × TMR$_A$
Dose$_A$ = Dose$_B$/TPR$_B$ × source calculation point dose (SCPD$_B$)^2/(SCPD$_A$)^2 × TPR$_A$

Step 4. The prescribed dose is 300 cGy per fraction (3000 cGy/10 fractions).

Step 5. The factors for the dose rate at a point are RDR, Sc, TAR, and tray factor:

$$\text{Reference Dose Rate} = 1.0 \text{ cGy/MU (see Table 22.3)}$$

$$\text{Sc } (15 \times 15 \text{ cm}) = 1.021 \text{ (see Table 22.4)}$$

$$\text{TAR } (5,8) = 0.941 \text{ (see Table 22.8)}$$

Step 6. Use the appropriate equation to determine the MU setting:

$$\text{MU Settings} = \text{Prescribed Dose/RDR} \times \text{ISCF} \\ \times \text{Sc}_{(CS)} \times \text{TAR}_{(EFS)}$$

$$\text{MU Settings} = 300 \text{ cGy/1.0 cGy/MU} \\ \times (100/100)^2 \times 1.021 \times 0.941$$

$$\text{MU Settings} = 312 \text{ MU}$$

with *ISCF* as the inverse square correction factor, *SCPD* as the source-to-calculation point distance, and *CS* as collimator setting.

Note that the ISCF used for isocentric calculations (with TAR, TMR, or TPR) can be determined with the following formula:

$$\text{ISCF} = (\text{Reference Distance/SCPD})^2$$

A patient is treated at 100 cm SAD. The SSD is 90 cm, and therefore the isocenter is located at a depth of 10 cm. Determine the ISCF for a depth of 10 cm and a depth of 15 cm.

$$\text{ISCF (for a Depth of 10 cm)} = (100 \text{ cm}/100 \text{ cm})^2$$

$$\text{ISCF (for a Depth of 15 cm)} = (100 \text{ cm}/105 \text{ cm})^2$$

In both cases, the reference distance is 100 cm (isocenter distance). The SCPD at a depth of 10 cm is equal to the 90 cm SSD + the 10 cm depth (100 cm). The SCPD at a depth of 15 cm is equal to the 90 cm SSD + 15 cm depth (105 cm).

Example 9: A patient is treated on the 6-MV linear accelerator treatment machine at 100 cm SAD. The treatment SSD is 90 cm. The collimator setting is 15 × 15 cm. The MLC reduces the treated area to an 8 × 8 cm EFS. The prescription states that a dose of 4000 cGy is to be delivered to a depth of 10 cm in 20 fractions with an AP/PA treatment field arrangement. Calculate the MU setting with use of TAR.

The factors for the dose rate:

$$\text{Reference Dose Rate} = 1.0 \text{ cGy/MU}$$

$$\text{Sc } (15 \times 15 \text{ cm}) = 1.021$$

$$\text{TAR } (10,8) = 0.787$$

$$\text{Prescribed Dose} = 100 \text{ cGy/Field}$$

$$MU \ Settings = Prescribed \ Dose/RDR \times ISCF \times Sc_{(CS)}$$
$$\times TAR_{EFS}$$

$$MU \ Settings = 100 \ cGy/1.0 \ cGy/MU \times (100/100)^2 \times 1.021$$
$$\times 0.787$$

$$MU \ Settings = 100 \ cGy/0.7794 \ cGy/MU$$

$$MU \ Setting = 124 \ MU/Field$$

Today, TMR and TPR have replaced TAR as the method of hand calculations for obtaining the MU setting or dose to a point.

When TMR or TPR is used for dose calculation, the output for the 10 × 10 cm field size is normally 1.0 cGy/MU. In the TMR calculations presented in this chapter, two scatter factors are used. One of the scatter factors corrects for Sc. The other scatter factor corrects for phantom or patient scatter (Sp). The total scatter factor is obtained by multiplying Sc by Sp.

For the following examples, TMR is used. However, because the depth of D_{max} changes slightly with changes in field size, many centers now use TPR, which is independent of the change in depth of D_{max} with changes in field size. When TPR is used, any depth may be chosen as the reference depth. This includes the depth of D_{max} for a 10 × 10 cm field. In other words, a 6-MV TMR table can become a TPR table by choosing the reference depth of 1.5 cm.

Example 10: A patient is treated on the 6-MV linear accelerator treatment machine at 100 cm SAD. The treatment SSD is 95 cm. The collimator setting is 15 × 15 cm. No beam shaping is used for this treatment. The prescription states that a dose of 3000 cGy is to be delivered to a depth of 5 cm in 10 fractions through a single field. Calculate the MU setting with use of TMR.

The factors for the dose rate at a point are RDR, Sc, Sp, and TMR:

$$Reference \ Dose \ Rate = 1.0 \ cGy/MU$$

$$Sc \ (15 \times 15 \ cm) = 1.021$$

$$Sp \ (15 \times 15 \ cm) = 1.014$$

$$TMR \ (5,15) = 0.937 \ (see \ Table \ 22.9)$$

$$Prescribed \ Dose = 300 \ cGy$$

$$MU \ Settings = Prescribed \ Dose/RDR \times Sc_{(CS)}$$
$$\times Sp_{(EFS)} \times TMR_{(EFS)}$$

$$MU \ Settings = 300 \ cGy/1.0 \ cGy/MU \times 1.021 \times 1.014 \times 0.937$$

$$MU \ Settings = 300 \ cGy/0.9701 \ cGy/MU$$

$$MU \ Setting = 309 \ MU$$

Example 11: A patient is treated on the 6-MV linear accelerator treatment machine at 100 cm SAD. The treatment SSD is 90 cm. The collimator setting is 15 × 15 cm. MLCs are used to create a 12 × 12 cm EFS. The prescription states that a dose of 4000 cGy is to be delivered to a depth of 10 cm in 20 fractions with an AP/PA treatment field arrangement. Calculate the MU setting with use of TMR.

The factors for the dose rate are:

$$Reference \ Dose \ Rate = 1.0 \ cGy/MU$$

$$Sc \ (15 \times 15 \ cm) = 1.021$$

$$Sp \ (12 \times 12 \ cm) = 1.006$$

$$TMR \ (10,12) = 0.797$$

$$Prescribed \ Dose = 100 \ cGy/Port$$

$$MU \ Settings = Prescribed \ Dose/RDR \times ISCF \times Sc_{(CS)}$$
$$\times Sp_{(EFS)} \times TMR_{(EFS)}$$

$$MU \ Settings = 100 \ cGy/1.0 \ cGy/MU \times (100/100)^2 \times 1.021$$
$$\times 1.006 \times 0.797$$

$$MU \ Settings = 100 \ cGy/0.8186 \ cGy/MU$$

$$MU \ Setting = 122 \ MU$$

Derivation of Given Dose and Dose to Points of Interest for Isocentric Problems

The given dose is the dose delivered at the depth of D_{max} for a single treatment field. In this example problem, each treatment field has its own given dose. Calculation of the given dose with TAR, TMR, or TPR is more complex than with PDD. For calculation of the given dose with TMR for this example, the prescribed dose for the field, the SCPD, and the TMR at the depth of the prescribed dose must be known.

As discussed previously, both measurements for the TMR are made at the same distance from the source. The field size increases because of divergence as the distance from the source increases. Therefore when TMR (or TAR or TPR) is used, the field size at the point of calculation must be known. To find the field size at any distance, the following relationship, based on similar triangles, can be used:

$$Field \ Size_A/Distance_A = Field \ Size_B/Distance_B$$

In practice, the ES of the rectangular field is used in place of the actual field size. For example, if the field size is 20 × 10 cm, its ES of 13.0 is used for the field size. For calculation of the given dose with TMR/TPR, the following equation is used:

$$Dose_A = Dose_B/TMR_B \times (SCPD_B)^2/(SCPD_A)^2 \times TMR_A$$

with $Dose_A$ as dose at point A, $Dose_B$ as dose at point B, TMR_A as TMR at point A, TMR_B as TMR at point B, $SCPD_A$ as source-to-calculation point distance for point A, and $SCPD_B$ as source-to-calculation point distance for point B.

Example 12: A patient is treated on the 6-MV linear accelerator at 100 cm SAD. The treatment SSD is 95 cm and the collimator setting is 10 × 10 cm. No field shaping is used. The prescription requires a dose of 300 cGy to be delivered to the isocenter daily. Calculate the given dose.

Use the following equation:

$$Dose_A = Dose_B/TMR_B \times (SCPD_B)^2/(SCPD_A)^2 \times TMR_A$$

with $Dose_A$ as dose at point A (given dose in this example), $Dose_B$ as dose at point B (isocenter in this example), TMR_A as TMR at point A (depth of D_{max}), TMR_B as TMR at point B (depth of isocenter), $SCPD_A$ as source-to-calculation point distance for point A (95 cm SSD + 1.5 cm depth), $SCPD_B$ as source-to-calculation point distance for point B (95 cm SSD + 5 cm depth), $Dose_A$ as 300 cGy/.929 × $(100/96.5)^2$ × 1.000, and $Dose_A$ as 346.8 cGy.

Note that the ratio of $SCPD_B$ and $SCPD_A$ is the application of the inverse square law. SCPD is found by adding the depth to the SSD for that point. The following table assists in the organization of data when calculating the dose to points with TAR, TMR, and TPR.

Chart for Organizing Data

Point	SSD	Depth	SCPD	Equivalent Square	TMR	Dose
A						
B						
C						
D						

Example 13: A patient is treated on the 6-MV linear accelerator treatment machine at 100 cm SAD. The treatment SSD is 90 cm. The collimator setting is 15 × 15 cm. MLCs are used to create a 12 × 12 cm EFS. The prescription states that a dose of 4000 cGy is to be delivered to a depth of 10 cm in 20 fractions with an AP/PA treatment field arrangement. Calculate the total dose to the depth of D_{max} and the total dose to the cord. For this example, the cord lies at a depth of 5 cm beneath the patient's posterior skin surface.

In Example 13, the total dose delivered to two points, at D_{max} and at the level of the spinal cord, must be calculated. A dose is contributed to each point from both the anterior and the posterior treatment fields (obtained with adding the dose delivered by the anterior field to the dose delivered by the posterior field). Derivation of this information is explained in the next series of steps. Note that derivation of this information can be done with TMR, TPR, and TAR.

Part 1: Calculate the Dose to Points From the Anterior Field.

Point A represents the depth of D_{max} beneath the skin surface. Point B represents the isocentric point, in this case at a depth of 10 cm at midplane. Point C represents the depth of the cord beneath the anterior skin surface. The cord depth below the skin surface is found by subtracting the depth of the cord beneath the posterior surface (5 cm) from the patient's total central axis separation. With that, we have the following:

Point	SSD	Depth	SCPD	Equivalent Square	TMR	Dose
A	90	1.5	91.5			
B	90	10	100	12.0	0.797	100 cGy (Rx dose to mid-plane)
C	90	15	105			
D	90	18.5	108.5			

With this the ES and TMR for points A, C, and D can be found:
Field size at point A:
$$Field\ Size_A/91.5\ cm = 12.0\ cm/100\ cm;\ therefore$$
$$11.0\ (10.98\ rounded\ off)\ cm$$

Now the TMR (1.5,100) can be found. Note that the exact numbers are not directly listed in the tables. Interpolation can be used to derive the exact numbers. In this case, TMR (1.5,100) = 1.000. (Note: If 6-MV TMR is used and the reference depth of the TMR is set to 1.5 cm depth, then the TMR at a depth of 1.5 cm is equal to 1.000 for all field sizes.)
Field size at point C:

$$Field\ Size_C/105\ cm = 12.0\ cm/100\ cm;\ therefore\ 12.6\ cm$$

$$TPR\ (15,12.6) = 0.6672$$

Field size at point D:

$$Field\ Size_D/108.5\ cm = 12.0\ cm/100\ cm$$

$$Field\ Size_D = 13.0$$

At this point, enough information is available to calculate the dose from the anterior field to points A, C, and D.
- The TMR at depth of D_{max} is 1.000.
- The TMR at a depth of 10 cm is 0.7970.
- The TMR at a depth of 15 cm is 0.6672.
- The TMR at a depth of 18.5 cm is 0.5880.

Further completing the chart is:

Point	SSD	Depth	SCPD	Equivalent Square	TMR	Dose
A	90	1.5	91.5	11.0	1.000	
B	90	10	100	12.0	0.797	100 cGy (Rx dose to mid-plane)
C	90	15	105	12.6	0.6672	
D	90	18.5	108.5	13.0	0.5880	

The midplane dose (depth, 10 cm) is known to be 100 cGy per field. With the previous information, the dose can be calculated to points A, C, and D from the anterior field.
Dose to point A (from anterior field):

$$Dose_A = Dose_B/TMR_B \times (SCPD_B)^2/(SCPD_A)^2 \times TMR_A$$

$$Dose_A = 100\ cGy/0.797 \times (100\ cm)^2/(91.5\ cm)^2 \times 1.000$$

$$Dose_A = 149.9\ cGy$$

Dose to point C (from anterior field):

$$Dose_C = Dose_B/TMR_B \times (SCPD_B)^2/(SCPD_C)^2 \times TMR_C$$

$$Dose_C = 100\ cGy/0.797 \times (100\ cm)^2/(105\ cm)^2 \times 0.6672$$

$$Dose_C = 75.9\ cGy$$

Dose to point D (from anterior field):
$$Dose_D = Dose_B/TMR_B \times SCPD_B/SCPD_D \times TMR_D$$

$$Dose_D = 100 \text{ cGy}/0.797 \times (100 \text{ cm})^2 / (108.5 \text{ cm})^2 \times 0.5880$$

$$Dose_D = 62.7 \text{ cGy}$$

At this point, the table for the anterior perspective can be completed.

Point	SSD	Depth	SCPD	Equivalent Square	TMR	Dose
A	90	1.5	91.5	11.0	1.000	149.9 cGy
B	90	10	100	12.0	0.797	100 cGy (Rx dose to midplane)
C	90	15	105	12.6	0.6672	75.9 cGy
D	90	18.5	108.5	13.0	0.5880	62.7 cGy

Note the confirmation of trends discussed previously in the chapter. As the depth of calculation increases, the TMR decreases (because of more attenuation). In addition, the dose is greater closer to the skin surface.

Part 2: Calculate the Dose to Points From the Posterior Field.
Again, point A represents the depth of D_{max} beneath the anterior skin surface. Point B represents the isocentric point, in this case at a depth of 10 cm at midplane. Point C represents the depth of the cord beneath the anterior skin surface. However, these points are now measured with respect to the posterior surface. Another grid can be produced. Because of the symmetry of the doses for parallel opposed treatment fields, the dose at the depth of D_{max} from the posterior field (point D) is the same as the dose at the depth of D_{max} from the anterior field (point A). The same relationship exists for the doses at the depth of 18.5 cm. Therefore the only calculation that is required from the posterior field is the dose to the depth of 5 cm.

Dose to point C (from posterior):

$$Dose_C = 100 \text{ cGy}/0.797 \times 100 \text{ (cm)}^2/95 \text{ (cm)}^2 \times 0.9308$$

$$Dose_C = 129.4 \text{ cGy}$$

Point	SSD	Depth	SCPD	Equivalent Square	TMR	Dose
A	90	18.5	108.5	13.0	5880	62.7 cGy
B	90	10	100	12.0	0.797	100 cGy (Rx dose to midplane)
C	90	5	95	11.4	0.9308	129.4 cGy
D	90	1.5	91.5	11.0	1.000	149.9 cGy

Part 3: Add the Doses to the Points From the AP/PA Fields to Finalize the Problem

Point	Anterior	Posterior	Total
A	149.9	62.7	212.6
B	100	100	200.0
C	75.9	129.4	205.3
D	62.7	149.9	212.6

This technique gives a perspective of the doses received at points other than the isocenter for SAD calculations. If calculations for several energies are performed for the parameters just given, a pattern is definitely noted. Lower energies deposit a higher dose at the outer aspects of the treatment volume. In other words, the D_{max} doses are higher for the lower energies, with all other parameters remaining the same. Conversely, as energy increases, the superficial doses are lower. In all cases, the dose to isocenter is the same. The higher energy beams exhibit more skin sparing (less superficial dose) and therefore are deemed to be better suited for treatment of deep-seated tumors.

Extended Distance Treatment

Example 14: A patient is treated on the 6-MV linear accelerator at 144 cm SSD. The collimator setting (field size at 100 cm) is 10 × 10 cm. The prescription calls for a dose of 100 cGy to be administered to a depth of 6 cm with a single anterior field.

In this example, the patient is being treated at an "extended" distance. For calculation of the MU setting, a correction must be made for the loss of intensity from the increased distance. Therefore an ISCF is applied.

The field size at the isocenter is 10 × 10 cm. However, the point of calculation is 150 cm (144 cm SSD + 6 cm depth). With use of similar triangles, the field size at 150 cm is 15 × 15 cm. Also in this calculation, the collimator scatter is based on the field size at 100 cm. Therefore Sc is used for a 10 × 10 cm field. In addition, Sp is calculated for a 15 × 15 cm field size (field size at the calculation depth). (Note: Other techniques are available for determination of Sp for extended distance calculations.)

$$\text{Reference Dose Rate} = 1.0 \text{ cGy/MU}$$

$$Sc = 1.000$$

$$Sp = 1.014$$

$$\text{TMR } (6,15) = 0.913$$

$$\text{ISCF} = (100/150)^2, \text{ which equals } 0.4444$$

$$\text{MU Setting} = \text{Prescribed Dose/RDR} \times \text{ISCF} \times Sc \times Sp \times \text{TMR}$$

$$\text{MU Setting} = 100 \text{ cGy}/1.0 \text{ cGy/MU} \times (100/150)^2 \times 1.00 \times 1.041 \times 0.913$$

$$\text{MU Setting} = 100 \text{ cGy}/0.4115 \text{ cGy/MU}$$

$$\text{MU Setting} = 243 \text{ MU}$$

Note the large increase in the MU setting necessary to administer 100 cGy at the increased distance (150 cm).

UNEQUAL BEAM WEIGHTING

Some radiation therapy cases use parallel opposed or multiple-beam arrangements, with different doses delivered to the treatment portals. This is commonly done when the tumor volume lies closer to the skin surface but can still benefit from multiportal treatment. The result is a greater dose near the entrance of the favored field and a lower dose in the tissue near the entrance of the opposing field.[2,3] Although uneven doses are administered in the outer tissues, the doses to the point of specification should remain consistent with the prescription. In other words, the isocenter in an SAD technique still receives the overall prescribed dose.

Look at the basic dose calculation equation:

$$\text{MU Setting} = \text{Dose/Dose Rate}$$

The component that is affected directly by the field weighting is the prescribed dose per port. If a prescription is written to deliver 200 cGy through two ports and the fields are equally weighted, each port delivers 100 cGy to the prescription point. However, if the prescription describes a treatment to be delivered from an AP/PA perspective and specifies that the AP field is to receive twice the amount of the PA field (written as 2 to 1 or 2:1), a different dose must be delivered through each field.

The total dose to be delivered through all ports (in this case, two) should be divided by the sum of the weighting. In this case, the weighting sum is 3 (2 + 1), and the total dose is divided by this number: 200 cGy/3 = 66.7 cGy. This defines the amount of each dose component. Then this component is multiplied by the weighting for each port, which provides the appropriate dosage to be delivered through each port as follows:

$$\text{AP Dose} = 66.7 \text{ cGy} \times 2 = 133.4 \text{ cGy}$$

$$\text{PA Dose} = 66.7 \text{ cGy} \times 1 = 66.7 \text{ cGy}$$

These numbers are used in the dose calculation to find the time or MU setting for each treatment portal. A quick check for accuracy is to add the individual port doses; they should be equal (or very close because of rounding off numbers) to the original dose prescribed.

This method can be used for any number of treatment ports and beam arrangements and can be used in all treatment calculations. Weighting does not affect the dose rate, only the dose to be administered through each port.

Example 15: A patient is treated on the 6-MV linear accelerator treatment machine at 100 cm SAD. The treatment SSD is 90 cm. The collimator setting is 15 × 15 cm. The EFS is 12 × 12. The prescription states that a dose of 180 cGy/fraction is to be delivered to a depth of 10 cm with an AP/PA treatment field arrangement. The fields are weighted 2:1 AP/PA. Calculate the MU setting with use of TMR.

The total dose is 180 cGy, and the total weights are 3 (2 + 1). Dividing 180 cGy by a total weight of 3 results in a dose of 60 cGy for a weight of 1. Therefore for a weight of 2, the dose is 60 cGy × 2, which equals 120 cGy. The next step is to calculate the MU setting for 120 cGy and 60 cGy.

$$\text{MU Setting} = \text{Prescribed Dose/RDR} \times \text{ISCF} \times \text{Sc} \times \text{Sp}$$
$$\times \text{TMR} \times \text{Other Factors}$$

$$\text{Anterior Field MU Setting} = 120 \text{ cGy/1.0 cGy/MU}$$
$$\times (100/100)^2 \times 1.021$$
$$\times 1.006 \times 0.797$$

$$\text{Anterior Field MU Setting} = 120 \text{ cGy/0.8186 cGy/MU}$$

$$\text{Anterior Field MU Setting} = 147 \text{ MU}$$

$$\text{Posterior Field MU Setting} = 60 \text{ cGy/1.0 cGy/MU}$$
$$\times (100/100)^2 \times 1.021$$
$$\times 1.006 \times 0.797$$

$$\text{Posterior Field MU Setting} = 60 \text{ cGy/0.8186 cGy/MU}$$

$$\text{Posterior Field MU Setting} = 73 \text{ MU}$$

Example 16: This example is of a calculation when a block tray is used. A patient is treated at 100 cm SAD with a 6-MV beam The

treatment SSD is 86 cm SSD. The collimator setting is 15 × 15 cm, and the field is blocked to a 12 × 12 cm EFS. A 5-mm solid tray is used to support the blocks. The prescription calls for 90 cGy to be delivered per field daily. Calculate the MU setting:

$$\text{MU Setting} = \text{Prescribed Dose/RDR} \times \text{ISCF} \times \text{Sc} \times \text{Sp}$$
$$\times \text{TMR} \times \text{Tray Factor}$$

$$\text{MU Setting} = 90 \text{ cGy/1.000 cGy/MU} \times (100 \text{ cm/100 cm})^2$$
$$\times 1.021 \times 1.006 \times 0.688 \times 0.98$$

$$\text{MU Setting} = 130 \text{ MU}$$

Alternative method: First calculate the MU setting without the tray factor. Second, multiply the MU setting by the reciprocal of the tray factor, 1/0.98 = 1.02

$$\text{MU Setting} = 90 \text{ cGy/1.000 cGy/MU} \times (100 \text{ cm/100 cm})^2$$
$$\times 1.021 \times 1.006 \times 0.688$$

$$\text{MU Setting Without Tray Factor} = 127.4 \text{ MU}$$

$$\text{MU Setting} = 127.4 \times 1.02 \text{ MU}$$

$$\text{MU Setting} = 130 \text{ MU}$$

Example 17: This example is of a calculation when a "hard" wedge is used. A patient is treated at 100 cm SAD with a 6-MV beam. The patient is treated with an anterior field and right and left lateral fields. A 30-degree wedge is used with each lateral field. The anterior field is set to 94 cm SSD. Each lateral field is set to 85 cm SSD. The anterior field collimator setting is 12 × 12 cm. The MLC is used to create a 10 × 10 cm EFS. The collimator setting is 6 × 12 cm. The MLC is used to create a 6 × 6 cm EFS. The prescription calls for 180 cGy to be delivered at 60 cGy per field daily. Calculate the MU settings.

Anterior field:

$$\text{MU Setting} = 60 \text{ cGy/1.000 cGy/MU} \times (100 \text{ cm/100 cm})^2$$
$$\times 1.008 \times 1.000 \times 0.900$$

$$\text{MU Setting} = 66 \text{ MU}$$

Each lateral field:

$$\text{MU Setting} = 60 \text{ cGy/1.000 cGy/MU} \times (100 \text{ cm/100 cm})^2$$
$$\times 0.987 \times 0.984 \times 0.613 \times 0.714 \text{ (WF)}$$

$$\text{MU Setting} = 141 \text{ MU}$$

$$\text{Anterior Field} = 66 \text{ MU}$$

$$\text{Right Lateral Field} = 141 \text{ MU}$$

$$\text{Left Lateral Field} = 141 \text{ MU}$$

SEPARATION OF ADJACENT FIELDS

Many treatment techniques involve the junction of fields with the adjoining margins either abutted or separated depending on various circumstances. This may be because of the need to break what is a very large, irregularly shaped field into two or more fields, which are better managed. It may also be necessary because of the need to use different beam energies over a large area that must also be continuous. Because of rapid "falloff" of the dose near the edge of each field, a small change in the relative spacing of the field borders can produce a large change in the dose distribution in the junction volume.

The hazard of having a "gap" or junction area may be a dose that (1) exceeds normal tissue tolerance, or (2) is inadequate to therapeutically treat the tumor.

Fields may be abutted or have a gap between them.

1. *Abutted fields.* If the adjacent fields are abutted on the surface, the fields overlap to an increasing degree with depth because of divergence.
2. *Separated fields.* The theory behind this is that field edges can be abutted at depth as opposed to on the skin surface. In this way, tissue can be spared at depth and overdose prevented because of overlapping fields. The fields then would be abutted at a desired depth, with a gap left on the skin surface.

Examples of abutting fields include lateral head and neck and supraclavicular fossa fields or tangential breast and supraclavicular fossa arrangements. Examples of separated fields are evident in craniospinal irradiation is sometimes found in lymphoma cases. In either case of abutting or separated fields, the medical dosimetrist and radiation therapist must be able to make sure that the area of overlap (or nonoverlap) occurs where it is intended.

Several common methods are used to obtain dose uniformity across field junctions, including dosimetric isodose matching, junction shifts, half-beam blocking, and geometric matching.

Dosimetric isodose matching. With the availability of modern treatment planning computers, separation of fields can easily be calculated and plotted for maximum dose uniformity. The hot and cold spots can easily be seen and compensated for. The accuracy of dosimetric isodose matching depends on the accuracy of the individual field isodose curves.

Junction shift. Fields that abut on the skin surface can be moved during the course of treatment so that any hot or cold spot inherently present can be spread, or feathered, over a distance. This technique calls for a shift in field sizes for the abutting fields. The fields are shifted one or more times during the course of the patient's treatment to move the areas of overlap. In this way, the overall dose in any areas of overlap is spread out over a greater volume and allows for a better opportunity of lowering side effects in that area.

Half-beam blocking. Specific shielding blocks can be designed to block out one side of a treatment field to produce a field that has no divergence along one side, most commonly along the central ray of the beam where there is no divergence. Two abutting fields can then be used to match field borders on the phantom surface and have no divergence at depth. Asymmetric jawed fields or MLCs can also accomplish this on modern treatment units.

Geometric matching. Dose uniformity can be achieved at the junction of two fields at depth through geometric means (Fig. 22.11). This is possible because the geometric boundary of each abutting field is defined by the 50% decrement line (at the edge of all fields, the dose to the very edge falls off to 50% of the dose at the central ray). With knowledge of the field sizes of adjacent fields, the treatment SSD, and the depths, the size of the gap on the patient can be calculated to ensure that the fields abut at the correct depth. Note that it is possible to have fields at different depths; the important aspect is that the fields abut at a depth and that the gap measurement on the skin surface can be calculated with the following equation:

$$Gap = \left(\frac{L_1}{2} \times \frac{d}{SSD_1} \right) \times \left(\frac{L_2}{2} \times \frac{d}{SSD_2} \right)$$

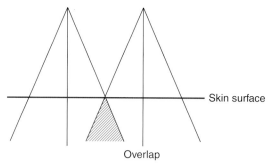

Fig. 22.11 Geometric matching at depth. Because of divergence, a gap on the patient's skin between two adjacent fields converges at a depth within the patient.

with L_1 as length of the first field, SSD_1 as treatment source-skin distance of the first field, L_2 as length of the second field, SSD_2 as treatment source-skin distance of the second field, and d as depth of abutment.

The following example demonstrates the calculation of a field gap.

Example 18: A patient is treated with two adjacent fields. The collimator setting for field 1 is 8 cm width × 12 cm length. The collimator setting for field 2 is 10 cm width × 20 cm length. Both fields are set up at 100 cm SSD. Calculate the gap on the skin surface for the fields to abut at a 5-cm depth.

The geometric gap calculation is based on the principles of similar triangles. An important consideration when performing a gap calculation is to ensure that the field size (L) is corrected for the SSD. In this example, the field size is defined at the skin surface that is 100 cm SSD. Therefore the field size is the same as the collimator setting. A second consideration is that the depth must be the same for both fields:

$$Gap = (12 \text{ cm}/2 \times 5 \text{ cm}/100 \text{ cm})$$
$$\times (20 \text{ cm}/2 \times 5 \text{ cm}/100 \text{ cm})$$

$$Gap = 0.3 \text{ cm} + 0.5 \text{ cm}$$

$$Gap = 0.8 \text{ cm}$$

The 0.8 cm calculated is the minimal skin gap between the two fields, which means that the distance between the inferior border of field 1 and superior border of field 2 must be at least 0.8 cm. Often, the gap is made slightly larger to allow for variations in the day-to-day setup.

Example 19: A patient is treated with two adjacent fields. The collimator setting for field 1 is 8 cm width × 16 cm length. The collimator setting for field 2 is 10 cm width × 26 cm length. Field 1 is set up at 95 cm SSD, and field 2 is set up at 90 cm SSD. Calculate the gap on the skin surface for the fields to abut at a 5-cm depth.

Because the collimator setting is the field size at 100 cm, the field sizes must be adjusted to the appropriate SSD. For field 1, this is 15.2 cm, and for field 2, it is 23.4 cm:

$$Gap = 15.2 \text{ cm}/2 \times 5 \text{ cm}/95.0 \text{ cm}$$
$$+ 23.4 \text{ cm}/2 \times 5 \text{ cm}/90.0 \text{ cm}$$

$$Gap = 0.400 \text{ cm} + 0.65 \text{ cm}$$

$$Gap = 1.05 \text{ cm}$$

Again, 1.05 cm is the minimum gap, and the treatment team can probably round up and measure 1.10 on the skin.

SUMMARY

- The methods used in most therapy centers reflect the treatment team's philosophy, as developed by the medical physics team and the radiation oncologists.
- The output of every treatment unit used to deliver a dose of radiation to a patient is the amount of radiation exposure that is produced by a treatment unit as defined by a reference field size and at a specified reference distance.
- Each time a variation from a standard is used to measure the reference beam, a correction is made with various output factors.

- Each time any item, be it a wedge, shielding tray, or compensating filter, is used, it must be accounted for in the beam calculation with a modifier that considers the attenuation of the beam through it.
- The time or number of MUs used to deliver a prescribed dose, no matter how complex treatment is, can be found by dividing dose by dose rate. The key is an understanding of all the components that modify each one.
- This material should provide the radiation therapist and medical dosimetrist with a good basis on which to further explore dosage treatment factors and concepts of treatment planning in radiation therapy.

REVIEW QUESTIONS

The answers to the Review Questions can be found by logging on to our website at: http://evolve.elsevier.com/Washington/principles

1. Percentage depth dose increases with increasing:
   I. Energy.
   II. Depth.
   III. SSD.
      a. I and II only.
      b. I and III only.
      c. II and III only.
      d. I, II, and III.
2. Tissue-air ratio decreases with decreasing:
   I. Field size.
   II. Depth.
   III. SSD.
      a. I.
      b. II.
      c. III.
      d. I, II, and III.
3. When MLC blocking is used in a treatment calculation, the area of the collimator is used in determining:
   I. TMR.
   II. Sc.
   III. PDD.
      a. I.
      b. II.
      c. III.
      d. I, II, and III.
4. Which of the following central axis depth dose quantities are most likely used to compute an accurate monitor unit setting on an 18-MV unit for an isocentric treatment?
   a. Percentage depth dose.
   b. Backscatter factor.
   c. TMR or TPR.
   d. All of the above.

5. Two parallel opposed equally weighted 6-MV fields are separated by 20 cm of tissue and treated with an SSD technique. The maximum dose occurs:
   a. Directly on the skin surface.
   b. At the midline of the patient.
   c. 1.5 cm under the skin surface.
   d. 5 cm under the skin surface.
6. What is the advantage of using parallel opposed isocentric fields for treatment delivery (compared with nonisocentric)?
   a. Less opportunity for movement error.
   b. Less overall dose to the skin surface.
   c. Both a and b.
   d. Neither a nor b.
7. A wedge filter _____ the output of the beam and thus must be taken into account in the treatment calculations.
   a. Increases.
   b. Decreases.
   c. Does not affect.
   d. There is not enough information given.
8. The Mayneord factor is used to convert:
   a. PDD with a change in SSD from the standard.
   b. TAR with a change in SSD from the standard.
   c. Exposure rate with a change in SSD from the standard.
   d. An Exposure in roentgens to cGy.
9. Any time an object is placed in the path of a therapeutic beam of radiation, it must be corrected for in the dose calculation to account for beam absorption.
   a. True.
   b. False.
10. The MU setting is calculated for opposed treatment fields with 45-degree wedges. The therapist does not use the wedges and uses the wedged field MU setting. This error could result in a severe overdose or serious complication to the patient.
   a. True.
   b. False.

QUESTIONS TO PONDER

1. Analyze how the collimator or field size can affect the output of a linear accelerator.
2. Describe how the SSD causes PDD to vary. (Hint: The correct answer is not related to scatter.)
3. A patient's larynx is to be treated with an isocentric technique on a linear accelerator; the patient's separation at the central axis is 9 cm and will be treated to midplane. The treatment will use parallel opposed right and left lateral fields. The isocenter of the machine is established at 100 cm.

   a. What is the SSD on the patient's skin?
   b. If a field size of 6 × 6 cm is set on the collimator, what is the field size on the skin surface?
4. Explain the relationship between beam quality (energy) and TMR.
5. A 20-cm-thick patient is to be treated with a 6-MV beam at 100 cm SAD. Two open (no MLC) opposed 15 × 15 cm ports are used to deliver a treatment dose of 180 cGy per day to the midline (midplane). Use TMR to determine the MU setting for each port.

6. A patient is to receive 5040 cGy to his lung in 28 fractions. The treatment will use 15×11 cm opposed 6-MV photons fields to midplane at 100 cm SAD. The separation is 21 cm. The field is blocked to an 11×11 cm equivalent field. A 5-mm solid tray is used to support the blocks. Use TMR to determine the MU setting for each port each day.

7. Calculate the MU setting to deliver 300 cGy to a depth of 12 cm on a 6-MV unit with a single-beam open field (i.e., no MLC) at 100 cm SSD with a field size of 15×8 cm. With this information, determine the dose at a depth of 6 cm.

8. A patient is treated at 100 cm SAD with a 6-MV beam. The patient is treated with an anterior field and right and left lateral fields. A 45-degree wedge is used with each lateral field. The anterior field is set to 94 cm SSD. Each lateral field is set to 85 cm SSD. The anterior field collimator setting is 12×12 cm. The MLC is used to create a 10×10 cm EFS. The collimator setting is 6×12 cm. The MLC is used to create a 6×6 cm EFS. The prescription calls for 180 cGy to be delivered daily. The fields are weighted 2:1:1 (anterior:right lateral:left lateral). Use TAR to calculate the MU setting for each field.

9. Compare and contrast the factors that influence PDD and TPR.

REFERENCES

1. Almond PR, Biggs PJ, Coursey BM, et al. AAPM's TG–51 protocol for clinical reference dosimetry of high–energy photon and electron beams. *Med Phys.* 1999;26:1847–1870.
2. Bentel GC. *Radiation Therapy Planning.* McGraw Hill Professional, New York, NY; 1996.
3. Bentel GC, Nelson CE, Noell KT. *Treatment Planning and Dose Calculation in Radiation Oncology.* Elmsford, NY: Elsevier; 2014.
4. Khan FM, Gibbons JP. *Khan's the Physics of Radiation Therapy.* Philadelphia, PA: Lippincott Williams & Wilkins; 2014.
5. McEwen M, DeWerd L, Ibbott G, et al. Addendum to the AAPM's TG–51 protocol for clinical reference dosimetry of high–energy photon beams. *Med Phys.* 2014;41(4):041501.
6. Paganetti H. *Proton Therapy Physics.* Boca Raton, FL: CRC Press; 2018.
7. Selman J. *Basic Physics of Radiation Therapy;* ed 3, Springfield, IL, Charles C Thomas Publishers, 1990.
8. Shahabi S. *Blackburn's Introduction to Clinical Radiation Therapy Physics.* Madison, WI: Medical Physics Publishing; 1989.
9. Stanton R, Stinson D, Mihailidis D. *Applied Physics for Radiation Oncology.* Madison, WI: Medical Physics Publishing; 2010.
10. Yan Y, Yadav P, Bassetti M, et al. Dosimetric differences in flattened and flattening filter-free beam treatment plans. *J Med Phys.* 2016;41:92.
11. Zhou S, Wu Q, Li X, et al. Using weighted power mean for ES estimation. *J Appl Clin Med Phys.* 2017;18:194–199.

23

Photon Dose Distributions

Charlotte M. Prado, Karl L. Prado, J. Mechalakos

OBJECTIVES

- Describe the nature and characteristics of isodose distributions of single-photon fields.
- Discuss the combination of multiple fields used to produce cumulative isodose distributions.
- Compare and contrast corrections made to isodose distributions to account for contour irregularities and tissue heterogeneities.
- Analyze the principles and types of algorithms used for photon dose calculations and treatment planning.
- Discuss the rationale for three-dimensional conformal radiation therapy, intensity-modulated radiation therapy, and volumetric modulated arc therapy.

- List and explain treatment planning concepts and definitions for target volumes, organs at risk, and margins to account for uncertainties.
- Describe the tools currently available for treatment planning and how these tools are used.
- Discuss the importance of treatment intent and planning objectives.
- Compare methods of quantitative treatment plan evaluation.
- Explain the treatment plan verification process needed before actual implementation.

OUTLINE

KEY TERMS

Beam's-eye view
Beam optimization
Contour corrections
Deformable registration
Digitally reconstructed radiograph
Dose calculation matrix
Dose clouds
Dose distributions
Dose-volume histogram
Dynamic wedge
Flatness
Flattening filter
Flattening filter free (FFF)
Forward planning

Heterogeneity corrections
Hinge angle
Image fusion
Inverse planning
Isodose curve
Isodose distributions
Normalization
Obliquity corrections
Organs at risk
Organ segmentation
Parallel-opposed field set
Parallel response tissues
Penumbra
Profile

The patient will benefit from a course of radiation therapy. Thus begins the treatment planning process. Radiation will be used to treat the patient. How is the patient best treated? What are the goals and constraints of treatment? Does the attained dose distribution meet these goals? Treatment planning can be defined as the process by which dose delivery is optimized for a given patient and clinical situation. The radiation therapy planning and delivery process is intricate. Radiation dose deposition and distribution methods must be properly understood and planned to ensure disease is treated and healthy structures are spared. The clinical picture is often variable, and decision-making is complex. The treatment planning method must be an effective tool in the decision-making process. It should simplify the definition of specific treatment goals and facilitate their implementation. In this chapter, clinical radiation dose distributions produced with external beams of photons are discussed, and photon beam treatment planning methods are reviewed.

PHOTON DOSE DISTRIBUTIONS

Single-Field Isodose Distributions

Dose distributions are spatial representations of the magnitude of the dose produced by a source of radiation. They describe the variation of dose with position within an irradiated volume. The percentage depth dose (PDD) curve (Fig. 23.1) is a one-dimensional representation of the variation of dose. Percent depth dose curves, explained in Chapter 22, describe dose variation with depth along the central axis of a beam. Computer displays of isodose distributions, on the other hand, are typically two-dimensional spatial representations of dose. The typical isodose distributions illustrate dose variation both along and across the direction of a beam of radiation. Three-dimensional dose distributions describe dose deposition in a volume. These concepts are illustrated in greater detail in subsequent sections of the chapter.

Treatment planning attempts dose distribution optimization for a given clinical goal in a given clinical situation. Treatment fields are arranged in ways that produce adequate tumor dose and minimal healthy tissue dose. Thus, an understanding of how dose distributions are both produced and then used is necessary. The discussion begins with simple, single fields and then progresses to more complex, multiple-field arrangements.

Open Fields: Profiles. A beam profile is another one-dimensional spatial representation of the variation of beam intensity. A profile describes radiation intensity as a function of position across the beam at a given depth. It depicts the beam's intensity in a direction perpendicular to the beam's direction. The concept of beam intensity variation as a function of position within the beam is best understood if one thinks about the response of a small radiation detector moving within a tank of water that is being irradiated. Fig. 23.2 illustrates this process, a common method of measurement of clinical beam data. As the radiation detector moves across the beam at some depth in the phantom, beam intensity (detector response) is plotted as a function of position within the beam. The resulting intensity curve as a function of position within the beam is called a profile. The intensity curves shown in Fig. 23.2 are typical of photon field profiles. They are characterized by a rapid increase in intensity (as the radiation detector enters the beam), followed by a region of relatively uniform intensity (characterizing the central portion of the beam) and then ending with a rapid decrease in intensity (as the detector exits the beam). The edges of the profile in

which there is a rapid increase or decrease in intensity are known as the penumbra region.

The shape of a beam's profile is a function of depth. At shallow depths, because scatter is less of a contributor to the total intensity of the beam than it is at deeper depths, the beam's profile better characterizes the beam's "primary" intensity. The depth of maximum equilibrium (D_{max}) profile, the profile of beam intensity at the depth of maximum dose, shown in the left panel of Fig. 23.3 (blue curve), illustrates the influence of the accelerator's flattening filter on the beam. Flattening filters are introduced into photon beams to reduce the increased photon intensity that exists in the center of the beam. Evidence for this effect is the somewhat reduced intensity shown in the center of the beam compared with that which exists away from the central axis. The flattening filter is designed to produce a "flat" intensity pattern at some predefined depth (normally 10 cm). Box 23.1 expands on this thought. Note the flatter shape of the 13-cm depth profile in the right panel of Fig. 23.3 compared with the D_{max} profile in the left panel. At deeper depths, scatter becomes a more significant component of dose, and a greater amount of scattered radiation exists along the center of the beam than along the periphery. This offsets the shape of the beam's primary profile, producing a relatively flat dose distribution.

The profile of the beam without the flattening filter present is also shown in both panels of Fig. 23.3 for comparison (Noted as FFF). The cost of using a flattening filter is that it attenuates the beam, therefore lowering the dose rate delivered by the treatment machine. Modern treatment planning systems are able to accurately model photon beams with the flattening filter out of the beam, known as "flattening filter free" (FFF) beams. This allows for a shorter delivery time. FFF beams are used for more complex treatment plans with intensity modulation (described later in this chapter) for which a treatment planning system is needed; they are not used for simple treatments such as parallel-opposed fields.

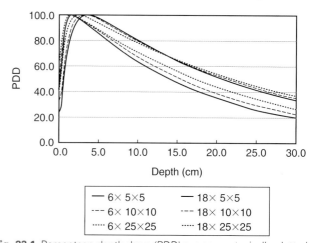

Varian Clinac 2100C SN 396 6-MV and 18-MV X-ray PDDs

— 6× 5×5	— 18× 5×5
--- 6× 10×10	--- 18× 10×10
····· 6× 25×25	····· 18× 25×25

Fig. 23.1 Percentage depth dose *(PDD)* curves are typically plotted as a function of depth and are normalized to the PDD at the depth of maximum dose. X-ray depth dose curves of 6 MV and 18 MV are shown. Note the variation of PDD with energy and field size. Note also the shift of the depth of maximum dose and the difference in PDD field size variation between 6-MV and 18-MV x-rays.

Open Fields: Isodose Distributions. Isodose distributions consist of a series of isodose curves or surfaces. The traditional isodose display is a two-dimensional representation of how dose varies with position in a plane within a beam along directions both parallel (coincident) and perpendicular to the beam's direction. It is a collection of points, all with the same dose (hence the term *iso*dose). Fig. 23.4 presents typical isodose distributions produced by photon beams of different energies.[1] The numeric values of the lines represent percentages of the dose that exist at a point along the central axis at the depth of D_{max}. Thus, the 90% isodose contains all points within the plane of presentation where the dose is equal to 90% of the dose at D_{max}. The dose at points between isodose curves lies between the doses represented by the curves.

Isodose distributions combine both the depth dose and off-axis profile characteristics of the beam. The numeric value of the isodose line along the central (depth) axis of the isodose curves is equal to the PDD at that depth. The shape of the isodose curve along a direction perpendicular to the central axis describes the off-axis characteristics (profile) of the beam. Isodose distributions vary with beam energy, source-skin distance (SSD), and field size. Note also from Fig. 23.4 that beams produced by accelerators are, in general, flatter than cobalt-60 or low-energy x-ray beams. As mentioned previously, this results from the introduction of flattening filters used in linear accelerators. Note the shape of the 90% isodose curve of the 4-MV beam shown in Fig. 23.4C. The flattening filter causes the "dip" in the central region of the curve.

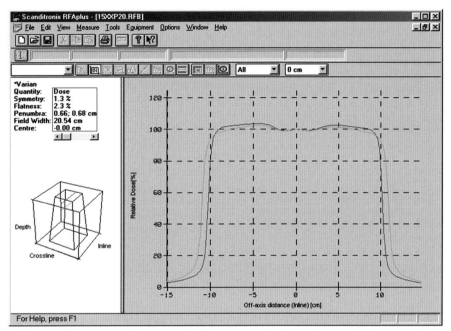

Fig. 23.2 Beam profiles are normally measured with a computerized beam data acquisition system that includes a water tank, radiation detector, and specialized software designed for radiation beam measurement and analysis. Note the beam data acquisition geometry shown on the *bottom left* of the screen showing the direction of ionization chamber travel within the water tank. Two in-plane scans were acquired, and the resulting profiles are displayed.

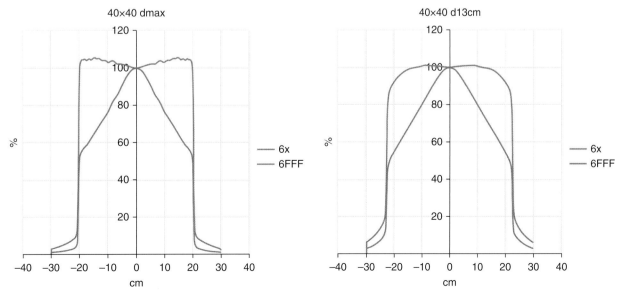

Fig. 23.3 Profiles of an 18-MV x-ray beam taken at two depths, depth of maximum equilibrium *(D_{max})* and 13.0 cm. Note the differences in shape and size. The deeper profile is wider because the field diverges and its size increases with depth. The deeper profile is also flatter than the shallower profile because the accelerator's flattening filter is designed to produce flat beams at a depth of approximately 10 cm (see Box 23.1).

In its simplest form, a given beam's isodose curve combines dose variation versus depth (percent-depth dose) with dose variation across the beam (profile) in a single two-dimensional graphic representation.

BOX 23.1 Photon Beam Shape Specifications

Quantitative analysis of beam profiles is often necessary to characterize the shape of photon beams. When profiles are measured along a direction parallel to the direction of electron motion along the accelerator's waveguide (parallel to the treatment couch), the profile is often termed a radial or in-plane profile. A profile measured along a direction perpendicular to the direction of the electron travel (perpendicular to the treatment couch) is often called a transverse or cross-plane profile.

Accelerator manufacturers provide specifications of the flatness and symmetry of photon beams. These specifications ensure that the accelerator produces beams that possess characteristics suitable for clinical use. The flatness and symmetry of clinical beams are checked periodically as a part of the accelerator's ongoing quality assurance program. A common way to define flatness is with noting the difference between the maximum and minimum intensity of the central 80% of the profile and specifying this difference as a percentage of the central axis intensity:

$$\text{Flatness}_{(\%)} = 100 \times [(I_{max} - I_{min}) / I_{CAX}]$$

with I_{max} and I_{min} as the maximum and minimum intensities of the central 80% of the profile, respectively, and I_{CAX} as the intensity of the profile on its central axis. Symmetry can also be quantified in a similar fashion by noting profile intensities on either side of the central axis:

$$\text{Symmetry}_{(\%)} = 100 \times [(I_{+x} - I_{-x})_{max} / I_{x0}]$$

with I_{+X} and I_{-X} as corresponding profile intensities at a distance x on either side of the profile's central axis, and I_{x0} as the central axis intensity. A common definition of symmetry specifies the maximum point-to-point difference. As before, symmetry is defined in the central 80% of the profile.

Wedged Fields: Isodose Distributions. It is sometimes desirable to produce beams of nonuniform intensity across the field. Introduction of an attenuator of varying thickness in the beam can produce the desired difference in intensity. Because of its shape, this variable-thickness attenuator is called a wedge. When a wedge is introduced into a beam, differential attenuation along the varying thickness of the wedge produces a dose gradient along the wedged dimension of the beam; that is, less dose exists under thicker portions of the wedge than exists along thinner portion. At a given depth within a wedged beam, and in a direction toward the toe or thinner portion of the wedge, the dose increases with distance from the central axis of the beam. Similarly, the values of isodoses toward the heel or thicker portion of the wedge decrease with increasing distance from the central axis.

Examples of wedged-field isodose distributions are shown in Fig. 23.5.[2] Note that wedged-field isodose lines are now "tilted"—a given-valued isodose penetrates to a greater depth along thinner portions of the wedge. The amount of incline of the isodose curves depends on the shape of the wedge. Wedges with a greater variation in thickness from heel to toe produce more inclined isodoses. The angle between the slanted isodose line and a line perpendicular to the central axis of the beam is called the wedge angle. Wedges are designed to produce certain discrete wedge angles. Traditionally, wedges supplied with the treatment machine are fabricated to produce discrete wedge angles of 15 degrees, 30 degrees, 45 degrees, and 60 degrees. Because the tilt of isodose lines varies slightly with depth (again because of the relative influence of scatter) for any given wedge, either the depth of the 80% depth dose or a depth of 10 cm is often chosen for wedge angle measurement and subsequent wedge attenuator design.[3,4]

Wedged-field isodose distributions have similar dependencies on beam energy, SSD, and field size as do open-field isodoses. Because of the presence of the wedge attenuator in the beam, the energy spectrum of wedged fields differs slightly from that of its nonwedged counterpart. This results in slight differences between open-field and wedged-field PDDs. The effect is more pronounced at lower beam energies and larger wedge angles. Table 23.1 shows data that illustrate this effect. The PDD at 20 cm depth in a 6-MV, 15 × 15 cm photon field increases by

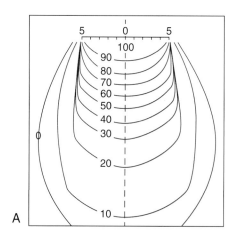

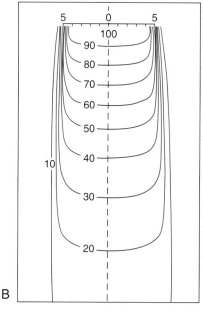

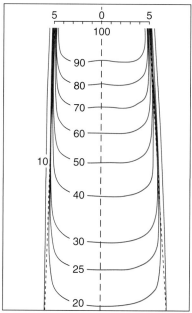

Fig. 23.4 Open 10 × 10 cm fields of different energies. (A) 200-kVp, 1-mm copper (Cu) half-value layer, source-skin distance (SSD): 50 cm. (B) Cobalt-60, SSD: 80 cm. (C) 4-MV SSD: 100 cm. (Modified from Khan FM. *The Physics of Radiation Therapy*. 2nd ed. Baltimore, MD: Williams & Wilkins; 1994.)

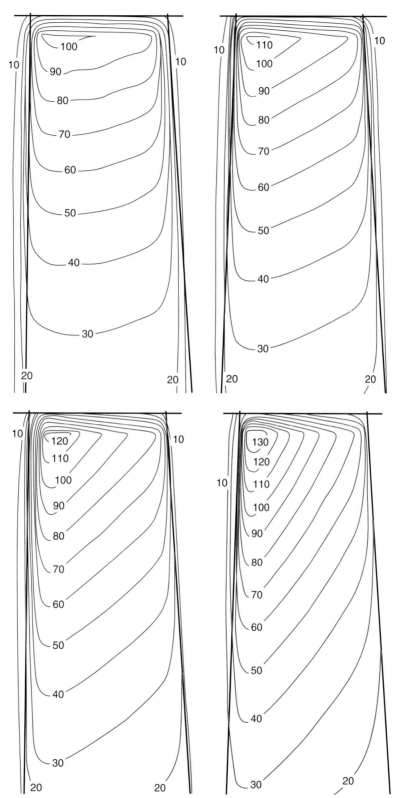

Fig. 23.5 The tilt of wedged-field isodose curves is dependent on the particular wedge filter used. This figure shows typical isodose distributions produced by conventional 15-degree, 30-degree, 45-degree, and 60-degree conventional wedge filters. (Modified from Bentel GC. *Radiation Therapy Planning.* 2nd ed. New York, NY: McGraw-Hill; 1996.)

TABLE 23.1	6-MV and 18-MV Open-Field and Wedged-Field Percent Depth Dose Data			
Percentage Depth Dose	6-MV Open	6-MV 45-Degree Wedge	18-MV Open	18-MV 45-Degree Wedge
Depth 10 cm	69.3	70.5	79.1	80.7
Depth 20 cm	41.8	43.5	53.7	54.7

Data for a Varian Clinac 2100C (Varian Medical, Palo Alto, CA), 15 × 15 cm fields, 100 cm source-skin distance.

4% when a 45-degree wedge is introduced; an 18-MV photon beam shows a 2% increase in depth dose in similar circumstances.

Wedged-field isodose distributions can also be produced without the use of physical wedge attenuators. If a collimator jaw is allowed to move across the beam during irradiation, a variation in intensity across the beam similar to that produced by a wedge can be achieved. The use of a moving collimator jaw to produce a wedged field is often termed *dynamic wedge.* Often, jaw movements during production of dynamic wedge fields are controlled to produce only fields that are equivalent to those produced by conventional wedges: 15-degree, 30-degree, 45-degree, and 60-degree wedged fields. More recently, dynamic wedge capability has been extended to produce a wider range of wedged fields not limited to the conventional wedge angles. This capability has been called *enhanced dynamic wedge.*[5]

Clinical use of dynamic wedges has far-reaching dosimetric consequences beyond the scope of this chapter. The traditional *wedge attenuation factor* of physical wedges, the ratio of the dose in the wedged field to the dose in the open field, no longer exists as such because the wedging function is no longer produced by differential attenuation through a physical attenuator. *Dynamic wedge factors*, also defined as the ratio of the dose in the wedged field to that in the open field, are more related to field size–dependent output factors because wedging is now produced by varying collimator jaw positions. In addition, because wedge attenuators are not used, the PDD of dynamic wedge fields is the same as that of their open-field counterparts.

Isodose distributions that are even more complex can be achieved by varying the field aperture with the unit's multileaf collimator during irradiation. Fields produced in this fashion are often termed intensity modulated.

Multiple-Field Isodose Distributions

Combined-field Isodose Distributions: Open Fields. Except for a few clinical situations in which the treatment depth is shallow, such as the treatment of supraclavicular nodes or portions of the spinal column, single-photon fields are rarely used for treatment. Often, multiple fields are used in combination to take advantage of the improved dose distribution that results from aiming multiple fields from different directions at a common target area. Multiple fields convergent on a shared target result in a concentrated dose in the common target area.

The simplest combined-field geometry is the parallel-opposed field set. In this field geometry, two treatment fields share common central axes, 180 degrees apart. A second field equal in size and mirrored in shape but opposite in direction compensates for the falloff in dose with depth from the first field. Parallel-opposed fields are often used to treat target volumes that are at middepth in the treatment area. Examples of clinical parallel-opposed fields are anteroposterior (AP) and posteroanterior thoracic fields and right lateral and left lateral whole-brain fields.

Parallel-opposed fields work best in situations in which beam energy and patient thickness can be matched to allow for a uniform dose within the irradiated volume. With proper selection of energy and with favorable patient thickness conditions, parallel-opposed fields can be used to deliver reasonably uniform doses, as seen in Fig. 23.6.[1] In this

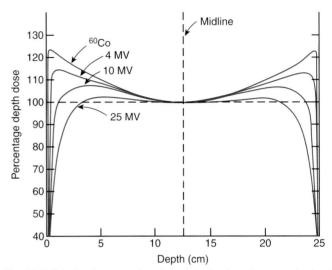

Fig. 23.6 Relative dose as a function of depth along the central axis of parallel-opposed fields incident on a patient 25 cm thick. Curves, showing dose relative to the dose existing at middepth, are representative of the dose produced by 10 × 10 cm² treatment fields of energies cobalt-60, 4 MV, 10 MV, and 25 MV. (Modified from Khan FM. *The Physics of Radiation Therapy.* 2nd ed. Baltimore, MD: Williams & Wilkins; 1994.)

figure, the doses at all points along the central axes of parallel-opposed beams 25 cm apart are shown for beams of different energies. (This figure is best understood if one thinks of the parallel-opposed beams as entering from the left and right of the figure.) Note that as beam energy increases, the dose along the central axes of the beams becomes more uniform. Lower-energy beams, because of their decreased penetrating ability, produce higher doses at their respective entrance depths, which creates a less uniform dose distribution as a function of depth. A similar situation occurs as patient thickness increases and the entrance-to-midline dose ratio becomes unacceptably high. In Fig. 23.7, for example, approximately 12% more dose exists at the entrance of 6-MV beams in a 25-cm-thick patient than at the patient's midline.[1] In these circumstances, other beam combinations may be more appropriate.

Multiple convergent beams are often used in situations in which parallel-opposed beams cannot produce acceptable dose distributions or in which further restriction of the high-dose region of the dose distribution may be desirable. In Fig. 23.8, the dose distributions that result from the use of a parallel-opposed field set, a three-field arrangement, and a four-field arrangement are contrasted. Note that as supplementary fields are added, the high-dose region conforms to the intersection of the beams, and the relative dose outside the beams' intersection decreases. When the angles between the fields are equal, the dose distribution is relatively uniform within the region of the beams' intersection.

Combined-Field Isodose Distributions: Wedged Fields. In some clinical situations, parallel-opposed or equally angled beams are not appropriate for the particular treatment scenario. An example is the treatment of disease on one side of the brain in which sparing of the

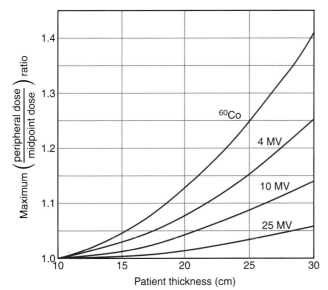

Fig. 23.7 A patient is treated with parallel-opposed fields. This figure shows the maximum dose along the central axes of the fields expressed as a ratio of dose at the patient's midline. The curves, plotted as a function of patient thickness, are representative of cobalt-60, 4-MV, 10-MV, and 25-MV 10 × 10 cm², 100-cm source-skin distance fields. Note that for a patient 25 cm thick, parallel-opposed cobalt-60 fields produce a maximum dose along the central axis 25% greater than that produced at the patient's midline. (Modified from Khan FM. *The Physics of Radiation Therapy.* 2nd ed. Baltimore, MD: Williams & Wilkins; 1994.)

opposite hemisphere is desired. In this situation, a pair of wedged beams can be used to produce a region of reasonably uniform dose. Recall that the isodoses of wedged fields are tilted at an angle characterized by the wedge angle. A region of uniform dose can be achieved in the area common to two wedged fields if the angles of the central axes of the fields bear an appropriate relationship to the wedge angles of the beams. If ø is the angle between the beams' central axes, called the hinge angle, and θ is the wedge angle of the beams, then the relationship between the hinge and wedge angles that produces a uniform dose distribution is as follows:

$$Ø = 180 \text{ degrees} - 2θ$$

or

$$θ = 90 \text{ degrees} - Ø/2$$

The previous relationship applies to pairs of wedged fields. The hinge angle can be adjusted slightly to accommodate clinical restraints, such as protection of healthy structures. Wedged-field combinations are not limited to only pairs of wedged fields. Wedged fields can be used with open or other wedged fields in other fashions. Fig. 23.9 shows examples of the use of wedged fields to achieve more uniform dose distributions in healthy structure–sparing constraints.

Corrections to Isodose Distributions

Beam data for treatment planning systems are almost always obtained from measurements acquired in water phantoms. These data represent dose distributions obtained when a flat-surfaced homogenous (water) medium is irradiated. When actual irradiation conditions differ from those in which standard isodose distributions were obtained, dose distributions are modified and corrections must be applied. Corrections for beam incidence onto surfaces other than flat surfaces and for

angles of incidence other than 90 degrees ("normal" incidence) are called obliquity corrections or contour corrections. Corrections that account for the presence of irradiated media other than water are called heterogeneity corrections.

Obliquity/Contour Corrections. Contour corrections can be made in several ways. The effective SSD method is a graphic contour correction method. It is exemplified with use of an isodose chart (a set of isodose curves). It entails "sliding" the isodose chart along the irregular contour such that its surface line is at the contour surface at a vertical line above the given point of interest. The PDD value at the point of interest is read and then corrected with an inverse square correction. In Fig. 23.10, the isodose chart is shifted from its position at the central axis (surface S″ – S″) to a position on the contour above the point A.[6] The PDD value *(P)* at point A is read off the chart and is then corrected by multiplying it by an inverse square factor to give the corrected PDD value *(P′)*. The inverse square correction factor *(CF)* to be applied is as follows:

$$P' = P \times \left(\frac{SSD + d_m}{SSD + d_m + h} \right)^2$$

where *h* is the tissue deficit or excess (either plus or minus) above the point of interest relative to the central axis.

Example: Suppose that (in Fig. 23.10) point A was located at a depth of 5 cm in a 10 × 10 cm field and that the gap above point A was 3 cm. A 10 × 10 cm isodose curve is slid down until the horizontal line representing the surface intersects the surface of the contour directly above the point of interest (i.e., point A). Suppose the isodose value now read *(solid line)* at *P* is 78%. This isodose value is corrected with the previously shown inverse square correction to yield the resultant depth dose:

$$P' = P \times \left(\frac{SSD + d_m}{SSD + d_m + h} \right)^2 = 78\% \left(\frac{100 + 1.5}{100 + 1.5 + 3} \right)^2 = 73.6\%$$

The dose at point A is 73.6% of the dose at the (preshift) D_{max} point.

The tissue-air ratio (TAR, or tissue-maximum ratio [TMR]) method is another contour correction method. In this method, PDD corrections to isodose values are obtained with ratios of TARs or TMRs:

$$P' = P \times [TAR(d) / TAR(d + h)]$$

Heterogeneity Corrections. Standard isodose charts and depth dose tables assume homogeneous unit density (water) media. However, within a patient are fat, bone, muscle, and air, which attenuate and scatter the beam differently than water does. Boundary interfaces can present additional (transitional zone) problems (i.e., near bone, air cavities, or metal prostheses).

In the megavoltage range of x-ray energies that are common in radiation therapy, the Compton effect is the predominant mode of interaction.[5,7] Thus, the attenuation of the beam in any medium is a function mostly of the electron density of the medium (number of electrons per cm³). The schematic representation in Fig. 23.11 explains some of the methods used to account for the presence of some material that is not water equivalent.[1]

Assume that dose is to be calculated at a point *P* at a depth *d* in a heterogeneous phantom. The radiation beam first traverses a depth d_1 of water-equivalent material, then passes through some other material

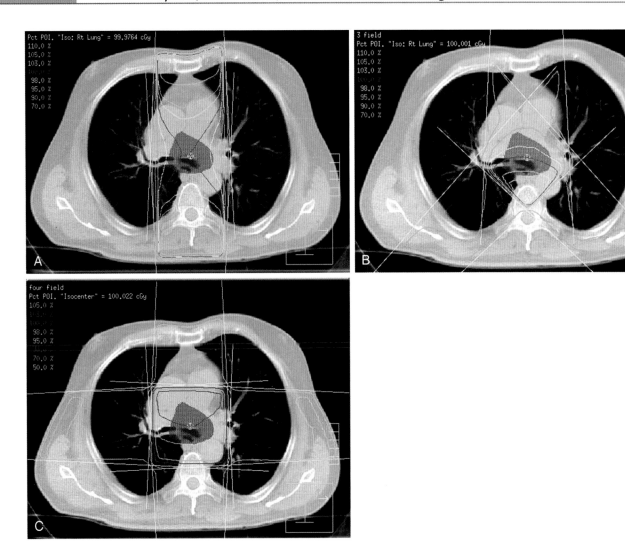

Fig. 23.8 Thorax isodose distributions produced by (A) a parallel-opposed field arrangement, (B) a three-field arrangement, and (C) a four-field arrangement. The *red shaded area* in the center of the computed tomographic scan image represents the target volume. The numeric values of the isodoses represent percentages of the dose at the isocenter of the fields.

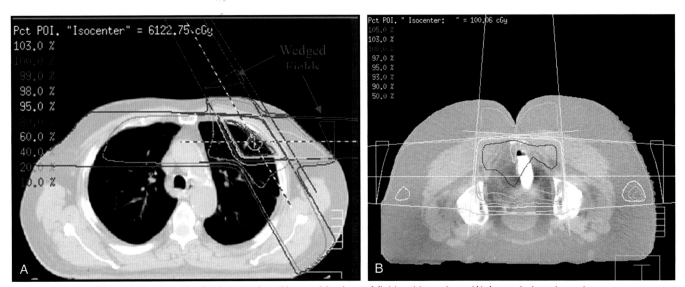

Fig. 23.9 Isodose distributions produced by combinations of fields with wedges. (A) An angled wedge pair. (B) A combination of a posterior open field with two lateral wedged fields.

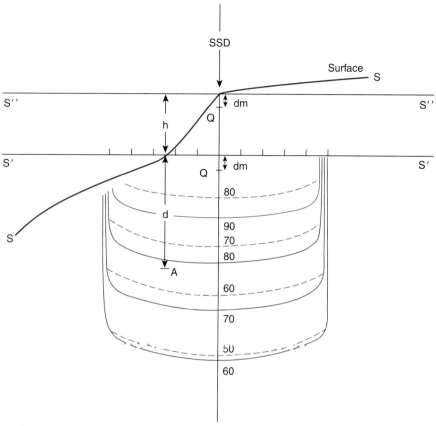

Fig. 23.10 Diagram illustrates methods of correcting dose distribution in an irregular surface such as $S - S$. The *solid* curves are from an isodose chart that assumes a flat surface located at $S' - S'$. The *dashed* isodose curves assume a flat surface at $S'' - S''$ without any air gap. *SSD,* Source-skin distance. (Modified from Khan FM. *The Physics of Radiation Therapy.* 2nd ed. Baltimore, MD: Williams & Wilkins; 1994.)

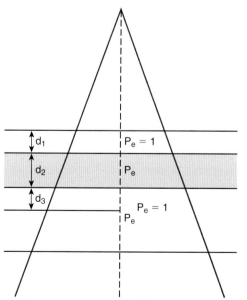

Fig. 23.11 Schematic diagram shows a water-equivalent phantom that contains an inhomogeneity of electron density P_e relative to that of water. P is the point of dose calculation. (From Khan FM. *The Physics of Radiation Therapy.* 2nd ed. Baltimore, MD: Williams & Wilkins; 1994.)

(inhomogeneity) with a depth d_2 and then again through a depth d_3 of water-equivalent material. If ρ_e represents the density of the heterogeneous material relative to water, then the total (uncorrected) depth d and the effective (corrected) depth d_{eff} are each given by the following equations:

$$d = d_1 + d_2 + d_3$$

$$d_{eff} = d_1 + \rho_e d_2 + d_3$$

The effective SSD method assumes that the corrected PDD is equal to the PDD for the effective depth d_{eff} multiplied by an inverse square correction. The effective depth is the equivalent radiologic path length, d_{eff}, previously:

$$PDD\,(FS,SSD,d)\;\text{corrected} = PDD\,(FS,SSD,d_{eff}) \times$$
$$(SSD + d_{eff}/SSD + d)^2$$

The TAR or TMR method applies an attenuation correction to the TAR (or TMR) based on the physical depth as opposed to the effective or radiologic depth:

$$CF = \frac{TAR\,(d_{eff},r_d)}{TAR\,(d,r_d)}\;or\;\frac{TMR\,(d_{eff},r_d)}{TMR\,(d,r_d)}$$

where d is the actual, physical depth to the point P; d_{eff} is the effective water depth, taking into account the relative electron densities of the materials ($d_{eff} = d_1 + r_e d_2 + d_3$); and r_d is the field size (FS) at the depth of calculation. The dose at point P (achieved with assumption of water-equivalent depths) is multiplied by the CF to get the inhomogeneity-corrected dose.[19] Note that TMRs can also be used in the same fashion as TARs.

Example: Consider the following as an illustration of the TAR method for heterogeneity corrections (see Fig. 23.11). Assume the phantom of Fig. 23.11 is irradiated with a 10 × 10 cm, 80-cm SSD, cobalt-60 field. Further assume that $d_1 = 5$ cm, $d_2 = 10$ cm, and $d_3 = 3$ cm and that the density ρ_e of the 10-cm-thick medium relative to water is 0.3. With those assumptions, $d_{actual} = 5 + 10 + 3 = 18$ cm, and $d_{eff} = (5 \times 1) + (10 \times 0.3) + (3 \times 1) = 11$ cm. The distance to the point P is 80 + 18 = 98 cm, and the field size at P is (98/80) × 10 = 12.25 × 12.25 cm. The CF to be applied is as follows:

$$CF = TAR\ (11, 12.25)/TAR\ (18, 12.25) = 0.704/0.487 = 1.45$$

The dose at P with the presence of the heterogeneity considered is 1.45 times the dose computed with the presence of the heterogeneity ignored. (Note that the previous correction produces the "effective" TAR that results as a consequence of the presence of the heterogeneity. The effective TAR at $P = 0.487 \times 1.45 = 0.487 \times [0.704/0.487] = 0.704$.)

The heterogeneity correction methods explained up to this point assume infinite slabs of heterogeneous media and do not take into account the relative location of the heterogeneity with respect to the point of calculation. As such, these methods yield only rough approximations of the effects of heterogeneities on dose calculations performed with assumptions of homogeneous media. More sophisticated calculations take these effects into account to varying degrees of accuracy.[8] Some of these methods are as follows:

1. *Power law TAR method:* A TAR correction method that accounts for the relative location of the point of calculation with respect to the inhomogeneity.
2. *Generalized Batho correction:* A generalization of the power law method to allow for dose calculations at points within the heterogeneity.
3. *Equivalent TAR method:* A method that considers the effects of heterogeneities on scatter, as well as on primary. In this method, both the field size and the depth are scaled to account for the presence of heterogeneities.
4. *Delta volume method:* In this method, primary and scatter are separated. The irradiated volume is broken into volume elements, and scatter is computed from a weighted summation of the scatter from each of the volume elements. This scatter is then added to the primary.

Typical Heterogeneity Corrections. Tables 23.2 and 23.3, modified from Anderson,[9] can be useful in estimating the dose or correction to the dose beyond a given heterogeneity.

Example (see Fig. 23.11): Assume that this phantom is irradiated with a single beam of 4-MV photons and that the dose is calculated at a point P assuming homogeneous media. The point P is located at a total physical depth of 6 cm. It is located beyond an inhomogeneity 2 cm thick. The homogenous dose at P from the single 10-MV beam is 100 cGy. If the inhomogeneity has a relative density of healthy lung (0.25), what is the radiologic depth, and what is the heterogeneity-corrected dose at P? If the heterogeneity has a relative density of bone (1.65), what is the radiologic depth, and what is the heterogeneity-corrected dose at P?

The physical depth is 6 cm, of which 2 cm consists of the heterogeneity. Thus, the radiologic (or effective) depth of the point P is 4 + (0.25 × 2.0) = 4.5 cm (with a healthy lung CF), and 4 + (1.65 × 2.0) = 7.3 cm (with a bone CF). The dose at P assuming lung heterogeneity is approximately 100 cGy + (100 × 0.02 × 2) = 104 cGy (an increase in dose of 3% per cm of lung). The dose at P assuming bone heterogeneity is approximately: 100 cGy − (100 × 0.02 × 2) = 96 cGy (a decrease in dose of 2% per cm of bone).

The previously described isodose-distribution corrections have been presented here to illustrate the fundamental processes underlying these corrections. In state-of-the-art treatment planning systems, modern dose calculation algorithms take into account tissue heterogeneities and contour irregularities explicitly.

TREATMENT PLANNING ESSENTIALS

Treatment planning systems, capable of handling large three-dimensional anatomy data sets from computed tomography (CT) or magnetic resonance imaging (MRI), accurately modeling treatment unit capabilities and offering visualization tools, have taken on the role of virtual patient simulators. Treatment planning tools allow for greater dose delivery precision. Greater use is being made of beam optimization, mathematic processes that iteratively modify beam parameters based on characteristics that are desirable in the plan. Optimization techniques permit more homogenous tumor volume irradiation while providing increased protection for organs at risk (OARs) in the irradiated volume. Algorithms have been developed to combine primary and scatter doses from across the radiation beam in all directions and at all points within the patient anatomy, which allows for more accurate dose evaluation within an irradiated area. This section provides an overview of current treatment planning capabilities and methods. Although three-dimensional conformal radiation therapy (3D-CRT), intensity-modulated radiation therapy (IMRT), and volumetric modulated arc therapy (VMAT) are addressed, the characteristics common to each technique are pointed out. Treatment planning fundamentals (including basic concepts), treatment planning algorithms, and the treatment planning process are emphasized.

Rationale for Three-Dimensional Conformal Radiation Therapy

The fact that radiation dose affects both tumor-bearing and healthy tissues is well known in radiation oncology. The degree of biologic effect is dependent on several factors, among them the magnitude of the dose

TABLE 23.2 **Increase in Dose to Tissues Beyond Healthy Lung**	
Beam Quality	**Correction Factor**
Orthovoltage	+10%/cm of lung
Cobalt-60	+4%/cm of lung
4 MV	+3%/cm of lung
10 MV	+2%/cm of lung
25 MV	+1%/cm of lung

Tissue-air ratio method and $\rho_{e\ lung} = 0.25$.

TABLE 23.3 **Reduction of Dose Beyond 1 cm of Hard Bone**	
Beam Quality	**Correction Factor**
1 mm Cu HVL	−15%
3 mm Cu HVL	−7%
Cobalt-60	−3.5%
4 MV	−3%
10 MV	−2%

Tissue-air ratio method and $\rho_{e\ bone} = 1.65$.
Cu, Copper; *HVL*, half-value layer.

and the radiosensitivity of the tissue. The desired outcome in radiation oncology is a high degree of tumor control with very little deleterious side effects. This is often achievable only to a certain degree.

Fig. 23.12 can be used to explain the compromise between probability of tumor control and the incidence of normal tissue complications.[6] Both tumor control probability and healthy tissue complication incidence increase with dose. When tumors are more radiosensitive than their surrounding healthy tissues, a relatively high degree of tumor control may be achievable, at some given dose, with a reasonably low healthy tissue complication probability (see Fig. 23.12A–C). When tissues of equivalent radiosensitivity surround tumors, any dose that produces a reasonable tumor control probability also induces healthy tissue complications with an equal probability. This is illustrated in Fig. 23.12A, where the dose that produces a reasonable tumor control probability also produces a high complication rate.

Greater tumor control probability and lower healthy tissue complication probability can be achieved simultaneously if tumor doses are maximized while healthy tissue doses are kept to a minimum. This is the rationale for conformal radiation therapy. In 3D-CRT, three-dimensional image visualization and treatment planning tools are used to conform isodose distributions to only target volumes while excluding healthy tissues as much as possible. This section discusses the tools and processes used during 3D-CRT.

Three-Dimensional Treatment Planning and Delivery Methods.

Three-dimensional treatment planning (3DTP) includes the processes with which three-dimensional visualization, dose calculation, and plan evaluation tools are used to produce optimized treatment field arrangements. Planning is image based, and patient anatomy is represented with CT data sets. Tumor volumes and OARs are identified and outlined with image-contouring tools. OARs are healthy tissues whose radiosensitivity and location in the vicinity of the planning target volume (PTV) may significantly influence treatment planning or the absorbed dose level to be used. Margins are established around tumor volumes to include disease microinvasion and allow for tumor volume and patient motion. Beams are arranged to target tumor volumes and to avoid OAR. Treatment plans are then objectively evaluated based on their volume-dose relationships.

Current 3DTP methods include both conventional 3D-CRT and intensity-modulated techniques. In both methods, target volumes and OARs are defined and beams are arranged in an attempt to maximize the dose to targets while minimizing the dose to critical structures.[10] In addition, intensity-modulation techniques such as IMRT or VMAT (described later) allow for the modification of the distribution of intensity within a treatment beam to achieve the stated goal.

The 3D-CRT technique uses conventional "forward planning," which requires that dose-altering parameters and beam modifiers be entered into the treatment plan by the planner. After the initial dose calculation is completed, the planner evaluates the dose distribution and edits the modifiers or other parameters to produce an improved plan. This process is repeated until an acceptable plan is achieved. "Intensity-modulated" techniques such as static field IMRT (usually referred to simply as "IMRT") are more sophisticated in that they are able to vary the intensity of the radiation *within the same beam*, which enables the system to create very conformal dose distributions. Such techniques are "inverse planned." In inverse planning, rather than having the planner manipulate the beam limiting devices manually and evaluate the resulting dose distribution as is done with forward planning, the desired dose objectives are first entered into the planning system, and the system calulates the delivery by creating multileaf collimator (MLC) patterns that satisfy the constraints. For IMRT, this is usually done in two steps: the "optimization" step in which the desired

dose objectives are entered into the system and intensity profiles are generated, followed by the "leaf sequencing" step in which the desired intensity profiles generated by the optimizer are turned into the final deliverable MLC patterns.

There are typically two types of MLC operation that are used to deliver IMRT fields, "step-and-shoot" and "sliding window." A step-and-shoot or "segmental MLC" delivery begins with an initial MLC

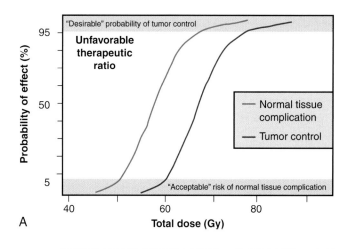

A

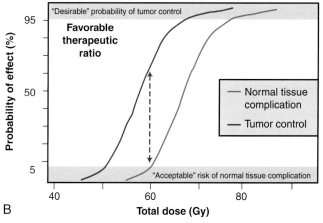

B

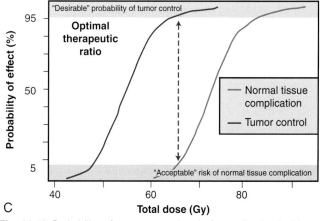

C

Fig. 23.12 Probability of tumor control and of complication incidence as a function of dose. (A) The ratio is unfavorable because the tissue tolerance dose is less than the tumor control dose. (B) The ratio is favorable because the tolerance dose is greater than the tumor control dose. (C) This is the optimal ratio that predicts low complication as shown by the curve separation. (From Gunderson LL, Tepper JE. *Clinical Radiation Oncology*, Philadelphia, PA: Elsevier; 2016.)

pattern. A portion of the dose is delivered through this leaf pattern or segment. (Beam is delivered *after* the MLC has achieved the shape that corresponds to its appropriate segment.) With the gantry in the same position, the beam is automatically interrupted, and the leaf pattern changes to that which corresponds to the second segment. The beam is then turned on for the second segment. This may occur several times to produce the desired intensity map, which represents different doses that are delivered across the shape of the treatment field. During "sliding window" or "dynamic MLC" (DMLC) delivery, the leaves of the MLC move during the delivery of the beam. After the dose of the first beam is delivered for either of these two types of IMRT techniques, the gantry is moved to the next position, and the treatment is delivered with the intensity map for the next beam.

The technique described earlier is referred to as static field IMRT because the gantry is stationary during delivery of each field. VMAT also uses inverse planning and DMLC delivery but differs from IMRT in that the beam is delivered *while the gantry rotates around the patient.* The MLC moves during the arc to alter the intensity of the beam according to the requirements of the treatment plan. The dose rate can also be modulated during delivery. The planner determines the angular extent of the arc and its direction. Some treatment plans require the gantry to arc through the same rotation to deliver the entire dose. Primary collimator openings are set by the planner to ensure the PTV is included throughout the entire arc. *The VMAT beam collimators are sometimes rotated if the arc repeats in the opposite direction to ensure no increased area of dose occurs from the leakage between collimators.*

Treatment Planning Algorithms

Treatment planning algorithms are the planning systems' mathematical dose calculation processes. They consist of a series of equations, and their associated input parameters, that produce values of dose as a function of position within the dose calculation matrix—a grid of points at which dose is computed and subsequently displayed.

Treatment planning algorithms can be categorized on the basis of their dose calculation methodology. Data-driven algorithms compute dose mainly from interpolations between measured beam data (depth dose data, off-axis profiles, and so forth). Correction factors are applied to account for differences between the measurement geometry and the geometry of the patient. Data-driven algorithms are now seldom used in modern planning systems, although they continue to be used in secondary check dose calculation programs.

Model-driven algorithms mainly use equations, "fit" to measured data, that are intended to predict the variation of dose with changes in parameters such as depth, distance off axis, and proximity to field edges. An example of a modern model-driven algorithm is the convolution algorithm.

Treatment planning algorithms can also be classified according to the dimensionality of the calculation methodology. A common classification is two-dimensional and three-dimensional algorithms. Although descriptions of two-dimensional and three-dimensional algorithms often differ, several distinguishing traits are salient. The three-dimensional algorithms make use of entire CT data sets that are treated as one comprehensive CT volume; two-dimensional algorithms often treat CT data as a series of independent CT planar contours. This is of particular importance during the dose calculation phase. The three-dimensional algorithms use the entire data set when estimating scatter to each point in the volume; two-dimensional algorithms assume that all CT image planes are of equal size, shape, and composition as the current calculation plane, and they compute scatter with that (inaccurate) presumption. Because of the availability of volume information, three-dimensional algorithms also permit evaluations of plan quality with a tool called the *dose-volume histogram (DVH)*. The DVH is discussed subsequently in the chapter.

Treatment planning algorithms can be evaluated based on several criteria. Algorithms differ in their ability to properly model beam intensities in different irradiation conditions. An ideal algorithm properly represents a beam's depth dose and off-axis intensity. It properly characterizes the irradiation geometry (gantry, collimator, and couch angles) and the effects of beam modifiers such as independent jaws, MLCs, wedges, compensators, and bolus. Treatment planning algorithms should also properly use patient data sets such as CT and MRI data. Dose calculation accuracy and speed are yet other considerations.

Calculation Algorithms: Scatter Integration. For a simplified explanation of the dose calculation process, it is often useful to consider dose as consisting of primary and scatter components.[9] In basic terms, at all points in the irradiated volume, dose from primary radiation is computed first, then the dose from scattered radiation is added. A scatter integration–like algorithm may use an equation similar to the schematic formula that is shown in the following:

$$D\ (f,r,d,x)\ =\ D_{ref} \times OF_{pri} \times ISF\ (f + d)\ \times OAF\ (x,d)\ \times T\ (r)\\ \times\ OF_{scat}(r)\ \times\ [TPR\ (0,\ d)\ +\ SPR_{avg}\ (r,d)]$$

where:

$D(f,r,d,x)$ = dose at some point *P* at a depth *d*, source-surface distance *f*, field size *r*, and off-axis distance *x*;

D_{ref} = a known reference dose (e.g., dose at D_{max}, 100 cm SSD, 10 × 10 cm field);

OF_{pri} = an output factor that describes the change in primary output as a function of collimator setting (akin to Khan Sc)[1];

$ISF(f + d)$ = an inverse square correction;

$OAF(x,d)$ = an off-axis factor that models the beam's profile;

$T(r)$ = beam transmission through wedges, trays, and other possible beam modifiers;

OF_{scat} = an output factor that describes the change in scatter contribution as a function of field size and shape (akin to Khan Sp);

$TPR(0,d)$ = the primary (0 × 0 field) TPR or TMR;

and $SPR_{avg}(r,d)$ = the average scatter-phantom (or scatter-maximum) ratio, a function of field size and shape, that is added to the primary TPR (or TMR) to produce an effective TPR (or TMR).

The product of $D_{ref} \times OF_{pri} \times ISF(f + d) \times OAF(x,d) \times T(r)$ describes the primary radiation intensity that is available at *P*. The remaining parameters OF_{scat}, $TPR(0,d)$, and $SPR_{avg}(r,d)$ are a function of the conditions within the attenuating media.

Example: The previous equation may seem complex, but in reality, it is not. The perceived complexity is because of the large number of variables and parameters that require definition. To illustrate the calculation method, consider the following situation. Suppose that a phantom is irradiated with a 12 × 12 cm field; the SSD is 90 cm, and dose is to be computed to a point *P* that is 10 cm deep. If the accelerator is calibrated so that 1 cGy/MU (D_{ref}) exists at D_{max}, 100 cm SSD, for a 10 × 10 cm field, then the dose at *P* is 1 cGy/MU × the output factors for a 12 ×12 cm field (OF_{pri}) and (OF_{scat}) × an inverse square correction for possible differences between calibration and calculation distances [$ISF(f + d)$] × the appropriate TMR [$TPR(r,d)$] and tray transmission factors [$T(r)$]. Remaining variables [such as $SPR_{avg}(r,d)$ and $OAF(x,d)$] are used when needed to account for situations such as irregular blocking or dose to points away from the central axis.

Calculation Algorithms: Convolution Algorithm. Convolution algorithms used in three-dimensional planning systems work in a similar way. Primary and scatter contributions are computed separately and then are summed. A three-dimensional convolution algorithm[11] may use a calculation methodology described by the following:

$$D(r) = \int \frac{\mu}{\rho}(r) \times \psi(r) \times K(r' \rightarrow r) \, dV$$

Here, $D(r)$ represents the dose at some point r. The primary fluence, $\psi(r)$, describes the primary dose that exists at the point r. The in-air fluence (photon intensity: photon number and energy) exits the head of the treatment unit, is moderated by beam modifiers, and is then attenuated by the patient. The $\psi(r)$ term contains all primary radiation output, inverse square, off-axis, and beam modifier corrections. (It is analogous to the product $D_{ref} \times OF_{pri} \times ISF[f + d] \times OAF[x,d] \times T[r] \times TPR[0,d]$ used in the description of the scatter integration algorithm.)

The product of $\psi(r)$ and $\mu/\rho(r)$ produces a quantity that represents the total radiation energy released at the point r *within the medium*. The incident fluence is projected onto the patient's CT data set and is attenuated.

The result is a matrix of radiation energy that is available for dose deposition.

The dose-spread kernel, $K(r' \rightarrow r)$, represents the energy distribution from the primary interaction site throughout the irradiated volume. $K(r' \rightarrow r)$ is a description of how dose is deposited in the vicinity of a primary interaction site (i.e., the relative amount of energy that is deposited in the vicinity of the primary interaction site). (It is, in some ways, analogous to the scatter terms OF_{scat}, and $SPR_{avg}[r,d]$ used to compute scattered dose in the scatter integration algorithm.)

Because the total dose at the point r is dependent on the total radiation energy released at all points r', the total dose at r is the superposition (a fluence and attenuation coefficient-weighted summation) of the function $\psi(r) \times \mu/\rho(r)$ and the dose-spread function $K(r' \rightarrow r)$. The integration sign, $\int$, represents the summation process.

> Although the mathematic description of these types of dose-calculation algorithms may seem intimidating, the concepts are relatively straightforward. The dose to all points from primary radiation is computed, and then scattered radiation from these primary dose depositions is added to obtain the total dose. The effects of contour irregularities and tissue heterogeneities are taken into account, as appropriate, in each step.

Calculation Algorithms: Monte Carlo.

The most accurate method of dose calculation is known as the *Monte Carlo method*. In Monte Carlo calculations, individual particle histories are tracked as they pass through the delivery system and patient, and the fundamental physics of each individual interaction is modeled based on its probability of occurrence. Hundreds of millions of particles or more must be traced to perform a Monte Carlo calculation of sufficient precision. It is for this reason that Monte Carlo calculations, although being extremely accurate compared with measurement, are computationally intensive and often not practical given the time constraints of treatment planning. As available computing power increases, so does the practicality of using Monte Carlo for clinical dose calculations.

Treatment Planning Concepts and Tools.

Treatment planning algorithms constitute the calculation engine of the treatment planning process. Calculation algorithms are only one piece of the entire three-dimensional planning process. Before dose is calculated, treatment beams must be established in a way that achieves the intent of

radiation therapy: maximization of tumor, or target, dose, and minimization of OAR dose.

Planning Volume and Margin Concepts. Because the 3D-CRT process seeks to conform dose to specific target volumes, these volumes must be accurately defined. The International Commission on Radiation Units and Measurements (ICRU) has recommended the use of specifically defined volumes[12]:

Gross tumor volume (GTV) is the gross palpable, visible, or demonstrable extent and location of malignant growth. It is the volume of known disease. Disease that is visible on CT scan is a common example of a GTV.

Clinical target volume (CTV) is a tissue volume that contains the GTV or subclinical microscopic malignant disease. The CTV includes gross visible or palpable disease *plus* any possible microscopic extensions of disease that may not be visible or palpable. The CTV is the volume that must always be enclosed by the treatment isodose. Untreated portions of the CTV could lead to local failure of therapy. *PTV* is a geometric volume; it has dimensions that are believed to always contain the CTV, taking into account all possible geometric uncertainties, such as patient setup uncertainties and patient or organ motion.

Treated volume is the volume enclosed by the isodose surface selected as appropriate to achieve the purpose of treatment (i.e., the volume enclosed by the prescription isodose surface).

Irradiated volume is the volume of tissue that receives a dose considered significant in relation to healthy tissue tolerance.

OAR and *planning OAR volumes (PRV)* represent volumes of tissue that may be at risk of damage. Similar to the PTV, the PRV places a margin around the OAR to account for uncertainties in OAR position. These volumes are shown schematically in Fig. 23.13.[12]

Margins are created around the CTV to ensure appropriate beam targeting. As previously stated, the margin that surrounds the GTV is devised to account for the uncertainties that exist in the precise definition of disease. The PTV includes a margin around the CTV to ensure that the CTV is always contained within the PTV. The exact definitions of these margins are evolving as newer technologies are introduced (Box 23.2). The GTV-to-CTV margin is mostly pathology driven. The margin of the PTV around the CTV is designed to make certain that the CTV is always contained within the treated volume. Note that the PTV margin around the CTV is not necessarily symmetric. The PTV allows for target motion and uncertainty in patient setup positioning.[13] Greater spatial uncertainties in the position of the target volume may exist in one dimension more than in another. For example, prostate motion in the AP direction is generally believed to potentially exceed lateral prostate motion.[14] Thus, the PTV margin around the CTV should be designed to account for these types of uncertainties.

> Newer target volume and margin descriptions have been introduced to better account for the specific uncertainties in target definition caused by motion. An internal margin (IM) is added around the CTV to account for the CTV's internal motion within the patient. Four-dimensional CT images allow this motion to be accounted for very precisely. The result is an internal target volume (ITV): ITV = CTV + IM. A setup margin (SM) is added around the ITV to account for the uncertainty in patient position. The final result is now the PTV: PTV = ITV + SM. If no GTV is visible, the CTV may include areas of possible disease after surgery or the potential involvement of lymphatics. Better immobilization devices and daily image guidance have allowed for smaller margins for the setup uncertainties.

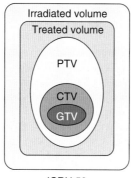
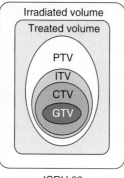

Fig. 23.13 Definition of target volumes used in radiation therapy from International Commission on Radiation Units and Measurements Reports 50 and 62. *CTV,* Clinical target volume; *GTV,* gross tumor volume; *ITV,* internal target volume; *PTV,* planning target volume.

BOX 23.2   The Quest to Better Define the Clinical Target Volume and the Planning Target Volume

Precise definitions of the clinical target volume (CTV) and planning target volume (PTV) have become areas of much attention and focus. For treatment of disease while sparing of organs at risk (OARs), gross tumor volumes (GTVs) should be expanded to CTVs and then to PTVs in insightful ways.

Molecular and functional imaging methods are used to better define diseased anatomy that was previously only suspected of containing disease. Positron emission tomography (PET) with ^{18}FDG (fluoro-2-deoxy-D-glucose), for example, is commonly used to stage non-small cell lung cancer because of its increased sensitivity to the metabolic activity associated with tumor cell proliferation. The first figure in this box clearly shows an increased concentration of ^{18}FDG in a mediastinal lymph node that could have been otherwise undetected in computed tomographic (CT) scan. With use of advanced functional imaging techniques such as this, population-based traditional expansions of GTVs to CTVs could be reduced.

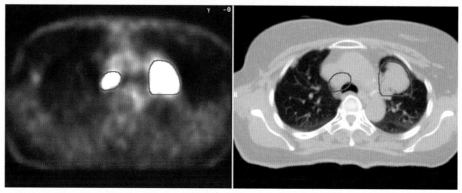

Increased concentration of ^{18}FDG in a mediastinal lymph node.

Image-guided radiotherapy (IGRT) techniques seek to further reduce expansions of target volumes by decreasing the uncertainty associated with daily patient positioning. If images of a patient's target volume are taken daily and the patient position is suitably adjusted, the CTV to PTV expansion can be fittingly modified. In the second figure in this box, the GTV, as seen on an image of a daily CT scan taken with an in-room CT scanner *(Daily),* is compared with the GTV defined on the treatment planning CT scan *(Ref).* With proper alignment of the target volumes of both image sets, corrections to the patient's position can be made, thus decreasing the uncertainty in patient position.

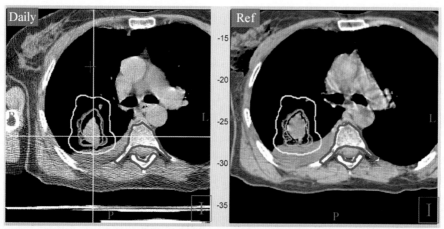

The GTV as seen on an image of a daily CT scan taken with (A) an in-room CT scanner *(Daily),* and compared with (B) the GTV defined on the treatment planning CT scan *(Ref).*

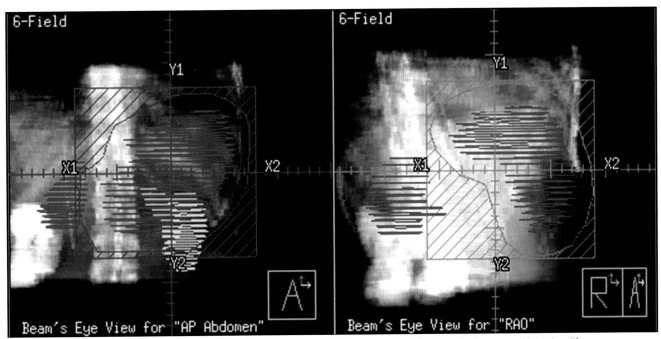

Fig. 23.14 Use of the beam's-eye view (BEV) tool for treatment-field design and placement. Note the differences between the anteroposterior *(AP)* and right anterior oblique *(RAO)* fields. The shape and spatial relationships of the tumor and the kidney volumes change as a function of gantry angle, which allows more favorable tumor volume targeting.

Treatment fields are often designed from beam's-eye view (BEV) of PTVs. (BEV images are images reconstructed from CT data that represent the patient's anatomy and defined volumes from the perspective of the treatment beam. BEV images are discussed in more detail in the next section.) BEV-designed three-dimensional and IMRT treatment fields should include a margin that allows for full dose coverage of the PTV and accounts for beam penumbral effects, the distance from the 50% to the 90% profile level. Although this margin accounts, primarily, for possible lateral radiation transport equilibrium losses, it should also allow for exclusion of critical structures.[15] Fig. 23.14 illustrates the volume and margin concepts that have just been discussed. The BEV of VMAT treatment fields should be evaluated throughout the entire arc to ensure that the PTV is included throughout the angles of the arc beams. The entire PTV may not be seen in each BEV if multiple arcs are used. Some may include the medial portion and some the lateral portion of the PTV, depending on the position of the gantry. Superior and inferior portions of the PTV are to be covered at all angles.

Treatment Planning Tools. Virtual simulation is a process by which treatment fields are defined with patient CT image data, identified targets and OARs, and treatment unit geometric information.[16] Specialized software is used to contour patient anatomy, set up the treatment beam arrangement, identify the location of patient markings, and design blocking for the treatment fields (Fig. 23.15). Commercially available treatment planning systems incorporate tools that facilitate the process of tailoring the delivery of the prescribed radiation dose to the specific clinical presentation of the patient.

Because the CT data set is used for all treatment planning and the patient is not present during the virtual simulation process, the patient must be set up in position for treatment, and all immobilization devices to be used must be included in the CT scan. The data set should include the area defined by the physician to be treated and include full volumes of the OARs. Anatomic landmarks to be visualized in a digital radiograph to evaluate the setup need to be included in the CT data set. Adjustment of the CT slice thickness and table indexing to small

increments increases the quality of the digital radiographs created from the CT data set. Radiopaque markers (small-bead fiducial markers) should be placed on the patient at the intersection of the coronal, transverse, and sagittal positioning lasers on the center slice of the scanned volume. Radiopaque markers should be placed to indicate the right or left side of the patient and any skin markings that the physician may want to identify in the treatment plan (i.e., scars). Documentation of setup parameters should be made at the time of the CT scan.

Treatment planning systems have drawing tools that allow the planner to outline structures and target volumes. The process of identifying structures, target volumes, OARs, and healthy tissues by creating contours around them is frequently called organ segmentation. The contouring process often makes use of auto-segmentation tools that help the planner identify the target or OAR. Segmented structures can be displayed graphically as outlines surrounding the structure or can be filled to create a solid volume. Segmented structures are commonly used to assist in field shaping and positioning and in isodose evaluation.

Anatomy that is to be identified for treatment planning may be better defined with use of other imaging modalities in addition to CT scan. Because of physical principles underlying their image production, MRI and positron emission tomography (PET) scans show anatomy differently than a CT scan. Both MRI and PET incorporate physiology in the production of images. This can be used to better differentiate between diseased and healthy tissues. Treatment planning systems are often capable of combining the images from the different modalities with the CT image. The process of geometrically combining the images is called image fusion or image registration. When image sets are fused or registered, a one-to-one correspondence exists between the positions of each element (voxel) of the images. Image registrations can be either **rigid** or **deformable**. Rigid registrations simply line the two images up with each other without making any modifications to either image. These are satisfactory when the anatomy is sufficiently identical in both images, such as a fusion in the brain where the skull bones of the CT and MRI are aligned. In some cases, the anatomy is not exactly the same such as when fusing in the neck region in a case where the

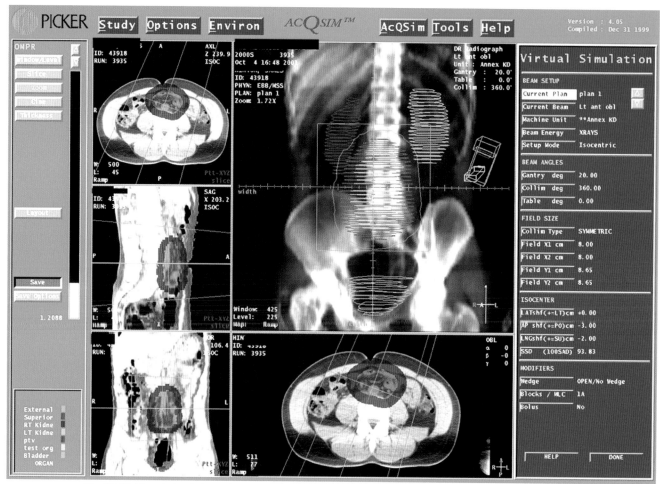

Fig. 23.15 Virtual simulation software sample screen. A "virtual" patient is created from computed tomographic scan data. The software supports healthy tissue and target volume definition and identification; treatment fields can then be designed and placed.

neck flexion is different in the CT and MRI. In this case, a deformable registration may be more accurate, in which one of the images, called the secondary, is warped to match the anatomy of the other image (the primary). Deformable registration algorithms are more sophisticated and must be tested thoroughly before use. Properly fused images can then combine the enhanced imaging capabilities of MRI or PET with the spatial accuracy of CT scan. Anatomy can be defined on any of the image data sets and can then be displayed on the CT image (Fig. 23.16). The CT data set is used for dose computations. All outlines should be evaluated by the clinician on the CT images.

Once a beam has been created, the clinician can view the patient as seen through the opening of the beam. As stated previously, this particular view of the patient anatomy from the perspective of the treatment field is called a *BEV*. The BEV changes in shape and size the same way the radiation beam diverges through the patient. Field size and blocking can be demonstrated according to their size and shape in relation to the plane of the body being viewed. Three-dimensional planning systems allow the clinician to rotate the data set to evaluate the beam path from all angles. When a BEV is reconstructed such that diverge-corrected patient anatomy from the CT data set is also included in an image that imitates a radiograph, the resulting image is called a digitally reconstructed radiograph (DRR). A typical DRR is shown in Fig. 23.17.

A room's-eye view shows the geometric relationship of the treatment machine to the patient. The room's-eye view allows clear visualization of the entrance and exit of the beam through the patient. This

view may also help prevent possible orientations of the equipment that could result in collisions with the patient or treatment table.

Other image-rendering techniques allow visualization of anatomic structures that have been highlighted. The skeleton of the body or the skin can be distinguished with image visualization techniques that display the specific ranges of CT density. Skin rendering allows the planner to see markers that were placed on the skin during the CT scan. Room lasers and field and block outlines can be displayed on the patient's skin (Fig. 23.18). This technique is similar to looking at the field light on the patient in a conventional simulator or on the treatment machine.

The three-dimensional treatment plans can be objectively evaluated with dose and volume information. An extremely useful evaluation tool is the DVH, a representation of dose received by an organ versus the volume of the organ. Lawrence and colleagues[17] have explained the fundamentals of DVHs and their clinical interpretations in detail. The DVH is a plot of target or OAR volume as a function of dose. It is, in essence, a frequency distribution of the number of target or OAR structure voxels (volume elements) receiving a certain dose. In its most common form (the cumulative DVH), it is a plot of volume versus the minimum dose absorbed within that volume. Fig. 23.19 presents a cumulative DVH for a hypothetical PTV, CTV, and GTV. The characteristics of an optimal target volume DVH are (1) high percentage volume at prescribed target dose (adequate target volume coverage), and (2) rapid decrease in volume beyond the prescribed dose (dose uniformity within target).

Interpretation of healthy tissue DVHs is somewhat more complex. Clearly, a desired trait of an OAR DVH is large volume maintained at lower dose. This is often not attainable, and DVHs such as those shown in Fig. 23.20 result.[8] Depending on their response to radiation, tissues can be characterized as either serial response tissues or parallel response tissues. The overall function of organs that consist of serial response tissues can be affected by the incapacitation of only one element. The spinal cord is such an organ. The high-dose region of a serial tissue DVH is of particular importance. The overall function of organs that consist of parallel response tissues, on the other hand, is affected by the injury of a number of elements of that organ above a certain minimum reserve. The liver is an example of such an organ. Interpretation of DVHs of organs of parallel response tissue is less clear. Site-specific DVH-based criteria are used for the evaluation of critical structures in treatment plans. In thoracic radiation therapy, for instance, a DVH-based constraint used for normal lung is V_{20} less than 40% (meaning less than 40% of normal lung should receive a dose in excess of 20 Gy). Another thoracic constraint is V_{50} less than 50% for the heart.

The Three-Dimensional Treatment Planning Process

Imaging and Anatomy Differentiation. The planning process begins with the CT data set taken for the virtual simulation. The images are sent to the planning system. Identification markers are evaluated along with quality of images and accuracy of data transfer. For reproduction of the treatment plan generated by the planner, a starting point needs to be identified that allows the therapist to reproduce the plan parameters on the patient in the treatment room. The planning system is designed to give coordinate information that translates from the CT data set to the treatment machine. For this to be done, there needs to be an origin in the plan. The point used as origin is commonly the intersection of the lasers in the coronal, sagittal, and transverse planes at the level of the small bead fiducial markers

placed on the patient at the time of the CT scan. This mark becomes the zero coordinate for the treatment plan in all directions (superior/inferior, anterior/posterior, right/left). All shifts for the beam coordinates start from this zero point when the isocenter for each treatment beam is verified (Fig. 23.21).

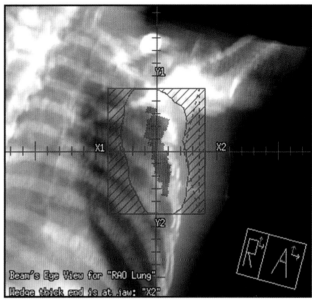

Fig. 23.17 Digitally reconstructed radiograph (DRR). A DRR is a two-dimensional radiograph-like image that is reconstructed from a computed tomography data set. The image of this figure was reconstructed from a thoracic data set to produce a view equivalent to that obtained if a radiographic image were obtained from the patient's right anterior side. Superimposed on the image is the projection of the contoured clinical target volume and the treatment field designed to cover the volume with a 2-cm margin.

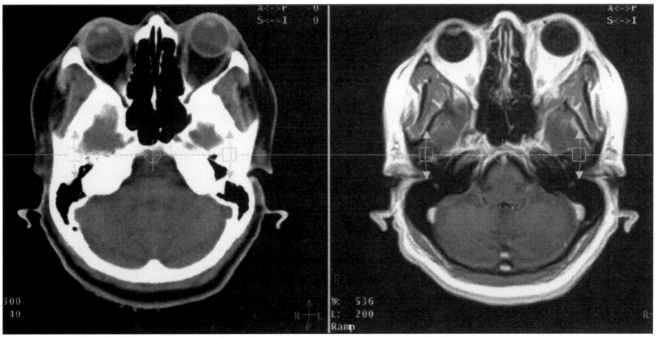

Fig. 23.16 Computed tomography (CT) and magnetic resonance imaging (MRI) image fusion. The superior soft tissue imaging ability of the MRI image on the right can be combined with the superior spatial accuracy of the CT image on the left to produce a composite correlated image. In the fusion process, common anatomic features are identified in each image, and these common features are then used to link the data sets so that they form a composite set. From that point on, features identified on an image of one modality are shown on its corresponding second modality image.

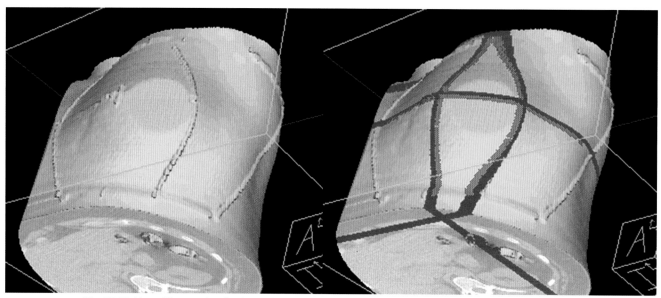

Fig. 23.18 Use of image visualization tools to aid in treatment-field placement during virtual simulation and treatment planning. The computed tomography (CT) data set can be visualized with an image rendering technique that emphasizes the patient's skin and any markers placed on the skin. In this figure, beams have been placed such that the lasers that indicate their isocenter coincide with catheters placed on the patient before CT scan.

Anatomy Delineation. Image fusion of the planning CT scan with the MRI or PET scan is completed to allow the clinician to toggle between or overlay images to outline the target volumes. GTV, CTV, and PTV are identified and outlined. OARs are outlined, and any healthy tissue for evaluation or for dosage control is also outlined. The clinician should review all anatomy before starting the treatment planning process. OARs that will have dose constraints defined in the intent of the treatment plan must be completely included in the CT data set. Partial structures can be identified if their maximum doses are the only constraint in the treatment plan or if the clinician is aware of the partial volume.

Why not simply plan using an MRI rather than having to take both the CT and MRI and fuse? It is possible but more complex. The CT is necessary for the dose calculation attributed to the fact that it imparts tissue density information to the treatment planning dose calculation engine. Brighter objects on the CT scan are higher density than darker objects, and part of the commissioning process of a treatment planning system is to input the relationship between the CT value associated with each pixel (known as the *Hounsfield number*) and tissue density. MRIs, while having superior tissue contrast compared with CTs, do not, in general, have a simple relationship between brightness and density; different MRI sequences render different types of tissue with varying brightness, so the treatment planning system would not know what the correct density was from the image. Therefore, the CT is fused with the MRI image so that CT information can be used for dose calculation, and the superior imaging characteristics of the MRI can be incorporated as well. Algorithms are becoming available, however, that convert MRI scans into "pseudo-CTs" that can be used for dose calculation using a variety of methods, thus making MRI-only simulations possible without the need for a CT.

During the treatment planning process for IMRT and VMAT, creation of structures that assist in controlling the intensity of the beam may be necessary. These structures can be identified as planning structures not for dose evaluation. Dose clouds are sometimes turned into structures to control high-dose areas. Another example is areas where the PTV overlaps an OAR and the OAR maximum dose needs to be less than the PTV dose. The intensity of the beam can be adjusted to control these objective doses.

Treatment Field Definition. After target and anatomy definition, the orientation of treatment beams is arranged. The center of the PTV is a recommended starting point for the placement of the beams' isocenter. Some treatment planning systems can automatically set the isocenter to the center of the PTV. If manual means are necessary for isocenter positioning, coronal, transverse, and sagittal views can be used to set the position of the isocenter to the center of the PTV.

With both two-dimensional and three-dimensional visualization techniques, the angles of the gantry and couch are adjusted to include the PTV in the beam while critical structures are excluded out of the path of the beam. The collimator size and rotation can be adjusted also to exclude structures from the beam. In three-dimensional and IMRT, the shape of the treatment field can be fashioned. *Autofielding*, a technique used to set an open area around the PTV from the perspective of the BEV, can be used to shape the field following the contour of the PTV. The autofield should include a margin around the PTV that allows for beam penumbra and block edge effects. The margin should be sufficient to allow isodose lines of 90% or greater to cover the PTV. A blocking technique called *autoblocking* can be used to create a block pattern or an MLC shield to decrease dose to critical structures. These structures can be covered with the block plus a margin of extra blocking if deemed necessary. Maximum collimator settings are determined by the planner. Dose limits are set for each beam. A point inside of the area to be treated is chosen to receive 100% of the dose. This normalization point is usually the beams' isocenter. If the isocenter of any of the beams is close to a block or near the surface of the patient, another point of normalization can be chosen. Each beam is then assigned a percentage of the total dose to be delivered. When the plan is normalized, numeric values of isodoses are equal to fractions of the dose existing at the point of normalization.

Prescription: Dose Intent. For a desirable treatment plan to be created in a timely manner, clear guidelines from the clinician for the treatment intent are essential. Prescriptions for the PTV volume should be conveyed to the planner, as well as the tolerances and allowable doses for the OAR. If the plan will have a boost or reduced treatment area plan after the primary plan, these treatment plans are best completed before therapy begins so that total dose plans and DVHs can be

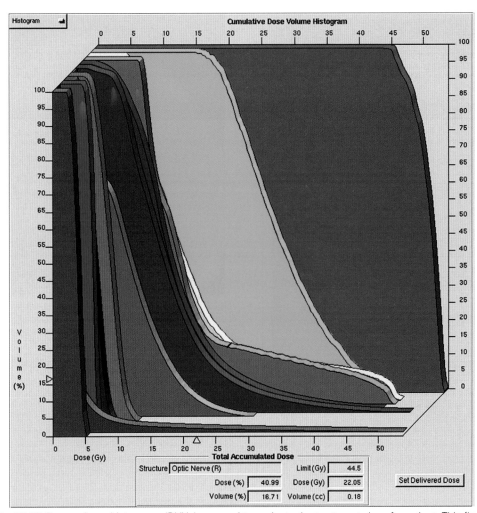

Fig. 23.19 Dose-volume histograms (DVHs) are used to evaluate the treatment plan of a patient. This figure shows a composite plot of the DVHs of the target volume and of critical structures within the irradiated volume. Dose is represented on the x-axis of the plots, and the y-axis represents the percentage of total volume enclosed by that dose level. To illustrate, note the x,y,z value of the target DVH on the upper right corner of the figure. It appears that 100% of the target volume will receive a dose of 45 Gy or greater. A move a little farther to the right on the target DVH shows that approximately 80% of the target volume will receive a dose of approximately 50 Gy or greater. The optic nerve (R) structure evaluation: V22 = 16.7. Intent of 44 Gy dose limit has been exceeded.

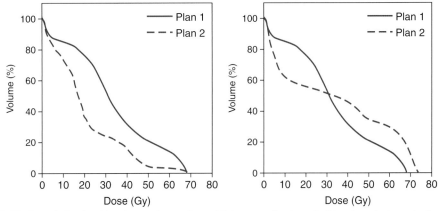

Fig. 23.20 Cumulative healthy tissue dose-volume histograms for two rival treatment plans. Left: Plan 2 is superior to plan 1 over the complete dose range. Right: The superior plan depends on how the organ responds to radiation damage. (Modified from Purdy JA, Starkschall G, eds. *A Practical Guide to 3-D Planning and Conformal Radiation Therapy*. Madison, WI: Advanced Medical Publishing; 1999.)

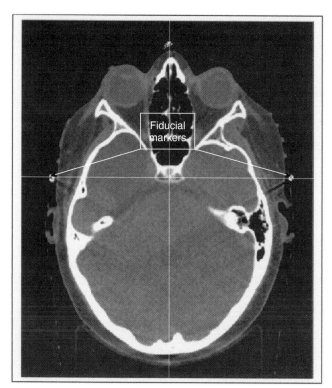

Fig. 23.21 Establishment of treatment plan coordinate system origin. External radiopaque markers, placed on the patient before computed tomographic scan, are routinely used to register the origin of the coordinate system of the treatment plan. This origin corresponds with the skin marks made on the patient. In this figure, markers placed on the immobilization mask of a patient are used to register the position of the plan origin. Any possible isocenter displacement from this point is noted as an isocenter shift.

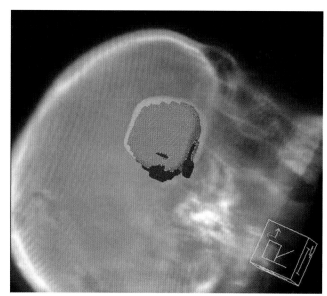

Fig. 23.22 An isodose cloud enclosing a target volume. The prescription isodose level can be seen in a three-dimensional visualization called an isodose *cloud*. If the cloud is shown semitransparent, the coverage of the target volume can be assessed. In this figure, a semitransparent isodose cloud produced by a three-field beam arrangement is superimposed on a hypothetical pituitary target volume. Shown are target areas not covered by the prescribed dose.

evaluated and edited if necessary. The OAR guidelines for the intent of treatment should also be conveyed to the planner. The maximum dose allowed to the structure and the percentage of volume allowed to receive a specific dose need to be specified. For documentation, these intents can be written in the format "V20 <40%," which means the volume receiving 20 Gy should be less than 40%. Multiple doses may need to be controlled within the structures. The intent should address each of these. The tolerance doses for the OARs should also be reported.

Whether the area has received previous radiation therapy treatments and the doses delivered from those treatments are very important to know. Reviews of previous treatments can range in complexity from simply reporting doses to relevant OARs from the previous and current treatment to performing image fusions and adding dose distributions from both treatments, if that information is available. The radiation dose received in the past will play a key role in determining what dose to prescribe and what OAR constraints to follow in the current treatment. Therefore, it is important to review all information carefully with the physician when preparing the current treatment plan.

For the intent for treatment to be incorporated into the treatment planning objectives, a form on which the intent can be written by the clinician and then reviewed with the planner can be created for the radiation oncology department. The clinician first enters the intent. After the plan has been completed and approved by the clinician, the final values for the dose limits can be entered into the form. This intent versus approved dose information allows for easy check of achieved objectives for OARs during the plan evaluation process.

The intended dose values for the objectives of the treatment plan are decided by the clinician. There are published guidelines for the OAR doses. The review of QUANTEC[18] (quantitative analysis of normal tissue effects in the clinic) summarizes the currently available three-dimensional dose/volume/outcome data to update and refine normal tissue/dose/volume tolerance guidelines. New technologies provide the treatment planner increased flexibility in determination of which normal tissue will be irradiated. IMRT and VMAT techniques allow portions of the dose to be delivered while the OAR is in the beam. One of the goals of QUANTEC is to summarize the available three-dimensional dose/volume/outcome data and to produce practical guidance, which allows the clinician to reasonably categorize toxicity based on dose/volume parameters or model results. These values are often posted in planning laboratory values and used as references.

The plan is evaluated after the dose calculations are completed, and the plan undergoes normalization such that isodose values represent percentages of a given dose. Although the beams are weighted to deliver 100% of the dose to a specific point, the plan may be normalized to deliver the prescription to a volume (e.g., 45 Gy to 95% of the PTV). This dose volume is a percent isodose that best covers the PTV while keeping the maximum dose to a predetermined percentage of dose above the prescription. Once the normalization of the plan is completed, the dose to the targets and OARs can be evaluated.

Treatment Plan Evaluations and Implementation. Each treatment plan is assessed to determine whether it can be used to deliver the prescribed dose to the PTV. Composite primary and boost plans allow the clinician to evaluate the DVHs for the entire treatment. Multiple plans can be compared with DVHs as bases for the comparison. Dose distributions can be displayed as isodose lines on two-dimensional planes or as clouds of dose for three-dimensional viewing (Fig. 23.22). The three-dimensional isodose clouds allow the planner to select an isodose value and then rotate the three-dimensional image of the PTV to view the distribution of dose around it. This technique shows whether any portion of the PTV extends outside of the isodose cloud and is not covered properly. Dose clouds allow for evaluation of doses that involve the OAR and their location within the structures. Maximum doses and hot spots are reviewed within each plan and within the composite plan to ensure that normal tissue constraints are not exceeded. Minimum doses to targets are evaluated to ensure that the disease is adequately treated. Mean doses to structures, such as mean lung dose, can also be reviewed in situations when response has been shown to vary with mean dose.

The complexity of the treatment plan is also reviewed. The number of fields used and the viability of the field arrangement are considered. Time of treatment delivery, setup reproducibility, setup complexity, and plan verification feasibility are important plan evaluation criteria.

Once the plan is approved, documentation is produced and filed in the patient's treatment record to clearly communicate plan parameters. Isodose distributions in transverse, coronal, and sagittal planes are printed. These should show the approved isodose distribution and the magnitude and location of hot spots. The use of heterogeneity corrections is documented. BEVs or, preferably, DRRs for each field are printed along with the corresponding MLC information if applicable. An orthogonal pair of DRRs can be printed to be used as a setup reference of the location of isocenter. Applicable DVHs should also be included in the documentation. Patient setup instructions should be clearly documented so that the position of the beams' isocenter and its relationship to patient markings are evident. Skin-rendering images (see Fig. 23.18) are often useful patient setup aids. If the patient is to be set up to original markings

and the isocenter is to be shifted to a new position, shift instructions should be clearly specified and properly verified. A record and verify system is highly recommended to be used because three-dimensional treatment plans are often complex and commonly have multiple beams with varying combinations of couch, gantry, and collimator positions.

The treatment plans of new patients should be verified as they are implemented clinically for the first time. As a part of the plan approval process for IMRT and VMAT plans, a phantom plan is generated. This type of plan transfers the beams that will be used for treatment into a plan that delivers the same treatment to a phantom. The plan is delivered to the phantom, and measurements are taken to ensure the doses can be delivered with the planned treatment parameters (i.e., MLC and intensity patterns). Treatment initiation is an extremely important last step of the planning process. Before delivery of the treatment, each field should be checked to ensure that there are no collisions between the machine and the treatment table or the patient. Beam paths are examined to ensure that the treatment couch does not adversely interfere with either beam delivery or portal imaging. Any delivery or imaging limitations should be identified and approved. Each field's blocks or MLC patterns are examined. DRRs should be used for comparisons with portal images. Patient SSDs are checked. The relationships between field blocking, collimator settings, and planned wedge orientations are also assessed. All documentation is reviewed to ensure consistent adherence to the plan. The treatment planning phase ends only when there is certainty that the plan can be consistently delivered accurately. Cone-beam CT scans are used to evaluate the position of the patient and internal structures and compare those with the treatment planning CT image. Clinics should establish guidelines to determine the policies for making shifts in patient setup.

▌ SUMMARY

The treatment planning process pulls together the entire radiation oncology team, both clinical and technical staffs. The sciences of radiation oncology, biology, therapy, dosimetry, and physics collaborate to optimize a patient's treatment. This chapter discussed the role of physics and dosimetry in the treatment planning process. The fundamental principles of photon beam treatment planning and the basics of the treatment planning process were described. Specifically addressed were the following points:

- Isodose distributions described, in graphic form, how radiation dose is deposited in an absorbing medium. In its simplest form, an isodose distribution describes the absorbed dose delivered to a rectangular phantom of water-equivalent material.
- Isodose distributions in a water phantom can be, and are, used to evaluate the characteristics of single beams of radiation. The effects of beam modifiers, such as wedges, can also be discerned.
- Combinations of multiple beams are also well characterized with isodose distributions.
- Corrections can be made to water phantom–based isodose distributions to account for the effects of patient contour irregularities and heterogeneous composition. These corrected dose distributions are then used to evaluate the appropriateness of a patient treatment plan.
- Treatment planning has evolved from a simple two-dimensional review of dose distributions to a process of identifying

three-dimensional target structures and OARs and then evaluating the three-dimensional dose to these volumes.

- Three-dimensional conformal radiation therapy has been made possible by the increased efficiency of three-dimensional dose calculation algorithms and by the increased capabilities of modern computer planning systems.
- Planning volumes have been precisely defined by the ICRU.
- Visualization tools have been packaged into software products collectively known as virtual simulation tools.
- Virtual simulation is the process by which a patient's treatment plan can be developed with the patient's CT data set—the "virtual patient." Targets and OARs are defined and visualized, and three-dimensional dose is evaluated.
- IMRT and VMAT treatment delivery with inverse planning has been introduced as an option. Treatment intent objectives are entered into the planning system, and intensity patterns are designed by the software.
- Dose prescriptions reflect dose to the PTV. OAR volume constraint guidelines have been identified with QUANTEC toxicity data.
- Treatment plan appropriateness is commonly evaluated with a tool known as the DVH. The DVH correlates target or organ volume to the dose received by that volume.
- Phantom plans have been introduced as a means for plan evaluation.

REVIEW QUESTIONS

The answers to the Review Questions can be found by logging on to our website at: http://evolve.elsevier.com/Washington/principles

1. Isodose distributions are _____-dimensional representations of the spatial distribution of dose.
   a. One.
   b. Two.
   c. Three.
   d. Four.

2. Wedged-field isodose distributions are characterized by increased radiation intensity under the _____ of the wedge.
   a. Heel (thicker portion).
   b. Toe (thinner portion).
   c. Both a and b.
   d. Neither a nor b.

3. Use of parallel-opposed fields only is contraindicated as beam energy _____ and patient thickness _____.
   a. Decreases; decreases.
   b. Increases; increases.
   c. Decreases; increases.
   d. Increases; decreases.

4. _____ corrections account for the dose effects produced by the presence of materials of density different from water or unit density.
   a. Homogeneity.
   b. Heterogeneity.
   c. Isocentric.
   d. None of the above.

5. In treatment planning, when dose delivery parameters are computed based on target dose delivery and normal tissue avoidance criteria, the process is termed _____ planning.
   a. Forward.
   b. Inverse.
   c. Reciprocal.
   d. Reverse.

6. IMRT is a treatment planning and delivery process that seeks to achieve treatment plan optimization by varying the _____ of treatment beams in addition to their position.
   a. Field size.
   b. Intensity.
   c. Area.
   d. Energy.

7. The CTV is a treatment planning volume that includes gross visible or palpable disease and _____ disease.
   a. Microscopic.
   b. Subclinical.
   c. Both a and b.
   d. Neither a nor b.

8. Image _____ is a process by which images produced by different modalities can be combined to use the best features of each modality.
   a. Production.
   b. Fusion.
   c. Manipulation.
   d. None of the above.

9. The quality of DRRs can be improved by _____ the thickness of CT slices.
   a. Increasing.
   b. Decreasing.
   c. Rotating.
   d. Multiplying.

10. A plan evaluation tool that simultaneously presents dose and volume information in a graphic form that allows objective plan assessment is the DVH.
    a. True.
    b. False.

QUESTIONS TO PONDER

1. The use of heterogeneity corrections in dose calculations is becoming more commonplace because these calculations are more accurate. Most clinical outcome data, on the other hand, are based on homogeneous dose calculations. What are the challenges associated with clinical heterogeneity correction implementation, if existing clinical outcomes data are to be preserved?

2. It is clear that use of the newer technology produces superior radiation dose distributions. It is also becoming apparent, however, that this technology comes at an increased cost in terms of resources needed per patient. How are these two apparently conflicting patient treatment perspectives to be reconciled?

3. Compromises between tumor control and normal tissue complication probabilities are often necessary in treatment planning. What factors need to be considered when these determinations are made?

4. Multimodality image fusion is becoming the standard of care for the definition of target volumes in specific disease sites. In what disease sites is multimodality fusion becoming the norm? What imaging modalities are commonly used, and why? Does the use of multimodality fusion affect traditional GTV to CTV expansions (margins)? Why?

5. Discuss the necessary features of an appropriate quality assurance review of a patient's treatment plan before initiation of treatment. Address in the discussion the specifics of ensuring that the prescription is fulfilled: dose to targets and OARs, appropriate transfer of information to the treatment unit, verification of position of anatomy, and so forth.

REFERENCES

1. Khan FM. *The Physics of Radiation Therapy.* 2nd ed. Baltimore, MD: Williams & Wilkins; 1994.
2. Bentel GC. *Radiation Therapy Planning.* 2nd ed. New York, NY: McGraw-Hill; 1996.
3. International Commission on Radiation Units and Measurements (ICRU). *Determination of Absorbed Dose in a Patient Irradiated by Beams of X or Gamma Rays in Radiotherapy Procedures.* Report 24, 1976. Bethesda, MD: ICRU.
4. International Electrotechnical Commission (IEC). *Medical Electron Accelerators—Functional Performance Characteristics.* Performance Standard 976, 1989. Geneva, Switzerland: IEC.
5. Varian Medical Systems. *C-Series Clinac: Enhanced Dynamic Wedge Implementation Guide.* Palo Alto, CA, 1996: Varian Medical Systems.
6. Perez CA, Brady LW. *Principles and Practice of Radiation Oncology.* Philadelphia, PA, 1998: Lippincott-Raven Publishers.
7. Hendee WR. *Medical Radiation Physics.* St. Louis, MO, 1970: Mosby.

8. Ten Haken RK, Kessler ML. 3-D RTP plan evaluation. In: Purdy JA, Starkschall G, eds. *A Practical Guide to 3D Planning and Conformal Radiation Therapy*. Madison, WI: Advanced Medical Publishing.

9. Anderson DW. *Absorption of Ionizing Radiation*. Baltimore, MD, 1984: University Park Press.

10. Starkschall G, Hogstrom KR. Dose-calculation algorithms used in 3-D radiation therapy treatment planning. In: Purdy JA, Starkschall G, eds. *A Practical Guide to 3-D Planning and Conformal Radiation Therapy*. Madison, WI, 1999: Advanced Medical Publishing.

11. Mackie TR, Liu HH, McCulough EC. Model-based photon dose calculation algorithms. In: Khan FM, Potish RA, eds. *Treatment Planning in Radiation Oncology*, 1998. Baltimore, MD: Williams & Wilkins.

12. International Commission on Radiation Units and Measurements (ICRU). *Prescribing, Recording, and Reporting Photon Beam Therapy*. Report 50. Bethesda, MD, 1993: ICRU.

13. Verhey L, Bentel G. Patient immobilization. In: Van Dyk J, ed. *The Modern Technology of Radiation Oncology*. Madison, WI, 1999: Medical Physics Publishing.

14. Antolak JA, Rosen II, Childress CH, et al. Prostate target volume variations during a course of radiotherapy. *Int J Radiat Oncol Biol Phys*. 1998;42:661–672.

15. Mohan R, Leibel SA, Pizzuto D, et al. Three-dimensional conformal radiotherapy. In: Khan FM, Potish RA, eds. *Treatment Planning in Radiation Oncology*. Baltimore, MD, 1998: Williams & Wilkins.

16. Coia LR, Schultheiss TE, Hanks GE. *A Practical Guide to CT Simulation*. Madison, WI, 1995: Advanced Medical Publishing.

17. Lawrence TS, Kessler ML, Ten Haken RK. Clinical interpretation of dose-volume histograms: the basis for normal tissue preservation and tumor dose escalation. In: Meyer JL, Purdy JA, eds. *3-D Conformal Radiotherapy*. Basel, Switzerland, 1996: Karger.

18. Bentzen SM, Constine LS, Deasy JO, et al. Quantitative analyses of normal tissue effects in the clinic (Quantec): an introduction to the scientific issues. *Int J Radiat Oncol Biol Phys*. 2010;76(suppl 3):S3–S9.

19. Wong JW, Purdy JA. On methods of inhomogeneity corrections for photon transport. *Med Phys*. 1990;17:807–814.

24

Electronic Charting and Image Management

Ana Weeks, Annette M. Coleman

OBJECTIVES

- Define electronic medical record (EMR).
- Identify the role of nonclinical information to the EMR.
- Define workflow and its role in the EMR.
- Describe unique aspects of radiation oncology necessitating a specialty EMR.
- Differentiate between proprietary and open standard communication protocols.

- Differentiate between connectivity and interoperability.
- Identify systems on which EMRs may be operated and the necessity for mechanisms securing system privacy, security, and stability.
- Discuss impact of human factors and EMR design on patient safety.
- State three potential goals of compilation of patient records.

OUTLINE

KEY TERMS

Analytics
Application service providers (ASPs)
Artificial intelligence
Biometric technology
Computerized physician online order entry (CPOE)
Connectivity
Data
Data mining
Digital Imaging and Communications in Medicine (DICOM)
Electronic health record (EHR)
Electronic medical record (EMR)
Electronic Prescribing (e-Prescribing or eRx)
Health Insurance Portability and Accountability Act of 1996 (HIPAA)

Information
Integrating the Healthcare Enterprise (IHE)
Interoperability
Medical informatics
Oncology information system (OIS)
Proprietary interface
Standards interface
Structured data
Usability
Use error
User interface
Workflow

INTRODUCTION

A medical record, or chart, chronicles the story of care for one patient. Essential for providers, the medical record serves a wider constituency, including referring clinicians and healthcare insurance carriers. It serves as documentation as to whether a patient received proper care in the event of litigation or as a source of information for retrospective research.[1]

Clinical care requires unambiguous information about a patient—information identifying the individual, their illness, comprehensive intervention plan, and response. Intensive coordination and communication must be managed across clinical and administrative teams, and the ability to interpret, apply, and author patient medical records is foundational to professional practice as a radiation therapist.[2,3]

Radiation oncology's unique information necessitates the existence of a radiation oncology–specific chart. Even when a clinic is housed within a larger institution, radiation oncology maintains an independent medical record designed to meet its distinct requirements. Led by the radiation oncologist, the care team, including radiation therapists, physicists, medical dosimetrists, nurses, tumor registrars, and administrative staff work together to execute a patient's treatment plan. Each caregiver is responsible for the development and character of a medical record, which unmistakably communicates an individual's treatment plan, execution of the plan, supportive care, and continuing patient status. Each contributes and applies shared information to deliver safe, efficient, and effective patient care. Errors, omissions, or otherwise poor documentation are potential sources of harm. Given the large number of handoffs and independent tasks that occur routinely during the planning and delivery of radiation therapy (RT), well-defined charting procedures, preferably electronic, are critical.[4]

With the information era came digitization of patient charting, the **electronic medical record (EMR)**. Capture of patient medical history in an EMR provides a foundation for improved safety and efficiency through fully informed decision-making. No longer tethered to a static form, the clinical care team can be provided with the most relevant information for the specific task or decision at hand. Facility operations, including demographic, scheduling, and billing, also came to leverage computerization to manage resources and processes. Awareness of efficiencies gained using these systems and universality of data across healthcare drove value into integration of the EMR with practice management systems. Thus, the radiation oncology EMR typically functions within a larger oncology information system (OIS). OISs facilitate data and information flow between administrative functions and medical equipment such as linear accelerators or treatment planning systems in addition to systems outside the specialty clinic.

A data-intensive medical specialty, oncologic care improves through study of past practices. Computerization offers potential beyond managing individual care and healthcare's response as the explosion of data in the modern age continues. Knowledge regarding cancer, an individual's diagnosis, and options for treatment are growing exponentially. An opportunity available today, artificial intelligence (AI), combs the breadth of published information presenting findings of relevance to the clinician. With such potential, the specialty EMR forms a comprehensive hub for information management in the modern radiation oncology facility.

Origins

The history of medical practice is one of leaps and incremental evolution. Hippocrates is credited with establishing medicine as a scientific practice based on observation and case recording. Observations, recorded in a purely chronological manner, created a time-oriented medical record. The model persisted, and physician records remained largely isolated, one-to-one chronicles of a caregiver regarding each patient. Centuries later, at the Mayo Clinic in Rochester, Minnesota, physicians forming the first group medical practice initially kept such individual records of patient encounters, making coordination of care difficult. In 1907, the Mayo Clinic pioneered the concept of one file for each *patient* with contributions across multiple clinicians, creating the patient-centered medical record. Although this system was an improvement, records continued to be somewhat disorganized, a mixture of notes, complaints, test results, and physician opinion on findings. In the 1960s, Lawrence Weed, MD, introduced standardization of patient records within a problem-oriented structure. SOAP, which stands for Subjective, Objective, Assessment, and Plan, created a better method to document the line of reasoning for diagnosis and treatment of patient problems.[5]

Growth of medical knowledge and increasing range of clinical specialties allow patients to consume care from a broad range of providers. As a result, there are generally as many medical records for an individual as there are specialties involved in his or her treatment. In such an ecosystem, reliance on hard copy systems poses persistent limitations to meeting healthcare objectives. When clinicians want to form a complete picture about a patient's health, they must consult records that are kept by other individuals or institutions. Paper records posed persistent limitations, handwriting may be poor or illegible, data missing, or notes too ambiguous to support interpretation. Manual searching for relevant information during the patient encounter and energy expended on the search rather than in the application of information is counterproductive. Access is limited to one person at a time, and such access must be on location. Paper records require physical storage space and must be organized for ready access. Security is limited, without the ability to log record of who accessed sensitive personal information or when. Paper is not a durable media and is susceptible to both water and fire. Records are often lost or missing, and backup of paper-based records is unwieldy, requiring time and resource-intensive effort to maintain.[5]

In contrast, an EMR captures, aggregates, and presents information relevant to patient care for a clinical group in digital form. Information can be legibly presented in varied contexts and disseminated within and between systems. The EMR may be defined as an application or applications in an environment composed of a clinical data repository, clinical decision support system, controlled medical vocabulary, computerized provider order entry, pharmacy, and clinical documentation applications. Patients' EMRs are supported across inpatient and outpatient environments, used by healthcare practitioners to document, monitor, and manage care delivery within the care facility. The data in the EMR are the legal record of what happened to the patient during encounters at the care facility.[6]

Sometimes confused with the provider centric EMR, the promise of electronic health records (EHRs) is mobility and sharing of an individual's overall health information across and between authorized individuals or facilities, with the patient controlling access to information. Although EMRs are computerized legal clinical records created in an individual care facility, the concept of the EHR proposes the ability to easily share a subset of medical information within a community, region, or state (or in some areas, the entire country). Beneficiaries include patients, healthcare providers, employers, and payers, including the government. For example, EHRs reduce repetitive testing and reduce time accessing critical information such as allergies or blood type in emergencies. Before effective EHRs are possible, however, provider organizations must not only install but effectively integrate complete EMR systems into their practices.

COMPUTERIZATION, THE EARLY ELECTRONIC MEDICAL RECORD

Radiation oncology adopted computerization early. Complex treatment planning and treatment delivery requirements drove advances in algorithms and necessitated technology integration. While optimization of planning and delivery systems progressed, EMR adoption struggled with overcoming legal and communication continuity concerns; thus, reliance on paper records predominated well into the first decade of the new millennium.

> EMR systems contain a record of all clinical, administrative, treatment planning, and laboratory encounters between a patient and a provider, including physician notes, examination results, billing and insurance information, and other related patient data typically linked with a unique patient identifier.

Governments globally recognized benefits and risks associated with data exchange and aggregation and increasingly enticed electronic charting adoption through legislation. The United States, for example, enacted the Health Information Technology for Economic and Clinical Health Act in 2009, providing incentives for EMR implementations. A set of standards defined by the Centers for Medicare & Medicaid Services incentive programs, Meaningful Use, governed the use of EHRs and allowed eligible providers and hospitals to earn incentive payments by meeting specific criteria.[7] The goal of Meaningful Use was to promote the spread of EHRs to improve healthcare in the United States.

In 2015, the US Health and Human Services demonstrated continuing commitment to improving healthcare delivery and information sharing through EMRs with the Medicare Access and CHIP Reauthorization Act (MACRA). MACRA changed the programs measuring and incentivizing EMR use by physicians under a new Merit-based Incentive Payment System (MIPS).[8]

Analog Imitation

As data sources expanded from treatment planning and treatment delivery systems to hospital information systems and external physicians or facilities such as laboratories or pharmacies, changing actual practice remained challenging. Familiarity initially won over radiation oncology EMR early adopters. Clinicians looked for information organized and displayed similarly to existing paper and film records (Fig. 24.1). Image

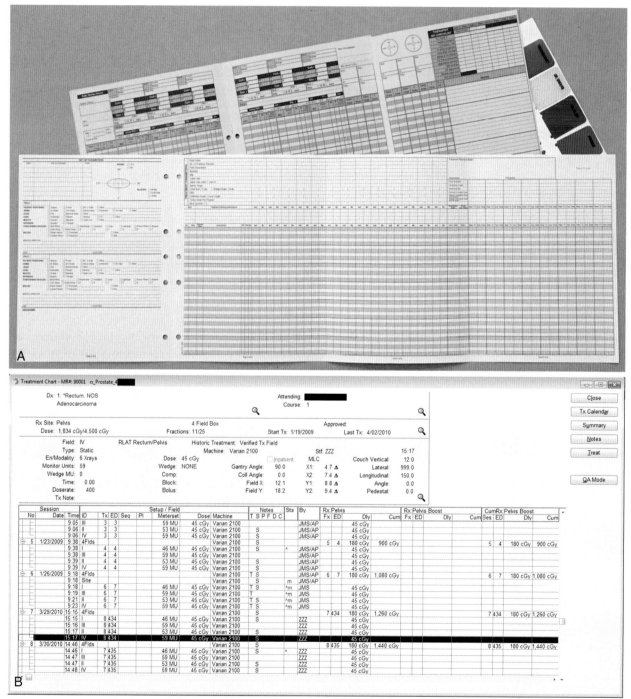

Fig. 24.1 Daily treatment record. (A) Paper 'trifold." (B) Electronic medical record corollary.

review mimicked traditional film and lightbox evaluation of treatment verification imaging. A high dependency on hard copy printouts and handwritten signatures persisted. The validity and legal security of electronic signatures was highly scrutinized. The advantages of information presentation in problem-oriented views and selectively presenting complex information applicable to a specific clinical focus or task remained underdeveloped. Simple alerting functions and concurrent access to information was most prized.

Workflow

Data on its own has little purpose or meaning. Presenting the right data in the right context generates information. Information fuels decision-making and activity coordination. More than a data repository, the EMR is a primary communication tool for the radiation oncology team. The EMR informs clinical tasks and workflows. Workflow is defined as sets of actions performed to generate results. Workflow management through contextual presentation of data may be the most defining feature of the EMR (Fig. 24.2).

Workflows may be described at very high levels, such as the general path a patient takes moving through the clinic, or very specific procedures such as the steps followed when the therapist tattoos a patient. Workflows may be simple, involving few steps or decisions, or very complex, with changing pathways as each decision is made. They may involve one or several individuals working at the same time or may require information passing between individuals who are separated by time or location.

A workflow example and core EMR component, computerized physician online order entry tracks and documents the entire clinical order process, from entry to return of results. A relatively linear process, one action follows another—the physician enters an order, another team member executes the order, and results are recorded. Many caregivers interact with the system, executing and documenting completion of tasks. Human hand offs are minimized, resulting in improved compliance and efficiency gains. For example, medication may be ordered using electronic prescribing (e-Prescribing or eRx), which writes and transmits medication orders. Computerization of this process improves efficiency and safety with the ability to include checks on drug interactions, patient health information such as allergies, and elimination of legibility risks associated with handwritten orders.

The typical series of events for the radiation oncology patient includes:

- consultation
- decision to treat
- simulation
- verification of treatment plan
- treatment delivery
- monitoring of response
- follow-up

Each event is further supported by complex processes involving information shared between the patient care team. On consultation, the oncology nurse may perform an initial functional assessment including vital signs and weight. The radiation oncologist, possibly with the assistance of a resident, a physician's assistant, or nurse practitioner, follows with an examination and so on. As is clear in the clinic, each of these events includes complex subevents with decision points, information moving in and out to proceed to the subsequent phases (Fig. 24.3).

How each event is executed will be designed to meet the specific needs of an individual facility and will change over time. Traditional records are relatively static and not responsive to changing workflows. Changing technology itself impacts process; the EMR's goal is not to replicate past practice—it is to optimize efficiency and accuracy through process formalization and single-source data capture. Electronic charts increasingly provide flexibility to rapidly adapt to evolving workflow and information needs.

Adoption/Continuing Use

Despite broad agreement on the benefits of EHRs and other forms of health information technology (IT), healthcare providers moved slowly to adopt these technologies. Lack of readiness caused weakness in organizations to undergo transformation during implementation.[9]

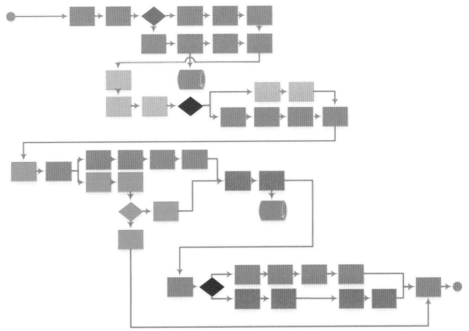

Fig. 24.2 Workflow diagramming.

Organizational transformation is very difficult. Twenty years ago, John Kotter reported the failure rate at around 70%. Major change also takes a long time to implement, usually between 5 and 7 years on average. In healthcare, change is even harder than in most industries. Although a desperate need for change and organizational performance improvement may be obvious to administration, clinical staff can view that premise as a threat.[32]

The EMR itself is only a tool to facilitate the process of patient care. Without a detailed understanding of clinical process, the transition was fraught with obstacles and challenges, and imitation and digitization of paper-analogous practices persisted for many years. Eventually, EMR champions and visionaries emerged for radiation oncology. Some organizations employed systems analysts to forward EMR selection and implementation. More frequently, existing clinical team members developed and applied the system analyst skill set. Charting practices and information flow across a facility were critically examined to identify opportunities to exploit the transformative technology.

A systems analyst evaluates patterns of information use and provides objective insight. They coordinate resources and often remain with the organization throughout the entire change process to manage purchases, installations, and workspace layouts; to produce new policies and procedures; and to measure results. Systems analysts perform the complex task of analyzing activities in an organization to precisely determine what must be accomplished and how it must be accomplished. The systems analyst may supervise or even have primary responsibility for system management, designing, implementing, and maintaining software configuration settings or configurable components.

EHR use requires the presence of certain user and system attributes, support from others, and numerous organizational and environment facilitators. Along with choosing the right EMR technology solution, the foundation for any successful implementation begins with involving stakeholders and developing a solid plan in advance. A team of key stakeholders (champions) who can establish and promote a long-range vision aligned with the goals of various constituencies and those of

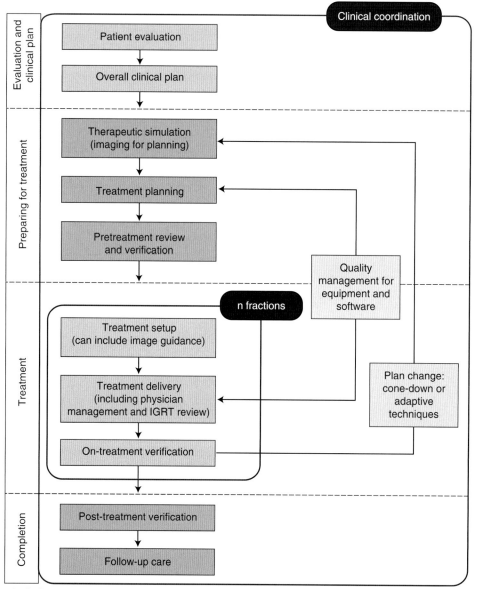

Fig. 24.3 Care process for external beam radiation therapy. *IGRT,* Image-guided radiation therapy. (From American Society of Radiation Oncology. *Safety is No Accident: A Framework for Quality Radiation Oncology and Care.* Albuquerque, NM: American Society of Radiation Oncology; 2012.)

the organization is the first step of implementation. A champion team should be truly cross-functional, representing each role in the department, and should thoroughly investigate current critical processes and develop expertise in the new technology to produce transition plans that fit with the organization. It should also examine adoption barriers with the goal of diminishing their effect, commit to bidirectional communication of plans and concerns, and provide and accept as much training as possible. Also critical is appointing clinical super users devoted to supporting others throughout the system implementation and into the early months of use.[10]

RADIATION ONCOLOGY ELECTRONIC MEDICAL RECORDS

A radiation oncology EMR is maintained independent of a hospital's charting records to capture radiation treatment rationale, objectives, delivery, and supporting care provided by the specialty facility.

Radiation Treatment: Verify and Record

As linear accelerator capabilities and treatment plans increased in complexity, limitations of traditional paper records became clear. The number of individual machine parameters became too large to manually set, confirm, and chart in the treatment history. When planned treatment machine settings are entered once to the EMR, they may then be represented across as many contexts as the information is needed. The radiation therapist applies them to assure accuracy in treatment setup and delivery. The physicist is assured the same parameters they authorized are applied at treatment and may review any deviations that took place. Following treatment, the physician has access to the summary of dose delivered using those settings.

Verify and record (V&R) systems assist and validate execution of a treatment plan as intended. Actual machine settings are compared against those most recently prescribed and prevent initiation of the treatment beam if settings vary outside a specified tolerance range. Settings during beam on are documented, including deviations from those planned. Machine parameters monitored include meterset (e.g., monitor units or time), gantry position, collimator and aperture settings, table position, arc versus fixed treatment, and use of beam modifiers. V&R systems can extend verification beyond the treatment machine, from patient identification to communication with secondary equipment attached to, but not integrated with, the treatment machine itself. Treatment sequences may be defined, automating treatment field selection and parameter setup.

Providing significant functionality to aid in the accurate and efficient delivery of RT, V&R, like the EMR, changed the medium but not the requirements of treatment delivery charting. The patient's complete course of external beam RT is defined and recorded online for access at any time, but the accuracy of the record remains the responsibility of each professional contributing to its development. Data are confirmed at entry, always associated with a login and often with password-protected electronic signatures. Questioning and reviewing information at the time of data entry and on a regular schedule through the treatment course remains a critical radiation therapist responsibility.

Imaging and the Radiation Oncology Electronic Medical Record

As complex imaging functions made their way to the megavoltage therapy room, so did demand for digital imaging. Radiation oncology heavily invests in imaging, from diagnosis to planning to treatment execution. From patient identification and treatment setup photographs to sophisticated planar and volumetric medical imaging, image-enabling radiation oncology EMRs produced more comprehensive care records

and optimized treatment planning and delivery workflow. With diagnostic and planning images readily transferable between systems, treatment accuracy and communication among the treatment team improve significantly. Advanced functions such as image registration and fusion provide rapid, accurate assessment of setup deviations, enabling increased precision in treatment technique.

ACCESS AND MOBILITY

EMR adoption changed information access expectations. The constraints of one hard copy in hand, on clinic premises, are undone. With digitization, concurrent access across a care team is possible, and a clinic's physical confines become virtual. Clinical decision making and care quality and efficiency improve as information regarding a patient and a facility is available when and where the care team needs it. Access to the EMR is limited only by the nature of the system on which it is installed and authorization of its users.

Patient safety and legal requirements dictate patient information access be secure, stable, and dependable. The complexity and criticality of the EMR's functions and the technical infrastructure to support them necessitate IT expertise. With responsibilities from installation and maintenance of secure IT networks, to organizing human and technical considerations for large-scale upgrades, to ensuring the EMR is used efficiently by clinicians and staff, IT departments employ professionals whose skill sets range from hardware and network management to systems analysts.

Traditional radiation oncology EMR hosting exists on a computer server connected to client workstations. A local area network (LAN) suffices for self-contained facilities, whereas multiple locations may be joined through a wired wide area network (WAN), enabling each location use of the same main server. WAN functional operation may be assisted at remote locations by "thin clients," software and equipment reducing network traffic, improving the experience of those using the system.

Increasing mobility demand in healthcare requires secure wireless network access. A wireless LAN (WLAN) provides the most common connection within buildings, supporting secure mobile connectivity to core business functions such as charting and facility management applications. Mobile technologies, such as laptops, smartphones, and tablets, connect and communicate via wireless access points, which are in turn connected to the building's hard-wired network. A WLAN requires appropriate hardware administration and security systems for protecting private patient information. Separate wireless networks can be broadcasted to allow patient and family members to connect to the internet within a building while maintaining security of clinical information. Connectivity across a WLAN network is limited to the areas covered by installed access points. Transmissions from various devices, however, can create interference, and walls can cause connection loss or create gaps in wireless coverage, interfering with reliability and availability of the network. It should be noted that the location and layout for radiation oncology centers may necessitate installing higher than average numbers of access points accommodating presence of shielded vaults (treatment rooms).

Wireless access can be extended further via mobile broadband, or cellular, services, allowing doctors and staff members secure access to patient information from a remote location—clinic, home office, or patient home. Public data networks operated by cellular service providers, eliminating hardware administration and management. A wireless network is delivered to users of smartphones and other handheld devices directly, allowing for mobility, portability, and remote access. Mobile operations or tasks operate most successfully when designed for specific tasks and the smaller format of a mobile device; for example, home health nurses use tablet devices to access patient records and test results securely, without having to connect to a wireless network.

As the complexity of maintaining networks strains resources, dedicated application service providers (ASPs) emerged, offering contracts to house and maintain healthcare organizations' EMRs in data centers with the clinic owning their data and leasing EMR licenses instead of installing them locally. With this model, IT expertise specific to the hosted products and optimal hardware are continually maintained with secure web access to the EMR assured by the ASP provider. From the point of view of the end user, models such as SaaS and "Cloud" function similarly[11]; technical distinctions are beyond the scope of this chapter. Regardless of hosting environment, EMR software is distributed to end user equipment, including laptops, stand-alone computers, and portable devices.

Connectivity and Interoperability

A patient's story forms from data collected outside and within the radiation oncology department. EMRs and EHRs can improve preventive medicine, patient-provider communication, and positive drug interactions as well as offer increased transparency and communication through patient portals. However, many blame systems for sucking the personal touch out of medicine and making many doctors feel like little more than data entry clerks.

Reliable data exchange between information systems improve EMR quality and clinic efficiency. Single points of data entry and electronic data transfer save time and reduce errors. Information ranging from demographics to concurrent medical state to laboratory, pathology, or imaging examination reports can be available on patient referral to the radiation oncology department. Information also flows outbound, requesting diagnostic examinations, supporting reimbursement claims, or communicating with external physicians and facilities.

Linking systems clearly improves information reliability and safety by eliminating the need to duplicate data entry, but this process is more complicated than it might seem. Although two systems may present similar information, underlying data might not match. Where a caregiver might interpret information presented in different formats, computers require explicit instructions to equate and transfer like information.

Multiple interfaces and interface models operate in healthcare to improve efficiency of systems and workflow. Interfaces common to radiation oncology practice include proprietary interfaces and standard-based interfaces such as HL7 (Health Level 7) and Digital Imaging and Communications in Medicine (DICOM).

Proprietary interface protocols are written and owned by private or commercial entities. In the absence or insufficiency of national or international standards, proprietary interface protocols provide much-needed tools for sharing data. These protocols may be retained for exclusive use or published for integration by others. In radiation oncology, innovative leaps and niche development evolve faster than community standards can be agreed upon, assuring an ongoing role for open proprietary interfaces, particularly for connectivity to treatment delivery devices. Community expectations encourage continued manufacturer sharing of interface specifications and maintenance of interoperability to meet clinician needs.

Drawbacks of proprietary protocols include duplication of effort when solving common problems in unique ways. Proprietary systems can be wasteful of time and resources during development and can add difficulty for users who must understand the variety of capabilities and operating procedures of resulting systems. These systems also offer little progress toward solving overriding difficulties of universal data access. Although proprietary interfaces remain widely in use in RT, the desire to streamline process from decision to planning to treatment, as

well as efforts to collect and analyze treatment information from clinical trials, drive expectations for interface standardization. Proprietary protocols may become or provide a basis for industry standards.

Standards interface specifications are generally developed by national and international committees accredited by organizations such as the American National Standards Institute (ANSI) or the International Standards Organization. Wide representation from the industry for which interoperability standards are being designed is included. Standards are subsequently published in the public domain. Agreement can be a long process, and latitude in interpretation persists. Commercial interfaces using standards often require compliance statements describing in detail how a system adheres to the published standard. Standard interfaces offer efficient development and vendor independence as connectivity requires less interaction between developers.

HL7 is an ANSI-accredited organization developing standards for exchanging clinical and administrative data. HL7 interfaces enable a single point of entry, including updates and corrections, for clinical and administrative (admission, transfer, demographics) patient data, and are useful across the entire healthcare facility. Information propagates throughout the connected organization. Specifically, HL7 defines a comprehensive framework and standards for the exchange, integration sharing, and retrieval of electronic health information that supports clinical practice and the management, delivery, and evaluation of healthcare services.[12]

> Founded in 1987, HL7 International is a not-for-profit organization dedicated to providing a framework and related standards for the exchange, integration, sharing, and retrieval of electronic health information that supports clinical practice and the management, delivery, and evaluation of health services. HL7 is supported by more than 1600 members from over 50 countries, including over 500 corporate members representing healthcare providers, government stakeholders, payers, pharmaceutical companies, vendors/suppliers, and consulting firms.[12]

FHIR (Fast Healthcare Interoperability Resources) is a next generation from HL7. HL7 has the underpinnings of the healthcare industry but requires a high level of configuration and can be costly and complex to implement. FHIR incorporates the best of HL7 while leveraging the latest web standards and applying a tight focus on implementation.[13] FHIR improves security and offers a more strongly defined model with easier customization.[14]

DICOM is the international standard for medical images and related information sharing. Whereas HL7 or FHIR facilitate transfer of general clinical and administrative patient data, DICOM standards address radiology and radiation oncology needs. Produced by a joint committee of the National Electrical Manufacturers Association and the American College of Radiology, DICOM initially facilitated distribution of diagnostic image–defined information.

In response to image-based volumetric treatment planning in radiation oncology, DICOM published the RT extension (DICOM RT) in 1996, adding volumetric and projection images, image segmentations, treatment plans, volumetric doses, and treatment delivery records. DICOM RT promised RT manufacturer a means to concentrate on a single internationally accepted format for connectivity.[15,16]

DICOM 3 describes each type of information that may be transferred. These information types describe formats for the exchange of image or textural information. The following are examples used in RT:

- RT image—conventional and virtual simulation images, digitally reconstructed radiographs, or portal images
- RT dose—dose distributions, isodose lines, dose-volume histograms
- RT structure set—volumetric contours drawn from computed tomography (CT) images

- RT plan—text information describing treatment plans including prescriptions and fractionation, beam definitions, and so forth
- RT beams and RT brachytherapy—treatment session reports for external beam or brachytherapy, may be used as part of a V&R system
- RT treatment summary—cumulative summary information, may be used after treatment to send information to a hospital EMR

DICOM's Radiotherapy Working Group's primary goal is enabling departmental workflow, improving safety through tighter standard definition, and opening DICOM to new technologies and processes in RT. Although DICOM RT addressed early treatment planning needs, the evolution of RT procedures and techniques is pushing existing boundaries. The working group is responding with second-generation radiotherapy definitions.[18] As this is a work in progress, objects are undergoing major rework adding treatment modalities, equipment, and techniques, such as adaptive RT.

It might seem, given open systems connectivity specifications, information transfer would be seamless, but connectivity does not guarantee ease of use between systems with different purposes. Although connectivity standards form a basis for information exchange between systems gaps, options and differing interpretations must be bridged. Integrating the Healthcare Enterprise (IHE) combines and interprets standards consistently, providing interoperability "maps" to clinical workflow objectives and the means for manufacturers to independently demonstrate compliance.[19] Formed in the late 1990s, IHE's mission was to improve interoperability between computerized systems in diagnostic radiology, expanding to almost a dozen specialty domains.

As connectivity improved in radiation oncology, expectations for productivity assistance and safety assurances developed. In 2004, the IHE for Radiation Oncology (IHE-RO) formed. Composed of leading radiation oncology professionals, international standards organizations, and industry representatives, IHE-RO defines "Integration Profiles" solving requirements for sharing data between component systems of a clinical workflow. Through coordinated use of established standards, particularly HL7 and DICOM, data entered once flows between CT, treatment planning, the EMR, and the linear accelerator. Manufacturers build products meeting requirements and gather in meetings called "Connectathons," where they test and refine interoperability. Once a product is successfully validated, vendors are then entitled to participate in demonstrations for the clinical community, typically held at major clinical association meetings.

With heavy reliance on specialized systems for planning and delivery, radiation oncology benefits greatly from IHE involvement. IHE-RO helps to ensure safe, efficient radiation treatments by improving system-to-system connections. It provides a platform for the radiation oncology team, administrators, and industry representatives to address these issues and develop solutions that ensure the clinic is delivering the most optimal care.

> See the following websites for more information on HL7 or FHIR (http://www.hl7.org), IHE (http://www.ihe.net), and DICOMRT (http://medical.nema.org).

Portability, Security, and Privacy

EMRs must incorporate the following components within their system security policies and procedures[20]:

- authorization
- authentication
- availability
- confidentiality
- data integrity
- nonrepudiation

Access to view and enter any personal data must be restricted to qualified and authorized individuals. Passwords are currently the most common method of restricting access to the electronic chart and are used in conjunction with security privileges; individuals may be assigned access to only portions of the chart necessary to performance in their role. Password security guidelines are designed to enforce sufficient uniqueness and complexity to avoid improper impersonation and may be extended to include biometric technology such as fingerprint, retinal scanning, or facial recognition for further security.

Sharing digital patient records across systems increases the potential to make private information accessible to unauthorized viewers, risking individual harm should it be used to make unfair employment, insurance coverage, or other decisions. Medical electronic information systems, like other computer systems, can be vulnerable to security breaches, potentially impacting the safety and effectiveness of the system. This vulnerability increases as medical devices are increasingly connected to the Internet, hospital networks, and to other medical devices.[21]

Although the ability to transfer large amounts of electronic data from one system to another holds great promise for streamlining healthcare and supporting clinical decision making, transferred data must be secured during transfer and accurately assigned in the receiving system.

The US Food and Drug Administration (FDA) issued final guidance on the postmarket cybersecurity of medical devices, outlining important steps that hospitals, clinics, and others must take to better protect patient data and keep patients safe. The FDA recommendations to medical device manufacturers and healthcare facilities to ensure appropriate safeguards for mitigating and managing cybersecurity threats include:

- Manufacturers are responsible for remaining vigilant about identifying risks and hazards associated with their medical devices, including risks related to cybersecurity. They are responsible for putting appropriate mitigations in place to address patient safety risks and ensure proper device performance.
- Hospitals and healthcare facilities should evaluate their network security and protect their hospital systems.[21]

Interest is increasing in the security of electronic medical information, or patient health information, that is digitally stored. Sometimes this information needs to be accessed, helping physicians to make the best decisions about patient care. Patients have the right to determine how and when their health information is shared. To facilitate the exchange of electronic patient information while protecting patient privacy, the US Congress passed the Health Insurance Portability and Accountability Act of 1996 (HIPAA). Regulations are developed under the provisions of this act to standardize information sets for healthcare reimbursement and to restrict access to the minimum needed to provide care. In general, access to information that is identifiable to an individual is restricted except to those caregivers to whom the patient has given consent. In addition to ethical obligations, breaching confidentiality of patient records now carries substantial legal consequences for the individual and the institution. Full disclosure is extended when the purpose of disclosure is to provide treatment decision making. Certain exceptions are included in the regulations for public health needs, certain law enforcement activities, general oversight of care (i.e., quality assurance procedures), and some research activities.[22]

Disaster Recovery

When the patient record is maintained electronically and critical systems such as V&R system are integrated, its continuous availability becomes integral to providing radiation oncology care. System administrators must defend against various threats providing fault tolerance for their systems (duplicated hardware, data archives, power and networking systems), physical safety of servers, and preventative virus and intrusion detection.[20]

Regardless of the network type and the location of the system, automatic and secure backup of file servers is essential to protecting patient records. EMR backup can be performed locally for rapid recovery, but full remote or online storage of backups is also appropriate or even required. Disasters in the United States, such as Hurricanes Katrina (2005) and Sandy (2012) proved the value of electronic systems' ability to support rapid resumption of patient treatment following devastation that would have made inaccessible, or even destroyed, hard copy records.[23]

The most effective backup protocol is a combination of two options, with automated online EMR backup software being one of the choices to protect your EMRs. An appropriate backup software must be HIPAA compliant, and the providers must be able to outline a detailed disaster recovery plan that ensure a speedy recovery after a disaster.[6]

ELECTRONIC MEDICAL RECORDS, THE NEXT GENERATION

User Interface, Human Factors, and Safety

The medical record, in any form, remains the clinician communication hub and thus is fundamental to patient care quality. Early EMRs reproduced familiar paper processes facilitating healthcare's transition to electronic charting. As software use norms evolved in every aspect of modern life, so, too, did expectations grow for data management and information presentation by the modern EMR. Given the data-intensive nature of radiation oncology, the necessity of selective and malleable information presentation increasingly challenges software design. Too much information clutters without improving decisions, whereas too little slows process completion as one searches elsewhere. Safety and efficiency improve as information required for a specific task distinctly presents from the general clinical picture. Consider setup verification as an opportunity for context-sensitive presentation in radiation oncology. Online verification imaging executed by a radiation therapist "standing" at the treatment machine before treatment depends primarily on active treatment session information and a limited set of tools, whereas offline, away from the treatment machine, the "sitting down" clinician frequently explores patterns of assessment more deeply using a full set of tools and patient data. Past imaging session data and trend analysis tools may be available "one click" away from the active screen.

User interface refers to graphic, textual, and auditory information presentation and the input methods employed by a person operating the program. Quite simply, it's a program's look and feel. Interface design influences perceptions of information and product quality. Usability describes how well target users accomplish intended purpose in the context of expected use, measured by efficiency, effectiveness, and satisfaction. EMR usability is the degree to which the design fits into the overall patient visit and the logic required to determine how to use it. The experience includes effort required for accurate interpretation, data input, and learning required to achieve both. The extent that usability is considered in the design of the system will have a significant effect on satisfaction.

Complexity and frequent hand offs preparing and delivering radiation treatment position the EMR squarely on the information trajectory. Thus, EMR design directly impacts radiation oncology patient safety. In any system, mistakes are inevitable. Technology provides important solutions to improving quality of care, yet technology changes the way work is performed and may introduce unintended new forms of error. Operators may adapt intended workflows to unique situations, or a single error in data entry might be propagated across an entire interconnected system, making it more difficult to detect and correct. Human-to-software interaction is just one layer of complex human interactions in healthcare delivery.[24] A primary EMR design objective is uncovering and limiting potential error sources.

Patient safety necessitates EMR design where levels of defense are identified and mitigated, not overlooked or bypassed, so treatment is delivered as intended. Uncovering potential sources of error is a complex process involving humans with ingenuity to adapt tools from their designed purposes. Human factors engineering (HFE) or usability engineering (UE) is a science including methods and tools helping healthcare teams and manufacturers perform patient safety analyses, such as root cause analyses. The literature on HFE over several decades contains theories and applied studies to help to solve difficult patient safety problems and design issues.

Usability testing measures more than consumer satisfaction with a user interface. The FDA requires software manufacturers provide evidence of systematic HFE/UE integration in design and testing of software products. HFE strives to eliminate use errors, particularly those with potential impact on patient safety. Use error is an action or lack of action differing from manufacturer expectations causing a result that (1) differs from the result expected by the user, (2) was not caused solely by device failure, and (3) did or could result in harm.[25]

One familiar human factors model, the Swiss cheese model of organizational accidents, hypothesizes that in any system, there are many levels of defense. Each of these levels of defense has little "holes" in it that are caused by poor design, senior management decision-making, procedures, lack of training, limited resources, etc. (Fig. 24.4). Often, multiple mitigations are necessary to effectively reduce overall risk, particularly in increasingly complex systems such as healthcare.[26] See Chapter 18 for more information.

The most reliable software mitigations cannot be overlooked, overridden, or worked around. Forcing functions, computerized automation, human-machine, or machine-machine redundant checks block users from proceeding or otherwise prevent incorrect actions. Somewhat reliable mitigations include prompts for user actions, checklists, reminders, multiuser confirmations, and forced pauses, such as The Joint Commission's "Time Out." Least reliable mitigations depend on education, training, or rules, policies, and procedures.[27]

Automation/Workflow Engines

As discussed earlier an efficient way of cutting down on patient safety issues is to eliminate repetitive manual entry. Manual entry can become a risk factor as distracted therapists and physicians can enter incorrect information into systems, leading to ordering errors and misinformation. Designing technology capable of entering data automatically removes the possibility for human error that often leads to additional costs and patient harm. This kind of automation also takes data entry off the provider's plate, freeing up time for physicians and therapists to focus more on patient care.[28]

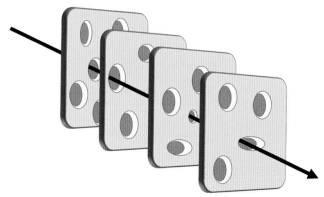

Fig. 24.4 Swiss cheese risk management model. (From Reason J: A system approach to organizational error. *Ergonomics* 38:1708-1721, 2005.)

Workflow engines and software automating repetitive tasks present yet another tool improving efficiency and reducing errors. A workflow engine automation uses preset rules specifying how tasks are to flow from one stage to another and then executes steps, pushing actions from one stage to the next. Note that the workflow engine does not make independent decisions; rather, it takes its direction from the workflow design.

Medical Informatics

Clinical decision making integrates clinical circumstances with practitioner knowledge and experience and patient preference. Options and decisions are based on historical knowledge of the disease's natural history and current understanding of available treatment interventions. Standards of care derive from compiling the customs and behavior of the members of the profession, and they reflect a consensus of how the profession is to be practiced. Standards cannot be fixed but must adapt to incorporate newly determined therapies and may define acceptable scales for judging individual variations. As treatment choices evolve, new information feeds continual improvement in care. The ability to review information across large populations can lead to in-depth analysis. Therefore, a course of care for an individual has the potential to contribute to our collective knowledge for future patients.

Optimal clinical decisions depend on optimal information and accessible and accurate analysis of patterns of care and outcomes. Systematic collection of the actions and responses of individuals contribute to collective knowledge, advancing care quality for future patients. Medical informatics optimizes organization, analysis, management, and use of healthcare information. The goal of informatics is to enable organizations to make more informed decisions based on data they have gathered. Computerization provides informatics a framework, and the EMR provides tools, accelerating information compilation and analysis. The challenge to optimize individual patient care is integral to ongoing EMR evolution.

The capture of the individual patient story may be effectively documented in several ways. Narratives, freely written stories, are the most flexible data entry method for clinical observations. Documents may be scanned, converting text into images. These simple methods for capturing patient encounters may add large amounts of data to a chart without adding equivalent information, and important details can be lost, buried within superfluous details. Freeform data also hinder analytics, as discrete information is difficult to compile across records. In contrast, explicit data entry—structured data—facilitates EMR presentation of the right data for a given patient care context and data integrity for later analysis and research (Fig. 24.5). Structured data will invariably facilitate better coordinated care for patients. It is the only way that physicians can truly "speak a common language" from physician to physician, between hospital departments, and even between health systems. It is truly the backbone to a world where a patient's complete health record can be shared and coordinated. Second, structured data will set the stage for big data and predictive health analytics. EHRs have the power to capture incredible amounts of data. So much data, in fact, which, if structured properly, we can begin to track, monitor, and even predict health outcomes.[29]

Data compilation measuring quality of care and clinical research is much more readily accomplished with computerized systems than through retrospective paper chart reviews, and organizations are collecting ever more data from their EMRs. Health systems have done a great job of acquiring data. But for the most part, the data just sit in a dark warehouse without creating value for those who store it.[30] Buried inside these mountains of data are veins of information that can uncover customer satisfaction, find the cause of errors for future prevention, fine-tune relationships with patients, and identify potential new business. Data mining can overcome many of the limitations of traditional statistics, discovering information and turning them into action. New hypotheses can be generated, observational studies conducted more rapidly, and clinical trial recruitment and conduct greatly facilitated. Such enhancements will be accomplished through secondary use of EMR data for research and the development of automated decision support systems that rely on EMR data.[31]

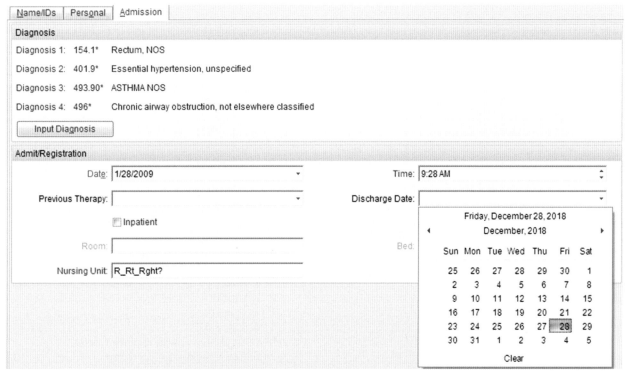

Fig. 24.5 Structured data, reusable and reducing ambiguity, in contrast to free-text sample entry.

The ability to review information across large populations can lead to in-depth analysis. Integration with clinical research systems has the potential to greatly enhance the efficiency, speed, and safety of cancer research. By providing links to research groups and literature sources, decision support systems aid the clinician by applying rules to the data collected and suggesting care actions. As recommendations are applied to an individual treatment plan, specific risks and response norms can be flagged for attention when the patient's response is inconsistent with expectations.

As the knowledge base for cancer management grows, accessibility to information becomes increasingly critical to the decision-making process of defining an individual course of treatment. EMRs increasingly integrate **AI** to suggest actions such as tests, medications, or treatment protocols based on consistency of patient information or findings matching identified criteria or triggers.

AI is an umbrella term for computer actions mimicking work traditionally requiring human intelligence. It is important to remember these tools augment, but do not replace, human assessment. Actions are suggested, not prescribed. Machine learning is a subset of AI where information is provided to a machine that learns patterns and rules to apply to new data, for example, using large sets of anatomic contours to autogenerate contours used for CT treatment planning. Machines can be expected to increasingly analyze outcomes from large data sets to identify patterns that will influence new standards of care. Treatment choices will evolve, and outcomes will be measured, feeding continual improvement in patient care.

SUMMARY

- The EMR captures, aggregates, and presents information relevant to patient care in digital form.
- The EMR improves on paper records, facilitating efficient, consistent, and legible access to patient data across multidisciplinary teams.
- The medical record is an evolving tool. Centralization of patient medical history in an EMR provides a foundation for improved safety and efficiency through communication and fully informed decision-making.
- The EMR should incorporate process flow and unique charting needs for a given patient population and their caregivers. To be useful in the complex medical environment, it must be flexible and configurable, yet provide structure that can be easily sorted and reported on.
- The EMR can improve workflow in a department and contribute to the EHR, simultaneously empowering the patient and improving overall quality of care.
- Nonclinical information, such as demographics, scheduling, and reimbursement information, is integral to the comprehensive medical record. Integration of systems leverages the benefits of centralization; shared information advances reliability and accuracy resulting from single point of entry.
- EMRs can provide benefits for providers and their patients, but the improvement depends on extent of use. Meaningful Use and MACRA promote deepening adoption to advance healthcare in the United States.
- The complexity and criticality of the EMR's functions and the technical infrastructure to support it necessitate information technology expertise.
- With all its potential benefits, implementation of an EMR is not without challenge. Software selection must balance privacy, security, and accessibility. Although information must be available to authorized individuals, it must be protected from loss or unsanctioned viewing.

- To facilitate the exchange of electronic patient information while protecting patient privacy, the US Congress passed HIPAA, which standardizes information sets for healthcare reimbursement and restricts access to the minimum needed to provide care.
- EMR software can be distributed in multiple ways, either on a main computer server, which is client based, or hosted elsewhere with an ASP and accessible through secure web access. In either case, the EMR software coordinates with other devices, including laptops, standalone computers, and portable information-sharing devices.
- The exchange of information between systems in radiation oncology is enabled through extensive use of interfaces. Interfaces improve efficiency and accuracy by reducing redundant data entry and resulting errors. Proprietary interfaces are designed and owned by commercial entities. Nonproprietary standards designed by professional organizations (HL7, FHIR, DICOM) are part of the public domain; these public standards are highly desirable yet can be the hardest to integrate and make available for use.
- Streamlining the flow of medical information between systems and among caregivers holds great promise for improving healthcare. Full access to the patient's medical history is invaluable to diagnosis and treatment of illnesses, and streamlining administrative processes enables better use of resources. Data from many patients can be more readily compiled, providing more accurate profiles of illness and response to treatment choices.
- Usability must be considered in the design of the system, as it will have a huge effect on how effective, efficient, and satisfying the user will "feel" about the software as well as in patient safety—the EMR levels of defense shouldn't be allowed to be overwritten, and the treatment can be delivered accurately.
- The efficiency, speed, and safety of cancer research can be furthered when full advantage is taken of the EMR.

REVIEW QUESTIONS

The answers to the Review Questions can be found by logging on to our website at: http://evolve.elsevier.com/Washington/principles

1. EMRs provide:
   I. Workflow management.
   II. One central record for a clinical team.
   III. Retrospective data analysis.
   a. I and II.
   b. I and III.
   c. II and III.
   d. I, II, and III.

2. Benefits of the Meaningful Use of EMRs are:
   I. Complete and accurate information.
   II. Better access to information.
   III. Patient empowerment.
   a. I and II.
   b. I and III.
   c. II and III.
   d. I, II, and III.

3. HIPAA regulations provide requirements for:
   a. Computerization of patient records.

b. Tracking of all individuals accessing patient information.

c. Government regulation of treatment methods.

d. Password access to patient records.

4. Nonproprietary data communication standards in medicine include:

 I. HL7.

 II. PACS.

 III. DICOM.

 a. I and II.

 b. I and III.

 c. II and III.

 d. I, II, and III.

5. Data collection and interpretation is not facilitated using:

 a. Templates.

 b. Radio button selections.

 c. Free text.

 d. Drop lists.

6. Standards of care are:

 a. Fixed compilation of the customs and behaviors of a professional group.

 b. Dynamic.

 c. An assumed activity that any person would demonstrate in a given situation.

 d. The result of improved treatment outcomes.

7. Which of the following information has a role in the radiation oncology EMR?

 I. Patient schedule.

 II. Positron emission tomography (PET) scans.

 III. Letters to the patient.

 a. I and II.

 b. I and III.

 c. II and III.

 d. I, II, and III.

8. Effective EMR backup protocol must be:

 I. HIPAA compliant .

 II. Stored in the care facility.

 III. Able to provide a detailed disaster recovery plan to ensure a speedy recovery.

 a. I and II.

 b. I and III.

 c. II and III.

 d. I, II, and III.

9. Multilevel defense in radiation oncology EMR safety design might include:

 I. Forcing functions to prevent the clinician from making a mistake.

 II. Protocols to stipulate the calculation of monitor units.

 III. Independent double checks.

 a. I and II.

 b. I and III.

 c. II and III.

 d. I, II, and III.

10. Data mining software used to examine radiation oncology patient information:

 a. Can uncover customer satisfaction.

 b. Can find the cause of errors for future prevention.

 c. Can fine-tune relationships with patients.

 d. All of the above.

QUESTIONS TO PONDER

1. What are unique characteristics of radiation oncology practice that encourage use of a specialty EMR in addition to an enterprise EMR in the hospital?

2. What do national and international standards organizations contribute to achievement of medical informatics goals through the EMR?

3. What are some examples you have observed of the difference between connectivity and interoperability in radiation oncology?

4. Discuss some relative advantages and disadvantages between proprietary and open system interfaces.

REFERENCES

1. Luo JS. Electronic medical records. *Prim Psychiatry*. 2006;13(2):20–23.

2. American Society of Radiologic Technologists. The practice standards for medical imaging and radiation therapy: radiation therapy practice standards. Albuquerque, NM: American Society of Radiologic Technologist; 2017.

3. American Registry of Radiologic Technologists Content Specifications. *ARRT Radiation Therapy Examination*. St Paul, MN. American Registry of Radiologic Technologists; 2017.

4. American Society of Radiation Oncology. *Safety Is No Accident: A Framework for Quality Radiation Oncology and Care*. Albuquerque, NM: American Society of Radiation Oncology; 2012.

5. Van Bemmel JH, Musen MA, eds. *Handbook of Medical Informatics*. Heidelberg, Germany: Springer; 1997.

6. How to protect your EMR: EMR backup storage and recovery. Medicalrecords.com website. http://www.medicalrecords.com/emr-backup-storage-and-recovery. Accessed January 2019.

7. Blumenthal D, Tavenner M. The "meaningful use" regulation for electronic health records. *N Engl J Med*. 2010;363(6):501–504.

8. The Medicare Access and CHIP Reauthorization Act of 2015, Path to Value. Centers for Medicare and Medicaid Services (CMS) website. https://www.cms.gov/Medicare/Quality-Initiatives-Patient-Assessment-Instruments/Value-Based-Programs/MACRA-MIPS-and-APMs/MACRA-LAN-PPT.pdf. Accessed November 2018.

9. Barriers for adopting electronic health records (EHRs) by physicians. https://www.ncbi.nlm.nih.gov/pmc/articles/PMC3766548/. Accessed October 12, 2019. Published online June 2013.

10. Hagstrom M. Best practices for successful EMR system implementations. Healthcare News website. April 5, 2013 https://www.amnhealthcare.com/latest-healthcare-news/best-practices-successful-emr-system-implementations/. Accessed October 12,2019.

11. Erel O. SaaS vs ASP—Understanding the difference. Dzone website https://dzone.com/articles/saas-vs-asp-%E2%80%93-understanding October 28, 2014. Accessed November 2018.

12. About HL7. HL7 website. http://www.hl7.org/about Accessed August 2018.

13. Introducing HL7 FHIR. HL7 website. https://www.hl7.org/fhir/summary.html. Accessed August 2018.

14. Musal S. The differences between HL7 and FHIR (and why you should care) (website). https://blog.interfaceware.com/what-is-fhir-and-why-should-you-care/. Accessed October 12, 2019.

15. History. DICOM. Digital Imaging and Communications in Medicine website. https://www.dicomstandard.org/history/. Accessed August 2018.

16. Supplements. DICOM. Digital Imaging and Communications in Medicine website. https://www.dicomstandard.org/supplements/. Accessed August 2018.

17. DICOM. Digital Imaging and Communications in Medicine website. http://medical.nema.org. Accessed August 2018.

18. WG-07. Radiotherapy. DICOM Digital Imaging and Communications in Medicine website. https://www.dicomstandard.org/wgs/wg-07/. Accessed August 2018.

19. Why is IHE Needed? IHE website. https://www.ihe.net/about_ihe/faq/#Why_is_IHE_needed? Accessed August 2018.

20. Patient privacy and security of electronic medical information. RadiologyInfo website. https://www.radiologyinfo.org/en/info.cfm?pg=article-patient-privacy. Accessed January 20, 2018.

21. Cybersecurity. US Food and Drug Administration website. https://www.fda.gov/MedicalDevices/DigitalHealth/ucm373213.htm. Accessed October 31, 2018.

22. Health information technology. US Department of Health and Human Services website. http://www.hhs.gov/ocr/privacy/hipaa/understanding/special/healthit/index.html. Clinical research systems and integration with medical system Revie.

23. Horahan K. Electronic health records access during a disaster. *Online J Public Health Inform*. 2014;5(3):232.

24. Carayon P, Wood K. Patient safety: the role of human factors and systems engineering. *Stud Health Technol Inform*. 2010;153:23–46.

25. *Applying Human Factors and Usability Engineering to Medical Devices Guidance for Industry and Food and Drug Administration Staff*. US Department of Health and Human Services, Food and Drug Administration, Center for Devices and Radiologic Health. Washington, DC; 2016.

26. US Department of Health and Human Services, Agency for Healthcare Research and Quality. Patient safety primer: systems approach. Patient Safety Network website https://psnet.ahrq.gov/primers/primer/21. Accessed October 12, 2019.

27. The Joint Commission. Human factors analysis in patient safety systems. *The Source*. 2015;13(4):10–12.

28. Monica K. Could automation solve the healthcare industry's EHR problem? EHR Intelligence website. https://ehrintelligence.com/news/could-automation-solve-the-healthcare-industrys-ehr-problem. Accessed October 12, 2019.

29. Clare B. I care about structured data, here's why you should too. KevinMD website. https://www.kevinmd.com/blog/2015/05/i-care-about-structured-data-heres-why-you-should-too.html. Accessed October 12, 2019.

30. Barlow S. Healthcare informatics: ready to unleash a new wave of advanced analytics? https://www.healthcatalyst.com/healthcare-informatics-close-analytics-loop. June 27, 2014. Accessed August 2018.

31. Niland JC, Rouse L. Clinical research systems and integration with medical systems. In: Ochs MF, Casagrande JT, Davuluri RV, eds. *Biomedical Informatics for Cancer Research*. New York: Springer; 2010.

32. Brickman J. How to get health care employees onboard with change. *Harvard Business Review*. https://hbr.org/2016/11/how-to-get-health-care-employees-onboard-with-change. November 23, 2016. Accessed January 18, 2019.

25

Bone, Cartilage, and Soft Tissue Sarcomas

Jana Koth, Lisa Bartenhagen

OBJECTIVES

- Recall epidemiologic trends associated with bone and soft tissue sarcomas.
- Sketch appropriate anatomy of bone and connective tissue.
- Discuss various pathology, staging, and grading systems for bone and soft tissue sarcomas.
- Identify the treatments of choice for a variety of bone and soft tissue sarcomas.
- Compare and contrast current procedures available for detection and diagnosis of diseases in this category.

- Support the idea that the degree of differentiation and aggression of tumor growth greatly affect the patient's prognosis.
- Recall generally accepted doses of radiation for various bone and soft tissue sarcomas.
- Simulate and help plan a bone or soft tissue sarcoma case as part of the cancer care team.
- Apply knowledge of radiobiology to educate patients on possible side effects of treatment.
- Discuss emerging treatments and technology for the management and cure of bone and soft tissue sarcomas.

OUTLINE

KEY TERMS

American Joint Committee on Cancer
Biopsy
Diaphysis
Epiphyses
Erythema
Etiologic factor

French Federation of Cancer Centers Sarcoma Group
Grade
Intraoperative radiation therapy
Limb-sparing surgery
Local control
Mesoderm

Multidisciplinary approach
Osteoblastic
Osteolytic
Pathologic staging
Periosteum
Postoperative radiation therapy
Preoperative radiation therapy

Primary site compartment
Pseudocapsule
Radionuclide
Radioresistant
Retroperitoneal sarcomas
Skip metastases

TABLE 25.1   Malignant Bone Tumors

Tumor	Age (Years)	Gender Ratio (Male/Female)	Treatment (5-Year Survival Rate)	Bones Commonly Involved	Location
Osteosarcoma	10–25	2:1	S C (60%–80%)	Metaphysis	Long bones of extremities (knee joint), jaws
Chondrosarcoma	35–60	2:1	S (variable, 45%–90%)	Diaphysis or metaphysis	Pelvis, ribs, vertebrae, long bones (proximal part)
Ewing sarcoma	10–20	2:1	C S (60%–78%%)	Diaphysis	Long bones; may be multiple
Giant cell tumor	20–40	1:1	S (95%)	Epiphysis	Long bones (knee joint)

C, Chemotherapy; *S*, surgery.
From Damjanov I. *Pathology for the Health Professions*. 5th ed. St. Louis, MO: Elsevier; 2017; and Ewing sarcoma treatment. National Cancer Institute website. https://www.cancer.gov/types/bone/hp/ewing–treatment-pdqhttp. Accessed November 10, 2018.

DISEASE MANAGEMENT PROFILE

Cancer of the bone and cancer of the soft tissue are challenging for the cancer care team because of their unique character, the infrequency of occurrence, and the difficulties in predicting outcomes. Connective tissue tumors represent one of the most morphologically heterogeneous classifications in human pathology. To date, clinical outcomes for bone and soft tissue tumors have been somewhat discouraging. The evolution of a multidisciplinary approach of surgery, radiation therapy, and chemotherapy to planning and treating these diseases has improved over the past 30 years, and clinical trials that involve gene therapy are currently underway. A comprehensive knowledge of this multifaceted disease is necessary for radiation therapists to provide the best quality care possible.

BONE AND CARTILAGE TUMORS

Natural History

The skeletal system is composed of bones or osseous and cartilaginous tissues. These tissues give the body its shape, form, and ability to move. Bones and cartilage possess the exceptional ability to support and protect softer tissues in the body. Bones also serve as a reservoir for fats, minerals (especially calcium), and other substances vital to blood cell production. The extraskeletal connective tissues include all those soft tissues that provide connection, support, and locomotion. Although bone tumors refer to malignancies that involve the bone, they may also frequently include tumors of a collective group of tissues, such as cartilage, joints, and blood vessels that surround the bone. Bone marrow, which is responsible for blood cell production, is not spared from the attack of malignant cells. Soft tissue tumors are limited to those sarcomas that arise in the extraskeletal connective tissues and are found throughout the human body.

Primary and metastatic tumors of the bone are examined in this chapter. An estimated 3450 new cases of primary bone cancers are projected each year, with an estimated 1590 fatalities from this disease.[1] Although the number of primary bone cancer cases has decreased over recent years, the number of metastatic bone cancers remains high.[1]

Tumors of the primary bone include osteosarcoma, chondrosarcoma, fibrosarcoma, malignant histiocytoma, malignant giant cell tumors (GCTs), multiple myeloma, and metastatic bone disease. Fibrosarcomas and malignant histiocytomas are often classified in a group of tumors known as *malignant fibrous histiocytoma* (MFH). These tumors, along with Ewing sarcoma, are unique among connective tissue cancers in that they affect both bone and soft tissue.

See the website of the American Academy of Orthopaedic Surgeons at https://orthoinfo.org/en/search/?q=Bone+tumors for additional information. This site provides information on bone tumors, images, and related articles.

Epidemiology

Primary bone tumors are rare; they account for less than 0.2% of all malignancies.[3] *Osteosarcoma*, the most common osseous malignant bone tumor in children, comprises an estimated 56% of all pediatric primary skeletal malignancies.[1] Children and young adults between 10 and 30 years are most commonly affected, with a peak incidence in the teens.[1] Osteosarcoma is more prevalent in young males (60%) than females. It is the second most common type of primary bone tumor in adults.[1] Table 25.1 and Fig. 25.1 depict the prevalence of various bone tumors.

Chondrosarcoma is a common primary bone tumor in adults but is fairly rare in children. It accounts for just 6% of all pediatric primary bone tumors but for more than 40% of all adult bone tumors.[1] Most chondrosarcomas are diagnosed in older adults with a mean age of approximately 60 years.[17] The overall incidence rate among men and women has been reported to be fairly equal.[7]

Fibrosarcoma may occur in bone or soft tissue. It is classified in the MFH group of tumors and accounts for less than approximately 6% of primary bone tumors.[1] Most cases are diagnosed in patients between the ages of 30 and 70 years. A slight male predominance has been reported.

Ewing sarcoma accounts for approximately 16% of bone tumors and approximately 3% of childhood cancers.[1] This disease can affect anyone from the age of 5 months to 60 years, with a peak incidence in children from 10 to 20 years of age. Occurrence in children younger than 5 years of age is rare. It is also unusual for this tumor to affect Asian or African children. Ewing sarcoma appears to be more predominant in males than in females.

Multiple myeloma is a malignant disease of the plasma cells.[7] Abnormal resorption of bone causes painful osseous lesions. This disease process arises in the B-cell lymphocytes of the bone marrow and makes up approximately 17% of all hematologic malignancies.[20] Multiple myeloma is usually seen in middle-aged and older adults, with a peak incidence in the seventh decade.[9] It is more common in men than in women, with a ratio of 1.5:1. It is also twice as common among black persons than white persons.

Additional risk factors for osteosarcoma include multiple genetic mutations, such as Rothmund-Thomson syndrome, Li Fraumeni syndrome, Bloom syndrome, and hereditary retinoblastoma.[23] Although no exact cause of Ewing sarcoma has been identified, there is a strong association with genetic alterations. In 40% to 70% of cases, patients with Ewing sarcoma have been found to have a loss of heterozygosity, which is caused by a chromosomal event. The next most common alteration affects a tumor protein, p53, which arises from the *TP53* gene. Approximately 10% to 39% of cases are linked to this event.[2]

General Anatomy and Physiology, Including Pertinent Lymphatic Considerations

Bone tumors have their embryologic origin in the mesoderm, the primitive mesenchyme, or the ectoderm cells, which give rise to the common connective tissues (Fig. 25.2).

The high incidence rate of bone tumors in children supports the assumption that these neoplasms arise in areas of rapid growth. The most common site of a primary bone sarcoma is near the growth plate. A typical long bone, as illustrated in Fig. 25.3, consists of the diaphysis (the main shaft of the bone), two epiphyses (the knoblike portions at either end of the bone), the cartilage cap (covers the articular surface), and the periosteum (the hard, dense covering of the bone). The growth (epiphyseal) plate is the area in long bones where rapid cell proliferation and remodeling activity takes place.[7] This area may appear as a "line" or lighter density than bone on a diagnostic radiograph, especially in those who are still growing. Because they possess large growth plates, the distal femur and proximal tibia are the two most common locations for bone tumors.

Osteosarcomas are most commonly found in the distal femur, followed by the proximal tibia and the proximal humerus. Lesions may appear in other areas, such as the proximal femur, distal tibia, and fibula, with rare occurrences in the vertebrae, ileum, facial bones, and mandible.

Chondrosarcomas are typically found in the pelvis and femur, although they can also involve the shoulder girdle and proximal humerus. They occur in the ribs more frequently than do osteosarcomas; however, both tumor types are rarely found in the distal extremities.

Fibrosarcomas (MFHs) and GCTBs typically arise in the metaphysis and epiphysis of long bones, including the distal femur, proximal tibia, and distal radius.

Ewing sarcoma is most frequently seen in the appendicular skeleton, with about 25% of tumors developing in the pelvis and about 17% of cases affecting the femur.[6] Ewing sarcoma can occur in any part of the bone but is most commonly seen in the diaphysis. Metaphyseal involvement occurs less often, and epiphyseal involvement is rare.

Multiple myeloma is the most common oncologic disease of bone. It can occur in any bone and is characterized by osteolytic lesions shown on diagnostic radiographs (similar to what is seen in Fig. 25.4 and 25.12). This feature limits the healing process in most patients, which commonly leads to pathologic fracture.

Metastatic bone disease most often involves the spine, pelvis, femur, and humerus. It is not uncommon for metastatic disease to affect the ribs and skull.[1] The most common cancers to metastasize to bone are advanced diseases of the lung, breast, and prostate. Nearly 40% of patients with non–small cell lung cancer with advanced disease have development of metastatic bone disease. Approximately 70% of patients with metastatic breast or prostate cancer are affected.[24]

Clinical Presentation

Pain is the most common presenting symptom of a bone tumor, which may occur even without a mass that can be felt.[23] Patients with osteosarcoma usually experience nonspecific pain and swelling that becomes

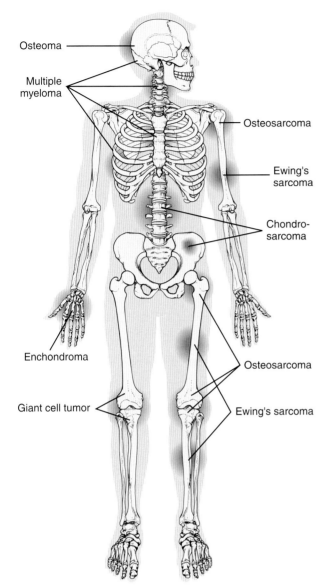

Fig. 25.1 A schematic representation of common sites of origin for primary bone tumors. (From Damjanov I. *Pathology for the Health Professions.* 5th ed. St. Louis, MO: Elsevier; 2017.)

GCT accounts for approximately 5% of primary bone tumors.[8] This tumor is typically benign, with only about 10% of cases being malignant.[1] It affects adults from 30 to 40 years of age, and the incidence rate is slightly higher in adult females.[8] GCT of bone (GCTB) arises in the metaphysis or epiphysis of long bones and has a high tendency to metastasize to the lungs, although most cases are benign.

Metastatic bone disease accounts for most malignant bone lesions.[1] It occurs most often in the spine and pelvis; lesions are less common farther from the trunk. Lung carcinoma is the most common primary site to metastasize to bone, followed by the prostate, breast, kidney, and thyroid.[7]

Etiology

Although an exact cause has not been identified, some known associations are related to the development of primary bone tumors. Genetics may contribute, with two common suppressor genes, *RB1* and *TP53*. An association appears to exist between these genes and the development of osteosarcoma. In addition, previous exposure to environmental elements, including radiation and chemicals, has been linked to osteosarcoma.[25]

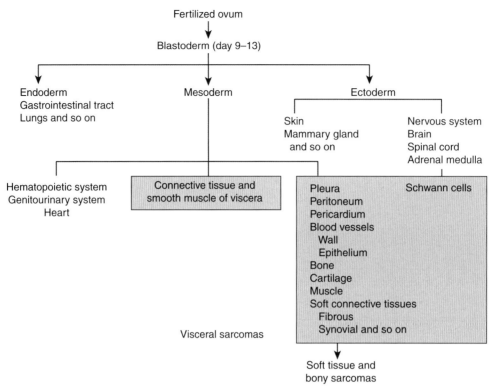

Fig. 25.2 Embryonic derivation of the soft tissue and bony sarcomas. Cells of origin determine designations as particular types of soft tissue sarcomas. (From Rosenberg SA, Suit HA, Baker LH. Sarcomas of soft tissues. In: DeVita VT, Hellman S, Rosenberg SA, eds. *Cancer: Principles and Practice of Oncology.* Vol 2. 2nd ed. Philadelphia, PA: JB Lippincott; 1982.)

progressively worse over several months.[23] Chondrosarcomas, fibrosarcomas, and GCTs cause symptoms similar to those of osteosarcomas, although the duration of the symptoms may be somewhat longer. Pain usually correlates with the degree of histologic aggressiveness of the disease, and rapid worsening of symptoms may indicate the histologic grade or cell type. Pathologic fractures are common with fibrosarcomas. Also seen are neurologic abnormalities in vertebral lesions, a decreased range of motion of the involved extremity, and muscular atrophy.

Patients with Ewing sarcoma typically have pain and swelling in the affected area. Other symptoms may include fever, weight loss, and generalized fatigue. Occasionally delays in diagnosis occur from an absence of pain. Patients may prolong seeking medical attention until the lesion changes in size.[17]

Multiple myeloma causes bone loss, which results in painful bony lesions. This loss of bone is caused by a disruption in the process of bone formation and resorption. Patients may also have pathologic fractures and hypercalcemia, which sets this disease apart from the other primary bone tumors. In fact, nearly 60% of patients with multiple myeloma have pathologic fracture at some point.

Metastatic bone disease causes increasing pain that develops gradually over a few weeks or months. Inflammation or the tumor itself is typically what causes the pain. The pain is often difficult to localize and becomes progressively worse. Left untreated, symptoms can be debilitating, which could result in pathologic fracture.[24]

Detection and Diagnosis

Patients generally have pain that tends not to be activity related and that may be worse at night. A complete history of the patient is important to determine the duration of symptoms. In addition, history of carcinoma may suggest a new metastatic lesion of a bone. An important consideration is that a sarcoma may develop in a previously irradiated

area. Chronic symptoms from a bone lesion may indicate a benign condition, whereas symptoms that rapidly progress over weeks or a few months usually signify a higher likelihood of a malignant process.

Primary bone tumors are rare. This low incidence is a contributing factor in making early detection extremely difficult. Persistent pain in a bone raises concern with physicians, especially if the pain occurs during sleep. Because of the rapid growth pattern of bone tumors, incidental discoveries of these lesions are rare.

The National Comprehensive Cancer Network (NCCN) is composed of a group of physicians who specialize in cancer treatment. They have established Clinical Practice Guidelines in Oncology, based on their observations of current recognized acceptable approaches to treatment. For the diagnosis of bone tumors, the following steps are advised:

- History and physical
- Imaging of primary tumor site
- Chest imaging (to rule out lung metastases)
- Bone or positron emission tomographic (PET) scan
- Biopsy for confirmation of diagnosis[3]

A radiograph is an important tool for the detection and diagnosis of a bone tumor. A variety of parameters are associated in accurate diagnosis of a bone lesion. Some of these parameters are the permeative pattern, the sunburst periosteal reaction, and the onionskin periosteal reaction and whether the lesion is osteolytic or **osteoblastic** (pertaining to bone-forming cells). All of these indicate the level of advancement, aggressiveness, and rate of growth. The key indicator of malignancy on a radiograph is the characteristic of the margin. A lesion with well-defined sclerotical borders is malignant in only 6% of cases. However, an osteolytic lesion with less defined edges on a radiograph has a 50% chance of being malignant. This chance increases to as high as 80% for lesions with a permeative pattern.[2a] Fig. 25.4 illustrates several lytic lesions of the humerus caused by metastatic renal

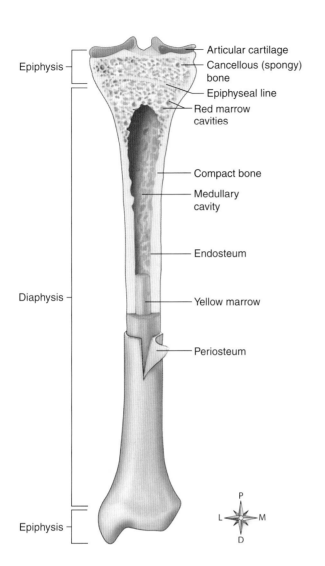

Fig. 25.3 A longitudinal section of long bone shows diaphysis, epiphyses, and articular cartilage. (From Patton KT, Thibodeau GA. *The Human Body in Health & Disease.* 7th ed. St. Louis, MO: Elsevier; 2018.)

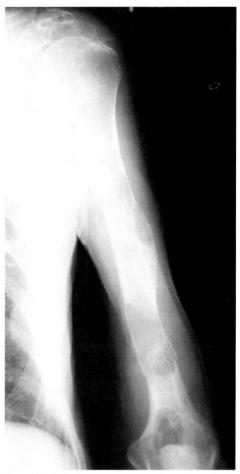

Fig. 25.4 Several lytic lesions are present throughout the humerus of this patient with metastatic renal cell carcinoma. Note the destruction of the periosteum along the midportion and lower portion of the shaft.

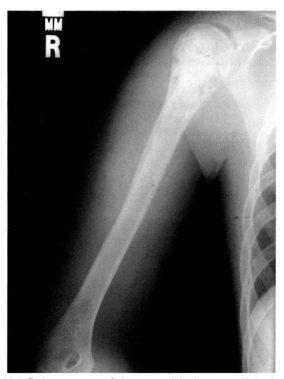

Fig. 25.5 Ewing sarcoma of the upper right humerus. Note the diffuse permeative destruction of the bone, with periosteal reaction that involves the proximal portion of the humerus.

cell carcinoma, and Fig. 25.5 shows the presence of an Ewing sarcoma of the upper humerus.

Computed tomography (CT) is useful for establishing the extent of the tumor in the bone and for determining the presence or absence of soft tissue masses. However, magnetic resonance imaging (MRI) has replaced CT scan in many instances (Fig. 25.6). MRI is used particularly in instances of aggressive bone tumors because of the accuracy in distinguishing healthy tissues and neurovascular structures from the tumor tissue. This is essential in planning a surgical biopsy and treatment. MRI is highly sensitive, demonstrating the reactive zone of the tumor in the bone while differentiating marrow edema adjacent to tumor tissue. PET/MRI will likely be used in the future in the diagnosis and staging of primary bone tumors. It is an excellent tool for evaluation of tumor size before surgery and can be used to monitor progress after neoadjuvant therapy.[4]

Bone scans are extremely sensitive and can detect tumor foci in bone that are not yet visualized on diagnostic radiographs. The extent of the tumor in the bone and the presence of skip metastases can be shown accurately. For multiple myeloma, however, bone scan results are often negative and may underestimate the extent of the disease. Fig. 25.7 shows a bone scan of a patient with osteosarcoma. This modality is useful, as with this case, to rule out distant metastases.

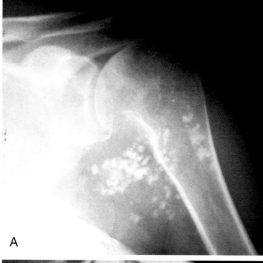

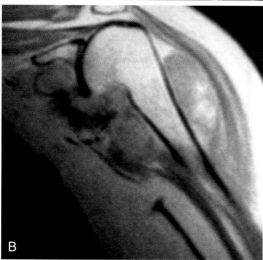

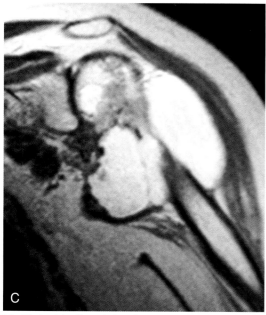

Fig. 25.6 (A) A plain film of the shoulder shows a partially calcified mass, which is eroding the medial aspect of the humerus. (B) and (C) Magnetic resonance imaging of the shoulder reveal a large mass encircling the humeral head, which was interpreted as a sarcoma. (From Helms CA. Fundamentals of Skeletal Radiology. 5th ed. Philadelphia, PA: Elsevier; 2020.)

Biopsy is the most important step in confirmation of a pathologic diagnosis. The biopsy site and approach must be discussed with the surgeon and radiation oncologist before the procedure is performed. Typically, a core needle biopsy or open biopsy is the preferred method.[12] One of the disadvantages of open biopsy is the risk for tumor cell seeding. This results from a larger exposed section of the tumor during the surgical procedure. For this reason, the needle biopsy is recommended over the open method.[12] Many patients have a considerable associated soft tissue mass; they can undergo a soft tissue biopsy rather than a biopsy of intraosseous tissue. A soft tissue biopsy avoids further weakening of the bone, the integrity of which may already be compromised by the tumor. This is especially true in patients who have lesions in weight-bearing bones, which have increased potential for pathologic fracture.

Metastatic disease necessitates a complete workup in order to accurately assess the extent of the disease. This workup may include CT scan and MRI, blood tests, and diagnostic radiographs. The sites most frequently involved include the vertebral bodies, pelvic bones, and ribs. In patients with widespread disease, lesions in the humerus, femur, scapula, sternum, skull, or clavicle are not uncommon. A radiograph is typically the first diagnostic image obtained. A useful practice is to rule out a pathologic fracture and determine whether surgical intervention is necessary.

The radiographic appearance of bony metastases can vary, depending on the type of lesion. Osteoblastic lesions appear as an increased density on a diagnostic radiograph. Fig. 25.8 demonstrates metastatic lesions on two separate images, each showing osteoblastic lesions, one in the female pelvis and another in the body of a lumbar vertebrae. Osteolytic lesions (generally show a decreased density on a radiograph, Figs. 25.4 and 25.12), have ragged margins and may appear as a granular, mottled-looking area on a radiograph. If the margins are smooth, a benign process must be considered. In a comparison of Fig. 25.9 with Fig. 25.10, a difference is evident between the ragged and smooth borders of the tumor, which generally indicate a benign or malignant process.

Patients with vertebral involvement or sacral metastases may have nerve pain that results from tumor expansion and pressure on the sciatic nerve. A careful and extensive neurologic workup is necessary because vertebral destruction is often associated with extradural spine disease, which can result in spinal cord compression. Early treatment of a partial or complete spinal cord blockage is crucial to prevent paralysis and sensory loss. This is one of the few emergency procedures encountered in radiation oncology.

Multiple myeloma creates osteolytic lesions of the bone, which are likely to cause a fracture. A radiograph may show the number of lesions and whether a pathologic fracture is present. If a patient has multiple bone lesions without a known primary tumor site, multiple myeloma must be considered.

Pathology

Osteosarcomas are generally classified as poorly differentiated tumors, with less than 1% diagnosed as a grade 1 (grade ranges from 1 to 4). Approximately 85% are categorized as grade 3 or 4. Predominant histologic subtypes of osteosarcomas are osteoblastic, chondroblastic, fibroblastic, or mixed chondroblastic. The most aggressive subtype is osteoblastic, which is considered high grade. Chondroblastic is considered intermediate grade, in which periosteal lesions are histologically classified. The low-grade subtype is fibroblastic, which commonly presents as a parosteal tumor.[23]

Chondrosarcomas arise from mesenchymal elements of the bone. The degree of cellularity and rate of mitosis are important in establishing a histologic grade, which ranges from 1 to 3. Low-grade tumors

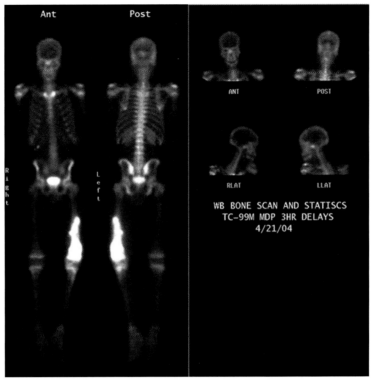

Fig. 25.7 This bone scan shows a large osteosarcoma in the left femur and rules out the presence of distant metastases.

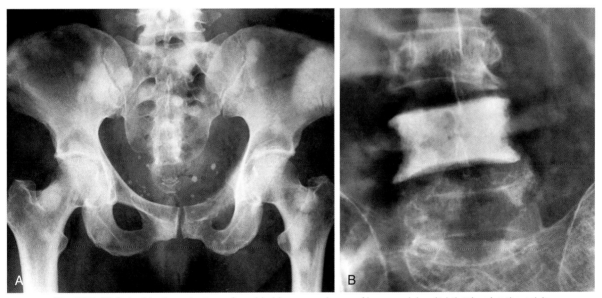

Fig. 25.8 (A) Osteoblastic metastases from bladder cancer (areas of increased density) that involve the pelvis and proximal femurs. (B) Osteoblastic lesion of L4 metastatic from prostate cancer. (From Eisenberg RL, Johnson NM. *Comprehensive Radiographic Pathology*. 6th ed. St. Louis, MO: Elsevier; 2016.)

may be clear cell or juxtacortical chondrosarcomas. Mesenchymal chondrosarcomas are usually undifferentiated and associated with a higher grade.

Fibrosarcomas originate in mesenchymal tissue and often have the appearance of normal fibroblasts but are malignant. Improvements in histologic classification have categorized low-grade fibrosarcomas as low-grade myxofibrosarcoma, low-grade fibromyxoid sarcoma, and sclerosing epithelioid fibrosarcoma.[10]

The cell of origin for MFH is the histiocyte or the macrophage. MFH is an undifferentiated pleomorphic sarcoma with histiocytic and fibroblastic differentiation.

The GCTBs are histologically composed of round or spindle-shaped mononuclear cells uniformly incorporated in with multinucleated giant cells. Grading for this type of tumor is not prognostically reliable.

Ewing sarcoma is composed of populations of small, blue, round cells with a high nuclear-to-cytoplasmic ratio. These cells are arrayed in

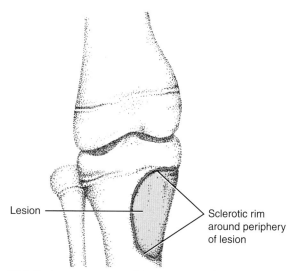

Fig. 25.9 Benign appearance of bone tumors shows a sclerotic rim around the periphery of the lesion.

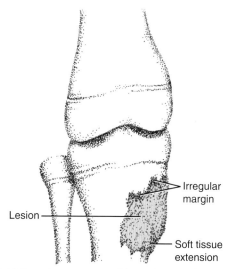

Fig. 25.10 Malignant appearance of bone tumors shows an irregular margin with soft tissue extension.

sheets.[2] Approximately 90% to 95% of Ewing tumors have a cytogenetic translocation between the *EWS* gene on chromosome 22 and the *FLI1* gene on chromosome 11. These alterations make a diagnosis of Ewing sarcoma definitive.[3]

Plasma cells originate from B-cell lymphocytes. They develop from stem cells found in all tissues of the body, which makes it possible for plasma cell tumors to manifest in any organ or tissue of the body. Multiple myeloma is characterized by neoplastic proliferation of a single clone of plasma cells. These cells produce a monoclonal protein that, along with the proliferation of plasma cells, leads to the destruction of bone.

Staging

Pathologic staging and grading of primary bone tumors are intimately associated with current anatomic staging systems. Grade is a significant prognostic factor; it is classified as either low (G1) or high (G2) and is nearly synonymous with early (I and II) or late (IIB and III) stage. Although staging of sarcomas is difficult because of low incidence and the various subtypes, the American Joint Committee on Cancer (AJCC) has established a Cancer Staging Handbook, now in

its eighth edition. The handbook incorporates grading, histology, and tumor size. The Enneking staging system was previously considered the standard classification system. It has been updated by the AJCC to replace compartmentalization with tumor size. Tumors are classified according to grade (low grade or high grade), tumor size (either greater than or less than 8 cm), and presence or absence of distant metastases. Table 25.2 shows this staging system.

Spread Patterns

Most sarcomas, especially high-grade sarcomas, metastasize through the blood to the lungs. Occasionally, osteosarcoma, MFH, and chondrosarcoma metastasize to other sites, including bone, liver, and brain. Lung metastases tend to occur in approximately 90% of patients with high-grade osteosarcoma within 2 to 3 years after the initial diagnosis. Typically, low-grade tumors do not readily metastasize, which makes them easier to control. However, a local or distant recurrence is common in about 30% to 40% of patients with localized osteosarcoma. When this occurs, growth continues and the tumor eventually evolves into a high-grade tumor. Skip metastases are another pattern of spread in osteosarcomas. A skip metastasis is a second, smaller focus of osteosarcoma in the same bone or a second bone lesion on the opposing side of a joint space. This phenomenon is attributed to the extensive spread by the lesion into the marrow cavity of the bone. The overall aggressiveness of bone tumors makes control difficult. Lymphatic spread of most bone tumors is not of great concern unless the tumor arises in the trunk of the body. There, the lymph vessels and nodes are more prominent, and a greater chance exists of the tumor invading the lymph system. If this occurs, the microscopic tumor cells can be carried to other parts of the body through the lymphatic system.

Treatment Considerations

In the following sections, specific treatment techniques are discussed regarding osteosarcoma, chondrosarcoma, fibrosarcoma (MFH), GCTs, multiple myeloma, Ewing sarcoma, and metastatic bone disease. The roles of surgery, chemotherapy, and radiation therapy are presented.

Osteosarcoma. The presence or absence of metastases at the time of diagnosis is the most important prognostic indicator. Approximately 15% to 20% of patients have distant metastasis at presentation.[23] Other factors include age, gender, tumor size and location, grade of the tumor, duration of symptoms, and the interval between chemotherapy and surgery. Prognosis is typically worse in males younger than 10 years of age and in those with a duration of symptoms less than 6 months. Patients with fewer of these indictors may respond well to aggressive surgical and chemotherapeutic treatment. Reason dictates that the smaller and less aggressive the tumor, the more easily it can be surgically removed and the less chance it has of metastasizing. In addition, lesions that occur in the lower extremities are more favorable because of easy accessibility for surgical removal of the tumor to obtain local control.

The treatment of osteosarcoma necessitates a multidisciplinary approach because it is relatively chemosensitive and radioresistant. The current accepted treatment consists of neoadjuvant, multiagent chemotherapy, surgical resection of the primary tumor, followed by additional chemotherapy.[23] Treatment according to a clinical trial protocol is optimal because these tumors are rare and difficult to manage.

Historically, treatment for the primary lesion was amputation. Amputation achieved excellent local control, but quality of life and functionality were unsatisfactory. Fortunately, amputation rates have declined over the years; currently only 5% to 10% of patients require this extensive surgery.[3] Often, this is performed because of inoperability or the inability to obtain clear margins. If positive margins are present, the risk for local recurrence rises significantly.[23] The evolution of new chemotherapy treatments has greatly affected the shift from amputation to limb-sparing surgery(LSS). In this procedure, the bone involved with the tumor is removed and reconstructed with an implant. Rotational and free flap techniques are used during surgery to aid in soft tissue coverage of the reconstruction. Improvements in techniques with soft tissue and implants rather than allograft bone have decreased the incidence of complications, such as wound necrosis, infection, and fracture.

Current surgical techniques and neoadjuvant chemotherapy have improved survival rates, with approximately 75% of localized cases disease free at 5 years.[3] In fact, patients who present with metastatic disease still have a chance for cure.[3]

The standard chemotherapy regimen involves the combination of several agents. The most widely used are cisplatin, doxorubicin, and high-dose methotrexate with leucovorin. Recent studies have shown a significant benefit to administering at least three of these agents compared with giving two. The addition of ifosfamide is not part of the standard regimen, as it increases toxicity and has not been proven to be that beneficial in terms of outcomes. In patients with early-stage disease, the administration of chemotherapy before surgical resection largely decreases the recurrence risk. The objective of this approach is to induce tumor necrosis by a minimum of 90% to improve surgical resection outcomes. No matter the clinical response to preoperative chemotherapy, additional rounds of chemotherapy are given following surgery.[23]

Radiation therapy is not part of the standard treatment regimen for patients with osteosarcomas. These tumors are radioresistant, and doses necessary for a clinical response often result in tissue damage and subsequent amputation. However, radiation can be administered before surgery with adjuvant chemotherapy, and may be an option for patients with unresectable tumors. According to the NCCN guidelines, external beam therapy is advised for patients with positive surgical margins and partial resections and for nonsurgical candidates. The recommended postoperative dose is 64 to 68 Gy to the high-risk anatomic site, and as high as 70 Gy for patients with unresectable tumors.[3] Complications from treatment of osteosarcoma include nephrotoxicity and neurotoxicities from chemotherapy. Side effects of radiation are site dependent and may include skin reaction, reduction in blood counts, and pathologic fractures. Note that more side effects are normally experienced when several modalities are used in a combined sequence.

A newer therapeutic approach being investigated is the use of immunotherapy. This therapy focuses to increase the tumor's immunogenicity, which would essentially cause tumor rejection in the body. Because osteosarcoma is difficult to treat as a result of the diverse molecular nature, these universal treatments may show more promise than targeted therapies.[23]

> Immunotherapy is treatment that uses certain parts of a person's immune system to fight diseases such as cancer. This can be done by stimulating a person's own immune system to work harder and smarter, attacking cancer cells, or by giving the immune system man-made proteins that help fight the cancer. In the last several decades, immunotherapy has become an important part of cancer treatment. Newer types of immunotherapy are now being studied, and they will impact how we treat cancer in the future.[1]

Chondrosarcoma. Chondrosarcomas are malignant mesenchymal neoplasms that produce cartilage, but no osteoid, and may occur in

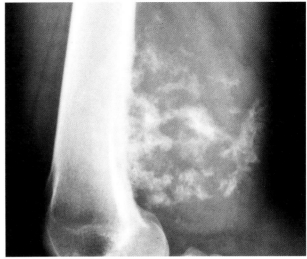

Fig. 25.11 Large chondrosarcoma located in the area of the distal femur. Note the prominent dense calcification of the lesion. (From Eisenberg RL, Johnson NM. *Comprehensive Radiographic Pathology.* 6th ed. St. Louis, MO: Elsevier; 2016.)

any cartilage-forming bone (Fig. 25.11). Remember, bones were, at one time, mostly cartilage before primary and secondary ossification centers began to encourage the deposit of bone early in life. The prognosis of patients with chondrosarcomas and benign chordomas depends on two factors. One factor is the histologic grade of the tumor. Lesions are graded on a scale of 1 to 3, with 3 being the most anaplastic (exhibiting a loss of cell differentiation). Low-grade tumors are locally invasive and do not tend to metastasize, which makes them easier to control. High-grade tumors, in contrast, often metastasize, typically to the lungs, giving the patient a poorer prognosis and making tumor control more difficult. The other prognostic indicator is the tumor's location. If the tumor is located peripherally, it is more surgically accessible. However, if it appears in the pelvis, sacral area, or head and neck, surgery may not be possible, or the tumor may be unable to be completely resected.

Surgical resection is the primary method of treatment for chondrosarcomas and chordomas; it includes removal of the entire mass, with adequate bone and soft tissue margins. Chemotherapy agents do not appear to have any substantial effect on the disease.

External beam radiation therapy (EBRT) is usually not part of the treatment because of the radioresistant qualities of this type of tumor. However, radiation therapy is used definitively when the tumor cannot be completely removed as a result of the proximity of critical structures. This is a common occurrence because of the aggressive nature of these tumors and how they invade critical structures. Total resection is often difficult. The NCCN guidelines suggest preoperative doses of 20 to 50 Gy and 70 Gy for unresectable tumors.[3] Newer forms of treatment, such as photon-based radiosurgery or charged particle (proton) radiotherapy has been used to improve tumor control rates. Stereotactic radiosurgery for the treatment of chordoma can produce local control rates as high as 72% for 5 years, with 5-year survival rates up to 80%.[19] Chondrosarcomas are even better controlled than chordomas, resulting in a better prognosis.[19]

> A lead wire, or radiopaque marker, that outlines the incision that must be treated is helpful during CT simulation. Remember that the marker gives information at the skin surface only and not at depth.

Fibrosarcomas. Treatment for fibrosarcomas that involve bone necessitates an aggressive surgical procedure with wide or radical excision. Postoperative radiation is advised because of the high rate of recurrence. Fibrosarcomas are not highly radiosensitive, but irradiation is recommended for inoperable tumors, postoperative residual disease, and palliation. Doses of 66 to 70 Gy with a shrinking-field technique are recommended if radiation therapy is prescribed to control a skeletal fibrosarcoma. The prognostic indicators for fibrosarcomas include the histologic grade, the location in the bone (medullary or periosteal), and whether the lesions arise de novo (anew) or are secondary to a preexisting bony condition.

Malignant Fibrous Histiocytoma. Treatment for MFH is similar to that of many bone tumors. The disease is extremely rare, making it difficult to find clinical trial data. However, the benefit of a complete local excision has been shown to prolong relapse-free survival. Skin grafts, amputation, and disarticulation are common methods of treatment as well.[13] Preoperative and postoperative chemotherapy clinical trials in conjunction with surgery to investigate limited surgical approaches are underway. Radiation therapy may be used as a definitive treatment for inoperable lesions or in cases with positive surgical margins. MFH of the bone carries a poorer prognosis than does MFH of soft tissue.[13]

Giant Cell Tumors. GCTs of bone can be challenging to control. Although rates of metastasis are low, the disease can recur. Current management of this disease is dependent on the anatomic site of the tumor and how much bone destruction has occurred. For most tumors, surgical curettage is most effective. However, the local control rate for curettage alone is approximately 61%; therefore additional therapies are frequently used. These include intracavitary high-speed burr drilling and locally applied liquid nitrogen, phenol, or hydrogen peroxide.

Radiation therapy is reserved for GCTs that occur in areas where complete surgical excision is not possible, as in the case of large or axially located tumors. Doses ranging from 50 to 60 Gy are recommended for cases when surgery is not an option. The same dose is given for recurrences and locally advanced disease.[27]

Multiple Myeloma. Myeloma is a low-growth fraction tumor with only a small percentage of tumor cells in cycle at any time, which means that the time before patients need treatment can range from 1 to 3 years, with the actual time of treatment ranging from 1 to 10 years or longer. Fig. 25.12 shows an abundance of lytic lesions on a lateral skull radiograph in a patient with multiple myeloma.

Patients who have advanced renal disease in addition to multiple myeloma have a poorer prognosis. Other findings associated with shortened median survival times or remission durations include age older than 65 years, severe anemia, hypercalcemia, elevated blood urea nitrogen values, elevated M protein, hypoalbuminemia, and a high tumor cell burden. In addition, patients with rapid response to treatment have shorter median survival times and shorter remission durations than do patients with slower responses. Patients diagnosed early in the disease process are much more likely to have a longer survival time or remission duration.

Treatment for multiple myeloma is typically a combination of chemotherapy and radiation therapy. Chemotherapy is given with a curative intent, whereas radiation is effective in controlling the pain from a bony lesion. Melphalan is a common chemotherapy agent and is often given with prednisone. The treatment may also include bortezomib, a proteasome inhibitor and radiosensitizer, or thalidomide, an

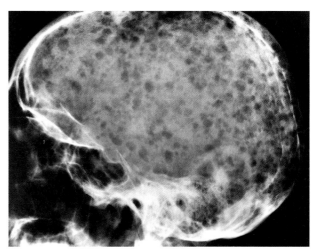

Fig. 25.12 Abundance of lytic lesions scattered throughout the skull in this patient with multiple myeloma. Flat bones (such as the skull, vertebrae, ribs, and pelvis) tend to be more affected. (From Eisenberg RL, Johnson NM. *Comprehensive Radiographic Pathology.* 6th ed. St. Louis, MO: Elsevier; 2016.)

immunomodulatory agent used to boost immune function. Response rates are higher with aggressive agents, such as lenalidomide-dexamethasone or thalidomide-dexamethasone; however, these do not improve survival rates compared with the traditional agents.

Autologous stem cell transplant after high-dose chemotherapy is also becoming a common treatment regimen. This treatment is currently preferred for patients younger than the age of 60 years. Cure is unlikely; however, the disease can be controlled for up to 3 years.

Radiation therapy is primarily used to help manage a symptomatic lesion associated with multiple myeloma. The lesion is usually painful and can result in fracture if not treated. A dose of 30 Gy is effective in controlling the pain and is typically administered in 10 to 15 treatments. With the use of irradiation to treat localized lesions, the field must be planned carefully so that the entire lesion is treated. In addition, generous margins should be used in the treatment of osteolytic lesions of the long bones. For these reasons, MRI has been supportive in guiding the location, planning, and treatment portals for a lesion. The objective should be to treat the entire lesion but spare as much healthy tissue as possible. Fig. 25.13 shows a single posterior treatment field for disease in the sacrum and lumbar vertebrae.

Surgery is uncommon in the treatment of multiple myeloma; however, it may be performed in certain instances. If a patient has a pending pathologic fracture, stabilization of the bone before radiation therapy is initiated, and may be appropriate. In addition, for paraspinal masses, which can be extremely large and can cause paralysis and pain, debulking the tumor before radiation therapy is initiated, and may be advised.

Supportive intervention for these patients is extremely important and should not be forgotten. This type of care includes treatment for anemia, hypercalcemia, azotemia (abnormal levels of urea, creatinine, body waste compounds, and other nitrogen-rich compounds in the blood), and frequent infections. These patients cannot be cured, so in addition to palliative therapies for the relief of pain, support care is necessary to sustain a desirable quality of life.

Ewing Sarcoma. Treatment of Ewing bone sarcoma includes surgery, chemotherapy, and radiation therapy. A combination of these modalities is most effective in achieving local control and improving long-term survival.[3] Overall survival rates near 70% may be achieved

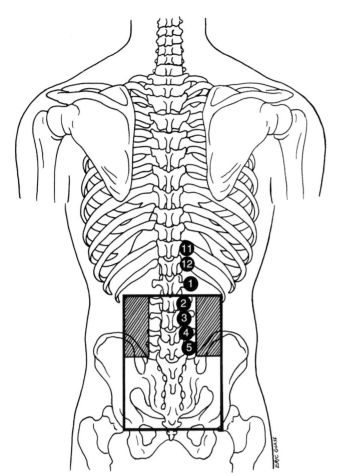

Fig. 25.13 Schematic representation of a single posterior treatment field for metastatic disease in the sacrum and lumbar vertebrae. Shaded areas represent shielding used to spare healthy tissue. Circled numbers correspond to thoracic and lumbar vertebrae.

in patients with localized disease.[3] Although a combination of surgery and radiation therapy is the standard of care, the disease is sensitive to chemotherapy, which may be given pre- or postoperatively. Shrinking the tumor before surgery increases the likelihood of achieving clear margins with complete resection. Chemotherapy is often used following surgery to improve overall survival. Common agents include vincristine, doxorubicin, cyclophosphamide, ifosfamide, and etoposide.[3] The ultimate goal for patients with Ewing bone sarcoma is the eradication of the entire tumor and the preservation of as much function as possible at the same time.

Radiation therapy is typically given postoperatively, especially in cases with positive surgical margins. However, if the tumor is unresectable, external beam therapy is the only option in conjunction with chemotherapy. Pelvic and spine tumors are typically more aggressive, and the use of surgery can be limited. In these cases, achieving local control with radiation therapy is necessary. Five-year local control rates of 95% are possible with surgery and external beam therapy.[3] The radiation treatment volume includes a 2-cm margin around the soft tissue component and the entire bone, to doses of 55 to 60 Gy for definitive cases. Preoperative and postoperative cases typically necessitate a lower dose, ranging from 36 to 45 Gy. In postoperative cases, it is recommended to start radiation therapy within 60 days of surgery for optimal response. Postoperative doses range from 45 to 55.8 Gy, depending on the level of resection.[3]

The most important prognostic factor for Ewing sarcoma is the extent of the disease at the time of the diagnosis. Patients with metastatic disease at the time of the diagnosis usually have a poor outcome. Early studies have shown that patients with bone or bone marrow involvement did not do as well as patients with limited pulmonary involvement. In addition, extension into the soft tissue is associated with a less favorable prognosis than that in patients with limited or no soft tissue involvement. Tumor size and location are other factors. Larger tumors and those that arise in the pelvis can negatively affect prognosis. Unfortunately, the recurrence rate is 30% to 40%, which includes local or distant disease.[3]

Metastatic Bone Disease. Most malignant bone lesions are metastatic. The radiation therapist treats more patients with metastatic bone disease than patients with primary bone lesions. For example, approximately 30% to 40% of patients with nonsmall cell lung cancer and up to 75% of patients with prostate cancer with advanced disease have bone metastases develop. Breast carcinoma also metastasizes to bone, with 70% of patients with breast cancer affected.[24] Bone metastases cause pain and skeletal-related events (SREs), including pathologic fractures, spinal cord compression, and forced immobility, which are associated with a significant decrease in the quality of life.

Metastatic bone disease is not curable; therefore maintenance of a certain quality of life for patients becomes important. The prognosis for those with metastatic bone disease depends on the primary site, histology, and degree of metastases at the time of diagnosis. Lung cancer patients with bone metastases live an average of 6 to 7 months after diagnosis. Breast cancer patients with bony involvement have a median survival of 19 to 25 months, and those prostate cancer patients with metastatic bone disease live an average of 12 to 53 months.[24]

The treatment goal of bone metastases is prevention and reduction of the occurrence of SREs. Palliation of pain and prevention of fractures to weight-bearing bones are very important. Approximately 10% to 30% of patients will suffer from a pathologic fracture. The most common fracture results from metastatic breast cancer, accounting for 60% of all pathologic fractures. This can occur in the spine and ribs; however, the long bones are most commonly affected. In over 50% of cases, the proximal femur is where the breakage occurs.[24]

Radiation therapy is effective in local control of the lesion, with relief of pain and prevention of the loss of function of the bone. In fact, over 50% of patients with bone metastases have significant pain relief after 5 to 10 fractions. Surgery is usually only necessary to stabilize a weight-bearing bone or to debulk an extradural mass to relieve excruciating pain. Radiation therapy may be given after the surgical procedure to obtain local control.[24]

Radiation fields need to include all involved bone but also spare uninvolved tissue when possible. If stabilization has been performed surgically, radiation therapy should be initiated as soon as the wound has healed. The portal should include the fixation device and any micrometastases that may have been dislodged during the surgical procedure. However, a strip of soft tissue should be left untreated to preserve lymphatic drainage. In the treatment of the spine, the fields should include the symptomatic vertebrae, with a one-vertebral-body margin above and below the involved vertebrae. If necessary, multileaf collimation can be used to shield healthy bone and reduce the amount of small bowel in the field.

Standard radiation dose for bone metastases palliation is 30 Gy in 10 fractions. However, optimal pain control is also achievable with lower total doses and higher dose per fraction. Clinical trials have shown no significant difference in pain control between the standard dose and other fractionation schemes, including 24 Gy given in 6 fractions and 20 Gy administered in 5 sessions. Treatment of the patient in 1 fraction with 8 Gy provides adequate pain relief as well and is now quite common in practice, saving the patient multiple trips to the oncology department.[24]

> Patients treated for malignancies in the lower extremities often need to be in reversed position on the treatment couch, with the feet toward the gantry. This position must be documented clearly in the simulation and treatment records.

Radiopharmaceutical agents can also be used for the palliation of metastatic bone disease. Strontium-89 (^{89}Sr), rhenium-186, and samarium-153 have been shown to provide pain relief for patients with metastatic prostate carcinoma and, in some cases, with breast cancer that is metastatic to bone.[24] Strontium-89 is a pure beta-emitter that causes minimal irradiation of healthy tissues. This agent localizes to osteoblastic areas or skeletal metastatic lesions from the primary cancer. It has a therapeutic half-life of 50.5 days; therefore its therapeutic effect may last up to 15 months. Radionuclide therapy is generally administered intravenously on an outpatient basis with minimal side effects.

The most recent advancement in radiopharmaceutical therapy is the use of radium-223, an alpha-emitter and calcium derivative.[24] Clinical trials have been in progress to establish the effectiveness of this agent and were recently published in *The New England Journal of Medicine*. Patients with prostate cancer having at least two metastatic bone lesions were included in the study ($n = 900$). Patients in the radium-223 group received six injections of the agent, and patients in the control group received five injections of a placebo. Results indicated that survival time was greater among the patients who had received the radium-223 injections compared with those in the control group. They lived about 3 months longer than the control group patients. In addition, prostatic specific antigen levels were significantly lower among the patients who received radium-223 compared with those who received the placebo.

As with any therapy, acute and chronic side effects and complications are possible with the treatment of bone tumors. Patients who undergo multimodality treatment with combined radiation therapy and chemotherapy are at higher risk for moderate to severe complications (Radiation Therapy Oncology Group Grade 3 and 4; see Chapter 4 for more information). Aggressive systemic treatment (chemotherapy) and local treatment (radiation) may cause acute problems, including erythema, fever, neutropenia, mucositis, nausea, vomiting, and diarrhea. Late or chronic effects of radiation to bone may lead to growth delays in pediatric patients, scoliosis after vertebral irradiation, increased sensitivity to chronic infection, fracture, and necrosis. Radiation-induced malignancies are also sequels of treatment. In general, the side effects experienced by patients with primary bone cancer are fairly well tolerated.

CASE I: Fibrous Dysplasia

A 26-year-old African-American woman presented with a growth in her hard palate/maxilla. She had a personal history of smoking and a family history of cancer; her father had been diagnosed with prostate cancer and osteosarcoma. She reported the lump growing rapidly, having tripled in size in 3 months. On examination, the clinical diagnosis was fibrous dysplasia. Surgical resection was performed.

The final pathology examination showed a chondroblastic osteosarcoma with positive margins at the left lateral and posterior resection margins.

Are the etiologic factors consistent with this patient's diagnosis?

She underwent 12 weeks of systemic chemotherapy, including ifosfamide and Adriamycin.

A second surgical resection was then performed with less than 50% necrosis of tumor remaining; therefore an additional three cycles of ifosfamide/VP-16 and three cycles of ifosfamide/Adriamycin were given.

Why was a second resection performed?

Side effects of chemotherapy included prolonged periods of pancytopenia. The patient had had a remission period of approximately 16 months when a 6-mm recurrence was found on a follow-up CT scan. She then underwent a maxillectomy and later extraction of teeth in preparation for radiation therapy.

In consultation with the radiation oncologist, the patient was informed that the role of radiation therapy in osteosarcoma of the head and neck was limited because of the relative radioresistance of bone tumors. Because standard treatment had failed for this patient, radiation therapy seemed reasonable in an effort to obtain local control.

What tumor characteristics make this case radioresistant in comparison with other histologies?

A CT simulation was performed to plan for an intensity-modulated radiation therapy (IMRT) treatment course. The patient was immobilized with an Aquaplast (Patterson Medical, Warrenville, IL), headrest, and standard bite block. Her arms were on her abdomen, with her hands holding a ring, and a sponge was placed under her knees. The prescription was written for a total dose of 66 Gy, with 50 Gy initially and 16 Gy to a boost field in a total of 33 fractions. Seven different 6-MV photons beams were used, prescribed to 90% isodose lines.

The volume treated was confined to the oral cavity and maxillary sinus, with an effort to spare one of the parotid glands. Regional lymphatics were not electively irradiated in light of low risk of lymphatic metastasis from well-differentiated osteosarcoma. The dose delivered to the cord was 11.6 Gy.

The patient had significant mucositis during and after therapy, with a total weight loss of 20.5 lb (12% of body weight).

What should be suggested to manage these side effects?

Pain management included a fentanyl (Duragesic [Janssen Pharmaceuticals, Titusville, NJ]) patch, viscous lidocaine, and morphine (MS Contin [Purdue Pharma, Stamford, CT]). The patient also was prescribed fluoxetine (Prozac [Eli Lilly & Company, Indianapolis, IN]) for depression. The course of radiation therapy was completed, and the patient underwent 40 hyperbaric chamber treatments to aid in the healing of osteoradionecrosis of the right maxilla.

At follow-up, the patient was disease-free, with necessary routine adjustments of her facial obturator. She was encouraged to continue mouth-opening exercises and strict oral hygiene. Overall, the patient was doing very well.

CASE II: Osteomyelitis

A 52-year-old Caucasian man, with an insignificant medical history, presented with flulike symptoms followed by pain in his right anterior thigh and groin. He was treated with a cortisone injection, which was not effective.

What conditions was the physician trying to treat with cortisone?

One week later, plain films and MRI were obtained. The studies showed a 7.3 × 7.6 cm destructive process in the subtrochanteric region of the upper thigh that could mimic either infection or malignancy. A biopsy was performed, and the final diagnosis showed acute osteomyelitis of the right hip and chondrosarcoma. The osteomyelitis was treated with cefazolin (Ancef [SmithKline Beecham, Philadelphia, PA]) and levofloxacin (Levaquin [Janssen Pharmaceuticals, Inc., Titusville, NJ]). The Levaquin was discontinued because of chills and considerable fatigue. The patient's condition was deemed stable; however, he could not undergo surgery for resection and reconstruction at that time because of the size of tumor, so neoadjuvant chemotherapy was ordered. The patient received three cycles of Adriamycin, ifosfamide, and mesna with excellent response. A resection and a right total hip arthroplasty were then performed. It was noteworthy that the preoperative MRI showed a lesion in the right sacral spine that was thought to be a separate chondrosarcoma primary, but this lesion was surgically unapproachable (Fig. 25.14).

After 3 months of healing and rehabilitation, the patient was seen in radiation oncology to treat the right hip surgical bed and give definitive radiation therapy to the sacral lesion. The patient was simulated with CT guidance, positioned supine in a Vac-Lok (Civco, Coralville, IA) with two pillows, no knee sponge, and toes together. His arms were on his abdomen, holding a ring with both hands.

What happens to the isocenter if the patient is treated with a knee sponge, considering the simulation notes did not include one?

The prescription was written to give 45 Gy in 25 fractions to an anteroposterior/posteroanterior (A/P) comprehensive field that encompassed the right hip and sacral spine (Fig. 25.15); 25-MV photons were used to deliver 1.8 Gy/fraction. A sacral boost was delivered via a six-field conformal technique. Again, 25-MV photons were used to deliver 1.8 Gy/fraction for a dose of 19.8 Gy, bringing the total dose to the sacrum to 64.8 Gy. The patient tolerated treatment well with no interruptions.

Why was the physician not concerned about exceeding the spinal cord dose of 45 Gy?

Approximately 16 months after radiation, the patient showed no evidence of disease. He stated that he had a slight clicking in his thigh from the prosthesis but could carry out most activities with minimal limitations. Otherwise, he was doing well.

SOFT TISSUE SARCOMAS

Soft tissue sarcomas (STSs) are part of the classification of solid tumors that arise from mesenchymal stem cells (cells that can differentiate into a variety of cell types, including osteoblasts, chondrocytes, and myocytes). They arise in connective tissues, including adipose tissue, muscle, nerve sheath, and blood vessels. Although they are rare, tumors that occur in soft tissue are more common than those in bone. They are

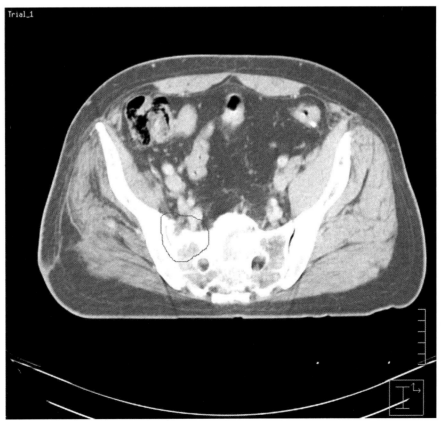

Fig. 25.14 Computed tomography treatment planning image denotes sacral mass.

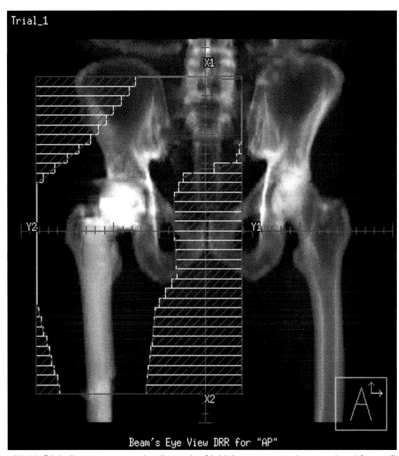

Fig. 25.15 Digitally reconstructed radiograph of initial anteroposterior sacral and femur field.

grouped in one classification because there are approximately 50 different pathologic subtypes. Approximately 43% occur in the extremities, followed by trunk (10%), viscera (19%), retroperitoneum (15%), and head and neck (9%).[28] The most common STS that affects children is rhabdomyosarcoma. The most common types among adults are liposarcoma and leiomyosarcoma.[11]

This section of the chapter presents fundamental information about the nature of this disease, including etiology, tissue derivation, histology, staging, grading, and patterns of spread. Treatment options, management of STS, and the role of the radiation therapist are also addressed.

Natural History

The natural history of STS is highly dependent on the site of the initial neoplasm and its grade. The local growth pattern of STS follows the lines of least resistance in the longitudinal axis of the primary site compartment. The primary site compartment consists of the natural anatomic boundaries that surround the STS primary. It is composed of common fascia plane(s) of muscles, bone, joint, skin, subcutaneous tissues, and major neurovascular structures.

As a tumor progresses and grows, it pushes away other structures and forms a pseudocapsule that is made of compressed healthy and fibrotic tissue. Trunk and head and neck primaries are generally high grade and tend to invade adjacent muscle groups, whereas extremity tumors spread along the longitudinal axis of muscular compartments. The likelihood of regional lymph node involvement is low. Intermediate-grade and high-grade lesions typically result in hematogenous metastases, primarily to the lungs. Retroperitoneal primaries also have

the potential for lung metastases; however, they usually spread to the liver and other abdominal structures.[28]

Epidemiology

In comparison with other malignancies, the incidence rate of STS is fairly low. Approximately 13,040 new diagnoses occur each year, accounting for 1% of malignancies in adults and 15% in children. Although the prevalence rate is low, the overall mortality rate is considerably high, with about 5150 deaths per year.[28]

Men have a slightly higher incidence rate of STS than women, with a ratio of approximately 1.5:1.[1] STS most commonly affects adults in the fifth and sixth decades of life; however, it can occur at any age. Rates of STS are generally highest in the African-American population. Rhabdomyosarcoma is most common among children around the age of 10 years. The two subtypes are embryonal and alveolar. Embryonal is more prevalent in children under 10 years, and the alveolar type tends to occur over the age of 10 years. As previously stated, STS can occur anywhere in the body, with the extremities the most frequent location, followed by the retroperitoneum. Of the STSs found in the extremities, most occur in the lower extremity, especially the thigh.

Etiology

The etiology of STS is unknown; however, associations are found with a variety of genetic and environmental factors. Prior exposure to radiation is a risk factor that has been identified, although it is only linked to fewer than 5% of cases.[1] For example, treatment for primary malignancies, including lymphoma, cervical, testicular, and breast cancers, may increase the risk for sarcoma years later.

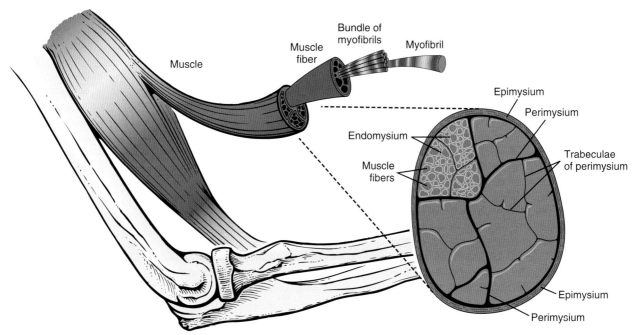

Fig. 25.16 Normal muscle anatomy. (From Damjanov I. *Pathology for the Health Professions*. 5th ed. St. Louis, MO: Elsevier; 2017.)

Several genetic conditions are associated with an increased risk of STS. The most common is neurofibromatosis, a familial disease that involves multiple benign tumors of the nerves. Peripheral nerve sheath tumors occur in approximately 5% of those with this condition.[1] Genetic defects in the *RB1* gene are associated with retinoblastoma, a pediatric eye tumor. The risk for STS increases with this condition, particularly in those who were treated with radiation therapy.[1] Patients with Li-Fraumeni syndrome are at high risk for development of multiple types of cancer, including sarcomas. They are very susceptible to secondary malignancies related to radiation therapy.[1] Additional genetic conditions that may increase STS risk are Gardner syndrome, Werner syndrome, tuberous sclerosis, and Gorlin syndrome.[1]

General Anatomy and Physiology, Including Pertinent Lymphatic Considerations

The embryonic origin of STS begins in the primitive mesoderm (middle layer). The loosely formed network of cells in the mesoderm, the primitive mesenchyme, and the ectoderm give rise to the most common connective tissues, such as the pleura, peritoneum, pericardium, walls and endothelium of blood vessels, bone, cartilage, muscles, and soft connective tissue. Visceral connective tissue, similar muscle organs, and smooth muscle organs (e.g., the kidney, ureters, uterus, gonads, heart, and a variety of hematopoietic tissues) all derive from the remainder of the primitive mesoderm. Refer to Fig. 25.2 for a schematic representation of tissue origin.

Skeletal muscle is composed of striated muscle fibers that vary from very large in size to extremely small. The compartmentalization of muscle fibers and the surrounding connective tissue coverings (epimysium, perimysium, and endomysium) can be seen in Fig. 25.16. Muscle cells are specialized, with their primary function being contraction. This allows the body to move, breathe, and maintain posture.[7] Lymphatic drainage is site specific and does not affect the management of STS. Skeletal muscle has a limited capacity to respond to tumor formation, so once symptoms present, detection and diagnosis should be evident.

Clinical Presentation

Symptoms of STS are often nonspecific. Most patients initially present with a painless, gradually enlarging mass. However, a tumor in the abdomen or pelvis may cause pain or bloating as it increases in size. Head and neck and distal extremities are often diagnosed earlier than are tumors of the thigh or retroperitoneum. Other presenting symptoms of site-specific STS are weakness, increased pressure such as paresthesia, distal edema, or presence of warmth or distended vascularity when fixed to other structures.[5]

Detection and Diagnosis

The initial physician consultation includes a detailed history and physical examination to exclude other conditions. For optimal visualization of tumor size and shape, an MRI is recommended. MRI is considered the diagnostic tool of choice for STS detection because of its exceptional soft tissue contrast and specificity (Figures 25.17 and 25.18)[21]. CT is still widely used, especially for retroperitoneal tumors. It is also useful in the staging process because most STS metastasize to the lungs. PET imaging is becoming an essential part of the staging and workup process as well. The maximum uptake value of the radionuclide may coincide with tumor grade and prognostic indicators. PET scans may also be used to predict the likelihood of recurrence or progression and evaluate chemotherapy response before surgery.[28]

After localization of the tumor, a biopsy is required to confirm the histology. Although various methods of biopsy exist, the core needle technique is the most widely used. Multiple samples are necessary to obtain an accurate diagnosis. Fine-needle biopsy often is not recommended because obtaining an adequate tissue sample is more difficult. Superficial lesions may be diagnosed with an excisional approach, especially with those less than 5 cm. An open biopsy has a relatively high risk of complications but a small likelihood of misdiagnosis and may be used in some cases. The open biopsy should be performed with consideration of subsequent definitive operative procedures because the biopsy route and scar must be resected during a future surgery.

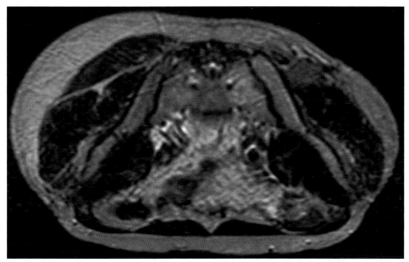

Fig. 25.17 Axial image of a soft tissue sarcoma of the buttock.

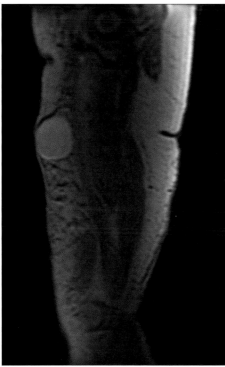

Fig. 25.18 Magnetic resonance imaging coronal view of soft tissue sarcoma in the lower extremity.

Pathology

Sarcomas are classified histologically and named according to the tissues in which they arise. Currently, more than 50 histologic types of STS are known. The most common in adults are liposarcoma and leiomyosarcoma. Less common subtypes are MFH, synovial sarcoma, and malignant peripheral nerve sheath tumors. Rhabdomyosarcoma is the most common histology in the pediatric population. The histologic distinction aids in the staging of STS.

Grading and Staging

Grading and staging are essential for determining prognosis and a treatment regimen, as recurrence and metastases are so common with different subtypes.[28] The two most commonly used primary

---

BOX 25.1   French Federation of Cancer Centers Sarcoma Group

Grades
- Grade 1: total score of 2 to 3 points
- Grade 2: total score of 4 to 5 points
- Grade 3: total score of 6 to 8 points

Tumor Differentiation
- **1 point**: resembles normal adult mesenchymal tissue, may be confused with a benign lesion, such as well-differentiated liposarcoma
- **2 points:** histologic typing is certain, such as myxoid liposarcoma
- **3 points:** synovial sarcoma, osteosarcoma, Ewing sarcoma/primitive neuroectodermal tumor (PNET), sarcomas of doubtful tumor type, embryonal and undifferentiated sarcomas

Mitotic Count (Count 10 Successive High Power Fields [Area of 0.17 mm Squared] in Most Mitotically Active Areas)
- **1 point:** 0 to 9 mitoses
- **2 points:** 10 to 19 mitoses
- **3 points:** 20 or more mitoses

Tumor Necrosis
- **0 points:** no necrosis on any slides
- **1 point:** less than 50% necrosis for all examined tumor surface
- **2 points:** tumor necrosis of 50% or more of examined tumor surface

From PathologyOutlines.com. http://www.pathologyoutlines.com/topic/softtissuegrading.html. Accessed November 14th, 2018. Originally from IARC Press on Soft Tissue.

systems for grading STS are the French Federation of Cancer Centers Sarcoma Group (FNCLCC) and the National Cancer Institute system.

The FNCLCC system provides scores for tumor differentiation, mitotic count, and tumor necrosis. The total score is then used to determine the histologic grade of the tumor. See Box 25.1 for category descriptions. The recommended staging system is the AJCC, or TNM, system. The primary tumor size is defined by T, extent of lymph node involvement N, and metastasis present M. It also includes the tumor grade and depth.

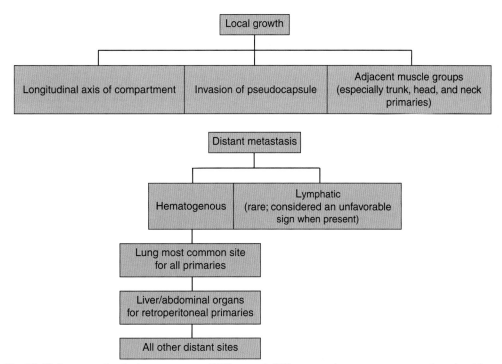

Fig. 25.19 Patterns of soft tissue sarcoma (STS) spread. STS metastatic patterns progress from local invasion to the early hematogenous extension to the lung, liver, abdominal organs, and all other distant sites. Lymphatic spread is rare.

Spread Patterns

The STSs are aggressive and invade along local, anatomically defined planes composed of neurovascular structures, fascia, and muscle bundles (Fig. 25.19). Lymphatic extension is not common. Hematologic pathways are the primary routes of spread; the lung is the most common site of metastasis, followed by the bones, liver, and skin.

Retroperitoneal sarcomas may have up to a 60% or greater local recurrence rate over 10 years, whereas extremity and other lesions recur at 20% during the same time interval.[27,26] On the other hand, the metastatic rate for high-grade extremity STS is approximately 30%. Thus death from STS is more likely to result from metastatic disease, most commonly to the lungs.[26]

Treatment Considerations

The treatment of STS requires a multidisciplinary team approach that involves a combination of surgery, chemotherapy, and radiation therapy. Treatment protocols are influenced by many factors, including size and site of the tumor, histologic stage and grade, its proximity to neurovascular or visceral structures, the patient's age and general health status, presence of metastases, and the desires of the patient and family.

Surgery. Surgical resection is the standard of care in the treatment of localized (stage 1A, 1B) STS. A wide excision (1 to 2 cm of healthy tissue) is necessary to achieve negative histologic margins in high-grade cases. A surgery is termed definitive when margins greater than 1 cm are achieved or when the fascial plane is left.[28] Surgical clips should remain in the surgical bed in cases in which positive margins are likely. This helps the radiation oncologist design an optimal treatment plan for postoperative radiation to the peritoneum or abdomen. For local control to be achieved in patients with STS of the extremity, limb-salvage (limb-sparing) surgery (LSS) is advised. This type of surgery may result in close or positive margins, which increases the risk for local recurrence. The NCCN recommends postoperative radiation in these cases, in cases in which the margin is less than 1

cm, and in cases in which positive margins microscopically involve bone.[28]

> A marginal surgical technique involves cutting through the surrounding fibrous membrane, often leaving microscopic foci of tumor. Wide excision is cutting outside the membrane and compartment, leaving only skip metastases, and a radical procedure involves amputation of the entire limb.

Radiation Therapy. Several different options are available for administration of adjuvant radiation therapy for STS. Treatment may be delivered with external beam radiation (including photon, electron, proton, and heavy particle beams), brachytherapy, intraoperative radiation therapy (IORT), or a combination of these modalities. Radiation therapy may be the only form of treatment if the patient is not a surgical candidate. The more common approach is either preoperative or postoperative therapy. Regardless of the method, the reason for treatment is local control and prolonged disease-free survival. The advantages and disadvantages of both are discussed subsequently.

Preoperative radiation therapy is becoming the standard of care, especially in the United States.[15] It is just as effective as postoperative treatment in achieving local control. In fact, radiation therapy before surgery is associated with a complete resection with negative margins.[28]

Advantages of preoperative radiation therapy include the following[15]:

- Radiation fields are smaller, which may result in less morbidity because of fracture, edema, and late effects, such as fibrosis.
- Lower total radiation dose is required, which results in improved overall function.
- A thickened pseudocapsule may make for a simpler resection, which reduces the recurrence risk.

There are several disadvantages to preoperative radiation. The primary one is reduced surgical wound healing, which can greatly affect the functionality of the limb. Another disadvantage is the gap of time necessary between the last radiation treatment and surgery. A minimum of 3 weeks is required for healing to occur and to reduce the surgical wound complication rate. Waiting longer than 6 weeks increases the chance for fibrotic changes, thereby hindering the surgical procedure.[15]

Total recommended dose for preoperative therapy is 50 Gy, with a radiation boost after surgery if the margins are close or positive. Because the evidence to support the long-term benefit of a postoperative boost is weak, it is recommended to evaluate on a case-by-case basis. The additional dose is delivered with brachytherapy, IORT, or EBRT. Recommended brachytherapy dose is 16 to 26 Gy about 3 days after resection, via catheters placed during surgery. The dose depends on whether a low-dose or high-dose rate technique is used. IORT involves a dose of 10 to 15 Gy delivered to the tumor bed immediately after tumor removal. The prescribed dose is dependent on the level of residual disease. Patients with microscopic disease receive 10 to 12.5 Gy, and in cases with gross disease, doses closer to 15 Gy are given. An advantage of this technique is that the surgeon displaces adjacent organs away from the radiation field. This is especially important in abdominal and pelvic sarcomas because of limited-tolerance doses for surrounding structures, such as the kidneys and small bowel.[28]

Postoperative radiation therapy is selected on more of an individual basis, rather than by margin status. The purpose is to eradicate any remaining cells following surgical resection. It is typically used in cases of high-grade STS with positive margins, particularly of an extremity. An advantage of surgery first is optimal tumor staging. In addition, wound healing is typically not compromised, as with preoperative treatment. However, the late effects are more likely, which is thought to result from a higher radiation dose and larger treatment volumes. The treatment options are brachytherapy, IORT, and EBRT, which should be administered between 3 and 8 weeks after surgery or when the patient's wound is healed. Low-dose-rate brachytherapy may be the only adjuvant therapy given, with a dose of 45 Gy for patients with negative margins. The NCCN recommends external beam therapy in addition to low-dose rate brachytherapy (16–20 Gy) in patients with positive surgical margins. Typical EBRT total doses are 45 Gy for STS of the abdomen or retroperitoneum and 50 Gy for other disease sites.[28] IORT local control rates have not been promising when it is used as the sole postoperative treatment. Therefore a recommended dose of 50 Gy delivered with EBRT should be given after the intraoperative dose of 10 to 16 Gy. Patients with positive surgical margins need an additional boost, up to 26 Gy for grossly positive margins. Boosting the primary tumor bed up to 16 Gy is even recommended in cases with negative margins.[28]

> With treatment of an extremity, the arm or leg must be extended away from the body to minimize scatter radiation to the body and to allow for any possible beam angle.

For delivery of an optimal therapeutic dose, dynamic treatments including IMRT, brachytherapy, and proton therapy are recommended.[15] These methods help to minimize the dose to healthy tissue. Proton beams are ideal because small amounts of energy are deposited initially, with the majority being deposited at end of the range, over a short distance. The result is a steep rise in absorbed dose known as the *Bragg peak*.[15] Several Bragg peaks of decreasing energies are superimposed on each other to achieve an optimal dose distribution. Doses of 74.4 to 81.6 Gy may be delivered with proton beam therapy and IMRT. Other charged particles that have been used for treatment of STS include neon, carbon, and fast neutrons. These particles have a high linear energy transfer, which affects the biologic effectiveness and

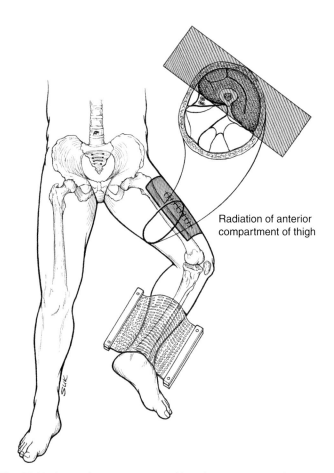

Fig. 25.20 Appropriate treatment position shows access to the tumor compartment.

has less reliance on cell cycle, DNA repair, and oxygen enhancement ratio than other forms of radiation. Although these particles seem ideal for treating radioresistant tumors, it is very costly and therefore not yet widely used.[15]

Postoperative radiation fields should include the full surgical bed with margins of 3 to 6 cm around the surgical site. The boost volume includes the primary tumor volume and a 2-cm to 3-cm margin. Regional lymph nodes are typically not included, except for rhabdomyosarcomas, synovial sarcomas, and epithelioid sarcomas. Total circumferential radiation of extremities must be avoided by leaving at least a 1-cm to 3-cm strip of skin and soft tissue to avoid future complications of fibrosis and edema. Fig. 25.20 illustrates a treatment setup for a lower extremity. This setup is also for patients with incomplete resection, with tumors in close proximity to critical structures, or with locally advanced or recurrent disease.

Overall, STSs require fairly high doses of radiation to achieve local control and long-term survival. With the technologic advances of conformal therapy and IMRT, total doses of 75 Gy are being reached.[15] As a result, better outcomes of long-term survival and limited morbidity from treatment have been seen. Local failures occur within 2 to 4 years without adjuvant radiation therapy.[16]

Chemotherapy. The overall benefit of chemotherapy in the treatment of STS remains unclear. Clinical studies suggest it is appropriate for patients with advanced, high-risk, recurrent, or metastatic disease. Survival rates are not significantly improved in most patients, likely because of the numerous histologic subtypes. The primary tumor is more difficult to target with systemic therapy because of its heterogeneity.[18] Chemosensitivity of a tumor depends on the tumor subtype. Therefore chemotherapy is typically given in conjunction with radiation therapy. Doxorubicin is currently the primary chemotherapy agent used in the treatment of STS; however, ongoing clinical trials are investigating whether the addition of other agents improves overall survival.[18]

A study of 119 adult patients at high risk with localized STS was conducted to see whether metastatic-free survival rates (MFS) could increase from 40% with the addition of ifosfamide to the standard chemotherapy agent, doxorubicin. Subjects received hyperfractionated radiation therapy with a dose of 1.8 Gy twice per day for a total dose of 36 Gy. Concurrent chemotherapy was given in six courses of doxorubicin and ifosfamide. This study was not randomized, but it showed promising results. Although 40% had development of metastases, the overall 5-year MFS rate was higher, at 59%. Overall survival rate was 68% at 5 years. Moderate levels of toxicity were noted.[18]

Chemotherapy has resulted in positive outcomes in the treatment of adolescents with Ewing soft tissue sarcoma and rhabdomyosarcoma. Aggressive therapy, including multiagent chemotherapy with adjuvant radiation therapy, is necessary. During the past 50 years, overall survival rates have improved from 20% to 80% in many cases of rhabdomyosarcoma and Ewing soft tissue sarcoma.[22] Recognized cytotoxic agents are vincristine, cyclophosphamide, etoposide, cisplatin, ifosfamide, and doxorubicin.

Despite the mixed views of the benefit of chemotherapy, progress is being made. New chemotherapy agents and dosing regimens paired with radiation therapy are supplementing surgical approaches for the treatment of STS. There are several new agents in the developmental stage, including aldoxorubicin, TH-302, and trabectedin. Aldoxorubicin is a derivative of doxorubicin, designed to increase the efficacy by serving as a carrier. TH-302 is drug designed to increase tumor response in areas that are hypoxic, thereby increasing the sensitivity in an otherwise resistant environment. Trabectedin is beneficial for advanced disease that does not respond to doxorubicin or ifosphomide.[22]

Role of Radiation Therapist

The radiation therapist should understand the clinical progression of connective tissue tumors and recognize the evidence-based results in the scientific literature. The therapist provides the best possible care to patients with this knowledge base. Caring for the patient as an individual, rather than just as a disease carrier, is also important. Critical thinking skills are implemented when positioning and immobilizing the patient for simulation before or after surgery. Careful transferring of the patient from the simulation table and treatment couch is vital because patients are often weak and in pain. Precision during treatment is critical to maintain the lymphatic drainage needed for the extremity or to minimize dose to the spine and kidneys for a retroperitoneal lesion. In addition, the use of IMRT requires precise positioning to ensure coverage of the tumor or surgical bed.

The therapist-patient relationship is based on trust, professionalism, and knowledge of the disease. Exhibiting confidence is very important, especially during the therapist's first encounter with the patient. Strong communication skills are one of the most important aspects of the care provided to patients. Delicate situations that involve younger patients with disfigurement may necessitate unique interactive skills. Bony metastases may occur in elderly patients, who also need specific care and patience. Everyone involved in the care of the patient must fully understand the treatment regimen and the nature and severity of expected side effects. The therapist assesses the patient's physical, emotional, and coping status during daily interactions. In this next section,

several specific roles of the radiation therapist are discussed, including education, communication, assessment, and management of accessory medical equipment.

Education. Knowledge is power. Studies indicate that patients often feel dissatisfied with the information received about their treatment and care. When given appropriate information about healthcare procedures, reports of anxiety, pain, and distressing side effects are generally reduced.

A study by Hawley and associates[14] investigated how patients with breast cancer perceived their coordination of care. Demographic factors such as health literacy and race/ethnicity were included. A large patient sample ($n = 2268$) completed a survey, either via mail or phone. Participants were asked about their perceptions and satisfaction with care coordination. Results indicated that those with lower levels of health knowledge were more dissatisfied with the coordination of care. In addition, patients with comorbidities were less satisfied than those with cancer alone. Younger patients were more likely to be dissatisfied with care compared with middle-age and older women.[14] Radiation therapists must use professional judgment when explaining procedures to patients and families. Check for understanding. If the patient seems unsure about receiving treatment and needs additional information, referring the patient to the physician may be necessary.

Communication. Effective communication with the patient involves attentive listening, human touch, and questioning. Therapists can enhance their communication with their patients by asking open-ended questions such as, "What are you feeling?" rather than "How are you feeling?" Openness and assertiveness offer the patient a comfortable invitation to talk. This applies to every patient, no matter the diagnosis. Because the patient sees the therapist on a daily basis, this communication channel is of utmost importance. Patients are often more comfortable discussing issues with their therapist because visiting with the physician can be intimidating.

Stability and control are important to the patient during treatment. Try to keep scheduled treatment times as prompt as possible and avoid rescheduling of treatments.

Assessment. Optimal cancer management includes a daily evaluation of the patient, both physiologically and emotionally. The therapist must be aware of changes in the patient's symptoms, especially if the patient already has metastatic bone disease. Regular assessment of skin changes is also important because many patients with bone tumors or STS have treatment after surgery. Monitoring of the anticipated erythema and dry or moist desquamation may necessitate a decision to withhold treatment until the radiation oncologist advises to resume therapy. Mood changes are also important to note; fatigue and depression are common among patients with cancer.

Immunosuppression may be common because of concurrent chemotherapy, which increases a patient's risk for infection, especially at the surgical site. Close observation for symptoms of infection and regular notation of blood values is the therapist's responsibility. An evaluation of the patient's nutritional status and performance rating may also indicate the need for an intervention referral. Recognition of and responding to medical emergencies such as allergic reactions, adverse drug interactions, and cardiac arrest are included in the radiation therapist's purview of professional obligations.

Monitoring of Medical Equipment. Patients treated for connective tissue cancers may range from the elderly with metastatic bone disease to a child with Ewing sarcoma. Accessory medical equipment may include intravenous fluids, oxygen, urinary catheter, chest tubes, and shunts. A pediatric patient recovering from radical surgery who is receiving adjuvant chemotherapy needs careful observation, evaluation, and interventions. Patients treated with sedation need additional intense monitoring and observation, including a pulse oximeter and blood pressure cuff. Attention to placement of these devices and monitoring of the patient during treatment are important for patient safety and accurate radiation dose delivery.

The radiation therapist's broad-based patient care responsibilities include the knowledge and understanding of connective tissue sarcomas as malignant processes and treatment delivery competency. The therapist is the patient's advocate in coordination of referrals for all aspects of conditions relevant to the patient's disease status and treatment.

CASE III: Metastatic Lesion

A 70-year-old Caucasian woman had swelling in her right forearm for several months' duration and then felt a palpable mass. The patient had a family history indicative of cancer: a mother with colon cancer, a paternal uncle with metastatic liver disease, and a paternal aunt with breast cancer. The patient had a history of uterine leiomyosarcoma 2 years previously, in which there were 35 to 40 small tumors studding the peritoneum, mesentery, and pelvic cul-de-sac. The uterus was enlarged to 12 weeks' gestational size with a tumor erupting from the uterus. At that point, the patient underwent a total abdominal hysterectomy and bilateral salpingo-oophorectomy with resection of the pelvic and abdominal tumor nodules. After surgery, gross residual disease was found in the abdomen, so the patient received six cycles of Adriamycin chemotherapy.

The patient was without evidence of disease until the symptoms of swelling, pain, and weakness in her arm made her seek medical attention 1 year later. MRI revealed a mass that involved the medial proximal forearm in the flexor muscle group that measured 4 × 3.2 × 5.2 cm. A pelvic CT scan also revealed a mass located to the left of the rectosigmoid area that measured 3.2 × 2.2 cm. Physicians believed the mass in the forearm to be metastatic disease versus a new primary and the pelvic lesion to be a recurrence. The recommendation was for the patient to have preoperative radiation therapy to the forearm and address the pelvic mass at a later date.

Knowing the characteristics of STS, why is the assumption that the forearm mass was a metastatic lesion reasonable?

The patient was simulated in the supine position, B-headrest, left arm at her side away from her body, and her affected right arm above her head. A sponge was placed under her knees. The treatment fields consisted of an AP and right anterior oblique. The prescription stated to deliver 50 Gy, 2.0 Gy/fraction for 25 fractions. Multileaf collimation was used for field shaping, and a 0.5-cm bolus was placed over the biopsy incision on the AP field. Calculation of monitor units were given to produce an approximate 55-degree wedge, with heels together for both fields. She did have some mild erythema and swelling in the treatment field but completed the treatments without interruption.

One month after radiation, the patient underwent surgical resection of the tumor and IORT. At the time of resection, the median nerve and ulnar nerve were visualized in the tumor bed. The median nerve was retracted with a Penrose drain and shielded with a strip of lead. The ulnar nerve was also shielded with a lead strip. A 6-cm-round intraoperative electron cone was docked using aseptic conditions. A dose of 15 Gy was delivered using 6-MeV electrons and a 0.5-cm bolus covering the treatment field. After the 5-minute procedure, the placement of the cone and shielding was verified and then removed. A small area of the median nerve, which measured less than 0.5 cm, may have been exposed during irradiation.

What long-term complications could arise from this?

Two months after treatment for the leiomyosarcoma of the forearm, the patient's pelvic mass was reassessed. Over a period of 6 months, the tumor appeared to be 1 mm larger. Because the mass had been fairly stable, the decision was made to let the patient further recuperate from her surgery. Three years after treatment, the patient continued to struggle with metastatic disease. The lesion near her sigmoid colon had grown, and additional masses were found in the right gluteus maximus muscle and left posterior ileum, both measuring greater than 3 cm. The patient was told she was not a candidate for further surgery, so she was being followed by her hometown physician for pain control.

CASE IV: Alveolar Rhabdomyosarcoma

An 8-year-old Latino boy had bilateral lower quadrant pain and decreased appetite. A large abdominal mass was palpated by his primary care physician, and a CT scan of the abdomen was obtained. The CT scan revealed a right-sided abdominal mass that measured 12 cm in greatest dimension. Also noted were enlarged periaortic lymph nodes. The patient underwent a CT scan–guided biopsy of the periaortic lymph node the following day, and pathology confirmed a diagnosis of alveolar rhabdomyosarcoma.

Medical history was unremarkable for this patient; however, he was born at 27 weeks' gestation. There was no family history of malignancies, and the patient had a healthy mother, father, and brother. The patient's parents both smoked cigarettes.

Immediately after his diagnosis, the patient was started on a chemotherapy treatment protocol, specifically for rhabdomyosarcomas. Weekly treatments included vincristine, cyclophosphamide, dactinomycin, and topotecan. He received 12 weeks of chemotherapy, followed by an exploratory laparotomy. Although the patient had a significant response to chemotherapy, residual disease was found (Fig. 25.21). The surgeon resected several 3 × 3 cm nodules surrounding the umbilical arteries, primarily right-sided. An additional mass in the right lower quadrant, which measured 1 × 3 cm, was also removed. On examination of the omentum, multiple nodules were found. A fine-needle aspiration was performed and confirmed these nodules to be residual rhabdomyosarcoma.

Because of the extent of this patient's disease, consolidative radiation therapy was suggested. The parents were informed about the benefits, risks, and acute and long-term side effects. Possible complications associated with abdominal treatment include damage to the small bowel, kidneys, and liver, along with the risk of acquiring a second malignancy.

What might be done in the planning process to minimize dose to critical structures?

The patient received whole abdominal radiation, with a total dose of 24 Gy in 16 fractions. The course of treatment was given through an opposing AP technique with 6-MV photons. Renal blocks were added after a prescribed dose of 13.5 Gy (Fig. 25.22). A boost was not given because of the diffuse peritoneal involvement. The patient tolerated the treatments well with no interruptions. On completion, he had no clinical evidence of disease progression.

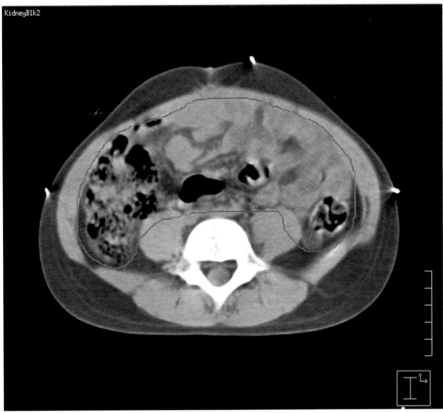

Fig. 25.21 Computed tomography treatment planning image contours the retroperitoneum, including large amounts of bowel.

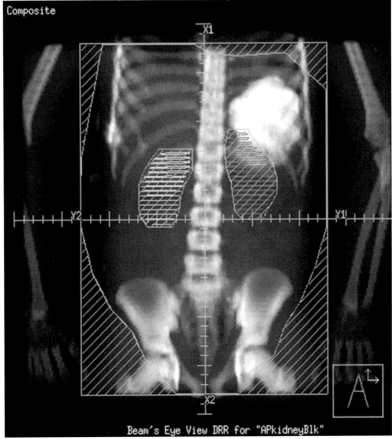

Fig. 25.22 Digitally reconstructed radiograph of anteroposterior abdomen field with kidney blocks.

SUMMARY

- Osteosarcoma is the most common osseous bone tumor; it occurs most often in patients 10 to 30 years of age. Chondrosarcomas and fibrosarcomas affect older adults with an average age of 60 years, whereas Ewing sarcoma is primarily a pediatric tumor that occurs in adolescents aged 10 to 20 years. Multiple myeloma tends to affect the middle-age and elderly population, with a peak in the seventh decade.
- The incidence rate of STS is fairly low. It is diagnosed most often in the fifth and sixth decades of life. Rhabdomyosarcoma, a form of STS, is most common in children, with the peak incidence in the first two decades of life and a median age at diagnosis of approximately 5 years old.
- A typical long bone consists of the diaphysis, two epiphyses, and the cartilage cap. A muscle is composed of the connective tissue coverings; perimysium, epimysium, endomysium, and the muscle fibers.
- Osteosarcomas are generally classified as poorly differentiated tumors. Chondrosarcomas arise from mesenchymal elements of the bone and are usually undifferentiated and associated with a higher grade. Fibrosarcomas originate in mesenchymal tissue. The cell of origin for MFH is the histiocyte or the macrophage. Ewing sarcoma is composed of populations of small, blue, round cells. Plasma cells associated with multiple myeloma originate from B-cell lymphocytes. No universally accepted staging system exists for primary bone sarcomas. Grade is determined to be either low or high grade.
- The standard treatment for bone and soft tissue sarcomas is surgery. With advancements in treatment options, chemotherapy and radiation therapy may become more widely used in some cases.

- MRI is becoming more widely used to detect bone and soft tissue sarcomas. Nuclear medicine scans, especially bone scans, are beneficial in detecting bone metastases. PET scans may be useful in the staging process. A biopsy must be performed to determine the diagnosis.
- The patient's prognosis is affected by the differentiation and aggression of the tumor. The more differentiated, the better the prognosis. Less aggressive tumors carry a better prognosis. Less differentiated, more aggressive tumors are associated with a worse prognosis.
- Average doses of radiation for most bone and soft tissue sarcomas are 50 to 60 Gy. However, in patients with gross disease, doses may be as high as 70 Gy to achieve local control. Intraoperative therapy may be used in conjunction with external beam therapy to give an additional dose of approximately 15 Gy in a single fraction. Patients with multiple myeloma need a lower total dose for pain control. Doses around 30 Gy are typically effective.
- The CT simulation process is extremely important to ensure proper treatment of bone and soft tissue sarcomas. The therapist must be sure the patient is in a reproducible position while kept as comfortable as possible. It is also important to work efficiently because these patients may be in pain.
- Most bone tumors are radioresistant because of their lower mitotic activity. The therapist must understand that these tumors are not extremely sensitive to radiation therapy, which makes them difficult to treat. This is primarily why sarcomas are treated with surgery.
- Emerging treatments include LSS, IORT, tumor suppressor gene therapy, new chemotherapy agents, stem cell transplant, and the use of radionuclides.

REVIEW QUESTIONS

The answers to the Review Questions can be found by logging on to our website at: http://evolve.elsevier.com/Washington/principles

1. The incidence rate of bone cancer is highest during what period?
   a. Infancy.
   b. Adulthood.
   c. Adolescence.
   d. Equal for all ages.
2. A nonosseous malignant tumor of the bone marrow is a(an):
   a. Fibrosarcoma.
   b. Chondrosarcoma.
   c. Osteosarcoma.
   d. Multiple myeloma.
3. A bone lesion that results from primary sites elsewhere in the body is a(n):
   a. Osteosarcoma.
   b. Multiple myeloma.
   c. Metastatic tumor.
   d. Chondrosarcoma.
4. The most common site of a primary bone sarcoma is:
   a. Epiphyseal.
   b. Metaphyseal.
   c. Diaphyseal.
   d. Shaft.
5. Emerging treatments for bone and STS include all of the following *except:*
   a. Cryotherapy.
   b. New chemotherapy agents.
   c. LSS.
   d. IORT.

6. The most common site of metastasis from primary bone cancer is:
   a. Brain.
   b. Bowel.
   c. Lung.
   d. Distal extremities.
7. _____ is most commonly used radionuclide in treating metastatic bone disease that results from primary prostate or breast cancer.
   a. Technetium-99m.
   b. Iodine-131m.
   c. Strontium-89m.
   d. Iodine-125m.
8. Although the exact cause of STS is unknown, a factor that has been implicated is:
   a. Prior sun exposure.
   b. Appearance as a second primary 3 to 15 years after high-dose radiation therapy for other cancers.
   c. Predisposition of Paget disease.
   d. Tobacco use.
9. Factors that are incorporated into the Federation of Cancer Centers Sarcoma Group histologic grading for STS include:
   I. Tumor differentiation.
   II. Mitotic count.
   III. Tumor necrosis.
      a. I and II.
      b. I and III.
      c. II and III.
      d. I, II, and III.

10. Regional lymph nodes are generally not included in the treatment portals for STS because:
    a. It is difficult to determine how STS spread.
    b. STS tend to spread via the blood.
    c. STS tend to spread via multiple lymph nodes.
    d. Edema is usually present, making it difficult to include lymph nodes in the treatment portal.
11. The rationale for leaving a 1-cm to 3-cm strip of skin and soft tissue rather than total circumferential irradiation of an extremity treated for STS is that it:
    a. Decreases excessive erythema.
    b. Promotes healing of the incision scar.
    c. Avoids future excessive fibrosis and edema.
    d. Increases future mobility for the treated limb.
12. Advantages of preoperative radiation therapy for STS include all of the following except:
    a. Radiation fields are smaller.
    b. Less morbidity, such as fracture, edema and fibrosis.
    c. Seeding may be less likely during tumor resection.
    d. Skin involvement increase when using postoperative radiation therapy.
13. Intraoperative radiation for STS usually involves doses in the range of _____ after tumor removal.
    a. 10 to 16 Gy.
    b. 20 to 25 Gy.
    c. 25 to 30 Gy.
    d. 30 to 40 Gy.
14. Which of the following bone tumors has the worst prognosis?
    a. Osteosarcoma.
    b. Chondrosarcoma.
    c. Metastatic bone tumor.
    d. Ewing sarcoma.
15. Radiation therapy doses for preoperative STS are generally in the range of:
    a. 20 Gy.
    b. 35 Gy.
    c. 50 Gy.
    d. 75 Gy.

QUESTIONS TO PONDER

1. Explain why patients with Ewing sarcoma of the pelvis carry a poorer prognosis than patients with the same tumor of an extremity.
2. Define skip metastases and explain how radiation therapy can be used to treat these lesions.
3. Explain the techniques involved in detecting primary bone tumors and the challenges associated with obtaining diagnoses of them.
4. Despite the evidence that lymphatic involvement of STS is rare, the radiation therapy technique selected for rhabdomyosarcomas, synovial sarcomas, and epithelioid sarcomas often includes the regional lymph nodes. Explain the rationale for this exception.
5. Why is a boost with bolus or electrons to the scar often necessary during radiation to bone and STS?

REFERENCES

1. American Cancer Society. American Cancer Society website. www.cancer.org. Accessed November 10, 2018.
2a. Bernard S, Walker E, Raghavan M. An approach to the evaluation of incidentally identified bone lesions encountered on imaging studies. *Am J Roentgenol.* 2017;208(5):960–970.
2. Bernstein M, Kovar H, Paulussen M, et al. Ewing's sarcoma family of tumors: current management. *Oncologist.* 2006;11(5):503–519.
3. Biermann JS, Chow W, Reed DR, et al. NCCN guidelines insights: bone cancer, version 2.2017. *J Natl Compr Canc Netw.* 2017;15(2):155–167.
4. Buchbender C, Heusner TA, Lauenstein TC, Bockisch A, Antoch G. Oncologic PET/MRI, part 2: bone tumors, soft-tissue tumors, melanoma, and lymphoma. *J Nucl Med.* 2012;53(8):1244–1252.
5. Clark MA, Fisher C, Judson I, Thomas JM. Soft-tissue sarcomas in adults. *N Engl J Med.* 2005;353(7):701–711.
6. Cote GM, Choy E. Update in treatment and targets in Ewing sarcoma. *Hematol Oncol Clin North Am.* 2013;27(5):1007–1019.
7. Damjanov I, ed. *Pathology for the Health Professions.* 5th ed. St. Louis: Elsevier Saunders; 2017.
8. Deveci MA, Paydas S, Gonlusen G, Ozkan C, Bicer OS, Tekin M. Clinical and pathological results of denosumab treatment for giant cell tumors of bone: prospective study of 14 cases. *Acta Orthop Traumatol Turc.* 2017;51(1):1–6.
9. Dispenzieri A, Kyle RA. Multiple myeloma: clinical features and indications for therapy. *Best Pract Res Clin Haematol.* 2005;18(4):553–568.
10. Folpe AL. Fibrosarcoma: a review and update. *Histopathology.* 2014;64(1):12–25.
11. George S. Evolving treatment of soft tissue sarcoma. *J Natl Compr Canc Netw.* 2017;15(5S):733–736.
12. Ghert M. CORR insights®: Are biopsy tracts a concern for seeding and local recurrence in sarcomas? *Clin Orthop Relat Res.* 2017;475(2):519–521.
13. Hardison SA, Davis PL 3rd, Browne JD. Malignant fibrous histiocytoma of the head and neck: a case series. *Am J Otolaryngol.* 2013;34(1):10–15.
14. Hawley ST, Janz NK, Lillie SE, et al. Perceptions of care coordination in a population-based sample of diverse breast cancer patients. *Patient Educ Couns.* 2010;81(suppl 1):S34–S40.
15. Hoefkens F, Dehandschutter C, Somville J, Meijnders P, Van Gestel D. Soft tissue sarcoma of the extremities: pending questions on surgery and radiotherapy. *Radiat Oncol.* 2016;11(1):136.
16. Horton JK, Gleason JF Jr, Klepin HD, Isom S, Fried DB, Geiger AM. Age-related disparities in the use of radiotherapy for treatment of localized soft tissue sarcoma. *Cancer.* 2011;117(17):4033–4040.
17. Ilaslan H, Schils J, Nageotte W, Lietman SA, Sundaram M. Clinical presentation and imaging of bone and soft-tissue sarcomas. *Cleve Clin J Med.* 2010;77(suppl 1):S2–S7.
18. Jebsen NL, Bruland OS, Eriksson M, et al. Five-year results from a Scandinavian sarcoma group study (SSG XIII) of adjuvant chemotherapy combined with accelerated radiotherapy in high-risk soft tissue sarcoma of extremities and trunk wall. *Int J Radiat Oncol Biol Phys.* 2011;81(5):1359–1366.
19. Kano H, Lunsford LD. Stereotactic radiosurgery of intracranial chordomas, chondrosarcomas, and glomus tumors. *Neurosurg Clin N Am.* 2013;24(4):553–560.
20. Kumar SK, Callander NS, Alsina M, et al. NCCN guidelines insights: multiple myeloma, version 3.2018. *J Natl Compr Canc Netw.* 2018;16(1):11–20.
21. Levy AD, Manning MA, Al-Refaie WB, Miettinen MM. Soft-tissue sarcomas of the abdomen and pelvis: Radiologic-pathologic features, part 1-common sarcomas: from the radiologic pathology archives. *Radiographics.* 2017;37(2):462–483.

22. Liebner DA. The indications and efficacy of conventional chemotherapy in primary and recurrent sarcoma. *J Surg Oncol.* 2015;111(5):622–631.

23. Lindsey BA, Markel JE, Kleinerman ES. Osteosarcoma overview. *Rheumatol Ther.* 2017;4(1):25–43.

24. Macedo F, Ladeira K, Pinho F, et al. Bone metastases: an overview. *Oncol Rev.* 2017;11(1):321.

25. Mehdinejad M, Sobhan MR, Mazaheri M, Zare Shehneh M, Neamatzadeh H, Kalantar SM. Genetic association between ERCC2, NBN, RAD51 gene variants and osteosarcoma risk: a systematic review and meta-analysis. *Asian Pac J Cancer Prev.* 2017;18(5):1315–1321.

26. Smith HG, Memos N, Thomas JM, Smith MJ, Strauss DC, Hayes AJ. Patterns of disease relapse in primary extremity soft-tissue sarcoma. *Br J Surg.* 2016;103(11):1487–1496.

27. Swallow CJ. Strategic delay: histology- and biology-driven decision-making in recurrent retroperitoneal sarcoma. *Ann Surg Oncol.* 2018;25(8):2117–2119.

28. von Mehren M, Randall RL, Benjamin RS, et al. Soft tissue sarcoma, version 2.2018, NCCN clinical practice guidelines in oncology. *J Natl Compr Canc Netw.* 2018;16(5):536–563.

26

Leukemias and Lymphomas

Amanda Sorg, Megan Trad

OBJECTIVES

- Differentiate between Hodgkin lymphoma and non-Hodgkin lymphoma.
- Identify lymph node areas and anatomy most often involved in Hodgkin and non-Hodgkin lymphomas.
- Explain A and B symptoms and their association with Hodgkin lymphoma.
- Explain the staging system used for Hodgkin lymphoma, including the differences between the four stages.
- Discuss the common treatment approaches for Hodgkin lymphoma and non-Hodgkin lymphomas.

- Identify the causes and distribution for Hodgkin and non-Hodgkin lymphomas.
- Compare and contrast the different classifications of Hodgkin lymphoma.
- Explain the importance of chemotherapy and radiation therapy and how they are applied in treatment.
- Discuss the prognosis and survival associated with Hodgkin and non-Hodgkin lymphoma.
- Differentiate between the four main types of leukemias.

OUTLINE

KEY TERMS

Agent Orange
Akimbo
Ann Arbor staging system
B symptoms
BCR-ABL
Contiguous
Extended field radiation
Indolent
Inverted Y

Involved field radiation
Mantle fields
Oophoropexy
Paraaortic fields
Philadelphia Chromosome
Reed-Sternberg cells
Total nodal radiation
Waldeyer ring

INTRODUCTION

Cancers of the lymphatic and hemopoietic system are unique in that unlike solid tumors that arise in a particular organ, leukemias and lymphomas are systemic diseases that require systemic treatment to achieve control. Although stem cells of both the hemopoietic system and lymphatic system are some of the most radiosensitive cells in the body, radiation therapy is a localized treatment method and so is not considered the first line of treatment for these diseases.[1] Radiation therapy, however, does play a part in the treatment of these diseases, and the treatment of leukemias and lymphomas are some of the most challenging and intricate treatments, as they require the management of large field sizes and can encompass a variety of critical structures that must be protected. This chapter is divided into two sections. The first section will cover lymphomas and describe all aspects of this disease, as it is more commonly treated with radiation therapy than leukemia. The second section will contain a brief description of the main types of leukemia and treatment rationale.

LYMPHOMAS

Hodgkin disease, also known as Hodgkin lymphoma, and non-Hodgkin lymphoma (NHL) are the predominant types of cancer that arise from the lymphatic system. Hodgkin lymphoma was first described by Thomas Hodgkin in 1832. NHL was introduced much later, around 1956 to 1966, as a need arose for further classification of other lymphomas. All types of lymphomas that are not Hodgkin lymphoma are classified as NHL.

HODGKIN LYMPHOMA

Hodgkin lymphoma is distinct from other lymphoma types. The presence of Hodgkin lymphoma is often determined by the existence of Reed-Sternberg cells (Fig. 26.1). Reed-Sternberg cells are large lymphoid cells that contain multiple nuclei. They have morphology unlike normal cells within the human body. Hodgkin lymphoma spreads in a systematic manner through the lymph nodes and lymph vessels. It is the result of abnormal growth of antibody-producing cells of the lymphatic system.

Anatomy and Lymphatics

The lymphatic system plays a major role in the immune system in conjunction with the circulatory system. The systems work together to transport nutrients and to remove wastes and are intertwined throughout the body. Red blood cells are eliminated by the lymphatic system, and portions of the blood help produce lymph. The lymphatic system consists of lymph fluid, lymph nodes, and lymphatic organs. Lymph fluid travels through the body via lymph nodes and vessels. Lymph fluid carries antibodies, nutrients, and lymphocytes throughout the body and provides protection while filtering harmful particles that may give rise to infection and disease. Lymph nodes become swollen when bacteria are present and when the body produces more lymphocytes to fight infection. Lymphocytes that grow abnormally are the origin of Hodgkin and NHL's and compromise the body's ability to fight infection. Knowledge of the major lymph node regions is important in the treatment of Hodgkin lymphomas. The major lymph nodes are as follows (Fig. 26.2):

1. Waldeyer ring (tonsillar lymphatic tissue that surrounds the nasopharynx and oropharynx) and cervical, preauricular, and occipital lymph nodes.
2. Supraclavicular and infraclavicular lymph nodes.
3. Axillary lymph nodes.
4. Thorax (includes hilar and mediastinal nodes).
5. Abdominal cavity (includes paraaortic nodes).

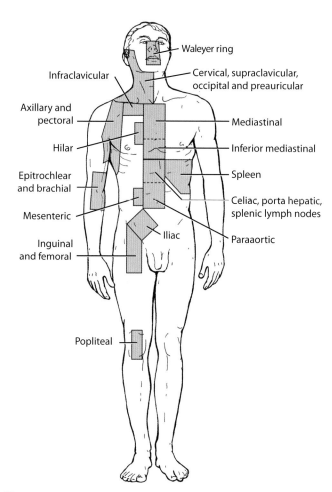

Fig. 26.2 Major lymphatic regions of the body. These regions play a significant role in the staging and treatment planning of Hodgkin lymphoma. After the lymphatic regions of known involvement are determined, the regions at risk for subclinical disease from contiguous spread may then be established. Identification of both the primary lymphatic region of involvement and the contiguous lymph node regions at risk is essential in treatment planning. (From Gunderson LL, Tepper JE. *Clinical Radiation Oncology*. Philadelphia, PA: Churchill Livingstone; 2000.)

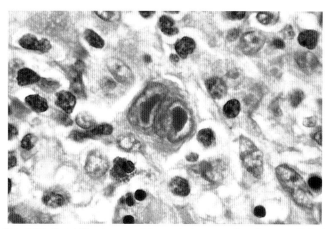

Fig. 26.1 Reed-Sternberg cell is a giant connective tissue cell that is characterized by one or two large nuclei. (Courtesy Dr. Robert W. McKenna, Department of Pathology, University of Texas Southwestern Medical School, Dallas; and from Kumar V, Abbas AK, Fausto N, Mitchell RN. *Robbins Basic Pathology*. 8th ed. Philadelphia, PA: Saunders; 2007.)

6. Pelvic cavity (includes iliac nodes and Peyer patches in the distal ileum).

7. Inguinal and femoral lymph nodes.

The spleen, thymus, tonsils, adenoids, and bone marrow are also part of the lymphatic system. The two types of lymphocytes, B and T cells, develop in the bone marrow and mature in the lymphatic organs. The spleen, the largest lymphatic organ, recycles red blood cells and houses lymphocytes that help contest certain types of bacteria.

Epidemiology

Hodgkin lymphoma can occur in any age group and in either gender. In 2018, 0.5% of all new cancer diagnoses were Hodgkin lymphoma. There are an estimated 8,500 new cases each year. Approximately 0.2% of the population will be diagnosed with Hodgkin lymphoma at some point during their lifetime. Hodgkin lymphoma rates are greatest in the age range from 20 to 34 years, a little more than 31% of all new cases. The median age at time of diagnosis is 39 years. Between 10% and 15% of cases involve children under the age of 17 years. Occurrence in children under the age of 5 years is rare. Hodgkin lymphoma is more prevalent in males, regardless of race. Whites, blacks, and non-Hispanics of both genders have slightly higher rates of occurrence.[2]

Etiology

The exact etiology of Hodgkin lymphoma remains unknown, although the correlation between the presence of the Reed-Sternberg cells and the disease has been established. Hodgkin lymphoma is also suspected to arise from interactions among an individual's genetic makeup, environmental exposures, and infectious agents.

Several risk factors that relate to the development of Hodgkin lymphoma have been identified. Previous infection with the Epstein-Barr virus, or infectious mononucleosis, has been linked to the development of Hodgkin lymphoma. Components of the Epstein-Barr virus have been found in the DNA of the Reed-Sternberg cells of some patients with Hodgkin lymphoma.

Family history has also been identified as a risk factor, with siblings of patients with Hodgkin lymphoma at a higher risk for development of the disease than the general population. Patients with human immunodeficiency virus (HIV) infection are also more likely to have development of Hodgkin lymphoma than are individuals without HIV.

Prognostic Indicators

The stage at diagnosis of Hodgkin lymphoma directly correlates with the prognosis. The prognosis is often worse in advanced stages of the disease. An advanced stage at diagnosis may be representative of bulky disease, a mass 10 cm or greater in size or with a transverse diameter that exceeds 33% of the transthoracic diameter. In advanced stages, distant spread and risk of relapse are increased.

Younger patients, such as teenagers and those in their 20s, tend to have better results in the treatment for Hodgkin lymphoma than do older adults. Hodgkin lymphoma death rates are highest in people aged 75 to 84 years.[2] Older patients tend to have more difficulty tolerating aggressive treatment because of other comorbidities.

Preservation of fertility may be of concern in younger patients and those treated in the lower pelvic regions. Fertility can often be preserved for men who undergo radiation therapy with the use of testicular shields and conformal treatment planning. However, the ovaries cannot always be shielded in the treatment of pelvic regions in women. Although fertility often can be salvaged with radiation therapy treatments, it also can be impaired from the toxicities of chemotherapy. As discussed, the stage at diagnosis and the presence of disease in the lower abdomen with or without splenic involvement influence the prognosis of patients. Patients who present with unexplained weight loss, night sweats, and fever are acknowledged to have a poorer prognosis.

Clinical Presentation

Most patients present with painless lymphadenopathy and are often asymptomatic. A painless mass is most often discovered in supraclavicular, cervical, and mediastinal lymph node areas. The spread of Hodgkin lymphoma is predictable; it mainly follows routes of lymphatic drainage before spreading to other organs. The routes of lymphatic drainage and knowledge of major lymphatic regions in the body play an important role in treatment planning. The areas surrounding known involvement become regions at risk for subclinical disease and must be treated accordingly.

Patients are assigned the letter A in their staging if they have no symptoms, or are asymptomatic. They will be assigned a letter B in their staging if they have specific symptoms associated with Hodgkin lymphoma that are known as B symptoms. B symptoms have been identified as: unexplained weight loss of more than 10% of their body weight in the 6 months before diagnosis; frequent, drenching night sweats; or unexplained fevers higher than 100.4°F. Generalized pruritus and pain with alcohol ingestion are additional symptoms that can also be defined under the B category.

Detection and Diagnosis

The most common sign of Hodgkin lymphoma is a painless mass found by the patient above the diaphragm. Mediastinal masses are often discovered on routine chest radiographs. These patients may have shortness of breath, cough, or chest discomfort. One-third of patients experience B symptoms before diagnosis. Patients with advanced Hodgkin lymphoma may have an enlarged spleen, tender abdomen, achy bones, and pleural effusion.

The diagnostic workup for Hodgkin lymphoma includes a thorough history and physical examination, radiographic examinations, and laboratory studies. Radiographic examinations may include a chest x-ray, computed tomography (CT), magnetic resonance imaging (MRI), and positron emission tomography (PET). These imaging modalities assist physicians in correctly staging the disease and in making decisions in the treatment planning process in radiation therapy.

Laboratory studies include a complete blood and platelet count and liver and renal function tests. Anemia, leukopenia, thrombocytosis, and lymphopenia can indicate bone marrow involvement. Few patients with Hodgkin lymphoma have bone marrow involvement, and bone marrow biopsies are reserved for those with later-stage disease and subdiaphragmatic disease. A liver biopsy should be done if splenic involvement is found.

Because the lymphatic system works in conjunction with the cardiovascular system, the following abnormal laboratory studies may indicate Hodgkin lymphoma as well:

- Low blood albumin level below 4
- High erythrocyte sedimentation rate
- High white blood cell count above 15,000
- Low red blood cell count, hemoglobin level below 10.5
- Low blood lymphocyte count below 600

Pathology

The presence of Reed-Sternberg cells is an indicator; however, it is not necessary to make a diagnosis of Hodgkin lymphoma. Pathologists use the World Health Organization (WHO) modification of the Revised European-American Lymphoma (REAL) classification for histologic classification of Hodgkin lymphoma. The WHO classification system includes morphology, immunophenotyping, and cytogenetics. It also considers a patient's age, gender, and medical history in classification of the disease. The characterizations of the cells and their appearances and the patterns of signs and symptoms have a direct correlation with the response to treatment. Therefore, these are used in determining a treatment plan.

The WHO classification system divides Hodgkin lymphoma into two categories and four subcategories:
1. Classic Hodgkin lymphoma
   About 95% of people diagnosed with Hodgkin lymphoma have one of the classic types. Presence of the Reed-Sternberg cells is the main characteristic of classic lymphomas. Nodular sclerosing and mixed cellularity lymphomas are the two most common types of classic Hodgkin lymphoma and account for 90% of cases.[3]
   A. Nodular sclerosing Hodgkin lymphoma
   This type usually involves nodes in the chest and neck and is typically diagnosed at an early stage. It is most common among people in their 20s and 30s.[3]
   B. Mixed cellularity Hodgkin lymphoma (MCHL)
   MCHL is less common than nodular sclerosing Hodgkin lymphoma, and the average age at diagnosis is 38 years old. It tends to be seen in those affected by HIV.[3] This type more commonly affects men than women and also tends to present in the abdomen and spleen.
   C. Lymphocyte-rich Hodgkin lymphoma
   This type is found in only 5% of cases, usually is found in the upper body, is more common in men, and typically doesn't occur in more than a few lymph nodes.[3]
   D. Lymphocyte-depleted Hodgkin lymphoma (LDHL)
   LDHL is the rarest of the four subtypes and usually presents with more advanced disease; thus, it carries the worst prognosis. It usually affects people in their 30s and those with HIV infection.[4]
2. Nodular lymphocyte predominant Hodgkin lymphoma (NLPHL)
   NLPHL is characterized by variants of the Reed-Sternberg cells that are termed "popcorn" cells because they closely resemble the look of popcorn. Men are more affected than women, as are people aged 30 to 50 years. This type accounts for 5% of Hodgkin lymphomas. It usually presents with disease in the lymph nodes of the neck and axilla. Ninety percent of patients have remission after surgery and radiation.[4]

Staging

The Ann Arbor staging system is a tool that has been used since 1971 to describe the features of Hodgkin lymphoma specific to each patient. The staging system aids physicians in treatment plans by categorizing the characteristics of the disease. The following letters may be included with the four stages when applicable:

A The patient does not have B symptoms.
B The patient has B symptoms.
E Extranodal disease is present.
S Disease is found in the spleen.

In addition to the stage assigned with the Ann Arbor staging system, patients are also designated as having favorable or unfavorable Hodgkin lymphoma, depending on the presence or absence of adverse risk factors. Early favorable Hodgkin lymphoma is designated if patients have clinical stage I or stage II disease without the presence of B symptoms, less than three sites of nodal involvement, and no markedly abnormal laboratory results, as mentioned previously. If patients have one or more of the previous risk factors, they are designated as having early unfavorable disease. Hodgkin lymphoma that is advanced can still be considered favorable with stage III or IV and three or fewer risk factors. Advanced unfavorable has stage III or IV and four or more risk factors.

Routes of Spread

Hodgkin lymphoma has a predictable, contiguous pattern of spread that mimics the route of the lymphatic system. If disease is found outside the lymphatic system, it is next to the involved site(s). The rate of progression is not predictable. In advanced stages, Hodgkin lymphoma may spread to the viscera, spleen, liver, bone marrow, or other organs.

Treatment Techniques

With the advancement of technology in radiation therapy and the discovery of chemotherapy drugs that produce less toxicity, patients with Hodgkin lymphoma have a high rate of curability with much more tolerability than before. Hodgkin lymphoma has also seemingly been found to be a more radiosensitive tumor, with the same effective tumor response but a smaller dosage than required by other forms of cancer. For those reasons, Hodgkin lymphoma is one of the most treatable types of cancer.

The primary treatment modality for early-stage disease is chemotherapy.

Chemotherapy is given initially, and patients may also receive radiation to the area of involvement to treat subclinical or residual disease. Patients with adverse reactions to chemotherapy may be treated with radiation therapy alone. Patients diagnosed with nodular lymphocyte predominant lymphoma may receive radiation after removal of the affected nodes without chemotherapy. Chemotherapy is also combined with radiation therapy to treat advanced stages.

For stages I and II, four cycles of the ABVD chemotherapy regimen (doxorubicin [Adriamycin], bleomycin, vincristine, and dacarbazine) is the standard treatment today.[5] The ABVD chemotherapy combination has proven more effective and less toxic than the initial chemotherapy regimen, MOPP (either mechlorethamine or methotrexate with oncovin, procarbazine, and prednisone). MOPP may be used for patients who are at risk for heart failure because Adriamycin has a risk factor of heart damage. A chemotherapy regimen may or may not be combined with radiation therapy in early stages and is most often prescribed when patients have bulky disease that may not quite disseminate with chemotherapy alone. When radiation therapy is used in the early stages, the fields are limited to treat the areas of known disease.[5]

Patients diagnosed with stage III or IV with bulky disease or with B symptoms are treated with a chemotherapy regimen and adjuvant radiation therapy. Combined modality therapy yields better results than chemotherapy alone. Radiation therapy can also be used for palliation to give the patient relief and prolong survival. Chemotherapy may also be used after the disease has reoccurred in an area already treated with radiation therapy, which is termed *salvage therapy*.[4]

Clinical trials regarding the effectiveness of monoclonal antibody therapy on Hodgkin lymphoma are in progress. Monoclonal antibodies are developed in a laboratory and infused into the patient. The antibodies are designed to attach to specific cancer-causing growths and either kill the cancer cells or prevent them from growing. Brentuximab vedotin (Adcetris [Seattle Genetics, Inc, Bothell, Wash.]) and Rituximab (Rituxan [Genentech, San Francisco, Calif.]) are two types of monoclonal antibodies that are currently used. These drugs are often combined with chemotherapy and radiation and may be used after recurrence.[3]

Radiation Therapy Techniques

Radiation therapy treatment is most often delivered to the neck, chest, and/or axilla or to paraaortic lymph nodes and the spleen. Some patients also receive treatment to the pelvic lymph nodes. Because of the predictable spread of Hodgkin lymphoma, the adjacent nodes surrounding the disease are also treated. Treatment fields to the neck, chest, and axilla combined are called mantle fields. If the pelvic and paraaortic fields are treated together, the treatment area is referred to as the inverted Y. When these three separate fields are treated together, they form total nodal radiation therapy. Patients receiving multiple treatment fields usually undergo sequential treatment for better tolerance. Treatment areas that only encompass the areas of known disease are called involved field radiation therapy (Fig. 26.3). Extended field radiation (Fig. 26.4) includes areas of known disease and contiguous uninvolved lymph nodes. For patients with a favorable prognosis, treatment to the pelvic region is avoided to preserve fertility.

If treatment with chemotherapy and radiation therapy fails, patients may undergo autologous bone marrow and peripheral blood stem cell transplants. These patients typically undergo high doses of radiation or chemotherapy to the whole body to destroy cancer cells and bone marrow tissue and to suppress the immune system. Immune system suppression helps prevent the body from rejecting the new stem cells.

Treatment Field Design and Techniques: Mantle. Most patients present with disease above the diaphragm. If the patient is treated with radiation therapy to this area, it is called a mantle. This field includes the cervical, submandibular, axillary, supraclavicular, infraclavicular, mediastinal, and hilar lymph nodes. With treatment of large areas, such as the mantle, as much healthy tissue as possible must be spared. A large field size is needed to encompass all of the lymph nodes in the neck, chest, and axilla. Patients are treated supine with their hands above their heads or akimbo with their hands on their hips and elbows turned outward, with chin extension to prevent exposure to the mouth. Body molds are used to ensure accurate daily setup with reduced patient movement. Mantle fields are treated in an anteroposterior/posteroanterior (AP/PA) approach. Lung, humeral head, occipital, anterior larynx, and posterior spinal cord blocks are used to minimize the dose to

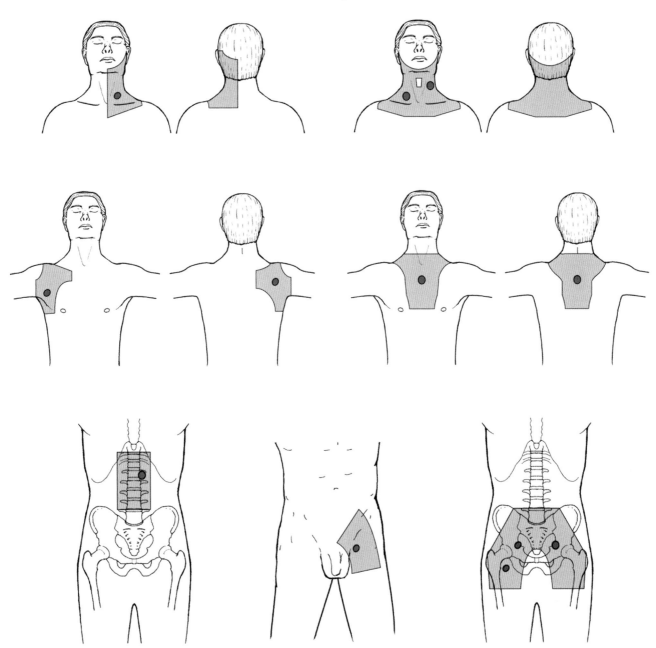

Fig. 26.3 Because of the high risk of subclinical involvement in adjacent lymph nodes within a region, the involved field treatment is the minimum field size typically used in radiation therapy for Hodgkin lymphomas. (Drawings by Louis Clark. From Gunderson LL, Tepper JE. *Clinical Radiation Oncology.* Philadelphia, PA: Churchill Livingstone; 2000.)

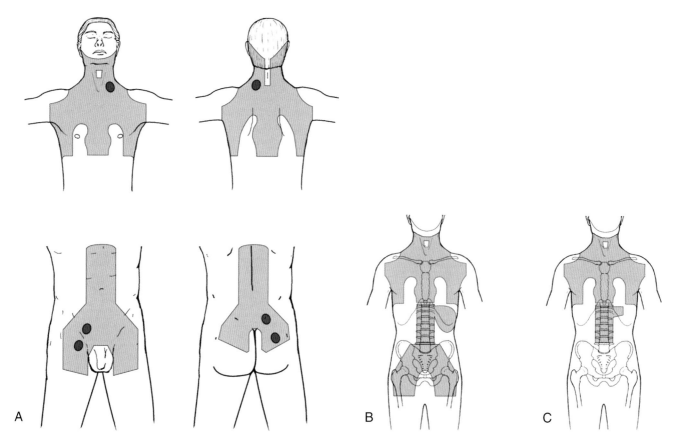

Fig. 26.4 (A) Extended fields include treatment of contiguous lymph node regions. (B) Total nodal irradiation; standard fields treat all lymph node areas typically involved with Hodgkin lymphoma. (C) Subtotal or modified total nodal irradiation, which excludes only the pelvic nodes. (Drawings by Louis Clark. From Gunderson LL, Tepper JE. *Clinical Radiation Oncology.* Philadelphia, PA: Churchill Livingstone; 2000.)

the surrounding healthy tissue. Typical borders for the mantle fields are:

Superior: Lower mandible and mastoid tips (chin is hyperextended so cervical and submandibular nodes can be treated while treatment of the mouth is avoided)

Inferior: T9-T10 interspace

Lateral: Flash beyond the axillary nodes[6]

Abdominal or Paraaortic Fields. The spleen, paraaortic, and retroperitoneal nodes are treated with an AP/PA abdominal field. Treatment of the mantle and abdominal fields without the pelvic portion is termed *subtotal nodal irradiation.* When the mantle field is treated, the patient position should remain the same for the other treatment ports. This aids in eliminating a change of position that may cause overlap. A spinal block may be added superiorly on the abdominal field to protect the spinal cord from overdose. The left kidney must be protected if the spleen is treated because the right one receives the dose. Borders for the abdominal field are:

Superior: Mid-T10–T11

Inferior: L4–L5

Lateral: 9-cm- to 10-cm-wide midline[6]

Pelvic Irradiation. The abdominal field and pelvic fields can be combined to form a field called the *inverted Y.* Shielding blocks are used to protect bone marrow, the bowel, and the bladder. Pelvic irradiation can cause concern for patients who desire to preserve fertility. In female patients, a pelvic midline block can be designed to shield the ovaries. Female patients can also undergo an oophoropexy, a procedure that

moves the ovaries midline or laterally to minimize exposure. A testicular shield may be used for male patients to reduce internal scatter radiation. Borders for AP/PA pelvic irradiation are:

Superior: L5

Inferior: 2 cm below ischial tuberosity

Lateral: 2 cm beyond pelvic inlet[6]

Patients receiving radiation therapy alone typically have been treated with 35 to 44 Gy to areas free of disease with 6-MV to 10-MV photons. The area of initial nodal involvement is treated from 25 to 30 Gy.[4] However, recent studies have shown that patients who are receiving chemotherapy and radiation may be treated to a lesser dose up of 20 Gy with the same results and less toxicity.[7] These results are important to the vast number of younger patients for preservation of fertility and prevention of second malignancies that may be caused from the initial treatment.

Keep in mind that because of the continual advancement in chemotherapy drugs and technologies in radiation therapy, often patients are treated with treatment fields that only involve the site of bulky disease (Figs. 26.5 to 26.7). This can eliminate toxicities and unnecessary treatment.

Pediatric Treatments

Hodgkin lymphoma accounts for 6% of childhood cancers. Hodgkin lymphoma in children closely resembles Hodgkin lymphoma in adults. The treatment procedure for pediatric cases is much like that for adults, but much emphasis is spent on minimizing lower doses for chemotherapy and radiation therapy to prevent toxicities and interruption in the growth process. Approximately 95% of patients with childhood Hodgkin lymphoma are cured.[4]

Radiation Side Effects

The side effects from radiation therapy treatment depend on the area and size treated. Patients may have the following acute side effects from radiation therapy treatments:

- Fatigue
- Alopecia
- Skin erythema
- Esophagitis
- Altered taste
- Dysphagia
- Dry cough
- Nausea
- Vomiting
- Diarrhea

Most side effects from radiation treatment for Hodgkin lymphoma subside soon after the completion of treatment. Because the radiation dose for Hodgkin lymphoma is much less than for other types of cancer, patients fare well with the management of side effects. Patients may use moisturizing skin creams and medications, such as antiemetics, analgesics, and anesthetics, during treatment. Adequate rest, protection from sunlight, and alterations in diet may also provide relief from radiation therapy reactions.

Late complications from radiation therapy may include:

- Hypothyroidism
- Cardiac disease
- Radiation pneumonitis
- Increased dental caries
- Xerostomia
- Lhermitte syndrome, which can be caused by the head flexion necessary for mantle fields. This syndrome is a temporary complication that consists of numbness or electrical sensations that run down the body to the limbs
- Second malignancies
- Xerospermia, loss of sperm production

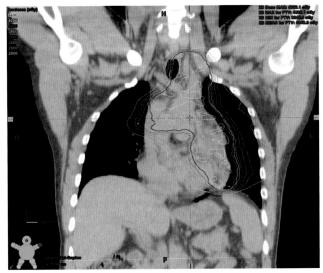

Fig. 26.5 This patient presented with a mediastinal and left peri-hilar mass. He was treated with a three-dimensional radiation therapy technique.

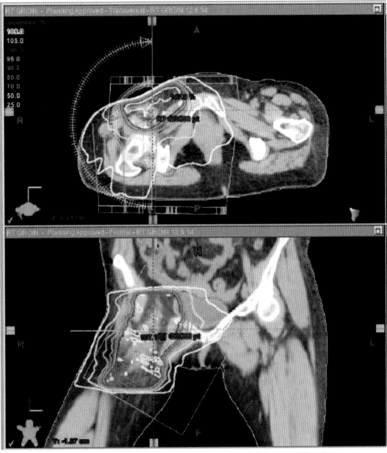

Fig. 26.6 This patient presented with an enlarged right-sided inguinal node.

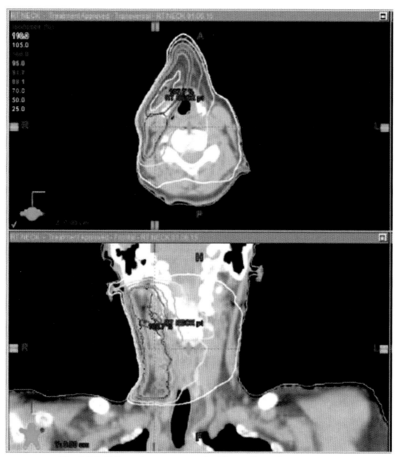

Fig. 26.7 This patient presented with a unilateral neck mass.

Proper dental care before radiation therapy begins and the use of custom mouth guards may help in dental care maintenance after treatment concludes. The use of daily kilovoltage (kV) images can ensure that treatment fields are being treated accurately and help prevent healthy tissue from being irradiated. Blocking of the lungs, heart, spinal cord, larynx, and humeral heads is also used to avoid late effects. Testicular shielding may be used in the treatment of pelvic and abdominal lymph nodes to preserve fertility in males.

Survival

Hodgkin lymphoma is one of the most curable types of cancer and has been proven to respond to chemotherapy and radiation therapy at a lower dose than other types of tumors. The overall survival rate for Hodgkin lymphoma is 86.6% per the National Cancer Institute's Surveillance, Epidemiology, and End Results Program.[5] The stage at diagnosis is inversely proportional to patient survival. As the stage increases, survival rates decrease. Age, overall health, and type of cancer can also affect decisions regarding treatment and survival. Generally, the later the stage at diagnosis, the more aggressive the treatment. However, patients who are older or have other health issues tend to fare worse with aggressive treatment. These patients tend to have lower survival rates than do younger patients and those who are healthy overall.

Other factors that may decrease a patient's survival and be a cause for more aggressive treatment may be:
- Male gender
- Age 45 years old or older
- B symptoms
- Markedly abnormal laboratory results

Box 26.1 from the National Cancer Institute's Surveillance, Epidemiology, and End Results Program website shows the percentage of cases and 5-year survival rates from the stage at diagnosis.

Role of the Radiation Therapist

As always, the quality of patient care should be the primary concern for the radiation therapist. Communication between the patient and the therapist is extremely important. The therapist is responsible for conveying the simulation and treatment process to the patient. When patients are fully aware of what is necessary to deliver the most ideal treatment, they are more likely to comply. The radiation therapist should take adequate time to ensure patient position is accurate and reproducible for optimal treatment. At the time of simulation, the therapist must take into account the treatment fields that will be irradiated and simulate accordingly. In most cases, the chin must be hyperextended for mantle fields, with arms akimbo. A body mold or thermoplastic mask that covers the head to the chest may be used to reproduce setup. Marks should be made on the mask or patient skin in stable areas for leveling. If the patient is being treated with a multiple fields, the therapist must ensure that the gap is verified to avoid overlap.

Therapists must also verify treatment parameters and accessories. Daily imaging can also be used to verify patient positioning before treatment. If daily imaging is not prescribed, then therapists must image the treatment fields when necessary. Knowledge of the healthy tissue being shielded helps the therapist confirm patient position and deliver the correct treatment. Daily treatments and any changes or discrepancies should be documented by the therapist to maintain current records.

Because radiation therapists see their patients on a daily basis, it is their responsibility to ensure that the patients are getting quality care

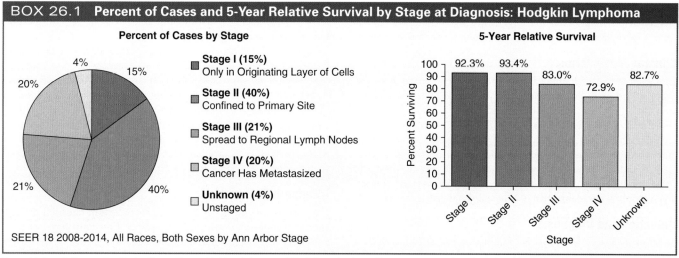

BOX 26.1   Percent of Cases and 5-Year Relative Survival by Stage at Diagnosis: Hodgkin Lymphoma

From National Cancer Institute. Surveillance Epidemiology and End Results. http://seer.cancer.gov/statfacts/html/hodg.html. Accessed November 22, 2019.

throughout treatment. They should be able to recognize a change in patient status and assess the need for further evaluation. Communicating, asking questions, and being an active participant in patient treatment allow for therapists to determine whether they need to advise the patient on certain subjects or refer to support staff. A general concern for patients and their well-being is an important attribute for a therapist to have.

NON-HODGKIN LYMPHOMA

Like Hodgkin lymphoma, Non-Hodgkin Lymphoma (NHL) can arise anywhere in the lymphatic system. The main distinction between Hodgkin lymphoma and NHL is the presence of Reed-Sternberg cells. If Reed-Sternberg cells are present, then the diagnosis of Hodgkin lymphoma is made. All other lymphomas are classified under the non-Hodgkin category. The WHO claims that there are at least 61 types of NHL. Several other disparities exist between Hodgkin and NHLs besides the presence or absence of the Reed-Sternberg cells. NHLs are more likely to spread randomly, involve extranodal tissue and multiple sites, and have a wide range of prognosis that depends on specific histologies.

Epidemiology

According to the National Cancer Institute's Surveillance, Epidemiology, and End Results Program, NHL represents 4.3% of all new cancer cases in the United States. White and non-Hispanic males have a higher incidence rate of diagnosis. The male predominance is more prevalent in NHL than in Hodgkin lymphoma. Nearly 25 males per 100,000 people are diagnosed, compared with 16.8 females. The median age at diagnosis for NHL is also higher at 67 years old. Although NHL can occur at any age, it affects people ages 65 to 74 most often. NHL is more common in the United States, Canada, and Europe and less likely to be diagnosed in Asian countries.[8]

Etiology

Like Hodgkin lymphoma, the exact etiology of NHL is unknown. That there are more than 61 types of NHL indicates the possibility of a considerable amount of risk factors. Researchers have found that NHL is not caused by inheritance but rather by DNA that has mutated during one's lifetime. Changes in the structure and function of B or T cells are

the source for the progression of cancer. Most changes that occur cannot be traced back to a specific origin, but some have been found to be associated with certain risk factors.

Many types of lymphomas have been traced back to immune system abnormalities. People with immune system deficiencies, autoimmune diseases, and chronic infections are more likely to develop NHL. For example, patients with immunosuppression who are awaiting organ or bone marrow transplant are at increased risk. Those who have been infected with viruses, such as Epstein-Barr, acquired immune deficiency syndrome (AIDS), HIV, hepatitis C, or human T-lymphotropic virus type 1 (HTLV-1), or with certain bacteria, such as *Helicobacter pylori*, are at a higher risk of development of NHL. Patients with Burkitt lymphoma have been found to have the Epstein-Barr virus. The Epstein-Barr virus infects B cells in the lymphatic system.

Overexposure to certain chemicals, most often occupation related, has to some extent been linked to the cancer. For example, industrial agents, such as solvents and vinyl chloride, and agricultural chemicals, such as pesticides and herbicides, are included. However, the research has not been consistent enough to make the correlation tangible. Ionizing radiation exposure also has shown a relationship with NHL. People who have had exposure to radiation during nuclear reactor accidents appear to have an increased risk for development of lymphomas. Some who have been treated with radiation therapy for previous conditions have been found to develop Non-Hodgkin lymphoma later in life. The risk is further increased when those patients also had chemotherapy.

Prognostic Indicators

Prognosis for NHL is more dependent on histology than is Hodgkin lymphoma. Vast amounts of histologies coincide with the large number of different lymphomas that exist. Identifying the histology can help in the determination of how aggressive the cancer is and help in the development of a treatment plan. Typically, the more the cancer cell deviates from a normal cell, the more aggressive it is.

NHL is divided into two groups: indolent and aggressive. An indolent lymphoma, like its meaning, is slow-growing and causes little problems at the time of diagnosis. This type of lymphoma has a median survival time from 10 to 20 years, depending on advancement. Aggressive NHL is faster growing and has an overall 5-year survival rate of 60%. The risk of relapse for both groups is the highest after the first 2 years of treatment.[2]

Patients with NHL are older at the time of diagnosis; therefore, they may have comorbidities that make aggressive treatment difficult to tolerate. A more advanced stage is also an indicator for decreased survival.

Clinical Presentation

The symptoms of NHL mimic those of Hodgkin lymphoma. Enlarged lymph nodes, night sweats, weight loss, fever, and itching are all common with diagnosis. NHL can be found in lymph nodes but is also found in a wide variety of locations in the body. Symptoms manifest according to the location of the disease, the surrounding organs, and the extent of the disease. The most common site for extranodal involvement is the gastrointestinal system, more specifically the stomach. Other common sites are Waldeyer ring, skin, bone marrow, sinuses, thyroid, central nervous system (CNS), and genitourinary system.

Detection and Diagnosis

A thorough history and physical examination can assist a physician in diagnosis. Knowledge of occupational risks and background on a patient's medical history can give a suggestion of NHL. Several imaging techniques can be used in the diagnosis of NHL. Chest radiographs, CT, PET, MRI, and ultrasound scans are all helpful in the assessment of the extent of disease and in initial staging. Laboratory studies that may be helpful in diagnosis include:

- Complete blood cell count: Anemia, thrombocytopenia, leukopenia, lymphocytosis, and thrombocytosis may be a sign of disease.
- Serum chemistry studies: Liver function tests, lactic acid dehydrogenase, and calcium levels may be abnormal.
- Serum beta-2 microglobulin level may be elevated.
- HIV serology.
- Human T-cell lymphotropic virus-1 serology.

Pathology

NHLs are separated into two groups: B-cell and T-cell lymphomas. B-cell lymphomas arise from abnormal B lymphocytes. B-cell lymphomas account for 85% of NHLs and include diffuse large B-cell lymphoma, follicular lymphoma, mantle cell lymphoma, and Burkitt lymphoma.[9] Peripheral T-cell lymphoma and cutaneous T-cell lymphoma are subtypes of T-cell lymphomas that develop from abnormal T lymphocytes. T-cell lymphomas account for 15% of NHLs.[9]

NHL is then further separated into two more groups: indolent and aggressive. Most indolent NHLs have nodular or follicular histology. NHL has the ability to transform from indolent to aggressive, most often within the first 2 years after treatment is finished. Because not all malignant cells make the transition, the patient is then diagnosed with both indolent and aggressive NHL.

The relapse of aggressive non-Hodgkin lymphoma (NHL) in the central nervous system (CNS) is a devastating event that is associated with a grim prognosis in most cases. In the highly aggressive subtypes of lymphoblastic and Burkitt lymphomas, CNS relapses tend to occur early after diagnosis, and its incidence is in the range of 30%. Therefore, a prophylactic treatment approach has been regularly incorporated into treatment protocols designed for these NHL subtypes as this has been proven to prolong survival and reduce the rate of early CNS relapse. However, in other aggressive lymphomas, the incidence of CNS relapse is low, ranging between 1% and 7%.[10]

Staging and Grading

The Ann Arbor staging system is most often used for NHLs. The Ann Arbor staging system is mostly concerned with lymphatic involvement associated with the diaphragm. However, it does not always encompass the variety that may come from the many different types of NHLs and

fails to classify extranodal sites. When this happens, physicians may choose to use staging systems that more relate to the specific location and pattern of that diagnosis.

Grading of the malignant cells is important in the determination of a treatment plan. Indolent, slow-growing cancers are low grade but tend to be more aggressive and recur over time. Aggressive tumors are referred to as high grade and grow at a much faster rate. Although aggressive tumor cells multiply more quickly than indolent lymphomas, they are often just as curable. Pathologists use the WHO modification of the REAL classification (Box 26.2) for histologic classification of NHL. The WHO classification system includes morphology, immunophenotyping, and cytogenetics for Hodgkin and NHLs.

Treatment Techniques

The primary treatments for NHL are chemotherapy, radiation therapy, immunotherapy, and stem cell transplants. Chemotherapy has been proven effective against NHL and is almost always given. One of the most common combinations of chemotherapy drugs is CHOP, which includes the drugs cyclophosphamide, doxorubicin, vincristine, and prednisone.[9]

Radiation therapy is used adjuvantly or in combination with chemotherapy. Like Hodgkin lymphoma, NHLs have been found to be radiosensitive, and radiation can also be used for treatment alone. However, NHL is more likely to emerge in various locations of the lymphatic system along with or in addition to extranodal sites. Because of this, radiation therapy treatments may differ a great deal among themselves and are more likely to be used in combination with chemotherapy.

When treatment with radiation therapy is indicated, the involved site is included along with the related drainage nodal clusters nearby. These treatment fields are treated to a dose of 35 to 45 Gy. Indolent NHL in early stages I or II can be treated with radiation alone. Aggressive lymphomas are treated with chemotherapy and radiation therapy combined. Patients with advanced or recurrent disease can benefit from aggressive chemotherapy and radiation treatment, followed by bone marrow transplant.[8]

One of the main risk factors for NHL is immune system deficiencies. Immunotherapy is used to boost the immune system into fighting off cancer cells. Once researchers identify the exact cause of cancer-causing growths, they are able to make drugs that can be aimed at those specific targets. Monoclonal antibodies, such as Rituximab (Rituxan), are currently being investigated for the treatment of non-Hodgkin disease and Hodgkin disease.[9]

Like Hodgkin lymphoma, bone marrow and stem cell transplants are reserved for those patients who have relapse or have an indolent lymphoma that has transformed into aggressive lymphoma. Patients can also be successfully retreated with chemotherapy and radiation depending on the histology, dose, and areas that were involved in any previous treatments.

Pediatric Non-Hodgkin Lymphoma

NHL accounts for 7% of all childhood cancers in children younger than 20 years old.[6] The signs and symptoms of childhood non-Hodgkin are the same as those of adult NHL. Most pediatric cases of NHL have been found to be associated with immune deficiencies. B-cell, diffuse large B-cell, lymphoblastic, and anaplastic large-cell lymphomas are the four most common types of NHLs. Treatment depends on site, histology, and stage of the lymphoma. Overall, children with NHL have a 5-year survival rate of more than 80%.[2]

Radiation Side Effects. Because NHL is found in many sites of the body, the treatment fields can vary a great deal. Side effects from radiation therapy are dependent on the area treated. Patients can expect to experience fatigue, alopecia, and skin erythema in any area treated. Avoidance of sunlight and application of skin cream to the treatment

BOX 26.2 The Revised European American Lymphoma Classification (REAL)

I. Precursor B-cell neoplasm
- Precursor B-lymphoblastic leukemia/lymphoma

II. Mature (peripheral) B-cell neoplasms
- B-cell chronic lymphocytic leukemia/small lymphocytic lymphoma
- B-cell prolymphocytic leukemia
- Lymphoplasmacytic lymphoma
- Splenic marginal zone B-cell lymphoma (± villous lymphocytes)
- Hairy cell leukemia
- Plasma cell myeloma/plasmacytoma
- Extranodal marginal zone B-cell lymphoma of mucosa-associated lymphoid tissue type
- Nodal marginal zone lymphoma (± monocytoid B cells)
- Follicle center lymphoma, follicular
- Mantle cell lymphoma
- Diffuse large cell B-cell lymphoma
  - Mediastinal large B-cell lymphoma
  - Primary effusion lymphoma
- Burkitt lymphoma/Burkitt's cell leukemia

T-Cell and Natural Killer Cell Neoplasms

I. Precursor T-cell neoplasm
- Precursor T-lymphoblastic lymphoma/leukemia

II. Mature (peripheral) T-cell and NK-cell neoplasms
- T-cell prolymphocytic leukemia
- T-cell granular lymphocytic leukemia
- Aggressive NK-cell leukemia
- Adult T-cell lymphoma/leukemia (HTLV-1+)
- Extranodal NK/T-cell lymphoma, nasal type
- Enteropathy-type T-cell lymphoma
- Hepatosplenic gamma-delta T-cell lymphoma
- Subcutaneous panniculitis-like T-cell lymphoma
- Mycosis fungoides/Sézary syndrome
- Anaplastic large cell lymphoma, T/null cell, primary cutaneous type
- Peripheral T-cell lymphoma, not otherwise characterized
- Angioimmunoblastic T-cell lymphoma
- Anaplastic large cell lymphoma, T/null–cell, primary systemic type

Hodgkin Lymphoma
- Nodular lymphocyte predominance Hodgkin lymphoma
- Classical Hodgkin lymphoma
  - Nodular sclerosis Hodgkin lymphoma
  - Lymphocyte-rich classic Hodgkin lymphoma
  - Mixed cellularity Hodgkin lymphoma
  - Lymphocyte depletion Hodgkin lymphoma

HTLV-1, Human T-lymphotropic virus type 1; *NK,* natural killer.
From National Cancer Institute. SEER training module: lymphoma. http://training.seer.cancer.gov/lymphoma/abstract-code-stage/morphology/real.html. Accessed November 22, 2018.

area can help manage and lessen skin reactions. Side effects from head and neck treatment are dry mouth, mouth sores, esophagitis, and dysphagia. An increase in fluids is encouraged to help with dry mouth. Good oral hygiene can reduce mouth sores as can the use of custom mouth guards. Esophagitis and dysphagia can be managed with analgesics and anesthetics during treatment.

If patients receive radiation therapy to the abdominal area, they may have nausea and vomiting. Antinausea medication may be given before treatment to avoid emesis. A reduction in appetite may also occur in patients receiving treatment in this area. The legalization of medical marijuana has proven beneficial in the treatment of nausea

and vomiting and can be prescribed in a number of states. It is also used as an appetite stimulant to maintain or help a patient gain weight.

Diarrhea may be an issue for those receiving radiation in the pelvic region. Antidiarrheal medication can ease gastroenteritis as can dietary changes. Patients can integrate a low-fiber diet to help manage diarrhea. Sufficient fluid intake for these patients can prevent dehydration.

Survival

The survival for NHL varies greatly among the different types. Generally, survival is dependent on age, stage, location, and histology at the time of diagnosis. The overall 5-year survival rate for patients diagnosed with NHL is 71%. The prevalent age group for people affected with NHL starts at 67 years old and extends to 74 years old.[2] Because NHL affects an older population, patients tend to fare worse than those with Hodgkin lymphoma because older populations may have other health issues and may not be able to tolerate aggressive treatment.

Box 26.3 from the National Cancer Institute's Surveillance, Epidemiology, and End Results Program website shows percent of cases and 5-year survival rates from stage at diagnosis of NHL.

Role of the Radiation Therapist

The role of the radiation therapist remains an important aspect in patient care from simulation throughout treatment. Precise daily treatments and adherence to the prescribed treatment plan allow the patient to have the highest possibility for effective treatment. The therapist must be aware of accurate blocking of critical structures and execute the treatment accordingly. The therapist must play an active role in communicating and providing patients with the information they need to understand what is involved in their treatment and to manage side effects. Patients diagnosed with NHL are generally older than patients with Hodgkin lymphoma, so they may need additional assistance in many regards. Older patients tend to have more comorbidities that may need to be addressed throughout their treatment as well. Leukemia patients, although not often seen in the radiation therapy clinic, pose challenges, as whole-body treatment, which can be used in preparing the patient for a stem cell transplant, requires atypical treatment and gantry setups, and therapists must work closely with the radiation oncologists and physicists to ensure accurate treatment delivery.

> Kaposi sarcoma is a cancer that can also develop in lymph node regions. Patients usually present with lesions on the skin. This type of cancer is commonly associated with patients diagnosed with human immunodeficiency virus (HIV) and acquired immune deficiency syndrome (AIDS). Radiation therapy is used in treatment of Kaposi sarcoma for skin lesions and lymph node regions.[11] Electrons are used for superficial areas and photons for deeper seated lymph node tumors.

LEUKEMIA

Leukemia is a cancer of the stem cells of the hematopoietic system, most commonly the white blood cells; however, cancer of the stem cells of other blood cell types is possible.[1,12] Leukemias are broadly divided into classifications based on if they are acute or chronic and if they derive from myeloid or lymphoid cells.[12] Most leukemias derive from precursor white blood cells; however, acute leukemias tend to show symptoms of disease quicker and spread more rapidly. Chronic leukemias manifest over a longer period of time, and individuals can even live with chronic leukemias for years before diagnosis as the cancer cells begin to change at a slower pace. Although this seems like a positive attribute, chronic leukemias are harder to treat and cure, as the cells are more resistant to treatment. Leukemias are classified as lymphocytic or myeloid dependent on the type

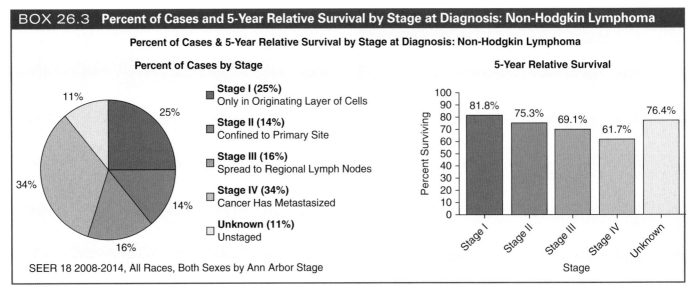

BOX 26.3 Percent of Cases and 5-Year Relative Survival by Stage at Diagnosis: Non-Hodgkin Lymphoma

Percent of Cases & 5-Year Relative Survival by Stage at Diagnosis: Non-Hodgkin Lymphoma

SEER 18 2008-2014, All Races, Both Sexes by Ann Arbor Stage

From National Cancer Institute. Surveillance Epidemiology and End Results. http://seer.cancer.gov/statfacts/html/nhl.html. Accessed November 22, 2019.

of cell they derive from. As each type of leukemia varies in behavior and prognosis, each classification will be covered individually below.

Acute Lymphocytic Leukemia

Acute lymphocytic leukemia, also called acute lymphoblastic leukemia (ALL), is a cancer that develops from lymphocytes, which are a type of white blood cell. ALL originates in the bone marrow where new blood is made but then can quickly spread to circulating blood and eventually metastasize, most commonly to the lymph nodes, liver, spleen, and CNS.[12] There are not many clearly identified factors that raise ones risk of developing ALL; however, previous exposure to ionizing radiation, exposure to benzene (a product used in cigarettes, some cleaning supplies, and detergents) can also increase ones risk. Infection of the human T-cell lymphoma/leukemia virus-1 (HTVL-1) is known to cause a rare form of T-cell leukemia; however, this virus is rare in the United States and more prominent in Japan and the Caribbean.[12] ALL is rare over the age of 50 years, and in fact, three out of four leukemias in children are ALL, with the peak incidence being among children ages 2 to 5 years. Symptoms of ALL include lethargy, dizziness, bruising easily, consistent infections that are hard to clear, and bleeding.[12] If a leukemia is suspected, physicians will begin testing by ordering a blood panel. ALL will present with a large number of lymphoblasts present in the blood and a diminished number of red blood cells and platelets, which is the cause of many of the symptoms, such as shortness of breath, bruising, and bleeding easily. The increased number of lymphoblasts crowd out circulating red blood cells and platelets. A bone marrow aspiration is also important in the diagnosis of all blood disorders, as well as a lumbar puncture because spread can occur through the CSF.

The mainstay of treatment for ALL is chemotherapy, as it is a systemic form of treatment. Vincristine and Daunorubicin are common drugs used for this type of disease. Much research has also been successful at identifying some targeted therapy drugs that work for patients who have specific genetic chromosome changes, which initiated the disease. For example, one out of four ALL patients have what is called a Philadelphia chromosome, or where the genetic information from chromosomes 9 and 22 has been swapped. In these specific patients, a targeted drug called Gleevec has shown promise.[12] Radiation therapy is not the main form of treatment for ALL, but it can be used to palliate symptoms, such as bone pain if spread has occurred, in the treatment of the brain or spine if it has spread to the CSF, or radiation therapy to the whole body plays a part in the process of a patient receiving a bone marrow or peripheral blood stem cell transplant.

Acute Myeloid Leukemia

Similar to ALL, acute myeloid leukemia (AML) starts in the bone marrow with the cells that are precursor cells to white blood cells and can quickly move into the bloodstream. Both ALL and AML are termed acute because they come on rapidly and have a quick disease progression. Smoking, exposure to ionizing radiation, and exposure to benzene are also risk factors for AML. In addition to previous use of alkylating agent chemotherapy drugs, increased age is also a factor as AML is more prevalent among older individuals, with the average age of diagnosis being 68 years.[12] AML is a relatively rare form of cancer, only accounting for 1% of all cancer diagnosed; however, the prognosis of AML is not as good as ALL, mainly because it occurs more commonly in the elderly who may not be able to withstand the vigorous chemotherapy regimens necessary to treat the disease. AML is typically treated with drugs consisting of Cytarabine and daunorubicin; however, there have been some targeted therapies identified for specific patients with genetic mutations, such as FLT-3 inhibitors and isocitrate dehydrogenase inhibitors. Radiation therapy is used for palliation and before bone marrow transplantation.

Chronic Lymphocytic Leukemia

Chronic lymphocytic leukemia (CLL) is the most common leukemia in adults. However, a person's lifetime risk of being diagnosed with CLL is only 1 in 175. It is a disease of older individuals, with it rarely occuring in individuals under 40 and virtually nonexistent in children. The average age of diagnosis is 70 years. CLL is also a leukemia derived from cells that would become white blood cells or lymphocytes; however, as opposed to ALL, the cells may still exhibit some characteristics of the lymphocyte and so are allowed to grow and manifest slowly over time. Because of this, many individuals are unaware of their disease for years before symptoms occur and after the disease has spread to the lymph nodes, liver, and/or spleen.

The major risk factors for CLL are age, exposure to Agent Orange (a powerful herbicide used by the US military during the Vietnam War in an effort to eliminate forest cover and crops), and having a family history of the disease. CLL is more common in North America and Europe. CLL is diagnosed using blood samples and bone marrow aspirations in addition to flow cytometry.

Chemotherapy is the treatment of choice in CLL, with purine analogs, alkylating agents, and corticosteroids being the drugs of choice.

These chemo drugs are given most commonly in the treatment of CLL, in addition to monoclonal antibodies, which are synthetic antibodies that target specific proteins on the cancer cells' surfaces. One commonly used monoclonal antibody is Rituximab, which specifically targets the CD20 protein found on the surface of B lymphocytes.[12] Radiation therapy is not often used in the treatment of CLL unless it is for palliative purposes or in preparation for a stem cell transplant.

Chronic Myeloid Leukemia

Chronic myeloid leukemia (CML) affects approximately one out of every 526 people in the United States, with an average age of diagnosis of 64 years. CML is identified as a genetic change to the myeloid stem cells, changing the normal gene into the identifying CML gene known as *BCR-ABL*.[12] It is unclear what causes this to occur, and the only risk factors associated with CML are previous radiation exposure, increased age, and a slight increase in males over females.

Many individuals with CML do not experience symptoms; the disease is typically found when testing for other illnesses. Further blood testing and bone marrow aspirations are then necessary after first identifying an elevated WBC; however, for a diagnosis of CML, genetic testing must be done to identify the Philadelphia chromosome or the *BCR-ABL* gene, which are the markers for CML. *BCR-ABL* is a protein known as a tyrosine kinase, and so targeted therapies, including tyrosine kinase inhibitors, are the main course of treatment. One common tyrosine kinase inhibitor is Gleevec, which needs to be taken for the rest of the patient's life.[12] Similar to the other forms of leukemia, radiation therapy does not play a large role in its treatment except for possibly treating bone pain or if pain occurs as a result of enlargement of the spleen. Radiation therapy may also play a role in preparing the patient for a stem cell transplant.

SUMMARY

- The major lymph node regions associated with Hodgkin and NHLs are the Waldeyer ring and supraclavicular, infraclavicular, axillary, hilar, mediastinal, paraaortic, iliac, Peyer's patches, inguinal, and femoral nodes.
- Although Hodgkin and NHLs both arise from the lymphatic system, they differ in histologic appearance, clinical presentation, and nodal involvement.
- The presence of Reed-Sternberg cells is an indication of Hodgkin lymphoma.
- B-cell lymphomas account for the majority of NHLs.
- In Hodgkin lymphoma staging, patients are classified as having A symptoms if they have no symptoms or B symptoms if they have unexplained weight loss, night sweats, and unexplained fevers higher than 100.4°F.
- Most patients present with painless, enlarged lymph nodes in both Hodgkin and NHLs.

- The Ann Arbor staging system is used for staging the lymphomas. The WHO modification of the REAL classification is used for histologic classification and grading.
- Hodgkin lymphoma has a contiguous pattern of spread that mimics the route of the lymphatic system, and NHL spread is less predictable and more often appears in extranodal sites.
- The mainstay treatment for lymphomas is chemotherapy often combined with radiation therapy. Lymphomas have been found to be radiosensitive and respond to chemotherapy with fewer doses than do other cancers.
- Communicating, monitoring, and delivering the prescribed treatment to the patient accurately is the responsibility of the radiation therapist. The therapist must have knowledge of the lymphatic system, surrounding critical organs, side effects, and technical skills to obtain optimal treatment results.
- Leukemias, which are not commonly treated with radiation therapy except in certain palliative instances, are divided into acute or chronic and whether they derive from myeloid or lymphoid cells.

REVIEW QUESTIONS

The answers to the Review Questions can be found by logging on to our website at: http://evolve.elsevier.com/Washington/principles

1. List the major lymph nodes and anatomy most often involved in Hodgkin and NHLs.
2. _____ are large lymphoid cells that contain multiple nuclei that are an indicator of Hodgkin lymphoma.
3. Explain A symptoms.
4. B symptoms include unexplained weight loss of more than 10% of body weight in the 6 months before diagnosis, night sweats, and unexplained fevers higher than 100.4°F.
   a. True.
   b. False.
5. The Ann Arbor staging system designates Hodgkin and NHLs to one of four stages. What are these stages?
6. Hodgkin lymphoma has an unpredictable, contiguous pattern of spread that mimics the route of the lymphatic system.
   a. True.
   b. False.
7. The primary treatment modality for early-stage Hodgkin lymphoma is:
   a. Chemotherapy.
   b. Radiation therapy.
   c. Surgery.

   d. None of the above.
8. Combined treatment fields to the neck, chest, and axilla are called _____ fields.
9. Treatment of pelvic and paraaortic fields together is referred to as the inverted Y.
   a. True.
   b. False.
10. Typical borders for the mantle fields are: *(Select all that apply.)*
    a. Superior: lower mandible and mastoid tips.
    b. Inferior: T9 to T10 interspace.
    c. Lateral: flash beyond the axillary nodes.
    d. Medial: flash beyond the axillary nodes.
11. List the radiation therapy side effects related to the treatment of HD.
12. Aggressive NHL tumors are referred to as:
    a. High grade.
    b. Low grade.
    c. Indolent.
    d. None of the above.
13. The most common type of NHL is:
    a. B cell.
    b. T cell.
    c. Splenic.
    d. All of the above.

14. The most common form of leukemia found in children is:
    1. ALL.
    2. AML.
    3. CLL.
    4. CML.

15. The specific gene used to identify CML is known as the:
    1. *BRCA-1.*
    2. *BCR-ABL.*
    3. *CML-2.*
    4. *BRCA-2.*

QUESTIONS TO PONDER

1. Explain the differences between Hodgkin lymphoma and NHL, including causes, clinical presentation, routes of spread, prognosis, and treatment modalities.
2. Why is the Ann Arbor staging system appropriate for Hodgkin disease but difficult to apply to NHL?
3. Compare involved field radiation with total-nodal radiation, and explain when each method is used.
4. What considerations must the therapist keep in mind when setting up a patient for a mantle field treatment? For a paraaortic field treatment?
5. Compare and contrast the four main types of leukemias, including risk factors, diagnostic techniques, and treatment.

REFERENCES

1. Dabaja B, Ha CS, Cox JD. Leukemias and lymphomas. In: Cox JK, Ang KK, eds. *Radiation Oncology: Rationale, Techniques, Results.* 9th ed. St. Louis, MO: Elsevier; 2010.
2. National Cancer Institute. SEER cancer statistics factsheets: Hodgkin lymphoma. http://seer.cancer.gov/statfacts/html/hodg.html. Accessed April 22, 2019.
3. American Cancer Society. Hodgkin disease. http://www.cancer.org/cancer/hodgkindisease/overviewguide/index. Accessed April 16, 2019.
4. Meyer RM, Gospodarowicz MK, Connors JM, et al. ABVD alone versus radiation-based therapy in limited-stage Hodgkin lymphoma. *N Engl J Med.* 2012;366(5):399–408.
5. Gunderson LL, Tepper JE. *Clinical Radiation Oncology.* Philadelphia, PA: Churchill Livingstone; 2000.
6. Sasse S, Klimm B, Görgen H, et al. Comparing long-term toxicity and efficacy of combined modality treatment including extended- or involved-field radiotherapy in early-stage Hodgkin lymphoma. *Ann Oncol.* 2012;23(11):2953–2959.
7. Engert A, Plütschow A, Eich HT, et al. Reduced treatment intensity in patients with early-stage Hodgkin lymphoma. *N Engl J Med.* 2010;363(7):640 652.
8. National Cancer Institute. PDQ adult Hodgkin lymphoma treatment. http://cancer.gov/cancertopics/pdq/treatment/adulthodgkins/HealthProfessional. Accessed November 22, 2018.
9. American Cancer Society. Non-Hodgkin lymphoma. http://www.cancer.org/cancer/non-hodgkinlymphoma/index. Accessed November 22, 2019.
10. National Cancer Institute. SEER cancer statistics factsheets: non-Hodgkin lymphoma. http://seer.cancer.gov/statfacts/html/nhl.html. Accessed November 22, 2018.
11. Vinjamaram S. Non-Hodgkin lymphoma. http://emedicine.medscape.com/article/203399. Accessed November 22, 2018.
12. American Cancer Society. Leukemia. https://www.cancer.org/cancer/leukemia.html. Accessed April 16, 2019.

27

Endocrine System Tumors

Jessica A. Church, Robert D. Adams

OBJECTIVES

- Discuss epidemiologic factors associated with endocrine tumors.
- Identify, list, and discuss etiologic factors that may be responsible for inducing endocrine tumors.
- Describe the hormones produced by the thyroid, pituitary, and adrenal glands and the clinical disorders associated with the overproduction and underproduction of them.
- Discuss the methods of detection and diagnosis for tumors in these anatomic regions.
- Differentiate between the histologic types of thyroid malignancies.

- Identify the treatments of choice for tumors of these anatomic sites.
- Discuss the healthy tissue tolerances and organs at risk for radiation therapy to these anatomic areas.
- Identify the side effects of radiation therapy to these anatomic regions.
- Describe the role of the radiation therapist in caring for patients with endocrine tumors.

OUTLINE

KEY TERMS

Acromegaly

Adenohypophysis

Alopecia

Amenorrhea

Bragg peak

Cortex

Dysphagia

Exophthalmos

Galactorrhea

Hyperthyroidism

Hypothyroidism

Infundibulum

Isthmus

Latent period

Macroadenoma

Medulla

Microadenoma

Negative feedback

Neurohypophysis

Stereotactic radiosurgery

The endocrine system is composed of multiple glandular organs responsible for complex metabolic regulatory functions. The principal organs of this system include the thyroid, pituitary, and adrenal glands. Also included are the parathyroid glands and specialized cells in the pancreas called the islets of Langerhans, which are referred to as the endocrine portions of the pancreas. Each of these organs (or specialized portions of them) produces hormones under complex feedback-control mechanisms that affect various functions to meet ongoing metabolic needs and stresses of the body.[1] The master regulatory gland of this system is the pituitary. This gland produces many hormones under the influence of the hypothalamus, which indirectly affects the function of other endocrine organs. This sophisticated mechanism of stimulation and inhibition of endocrine organ function, which is called a negative feedback loop, is critical for maintaining metabolic homeostasis (stability) and providing the body with the ability to respond to various stresses.[2]

Many disorders of the endocrine organs can result in disruption of this complex surveillance and response system. These disorders are related to benign, malignant, congenital, degenerative, autoimmune, or infectious processes that affect the function of one or many organs in the endocrine system. The result can range from minor to potentially life-threatening dysfunction. Probably the most widely recognized endocrine dysfunction is insufficient insulin production by the islet cells of the pancreas, or diabetes mellitus. Although this is a complex multisystem disease, the abnormality in glucose metabolism caused by insulin deficiency can be disastrous. This situation is remedied through the supply of insulin via an injection or oral medication to reestablish homeostasis of glucose metabolism.[2]

The function of the endocrine system also may be affected by neoplastic change in the various glands. Although true primary malignancies of these organs are rare, they are important to consider because of the wide-ranging effects they can have on the organism as a whole. Metabolic function altered by neoplastic change in various endocrine organs can produce classic paraneoplastic syndromes. These syndromes can lead the clinician to perform diagnostic studies to confirm the diagnosis of an endocrine gland tumor.[2] This chapter discusses neoplastic lesions of the thyroid, pituitary, and adrenal glands. Pancreatic tumors, which can display endocrine and exocrine function, are discussed in Chapter 31.

THYROID CANCER

Epidemiology

Although thyroid cancers are the most common of the endocrine malignancies (accounting for approximately 96% of all new cases and 67% of deaths), they represent only 2% of all cancers.[3]

Etiology

Unlike other endocrine glands for which malignancies are rare, thyroid cancer has several recognized risk factors.

External radiation to the thyroid gland, particularly before puberty, is the only well-documented etiologic factor. A patient who receives 1 Gy of external radiation to the thyroid gland has an attributable risk (the proportion of thyroid cancer that occurred because of radiation exposure) of 88%. These carcinomas are usually a low-grade papillary subtype.[4]

Many studies have been conducted on the inhabitants of Nagasaki and Hiroshima after the explosion of the atomic bombs in 1945. Of 105,401 exposed individuals examined between 1958 and 2005, 371 (0.3%) have had thyroid cancer develop. Again, most of these cancers have been papillary.[5]

After the radioactive fallout from a nuclear test in the Marshall Islands, the inhabitants have been systematically studied annually and compared with an unexposed population. Of 3709 exposed persons screened between 1993 and 1997, 57 (1.5%) had development of thyroid cancer.[6]

> The Marshall Islands Program was established in 1954 by the Department of Energy (DOE) after the accidental exposure of people in the Marshall Islands to fallout from the U.S. nuclear test at Bikini Atoll. More information is available at https://marshallislands.llnl.gov/.

The Chernobyl incident of 1986 has produced conflicting studies on the increase of thyroid cancer, probably because of the extremely short interval between radiation exposure and tumor occurrence. One study conducted 4.5 years after the Chernobyl reactor accident showed no significant difference in thyroid nodularity between persons residing in highly contaminated villages and those in control villages.[7] However, another study's data confirmed that the neoplasms increasingly diagnosed among children in Ukraine and Belarus were thyroid carcinomas.[8] The Cancer Registry of Belarus confirms this, detailing 101 instances of thyroid cancer in children younger than 15 years between 1986 and 1991, in contrast to only 9 cases between 1976 and 1985.[9]

External radiation for benign disease, especially in young patients, was a widespread practice in the United States in the 1930s, 1940s, and 1950s. X-rays and radium were used to treat benign conditions such as acne, tonsillitis, hemangiomas, and thymic enlargement. Young patients who received radiation for malignant conditions, such as mantle (involved field) irradiation for Hodgkin disease, also had an increased risk of development of thyroid cancer.[3]

The latent (time) period between exposure and incidence of abnormalities varies with age. The minimum latent period in infants is 4 years[10]; in adolescents, the average is 10 years.[11] Whether adults have development of cancer at a higher rate after exposure is questionable.

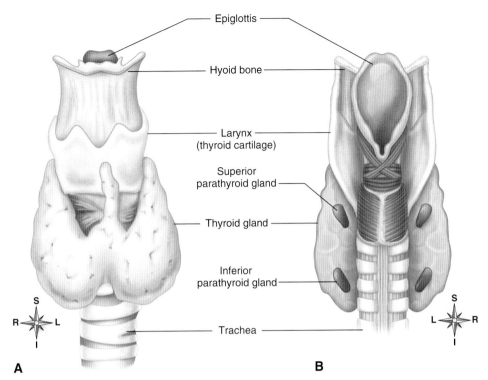

Fig. 27.1 Thyroid and parathyroid glands. Note their relationship to each other and to the larynx (voice box) and trachea. (A) Anterior view. (B) Posterior view. (From Patton KT, Thibodeau GA, eds. *The Human Body in Health and Disease*. 7th ed. St. Louis, MO: Elsevier; 2018.)

Prognostic Indicators

Age, gender, histologic subtype, and capsular invasion are prognostic indicators. Lesions confined to the gland have an overall better prognosis than those with capsular invasion. Patients with well-differentiated (papillary and follicular) thyroid carcinoma have a better prognosis than do those with undifferentiated (anaplastic) carcinoma.[12]

Anatomy

The thyroid gland, which consists of a right and left lobe, lies over the deep structures of the neck. It is close to the larynx, trachea, parathyroid glands, and esophagus and is anterior and medial to the carotid artery, jugular vein, and vagus nerve. Fig. 27.1 depicts the anatomy of the thyroid gland and its anatomic relationships to surrounding structures.

The two large lateral lobes are approximately 5 cm in length and extend to the level of the midthyroid cartilage superiorly and the sixth tracheal ring inferiorly. These lobes are connected in the midline by the isthmus at the level of the second to fourth tracheal rings. The thyroid gland weighs approximately 30 grams.[13]

Lymphatic capillaries are arranged throughout the gland and drain to many nodal sites. These sites include the internal jugular chain, Delphian node (anterior cervical node), pretracheal nodes, and paratracheal nodes in the lower neck. Superior mediastinal lymphatics can be considered the lowest part of the cervical lymphatic chain. Involvement of this represents significant regional spread of disease.[3]

Physiology

The thyroid gland produces several hormones, including triiodothyronine (T_3) and thyroxine (T_4), which are responsible for metabolic regulation. Thyroid function is regulated by pituitary and hypothalamic hormones, which respond to complex systemic negative feedback mechanisms based on metabolic needs. The thyroid-stimulating hormone (TSH) produced in the pituitary gland causes direct stimulation of thyroid cells to produce and release hormones that are critical for carbohydrate and protein metabolism.[2]

The production of these hormones relies on the thyroid gland's ability to remove iodine from the blood. Without sufficient amounts of iodine, the resultant deficiency in thyroid hormone production can cause several clinical disorders. Functional disorders of the thyroid gland are characterized by hyperactivity (hyperthyroidism) or underactivity (hypothyroidism).[2]

Disorders from hypothyroidism can include the following:
- Cretinism. This disorder appears in infants shortly after birth. It is a congenital condition characterized by dwarfism. Symptoms include stunted growth, abnormal bone formation, retarded mental development, lack of muscle coordination, low body temperature, and sluggishness.
- Myxedema. This disorder occurs if hypothyroidism develops later in life. Symptoms include a low metabolic rate, mental slowness, weight gain, and edema of the face and extremities, which often progress to coma and death.[2]

Disorders from hyperthyroidism can include the following:
- Graves disease. This inherited, possibly autoimmune disease is characterized by an elevated metabolic rate, abnormal weight loss, excessive perspiration, muscular weakness, emotional instability, and exophthalmos (abnormal protrusion of the eyeball). Graves disease is the leading cause of hyperthyroidism and often has no long-term adverse health consequences if the patient receives prompt and proper medical attention.
- Goiter. This disorder is a physical sign of an enlarged thyroid gland. Overstimulation by TSH causes an enlargement of thyroid cells. If the condition is associated with increased hormone production, it is referred to as toxic goiter.[2]

TABLE 27.1	Clinical Symptoms and Signs in 106 Patients With Thyroid Cancer		
Symptoms and Signs	Patients (*n* = 66) With Papillary Carcinoma (%)	Patients (*n* = 33) With Follicular Carcinoma (%)	Patients (*n* = 7) With Anaplastic Carcinoma (%)
Found in routine examination	27	30	0
Solitary nodule	60	65	14
Multinodular	33	20	70
Increasing size	56	75	85
Pain and pressure	8	6	28
Dysphagia	11	12	28
Dyspnea	3	6	43
Hoarseness	9	15	55

Modified from Ureles AL. Cancer of the endocrine glands. In: Rubin P, ed. *Clinical Oncology: A Multidisciplinary Approach for Physicians and Students*. 7th ed. Philadelphia, PA: Saunders; 1993.

Lastly, a specialized subgroup of cells within the thyroid is known as C cells. These cells produce calcitonin, which is a hormone involved in calcium metabolism.[2]

Clinical Presentation

Most patients with thyroid cancer have a palpable neck mass, which is often detected during a routine physical examination. Almost 25% of young people with differentiated thyroid carcinoma present because of a palpable cervical lymph node metastasis as a result of occult primary thyroid cancer. These occult, differentiated thyroid cancers can go undetected for years because of their indolent nature.[14] A biopsy should be performed on persistent, enlarged lymph nodes found in children, teenagers, and young adults, with a clinical differential of Hodgkin disease, benign inflammatory disease, or papillary carcinoma of the thyroid gland.[3]

Lesions in the thyroid gland should arouse suspicion if they exhibit extreme hardness, appear fixed to deep structures or skin, or are associated with hoarseness from recurrent laryngeal nerve paralysis.[12]

Most patients with medullary carcinoma initially have an asymptomatic painless mass. They may appear with systemic symptoms of diarrhea related to vasoactive substances (calcitonin) produced by the tumor. This usually represents an advanced stage of the disease.[15]

Anaplastic carcinomas are usually large, hard, and fixed; grow rapidly; and occur in older patients. Patients can appear with symptoms related to compression or invasion of the esophagus, airway, or recurrent laryngeal nerves. Symptoms include pain, dysphagia (difficulty swallowing), dyspnea, stridor, and hoarseness.[16]

Table 27.1 presents clinical symptoms and signs of patients with thyroid carcinoma.

Detection and Diagnosis

Clinical presentation cannot determine a diagnosis of carcinoma. For confirmation of the diagnostic suspicion of cancer, a biopsy (most important), specialized imaging studies, and laboratory testing are necessary.

Laboratory testing includes an analysis of the thyroglobulin and calcitonin levels. After surgery, however, elevated levels indicate residual, recurrent, or metastatic thyroid cancer and can be correlated with iodine-131 (I-131) imaging for the detection of thyroid cancer. As such, thyroglobulin levels may be useful for monitoring patients who have an established diagnosis of thyroid cancer. Calcitonin levels that are elevated before surgery indicate C-cell hyperplasia or medullary thyroid cancer. Postoperative elevated levels indicate residual, recurrent, or metastatic medullary thyroid carcinoma.[17]

Imaging studies include radionuclide imaging, sonography (ultrasound), computed tomography (CT), and magnetic resonance imaging (MRI).[3,12] Each examination can provide useful information for the diagnosis of thyroid cancer.

Radionuclide thyroid imaging is commonly used to evaluate the function and anatomic location of a palpable thyroid nodule through the localization of "hot" or "cold" spots in the gland. This imaging allows for improved detection of occult cancers in patients at high risk. It also permits detection of locoregional or distant metastatic disease, both at the time of diagnosis and in the setting of posttreatment surveillance.

Patients previously treated for thyroid cancer are typically monitored with repeat radionuclide-based imaging.[17]

The four radiopharmaceuticals most commonly used for radionuclide imaging of the thyroid are I-131, I-125, I-123, and technetium-99m (Tc-99m).[17] A thyroid nodule can be imaged in three ways: (1) cold thyroid nodule (no radionuclide uptake), (2) warm thyroid nodule (slightly higher concentration than the rest of the thyroid gland), and (3) hot thyroid nodule (radionuclide uptake much higher than the rest of the thyroid gland). Fig. 27.2 shows abnormal thyroid uptake. Most cold nodules are thyroid adenomas or colloid cysts, with only 5% to 20% representing thyroid cancers.[18]

The incidence of cancer in warm or hot nodules is low and usually represents a functioning adenoma or areas of healthy tissue in an otherwise diseased gland.[18] Some metastatic, well-differentiated follicular carcinomas accumulate radioiodine. Most metastatic, differentiated thyroid tumors do not accumulate radioiodine until all healthy thyroid tissue has been ablated because normally functioning thyroid tissue preferentially accumulates iodinated radiopharmaceuticals relative to the tumor.[19]

Sonography can determine whether a nodule is solid or cystic. This technique is used as a complementary test to radionuclide imaging. A nodule found to be solid with ultrasound has an up to 50% probability of being a cancer.[18]

CT cannot differentiate between a benign or malignant lesion. However, it can show the local and regional extent of advanced or recurrent cancer.[20] CT can also help a radiation oncologist in treatment planning if external beam radiation treatment is anticipated.

MRI can be useful in depicting lesion margins, lesion extent, tissue heterogeneity, cystic or hemorrhagic regions, cervical lymphadenopathy, invasion of adjacent structures, and additional, nonpalpable thyroid nodules.[20]

A needle biopsy in some circumstances can obviate surgery by differentiating malignant from nonmalignant lesions. Two types of needle biopsies are needle aspiration cytology (performed with a small-gauge needle) and core needle biopsy (performed with a large, cutting biopsy needle).

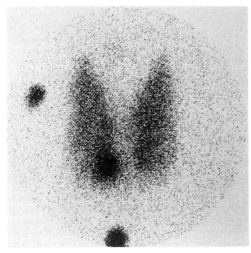

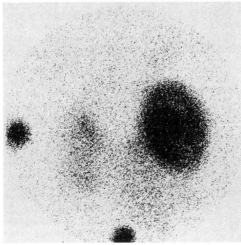

Fig. 27.2 Abnormal thyroid imaging with both images showing a hot nodule. (From Christian PE, Waterstram-Rich KM. *Nuclear Medicine and PET/CT, Technology and Technique.* 7th ed. St. Louis, MO: Mosby; 2012.)

The accuracy of the biopsy depends on the skill and experience of the physician performing and interpreting the sample.[12] A needle biopsy is indeterminate for follicular carcinoma because that diagnosis is made on the basis of capsular or vascular invasion, which can only be determined on a surgical specimen (i.e., it necessitates a larger piece of tissue than a needle biopsy can provide). However, a needle biopsy may play a role in the management of anaplastic thyroid malignancies and lymphomas because the diagnosis is more obvious.[3]

Pathology

Malignant thyroid neoplasms are divided into four categories: (1) papillary, (2) follicular, (3) medullary, and (4) anaplastic. Rare tumors that account for less than 5% of thyroid malignancies include the following:

- Lymphoma and plasmacytoma
- Squamous cell and mucin-producing carcinoma
- Teratoma and mixed tumors
- Sarcoma, carcinosarcoma, and hemangioendothelioma
- Metastatic carcinoma to the thyroid[17]

Differentiated thyroid cancers include papillary, mixed papillary-follicular, and follicular carcinomas. These tumors arise from the thyroid follicle cell and can usually be treated with surgical resection, radioactive iodine (I-131), or other hormone-suppressive therapy.[17]

Papillary cancers are the most common types of thyroid cancer; they represent 80% to 90% of all malignant thyroid lesions.[12] As previously mentioned, papillary carcinoma is the type most frequently seen in individuals with previous irradiation. These tumors are slow growing and nonaggressive and have an excellent prognosis. This type of cancer is two to four times more common in females than in males. The peak incidence is in the third to fifth decade of life, although the cancer may occur at any age. In children younger than 15 years, papillary carcinoma accounts for 80% of thyroid cancers.[17]

Follicular carcinoma accounts for 15% to 30% of all thyroid cancers.[12] These tumors have the greatest propensity to concentrate I-131. They are two to three times more common in women than in men, with the average age for a diagnosis from 50 to 58 years. They rarely occur in children. Follicular carcinoma has a worse overall prognosis than papillary carcinoma.[17]

Medullary thyroid cancer represents less than 5% to 10% of all thyroid cancers. About 80% of medullary thyroid cancers appear spontaneously, with 20% occurring as part of familial multiple endocrine neoplasia (MEN) syndromes MEN 1, MEN 2.[12] No gender differentiation is seen between spontaneous and familial forms. With regard to age, however, spontaneous forms occur from the fifth decade on, whereas familial forms have been seen in patients younger than 20 years.[21] Medullary carcinoma has a worse prognosis than papillary, mixed papillary-follicular, and possibly follicular cancers, although it has a better prognosis than anaplastic carcinoma.

Anaplastic carcinoma is the least common and carries the worst overall prognosis. It is more aggressive than the previously mentioned types, and a patient's life expectancy is typically 1 year or less.[17]

Staging

The American Joint Committee on Cancer has staged thyroid cancers according to the histologic type and age of the patient.

Routes of Spread

Each pathologic classification has its own route of spread, which ranges from slow growing to extremely aggressive.

Papillary and mixed papillary-follicular carcinomas metastasize to regional lymph nodes through lymphatic channels. Metastasis occurs early in the development of the disease, and nodal metastases are associated with poorer outcomes in older patients.[22] Hematogenous metastases can also occur.[3]

Follicular cancers have a tendency to invade vascular channels and metastasize via the bloodstream to distant sites, including the bone, lung, liver, and brain. Lymph node metastases are uncommon.[3]

Medullary thyroid cancer can vary from indolent to rapidly fatal growth patterns. Medullary carcinoma spreads regionally before displaying distant metastases. Metastases occur hematogenously and through lymphatic routes, with the main sites of spread the cervical nodes, lung, liver, and bone.[21]

Anaplastic carcinoma displays local invasion of structures like the trachea. Skin invasion is also seen, which gives rise to dermal lymphatic metastases on the chest and abdominal walls. Regional neck nodes are often involved, although the primary tumor is often so extensive that the regional node status is difficult to assess.[17]

Treatment Techniques

Surgery. Papillary carcinoma and mixed papillary-follicular carcinoma are rarely invasive, with surgical resection focused on the thyroid. Resection of the muscles of the neck, internal jugular vein, esophagus, or trachea is seldom necessary. Radical neck dissections are warranted only if nodes are grossly involved with metastatic disease. Because papillary and mixed papillary-follicular carcinomas are usually indolent diseases, prophylactic or elective neck dissections are no longer performed.[17] If a radical neck dissection is performed, special care is taken to spare the recurrent laryngeal, vagus, spinal accessory, and phrenic nerves. Care is also taken to preserve the parathyroid glands.

For small lesions that do not show extrathyroidal involvement or lymph node metastasis, lobectomy (partial thyroidectomy), including removal of the isthmus, is necessary.[3] Surgery for mixed papillary-follicular carcinoma is the same as that for papillary carcinoma, unless vascular invasion or hematogenous metastases are present, in which case the lesion is treated like follicular cancer.

For organ-confined follicular carcinoma, a lobectomy that includes the isthmus can often successfully control the disease. Early-stage disease has a low risk of nodal spread, so prophylactic neck dissection is not necessary. If a second lesion is present in the contralateral lobe, a total or near-total thyroidectomy may be performed. If follicular carcinoma is extrathyroidal or metastatic disease is present, a bilateral total thyroidectomy is necessary.[3]

All patients with familial medullary carcinoma and up to 30% of those with the spontaneous form have bilateral or multifocal disease, so the initial treatment is typically total thyroidectomy and central compartment lymph node removal. A modified radical neck dissection is warranted when the lymph nodes are clinically involved.[17]

For anaplastic carcinoma, surgery is effective in specific circumstances. Surgery is often necessary to alleviate a central airway obstruction that results from extrinsic compression of the larynx and upper trachea caused by this aggressive malignancy. A tracheotomy is usually necessary to preserve a patient's airway. Radical surgical attempts are not always justified or technically possible because growth into soft tissue and deeper structures of the neck is often present.[17]

For malignancies that metastasize to the thyroid (an extremely rare situation), the treatment varies with primary sites, including the larynx, esophagus, lung, kidney, rectum, and skin. A biopsy is usually needed to differentiate a metastasis from a primary thyroid cancer.

Side effects of surgery can include tumor hemorrhage, damage to the parathyroid gland that results in temporary or permanent hypoparathyroidism, and temporary or permanent vocal cord paralysis.

Radioactive Iodine. I-131 is used to treat papillary and follicular cancers. Indications for I-131 include the following:

- Inoperable primary tumor
- Thyroid capsular invasion
- Thyroid ablation after a partial or subtotal thyroidectomy
- Postoperative residual disease in the neck and recurrent disease
- Cervical or mediastinal nodal metastasis
- Distant metastasis[17]

The routine use of I-131 after surgery in small, well-differentiated cancers is debatable; thyroid suppression therapy alone may be adequate. Because healthy thyroid tissue has a greater propensity to absorb iodine than does differentiated thyroid cancer, the consensus seems to be that all healthy tissue should be ablated to allow residual or metastatic disease to accumulate I-131. An ablation dose administered after a thyroidectomy may vary from 30 to 100 mCi. If a tracer dose of radioiodine reveals persistent thyroid activity after this procedure, a second ablation dose is needed.[17]

After all healthy thyroid tissue is ablated, I-131 can be used to treat local and regional disease and distant metastases for differentiated thyroid cancers. Side effects are listed in Box 27.1.

BOX 27.1 Side Effects of Iodine-131 Treatment

- Nausea
- Change in taste
- Salivary gland edema
- Dry mouth with/without dental issues
- Male and female reproductive issues
- Change in female menstrual cycle
- Early menopause
- Second malignancy

Modified from Dagan R, Amdur RJ. Thyroid cancer. In: Halperin EC, et al, eds. *Perez and Brady's Principles and Practice of Radiation Oncology.* 6th ed. Philadelphia, PA: Lippincott Williams & Wilkins; 2013.

Two important thyroid hormones that regulate the metabolism of lipids, proteins, and carbohydrates are tri-iodothyronine and thyroxine. Tri-iodothyronine is referred to as T_3 because it contains three atoms of iodine; thyroxine is known as T_4 because it contains four atoms of iodine.[2] What do you conclude occurs when radioactive iodine (I-131) is administered to a patient with incompletely resected thyroid cancer or distant metastases?

Thyroid Hormonal Therapy. Thyroid hormone suppression therapy is routinely given for differentiated thyroid cancers, although its effectiveness remains unproven. Differentiated thyroid carcinoma grows under the stimulation of TSH. Thus, through the lowering of TSH levels, tumor activity should be decreased.[17]

External Beam Radiation. Responsiveness to external beam radiation varies according to histologic type. Among differentiated thyroid cancers, papillary and mixed papillary-follicular carcinomas are more radiosensitive than follicular carcinomas. Medullary thyroid cancer is less radiosensitive than papillary carcinoma. In general, anaplastic carcinomas are not responsive to any treatment.[17]

External beam radiation can be used alone or in conjunction with I-131 and surgery. The following are several indications for its use:

- Inoperable lesion
- Patient physically unfit for surgery
- Incomplete surgical removal of thyroid carcinoma
- Superior vena cava syndrome
- Skeletal metastases in which minimal accumulation of I-131 occurred
- Residual disease involving the trachea, larynx, or esophagus[17]

CT simulation of a patient with thyroid cancer should involve extension of the neck and careful immobilization of the head. Extension of the neck allows avoidance of more of the oral cavity, and immobilization assists with daily setup reproducibility.[3] The CT simulation typically begins at the apex of the skull and extends inferiorly to the carina, or even includes all of the lungs, because mediastinal lymph nodes are often treated, and dose to healthy lung tissue is an important consideration. The authors recommend scanning from the top of the skull down through the midabdomen to ensure complete coverage of the lungs, especially when central compartment lymph nodes are treated. Spinal cord dose also is an important consideration but is becoming secondary to lung tissue dose because intensity-modulated radiation therapy (IMRT) can effectively shape the dose off of the spinal cord.

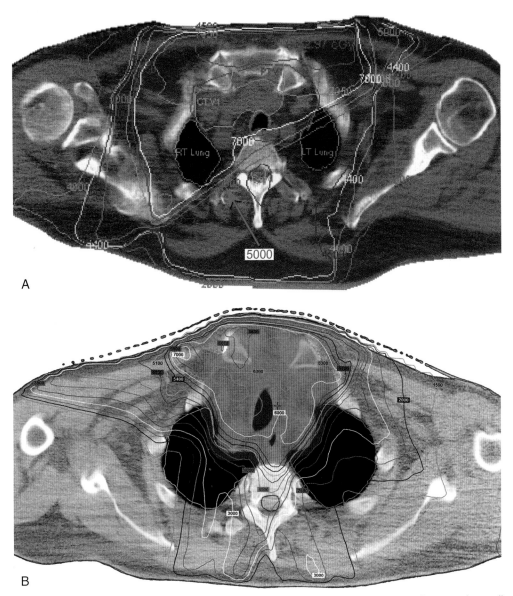

Fig. 27.3 (A) Three-dimensional treatment planning for a patient with locally recurrent and progressive papillary thyroid cancer. (B) Intensity-modulated radiation therapy (IMRT) plan for a patient with thyroid cancer with nine IMRT fields to a total dose of 60 Gy to the low neck and 54 Gy to the lateral upper neck and mediastinum. (From Hay ID, Peterson IA. Thyroid cancer. In: Gunderson LL, Tepper JE, eds. *Clinical Radiation Oncology*. 3rd ed. Philadelphia, PA: Churchill Livingstone; 2012.)

In differentiated thyroid cancer for the curative treatment of inoperable localized disease or in patients with gross residual disease, tumor doses should be in the range of 6000 to 7000 cGy at 180 to 200 cGy per fraction.[17] The radiation field should include the entire thyroid gland, neck, and superior mediastinum with three-dimensional (3D) treatment planning techniques, including IMRT.[3] Treatment planning should include the use of CT for simulation and any additional information available from diagnostic CT, positron emission tomography with CT (PET-CT), or MRI to evaluate anatomy, disease extent, and the treatment plan. IMRT is an increasingly attractive technique used to improve dose delivered to the target volume with better sparing of healthy structures, such as the spinal cord (Fig. 27.3).[17]

For medullary carcinoma that has not extended below the clavicles, radiation therapy can be considered. Dose ranges from 5000 cGy to 7000 cGy, depending on the clinical features of the case (i.e., microscopic versus gross residual disease present). The treatment fields typically encompass the primary lesion, bilateral cervical node chains, and superior mediastinum.[17]

Anaplastic carcinoma is the least radiosensitive of all the thyroid cancers. Tumor control is seldom accomplished, even after a dose of 6000 cGy to the primary lesion, neck, and superior mediastinum.[17]

Case I

Thyroidectomy. A 34-year-old woman presented to her primary care physician with a persistent left-sided nodule on her anterior neck. Other than the nodule, the patient had no other signs or symptoms of disease. She underwent radionuclide imaging in the form of a thyroid scan that showed a warm thyroid nodule. This left-sided nodule was excised. Pathology results showed follicular carcinoma with capsular invasion. No obvious vascular or lymphatic invasion was present. The patient was advised to have a complete lobectomy or an I-131 ablation of the left thyroid gland. The patient elected surgery.

Histopathologically, the resected lobe showed focal areas of residual follicular carcinoma. A thyroid scan after surgery showed no uptake in the neck. The patient had hypothyroidism for several weeks after the surgery and then underwent an I-125 scan that showed residual uptake in the left neck, which corresponded with the bed of the left thyroid nodule. No uptake was present on the right side, and no other activity was seen on a body scan. The patient was referred for I-131 treatment to the residual nodule in the left neck.

The acute risks of nausea and potential long-term risks of solid and hematologic cancer induction were discussed with the patient. The precautions to be taken by the patient and her family, with specific regard to exposure to her children, were carefully outlined.

With her consent, the patient was given 30 mCi of I-131 via a capsule. The dose was relatively low because the patient had a partial thyroidectomy and was young. After observation for 1 hour without any nausea, and the exposure rate measured and recorded, the patient was discharged. A 6-month repeat thyroid scan showed no residual uptake in the left neck.

Pituitary Tumors

Pituitary tumors are less aggressive than many central nervous system tumors, although pituitary neoplasms still pose problems as a result of local growth that causes compressive and destructive effects and endocrine abnormalities caused by pituitary hormone dysfunction.[23] Most pituitary tumors are benign adenomas. The pituitary is composed of an anterior, a posterior, and an intermediate lobe. Tumors of the posterior and intermediate portion are very rare.[24] This section addresses tumors that arise from the anterior pituitary gland, or adenohypophysis.

Epidemiology

Pituitary tumors are benign tumors and comprise the majority of tumors that arise in the sella turcica. These neoplasms represent about 10% to 15% of all intracranial tumors, although asymptomatic adenomas appear in approximately 14% of pituitary glands examined at autopsy and in 23% from radiography studies.[23]

Pituitary adenomas can be classified as functioning or nonfunctioning, as related to the hormones they produce. Hormone production often serves as a diagnostic and treatment-response marker. The frequency of the various types of pituitary adenomas differs widely according to age, gender, and type of hormone secretion.[23] The most common hypersecretory tumor type is prolactinoma. This tumor causes amenorrhea (the absence of menstruation) and galactorrhea (the discharge of milk when a woman is not pregnant or breastfeeding) in women and impotence and infertility in men. The second most common functioning pituitary tumor is growth hormone (GH)–secreting adenoma, which results in acromegaly (enlarged extremities) in adults and gigantism in children. The third most common functioning pituitary tumor results in an oversecretion of cortisol as a result of an adrenocorticotrophic hormone (ACTH)–secreting tumor. Cortisol is released by the adrenal glands, and its action helps maintain blood glucose levels within the normal range between meals. It also acts as to reduce inflammation in the body. TSH-secreting adenomas are rare.[23]

Nonfunctioning pituitary adenomas that arise from the gonadotropin-producing cells are not associated with the classical hypersecretion syndrome. These syndromes are listed in Table 27.2. Tumor extension beyond the sella turcica may cause pressure or invasion into surrounding structures. Patients may have a headache, diplopia, or other visual symptoms caused by the compression of the optic chiasm rather than syndromes associated with the hypersecretion of pituitary hormones.[23]

TABLE 27.2 Clinical Syndromes Associated With Hormonally Functional Pituitary Adenomas

Hormone	Target Tissue	Clinical Syndrome
Prolactin	Gonads	Amenorrhea, galactorrhea in women Impotence, infertility in men
GH	Bones, muscles, organs	Acromegaly in adults Gigantism in children
ACTH	Adrenal cortex	Cushing disease Nelson syndrome (after adrenalectomy)
TSH	Thyroid	Hypothyroidism

ACTH, Adrenocorticotrophic hormone; *GH,* growth hormone; *TSH,* thyroid-stimulating hormone.
Modified from Gibbs IC, et al. Pituitary tumors. In: Phillips TL, et al, eds. *Leibel and Phillips Textbook of Radiation Oncology.* 3rd ed. Elsevier; 2010.

Prognostic Indicators

The prognosis depends on the type of adenoma and a combination of other factors, including the following: (1) the extent of the abnormalities (through mass effect or hormonal alterations), (2) the success of the treatment in normalizing endocrine activity or relieving pressure effects, (3) the morbidity caused by the treatment, and (4) the effectiveness of the treatment in preventing a recurrence.[25]

Anatomy

The pituitary gland is about 1.3 cm in diameter and is located at the base of the brain. Attached to the hypothalamus by a stalklike structure (the infundibulum), the pituitary gland lies in the sella turcica of the sphenoid bone. The gland is divided structurally and functionally into an anterior lobe (adenohypophysis), a posterior lobe (neurohypophysis), and an intermediate lobe.[13] The blood supply to the adenohypophysis is from several superior hypophyseal arteries, and the blood supply to the neurohypophysis is from the inferior hypophyseal arteries. The pituitary gland is close to critical structures of the central nervous system, such as the optic chiasm (superiorly). The anatomic relationships are shown in Fig. 27.4. Related to topographic anatomy, the pituitary gland is positioned behind the temporomandibular joint and midplane behind the nasal bone (i.e., between the eyes).

Physiology

Derived from the endoderm, the adenohypophysis forms the glandular part of the pituitary. The glandular cells (acidophils and basophils) are responsible for the secretion of seven hormones.

Acidophils secrete the following two hormones:
- Prolactin (PRL): Initiates milk production.
- GH: Controls body growth.
  Basophils secrete the following five hormones:
- ACTH: Influences the action of the adrenal cortex.
- TSH: Controls the thyroid gland.
- Follicle-stimulating hormone (FSH): Stimulates egg and sperm production.
- Luteinizing hormone (LH): Stimulates other sexual and reproductive activity.
- Melanocyte-stimulating hormone: Relates to skin pigmentation.[13]

The release of these hormones is stimulated or inhibited by the chemical secretions from the hypothalamus, which are called regulatory, or releasing, factors. The posterior lobe, or neurohypophysis, secretes oxytocin, which causes smooth muscle contractions, and antidiuretic hormone (ADH), or vasopressin, which regulates free water resorption in the kidneys.[13]

Patients who have had their pituitary gland removed via surgery (hypophysectomy) or treated with high-dose radiation therapy must be put on hormone replacement for the rest of their lives.[23] Specific hormone deficiencies from the anterior and posterior pituitary gland include prolactin, growth, adrenocortical, thyroid, gonadotropin, and antidiuretic hormones.

Clinical Presentation

Hormonal Effects. Functioning pituitary tumors retain hormone-producing capabilities, although they are unresponsive to regulatory mechanisms and produce hormones regardless of metabolic needs. Hypersecretion of pituitary hormones results in varied clinical presentations, depending on the type of secreting tumor. The hypersecretion of GH produces clinical symptoms such as weight gain; thickening of the bones and soft tissues of the hands, feet, and cheeks; and overgrowth of the jaw and tongue. Patients are hypertensive and commonly report headaches and lack of energy. This clinical syndrome is referred to as acromegaly if hypersecretion occurs after puberty and as giantism if it happens before puberty.[24]

In some instances, local compressive effects of the tumor in the pituitary itself may cause deficient production of hormones normally synthesized in the gland. Hormones that have target organs (such as ACTH [adrenals], TSH [thyroid], and FSH [ovaries and testes]) can cause an array of abnormalities that result from a loss of pituitary hormonal action. These clinical manifestations are listed in Table 27.2.

Pressure Effects. The most common manifestation of an expanding pituitary lesion is headache and visual field defects. Local pressure on the lining of the sphenoid sinus can produce headaches.[26]

Visual acuity and field defects are clinical manifestations and signify extension beyond the sella turcica. Suprasellar extension of these tumors causes pressure effects on the inferior aspect of the optic chiasm, which results in visual symptomatology, and is usually progressive. The presentation may be altered visual acuity, but more commonly, visual field defects are observed. The most common field defect is bitemporal hemianopsia (loss of peripheral vision bilaterally). If pressure effects on the optic chiasm persist for significant periods, the result can be permanent visual field defects or blindness. In rare instances, these tumors can extend laterally into the cavernous sinuses (see Fig. 27.4) and cause characteristic cranial nerve deficits.[27]

Detection and Diagnosis

Patients with functional tumors have characteristic endocrine abnormalities that are associated with the hypersecretion of hormones. The clinical syndromes from Table 27.2 prompt medical attention. Laboratory testing, which can directly measure hormone levels, can confirm pituitary hormone dysfunction and strongly suggest the diagnosis. The expanding growth of nonfunctioning tumors into the suprasellar area causes pressure symptoms such as headache, visual disturbances, and impairment of various cranial nerves. These symptoms often bring the patient to medical attention and prompt diagnostic studies.

The principal imaging study for the pituitary gland is CT or MRI. MRI is superior to CT in delineating the extent of the tumor process relative to normal critical structures such as the optic chiasm, vascular structures, cranial nerves, and cavernous sinuses just lateral to the pituitary gland (see Fig. 27.4). Both MRI and CT provide detailed anatomic information in transverse, sagittal, and coronal projections. This information is invaluable to the neurosurgeon and radiation oncologist in determining a therapeutic approach.[27]

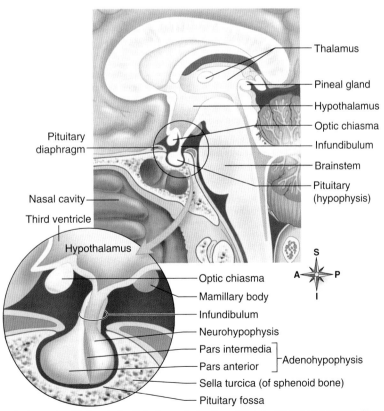

Fig. 27.4 The pituitary gland is located within the sella turcica of the skull's sphenoid bone. Note the location of the optic chiasm, superior to the pituitary gland. (From Thibodeau GA, Patton KT. *Anatomy and Physiology.* 7th ed. St. Louis, MO: Elsevier; 2009.)

Pathology

Neoplasms are formed of tightly packed cells that remain separate from healthy tissue without a membrane and are classified according to size. Microadenomas are less than 10 mm, and macroadenomas are greater than 10 mm.[25] This classification is important because predictions of the prognosis can be made from the tumor size. Larger adenomas are surgically more difficult to remove with complete resections, and recurrence is more common in this group.[27]

Pituitary tumors can also be classified according to their growth patterns (by expansion or invasion) and are separated into intrahypophyseal, intrasellar, diffuse, and invasive adenomas. Intrahypophyseal tumors stay in the pituitary gland, whereas intrasellar lesions grow within the confines of the sella turcica. Diffuse adenomas usually fill the entire sella turcica and can erode its wall. Invasive neoplasms have a more rapid growth rate and tend to erode outside the sella turcica to invade neighboring tissues, such as the posterior pituitary gland, sphenoid bone, and cavernous sinus. These neoplasms may even penetrate into the brain and third ventricle. Invasive adenomas are classified as malignant adenomas when metastases are present. Malignant adenomas metastasize via cerebrospinal fluid (CSF) or vascular pathways, but this is an extremely rare event.[28]

Staging

Because most tumors are benign, no true staging exists. However, pituitary tumors have been classified into four grades developed by Hardy and Vezina, according to the extent of expansion or erosion of the sella turcica. The system is based primarily on the presence of microadenomas (< 1 cm) and macroadenomas (> 1 cm) and the amount of tumor invasion. (Box 27.2).

Treatment Techniques

The primary goal of treatment is to normalize pituitary hormonal function or relieve local compressive or destructive effects of the tumor. In some instances, both factors must be improved. This can be accomplished surgically, therapeutically with radiation, medically, or with a combination of these modalities. An obvious secondary goal is prevention of recurrence.

Surgery. Surgery plays a significant role in the management of pituitary tumors. Before 1970, craniotomies were performed with an associated operative mortality rate of 2% to 25%. Currently, the less invasive transsphenoidal approach is widely used, which decreases the mortality rate to 0.6%. Complications of this surgery are CSF leakage (2%), infection (meningitis; 2%), and visual pathway defects, with have a combined morbidity rate of about 9%.[29] Fig. 27.5 is a depiction of the transsphenoidal approach. In summary, the two main surgical approaches are the transfrontal approach (transfrontal craniotomy) and the transsphenoidal approach, which allows direct access to the pituitary gland without disturbance of the central nervous system structures.[27]

Characteristic hormonal abnormalities show favorable responses after surgery. If surgical intervention of functioning adenomas is successful, the response in terms of the normalization of hormone levels is almost immediate. Symptomatic relief is seen in 80% to 90% of patients with acromegaly, although the recurrence rate is 20%. Results are generally satisfactory for patients with Cushing syndrome (ACTH-producing adenomas). Although results vary, remission occurs in 70% of patients, with a recurrence rate over 10 years of 15%. Similarly, excellent results are achieved with PRL-secreting adenomas.[27]

Radiation Therapy. Surgery is often only one part of the overall management for a pituitary adenoma. Although the role of postoperative radiation therapy is controversial, it has been shown in various series to reduce recurrence rates compared with surgery alone.[25] Radiation therapy alone has also been used to control pituitary tumors in patients who refuse surgery and in those who are medically unfit.[30]

Postoperative radiation therapy is used as an adjunctive modality in the following circumstances:
- An incompletely resected invasive tumor
- Tumors with suprasellar extension with an associated visual field defect
- Large tumors in which the risk of attempted removal is relatively high
- Persistent hormonal elevation after surgery[31]

Radiation Therapy Techniques. Sometimes the effect of radiation therapy on pituitary tumor control or hormone suppression may take years, which makes evaluation of the effectiveness of the treatment difficult.[25] The use of external beam radiation therapy and stereotactic radiosurgery (SRS) techniques may vary considerably among radiation therapy departments. At many institutions, conventional radiation therapy techniques with simple immobilization and limited beam angles (such as two to three fixed fields) have been replaced with advanced radiation therapy techniques that incorporate sophisticated treatment planning systems with CT and MRI studies, improvement in immobilization techniques, IMRT with micromultileaf collimators, and image-guided radiation therapy (IGRT). Modern radiation therapy techniques, such as 3D conformal therapy, stereotactic radiation therapy, SRS, and proton therapy, have allowed more focused delivery of the prescribed dose to the tumor and a reduced dose to healthy brain tissue.[27]

BOX 27.2   Hardy and Vezina's Pituitary Tumor Classification

Grade 0: Complete intraselar microadenoma
Grade I: Intrasellar microadenoma with local sellar turcica distortion
Grade II: Macroadenoma with local expansion of the floor of the sella turcica
Grade III: Macroadenoma with local destruction of the floor of the sella turcica and invasion of sphenoid sinus or cavernous sinuses
Grade IV: Macroadenoma with total sellar turcica destruction and local invasion

Courtesy of Jules Hardy, MD, and Jean L. Vézina, MD.

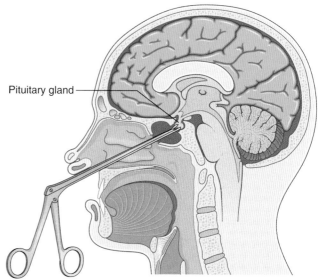

Pituitary gland

Fig. 27.5 Anatomic route for a transsphenoidal hypophysectomy. (From Chabner D. *The Language of Medicine.* 11th ed. St. Louis, MO: Elsevier; 2017.)

For the initial CT simulation procedure, the patient's neck is flexed, with chin down toward the chest, to minimize radiation exposure to the eyes. Bite blocks or intraoral stents are also used to fixate the position of the chin, mouth, and head and neck. Immobilization devices provide an accurate and reproducible patient positioning for 3D-conformal radiation therapy in the head and neck area.

Improvements in immobilization with more precise thermoplastic masks and fixed or relocatable (SRS) frames may allow a reduction in planning margin from 1.5 to 2.0 cm down to 0.5 to 1.0 cm.[25] Fig. 27.6

shows an example of an IMRT dose plan, and Fig. 27.7 shows a SRS plan for a patient with pituitary adenoma.

Proton Beam Therapy. Because of the proton beam's physical characteristics (i.e., a Bragg peak with a rapid dose falloff at depth), the dose can be precisely delivered within millimeters of a defined target directly related to the beam's energy.[30] This is a particularly attractive feature for treatment near critical structures such as the optic chiasm and the temporal lobe, areas in which an excessive radiation dose can produce devastating clinical consequences.

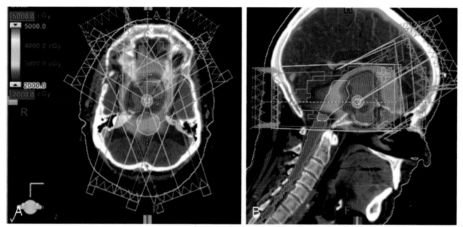

Fig. 27.6 Intensity-modulated radiation therapy (IMRT) isodose plan for a residual nonsecretory pituitary adenoma. Axial (A) and sagittal (B) images show a seven-field IMRT radiation plan for pituitary adenoma. (From Gibbs IC, et al. Pituitary tumors. In: Hoppe R, Phillips TL, Roach M. eds. *Leibel and Phillips Textbook of Radiation Oncology.* 3rd ed. Elsevier; 2010.)

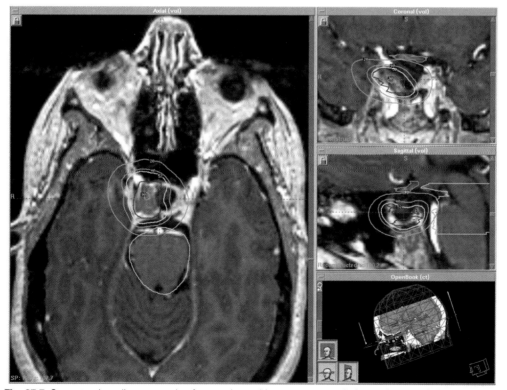

Fig. 27.7 Stereotactic radiosurgery plan for a patient with nonsecretory pituitary adenoma. A dose of 16 Gy was prescribed to the 50% isodose line. The maximum dose to the optic chiasm was 6.4 Gy. (From Suh JH, et al. Pituitary tumors and craniopharyngiomas. In: in Gunderson, L. L., & Tepper, J. E. (2015). Clinical radiation oncology. Elsevier Health Sciences.)

Protons are a valuable tool for clinical use for the following reasons: (1) they are precision controlled; (2) scattering is minimal compared with that from x-rays, neutrons, and cobalt radiation; (3) they have a characteristic distribution of dose with depth; and (4) most of their energy is deposited near the end of their range, where the dose peaks to a high value and then drops rapidly to zero. This sudden change in dose distribution with depth is called the Bragg peak. More information about proton therapy can be found in Chapter 15 and Chapter 16.

Stereotactic Radiosurgery. SRS uses a high-energy photon beam with multiple ports of entry convergent on the target tissue. This procedure is typically done as a single, large fraction of treatment with the patient immobilized in a stereotactic head frame. After rigid positioning, the patient undergoes a planning CT scan to define the tumor volume and determine the multiple ports of entry. With the patient immobilized the entire time, this procedure takes several hours and requires multiple images on the treatment unit to ensure accuracy.

This technique may not be an optimal approach to this particular disease because pituitary neoplasms are benign, and high single-fraction treatment can produce significant healthy-tissue morbidity if an uncertainty exists regarding the target volume treated. Fractionated SRS may be one means to reduce the risk of healthy tissue injury because it reduces the dose per fraction.[27]

Results of Treatment

Pituitary adenoma treatment outcomes are favorable. Surgery for microadenomas is generally curative. Series with radiation therapy alone have shown excellent disease-free survival rates of up to 95% at 10 years and more than 90% at 20 years.[25] A direct comparison between the results of different treatment approaches is difficult to make because of the various criteria used to select the optimal treatment, as previously described. However, surgery and radiation therapy alone or in combination clearly produce excellent results.

Case II

Pituitary Macroadenoma. A 32-year-old woman presented to the emergency department with a medical history of headaches. During physical examination, the patient was found to have features of acromegaly. She had a 2-year history of progressively enlarging hands and feet and pain in the joints of her extremities. She denied any visual symptoms.

As part of her workup, a brain MRI scan showed findings consistent with a pituitary macroadenoma that measured about 1.5 cm in diameter and extended suprasellarly into the optic chiasm. Slight elevation of the chiasm was present. The floor of the sella turcica was also eroded, and the tumor appeared to extend partially into the sphenoid sinus. Laboratory studies showed elevated GH levels (150 ng/mL; normal range, 1-10 ng/mL). A transsphenoidal hypophysectomy was advised.

After surgery, the patient had a remarkable reduction in her GH level and reversal of some of her acromegaly. However, because of the radiographic findings (erosion of the sella turcica and invasion into the sphenoid sinus), the patient was believed to be at high risk for recurrence. A course of radiation therapy to the pituitary fossa and sphenoid sinus was recommended to improve the probability of local control.

In a supine, immobilized position, the patient was treated via a seven-field IMRT technique with 6-MV photons. CT and MRI scans were performed to aid with the treatment planning. This seven-field IMRT arrangement was treated at 180 cGy/fraction for 25 treatments to 4500 cGy.

The patient tolerated the therapy well but still reported headaches at the end of radiation therapy. Approximately 6 months later, the patient continued to show regression of the acromegaly features. This regression was characterized by smaller hands and feet. An MRI scan at that time showed no evidence of disease. During subsequent follow-up visits, the patient continued to do well, with decreasing GH levels. Approximately 2 years after the therapy, the patient's GH level was 3.0 ng/mL.

ADRENAL CORTEX TUMORS

Neoplasms of the adrenal glands are rare, with malignant tumors accounting for only 75 to 115 new cases per year.[32] Tumors that arise in the adrenal glands are classified according to the portion of the gland from which they arise. This includes tumors that arise from the cortex (outer portion of the gland) and those from the medulla (inner portion of the gland). The cortex and the medulla, which make up the adrenal gland (Fig. 27.8), have distinct histologic features and physiologic

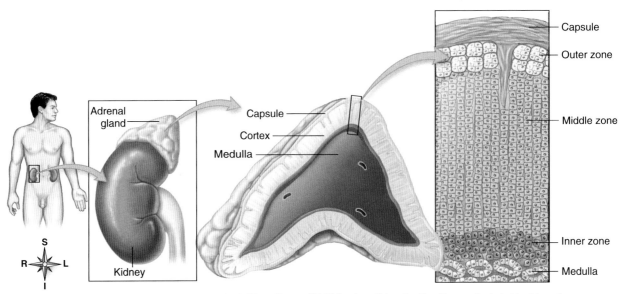

Fig. 27.8 Anatomy of the adrenal gland. (From Patton KT, Thibodeau GA, eds. *The Human Body in Health and Disease.* 7th ed. St. Louis, MO: Elsevier; 2018.)

TABLE 27.3 Clinical Manifestations of Adrenocortical Hormone Excess

Hormone	Syndrome	Clinical Manifestations
Cortisol (ACTH)	Cushing syndrome	Acid-base imbalance, hypertension, obesity, osteoporosis, hyperglycemia, psychoses, excessive bruising, renal calculi
Aldosterone	Conn syndrome (aldosteronism)	Hypernatremia, hypokalemia, hypertension, neuromuscular weakness and paresthesias, electrocardiographic and renal function abnormalities
Sex hormones (estrogen, testosterone, and progesterone)	Virilization (in women)	Male pattern baldness, hirsutism, deepening voice, breast atrophy, decreased libido, oligomenorrhea
	Feminization (in men)	Gynecomastia, breast tenderness, testicular atrophy, decreased libido

ACTH, Adrenocorticotrophic hormone.
From Donehower MG. Endocrine cancers. In: in Baird SB, Mccorkle R, and Grant MM. eds. *Cancer Nursing: A Comprehensive Textbook*. Saunders: Elsevier; 1991.

functions. In general, the cortex manufactures steroid hormones that are critical in metabolic regulation, and the medulla produces epinephrine (adrenaline) under the regulation of the autonomic nervous system.[13]

Epidemiology

As mentioned, adrenocortical tumors are extremely rare. Women are affected slightly more than men, and hyperfunctioning malignancies are also more common in women. Tumors arise as commonly in the left gland as the right. There is a bimodal age distribution, with peaks before age 5 years and in the 40s and 50s.[32]

Adrenal adenomas are benign neoplasms and are rarely associated with serious medical illness. However, in some circumstances, these can cause hypersecretion of normally produced steroid hormones, giving rise to various clinical syndromes. Many adrenal masses represent metastatic disease typically from lung cancer.[33]

Prognostic Indicators

The stage of the disease at the time of diagnosis closely parallels survival rates. Most patients have advanced disease at the time of presentation.[33]

The ability of the surgeon to achieve curative resection is another prognostic factor because surgery is the only modality that has shown a significant effect on survival rates. All patients should have close postoperative surveillance for the detection of abdominal and distant metastases while they are still resectable.[32]

Anatomy

The adrenal glands are paired organs located on the superior pole of the kidneys. These glands have a yellow cortex and dark brown medulla. They derive their blood supply from the adrenal branches of the inferior phrenic artery, aorta, and renal artery. The lymphatic drainage is to the paraaortic nodes. The normal adrenal gland weighs approximately 5 grams.[32]

Physiology

The adrenal cortex produces steroid hormones, including glucocorticoids, mineralocorticoids, and sex hormones, which are responsible for metabolic regulation. These hormones include cortisol, aldosterone, estrogen, and androgen.[13] The cells of the adrenal cortex that manufacture these hormones are regulated by the ongoing stresses and needs of an individual's metabolism. The normal functioning adrenal cortex can respond instantaneously to meet metabolic demands and maintain homeostasis.[2]

Clinical Presentation

Because of the location of adrenal cortex tumors in the abdomen and the inaccessibility for physical examination, many patients have symptoms of pain develop from advanced cancer. Alternatively, clinical manifestations of symptoms related to excess hormone production may prompt medical attention. Well-described syndromes are associated with the excessive production of hormones from the adrenal cortex. These are listed in Table 27.3.

In a series of 47 patients with adrenocortical carcinoma reported by Cohn and colleagues, symptoms relating to a nonfunctioning tumor included an abdominal mass in 77% of patients, weight loss in 46%, fever in 15%, and distant metastases in 15%.[11] Many patients have more than one symptom at the time of diagnosis. In the same series, symptoms relating to functional tumors included Cushing syndrome in 26% of patients, mixed Cushing syndrome and virilization in 24%, virilization in 15%, and feminization in 9%.[34]

Detection and Diagnosis

Patients may have functioning or nonfunctioning tumors. With functioning tumors, the clinical syndromes from Table 27.3 often lead to the diagnosis and can be easily confirmed with laboratory testing. In nonfunctioning tumors, pain is the presenting symptom and is often associated with locally advanced disease.

The initial imaging study for the adrenal gland is CT or MRI. These scans often suggest the diagnosis of an adrenal neoplasm and show the local and regional extent of the disease.[32] Fig. 27.9 shows an abdominal CT scan of a suspected adrenal neoplasm. A definitive tissue diagnosis requires a needle biopsy with CT guidance.

Pathology

Adrenocortical tumors are usually large, single, rounded masses of yellow-orange adrenocortical tissue. Because they are usually large at the time of diagnosis, they have considerable hemorrhage, necrosis, and calcification. In a series of 38 patients reviewed by Karakousis and associates, tumors were graded according to the cells' resemblance to healthy adrenal cortical cells. Well-differentiated (grade I) tumors were distinguished from adenomas by the presence of capsular and vascular invasion and abnormal mitoses. The survival rate for patients with grade I or II tumors is significantly greater than that for patients with grade III tumors.[35]

Staging

No true staging system exists because so few cases are reported. However, an example of a conventional staging system for adrenocortical carcinoma is presented in Box 27.3. This system stages according to the size of the tumor and the extent to which it has advanced locally or distantly.

Routes of Spread

Adrenocortical carcinomas can grow locally into surrounding tissues. However, these carcinomas may also spread to regional

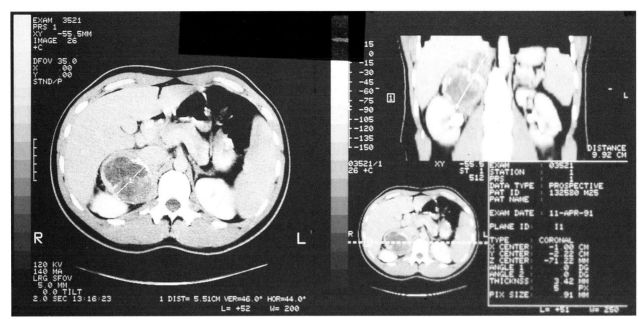

Fig. 27.9 An abdominal computed tomography scan of a suspected adrenal neoplasm.

BOX 27.3   Staging System for Adrenal Cancer

T Categories for Adrenal Cancer

T1: The tumor is 5 cm (about 2 inches) or less in size and has not grown into tissues outside the adrenal gland.

T2: The tumor is greater than 5 cm (2 inches) in size and has not grown into tissues outside the adrenal gland.

T3: The tumor is growing in the fat that surrounds the adrenal gland. The tumor can be any size.

T4: The tumor is growing into nearby organs, such as the kidney, pancreas, spleen, and liver. The tumor can be any size.

N Categories

N0: The cancer has not spread to nearby lymph nodes.

N1: The cancer has spread to nearby lymph nodes.

M Categories

M0: The cancer has not spread to distant organs or tissues (like liver, bone, brain).

M1: The cancer has spread to distant sites.

Stage Groupings for Adrenal Cancer in the AJCC System
Stage I

T1, N0, M0: The cancer is smaller than 5 cm (2 inches) and has not grown into surrounding tissues or organs. The cancer has not spread to lymph nodes (N0) or other body parts (M0).

Stage II

T2, N0, M0: The cancer is larger than 5 cm (2 inches) but still has not grown into surrounding tissues or organs. The cancer has not spread to lymph nodes (N0) or other body parts (M0).

Stage III
Either of the following:

T1 or T2, N1, M0: The tumor can be any size, but it has not started growing outside the adrenal gland (T1 or T2). The cancer has spread to nearby lymph nodes (N1) but not to distant sites (M0)
or

T3, N0, M0: The cancer has grown into the fat outside the adrenal gland (T3). It has not spread to nearby lymph nodes (N0) or to distant sites (M0).

Stage IV
Either of the following:

T3, N1, M0: The cancer has grown into the fat outside of the adrenal gland (T3), and it has spread to nearby lymph nodes (N1); it has not spread to distant body sites (M0),
or

T4, N0 or N1, M0: The cancer has grown from the adrenal gland into organs or tissues nearby (T4). It may (N1) or may not (N0) have spread to nearby lymph nodes, but it has not spread to distant sites (M0),
or

Any T, any N, M1: The cancer has spread to distant sites (M1). It can be any size and may or may not have spread to nearby tissues or lymph nodes.

From American Cancer Society. Adrenal cancer stages. http://www.cancer.org/cancer/adrenalcorticalcancer/detailedguide/adrenal-cortical-cancer-staging. Accessed June 22, 2018.

---

paraaortic nodes and distantly to the lung, liver, or brain.[32] Local invasion or distant metastases are often present at the time of diagnosis. Tumors on the right side involve the kidney, liver, and vena cava (often by direct extension of the tumor). Tumors on the left side often involve the kidney, pancreas, and diaphragm.

Treatment Techniques

Surgery is the treatment of choice. A complete resection is not always feasible because of invasion to adjacent vital structures, such as the spleen, kidney, and parts of the pancreas. Although the resection of adrenal carcinomas is not always for cure, debulking results in decreased pain. Radiation therapy has a limited role, but it may be used as an adjunct to surgery to improve local control and for the palliative treatment of metastatic disease.[32]

Because of the rarity of this malignancy, cytotoxic chemotherapy has not been widely studied. However, some evidence suggests that agents that have activity alone or in combination against adrenocortical carcinoma include etoposide, doxorubicin, cisplatin, and mitotane.[32] The role of these agents in an adjuvant setting is far from clear.

RESULTS OF TREATMENT

The outcome for patients treated with this disease is poor. The 5-year survival rates for all stages range between 20% and 25%.[32] The stage at diagnosis and the ability to resect the disease have a significant effect on its outcome. Because most patients (70%) have advanced-stage disease, the ability to accomplish a curative resection is minimized, and survival rates decrease.[34]

ADRENAL MEDULLA TUMORS

Epidemiology

Approximately 400 medullary tumors called *pheochromocytomas* are diagnosed in the United States per year. The peak incidence of this tumor is in the fourth and fifth decades of life, but it can be seen at any age. These tumors may be bilateral in various familial syndromes and can be associated with MEN syndromes. In addition, this type of tumor has been observed in patients with von Recklinghausen disease (type I neurofibromatosis).[32]

Anatomy

The anatomy of adrenal medulla tumors is discussed in the section on adrenal cortex tumors.

Clinical Presentation

A well-recognized clinical syndrome is associated with pheochromocytomas. The symptoms include hypertension, severe headache, nervousness, palpitations, excessive perspiration, angina, blurred vision, and abdominal pain. These are mediated by the excessive production of epinephrine associated with these tumors. Symptoms vary little among benign and malignant tumors and are often sporadic.[32]

Detection and Diagnosis

These tumors are suspected based on the clinical presentation. CT or MRI is used to assess the extent of disease. Laboratory testing, which measures urinary or plasma catecholamines (vanillylmandelic acid and precursors of epinephrine), can help confirm the diagnosis.[32] A needle biopsy can establish a tissue diagnosis but may not be necessary if the clinical, radiographic, and laboratory findings support the diagnosis.

Pathology

Adrenal medulla tumors are well-delineated, circumscribed tumors that range from dark red to gelatinous pink to gray-brown or gray. The tumor size varies from 1 cm to 30 cm, with areas of hemorrhage and necrosis.[32]

Routes of Spread

The metastatic pattern of malignant pheochromocytomas is similar to that of adrenocortical carcinoma. These tumors can grow locally into surrounding tissues and may also spread to regional lymph nodes, or distantly to the lung, liver, brain, or bone.[32]

Treatment Techniques

Surgery is the treatment of choice for these tumors. Malignant tumors may grow extensively into surrounding structures, which makes a complete resection impossible. Persistent elevation of blood pressure indicates residual tumor or metastatic disease.[32]

Results of Treatment

The surgical resection of benign pheochromocytomas results in a normal life expectancy, and patients with malignant pheochromocytomas can be maintained for many years. Patients with extra-adrenal malignancy have a poorer prognosis.

Case III

Adrenocortical Carcinoma. A 50-year-old man was in a normal state of health until approximately 3 months before presentation, at which time he experienced right flank pain and sought medical attention. His medical history was unremarkable. Physical examination showed no evidence of a functioning tumor (Cushingoid changes, hyperaldosteronism, or virilism). His blood pressure was normal, and he had no flushing, sweats, or palpitations.

As part of his initial workup, a CT scan was performed and showed a 6-cm mass that appeared to involve the right adrenal gland. There was obvious extrinsic compression of the right kidney. Neither adenopathy nor liver metastases were present. A preoperative chest x-ray was also unremarkable.

At the time of surgery, a clear plane was established between the mass and the kidney. However, adherence was encountered over the inferior vena cava, which required a resection of a portion of the cava to remove the mass. A lymph node overlying the right renal vein was also encountered and surgically resected.

The patient had an uneventful surgical recovery. Histopathologically, this case proved to be a low-grade adrenocortical carcinoma. Because of concern for residual tumor overlying the vena cava, the patient was sent for a radiation oncology consult. The radiation oncologist thought that because there may be gross residual disease, the patient was indeed at risk for locoregional recurrence. Postoperative external beam treatment was indicated to secure the optimal probability of local control.

The patient was treated in the supine position with 15 MV photons, receiving 6000 cGy using a volume-modulated arc therapy technique and daily IGRT to check the patient's position. A contrast-enhanced CT scan was performed at the time of simulation to delineate the primary target volume and neighboring critical structures. The dose to the spinal cord was 4600 cGy; two-thirds of the right kidney received less than 3000 cGy, and the left kidney received less than 1500 cGy (Table 27.4).

Other than mild fatigue and intermittent nausea and vomiting, the patient tolerated treatment well. He was sent to a medical oncologist to discuss an adjuvant chemotherapy program. The patient received four cycles of adjuvant chemotherapy with doxorubicin and cisplatin over a 4-month period. Other than minimal weight loss, the patient tolerated this treatment well.

Approximately 18 months have passed since the completion of the postoperative external beam radiation therapy. Since that time, the patient has undergone complete radiographic follow-up with a CT scan of the chest, abdomen, and pelvis and a PET scan. There is no evidence of recurrence.

ROLE OF THE RADIATION THERAPIST

Education of the patient and family members during radiation therapy is aimed at helping the patient understand the importance and goals of treatment and the potential side effects. Symptoms experienced during treatment are often difficult to endure and affect the patient's ability to consent to the completion of treatment. However, with the support of family and healthcare professionals and with information for controlling

TABLE 27.4 Tissues Tolerances for Organs at Risk

Organ	TD 5/5 (cGy) FOR CONVENTIONAL FRACTIONATION		
	Whole	2/3	1/3
Thyroid			
Larynx (edema)	4500	4500	—
Esophagus (stricture, perforation)	5500	5800	6000
Pituitary			
Optic chiasm	5000	—	—
Parotid gland	3200[a]	3200[a]	—
Lens of eye	1000	—	—
Optic nerve	5000	—	—
Adrenal			
Kidney	2300[b]	3000	5000
Liver	3000	3500	5000
Spinal cord	4700 (20 cm)	5000 (10 cm)	5000 (5 cm)

[a]Qualitative Analysis of Normal Tissue Effects in the Clinic (QUANTEC) data indicate that the mean dose after conventional fractionation should not exceed 2000 cGy when sparing one parotid gland, and the mean dose should not exceed 2500 cGy when both parotid glands are spared when included in three-dimensional-conformal radiation therapy (3D-CRT) volume.
[b]Qualitative Analysis of Normal Tissue Effects in the Clinic (QUANTEC) data indicate that the mean dose after conventional fractionation should not exceed 1500 cGy to 1800 cGy when bilateral whole kidney is included in 3D-CRT volume.
Modified from Emami B, Brown LJ, Coia L, et al. Tolerance of normal tissue to therapeutic irradiation. *Int J Radiat Oncol Biol Phys.* 1991;21:109–122, and Marks LB, Yorke ED, Jackson A, et al. The use of normal tissue complication probability (NTCP) models in the clinic. *Int J Radiat Oncol Biol Phys.* 2010;76(3):S1–S19.

side effects, the patient can successfully complete a course of therapy. Open communication between the patient and supporting staff members (nursing, dietary, and social services) is of utmost importance in abating and controlling symptoms during and after a course of treatment.

The following are some potential side effects patients may experience while receiving radiation to glands of the endocrine system:

1. Fatigue is a common side effect of most patients receiving radiation therapy. Daily treatments and the biologic effects of the disease and radiation can cause fatigue. Poor nutrition, depression, and family and financial worries are all contributing factors. Scheduling appointments around rest or mealtimes can aid in combating fatigue. The therapist should discuss the daily activity level with the patient to assess potential problems, and family members should be encouraged to assist in daily activities (e.g., meal preparation) to allow for rest time.

2. Appointments with the social services department can reduce financial worries and aid in emotional support. The therapist should encourage patients and family members to discuss their concerns and fears with each other.

3. Skin reactions can be painful and irritating to the patient. The therapist should advise the patient to avoid harsh creams, soaps, and lotions in the irradiated area. Hot water and sun exposure to the treated area should also be avoided. After a reaction starts, the therapist should communicate with the physician, and depending on the degree of desquamation (dry or moist), a treatment break may be warranted.

4. For patients who may have a tracheostomy, a plastic cannula should replace a metal one to allow it to stay in place during treatments. This aids in preventing the enhancement of a skin reaction at the tracheostomy site for the treatment of thyroid tumors.

5. Loose-fitting clothes, especially cotton, should be worn to prevent rubbing and further irritation.

6. Hair loss (alopecia) can occur in the irradiated field for pituitary adenomas as a result of the high mitotic activity of hair follicles. High-dose radiation may cause alopecia or delayed hair regrowth. The therapist should try to give the patient and family an appraisal for the potential and degree of hair loss and a time frame for its approximate occurrence. The therapist should inform patients to use mild shampoo and avoid excessive hair washing, which only dries and irritates the skin. In addition, the therapist should inform the patient and family that the new hair may have a different quality, texture, and color. If hair loss becomes significant, the use of a wig or a head wrap may be indicated. Therapists should inform patients of national programs (e.g., "Look Good... Feel Better" available at http://lookgoodfeelbetter.org/) that promote positive feelings and attitudes.

7. Dysphagia is often present in patients with thyroid cancers before the start of treatment as a result of the disease process. Early in the treatment, the patient may describe the feeling of "a lump in the throat." The therapist should encourage the patient to eat frequent meals that consist of high-protein and caloric foods. Eggnog, frappes, Ensure (Abbott Laboratories, Abbott Park, IL), and shakes supply high-protein and caloric intake and are soothing and easy to swallow.

8. The patient with thyroid cancer should be advised to avoid commercial mouthwash, hot food and drinks, smoking, spicy food, and alcoholic beverages. If available, a dietary consultation should be scheduled within 1 week of the start of treatment.

Visual changes that result from pituitary disease can also cause a patient to be depressed. Simple pleasures such as reading or watching television can no longer be enjoyed. Unfortunately, little can be done to alter these effects caused by damage to the optic nerve; even treatment may not reverse the damage already inflicted on the nerve. However, audiotapes of books are available and may offer some enjoyment to the patient. The therapist can also encourage a family member to take time out to read the daily paper or a novel to the patient. The therapist should try to encourage family participation so that the patient does not feel left out.

Endocrine neoplasms can cause an array of previously discussed hormonal upsets, which can result in changes in emotions, appearance, and abilities. An altered body image can lower a patient's self-esteem. Patients with hair loss, hormonal syndromes, or acromegalic features may have misconceived notions of the way others perceive them. The therapist should be alert to these changes, allowing patients to express their feelings, promoting support from family members, and offering support to the family. Illness not only affects the patient but also the family because aggression and anger is often directed toward the family members.

The therapist should offer outside counseling (e.g., online communities and support via the American Cancer Society) that is aimed at supporting families and patients through difficult times. Seeing other patients in similar circumstances lets patients know that they are not alone, that their feelings are normal, and that help is available.

Before the initiation of radiation therapy, the therapist should discuss the treatment process with the patient and family. The therapist should inform them that holding still is of the utmost importance for the delivery of proper treatment. In addition, the therapist should assure them that, although alone in the room, the patient is being carefully monitored. Before treatment, the therapist should take them into the room, explain positioning procedures, show them the monitors and intercom, and clearly explain that the machine will stop and someone will come in if help is needed. The therapist must give them a sense of control. The more patients understand, the less anxiety they feel, which makes the overall treatment process more tolerable.

Before educating patients and their families, therapists should educate themselves. Therapists should read the consultation notes, know the basics, and be prepared to address any specific questions or concerns a patient may wish to discuss. The patient must feel comfortable with and confident in the therapist, allowing for open communication and trust throughout the duration of the treatment. A lack of trust can inhibit communication and cause undue stress for the patient and family.

Therapists must present themselves in a professional manner. After all, patients are entrusting themselves to the therapist, with little understanding and with much apprehension for what is before them.

SUMMARY

- Endocrine tumors have a wide variety of epidemiologic factors. Thyroid cancers are the most common and account for approximately 96% of all new endocrine cases.[3]
- Thyroid cancer has several recognized etiologic factors, including:
  - External radiation to the thyroid gland, particularly before puberty. Historically, radiation treatment for benign conditions included that for acne, tonsillitis, hemangiomas, and thymic enlargement.
  - Thyroid cancer is more prevalent among inhabitants of Nagasaki and Hiroshima who were present after the explosion of the atomic bombs in 1945.
  - Fallout from a nuclear test in the Marshall Islands in the 1950s led to studies that showed a higher incidence in thyroid changes, including cancer, in those exposed to the radioactive fallout.
  - The Chernobyl incident of 1986 produced conflicting studies on the increase of thyroid cancer, probably because of the extremely short interval between radiation exposure and tumor occurrence.
  - Malignant thyroid neoplasms are divided into four categories: (1) papillary, (2) follicular, (3) medullary, and (4) anaplastic.
- Detection and diagnosis for endocrine tumors relies heavily on laboratory test results, physical examination, diagnostic imaging studies, and biopsy results. Radionuclide thyroid imaging can be used to evaluate the function and anatomic location of a palpable thyroid nodule through the localization of hot or cold spots in the gland.
- Pituitary adenomas can be classified as functioning or nonfunctioning as related to the hormones they produce. Hormone production often serves as a diagnostic and treatment-response marker. Pituitary adenomas categorized as functioning secrete the following hormones: PRL, GH, ACTH, and TSH.

- The rationale for treatment, regarding treatment choice, histologic subtype, and stage of the disease, varies for thyroid, pituitary, and adrenal gland tumors. Thyroid tumors are generally treated with surgery and radioactive I-131. Treatment for pituitary adenomas is controversial and may include surgery and external beam treatment, including IMRT, SRS, and proton therapy. Surgery is the treatment of choice for adrenal gland tumors.
- Radiation reactions for the treatment of tumors of the endocrine system vary.
  - Fatigue is a common side effect of most patients receiving radiation therapy.
  - Skin reactions can be painful and irritating to the patient. The therapist should advise the patient to avoid harsh creams, soaps, and lotions in the irradiated area. Hot water and sun exposure to the treated area should also be avoided.
  - Hair loss (alopecia) can occur in the irradiated field as a result of the radiosensitivity of hair follicles.
  - Dysphagia (difficulty swallowing) is often present in patients with thyroid cancers before the start of treatment as a result of the disease process.
- Organs at risk for external beam radiation therapy include the larynx and esophagus for thyroid cancers; the optic chiasm, parotid glands, lens of the eye, and optic nerve for pituitary adenomas; and the kidney, liver, and spinal cord for adrenal tumors. Dose to these critical structures depends on the type of external beam treatment plan and the total dose given (see Table 27.4).

REVIEW QUESTIONS

The answers to the Review Questions can be found by logging on to our website at: http://evolve.elsevier.com/Washington/principles

1. Which of the following is the most common endocrine system tumor?
   a. Thyroid.
   b. Pituitary.
   c. Adrenal cortex.
   d. Adrenal medulla.
2. Exposure to radiation is a well-documented etiologic factor for _____ tumors.
   a. Thyroid.
   b. Pituitary.
   c. Adrenal cortex.
   d. Adrenal medulla.

3. Thyroid cancer is generally treated with:
   a. Surgery alone.
   b. Surgery and I-131.
   c. I-131 alone.
   d. I-131 and chemotherapy.
4. Tumor control is seldom accomplished for _____ thyroid tumors.
   a. Papillary.
   b. Follicular.
   c. Medullary.
   d. Anaplastic.
5. The pituitary gland is close to critical structures of the central nervous system, such as the _____ (superiorly).
   a. Sella turcica.
   b. Optic chiasm.
   c. Occipital lobe of the brain.
   d. Parotid gland.

6. Pituitary adenomas characterized as functioning secrete which of the following hormones?
   a. T3.
   b. T4.
   c. TSH.
   d. Epinephrine.

7. Proton therapy is sometimes used in the treatment of _____ tumors.
   a. Thyroid.
   b. Pituitary.
   c. Adrenal cortex.
   d. Adrenal medulla.

8. _____ is often a presenting symptom for patients with advanced adrenal cortex tumors.
   a. Headache.
   b. Weight loss.
   c. Fatigue.
   d. Pain.

9. Organs at risk in the treatment of the adrenal gland with external beam radiation therapy include the:
   a. Esophagus.
   b. Lung.
   c. Spinal cord.
   d. Parotid.

10. The radiation therapist should be alert to _____ when treating patients with endocrine tumors.
    a. Fatigue.
    b. Hormonal upsets.
    c. Memory loss.
    d. Both A and B.

■ QUESTIONS TO PONDER

1. Describe symptoms a patient with a pituitary adenoma might have that may prompt him or her to seek medical attention.
2. Discuss the workup for a patient suspected of having an adrenal gland tumor.
3. Discuss the role of I-131 in the treatment of thyroid cancer. Why is this pharmaceutical useful in this disease?
4. Discuss clinical disorders associated with thyroid, pituitary, and adrenal gland tumors.
5. Discuss organs at risk and healthy tissue tolerances in the treatment of thyroid, pituitary, and adrenal gland tumors.
6. Discuss the ways you, as a radiation therapist, can help patients and their families deal with the physical and emotional changes brought on by an endocrine tumor.

REFERENCES

1. Endocrine system. In: Patton KT, Thibodeau GA, eds. *The Human Body in Health & Disease*. 7th ed. St. Louis, MO: Elsevier; 2018.
2. Brashers VL, Jones RE, Huether SE. Mechanisms of hormonal regulation. In: McCance KL, Huether SE, eds. *Pathophysiology: The Biologic Basis for Disease in Adults and Children*. 7th ed. St. Louis, MO: Elsevier; 2014.
3. Brito JP, Hay ID, Foote RL. Thyroid cancer. In: Gunderson LL, Tepper JE, eds. *Clinical Radiation Oncology*. 4th ed. Philadelphia, PA: Elsevier; 2016.
4. Sinnott B, et al. Exposing the thyroid to radiation: a review of its current extent, risks, and implications. *Endocr Rev*. 2010;31(5):756–773.
5. Furukawa K, et al. Long-term trend of thyroid cancer risk among Japanese atomic-bomb survivors: 60 years after exposure. *Int J Cancer*. 2013;132(5):1222–1226.
6. Takahashi T, et al. The relationship of thyroid cancer with radiation exposure from nuclear weapon testing in the Marshall Islands. *J Epidemiol*. 2003;13(2):99–107.
7. Mettler FA, et al. Thyroid nodules in the population living around Chernobyl. *J Am Med Assoc*. 1992;268(5):616–619.
8. Cardis E, Hatch M. The Chernobyl accident—an epidemiological perspective. *Clin Oncol*. 2011;23(4):251–260.
9. Furmanchuck A, et al. Pathomorphological findings in thyroid cancers of children from the republic of Belarus: a study of 86 cases occurring between 1986 ('post-Chernobyl') and 1991. *Histopathology*. 1992;21(5):401–408.
10. Nikiforov YE. Radiation-induced thyroid cancer: what we have learned from Chernobyl. *Endocr Pathol*. 2006;17(4):307–318.
11. Williams ED. Chernobyl and thyroid cancer. *J Surg Oncol*. 2006;94(8):670–677.
12. Dagan R, Amdur RJ. Thyroid cancer. In: Halperin EC, Wazer DE, Perez CA. 6th ed. *Perez and Brady's Principles and Practice of Radiation Oncology*. 6th ed. Philadelphia, PA: Lippincott Williams & Wilkins; 2013.
13. Endocrine glands. In: Patton KT, Thibodeau GA, eds. *Anatomy and Physiology*. 9th ed. St. Louis, MO: Elsevier; 2016.
14. Coleman SC, et al. Long-standing lateral neck mass as the initial manifestation of well-differentiated thyroid carcinoma. *The Laryngoscope*. 2000;110(2):204–209.
15. Hejna M, et al. Medullary thyroid carcinoma. *Oncol Res Treat*. 1998;21(4):334–337.
16. Keutgen XM, et al. Management of anaplastic thyroid cancer. *Gland Surg*. 2015;4(1):44–51.
17. Weiss TE, Grigsby PW. Thyroid. In: Halperin EC, et al., ed. *Perez and Brady's Principles and Practice of Radiation Oncology*. 5th ed. Philadelphia, PA: Lippincott Williams & Wilkins; 2008.
18. Hoang J. Thyroid nodules and evaluation of thyroid cancer risk. *Australas J Ultrasound Med*. 2010;13(4):33–36.
19. Freitas JE, et al. Radionuclide diagnosis and therapy of thyroid cancer: current status report. *Semin Nucl Med*. 1985;15(2):106–131.
20. Hoang JK, et al. Imaging of thyroid carcinoma with CT and MRI: approaches to common scenarios. *Cancer Image*. 2013;13(1):128–139.
21. Madhuchhanda R, et al. Current understanding and management of medullary thyroid cancer. *The Oncologist*. 2013;18(10):1093–1100.
22. Wang LY, Ganly I. Nodal metastases in thyroid cancer: prognostic implications and management. *Future Oncol*. 2016;12(7):981–994.
23. Varia MA. Pituitary tumors. In: Gunderson LL, Tepper JE, eds. *Clinical Radiation Oncology*. 1st ed. Philadelphia, PA: Churchill Livingstone; 2000.
24. Roberge D, et al. Pituitary. In: Halperin EC, et al., ed. *Perez and Brady's Principles and Practice of Radiation Oncology.*. 5th ed. Philadelphia, PA: Lippincott Williams & Wilkins; 2008.
25. Gibbs IC, et al. Pituitary tumors. In: Hoppe R, Phillips, TL, Roach M. Leibel and Phillips Textbook of Radiation Oncology-E-Book: Expert Consult-Online and Print. 3rd ed. Philadelphia, PA: Elsevier Health Sciences; 2010.
26. Levy MJ, et al. The clinical characteristics of headache in patients with pituitary tumours. *Brain*. 2005;128(8):1921–1930.
27. Suh JH, et al. Pituitary tumors and craniopharyngiomas. In: Gunderson LL, Tepper JE, eds. *Clinical Radiation Oncology*. 4th ed. Elsevier; 2016.
28. Kovacs K, et al. Classification of pituitary adenomas. *J Neuro Oncol*. 2001;54(2):121–127.
29. Halvorsen H, et al. Surgical complications after transsphenoidal microscopic and endoscopic surgery for pituitary adenoma: a consecutive series of 506 procedures. *Acta Neurochir*. 2013;156(3):441–449.
30. Yaeger TE. Pituitary gland cancer. In: Halperin EC, et al., ed. *Perez and Brady's Principles and Practice of Radiation Oncology*. 6th ed. Lippincott Williams & Wilkins; 2013.

31. Hansen EK, Roach III M. eds. Pituitary tumors. In: *Handbook of Evidence-Based Radiation Oncology*. 3rd ed. Cham, Switzerland: Springer; 2018.

32. Troicki FT, Coen JJ. Adrenal cancer. In: Halperin EC, et al., ed. *Perez and Brady's Principles and Practice of Radiation Oncology*. 6th ed. Philadelphia, PA: Lippincott Williams & Wilkins; 2013.

33. Altun E, et al. Imaging in oncology. In: Gunderson LL, Tepper JE, eds. *Clinical Radiation Oncology*. 4th ed. Philadelphia, PA: Elsevier; 2016.

34. Cohn K, et al. Adrenocortical carcinoma. *Surgery*. 1986;100(6):1170–1177.

35. Karakousis CP, et al. Adrenocarcinomas: histologic grading and survival. *J Surg Oncol*. 1985;29(2):105–111.

Respiratory System Tumors

Jessica A. Church

OBJECTIVES

- Identify the relationship between the natural history of lung cancer and prognosis.
- Describe the incidence and mortality rates associated with lung cancer.
- List the risk factors for developing lung cancer.
- Identify the anatomic and radiographic features of the lower respiratory tract, including the carina, mediastinum, and hilum.
- Describe the signs and symptoms of lung cancer.
- Explain how lung cancer is detected and diagnosed.

- Differentiate nonsmall cell lung cancer (NSCLC) from small cell lung cancer (SCLC).
- Examine the staging of lung cancer.
- Trace the patterns of spread for lung cancer, including lymphatic spread.
- Describe the roles of surgery, radiation therapy, and chemotherapy in the treatment of lung cancer.
- Define the role of the radiation therapist in the care of patients with lung cancer.

OUTLINE

KEY TERMS

Atelectasis
Carina
Dyspnea
Eastern Cooperative Oncology Group (ECOG) performance status
Hemoptysis
Horner syndrome
Hypertrophic osteoarthropathy
Internal tumor volume (ITV)

Karnofsky Performance Status (KPS)
Orthopnea
Pancoast tumor
Paraneoplastic syndrome
Pneumonitis
Prophylactic cranial irradiation (PCI)
Superior vena cava (SVC) syndrome

CANCER OF THE RESPIRATORY SYSTEM

The respiratory system is divided into the upper respiratory tract and the lower respiratory tract. The upper respiratory tract includes the nose, nasopharynx, oropharynx, laryngopharynx (hypopharynx), and larynx, and the lower respiratory tract includes the trachea, bronchial tree, and lungs. This chapter focuses on cancer of the lungs. The main types of lung cancer, nonsmall cell lung cancer (NSCLC) and small cell lung cancer (SCLC), are discussed. Mesothelioma, cancer of the pleura, which is the lining of the thoracic cavity and lungs, is also mentioned. Cancer of the upper respiratory tract is discussed in Chapter 29.

NATURAL HISTORY

The usual course of the development of lung cancer, especially without treatment, is influenced by several factors. The most significant factors, indicative of an individual's prognosis, are performance status, stage, and weight loss (defined as greater than 10% of an individual's body weight over 6 months' time).[1]

Performance status is indicated by an individual's ability to perform daily tasks, including self-care. It is measured using one of two scales, the Karnofsky Performance Status (KPS) or the Eastern Cooperative Oncology Group (ECOG) performance status. KPS scores range from 0 to 100, with an increasing score meaning an

TABLE 28.1	Karnofsky Performance Status
Score	Condition
100	Normal; no complaints; no evidence of disease
90	Able to carry on normal activity; minor signs or symptoms of disease
80	Normal activity with effort; some signs or symptoms of disease
70	Cares for self; unable to carry on normal activity or to do active work
60	Requires occasional assistance, but is able to care for most of their personal needs
50	Requires considerable assistance and frequent medical care
40	Disabled; requires special care and assistance
30	Severely disabled; hospital admission is indicated although death not imminent
20	Very sick; hospital admission necessary; active supportive treatment necessary
10	Moribund; fatal processes progressing rapidly
0	Dead

TABLE 28.2	Eastern Cooperative Oncology Group Performance Status
Score	Condition
0	Fully active, able to carry on all predisease performance without restriction
1	Restricted in physically strenuous activity but ambulatory and able to carry out work of a light or sedentary nature; e.g., light housework, office work
2	Ambulatory and capable of all self-care but unable to carry out any work activities; up and about more than 50% of waking hours
3	Capable of only limited self-care; confined to bed or chair more than 50% of waking hours
4	Completely disabled; cannot carry on any self-care; totally confined to bed or chair
5	Dead

From Oken MM, Creech RH, Tormey DC, et al. Toxicity and response criteria of the Eastern Cooperative Oncology Group. *Am J Clin Oncol.* 1982;5:649–655.

individual is able to carry out daily tasks (Table 28.1).[2] Conversely, ECOG performance status scores range from 0 to 5, with a decreasing score indicating an individual is highly functioning (Table 28.2).[3] An individual with a high KPS score or a low ECOG performance status score is predicted to have a better prognosis than a patient with a low KPS score or a high ECOG performance status score. Patients with early-stage disease and little weight loss are also predicted to have a more favorable outcome.

Together, the prognostic factors are used in determining a patient's course of treatment, if a patient is eligible for or would benefit from a clinical trial, and in predicting a patient's response to treatment.

Prognosis. Overall, the 5-year relative survival rate for patients with lung cancer is 16%. The prognosis is better for patients with early-stage cancers. The 5-year survival rates increase from 2% for patients with distant metastasis to 16% for patients with regional spread to 49% for patients with localized disease.[4] The outlook for patients with NSCLC is also better, as SCLC is prone to metastasize.

EPIDEMIOLOGY

Worldwide, lung cancer is the most common form of cancer. In the United States, it is the second most common form of cancer in both men and women. It accounts for about 13% of all new cancer cases each year; it is estimated that about 234,000 new cases are diagnosed each year.[5] More than 430,000 individuals living in the United States have been diagnosed with lung cancer at some point in their lives.[5]

The risk of developing lung cancer increases with age. Most of the individuals diagnosed with lung cancer are over the age of 65 years. The risk of developing lung cancer is also higher in women than in men (1:17 to 1:15, respectively). Blacks have a higher risk of developing lung cancer than whites.[5] For smokers, the risk increases.

Overall, the incidence of lung cancer is declining. In the 1990s, the incidence decreased dramatically in men but rose by a small percentage in women. Since 2000, the incidence in women has slowly decreased.[6] The difference in the decline can be attributed to trends in cigarette smoking between the genders, as the peak for women occurred 20 years later than the peak for men.[7]

Still, lung cancer is the leading cause of cancer death in the United States among men and women. It is estimated that about 154,000 deaths are attributed to lung cancer annually.[8]

ETIOLOGY

The leading risk factor for lung cancer, other than age, is smoking. Approximately 80% of lung cancers can be attributed to cigarette smoking.[2] A causal relationship is also suggested for secondhand smoking.[9]

The risk for lung cancer increases with the number of cigarettes smoked per day and the duration of smoking. Therefore, antismoking campaigns are aimed at teenagers and young adults. It is important to remember, however, that cigarette smokers can decrease their risk of developing lung cancer by quitting smoking at any age.[9]

Current smoking rates have declined from 21% in 2005 to 14% in 2017.[10] This trend corresponds with the decline in lung cancer incidence. Individuals with a history of lung cancer are at higher risk for developing a second lung cancer.[11] The risk increases for those who continue to smoke.

There is no difference in risk for individuals who smoke filtered cigarettes, but the reduced tar and nicotine in filtered cigarettes may be the cause of the recent shift in the predominant cell type from squamous cell carcinoma to adenocarcinoma.[12] The effects of electronic cigarettes are under investigation.

Cigar smoking and pipe smoking are risk factors for lung cancer; however, these activities are more associated with cancers of the upper aerodigestive tract than the lung.[13]

Additional risk factors for lung cancer include environmental and occupational exposures such as air pollution, radon, and asbestos. The association with air pollution is difficult to prove; however, studies have shown that long-term exposure to fumes from factories and automobiles may increase an individual's risk for lung cancer, especially in urban areas.[9] Radon is a naturally occurring radioactive gas, found in homes from soil and building materials, and a well-known risk factor. It is the second leading cause of lung cancer and the leading cause among nonsmokers.[5] Exposure to asbestos is linked to mesothelioma. Other environmental and occupational exposures include aluminum, arsenic, beryllium, cadmium, chromium, nickel, and soot.[9] Each of these risk factors has a synergistic effect with smoking.

ANATOMY AND PHYSIOLOGY

Structures. The respiratory system is divided into the upper respiratory tract and the lower respiratory tract. The lower respiratory tract includes the trachea, bronchial tree, and lungs. The anatomy of the upper respiratory tract is discussed in Chapter 29.

The trachea is a cartilaginous tube that provides a pathway for air from the laryngopharynx to the lungs. It extends from the inferior border of the larynx to the level of T5, where it bifurcates, or divides, into the primary bronchi. The bifurcation of the trachea is called the carina. The carina serves as an important radiographic landmark in radiation therapy (Fig. 28.1).

The primary bronchi, also called the right and left mainstem bronchi, branch into smaller airways, forming the bronchial tree. The primary bronchi branch into the secondary bronchi followed by the tertiary bronchi (or segmental bronchi). The tertiary bronchi branch into the bronchioles and further divide into tiny air sacs called alveoli.

The bronchi enter the lung at the hilum. This is also the area where the blood, lymphatics, and nerves enter and exit each lung. The mediastinum is the region between the lungs containing the trachea, esophagus, thymus gland, lymph nodes, heart, and great vessels. The hilum and mediastinum provide pathways for tumor cells to gain access to the lymphatic and circulatory systems.

The lungs are found within the thoracic cavity, or thorax. The thorax consists of the sternum, ribs, and thoracic vertebrae and provides protection for the lungs. The thoracic cavity is lined by the parietal pleura, and the visceral pleura is attached to the outer surface of each lung. The pleural cavity contains a small amount of fluid that lubricates the lungs. The visceral pleura extends into the fissures separating the lobes of each lung. The right lung has three lobes: upper, middle, and lower, and the left lung has two lobes: upper and lower. The apex, or top, of the lung is located a few centimeters above the clavicle, and the base, or bottom, of the lung is situated on the diaphragm.[22] When an individual inhales, the diaphragm moves in the inferior direction, allowing more air into the lungs; when an individual exhales, the diaphragm moves in the superior direction, pushing air out.

Function. The respiratory system transports oxygen from the air into the blood and removes carbon dioxide from the blood. Air is inhaled through the nose or mouth and travels through the pharynx and trachea to the bronchial tree. The bronchi continue to branch into the tiny air sacs at the distal end of the bronchioles called alveoli. Gas exchange occurs within the alveoli. The alveoli exchange the oxygen from the inhaled air and remove the carbon dioxide from the blood. The carbon dioxide is expelled during exhalation.

Blood supply and lymphatics. The location of the lungs in relation to the circulatory and lymphatic systems is important, as all of the systems are linked. Blood vessels and lymphatics are found throughout the respiratory system. Many of the blood vessels, lymphatics, and airways have similar names.

Blood supply to the lungs comes from the pulmonary and bronchial arteries, which branch from the thoracic aorta. The lymphatics follow the vasculature to the hilum and then to the mediastinum. The lymphatics can be divided into the following groups: intrapulmonary nodes, bronchopulmonary (hilar) nodes, mediastinal nodes, and supraclavicular (or scalene) nodes. The mediastinal nodes are divided into two groups: (1) superior, located above the carina, including the upper paratracheal, pretracheal, retrotracheal, and lower paratracheal (azygos) nodes, and a group of nodes located in the aortic window; and (2) inferior, located below the carina, including the subcarinal, paraesophageal, and pulmonary ligament nodes (Fig. 28.1).

Involvement of the lymphatics tends to follow the branches of the bronchial tree. The intrapulmonary nodes are involved first, followed by spread to the bronchopulmonary (hilar) nodes, then to the mediastinal nodes, and ultimately, the supraclavicular nodes. Overall, ipsilateral hilar nodes are involved in 50% of patients, mediastinal nodes in 40% to 50% of patients, and supraclavicular nodes in 5% to 30% of patients.[14] The lymphatic drainage joins the blood flow at the subclavian vein, where it gains access to the circulatory system as the flow enters from the thoracic duct.

CLINICAL PRESENTATION

Occasionally, an individual presents with an asymptomatic tumor that is incidentally detected on a chest radiograph. More often, an individual presents with a new or worsening sign or symptom. The signs and symptoms of lung cancer are frequently attributed to respiratory disease or the effects of smoking, so an individual may not present until the cancer is well advanced.

The signs and symptoms of lung cancer can be grouped into four categories: (1) signs and symptoms because of local disease, (2) signs and symptoms because of regional disease, (3) signs and symptoms because of distant metastasis, and (4) nonspecific signs and symptoms, or paraneoplastic syndromes.

The signs and symptoms of lung cancer related to local disease vary depending on the location and size of the cancer. A centrally located tumor may produce persistent cough, hemoptysis (blood in the sputum), and signs and symptoms of airway obstruction or pneumonia (e.g., dyspnea [shortness of breath]). A peripherally located tumor is more likely to be asymptomatic, but cough and chest pain may be apparent.[7] A small tumor may be asymptomatic, whereas the signs and symptoms of a large tumor may be more pronounced.

Regional spread is also associated with a variety of signs and symptoms. Mediastinal involvement may be indicated by chest pain, as well as nerve entrapment, vascular obstruction, or dysphagia (difficulty swallowing) because of esophageal compression. One of the most common symptoms is hoarseness because of entrapment of the recurrent laryngeal nerve, which is a branch of the vagus nerve.

Regional spread may also be indicated by superior vena cava (SVC) syndrome. The SVC is a large vein that carries blood from the head and upper extremities to the right atrium of the heart. A tumor in this area may compress the SVC and cause blood to pool in the vein. SVC syndrome may be indicated by swelling in the face and arms, distended veins in the upper chest, dyspnea, and orthopnea (shortness of breath that occurs when lying flat). SVC syndrome is considered an oncologic emergency and should be treated quickly. Usual treatment includes high-dose corticosteroid therapy as well as radiation therapy. A typical radiation technique includes three to four fractions of 3 to 4 Gy followed by a reduction of the daily dose to 1.8 to 2 Gy. Depending on the patient's condition, the total dose is 45 to 60 Gy.[15]

The location of the tumor can also alter the signs and symptoms of the disease. For example, a cancer that presents in the apex of the lung and often involves the brachial plexus is termed a Pancoast tumor. A Pancoast tumor is a tumor found in the superior sulcus and presents with pain in the shoulder and down the arm, atrophy of the hand muscles, erosion of the ribs and/or the vertebrae, or a specific set of symptoms called Horner syndrome. Horner syndrome is characterized by weakness or drooping of one eyelid, decrease in pupil size of the same eye, and decreased or absent sweating on the same side of the face. It should be noted that not all apical tumors have these signs and symptoms and are therefore not classified as Pancoast tumors.[16]

Signs and symptoms from distant metastasis may also be present and include headaches, visual changes, neurological deficit, or personality change from brain metastases or pain from bone metastases.

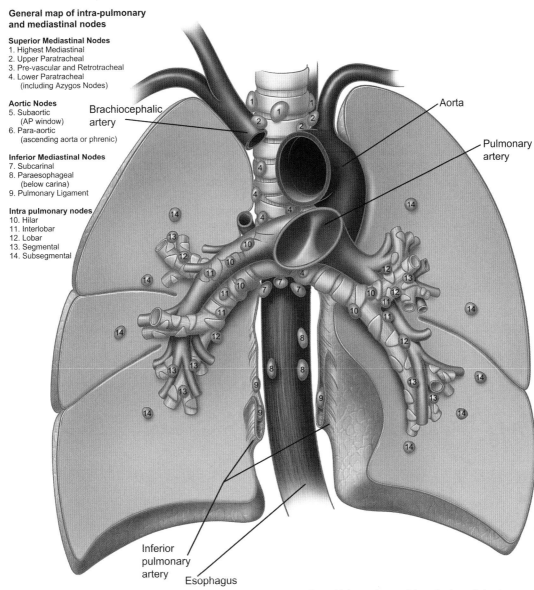

General map of intra-pulmonary and mediastinal nodes

Superior Mediastinal Nodes
1. Highest Mediastinal
2. Upper Paratracheal
3. Pre-vascular and Retrotracheal
4. Lower Paratracheal
   (including Azygos Nodes)

Aortic Nodes
5. Subaortic
   (AP window)
6. Para-aortic
   (ascending aorta or phrenic)

Inferior Mediastinal Nodes
7. Subcarinal
8. Paraesophageal
   (below carina)
9. Pulmonary Ligament

Intra pulmonary nodes
10. Hilar
11. Interlobar
12. Lobar
13. Segmental
14. Subsegmental

Brachiocephalic artery

Aorta

Pulmonary artery

Inferior pulmonary artery

Esophagus

Fig. 28.1 Respiratory system lymphatics. (From Riquet M. Bronchial arteries and lymphatics of the lung. *Thoracic Surgery Clinics* 17(4): 619–638.)

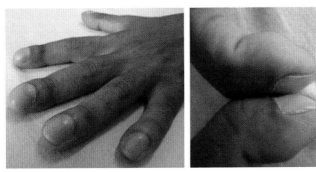

Fig. 28.2 Hypertrophic pulmonary osteoarthropathy (clubbing). (Published with permission of Elsevier. Muñoz Carlos Horacio, Vásquez Gloria María, González Luis Alonso. Hypertrophic osteoarthropathy as a complication of pulmonary tuberculosis. Reumatología Clínica 11(4),255-257. © 2014 Elsevier España, S.L.U. All rights reserved.)

Nonspecific signs and symptoms are common to cancer. Fatigue and weakness occur in approximately one-third of patients and weight loss, with or without anorexia (loss of appetite), in approximately one-half of patients.[7] Somewhat unusual are paraneoplastic syndromes. A paraneoplastic syndrome occurs when hormone-like substances are released into the blood and cause issues in areas away from the site of the cancer. Paraneoplastic syndromes associated with lung cancer include hypercalcemia, hypertrophic osteoarthropathy with clubbing of the fingers (Fig. 28.2), blood clots, and gynecomastia. Associated with some lung cancers are syndrome of inappropriate antidiuretic hormone secretion and adrenocorticotrophic hormone production syndrome. Paraneoplastic syndromes are more often present in patients with SCLC.[7]

DETECTION AND DIAGNOSIS

Screening. Individuals at high risk for lung cancer may benefit from screening. The National Lung Screening Trial compared lung cancer screening with chest radiography to low-dose computed tomography (CT). The study demonstrated a reduction in mortality with low-dose CT.[17] The American Cancer Society recommends low-dose CT for

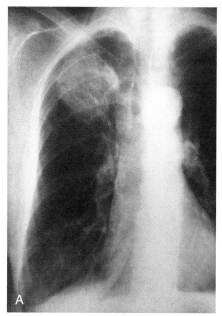

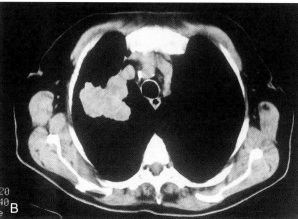

Fig. 28.3 (A) Posteroanterior chest radiograph shows right upper lobe tumor. (B) Computed tomography (CT) scan shows involvement of midline structures. Published with permission of Elsevier. Muñoz Carlos Horacio, Vásquez Gloria María, González Luis Alonso. Hypertrophic osteoarthropathy as a complication of pulmonary tuberculosis. *Reumatología Clínica* 11(4),255-257. © 2014 Elsevier España, S.L.U. All rights reserved.

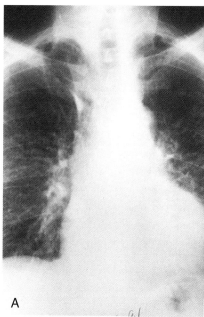

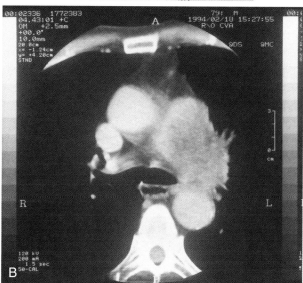

Fig. 28.4 (A) Posteroanterior chest radiograph shows midline disease. (B) Computed tomography scan shows involvement of the mediastinum.

individuals age 55 to 74, in otherwise good health, who are current smokers or have quit smoking in the past 15 years, who have at least a 30-pack year history (number of years smoked × number of packs of cigarettes/day), and who are willing to attend a smoking cessation program.[18] Routine chest radiography has not shown to increase survival.

Patient History and Physical Examination. As part of the initial workup, a physician gathers information on the patient's medical and social past, including information concerning his or her smoking and occupational history.

Imaging Tests. Imaging tests used to detect lung cancer include chest radiography, CT, magnetic resonance imaging (MRI), and positron emission tomography (PET). Chest radiography is preferred, as it is readily available, of lower cost, and of lower radiation dose than other modalities. Chest radiography may reveal lung tumors greater than 5 mm in size, atelectasis (complete or partial collapse of a lung), pneumonitis (inflammation of the lung), bronchitis, abscess, pleural reaction or effusion, rib erosion, or bulky disease in the mediastinum.[7] Figs. 28.3A and 28.4A show radiographs of upper lobe and midline disease, respectively. Much of the natural history of the disease may have occurred by the time the lung cancer is visible.

Chest radiography that reveals a suspicious lesion may lead to further investigation. CT may be used to evaluate the lesion, identify other lesions, examine the involvement of the hilum and/or mediastinum, and involvement of the chest wall and/or pleura.[13] Fig. 28.3B and Fig. 28.4B show CT scans of midline and mediastinal involvement, respectively. Contrast media may be helpful in highlighting variations. The inferior portion of the scan may include the abdomen to rule out adrenal or liver metastasis. CT may also be used to evaluate the brain, as individuals with lung cancer are at high risk for brain metastasis.

MRI may be used to better evaluate the soft tissue anatomy of the superior sulcus in Pancoast tumors and to evaluate brain metastasis.

PET may be used to determine if the lesion is benign or malignant. A PET-positive lesion is metabolically active and more than likely malignant. Additional uses of PET include staging and follow-up to evaluate tumor response to treatment. The combination of PET and CT is more accurate, sensitive, and specific than PET or CT alone. It is particularly useful in differentiating cancer from atelectasis and has proven to change the stage in 30% of cases compared with CT alone.[7]

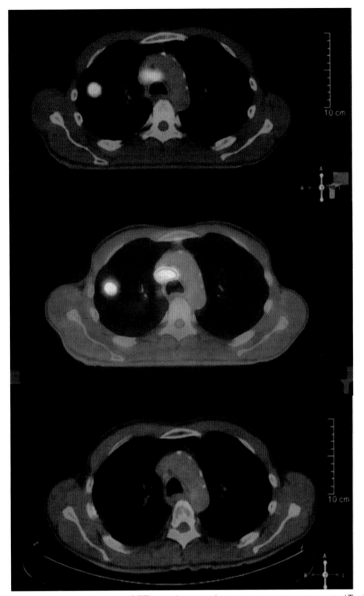

Fig. 28.5 Positron emission tomography (PET) used to monitor response to treatment. (*Top*) Pretreatment PET-computed tomography (CT) scan demonstrating irregular right upper lobe mass and right paratracheal node. Subsequent biopsy confirmed adenocarcinoma of lung origin. (*Middle*) Radiation therapy treatment planning PET-CT blended between the PET images and the CT images. (*Bottom*) Posttreatment PET/CT scan obtained 3 months after the completion of concurrent chemoradiation with cisplatin, etoposide, and proton therapy. (From Simone CB, Houshmand S, Kalbasi A, et al. PET-based thoracic radiation oncology. *PET Clinics* 2016;11(3):319–332.)

Fig. 28.5 shows a PET-CT scan with a positive right upper lobe mass and paratracheal node.

Laboratory Tests. An individual may have compromised lung function from existing respiratory disease, so pulmonary function tests are beneficial in determining whether a patient can tolerate treatment. Spirometry is a common test used to measure pulmonary volume and airflow.

Evaluation of the blood is also valuable and should include a complete blood count and serum calcium, alkaline phosphatase, lactic dehydrogenase (LDH), and serum glutamic oxaloacetic transaminase (SGOT) levels. Elevation of serum calcium is indicative of bony disease. Abnormal alkaline phosphatase, LDH, and SGOT values may indicate bony or liver involvement.[13]

Diagnosis. Sputum cytology is a noninvasive method to obtain a diagnosis. Sputum cytology involves obtaining a sample of mucus (expectorant) and examining it under a microscope. The results of sputum cytology are of limited significance because of the difficulty of determining the specific site of disease and the histology of the sample.[13]

A more reliable histologic evaluation may be obtained through bronchoscopy or surgical interventions such as mediastinoscopy. The sample obtained can be examined to determine the histology.

Bronchoscopy provides a means to examine the airway, identify an obstruction, visualize the lesion, and obtain a tissue sample. During the procedure, a flexible bronchoscope is inserted into the airway (trachea and primary bronchi), and an instrument is used to obtain the sample. Endoscopic bronchial ultrasound scan is another way to examine the airway and obtain a tissue sample. A bronchoscope is inserted into the airway, and when the tube is in place, an ultrasound probe at the end of the bronchoscope is used to visualize the area. If a suspicious lesion or lymph nodes are visualized, a sample can be obtained using ultrasound guidance.[13]

If a lesion is too peripheral for bronchoscopy, a CT-guided fine needle aspiration may be performed.[13] During this procedure, a thin, hollow needle is inserted percutaneously to obtain a tissue sample. A core biopsy uses a larger needle to remove a larger sample. Thoracentesis, inserting a needle to drain the fluid, may be used if an individual has a pleural effusion. A pleural biopsy may be necessary to diagnose cancers such as mesothelioma.

Mediastinoscopy is often used to evaluate the superior mediastinum. In this procedure, an incision is made at the top of the sternum, and a mediastinoscope is inserted to visualize and obtain tissue samples from the area. Similarly, video-assisted thoracoscopy is a procedure during which an incision is made between the ribs, and a thoroscope is inserted into the chest for viewing and tissue removal.

PATHOLOGY

Lung cancer arises from the epithelium of the respiratory tract. The histologic type of lung cancer corresponds with the site of origin.

The World Health Organization recognizes 12 different types of lung cancer as well as many subtypes. For ease in clinical practice, the types are classified into two main types, NSCLC and SCLC, based on the subtypes' clinical behavior. Approximately 80-85% of lung cancers are NSCLC, and 10% are SCLC.[5]

Within NSCLC, there are several subtypes, including adenocarcinoma, squamous cell carcinoma, and large cell carcinoma. The most common is adenocarcinoma. Adenocarcinoma arises from cells that secrete mucus and is usually found in the periphery of the lung. It is commonly found in smokers, but it is the most common type in nonsmokers. It is also more common in women than in men and is more likely to occur in younger individuals. It grows slower than other subtypes. Squamous cell carcinoma arises from cells that line the airway and is usually found in the central parts of the lung near the bronchi. It is usually found in smokers and is more common in men than in women. Large cell carcinoma is the least common subtype and can appear in any part of the lung but may appear in the periphery. It tends to grow quickly and has a high tendency to metastasize, especially to the brain.[5,13]

SCLC, also called "oat cell," tends to occur more centrally and behave similarly to large cell carcinoma. It is prone to metastasize early and have a poorer prognosis.[19]

Mesothelioma. Mesothelioma is a separate and distinct type of lung cancer which is caused by asbestos exposure. Mesothelioma is rare, accounting for 2,000 to 3,000 cases per year in the United States.[20] It arises from the mesothelial cells that line the pleural cavity and can affect the visceral or parietal pleura. An individual with mesothelioma may present with pleural thickening, dyspnea, and chest pain as a result of pleural fluid and invasion of the chest wall. It is detected using both chest radiography and CT, and diagnosed using thoracentesis with examination of the pleural fluid.[21] Most tumors are aggressive, and treatment options include surgery, radiation therapy, and chemotherapy. Surgical options include pleurectomy, the complete removal of the pleura and gross tumor, or extrapleural pneumonectomy, resection of the pleura, ipsilateral lung, mediastinal lymph nodes, ipsilateral diaphragm, and in some cases, the pericardium. Adjuvant radiation therapy is controversial because of lung toxicity. Platinum-based and pemetrexed chemotherapy may be offered. The prognosis is poor, with the 5-year survival rate for stage IA cancers at 16% and stage IV cancers at less than 1%.[20]

STAGING

Tumor staging is important in determining a patient's treatment options and estimating his or her prognosis. In most cases, staging is based on four factors: (1) location of the primary tumor, (2) tumor size, (3) lymph node involvement, and (4) presence or absence of distant metastasis.

The American Joint Committee on Cancer (AJCC) TNM system is most commonly used for lung cancer. The system describes the size and extent of the tumor (T), the spread to lymph nodes (N), and the spread to distant sites (M), (For more information on staging lung cancer, see: https://www.jtcvs.org/article/S0022-5223(17)32136-0/pdf.)

To describe SCLC, physicians also use a two-stage system, limited and extensive stage. Limited stage means the cancer is only on one side of the chest and can be treated with a single radiation portal. With modern radiation therapy techniques, limited stage is considered as stage I to III disease that can be treated with definitive radiation therapy.[11] Approximately one-third of patients have limited-stage cancer.[5,11] Extensive stage means the cancer has spread widely throughout the lung or to other parts of the body.

PATTERNS OF SPREAD

Lung cancer spreads locally by direct extension, regionally by the lymphatics, and distantly through hematogenous routes. At the time of diagnosis, approximately 15% of lung cancers are localized, 22% have regional spread, and 56% have distant metastases.[7]

Local extension occurs as the tumor cells continue to proliferate and the size of the tumor increases. The mass may compress or invade other structures such as other parts of the lung, the ribs, nerves, heart, esophagus and vertebrae. Tumors may also invade the chest wall, diaphragm, and pleura. A tumor in or near the hilum may grow directly into the hilum of the contralateral lung.[13]

With regional spread, cancer cells break off from the tumor and invade the local lymphatics. The primary lymphatics that drain the lungs are the intrapulmonary (hilar) and mediastinal lymph nodes. The lymph moves from the left lung into the thoracic duct and then into the left subclavian vein. From the right lung, the lymph moves into the right lymphatic duct and then into the right subclavian vein. The pleurae are also rich in lymphatics. They drain into the hilum.

Distant metastases occur as the cancer cells gain access to the blood vessels that supply the tumor. Alternatively, they pass through the vessels that supply the lymphatics. The most common sites of metastatic spread are the brain, bone (most commonly the vertebral bodies), liver, and adrenal glands, as well as the contralateral lung. Metastatic cancer to the lung is also common.[7]

TREATMENT CONSIDERATIONS

Smoking Cessation. Smoking cessation is an important part of the treatment of lung cancer. As stated, smoking is the leading risk factor for lung cancer, and many patients are smokers at the time of diagnosis. Studies suggest that up to 83% of patients continue to smoke after diagnosis.[23] This decreases the effectiveness of treatment and worsens a patient's prognosis. Smoking cessation programs should be tailored to individual patient needs.

Treatment. Despite extensive research and clinical trials, there is controversy over the appropriate treatment of lung cancer. The conventional treatment modalities—surgery, chemotherapy, and radiation therapy—may be used, alone or in combination. Newer modalities such as targeted therapy and immunotherapy may also be appropriate.

Overall, patients with early-stage (I and II) disease should be considered for surgery. Attention must be given to pre- and postoperative pulmonary function to prevent lung complications. Lobectomy, where an entire lobe is removed, is the preferred procedure; however, pneumonectomy, where the entire lung is removed, may be necessary for centrally located lesions.

The most effective chemotherapy agent for lung cancer is cisplatin. Agents such as paclitaxel, docetaxel, gemcitabine, irinotecan, and etoposide can be used in combination with cisplatin for improved response and survival. Radiation may be added for patients with residual disease after surgery or for patients who are not candidates for definitive surgery. Standard of care includes concurrent or sequential chemotherapy and radiation with radiation doses of 45 to 60 Gy using standard fractionation.[13]

Patients with advanced disease should be considered for palliation. Palliative radiation therapy is effective in controlling hemoptysis, as well as brain and bone metastases. Usually, radiation doses of 30 to 40 Gy are sufficient for pain and symptom relief. Short-course palliative radiation therapy, such as 8 Gy in one fraction, has been shown to be effective, but results in more frequent treatment.[24] In the case of solitary brain metastases, patients may benefit from surgery followed by whole brain radiation therapy or stereotactic radiosurgery.

NSCLC. Treatment of NSCLC may include surgery, radiofrequency ablation (RFA), radiation therapy, chemotherapy, targeted therapy, immunotherapy, or palliation.

In the early stages of NSCLC, surgery is the treatment of choice. Surgical options include wedge resection, where a part of a lobe is removed, lobectomy, pneumonectomy, or sleeve resection if the tumor is in the airway. The surgical standard of care for patients with early-stage NSCLC is lobectomy.[24]

RFA may be an option for patients with small tumors in the periphery of the lung. RFA uses radio waves to heat the tumor. A probe is inserted percutaneously, under CT guidance, into the tumor to destroy the tumor.

If a patient with NSCLC cannot undergo surgery, the patient should be considered for definitive radiation therapy. Typically, these patients have localized tumors that could be resected but are medically inoperable because of comorbidities or are patients with larger unresectable tumors. Most of the patients have stage III disease. Definitive radiation therapy includes a dose of 60 to 66 Gy to the gross disease and 50 Gy to the microscopic disease using standard fractionation.

Stereotactic body radiation therapy (SBRT) has been effective in early-stage NSCLC patients. It is most effective in patients with small tumors. The use of SBRT demands a high level of precision and accuracy throughout the treatment process. This is accomplished with the use of modern imaging techniques, CT simulation, precise treatment planning, and modern dose delivery technologies. Effective immobilization is essential. In recent years, SBRT has been considered the treatment of choice for medically inoperable patients with early-stage NSCLC.

Postoperative radiation therapy is indicated in patients with incomplete resections or positive mediastinal metastases. Patients should receive concurrent chemotherapy and radiation therapy. Common drugs used to treat NSCLC are cisplatin, carboplatin, and paclitaxel. Most commonly, a combination of drugs is used.

For advanced NSCLC, targeted therapy such as bevacizumab (Avastin) may be added. Drugs that target tumor blood vessel growth, epidermal growth factor receptor changes, *ALK* gene changes, or *BRAF* gene changes, may also be used. Immunotherapy is gaining popularity in stimulating the patient's immune system (i.e., antibodies) to destroy the cancer cells.

SCLC. Treatment of SCLC may include radiation therapy, chemotherapy, immunotherapy, or palliation. Most patients present with advanced disease, so surgery is not a common option.

For limited-stage SCLC, radiation therapy and concurrent chemotherapy should be considered. Standard practice includes the delivery of chemotherapy during accelerated hyperfractionated radiation therapy (1.5 Gy BID [twice daily] to 45 Gy over 3 weeks). Intensifying the radiation therapy course by accelerating the time has proven to be an effective strategy.[24] The results of an Intergroup trial favored the accelerated course over a course of 45 Gy with conventional fractionation. The increased toxicity was the doubling of acute esophagitis from 16% to 32%.[25] The most common chemotherapy drugs are cisplatin and etoposide, carboplatin and etoposide, and cisplatin and irinotecan.

Extensive SCLC is often treated with palliative radiation therapy to symptomatic sites and platinum-based chemotherapy.

SCLC often spreads to the brain, with 10% to 15% of patients presenting with brain metastases and 50% to 80% developing brain metastasis 2 years after radiation and chemotherapy.[11] Radiation can be given to the brain to help decrease the chance of metastasis. This is called prophylactic cranial irradiation (PCI). PCI is delivered with a dose of 25 Gy in 10 fractions and is indicated after the completion of radiation therapy and chemotherapy for patients with a good response. A study by the Prophylactic Cranial Irradiation Overview Collaborative Group revealed a survival benefit for the addition of PCI following positive response to therapy.[26]

SIMULATION AND TREATMENT PLANNING

Simulation. Accurate treatment planning and delivery depend on reproducible patient setup and tumor localization.

To obtain a reproducible setup, immobilization devices and positioning aids are needed. Typically, a wingboard with headrest and cradle (Vac-Lok, Alpha cradle) are used. A slanted support device may be used to elevate the upper half of the body if the patient has difficulty breathing. A cushion may be placed under the knees for lumbar support.

The patient is usually in the supine position, with the head neutral and both arms over the head, holding the pegs of the wingboard. Placing the arms above the head allows for a number of beam angles and arrangements to be considered during treatment planning. The sagittal laser should align with the suprasternal notch, xiphoid process, and pubic symphysis to ensure the patient is lying straight on the CT table.

CT images are acquired with the patient in the same position, from the level of the cricoid cartilage to approximately the L2 vertebral body. Contrast media is usually not required to identify the tumor, unless it is near the hilum or mediastinum. It may, however, be beneficial to identify nodal involvement.

After the CT images are acquired, the isocenter is determined, and the coordinates of the isocenter are transferred to the room lasers. An anterior and two lateral marks/tattoos, corresponding to the coordinates, are placed on the patient to assist in daily positioning and alignment.

Treatment Planning. In treatment planning for lung cancer, the tumor volumes and critical structures are defined, and an optimal beam arrangement is selected. The goal is to deliver the prescribed dose to the tumor while sparing the normal tissues.

The gross tumor volume (GTV) is defined as the volume of clinically evident macroscopic disease. The size of the GTV depends on the window and level settings of the CT scan. Ideally, the GTV should be contoured on the "lung" window setting. Fusion of a diagnostic

TABLE 28.3   Tolerance Doses of Critical Structures Related to Radiation Therapy for Lung Cancer

TD 5/5 (Gy); CONVENTIONAL FRACTIONATION				
Organ at Risk (OAR)	1/3	2/3	3/3	Consequence of Exceeding Tolerance
Lungs	45	30	17	Pneumonitis
Spinal cord	50 (5 cm)	50 (10 cm)	47 (20 cm)	Myelitis
Heart	60	45	40	Pericarditis
Esophagus	60	58	55	Stricture

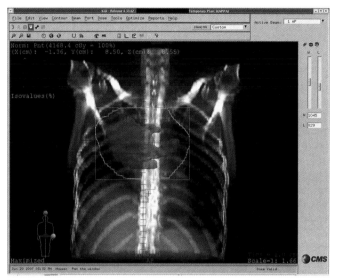

Fig. 28.6 Digitally reconstructed radiograph for parallel-opposed fields for right lung tumor with extension across midline. (Courtesy Bayhealth Medical Center at Kent General Hospital, Dover, DE.)

PET-CT scan may add additional information and help in distinguishing tumor versus atelectasis (Fig. 28.5). If the patient has nodal involvement, the initial diagnostic CT scan, before chemotherapy, should be used to delineate the volume.

The clinical target volume (CTV) is defined as the GTV and surrounding microscopic disease. Usually it is delineated as the GTV plus an additional 5- to 10-mm margin.

The planning target volume (PTV) is defined as the CTV with a margin to account for patient setup error and tumor motion.

The critical structures of primary concern are the healthy lung, spinal cord, heart, and esophagus. Doses to the structures are carefully monitored to ensure that tolerance is not exceeded (Table 28.3). Usually, definitive doses are higher than the tolerance doses, so this is very important. Additional scrutiny is needed for patients with respiratory disease and patients undergoing concurrent chemotherapy.

The right and left lung are delineated separately, and an additional volume of "combined lung" (excluding the GTV) is used to evaluate the V20, the volume (%) of lung receiving 20 Gy. The risk of pneumonitis increases with increasing V20 values. V5 and V10, the volume of lung receiving 5 Gy and 10 Gy, respectively, are also evaluated. Chang et al recommend the use of a mean lung dose of 20 Gy and V5, V10, and

V20 of 65%, 45%, and 35%, respectively, when concurrent chemotherapy is given.[7]

Dose to the spinal cord is typically limited to 45 to 50 Gy. Radiation oncologists generally err on the side of caution and limit the dose to the spinal cord to 45 Gy. If not already considered, there should be a change in technique when the dose to the spinal cord approaches 40 Gy. Exceeding the dose tolerance of the spinal cord can cause myelitis and paralysis. Depending on the level of the spinal cord affected, quadriplegia or paraplegia are possible.

When a significant portion of the heart is treated, there is an increased risk of pericarditis. Likewise, when much of the esophagus is the field, the risk of stricture or perforation increases. Chang et al. recommend a V55 volume of esophagus receiving 55 Gy, less than 50% if concurrent chemotherapy is given.[7]

Treatment field design is based on the size of the primary tumor, its location and proximity to critical structures, as well as the lymphatic drainage. Typically, there is a 2-cm margin around the primary tumor and the lymph nodes that are involved or at risk. Traditional field borders are as follows: If there is disease in the upper lobe, the field includes the primary tumor, hila, superior mediastinum, and both supraclavicular areas. The same areas are included if there is disease in the middle lobes with mediastinal involvement. If there is disease in the middle lobes without mediastinal involvement, the primary tumor, hila, and superior mediastinum are covered. The treatment field for the lower lobes without mediastinal involvement includes the primary tumor and mediastinum. Generally, if there is mediastinal adenopathy, both supraclavicular areas are covered.[14] A beam energy of 6 to 10 megavolts (MV) is used.

Initially, the treatment fields are treated anteroposterior/posteroanterior to a dose of 40 to 45 Gy (Figs. 28.6 to 28.8). To avoid exceeding the dose tolerance of the spinal cord, oblique fields are used to boost the tumor to the definitive radiation dose (Fig. 28.9). Total doses of 60 Gy using conventional fractionation are used to treat the gross disease. Collimator rotations, beam weighting, wedges, etc., may be needed to optimize the dose distribution (Fig. 28.10). Image-guided radiation therapy (IGRT), using MV or kilovolt (kV)-level two-dimensional imaging, or cone-beam CT three-dimensional imaging is recommended.

Patients with tumors close to critical structures or that have nodal disease may benefit from intensity-modulated radiation therapy (IMRT) or volumetric-modulated arc therapy (VMAT) (Fig. 28.11). IMRT allows the radiation dose to conform to the area of interest by modulating, or changing, the intensity of the radiation beam within smaller fields. Because patients with lung cancer typically have compromised respiratory function before radiation therapy, the use of smaller field sizes is essential. VMAT is comparable to IMRT with the benefit of reduced treatment time.[7]

SBRT is another option to deliver a high dose to the tumor while minimizing normal tissue toxicity (Fig. 28.12). SBRT incorporates a variety of systems to take tumor motion into account and decrease setup uncertainty using IGRT. SBRT allows reduction of treatment volumes, which facilitates hypofractionation to increase daily dose and significantly reduces overall treatment time. SBRT is typically delivered in five or fewer fractions.

If a patient has a pacemaker or internal cardiac defibrillator, there is increased risk for malfunction. Before simulation, the patient's need for the device should be evaluated. If the total dose to the device is greater than 2 Gy, it should be moved out of the field, when possible.[11]

Motion management. Lung motion can have a dramatic effect on radiation therapy simulation and treatment planning. A lung tumor can move more than 1 cm during a single treatment fraction.[13] Motion

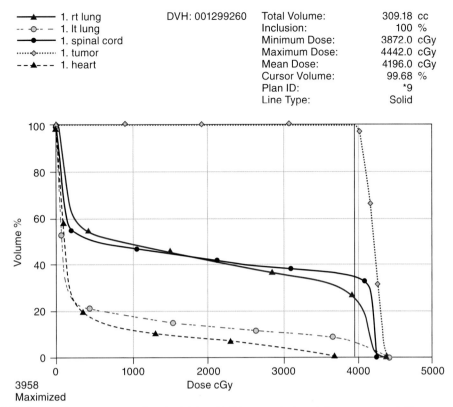

—▲— 1. rt lung	DVH: 001299260	Total Volume: 309.18 cc
-- -○- -- 1. lt lung		Inclusion: 100 %
—●— 1. spinal cord		Minimum Dose: 3872.0 cGy
···◇··· 1. tumor		Maximum Dose: 4442.0 cGy
-- -▲- -- 1. heart		Mean Dose: 4196.0 cGy
		Cursor Volume: 99.68 %
		Plan ID: *9
		Line Type: Solid

3958
Maximized

Fig. 28.7 Dose-volume measures dose to right and left lungs, spinal cord, tumor, and heart. Tumor received a maximum of 4442 cGy; spinal cord and heart received less than tolerance. See Fig. 28.6 for digitally reconstructed radiograph of fields. (Courtesy Bayhealth Medical Center at Kent General Hospital, Dover, DE.)

management should be considered when the range of tumor motion is greater than 5 mm in any direction.

The simplest method to reduce tumor motion is breath hold; however, this is problematic and not reliable for patients with respiratory disease. Alternative methods include abdominal compression (if the patient is cooperative), active breathing control, deep-inspiration breath hold, and respiratory gating with tumor tracking.

Active breathing control and deep-inspiration breath hold are two methods that help patients hold their breaths at specific times in the respiratory cycle. At certain times, the radiation beam is initiated. The use of these techniques is limited to patients who can hold their breath for up to 15 seconds.

Various commercial systems are available for respiratory gating. The method uses an externally placed fiducial that is tracked as the patient breathes. The beam can be triggered at a chosen point in the respiratory cycle, typically at the end of expiration, as this is the longest and most reproducible portion of the respiratory cycle.

When using respiratory gating, a four dimensional (4D)-CT scan is obtained during simulation. The CT scan is broken into groups of images that correspond with the patient's respiratory cycle. This allows the treatment planning team to assess the extent of tumor motion as the patient breathes. During treatment planning, an internal tumor volume, as defined by the International Commission of Radiation Units and Measurements Report 62, is delineated.

Side effects of radiation therapy. General side effects of radiation therapy include fatigue, anorexia, weight loss, skin changes, and hair loss in the area of treatment. These side effects are expected and may occur during or after treatment.

Side effects of radiation therapy to the lung include pneumonitis, esophagitis, dysphagia, and odynophagia (painful swallowing). Side effects related to the esophagus can be addressed with medication and monitored diet. These acute side effects can be severe and lead to treatment disruptions. Patients should be continually monitored for the side effects to be appropriately managed.

Radiation-induced pneumonitis typically occurs after the completion of radiation therapy, peaks at 2 months, and stabilizes or resolves 6 to 12 months after treatment. It manifests as cough, dyspnea, fever, and fatigue, and can be treated with corticosteroids, such as prednisone.

After 2 to 3 weeks of conventionally fractionated radiation therapy, patients may experience dysphagia or odynophagia that worsens toward the end of treatment and peaks at the first week after the completion of radiation therapy. This acute reaction can affect a patient's quality of life because of dehydration and weight loss. Late reactions generally involve fibrosis that can lead to strictures. Rarely, perforation or fistula formation occurs.

Complications differ from side effects and are frequently unexpected. These effects usually result from radiation doses that exceed critical structure tolerance (e.g., radiation pneumonitis, pulmonary fibrosis, myelopathy, or esophageal stricture or perforation). In some cases, they may be life-threatening. Distinguishing the effects of the disease from those of treatment is sometimes difficult.

ROLE OF THE RADIATION THERAPIST

The radiation therapist plays a major role in patient education, communication, and assessment. Unlike the physician or nurse, the radiation

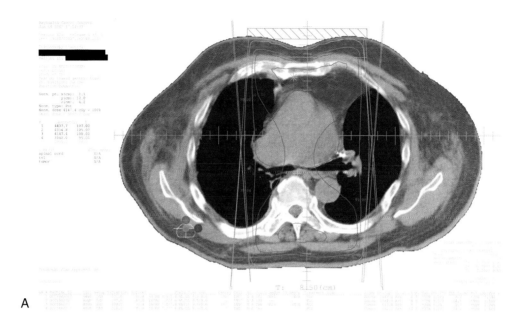

A

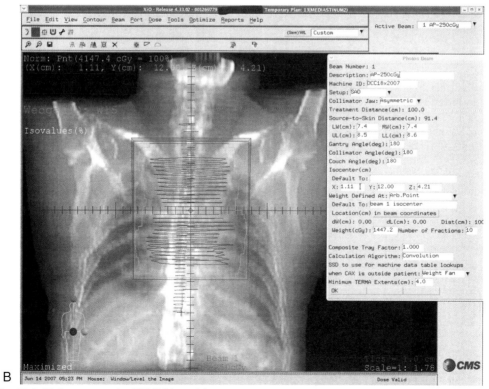

B

Fig. 28.8 (A) Anteroposterior (AP) fields to right upper lobe and mediastinum. (B) Beam's-eye view (BEV) of AP field. (Courtesy Bayhealth Medical Center at Kent General Hospital, Dover, DE.)

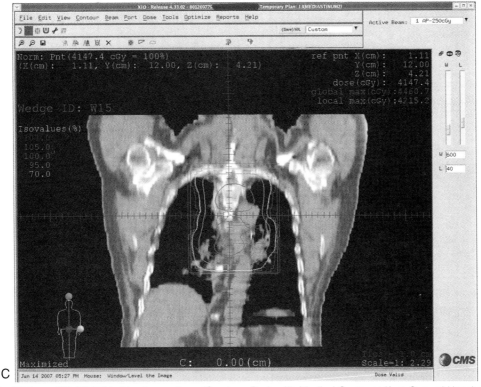

Fig. 28.8, cont'd (C) BEV of isodose values. (Courtesy Bayhealth Medical Center at Kent General Hospital, Dover, DE.)

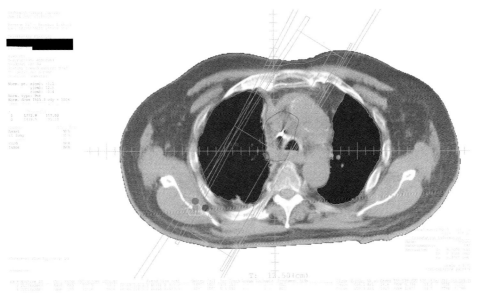

Fig. 28.9 Parallel-opposed off-cord oblique fields. (Courtesy Bayhealth Medical Center at Kent General Hospital, Dover, DE.)

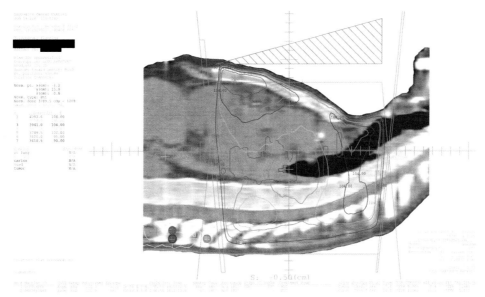

Fig. 28.10 Use of compensating wedge to address dose distribution across sloping chest. (Courtesy Bayhealth Medical Center at Kent General Hospital, Dover, DE.)

therapist interacts with the patient daily and often develops a rapport with the patient, family members, and/or friends that accompany the patient to the radiation oncology department for each treatment.

As part of the radiation oncology team, the radiation therapist informs the patient of the simulation, treatment planning, and treatment procedures. It is important for the patient to know the steps of each procedure, how long each procedure may take, and the risks and/or benefits of each procedure. The radiation therapist must present the information in a way that is understandable to the patient, avoiding jargon and recognizing that the patient may be fearful or distracted by other information. The patient should be given time to ask questions and to confirm his or her understanding. This is especially important in conveying appointment times because this may need reinforcement.

It is important for the radiation therapist to communicate clearly with the patient and his or her family members. The radiation therapist should use a volume and tone that is appropriate for the patient and concisely convey his or her expectations. The patient is more likely to cooperate if he or she is aware of the radiation therapist's expectations. Overall, patient compliance is a key to accomplishing the goals

of treatment. Clear communication also helps in the building of the radiation therapist-patient relationship. Patients are usually trusting of healthcare professionals and are more open to sharing questions or concerns when there is an established rapport.

The radiation therapist must monitor the patient throughout his or her treatment for side effects and/or complications. In the treatment of lung cancer, the patient's skin, ability to swallow, and breathing should be monitored before daily treatment. By consistently monitoring the patient, the radiation therapist is able to recognize the side effects, assist the patient with managing the side effect, and, if needed, refer the patient to the appropriate support personnel and services. The radiation therapist should be familiar with the radiation doses at which each side effect occurs and recognize when the effect is abnormal. The radiation therapist should also monitor the patient for signs of progressive disease. As previously stated, lung cancer often metastasizes to the brain or bone. Clinical evidence of brain metastasis may include headaches, problems with gait, visual changes, and personality changes. Bone metastasis may include pain or changes in gait. Such changes should be discussed with the radiation oncologist for further evaluation.

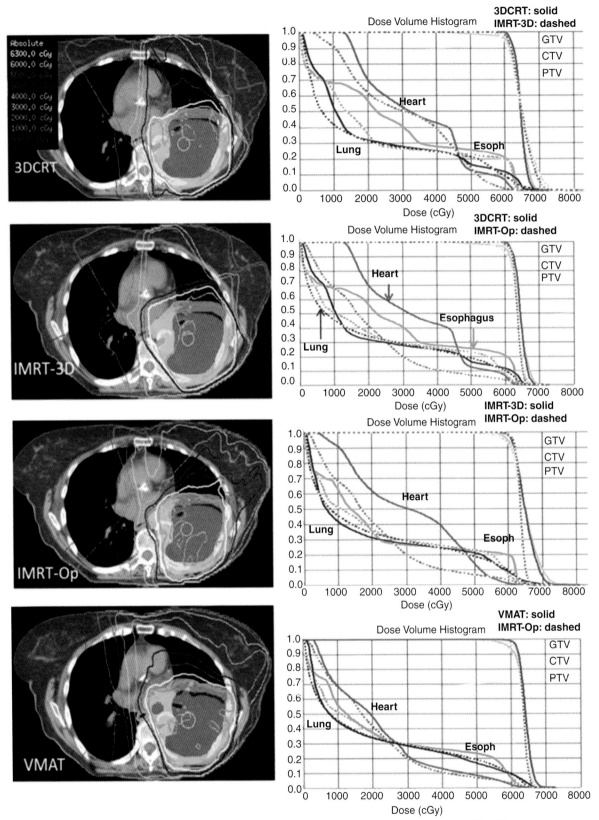

Fig. 28.11 Intensity-modulated radiotherapy *(IMRT)* or volumetric-modulated arc therapy *(VMAT)* can spare more critical structures better than three-dimensional conformal radiotherapy *(3DCRT)* in the treatment of a bulky stage III nonsmall cell lung cancer tumor located near the esophagus and the heart. (From Chang JY. Intensity-modulated radiotherapy, not 3 dimensional conformal, is the preferred technique for treating locally advanced lung cancer. *Semin Radiat Oncol.* 2015;25(2):110–116.)

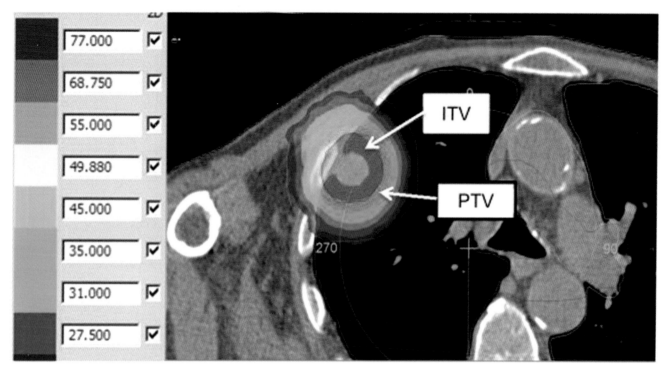

Fig. 28.12 Example of stereotactic body radiation therapy (SBRT) plan for a right upper lobe tumor receiving 55 Gy in five fractions with doses shown on the right in Gy. The planning target volume *(PTV)* is created by a 5-mm universal expansion margin. Immobilization is essential to make the patient comfortable and stable. This is usually achieved by a number of methods, either with specific SBRT immobilization devices or customization of existing methods, for example, addition of customized vacuum bags to more standard immobilization systems (wing, thoracic, or breast boards). *ITV,* Internal tumor volume. (From KN, Jain P, Snee MP. Stereotactic ablative body radiotherapy for lung cancer. *Clin Oncol (R Coll Radiol).* 2015;27(5):280–289.)

SUMMARY

- Lung cancer is the second most common form of cancer in the United States.
- The leading risk factors for lung cancer are smoking and radon exposure.
- The anatomy of the lower respiratory tract includes the trachea, bronchial tree, and lungs. The bifurcation of the trachea, the carina, is an important radiographic landmark.
- The lymphatics of the respiratory system include the intrapulmonary, bronchopulmonary (hilar), mediastinal, and supraclavicular nodes. Lymphatic spread is common.
- Signs and symptoms of lung cancer depend on the extent of disease. Local signs and symptoms include cough and hemoptysis, while regional spread may include chest pain, dysphagia, or hoarseness.
- Superior vena cava (SVC) syndrome is characterized by swelling in the face and arms, distended veins in the upper chest, dyspnea, and orthopnea. SVC syndrome is considered an oncologic emergency.
- A Pancoast tumor arises in the superior sulcus and presents with pain in the shoulder and arm, atrophy of the hand muscles, erosion of the ribs or vertebrae, or Horner syndrome.

- A paraneoplastic syndrome occurs when hormone-like substances are secreted into the blood and cause issues in a site away from the cancer.
- Imaging tests, particularly CT, are useful in detecting lung cancer. A diagnosis may be made through surgical procedures, including bronchoscopy.
- The most common types of lung cancer are NSCLC and SCLC.
- The AJCC TNM system is used in the staging of lung cancer.
- Lung cancer spreads through direct extension or by lymphatic or hematogenous routes.
- Treatment for early-stage lung cancer includes surgery. Radiation therapy and chemotherapy may also be prescribed.
- Total radiation dose is 60 Gy. Careful attention must be paid to ensure the tolerances of the healthy lung, spinal cord, heart, and esophagus are not exceeded. Motion management is an effective dose-limiting strategy.
- Side effects of treatment may include pneumonitis, dysphagia, and odynophagia.
- The radiation therapist plays a key role in educating, communicating with, and assessing the patient.

REVIEW QUESTIONS

The answers to the Review Questions can be found by logging on to our website at: http://evolve.elsevier.com/Washington/principles

1. The leading risk factor for lung cancer among nonsmokers is:
   a. Air pollution.
   b. Asbestos exposure.
   c. Radon exposure.
   d. Personal history of lung cancer.

2. The carina is found at the level of:
   a. C5.
   b. T2.
   c. T5.
   d. T10.

3. Local signs and symptoms of lung cancer include:
   a. Cough and dyspnea.
   b. Cough and hemoptysis.
   c. Dyspnea and hemoptysis.
   d. Cough and dysphagia.

4. A Pancoast tumor arises in the:
   a. Apex of the lung.
   b. Base of the lung.
   c. Mediastinum.
   d. Hilum.

5. In treating lung cancer, stereotactic body radiation therapy is reserved for:
   a. Patients with small tumors.
   b. Medically inoperable patients with early-stage NSCLC.
   c. Patients with SVC syndrome.
   d. Both a and b.

6. Mesothelioma is a cancer of the:
   a. Trachea.
   b. Bronchi.
   c. Alveoli.
   d. Pleura.

7. The treatment of choice for early-stage lung cancer is:
   a. Lobectomy.
   b. Pneumonectomy.
   c. Pleurectomy.
   d. Chemotherapy.

8. The total dose used in the definitive treatment of lung cancer is:
   a. 40 Gy.
   b. 50 Gy.
   c. 60 Gy.
   d. 75 Gy.

9. Critical structures considered in the treatment of lung cancer are:
   a. Trachea and esophagus.
   b. Esophagus and liver.
   c. Spinal cord and heart.
   d. Spinal cord and liver.

10. SCLC most commonly spreads to the:
    a. Brain.
    b. Bone.
    c. Liver.
    d. Adrenal glands.

QUESTIONS TO PONDER

1. Which factors related to smoking increase the risk of developing lung cancer?

2. Which lymph node groups are involved in the regional spread of lung cancer?

3. Discuss strategies to limit radiation dose to critical structures in the treatment of lung cancer.

4. Describe the side effects of radiation therapy for lung cancer.

5. Name the prognostic factors associated with lung cancer.

REFERENCES

1. Simmons CP, Koinis F, Fallon MT, et al. Prognosis in advanced lung cancer—a prospective study examining key clinicopathological factors. *Lung Cancer*. 2015;88:304–309.

2. Conill C, Verger E, Salamero M. Performance status assessment in cancer patients. *Cancer*. 1990;65:1864–1866.

3. Oken MM, Creech RH, Tormey DS, et al. Toxicity and response criteria of the eastern cooperative oncology group. *Am J Clin Oncol*. 1982;5:649–655.

4. National Cancer Institute. Non-Small Cell Lung Cancer Treatment (PDQ) – Health Professional Version. https://www.cancer.gov/types/lung/hp/non-small-cell-lung-treatment-pdq#link/_48499_toc. Accessed February 5, 2019.

5. American Cancer Society. Lung cancer. https://www.cancer.org/cancer/lung-cancer.html. Accessed January 22, 2019.

6. Dela Cruz CS, Tonoue LT, Matthay RA. Lung cancer: epidemiology, etiology, and prevention. *Clin Chest Med*. 2011;32:605–644.

7. Halperin EC, Wazer DE, Perez CA, et al., eds. *Perez & Brady's Principles and Practice of Radiation Oncology*. 7th ed. Philadelphia, PA: Wolters Kluwer; 2019.

8. American Cancer Society. Cancer facts and figures 2018. https://www.cancer.org/content/dam/cancer-org/research/cancer-facts-and-statistics/annual-cancer-facts-and-figures/2018/cancer-facts-and-figures-2018.pdf. Accessed February 5, 2019.

9. Mao Y, Yang D, He J, Krasna MJ. Epidemiology of lung cancer. *Surg Oncol Clin N Am*. 2016;25:439–445.

10. Centers for Disease Control and Prevention. Current cigarette smoking among adults in the United States. https://www.cdc.gov/tobacco/data_statistics/fact_sheets/adult_data/cig_smoking/index.htm. Accessed January 30, 2019.

11. Hansen EK, Roach III M, eds. *Handbook of Evidence-Based Radiation Oncology*. 3rd ed. New York, NY: Springer; 2018.

12. Ridge CA, McErlean AM, Ginsberg MS. Epidemiology of lung cancer. *Semin Intervent Radiol*. 2013;30:93–98.

13. Washington CM, Leaver D, eds. *Principles and Practice of Radiation Therapy*. 4th ed. St. Louis, MO: Elsevier; 2016.

14. Vann AM, Dasher BG, Chestnut SK, et al. *Portal Design in Radiation Therapy*. 2nd ed. Columbia, SC: The R.L. Bryan Company; 2006.

15. Straka C, Ying J, Kong FM, et al. Review of evolving etiologies, implications and treatment strategies for the superior vena cava syndrome. *Springerplus*. 2016;5:229.

16. Marulli G, Battistella L, Mammana M, et al. Superior sulcus tumors (Pancoast tumors). *Ann Transl Med*. 2016;4:239.

17. The National Lung Screening Trial Research Team. Reduced lung-cancer mortality with low-dose computed tomographic screening. *N Engl J Med.* 2011;365:395–409.

18. American Cancer Society. Lung cancer screening guidelines. https://www.cancer.org/health-care-professionals/american-cancer-society-prevention-early-detection-guidelines/lung-cancer-screening-guidelines.html. Accessed February 6, 2019.

19. Gould RJ, VanMeter KC, eds. *Gould's Pathophysiology for the Health Professions.* 6th ed. St. Louis, MO: Elsevier; 2018.

20. American Cancer Society. Malignant mesothelioma. https://www.cancer.org/cancer/malignant-mesothelioma.html. Accessed February 6, 2019.

21. McCance KL, Huether SE, eds. *Pathophysiology: The Biologic Basis for Disease in Adults and Children.* 7th ed. St. Louis, MO: Mosby; 2014.

22. Patton KT. *Anatomy and Physiology.* 10th ed. St. Louis, MO: Elsevier; 2019.

23. Cataldo JK, Dubey S, Prochaska JJ. Smoking cessation: an integral part of lung cancer treatment. *Oncology.* 2010;78:289–301.

24. Gunderson LL, Tepper JE, eds. *Clinical Radiation Oncology.* 4th ed. Philadelphia, PA: Elsevier; 2016.

25. Fietkau R. Which fractionation of radiotherapy is best for limited-stage small-cell lung cancer? *Lancet Oncol.* 2017;18:994–995.

26. Aupérin A, Arriagada R, Pignon JP, et al. Prophylactic cranial irradiation for patients with small-cell lung cancer in complete remission. *N Engl J Med.* 1999;341:476–484.

29

Head and Neck Cancers

Ronnie G. Lozano

OBJECTIVES

- Identify the medical professionals involved in the multidisciplinary care and treatment of the patient with head and neck disease.
- Name some of the advances that have had an impact on the localization and treatment of head and neck cancers.
- Identify the most common site of distant metastasis and other common sites of distant metastasis.
- Describe the use of intensity-modulated radiation therapy for the treatment of head and neck cancers.
- Name the specific head and neck cancer that consistently shows the greatest positive trend in the Surveillance Epidemiology and End Results reports.
- Identify four general etiologic risk factors for head and neck cancer.
- Name three occupations associated with a greater risk of head and neck cancers.
- Name the virus associated with nasopharyngeal cancer in all races.
- Identify the histopathology that is present in 80% of the head and neck cancers.
- Describe the various distinctive functions of a mouth stent (tongue blade and cork or other similar device).
- Describe the general radiation therapy treatment techniques for each of the head and neck sites.
- Discuss the management of symptoms and morbidity for head and neck cancers treated with radiation therapy.

OUTLINE

KEY TERMS

Accelerated fractionation

Cryotherapy

Digestive tubes

External auditory meatus

Electrocautery

Endophytic

Erythroplasia

Exophytic

Hemiglossectomy

Heterogeneity

Hyperfractionation

Jugulodigastric lymph node

Keratosis

Leukoplakia

Node of Rouvière

Percutaneous gastrostomy tube

Posterior cervical lymph node chain

Radical neck dissection

Retroauricular node

Otalgia

The management of head and neck malignancy requires a multidisciplinary team approach, with an understanding that this disease can produce significant morbidity. Survival cannot be measured only in terms of mortality. Reduction of deformity and restoration of function are essential to the management of head and neck cancer. The cure of cancer, with preservation of structure and function (with good cosmetic results), has become more evident with advances in modern radiation oncology because of technologic gains in radiation physics and insights into radiation biology and pathophysiology.[1] Treatment that causes the permanent loss of vision, smell, taste, or hearing should be evaluated concerning its effect on quality of life and survival. Maintenance of food passageways and airways is vital. Treatment decisions should also consider the patient's ability to speak. The loss of speech results in significant changes in the patient's lifestyle and therefore lowers the patient's quality of life. With early detection techniques, head and neck cancers treated with radiation therapy (RT) allow for greater preservation of voice and swallowing. The effective management of head and neck cancer involves the close cooperation of radiation oncologists, medical oncologists, dentists, maxillofacial prosthodontists, nutritionists, head and neck surgeons, neurosurgeons, plastic surgeons, oral surgeons, pathologists, oncology nurses, radiologists, social workers, radiation therapists, speech therapists, pain service, neurology service, and of course, the patient. The patient may decide to select a treatment approach that offers a slightly lower probability of survival in return for a better functional or cosmetic result if the treatment is successful.[1] This is an important reason to bring the patient into the decision-making process regarding treatment. Despite many major advances, the treatment of locoregional recurrence remains a major challenge, as indicated by low success rates for salvage therapy. Most patients with locoregional recurrence have progressive disease that results in a high degree of suffering.

With the continued improvements in imaging and the increasing accuracy of treatment techniques, tumors that involve critical structures and selected parts of the brain can be eliminated with preservation of vision and minimal neurologic impairment.[1] Current inverse planning processes (intensity-modulated radiation therapy [IMRT]) deliver nonuniform dose distributions on the basis of detailed tissue metabolic information. Our predecessors could not even imagine this technology before the advent of the computer. With systematic monitoring of treatment variations, adaptive RT allows reoptimization of the treatment plan during the course of treatment. This process adjusts field margin and treatment dose with routine customization to each individual patient to achieve a safe dose escalation. Integration of image-guided RT (IGRT) with IMRT and use of functional image information with positron emission tomography (PET) fused with treatment planning have the potential to improve both tumor control and healthy tissue sparing. The integration of robotics and new accelerator design coupled with image-guided tracking of bony landmarks or implanted fiducial markers has surpassed a degree of beam angle versatility and level of "exactitude" in treatment delivery.

NATURAL HISTORY

Head and neck cancer was marked in American history by public accounts and newspaper articles that described the extensive suffering and death of Ulysses S. Grant in the late 1800s. This event significantly added to the public fears of cancers and the inferior treatments of that era. Another historic figure was Sigmund Freud, who had malignancy of the jaw with spread through the hard palate and the sinuses to the base of the orbits. Contemporary figures include Sammy Davis, Jr, who reportedly said he would rather keep his voice than have a part of his throat removed after being diagnosed with laryngeal cancer, and film critic Roger Ebert, who had part of the mandible removed because of spread from cancer of the salivary gland. Others impacted by head and neck cancer include Sean Connery, Michael Douglas, Elton John, Rod Stewart, Eddie Van Halen, and too many others to name.

The Surveillance Epidemiology and End Results (SEER) program estimated that 51,540 men and women would be diagnosed with oral cavity and pharynx cancer by the end of 2018, and among those, 10,030 are expected to die of the disease.[2,3] The American Cancer Society (ACS) reports that incident rates for men are more than twice as high as those for women. Males will account for 37,160 new cases in 2018 as compared with the estimated 14,380 new cases for females.[2]

The ACS also reports the following trend: from 2005 to 2014, incidence rates decreased by more than 2% annually among African Americans but increased by about 1% annually among Caucasians.[3] This is largely driven by the rising rates of a subset of cancers associated with human papillomavirus (HPV) infection within the oropharynx. HPV infection is also associated with cancers of the tonsil, base of the tongue, and some other sites within the oropharynx.

The lungs are the most common site of distant metastasis. Other sites of distant metastasis include the mediastinal lymph nodes, liver, brain, and bones. The incidence of distant metastasis is greatest with tumors of the nasopharynx and hypopharynx. A direct correlation appears to exist between the bulk of cervical neck nodal disease and the development of distant metastasis. Atypical metastatic spread may occur in patients who have had a radical neck dissection (RND) or previous RT. These patients are at high risk for development of atypical metastasis to the neck and to subcutaneous and cutaneous sites. Tumors may also spread along the nerves. Direct nerve invasion may occur from tumors in the affected area. Nerve routes are an important consideration in treatment planning. High-grade parotid tumors are known to involve the facial nerves and to cause paralysis. The standard treatment for these patients is either surgery with preoperative or, more commonly, postoperative RT or primary RT followed by surgery. A combination of chemotherapy and RT is used in patients with inoperable or unresectable (stages III and IV) disease in an attempt to increase cure rates over RT alone. The advantage of multi modality treatment is the preservation of cosmesis and function that results compared with radical surgeries. A challenge of another form involves *cancerization*, which refers to the higher risk for formation of a second primary tumor (SPT) in the same anatomic field of a previous treatment. Patients who were cured of their first head and neck cancer have been shown to have a greater than 20% lifetime risk of development of a second cancer. SPTs are the leading cause of death among patients with early tumors of the head and neck. This finding has stimulated research on adjuvant chemoprevention regimens in prevention of SPTs. Targeted therapy is used initially or may be used to treat recurrent cancer. Immunotherapy is an option for advanced disease. The 5-year relative survival rate for oral cavity and pharynx is 65%. Caucasians have a 66% relative 5-year survival rate, whereas African Americans have a 48% 5-year relative survival rate. For patients diagnosed within the local stage, the survival rate increases to 84%; however, that accounts for less than one-third of cases.[3]

Epidemiology

Trends for new oral cavity and pharynx cancer cases show a constant rising of an average of 0.7% each year for the last 10 years.[4] The 2018 Cancer Facts and Figures by the ACS reports that about 1.7 million cancers are expected to be diagnosed in the United States in 2018. Incidence rates for oral cavity and pharynx are more than twice as high in men as in women. However, among white men and women, incidence rates are increasing for cancers in the oropharynx (the middle part of

the pharynx that includes the back of the mouth, base of the tongue, and tonsils) that are associated with HPV infection.[3] HPV-related head and neck cancers generally have a better prognosis. The most recent figures presented show increasing rates of all cancers of the oral cavity and oropharynx (Table 29.1).

The SEER program advises that survival rates can be calculated with different methods for different purposes. The survival rates presented by the SEER Stat Fact Sheets are based on the relative survival rate, which measures the survival of patients with cancer in comparison with the general population to estimate the effect of cancer. The overall 5-year relative survival rates for 2008 to 2014 for the SEER 18 geographic areas were reported to be 64.8% for oral cavity and pharynx cancer and 60.9% for cancer of the larynx. Table 29.2 presents the breakdown of the 5-year relative survival rates by race and by stage.[4]

Cancers of the nasopharynx are uncommon in the United States in comparison with Hong Kong and southern China; areas of southeast Asia including Taiwan, Vietnam, and Thailand; the Philippines and Malaysia; and some Mediterranean, North African, and Eskimo populations.[5,6] These areas are considered to be endemic for nasopharyngeal cancer (NPC). The incidence rate outside these areas is much lower and considered to be associated with tobacco.[6] A decreased incidence of NPC in successive generations of Chinese born in America suggests an etiologic role for environmental factors.[5,6] Tumors of the oral cavity and base of the tongue are more common in India, which also indicates a strong environmental and cultural influence in the prevalence of this type of disease. In the Indian subcontinent, oral squamous cell carcinoma (SCC) may account for 50% of all cancers. The high incidence rate of buccal mucosal cancer in particular is a result of the chewing of betel nuts, or pan, a mixture of betel leaf, lime, catechu, and areca nut.[5] Betel nuts or chewing betel quid alone or with tobacco known as gutka increases the risk of both oral cavity and oropharyngeal cancers. Of these types of chewing combinations, the areca nut is the only one considered to be carcinogenic when chewed, but both gutka and betel quid are related to a statistically significant increase in risk of oropharyngeal cancer.[7]

The alkaloids released when the nut is chewed provoke excessive and abnormal synthesis of collagen by cultured fibroblasts, which causes submucous fibrosis. Environmental and genetic predisposition results in nasopharynx cancer being the most common tumor in the Kwantung province of southern China. Recurrences usually occur within the first 2 years and rarely after 4 years; thus, a 5-year follow-up period is established for most sites.

Etiology and Predisposing Factors

The large number of disease processes that can affect the head and neck region can have a multitude of histologies, a reflection of the

TABLE. 29.1	National Cancer Institute Surveillance Epidemiology and End Results		
	Men	Women	Total
2018 Estimates			
Oral Cavity and Pharynx			
New cases	37,160	14,380	51,540
Deaths	72,80	2,750	10,030
Larynx			
New cases	10,490	2,660	13,150
Deaths	2,970	740	3,710

TABLE. 29.2 **National Cancer Institute Surveillance Epidemiology and End Results**		
	SURVIVAL	**PERCENT OF CASES**
	Men	**Women**
Overall 5-Year Relative Survival Rates by Race		
Oral Cavity and Pharynx		
White	69.4%	72.4&%
Black	50.4%	59.4%
Larynx		
White	61.0%	57.7%
Black	62.0%	33.8%
Overall 5-Year Relative Survival Rates By Stage SEER 18 2008–2014, All Races, Both Sexes by Seer Summary Stage 2000		
Oral Cavity and Pharynx		
Localized	83.7%	29%
Regional	65%	47%
Distant	39.1%	20%
Unstaged	49.2%	4%
Larynx		
Localized	77.5%	55%
Regional	45.6%	23%
Distant	33.5%	19%
Unstaged	54.6%	3%

National Cancer Institute Surveillance, Epidemiology and End Results Program. Cancer stat facts: oral cavity and pharynx cancer 2018. https://seer.cancer.gov/statfacts/html/oralcav.html. Accessed July 17, 2018.

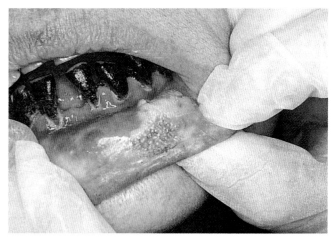

Fig. 29.1 Leukoplakia of the lower labial mucosa at site where patient held tobacco during a 27-year habit. Microscopic epithelial dysplasia and intense dental staining occurred. (From Silverman S. *Oral Cancer.* 5th ed. Hamilton, Ontario, Canada: BC Decker; 2003. Reprinted by the permission of the American Cancer Society, Inc.)

many specialized tissues present and at risk for specific diseases. This chapter refers to those tumors of an epithelial character that arise from the mucosal lining of the aerodigestive tract. The most common sites affected are the oral cavity, pharynx, paranasal sinuses, larynx, thyroid gland, and salivary glands. General etiologic risk factors for head and neck cancer include (1) tobacco and alcohol use, (2) ultraviolet (UV) light exposure, (3) viral infection, and (4) environmental exposures.

Smoking. Tobacco was first introduced to Western civilization by the Spanish explorers of America in the early 16th century. At first, tobacco was simply smoked in pipes, but as it became more popular, it was also chewed and snuffed. Cigarettes were first made in Spain in the mid-17th century, and in the 20th century, they became the most popular form of the tobacco habit. The incidence of head and neck cancers correlates most closely with the use of tobacco and alcohol.[1]

People who consume large amounts of both alcohol and tobacco incur the highest risk for cancers of the oral cavity, oropharynx, hypopharynx, and the larynx. The risks are about 35-fold for those who smoke and drink heavily than for those who never smoke or drink.[8,9,10]

Head and neck tumors occur six times more often among cigarette smokers than among nonsmokers. The mortality from laryngeal cancer appears to rise with increased cigarette consumption. For the heaviest smokers, death from laryngeal cancer is 20 times more likely than for

nonsmokers.[11] Pipe and cigar smoking results in extensive intraoral keratosis. Unfiltered cigarettes cause lip carcinoma, especially when habitually held in the same place. The use of unfiltered cigarettes or dark, air-cured tobacco is associated with further increases in risk. Certain cancers like oropharynx cases, closer to the esophagus, are associated with the pooling of saliva carrying carcinogens related to tobacco.[11]

Alcohol. Alcohol consumption alone is a risk factor for the development of pharyngeal and laryngeal tumors.[11] Alcohol has been known to damage mucosa, making it more permeable to contaminants. Secondary etiologic factors of head and neck cancers that have been related to chronic drinking include factors that fit the usual characteristics of alcoholism, such as nutritional deficiencies and environmental carcinogens (from smoking) that increase susceptibility to cancer in general.

Smoking Tobacco and Alcohol. This combination has been regarded as the most important risk factor for this disease.[1,6] Alcohol seems to have a synergistic effect on the carcinogenic potential of tobacco. This combination facilitates the pathogenic effects of the thousands of substances produced in the combustion process of smoking. These include tars (the basis for the tobacco taste) and aromatic hydrocarbons that contain the most potent carcinogens. Evidence suggests that ethanol suppresses the efficiency of DNA repair after exposure to nitrosamine compounds. Nitrosamines (*N*-nitrosonornicotine) have been identified as the most potent noncombustible product in snuff and chewing tobacco that possesses carcinogenic activity.[6]

Smokeless Tobacco. A higher frequency of premalignant and malignant oral lesions is found in young Americans because of the increasing use of smokeless tobacco.[7] Smokeless tobacco users frequently have development of premalignant lesions, such as oral leukoplakia, at the site where the tobacco quid rests against the mucosa (Fig. 29.1). Over time, these lesions may progress to invasive carcinomas.[11] Tobacco may clearly induce a benign clinical condition that involves the oral mucosa into malignant tumor. The most common conditions found with the use of smokeless tobacco are gingival recession, hyperkeratosis, and staining. The risk of oral epithelial dysplasia or carcinoma increases with long-term use.[1]

Ultraviolet Light. Exposure to UV light is a risk factor for the development of lip cancer. At least 31% of patients with lip cancer have outdoor occupations.

Occupational Exposures. Occupations associated with greater risk include (1) nickel refining, (2) furniture and woodworking (cancers of the larynx, nasal cavity, and paranasal sinuses), and (3) steel and textile work (oral cancer).[6] Exposure to dust, fumes, and formaldehyde has been associated with NPC.[12] Carpenters and sawmill workers who are exposed to dust of mainly hard and exotic woods have development of adenocarcinoma of the nasal cavity and ethmoid sinus. Other carcinogens include synthetic wood, binding agents, and glues.

Radiation Exposure. Exposure to radiation, particularly in childhood, is implicated in the development of thyroid cancer and salivary gland tumors.[7] Salivary gland malignancies have been radiation induced in patients treated for benign conditions like acne, tinea capitis, infected tonsils, etc. Radiation-induced salivary gland tumors have also been reported among survivors of the atomic bomb in Hiroshima and Nagasaki.[13] Cancer of the maxillary sinus has been associated with the radioactive contrast medium, Thorotrast, used for imaging of the maxillary sinus during the 1960s.[14]

Viruses. Increasing evidence suggests a role for viruses in the development of head and neck cancer. Epstein-Barr virus (EBV) has been identified in nasopharyngeal tissue in this type of cancer.[15] EBV has also been associated with NPC in all races.[7]

Herpes simplex virus 1 (HSV-1) is the well-known cause of primary herpetic stomatitis and of recurrent herpes labialis (cold sores). The virus remains latent in the trigeminal or other sensory ganglion for an entire lifetime. Reactivation occurs to produce recurrent lesions or to be shed asymptomatically in the saliva. The virus has the ability to transform cells to a malignant phenotype under certain conditions. In an experimental situation, the infected cells can become immortal in cell culture and invade and metastasize if they are injected into an experimental animal. Experiments with hamsters show that if tissue is exposed to low doses of the tobacco carcinogen benzo(a)pyrene and to HSV-1 simultaneously, tumors can be produced. This may have implications for a population of smokers with HSV-1 and oral cancer.

HPV has also been linked to head and neck carcinogenesis.[6] HPV has been found in oral papillomas, in leukoplakia lesions, and in oral carcinomas. Laryngeal papillomatosis and carcinoma of the larynx have been linked with HPV.[7,16] Cell studies show that high-risk HPVs can transform epithelial cells from cervix, foreskin, and the oral cavity to produce malignancy. Carcinomas of the tonsil, oral tongue, and floor of the mouth have been found to have a high prevalence of HPV DNA. Garden, Morrison, and Ang[17] describe a study that suggests that HPV is found frequently in patients with oropharyngeal carcinoma (OPC) with no history of smoking or alcohol use. An increasing number of younger patients with SCCs of the upper aerodigestive track without the typical social history of smoking and alcohol has been observed. Evidence suggests that viruses such as HPV may be linked to these cases.

Diet. Dietary factors that lead to hypopharyngeal cancer include nutritional deficiency (vitamins A and E), especially in alcoholics and females.[18] The ACS reports that heavy drinkers often have vitamin deficiencies, which may help explain the role of alcohol in increasing risk of these cancers. Eating fewer fried and processed foods and eating more plant-based foods might help reduce laryngeal cancer risk.[19] Iron-deficiency anemia has been associated with postcricoid cancers in women in Scandinavia and Great Britain who usually present with dysphagia from hypopharyngeal webs and atrophy of the oral mucosa.[16] Plummer-Vinson syndrome (esophageal web, iron-deficiency anemia, dysphasia from glossitis) is associated with a high incidence of postcricoid and tongue carcinoma and is most prevalent in Europe. *Web* refers to an inflammation condition associated with a weblike formation on the wall of the esophagus or hypopharynx. It consists of a thin mucosal membrane covered by normal squamous epithelium. The term *Plummer-Vinson syndrome* originates from Scandinavia; the condition is referred to as *Paterson-Brown-Kelly syndrome* in Great Britain.[16] Epidemiologic data suggest that fruits, vegetables, and carotenoids have a preventive role.[6] Nasopharyngeal cases among southern Chinese and Hong Kong populations have been associated with ingestion of salted fish since childhood. Dimethylnitrosamine, a carcinogen in the nitrosamine group found in snuff and chewing tobacco, has also been found in salted fish. This compound has induced carcinoma of the upper respiratory tract in rats.[17,20]

Marijuana. Chronic abuse of marijuana has been linked to head and neck cancer. Although some literature report that the degree of risk is unknown,[6,11] other publications make the comparison of smokers using filtered cigarettes and the lack of such filter in smoking marijuana. An increased risk is established because of a higher concentration of tar and aromatic hydrocarbons.[16] Some researchers believe that marijuana smoke contains known carcinogens, much like those in tobacco smoke. Several studies have shown changes in the lining of the respiratory tract in marijuana smokers. Results of epidemiologic studies of marijuana and cancer risk have been inconsistent, and most recent epidemiologic studies have not found a consistent link on cancer risk. Interestingly, medical marijuana use has gained attention in some states. The tetrahydrocannabinol (THC) and **cannabidiol** (CBD) in marijuana is known to relieve pain, control nausea and vomiting, and stimulate appetite in people with cancer, acquired immunodeficiency syndrome, and other diseases. Researchers also report that THC decreases pressure within the eyes, therefore reducing the severity of glaucoma.[3,16]

Dentures, Fillings, and Poor Oral Hygiene. Although studies with conclusive evidence are lacking, cases exist in which some carcinomas develop in areas covered by or adjacent to a prosthetic device. The risk is low, but chronic denture irritation in addition to other unidentified factors may possibly promote neoplastic activity. The same principle may apply to patients who have poor oral hygiene or jagged teeth or fillings that may act as irritants (Figs. 29.2 and 29.3). Denture material per se has not been shown to be carcinogenic.[1]

Genetics. Genetic predisposition to head and neck cancer has been suggested by its sporadic occurrence in unexpected populations like young adults and nonusers of tobacco and alcohol.[3] Increased susceptibility to environmental carcinogens has been attributed to genetic anomalies and other cofactors like viral infections. Current studies have identified at least 10 genetic alterations that generate an invasive tumor phenotype in cells. The research focuses on the inactivation of tumor suppressor genes and oncogene amplification. These types of studies continue to provide a greater understanding of the influence of genes and may be used in the future of screening. Chemoprevention of malignant transformation is a strategy that may be implemented on identification of high risk based on key genetic changes and markers of carcinogenesis.[1]

An association with the Bloom syndrome and the Li-Fraumeni syndrome has been implicated in head and neck cancers.[1] Bloom syndrome is a rare autosomal recessive disorder characterized by telangiectasia (erythema that appears as macules or plaques in a butterfly distribution

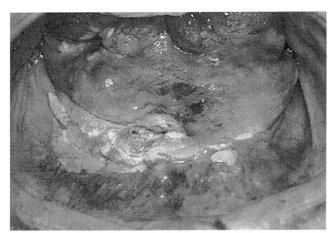

Fig. 29.2 Carcinoma developed under a lower denture in anterior alveolar mucosa after 15-year history of leukoplakia. (From Silverman S. *Oral Cancer*. 5th ed. Hamilton, Ontario, Canada: BC Decker; 2003. Reprinted by the permission of the American Cancer Society, Inc.)

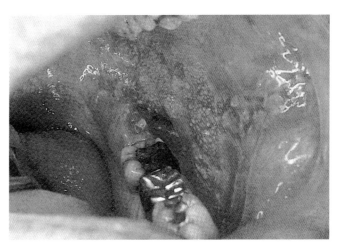

Fig. 29.3 Atrophic lichen planus, an inflammatory disease. Buccal oral lesion is transforming to carcinoma in posterior buccal after 13 years. (From Silverman S. *Oral Cancer*. 5th ed. Hamilton, Ontario, Canada: BC Decker; 2003. Reprinted by the permission of the American Cancer Society, Inc.)

on the face and other areas exposed to the sun), photosensitivity, and growth abnormalities. Patients with Bloom syndrome have an overall 150 to 300 times increased risk of malignancy compared with the general population. Li-Fraumeni syndrome, an autosomal dominant disorder, has been linked to germline mutations of the tumor suppressor gene *p53*. Several types of cancers have been associated with these genetic disorders. SCC of the head and neck is estimated to require the accumulation of 8 to 11 mutations, and 4 to 7 genetic mutations may be sufficient for the development of salivary gland malignancies.[7]

Prognostic Indicators

In general, the morbidity of treatment increases and the prognosis decreases as the affected area progresses backward from the lips to the hypopharynx, with the exclusion of the larynx. Common characteristics of advanced stages and unfavorable prognosis include tumors that cross the midline, exhibit endophytic growth (invasion of the lamina propria and submucosa), are poorly differentiated, and are non-SCCs. Advanced stages also involve cases that have fixed lymph nodes, a fixed lesion, or cranial nerve involvement. As with all cancer cases, the extent of lymph node involvement directly impacts prognosis. Vascular invasion may identify tumors with an aggressive biologic nature in their ability to invade healthy anatomic structures. An established association of vascular invasion in primary tumors, presence of cervical metastases, and an increased risk for subsequent locoregional recurrence indicates a poor prognosis. Kim, Smith, and Haffty[21] report that postoperative RT may mitigate the poor prognosis associated with vascular invasion.

Anatomy and Physiology

The organs that comprise the head and neck region serve dual purposes related to the respiratory and digestive systems. For a better appreciation of this complex system, a brief anatomic review is necessary.

The staging and classification of head and neck tumors are based on involvement of subsites. An understanding of the structure and physiologic relationships of these adjacent structures is important. The opening of the nasal cavities into the nasopharynx (Fig. 29.4) provides a natural pathway for tumor spread. During the act of swallowing, the soft palate elevates and prevents food from entering the nasopharynx. Tumors in this location do not allow this activity to occur. An enlargement of the pharyngeal tonsil can obstruct the upper air passage and allow breathing only through the mouth, which results in the passing of unfiltered, cool, dry air to the lungs. Collectively, the tonsils are bands

of lymphoid tissue that provide protection against airway infections and form a barrier between the respiratory tubes (nasopharynx) and digestive tubes (oropharynx and hypopharynx). This anatomy may be referred to as the *aerodigestive tract*. In addition, knowledge of the location of a cervical vertebral body provides boundary locations of the soft tissue aspects of the head and neck region. The first cervical vertebra (C1) lies at the inferior margin of the nasopharynx, whereas the second and third cervical vertebrae (C2 to C3) contain the oropharynx. The epiglottis is in line with C3, whereas the true vocal cords lie opposite the fourth cervical vertebra (C4; see Fig. 29.4).

Salivary gland tumors can involve facial nerves, major cranial nerves, arterial neck blood flow, and several lymph node groups (Fig. 29.5). Tumors in this area can cause facial paralysis, nerve pain, and interruption of the neck muscles' blood supply (Fig. 29.6).

Because tumors can damage the cranial nerves, which control the major senses, involvement of the cranial nerves leads to signs and symptoms that can point to a possible location of a tumor. Table 29.3 lists the 12 cranial nerves and their associated functions.

Lymphatics

Nearly one-third of the body's lymph nodes are located in the head and neck area. Lymphatic drainage is mainly ipsilateral, but structures like the soft palate, the tonsils, the base of the tongue, the posterior pharyngeal wall, and especially the nasopharynx have bilateral drainage. However, sites like the true vocal cord, the paranasal sinuses, and the middle ear have few or no lymphatic vessels at all. Lymphatic drainage of the neck was described by Rouvière in 1938. Variations exist in lymph node group level classifications.[22,23] Variation is based on specific objectives of standardizing the terminology. The six-level classifications were developed to standardize terminology for neck dissection procedures, and only the node groups routinely removed during surgical neck dissection are considered.[23] The six (surgical oncology) levels of classification and node groups have been identified and illustrated in Fig. 29.7. Lymph node levels have also been defined according to anatomic landmarks and regarded as an imaging-based nodal classification. Fig. 29.8B illustrates seven category levels, and Table 29.4 defines the category landmarks and depicts the major chains of the head and neck. Fig. 29.9 provides multiple views of anatomic lymph node levels of the neck based on a surgical and computed tomographic (CT) image–based nodal classification.

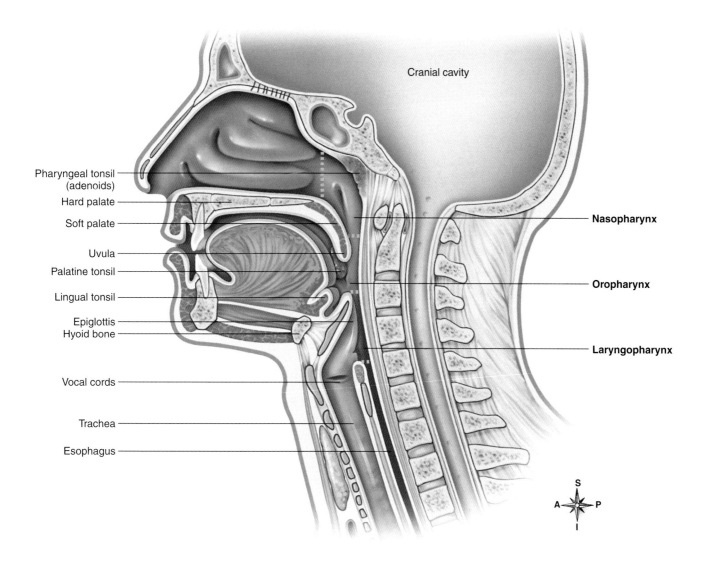

Fig. 29.4 Pharynx. This midsagittal section shows the three divisions of the pharynx (nasopharynx, oropharynx, and laryngopharynx) and nearby structures. (From Thibodeau GA, Patton KT: *The Human Body in Health & Disease* , ed 7, St. Louis, 2018, Mosby, Copyright Elsevier (2018).)

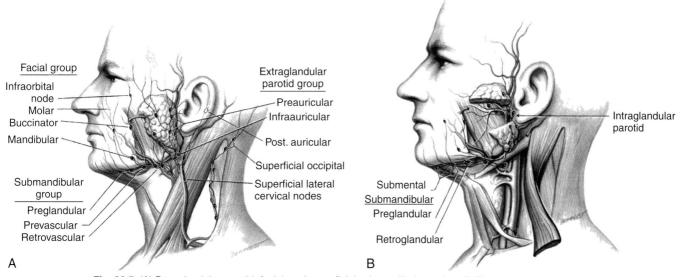

Fig. 29.5 (A) Extraglandular parotid, facial, and superficial submandibular nodes. (B) The deep submandibular and parotid lymph nodes. (From Haagensen CD. *The Lymphatics in Cancer*. Philadelphia, PA: Saunders; 1972.)

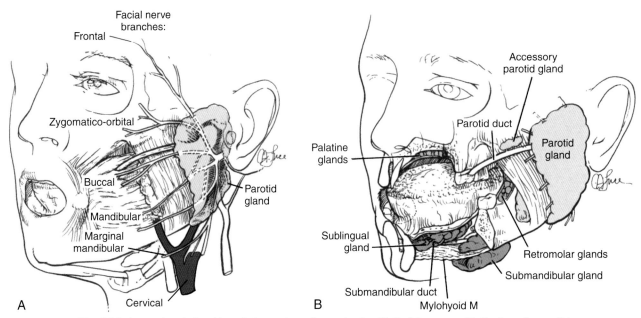

Fig. 29.6 Anatomic relationships of the major salivary glands. (A) Facial nerves. (B) Portion of mandible removed to show minor salivary glands in the palate. (From McCarthy JG. *Plastic Surgery: Tumors of the Head and Neck and Skin.* Vol 5. Philadelphia, PA: Saunders; 1990.)

TABLE. 29.3	Cranial Nerves and Their Functions		
Name	**Number**	**Function**	**Classification**
Olfactory	I	Smell	Sensory
Optic	II	Sight	Sensory
Oculomotor	III	Eye movement (up and down)	Motor
Trochlear	IV	Eye movement (rotation)	Motor
Trigeminal	V	Sensory (facial) and motor (jaw)	Mixed
Abducens	VI	Eye movement (lateral)	Motor
Facial (masticator)	VII	Expressions, muscle contractions, and mouthing	Mixed
Acoustic	VIII	Hearing	Sensory
Glossopharyngeal	IX	Tongue and throat movement	Mixed
Vagus	X	Talking and sounds	Mixed
Spinal accessory	XI	Movement of shoulders and head	Motor
Hypoglossal	XII	Movement of tongue and chewing	Motor

Clinical Presentation

Most head and neck cancers are infiltrative lesions found in the epithelial lining. They can be raised or indurated (hard and firm). These growths are sometimes classified as endophytic tumors, which are more aggressive in spread and harder to control locally. Exophytic tumors are noninvasive neoplasms characterized by raised, elevated borders. Symptoms usually center on the anatomic area affected, with 60% of patients reporting otalgia (ear pain).[24]

The glossopharyngeal nerve or cranial nerve IX (see Table 29.3) directly innervates the ear but also has pharyngeal, lingual, and tonsillar branches to supply the posterior one-third portion of the tongue, tonsillar fossa/pillars, pharynx, and parapharyngeal and retropharyngeal spaces. Any pathologic process involving these areas can result in referred otalgia. Oropharyngeal cancer most commonly produces referred pain to the ear. Otalgia may be the only presenting complaint but is usually accompanied by soreness or discomfort in the throat. The opposite is true for cancer of the nasopharynx, presenting this symptom in about 14% of patients. The usual presentation is a neck mass from metastatic adenopathy, conductive hearing loss, and bloody nasal discharge.[25]

Specific signs and symptoms correlate with anatomic sites. Box 29.1 provides a list of the common symptoms by site. A cervical lymph node mass can be present clinically from any of these sites. In an adult, any enlarged cervical node that persists for 1 week or more should be regarded as suspicious and should be evaluated for a malignancy.

Detection and Diagnosis

Most of the structures of the aerodigestive track and the soft tissue within the facial/cervical regions can be directly examined with palpation, direct inspection, or biopsy. Frequently, findings correlate with presenting symptoms during the physical examination, although accurate detection and staging requires radiographic evaluation.

Hornig and colleagues[26] indicate that the combination of traditional laying on of the hands and contemporary technology leads to accurate assessment and appropriate therapy. A similar message is delivered by

Some nodes have two names. The jugulodigastric lymph node is also called the *subdigastric node*; the node of Rouvière is also called the *lateral retropharyngeal node*; the *spinal accessory chain* is also referred to as the posterior cervical lymph node chain; and the *mastoid node* is also called the retroauricular node. The degree of lymph node involvement dictates the size of the radiation portal and the treatment plan. Fig. 29.10 illustrates the major lymph node chains of the head and neck.

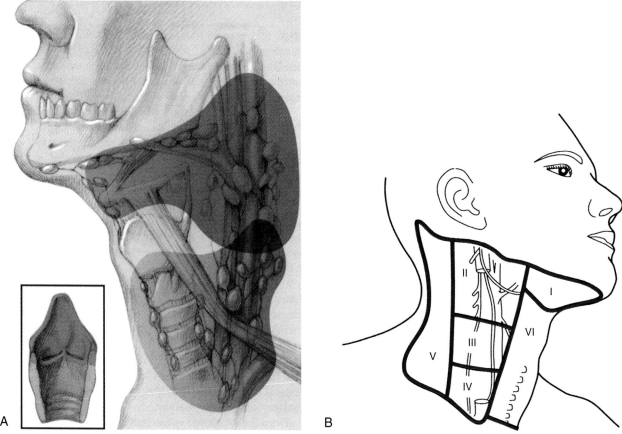

Fig. 29.7 (A) Lateral view of the superficial and deep node groups. (B) Lymphatic groups include the I, Submental; II, upper jugular; III, middle jugular; IV, lower jugular; V, posterior triangle; VI, anterior compartment. (From Werner JA, Davis KR. *Metastases in Head and Neck Cancer.* Berlin, Germany: Springer; 2004.)

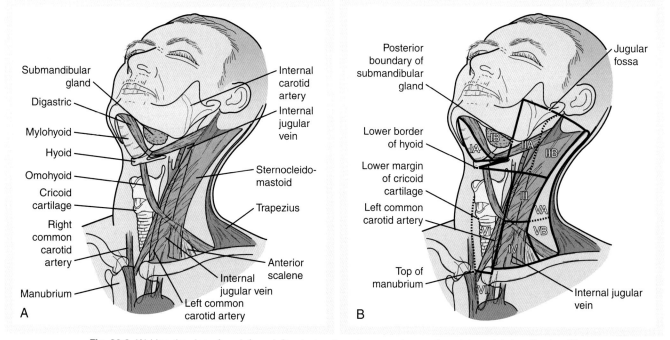

Fig. 29.8 (A) Line drawing of neck from left anterior view shows anatomy relevant to nodal classification.(B) Nodal classification levels are indicated with regard to anatomic landmarks. Posterior margin of the submandibular gland separates levels I and II, and the separation of levels II and III from level V is the posterior edge of the sternocleidomastoid muscle. The posterior edge of the internal jugular vein separates level IIA and IIB nodes. (From Hoppe RT, Phillips TL, Roach M. *Leibel and Phillips Textbook of Radiation Oncology.* 3rd ed. Philadelphia, PA: Saunders; 2010.)

TABLE. 29.4 Imaging-Based Nodal Classification

Nodes	Anatomic Boundaries	Subcategories	Anatomy and Lymphatic Drainage Patterns
Level I	Above hyoid bone, below mylohyoid muscle, anterior to back of submandibular gland	IA: Between medial margins of anterior bellies of digastric muscles IB: Posterolateral to level IA	Includes the submental and submandibular triangles
Level II	From skull base to lower body of hyoid bone, posterior to back of submandibular gland, and anterior to back of sternocleidomastoid muscle	IIA: Anterior, lateral, medial, or posterior to internal jugular vein IIB: Posterior to internal jugular vein with a fat plane separating nodes and vein	Includes the superior jugular chain nodes extending from the mandible down to the carotid bifurcation and posteriorly to the posterior border of the sternocleidomastoid muscle
Level III	From lower body of hyoid to lower cricoid cartilage arch, anterior to back of sternocleidomastoid muscle		Consists of the middle jugular nodes from the carotid bulb inferiorly to the omohyoid muscle
Level IV	From lower cricoid arch to level of clavicle, anterior to line connecting back of sternocleidomastoid and posterolateral margin of anterior scalene muscle, lateral to carotid arteries		Continues from the omohyoid muscle inferiorly to the clavicle including the lower jugular nodes The posterior border of regions II, III, and IV is the posterior border of the sternocleidomastoid muscle, which is the anterior border of the level V group
Level V	Posterior to back of sternocleidomastoid from skull base to clavicle Below cricoid arch, posterior to line connecting back of sternocleidomastoid muscle and posterolateral margin of anterior scalene muscle	VA: From skull base to bottom of cricoid arch, posterior to sternocleidomastoid muscle VB: From cricoid arch to clavicle, posterior to line connecting back of sternocleidomastoid muscle and posterolateral margin of anterior scalene muscle	Includes the spinal accessory group and represents the posterior triangle bounded by the sternocleidomastoid anteriorly, the trapezius posteriorly, and the omohyoid inferiorly Few lesions metastasize to level V without involvement of more central nodes
Level VI	Between carotid arteries from level of lower body of hyoid bone to top of manubrium		Denotes the anterior nodal compartment consisting of the pretracheal and paratracheal nodes, the Delphian node, and the perithyroid nodes
Level VII	Between carotid arteries below level of top of manubrium, caudal to level of innominate vein		Sometimes level VII is used to indicate the upper mediastinal nodes, although this designation is less common

Modified from Zeidan OA, Langen KM, Meeks SL, et al. Evaluation of image-guidance protocols in the treatment of head and neck cancers. *Int J Radiat Oncol Biol Phys.* 2007;67:670–677.

Beitler, Amdur, and Mendenhall,[27] who indicate that, despite increasingly sophisticated imaging, the cancer-directed physical examination is essential. Tumor diagrams and photographs of the lesions are an important resource for the patient record. Without dismissing the effectiveness of contemporary technology, a well-executed basic physical examination along with good old-fashioned documentation with diagrams and digital images clearly still holds much value among practices of RT.

Careful examination and inspection of the head and neck via indirect laryngoscopy, palpation, and fiberoptic endoscopy are important. A systemic, step-by-step examination of all the anatomic compartments for any suspicious growths or nodes is needed. Nodes that are hard, greater than 1 cm, nontender, nonmobile, and raised suggest characteristics of metastasis. The number of nodes should also be assessed. The location of neck masses can often suggest the site of the primary tumor.

Box 29.2 lists common clinical presentations relative to the origin of the head and neck primary cancers. Biopsies are performed on all suspicious lesions to determine a precursor benign condition or to evaluate the predominant malignant growth pattern (grading). A fine-needle aspiration biopsy (FNAB) is performed for neck masses. Anti-EBV antibody titers, immunoglobulin G and immunoglobulin A, are fairly specific for NPC and may aid in the diagnosis of cervical node cancer with unknown primary cancer.

Image Acquisition

Advances in imaging have transformed the diagnosis and treatment of malignancies of the head and neck. Imaging studies performed routinely include CT scan, magnetic resonance imaging (MRI), PET, and x-ray examinations of the skull, sinuses, and soft tissue. For symptomatic patients, barium swallow may be recommended, along with images of the chest and bone scans to rule out metastases. PET may be useful in locating occult tumor in situations of an unknown primary setting and in ascertaining tumor recurrence after treatment. PET has been shown to have advantages over physical examination and CT imaging in follow-up of patients. PET has been reported to accurately assess treatment response after IMRT; however, the newest studies regarding PET scanning show promising results in many other biological and functional variables involving tumor characteristics that impact the effectiveness of targeted and adaptive RT. The utilization of PET scanning to determine various treatment considerations follow.

Positron Emission Tomography Imaging for Hypoxia

Tumor hypoxia remains one of the leading causes of failure of tumor control and treatment success. Dose-response relationships for hypoxic tissue illustrates a poor response related to its radioresistance as compared with nonhypoxic tissue. Hypoxia is also known to promote

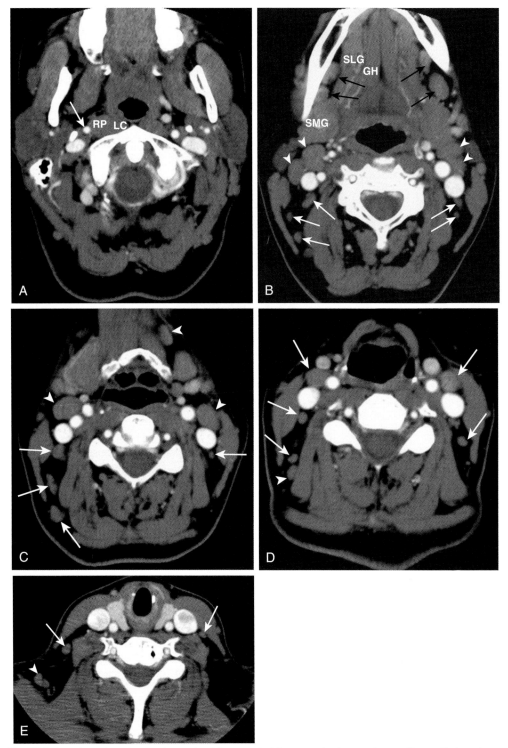

Fig 29.9 A series of contrast-enhanced axial computed tomography images in a patient with lymphoma shows the image-based nodal classification. (A) A retropharyngeal *(RP)* node is seen within 2 cm of the skull base, anterolateral to the longus colli muscle *(LC)* and medial to the internal carotid artery *(white arrow)*. (B) A scan through the suprahyoid neck shows level IB (black arrows), level IIA *(white arrowheads)*, and level IIB *(white arrows)* lymph nodes. Also shown are the submandibular *(SMG)* and sublingual salivary glands *(SLG)* and the geniohyoid muscle *(GH)*. (C) A scan at the level of the hyoid bone shows a level IA node *(large white arrowhead)*, level IIA (small white arrowheads) and level IIB (short white arrows) nodes, and level VA node *(long white arrow)*. (D) A scan of the infrahyoid neck above the level of the cricoid cartilage shows multiple level III lymph nodes *(white arrows)*. A level VA node *(white arrowhead)* is also seen. (E) A scan below the level of the cricoid cartilage shows level IV nodes *(white arrows)* and a level VB node *(white arrowhead)*. (See Table 29.4 for additional descriptive information.) (From Hoppe RT, Phillips TL, Roach M. *Leibel and Phillips Textbook of Radiation Oncology*. 3rd ed. Philadelphia, PA: Saunders; 2010: p 350, Fig. 17.28.)

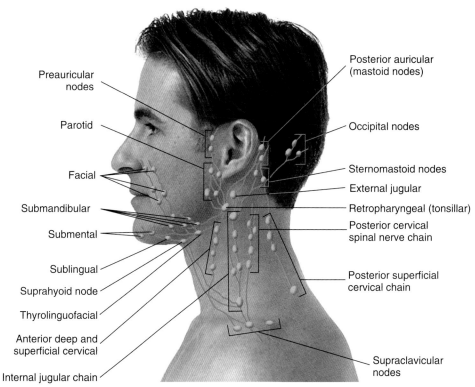

Fig. 29.10 Lymphatic drainage of the head and neck. (From Ball JW, et al. *Seidel's Guide to Physical Examination*. 9th ed. St. Louis, MO: Mosby; 2019.)

BOX. 29.1 Common Symptoms by Site

Oral Cavity
• Swelling or an ulcer that fails to heal

Oropharynx
• Painful swallowing and referred otalgia

Nasopharynx
• Bloody discharge
• Difficulty with hearing

Larynx
• Hoarseness and stridor

Hypopharynx
• Dysphagia
• Painful neck node

Nose/Sinuses
• Obstruction
• Discharge
• Facial pain
• Diplopia
• Local swelling

BOX. 29.2 Common Clinical Presentation by Site

• A high cervical neck mass often represents metastases from the nasopharynx
• Positive subdigastric nodes are often the site of metastases from the oral cavity, oropharynx, or hypopharynx
• Positive submandibular triangle nodes arise from the oral cavity
• Midcervical neck masses are associated with tumors of the hypopharynx, base of the tongue, and larynx
• Preauricular nodes frequently arise from tumors found in the salivary glands

angiogenesis leading to distant metastasis. This makes the identification and quantification of hypoxia within tumor masses critical for personalized treatment and patient selection. To understand the impact of solid tumors upon treatment outcomes, let us examine some basic tumor biology. Studies show that a characteristic of solid tumors is their heterogeneous (nonuniform or uneven) distribution of blood flow, with significant hypoxia and acidity in low-blood flow regions, regarded as areas of low perfusion. Solid tumors can have *high* local "microvessel density" because of uncontrolled angiogenesis, with significant regions of hypoxia and acidosis. Despite new blood vessels, its density demonstrates a low perfusion rate of agents and increasingly poorer blood flow and oxygenation. As the tumor continues to grow, the lack of blood flow and oxygen reaching the center produces cell death. This forms a necrotic center adding to the hypoxic characteristic of the solid tumor. From radiobiology and recent studies on transvascular exchange and extravascular transport of fluid and macromolecules like certain compounds and agents injected in tumors, we know that interstitial pressure is a major contributing factor to the heterogeneous (nonuniform) distribution of macromolecules within solid tumors. AS noted earlier, one factor related to the hypoxic center of a tumor is necrosis. Necrosis does not reduce the central interstitial pressure in a tumor. Recent studies show that macromolecules, and therefore PET radiotracers, do not penetrate a necrotic core at early times after injection. Repeated injections or longer time periods after injection are required.

Although FDG is the most commonly used PET tracer in oncology, it is not effective as a hypoxia-specific radiotracer. F-fluoromisonidazole (F-MISO) is considered the most studied hypoxia-specific PET radiotracer. F-MISO PET imaging of hypoxia can reveal the degree of tumor perfusion through the evaluation of perfused blood vessel density and blood flow. PET scans of head and neck patients with this agent reveals that tumors that exhibit high tracer uptake and low perfusion are at the highest risk of treatment failure. This dictates the consideration for a different treatment approach with varying fractionation or proton therapy among selected patients.[28,29]

Since the identification of limitations of FDG, such as slow uptake and low tracer accumulation, a successor has been located, F-fluoroazomycin-arabinofuranoside, which exhibits better pharmacokinetics.

Positron Emission Tomography Imaging for the Assessment of Angiogenesis

Having discussed the impact of solid tumors and characteristics that include angiogenesis, hypoxia, and necrosis leading to the failure of tumor control under standard treatment, identifying patients with high potential for these traits within tumor masses is critical for personalized treatment and patient selection. The treatment plan may target growth factors responsible for angiogenesis, and PET scanning with a specific radiotracer, Zr-bevacizumab, can identify their levels. Marcu et al and Oosting et al express the importance of personalized treatment because of the highly heterogeneous tracer uptake of this specific radiotracer by tumors.[29,30]

Tumors express a high level of what is referred to as vascular endothelial growth factor (VEGF) proangiogenic factor. This factor signals a protein to stimulat proliferation and migration of endothelia cells critical in pathological angiogenesis. Specific imaging is useful in patient selection and treatment guidance, as well as evaluation of treatment response to antiangiogenic therapy.[29,30]

Imaging of the Head and Neck with Computed Tomography and Magnetic Resonance Imaging

Staging entails a history and physical examination with CT scan or MRI of the head and neck, a chest radiograph, and routine blood cell counts and serum chemistries. Advanced nodal disease indicates a chest CT scan. CT scan with intravenous contrast is the main imaging modality,[27] although MRI can provide important supplemental information. Some patients with advanced disease may benefit from PET/CT scanning to precisely define locoregional disease and detect distant metastases (Fig. 29.11). However, Beitler, Amdur, and Mendenhall[27] report that PET may underestimate the extent of locoregional disease that is apparent in the CT scan. CT scans are performed for a number of reasons, including determining the extent of disease, especially deep invasion; for determination of bone invasion; and for regional lymph nodes assessment. MRI is useful to assess muscle invasion with retromolar trigone lesions. Mendenhall and associates[31] write that regular chest radiography is used to detect pulmonary metastases. The authors also state that routine use of PET is not recommended in cancers of the oral cavity.

Studies done in 2018 emphasize that accurate personalized therapy is possible because of advances in molecular imaging and imaging of biological processes referring to PET. Recent studies report that PET is the most specific and sensitive imaging technique for in vivo molecular targets and biological pathways. This provides highly detailed functional properties of target anatomy to pursue specific targeted therapy. This type of progress in functional imaging is expected to increase tumor control.[29] PET scans are, overall, most helpful in patients with locally advanced disease. In initial staging, PET has a sensitivity and specificity of about 90% for nodal staging, which makes PET more sensitive and specific than CT or MRI. Although a high specificity has been reported, a limitation has been identified with early-stage tumors (clinically N0 stages) because of its lower sensitivity of nodal disease at this early stage.

CT and MRI can identify up to 50% of primary tumors that show no clinical evidence of tumor on physical examination. Tumors that are not identified with CT scan or MRI are detected with a stand-alone PET scan (without fusion with CT). Stand-alone PET has a detection rate of 25% for localizing undetected tumors with these other two imaging modalities and an endoscopy examination. Fusion studies with CT are expected to produce a higher detection rate and should be performed instead of MRI or CT and before endoscopy.[32] PET demonstrates high sensitivity for restaging after RT; however, the optimal time for a PET study has been controversial. The recommended time is 3 months after treatment. A PET study before that time produces a higher chance of false-positive findings.[32]

Pathology

More than 80% of head and neck cancers arise from the surface epithelium of the mucosal linings of the upper digestive tract. These cancers are mostly SCCs. Adenocarcinomas are found to a lesser extent in the salivary glands. SCCs seen in the head and neck region include lymphoepithelioma, spindle cell carcinoma, verrucous carcinoma, and undifferentiated carcinoma. Lymphoepithelioma occurs in places of abundant lymphoid tissue (i.e., the nasopharynx, tonsil, and base of the tongue). Patients with this histologic type have a better cure rate than do patients with SCC.[1]

Undifferentiated lymphomas are similar histopathologically to undifferentiated carcinomas and should be treated as carcinomas if doubt exists after a microscopic evaluation. Box 29.3 lists some cell types found in the head and neck region. Tumor grading is classified as G1 (well differentiated), G2 (moderately well differentiated), or G3 (poorly differentiated). Well differentiated tumors generally have a lower cell proliferation rate and are less likely to have aggressive behavior.[33] A variety of nonepithelial malignancies, melanomas, soft tissue sarcomas (STSs), and plasmacytomas can also occur in the head and neck region.

Staging

Staging criteria is based on the combination of the American Joint Committee on Cancer (AJCC) *Cancer Staging Manual* and the Union for International Cancer Control (UICC) TNM (tumor, nodal, metastasis) classification. Recent work reflects significant changes of the 8th edition of the TNM classification for head and neck cancer, effective 2018. One notable change for oropharyngeal cancer is based on the HPV. Research has shown that HPV-positive cases are distinctly different from HPV-negative oropharyngeal cases. The new clinical and pathological TNM classification for HPV-positive cases was formed because of a better understanding of the disease behavior.[35,37]

The updates also reflect improved treatment outcomes because of technical advances in diagnostic imaging (MR, PET, CT) and radiotherapy planning (IMRT) as well as IGRT. What follows is a brief summary of the recent changes as described by Huang and O'Sullivan.[37]

In the newly published 8th edition TNM, the following changes have been made to the overall schema: (1) introduction of three new TNM classifications: HPV/ p16 immunostaining positive-mediated OPC, Head and Neck (HN)-STS, and HN unknown primary—cervical nodes (HN-CUP); (2) modification of the definition of the T and/or N categories in NPC; (3) modification of the T category by inclusion of

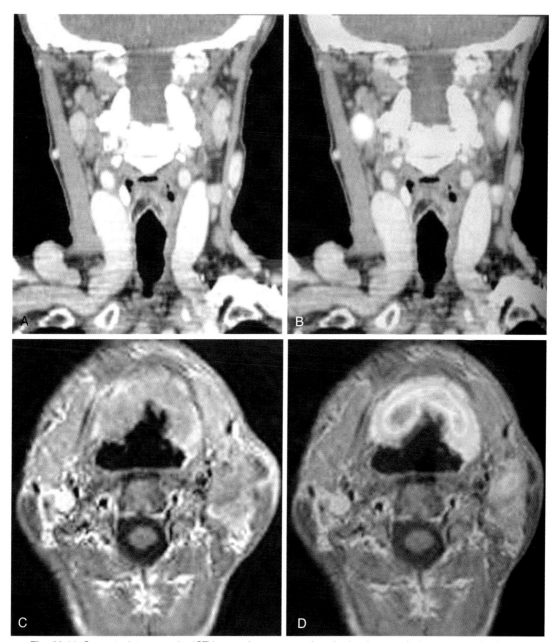

Fig. 29.11 Computed tomography (CT)/magnetic resonance imaging/positron emission tomography image fusion. (A) Postcontrast, reformatted CT image in the coronal plane shows bilateral, mildly enlarged metastatic modes in the carotid-jugular chains. Tumoral involvement of the nodes remains speculative because of borderline short-axis diameter and absence of obvious necrotic changes. (B) Superimposition of fluorodeoxyglucose positron emission tomography data on a CT image shows increased glucose uptake within the nodes. (C) transverse image of same anatomy in image A. (D) transverse image PET CT image fustion from image B. (From Gregoire V, Duprez T, Lengele B, et al. Management of the neck. In: Gunderson LL, Tepper JE, eds. *Clinical Radiation Oncology.* 3rd ed. Philadelphia, PA: Elsevier Saunders; 2012.)

the "depth of invasion" variable for oral cavity SCC; (4) modification of the N category by inclusion of the "extranodal extension" variable for nonviral-related mucosal HNC including salivary gland malignancies; and (5) reintroduction of size in the T categories for non-Merkel cell cutaneous carcinoma of the head and neck.[37–41]

A significant change from the 2018, 8th edition TNM classification for head and neck cancer is the separate clinical and pathological N definitions and T-N groupings. This is the first time both types of staging systems are introduced in the HNC classification.

The clinical staging system (cTNM) for head and neck cancers is based mostly on clinical diagnostic information that determines the size, extent, and presence of positive nodes. CT scan, MRI, and ultrasound scan have added to the accuracy of tumor (T) and nodal (N) staging in advanced stages, especially in cases that involve the nasopharynx, paranasal sinuses, and regional lymph nodes. Endoscopic evaluation also assures accuracy of the primary tumor staging. Any diagnostic information that contributes to the overall accuracy of the pretreatment assessment should be considered. Fine-needle

BOX. 29.3 Head and Neck Cancer Cell Types

- Squamous cell carcinoma
- Lymphoepithelioma
- Spindle cell carcinoma
- Verrucous carcinoma
- Undifferentiated carcinoma
- Non-Hodgkin lymphoma (NHL)
- Keratinized carcinoma
- Nonkeratinized carcinoma
- Adenocarcinoma
- Malignant mixed carcinoma
- Adenocystic carcinoma
- Mucoepidermoid carcinoma
- Acinic cell carcinoma

BOX. 29.4 Lymphatic Drainage by Site

Oral Cavity
- Lips into the submandibular, preauricular, and facial nodes
- Buccal mucosa into the submaxillary and submental nodes
- Gingiva into the submaxillary and jugulodigastric nodes
- Retromolar trigone into the submaxillary and jugulodigastric nodes
- Hard palate into the submaxillary and upper jugular nodes
- Floor of mouth into the submaxillary and jugular (middle and upper) nodes
- Anterior two thirds of the tongue into the submaxillary and upper jugular nodes

Oropharynx
- Base of the tongue into the jugulodigastric, low cervical, and retropharyngeal nodes
- Tonsillar fossa into the jugulodigastric and submaxillary nodes
- Soft palate into the jugulodigastric, submaxillary, and spinal accessory nodes
- Pharyngeal walls into the retropharyngeal nodes, pharyngeal nodes, and jugulodigastric nodes

Nasopharynx
- Retropharyngeal nodes into the superior jugular and posterior cervical nodes

Sinuses
- Retropharyngeal and superior cervical nodes

Larynx
- Glottis, extremely rare nodal involvement
- Subglottis into the peritracheal and low cervical nodes
- Supraglottis into the peritracheal, cervical submental, and submaxillary nodes

biopsy may confirm the presence of tumor and its histopathologic nature. This clinical staging system is based on the best possible estimate of the extent of disease before the first treatment. According to the AJCC handbook, when surgery is conducted, the cancer can be staged following pathologic staging (pTNM). This adds the pathologic findings of the resected specimen to the clinical staging but does not replace it.[18]

Staging criteria for the primary lesion are site specific. However, except for tumors in the nasopharynx, there is more uniformity in the nodal staging criteria and stage grouping for the system. NPCs are designated according to modified Union for International Committee on Cancer (UICC) staging. The staging categories provide a uniform description of advanced tumors whereby T4 lesions are divided into T4a (resectable) and T4b (unresectable). This allows descriptions of patients with advanced-stage disease to be grouped into three categories: stage IVA, advanced resectable disease; stage IVB, advanced unresectable disease; and stage IVC, advanced distant metastatic disease. Careful attention is given to the mobility of the nodes. Fixed nodes result in a poor prognosis. Contrast-enhanced CT and MRI scans can define the size and shape of the tumor better than a clinical evaluation. Three-dimensional (3D) multiplanar imaging has made staging much more precise and accurate for deeply invading disease and in the assessment of inaccessible neck nodes.

> The three basic descriptors—tumor, node, metastasis (TNM)—are grouped into stage categories. Refer to https://www.uicc.org/sites/main/files/atoms/files/TNM_Classification_of_Malignant_%20Tumours_8th_edition_24%20Jan%202018.pptx for a review of the UICC TNM Classification of Malignant Tumors.

Spread Patterns

The volume of the irradiated fields in the head and neck area is large because of the risk of nodal spread. The inferior cervical nodes are clinically positive in 6% to 23% of the cases for NPC. For this reason, the supraclavicular area necessitates treatment with an anterior port. Generally, hematogenous spread below the neck is rare, except in NPC or in the parotid gland. More than 75% of all head and neck cancers recur locally or regionally above the clavicle.[20]

NPC with known bilateral cervical node involvement has shown a 25% chance of bloodborne distant spread first to bone and then to lung. The normal lymphatic drainage by site is listed in Box 29.4. Box 29.5 lists areas of the head and neck region and the expected direct spread of a tumor in each area.

TREATMENT CONSIDERATIONS

General Principles

Radiation therapy and surgery are major curative modalities for head and neck cancers with adjuvant chemotherapy for advanced stages. The eradication of the disease, maintenance of physiologic function, and preservation of social cosmesis determine the best modality. The ability to cure and eradicate the disease without severe complications necessitates extremely selective treatment criteria. RT is indicated in most head and neck cancers because the tumors located in this region are often inaccessible for surgery. The goals of treatment, however, can only be achieved through a multidisciplinary approach that involves many specialists, as described in the first part of this chapter; the patient plays an important role. Emphasis is given to age and general condition, comorbidity factors (associated diseases, i.e., emphysema, cardiovascular disease), habits and lifestyle, occupation, and the patient's desires. It is pleasing to see that new editions of mainstream textbooks have now included sections devoted to quality of life, a new emphasis of the posttreatment aspect of care. Generally, small primary lesions with negative nodes are treated with one modality (surgery or radiotherapy). Small lesions with involved nodes may need both surgery and radiotherapy for control of neck disease. Large primary lesions (T3

BOX. 29.5 Expected Direct Spread of a Tumor

1. Lips
   a. Skin
   b. Commissure
   c. Mucosa
   d. Muscle
2. Gingiva
   a. Soft tissue and buccal mucosa
   b. Periosteum
   c. Bone and maxillary antrum
   d. Dental nerves
3. Buccal mucosa
   a. Side walls of the oral cavity
   b. Lips
   c. Retromolar trigone
   d. Muscles
4. Hard palate
   a. Soft palate
   b. Bone and maxillary antrum
   c. Nasal cavity
5. Trigone
   a. Buccal mucosa
   b. Anterior pillar
   c. Gingiva
   d. Pterygoid muscle
6. Floor of mouth
   a. Soft tissue, tonsils, and salivary glands
   b. Root of tongue
   c. Base of tongue
   d. Geniohyoid-mylohyoid muscles
7. Tongue
   a. Anterior two-thirds of tongue
   b. Lateral borders

c. Base and underside of tongue
d. Floor of mouth
8. Soft palate
   a. Tonsillar pillars
   b. Pharyngeal walls
   c. Hard palate
   d. Nasopharynx
9. Larynx
   a. True cords
   b. False cords
   c. Arytenoid muscles
   d. Epiglottis
   e. Hypopharynx
   f. Aryepiglottic folds
   g. Ventricles
10. Pharynx
    a. Anterior walls
    b. Posterior tongue
    c. Base of tongue
    d. Lateral walls
    e. Tonsillar pillars
    f. Uvula
    g. Soft palate
    h. Posterior walls
    i. Muscles and epiglottis
11. Tonsils
    a. Palatine-lingual tonsil
    b. Tonsillar pillars
    c. Base of tongue
    d. Soft palate
    e. Pharyngeal wall

---

and T4), extensive cervical node disease, or both, usually need surgery and irradiation and chemotherapy. Follow-up examinations at regular intervals to detect early recurrence, extension, or complications are important. Cases can often be salvaged if tumor recurrence is detected early.

Surgery

Surgical oncologists play a crucial role in staging. Although clinical staging is based on the results of a noninvasive physical examination and radiology, pathologic staging is based on findings in resected tumor specimens and biopsies. These findings reveal microscopic disease that is undetectable with imaging and serves to enhance the accuracy of the evaluation. Sabel[34] writes that clinical and pathologic staging may have two dramatically different outcomes. Fakhry, Zevallos, and Eisele[35] write that clinical stages N1, N2, and N3 are determined on the basis of size of lymph node and position, whereas in pathologic staging, only the number of lymph nodes is considered. Significant differences in overall survival estimates exist between the two staging methods. One example provided by Fakhry et al includes overall survival estimates for stages I, II, and III. With clinical staging, the estimate is 90%, whereas with pathologic staging, the estimate is 84%. Various factors that are beyond the scope of this chapter are accounted for in these differing results. However, overall, it is expressed that

pathological staging is a refinement of clinical staging, and both methods should provide prognostic information that is similar and used reliably.[35]

Surgical resection and reconstructive techniques produce good outcomes in most patients with early-stage tumors. The use of surgery as a curative modality is correlated to the possibility of an en bloc resection. Partial resections involve a high risk of recurrence. Wide margins (>2 cm) are usually necessary. A biopsy of the cervical nodes and lesion is mandatory and should be performed by experienced oncologic surgeons. Surgery is the mode of treatment for early-stage lesions of the oral cavity and floor of the mouth if no clinically positive nodes are present or if the risk of deep cervical node involvement is low. Surgery reduces the risk of dental or salivary damage seen with RT. Laser therapy, cryotherapy, and electrocautery are conventional curative surgical modalities.

Surgery has a higher success rate for palliative salvage therapy in the event of failure after RT. This holds true for conventional treatment only; accelerated treatments result in severe acute toxic effects that often require a feeding tube and mucosal healing time that takes several months. Salvage surgery in these cases is often challenging, especially in cases of oropharyngeal cancers treated via accelerated fractionation, where results include high incidence rates of complications and poor survival rates.[36]

Surgery offers better local control of disease that has invaded bone because curative RT doses have shown a high risk of necrosis. Microsurgery has revolutionized the approach to reconstruction of head and neck defects. Reconstructive procedures involve microvascular free flaps (a unit of tissue transferred en bloc from a donor to another recipient site) that consist of skin, myocutaneous tissue, the jejunum for replacement of the cervical esophagus, and bone grafts. Reconstruction of the midface, the oral cavity including the mandible, the base of tongue, and the hypopharynx has made the plastic surgeon an essential member of the head and neck disease management team.

Neck Dissection

Crile described the first removal of the regional neck nodes in 1906 for treatment of metastatic spread. Some form of a neck dissection has been included in most treatment plans since then. The radical neck dissection or **RND** is regarded as the gold standard for the treatment of neck disease.[24] RND removes the lymph nodes from levels I through V, the sternocleidomastoid muscle (SCM), the internal jugular (IJ) vein, and the spinal accessory/eleventh cranial nerve. The modified RND attempts to decrease morbidity by sparing the SCM, the IJ vein, and the 11th cranial nerve, depending on the location of the metastatic nodes. Various selective neck dissections preserve whole nodal levels to reduce morbidity further.[24] Fig. 29.12 illustrates steps of an RND.

The relation between wound healing and RT is not favorable after high doses. Both acute inflammatory changes in tissues and late radiation changes that include fibrosis and decreased vascularity require careful consideration. Wound healing is impaired by factors that include diminished blood supply, impaired collagen formation, and increased risk of infection in part from decreased leukocyte function. Healing complications are common in cases of myocutaneous flaps that involve tissue that is considered to be "severely injured" by high doses of radiation. An interesting note involves an irradiated hollow organ such as the trachea that requires resection and anastomosis. It is suggested that sparing one side from radiation exposure maintains a path of vascularity for better blood supply to the healing anastomosis and reduces fistula formation and leakage.[42]

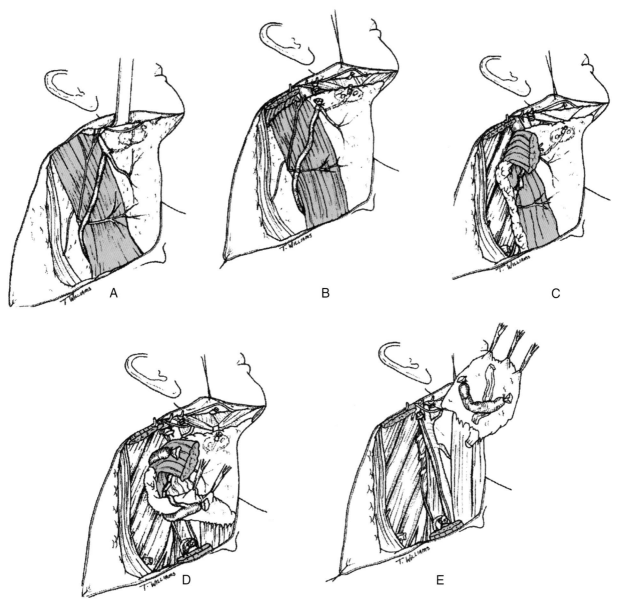

Fig. 29.12 Steps in a radical neck dissection. (A) Skin flaps are raised. The sternocleidomastoid muscle (SCM) is exposed, along with cranial nerves. (B) A flap is raised to protect the marginal mandibular nerve. (C) The SCM is detached from the mastoid, and the posterior border is delineated. (D) The internal jugular vein is ligated, and the neck-dissection specimen is raised from posterior to anterior. (E) The specimen is removed from the carotid sheath and medial attachment. (From Wolfe MJ, Wilson K. Head and neck cancer. In: Sabel MS, Sondak VK, Sussman JJ, eds. *Surgical Foundations: Essentials of Surgical Oncology.* Philadelphia, PA: Mosby; 2007.)

General Overview of Chemotherapy

Induction or neoadjuvant chemotherapy is useful in cases such as treatment of advanced NPCs before RT, as a radiosensitizer during treatment, or as an adjuvant after treatment. Combination chemotherapy for palliation of recurrence or metastases of NPC produces complete response rates up to 44%.[43]

The role of chemotherapy in head and neck cancer is standard for metastatic disease, locally recurrent disease, or salvage therapy for which surgery and RT can no longer be used. Chemotherapy's role is in primary head and neck cancer limited, but evolving. Single-agent therapy with methotrexate, cisplatin, carboplatin, bleomycin,

5-fluorouracil (5-FU), hydroxyurea, ifosfamide, and the taxanes paclitaxel and docetaxel produces responses that last from 2 to 6 months. Combination drug therapy has produced higher response rates, but the prognosis has not improved, and the toxicity to the patient is higher. Cisplatin-containing combinations have produced the highest overall and complete remission rates. The average duration of response has been 11.3 months for patients with complete remission. Cisplatin and 5-FU continue to be the most frequently used combination regimen. Among the newer multiagent chemotherapeutic regimens are those that combine cisplatin with agents such as the taxanes or ifosfamide. Overall survival rates for combination chemotherapy have been similar to those of single-agent therapy.[3] Neoadjuvant (induction) chemotherapy is the initial utilization of chemotherapy before local therapy, as a first-line modality. Neither induction chemotherapy nor adjuvant chemotherapy has improved survival when added to locoregional therapy; this includes multiagent regimens. Concurrent irradiation and chemotherapy yields a small increase in survival rate relative to irradiation alone, but complication rates also increased.[1] Because of the poor health and nutritional status of patients with head and neck cancer, the use of chemotherapy as a frontline modality has not been favorable.

Recent studies have involved the comparison of survival and overall outcome of concomitant relative to induction chemotherapy. In a study of locally advanced larynx cancer with the objective to preserve the larynx (no surgery), patients received induction cisplatin with fluorouracil (PF) followed by RT, concomitant cisplatin with RT, or RT alone. Overall survival did not differ significantly, although there was the possibility of worse outcome with concomitant relative to induction chemotherapy. Concomitant cisplatin with RT significantly improved the larynx preservation rate over that of induction PF followed by RT, as well as over RT alone; however, induction PF followed by RT was not better than treatment with RT alone. No differences in late effects were detected, but deaths not attributed to laryngeal cancer or treatment were higher with concomitant chemotherapy. After a 10.8-year follow-up period, conclusions still suggest no significant difference in locoregional control and larynx preservation. What was significant was the finding that the advantage of preservation by concomitant treatment was offset by extra mortality of that group. Both concomitant and induction chemotherapy followed by RT were deemed reasonable options for the patient whose surgical alternative is total laryngectomy. Suggestions have been made that concomitant chemotherapy may be offered to the fit patient who wants to maximize the chance to skip a (major) surgical operation and induction reserved for the patient with borderline fitness (acute toxicity during RT is lower with induction). Studies continue to clarify the cause of death and to help select patients accordingly.[45,45]

One institution's policy is to place a percutaneous endoscopic gastrostomy tube before the start of treatment in patients with head and neck cancers who will undergo concomitant chemoradiotherapy.[46]

General Overview of Proton Beam Radiation Therapy

Much has been written about the advantages of proton beam RT (PBRT). With the increasing numbers of proton therapy centers, access to PBRT is becoming a greater reality as an alternate treatment option today, the basis of which is the unique physical properties that deliver higher doses to tumor while minimizing the dose to surrounding tissue. The outcome achieves our classic goal for RT. As a quick review, we know that protons enter the body with low energy being deposited until a rapid increase in the deposit occurs with the Bragg peak. This follows a minimal exit dose, unlike a photon beam. The outcome allows the sparing of normal tissue while delivering a relatively higher dose to the tumor. The physical properties of this type of beam result in decreased acute toxicity and late reactions. This also provides benefits to sparing contralateral areas such as the treatment of the salivary gland. Many other applications for the treatment of head and neck cancer have been noted within the body of literature. The more recent studies focus on the use of PBRT to reirradiate recurrent disease. This modality of reirradiation therapy has specific benefits because of the specific morbidity that treating an already irradiated area

can cause. Despite advances in treatment of head and neck cancer, locoregional recurrences will develop in a high percent of patients. Recurrent disease is typically treated with surgery or chemotherapy because of the high degree of toxicity a second course of RT will produce, although a lower rate of toxicity has been reported with conformal radiation techniques.[47]

Radiation Therapy

The use of radiation is considered the mainstay of cancer management for the treatment of choice in the head and neck region. The choice of external beam RT or brachytherapy depends on the individual and the location of the tumor. Customization of the treatment technique is essential, although Khan[48] reports that the simple electron beam provides a useful ancillary technique for boosting doses to superficial regions in the head and neck area and is still in use today in some centers.

Contemporary treatment planning allows 3D planning with patient data obtained from CT, MRI, and PET. Advances in software provide complex treatments such as 3D conformal RT (3D-CRT), IMRT, IGRT, and high-dose-rate (HDR) brachytherapy. Sophisticated computer and imaging technology make inverse treatment planning the basis for IMRT. Standard fractionation schedules use daily treatments, 5 days per week, for approximately 6.5 to 7.5 weeks. Altered fraction schedules show improvement in tumor control; however, accelerated treatments also show a higher incidence of morbidity. SCCs with long doubling times are treated effectively with standard fractionation (200 cGy per day, 5 days a week). SCCs vary in doubling times; those with shorter doubling times show poorer control and may be treated more effectively with accelerated hyperfractionation (120 cGy, twice daily).

Attention to healthy tissue tolerance for clinicians, radiation therapists, and treatment planners is essential in delivery of a prescribed dose of RT. The Quantitative Analysis of Normal Tissue Effects in the Clinic (QUANTEC) report summarizes the currently available 3D dose/volume/outcome data.[49]

Table 29.5 provides the tolerance doses for several organs after conventional fractionation in the head and neck area.

Patient Positioning and Immobilization

Accurate and reproducible treatment has always been an important aspect of high-quality RT. The importance of precise reproducibility has grown with increased interest in 3D conformal therapy and dose escalation. The objective of tumor control with these new techniques involves higher doses with use of tighter target margins to limit the dose to adjacent healthy tissues. Precision calls for the use of numerous noninvasive immobilization techniques based on thermoplastic mask immobilization, customized polyurethane cradles and extended head to shoulder/upper thorax immobilization, and longer headboards that extend from the head to the upper thorax for additional support of the head and shoulders. The S-frame secures the shoulders in addition to the head and neck.[50] IGRT systems have been useful as an effective tool for confirmation of reproducibility once the patient has been immobilized.

The treatment of head and neck cancers involves the following general patient positioning principles for many cases. Patient positioning for the treatment of head and neck cancers, however, may be dependent on the specific type of cancer treated and the radiation oncologist's objectives regarding tumor volume and the sparing of healthy tissue. For instance, the treatment of a maxillary antrum usually necessitates that the patient's head be positioned

TABLE. 29.5 The Quantitative Analysis of Normal Tissue Effects in the Clinic Report for Tissue Complication Probability for Several Organs After Conventional Fractionation in the Head and Neck Region

Organ	Whole/Partial Organ	Dose (Cgy) Or Dose/ Volume Paremeters	Rate (%)	End Point
Optic nerve/chiasm	Whole organ	<5500	<3	Optic neuropathy
	Whole organ	5500–6000	3-7	Optic neuropathy
	Whole organ	>6000	>7–20	Optic neuropathy
Spinal cord	Partial organ	5000	0.2	Myelopathy
	Partial organ	6000	6	Myelopathy
	Partial organ	6900	50	Myelopathy
Cochlea	Whole organ	Mean dose less than or equal to 4500	<30	Sensory neural hearing loss
Parotid	Unilateral whole parotid gland	Mean dose >2000	<20	Long-term parotid salivary function reduced to <25% of preradiation therapy level
	Bilateral whole parotid glands	Mean dose <2500	<20	Long-term parotid salivary function reduced to <25% of preradiation therapy level
	Bilateral whole parotid glands	Mean dose <3900	<50	Long-term parotid salivary function reduced to <25% of preradiation therapy level
Pharynx	Pharyngeal constrictors	Mean dose <5000	<20	Symptomatic dysphagia and aspiration
Larynx	Whole organ	<6600	<20	Vocal dysfunction
	Whole organ	<5000	<30	Aspiration
	Whole organ	<4400	<20	Edema
	Whole organ	50 volume receiving <27%	<20	Edema
Brain	Whole organ	<6000	<3	Symptomatic necrosis
	Whole organ	7200	5	Symptomatic necrosis
	Whole organ	9000	10	Symptomatic necrosis
Brainstem	Whole organ	<6400	<5	Permanent cranial neuropathy or necrosis

Modified from Marks LB, Yorke ED, Jackson A, et al. Use of normal tissue complication probability models in the clinic, *Int J Radiat Oncol Biol Phys.* 2010;76(3):S10–S19.

with the chin extended to include the cephalad extent of the maxillary antrum in an anterior field without also including the eye. For most cases, the patient is in the supine position with the neck extended and the head resting on an appropriate headrest.[51,52] Tumor cells trapped in the surgical scars are generally believed to be less well oxygenated and therefore more radioresistant; higher radiation doses are believed necessary to eradicate them.[30] This may be achieved with an additional electron boost field or with maximization of the dose to the skin in the area with tissue-equivalent bolus material. A tongue blade with a cork attached to one end, or another similar device, may be inserted between the incisor teeth to depress the tongue, displace the tongue from the treatment volume, or displace the palate (Fig. 29.13). The head is immobilized with a customized thermoplastic face mask that is fixed to a base plate under the patient's head, which, in turn, may or may not be indexed to the treatment couch. A small hole may be made in the mask when a bite block, positional stent, or nasogastric tube is used (Fig. 29.14).[48]

If lateral photon portals are used, the shoulders should be displaced inferiorly as much as possible to maximize the utility of the lateral portals. Inferior displacement of the shoulders can be accomplished with the patient's arms being pulled by two ends of a strap wrapped around a footboard.[20] A strap with Velcro at two ends may secure the strap around the patient's wrists, routing the strap from one wrist, to both feet, to the other wrist while the knees are bent.

Straightening the knees pulls the shoulders down. Contemporary methods also use thermoplastic facemask-customized headrests. The shoulders are immobilized with either an extended mask or with a customized indexed handholding system.[53] Patients with short necks or those unable to displace their shoulders inferiorly pose a treatment planning problem. Another solution involves the use of lateral fields that are angled inferiorly to obtain better inferior coverage. This is done by rotating the foot of the treatment table 10 to 20 degrees away from the gantry.

A mouth stent or tongue blade may serve more than one purpose. Mouth stents may separate or displace the palate, thereby sparing it from treatment. A tongue blade may serve to either depress and fix the tongue within a field or displace it out of the field.

Treatment Data Capture and Treatment Planning

Imaging and modern treatment planning are inseparable. The most useful modalities are CT scan and MRI. Often a diagnostic MRI or a PET scan is fused to the treatment planning CT scan. Meticulous communication and a supervising form of continuity of care must exist from aspects of proper patient positioning as the process goes from initial image acquisition and localization to actual treatment delivery. Factors of error typically include imaging without a flat table and inconsistency in shape, form, and thickness or placement

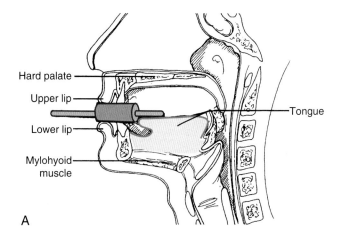

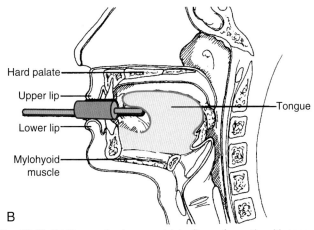

Fig. 29.13 (A) Tongue is depressed into floor of mouth with tongue blade and cork or bite block if tumor invasion includes the tongue. (B) Tip of tongue is displaced from treatment field when a lesion is limited to the anterior floor of the mouth. Tongue blade is positioned under the tongue.

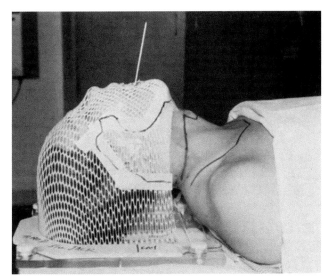

Fig. 29.14 Treatment position of a patient with nasopharyngeal carcinoma. (From Hoppe RT, Phillips TL, Roach M. *Leibel and Phillips Textbook of Radiation Oncology.* 3rd ed. Philadelphia, PA: Saunders; 2010.)

of positioning aids as the patient moves from the planning to the treatment stage. Hong et al report that highly conformal techniques referring to IMRT have revolutionized the treatment of head and neck cancers significantly, reducing toxicity to normal tissues. However, in studying types of variances among 20 institutions who were asked to contour an identical case, "substantial heterogeneity" was observed, with the "largest uncertainty" in target delineation because of "interobserver variability." The risk posed to patient delivery by the variability in treatment planning was risking a systematic error in dose delivery because of variation in contour delineation among staff.[54]

Improvement has been shown with more sophisticated and patient-dedicated devices and with dedicated imaging staff within the RT department. Dedicated staff for imaging capabilities integrated within the RT department have become the standard for progressive treatment planning. Conventional simulators, equipped with fluoroscopy, have, for the most part, disappeared from the forefront. Although they were once useful for final verification of a CT simulation, the development of digitally reproduced radiographs, special CT simulation software, portal imaging systems, and especially IGRT have made the conventional simulator outdated. A dedicated CT scanner with wide apertures and flat tabletops and accessories to accurately reproduce treatment conditions is now standard for the department. CT data sets to view images in any plane marks only one of the many advances in technology for treatment planning and delivery. Added information for treatment planning heterogeneity corrections is also provided. Beam arrangements can be either coplanar or noncoplanar. Field-in-field boost techniques may be facilitated with multileaf collimation (MLC) to deliver additional dose to a subset of a larger treatment field. The manual beam patching technique referred to as the *field-in-field technique* is a forward-planning technique to achieve a more desirable dose distribution.[17]

Most advanced conformal RT is designed with treatment planning by means of prescribing a target dose and letting the computer generate the optimal plan. Inverse treatment planning systems work with the defined target dose and programmed healthy tissue tolerance doses to optimize the number of beam portals and the beam intensity pattern within each portal to generate the best dose distribution to fit the prescription. IMRT is based on this inverse approach to treatment planning. There are multiple treatment planning systems today applying very sophisticated techniques.[55]

These techniques include a new version of helical tomotherapy that uses more sophisticated equipment: RapidArc (Varian Medical Systems, Palo Alto, CA), a volumetric-modulated arc therapy (VMAT) that permits the delivery of highly conformal dose distributions via rotational delivery, as opposed to classic IMRT, which uses fixed gantry beams, or the sliding window technique for IMRT and other techniques.[46]

SITE-SPECIFIC STUDY OF CANCERS OF THE HEAD AND NECK

The Oral Cavity Region

Anatomy. The oral cavity extends from the skin-vermilion junction of the lip to the posterior border of the hard palate superiorly and to the circumvallate papillae inferiorly. Subdivisions within the oral cavity include the anterior two-thirds of the tongue (anterior to the circumvallate papillae), lip, buccal mucosa, lower alveolar ridge, upper alveolar ridge, retromolar trigone, floor of mouth, and hard palate (Figs. 29.15 and 29.16).

Clinical Presentation. Patients who have oral cavity cancer often have poor oral and dental hygiene. In females, Plummer-Vinson syndrome (iron-deficiency anemia) is considered an important etiologic factor. Because premalignant conditions are usually asymptomatic, the general practitioner or dentist is responsible for clinical detection. Early diagnosis is essential for a good prognosis. The areas cited to be least commonly examined are the paralingual gutters.

As previously stated, leukoplakia and erythroplasia represent severe dysplastic changes and should be regarded as serious pathologic problems. Most often, oral cavity cancers appear as nonhealing ulcers with little pain. Localized pain is considered a symptom of advanced disease.

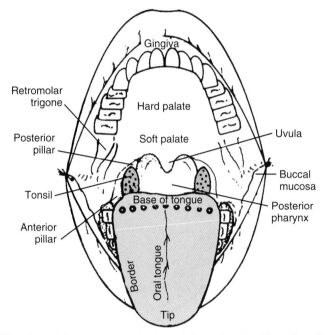

Fig. 29.15 A front open-mouth view of the oral cavity. (From Cox JD. *Moss' Radiation Oncology: Rationale, Technique, Results.* 7th ed. St. Louis, MO: Mosby; 1994.)

Diagnostic Procedures and Staging. Institutions commonly include the multidisciplinary tumor board, which comprises radiologists, surgeons, pathologists, and oncologists, in the review of diagnostic studies before or shortly after target delineation. Clinical target volumes are then defined as determined from preoperative diagnostic imaging studies, surgical and pathologic findings, and surgical defects and postoperative changes on the postoperative CT scan. Inspection and palpation are important first steps. The malignant ulcer is typically raised and centrally ulcerated, with indurated edges and an infiltrated base. Biopsy is mandatory. Clinical examination and imaging modalities include both CT and MRI and other modalities for staging of disease and for posttreatment follow-up. Physical examination, including fiberoptic laryngoscopy when possible, and PET and CT are obtained 3 to 4 months after treatment for assessment of treatment response and then 1 year after treatment for surveillance. For patients with suspicious findings on physical examination, CT scan, PET imaging, or biopsies are obtained to confirm the recurrence with fine-needle aspiration with ultrasound or CT guidance or with panendoscopy and directed biopsies performed with general anesthesia. If biopsy results are positive, salvage surgery may be performed if the patient is a suitable surgical candidate. Treatment outcome is determined with comparison of imaging studies, including CT, MRI, and PET.[56]

Histopathology. SCC accounts for 90% to 95% of the histopathologic types, either well differentiated or moderately well differentiated. Unusual variants of SCC include verrucous carcinoma and spindle cell SCC. Adenocarcinomas of the salivary gland may be identified.

Staging. Refer to the *UICC TNM Classification of Malignant Tumors.*

Metastatic Behavior. Cervical lymph node involvement at the time of presentation is uncommon, and oral cavity cancer has the lowest incidence (except glottic cancer) of nodal metastasis in the head and neck region. Bloodborne spread occurs in fewer than 20% of patients. Of those patients, most have cervical node involvement at the time of presentation and advanced-stage disease.

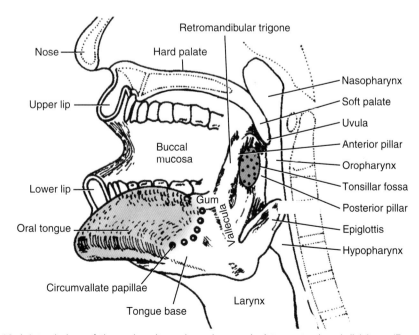

Fig. 29.16 A lateral view of the oral cavity and oropharynx depicts anatomic subdivisions. (From Cox JD. *Moss' Radiation Oncology: Rationale, Technique, Results.* 7th ed. St. Louis, MO: Mosby; 1994.)

Early-stage (<1 to 1.5 cm) and premalignant lesions are candidates for surgery alone. If inadequate surgical margins and neck node involvement are present, combination RT and surgery is indicated. The sequence of the therapy is usually dictated by the first treatment's design. If radical surgery is planned, the RT should not be given before surgery. Elective irradiation of the lymph nodes is included if a lesion has a high rate of spread or has a history of bilateral spread (anatomically) via the lymphatics. A 5-year follow-up plan is recommended because lesions in most sites recur within 2 years and rarely after 4 years.

RADIATION THERAPY FOR REGIONS OF THE ORAL CAVITY

Local regional control depends on accurate, consistent treatment delivery after a treatment plan with sharp dose gradients from the target volume to neighboring healthy tissue. IMRT, as a highly conformal modality of treatment, involves a degree of risk that may compromise local regional control in the treatment of targets within the oral cavity given the potential for significant movement. The challenge of contouring a postoperative tumor bed adds to the complexity. However, the Dana Farber Cancer Institute reports data that suggest that IMRT is safe and efficacious in the adjuvant setting for carcinomas of the oral cavity.[50] Induction therapy is considered for patients with T4 tumors or N3 nodal disease. After induction chemotherapy, concurrent chemoradiotherapy is delivered in all cases, typically with a platinum-based regimen. Patients are then strongly urged to undergo prophylactic percutaneous gastrostomy (PEG) tube placement before starting radiotherapy.

During IMRT, all gross disease receives a dose of 70 Gy, with a 0-mm to 5-mm expansion for the planning tumor volume (PTV). Volumes at high risk for microscopic disease (i.e., primary tumor clinical tumor volume [CTV] and high-risk lymph node CTV) receive a dose of 64 Gy with a 5-mm expansion for PTV. The lowest-risk CTV, which primarily encompasses the contralateral or low neck, is treated to 60 Gy. Patients may be treated to a total of 72 Gy to the primary lesion, with 66 Gy to high-risk CTV and 60 Gy to the low-risk CTV; the final 6 Gy is delivered with an en face electron field. For patients who receive induction chemotherapy, the original extent of tumor is used to define the target volumes.[50]

Recent studies that describe IMRT techniques for the oral cavity include patient populations with various disease sites within the oral cavity. Although the sites targeted within the oral cavity differ, the high level of beam sculpting with specific customized beam conformity is unique to each individual. The general techniques and doses described for carcinomas of the oral cavity have been reported in studies involving the following regions: the oral tongue, buccal mucosa, hard palate, retromolar trigone, floor of mouth, mandible, lip, and a few other sites within the oral cavity.[50,56,57]

The Oral Cavity: The Lip. The lymphatics of the upper lip drain into the submandibular and preauricular nodal beds (Fig. 29.17). Lymphatics from the midlower lip and anterior floor of the mouth drain into the submental nodal group (Fig. 29.18). Lymphatics from the oral tongue drain into the anterior cervical chain; more anteriorly placed lesions drain lower in the neck than do lesions placed more posteriorly (Fig. 29.19).

Lip cancer is treated with RT in the same manner as skin cancer; however, most cases can be surgically removed. Tumors that should be treated with RT are those that involve a commissure to obtain better cosmesis and local control in cases of more advanced disease.

Successful control is achievable, though, with electron beam RT, interstitial implants, or both. Single, anterior source-to-skin distance

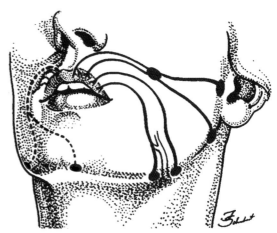

Fig. 29.17 Lymphatics of the upper lip drain into buccal, parotid, upper cervical, and submandibular nodes. Lymphatics of the skin of the upper lip *(dotted line)* may cross midline to terminate in submental and submandibular nodes of the contralateral side. (From Cox JD. *Moss' Radiation Oncology: Rationale, Technique, Results.* 7th ed. St. Louis, MO: Mosby; 1994.)

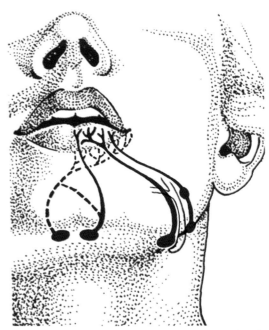

Fig. 29.18 Lymphatics of the lower lip drain to submental and submandibular nodes. Sometimes disease involves facial nodes. Lymphatics of the skin of the lower lip *(dotted line)* may cross midline to end in submental or submandibular nodes on the contralateral side. (From Cox JD. *Moss' Radiation Oncology: Rationale, Technique, Results.* 7th ed. St. Louis, MO: Mosby; 1994.)

ports, 100-kVp to 200-kVp x-rays, or 3-MeV to 7-MeV electrons at the 100% isodose line, are a common regimen. Protracted treatment schedules (4 to 6 weeks) with deliveries of 200 to 300 cGy per day can be given for lesions less than 2 cm. Larger, bulkier lesions need doses of 5000 to 6000 cGy. Regional (submental) lymphatics are rarely treated, whereas patients with advanced-stage or recurrent disease should have neck irradiation. Face shielding must be constructed to delineate the target volume and thus only expose 1 to 2 cm of healthy tissue. A lead shield is designed and positioned in place to expose the lip lesion. The lesion may be treated with 100-kVp x-rays through a cone. To reduce complications to teeth and gums, a stent coated with wax or a

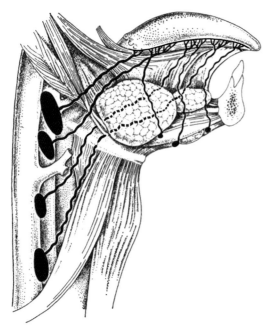

Fig. 29.19 Lymphatics of the tongue, illustrating that the more anteriorly they originate in the tongue, the lower in the neck their draining nodes may lie. (From Cox JD. *Moss' Radiation Oncology: Rationale, Technique, Results.* 7th ed. St. Louis, MO: Mosby; 1994.)

low-atomic-number compound (tissue equivalent) can be made to fit over the teeth. A stent is a lead shield that may consist of two sheets of lead (each one-eighth inch thick) overlaid with one sheet of aluminum and coated with wax or vinyl. The facemask shielding should also be coated with wax to reduce the electron scatter to the adjacent tissues. Exit radiation to the bone and gums needs to be controlled at safe levels to prevent progressive, long-term physiologic changes. With megavoltage electron energies, a tissue compensator is sometimes used to make the dose more uniform. Local control with interstitial implant is comparable with that achieved with electron beam treatment. For larger lesions, better cosmetic results are obtained with electron beam treatment.

If the tumor is less than 1 cm and lip function can be preserved, surgery is regarded as the best option. In larger tumors, brachytherapy can be a good alternative to surgery. Treatment with low-dose-rate (LDR) brachytherapy may be performed with iridium 192 (^{192}Ir) wires, and a HDR afterloading system with a ^{192}Ir stepping source may be used for HDR brachytherapy. Compared results of treatment have shown the equality of HDR brachytherapy and LDR brachytherapy in the treatment of lip cancer in terms of local and regional control. In addition, the observed acute and late toxicity rates are not significantly different between the two treatments.[58]

LDR brachytherapy in the treatment of lip cancer may deliver a mean total dose of 65 Gy for superficial tumors (thickness, <5 mm) and 68 Gy for more infiltrating lesions, according to the Paris system rules. HDR may consist of a total dose of 45 Gy within 5 days.[58]

The Oral Cavity: The Floor of the Mouth.
Historically, the medical literature has suggested that most cancers of the floor of the mouth are treated with resection. The optimal management of oral cavity SCCs typically involves primary surgical resection and adjuvant radiotherapy. On the basis of work by the Dana Farber Cancer and Brigham and Women's Hospital over the last 10 years, IMRT has become the standard technique in the treatment of oral cavity cancers, including the floor of the mouth.[43] However, megavoltage external beam alone gives

inferior control results, even for T1 lesions. Surgical techniques and reconstruction have improved over time and currently show improved functional outcomes; however, the only treatment approach that has enhanced locoregional control and overall survival has been the use of adjuvant chemoradiotherapy. Reports of several studies show that good local control may also be achieved with a combination of external irradiation interstitial implants or intraoral cone.[20]

Cancers in this area arise on the anterior surface on either side of the midline. They can spread to the bone and tongue. About 30% of these cancers have positive submaxillary and subdigastric nodes. Therefore, opposed lateral ports can be used. If the lesion is small and confined to the floor of the mouth, the tip of the tongue is elevated out of the portal with a cork or bite block. If the lesion has grown into the tongue, the tongue is flattened with a bite block to reduce the superior border of the portal (see Fig. 29.13A,B). A small stainless steel fiducial marker may be inserted into the posterior border of the tumor and serves as a marker for treatment planning (simulation) and brachytherapy.

The Oral Cavity: The Tongue.
Both the anterior tongue and the base of tongue are discussed in this section. Note that only the anterior two-thirds are included in the oral cavity. The base of tongue is considered to be in the oropharynx. The oral tongue is the freely mobile portion of the tongue that extends anteriorly from the line of circumvallate papillae to the undersurface of the tongue at the junction of the floor of the mouth. It is composed of four areas: the tip, the lateral borders, the dorsum, and the undersurface (nonvillous surface of the tongue).

Small tumors that arise in the anterior two-thirds of the tongue, also known as the oral tongue, are usually resected. RT is used in patients who are medically inoperable. Postoperative RT to the primary site and the cervical lymph nodes is used to cover positive margins, extensive primary tumor with bone or skin invasion, and multiple positive nodes. The anterior tongue drains into the submandibular lymph nodes, and the posterior portion of the tongue drains more to the jugulodigastric, posterior pharyngeal, and upper cervical lymph nodes (Fig. 20.19).

Lesions of the tongue usually appear on the lateral borders near the middle and posterior third section. The lesions can be quite large and still confined to the tongue (Fig. 29.20). Only a limited number of tongue cancers can be completely excised. Lesions on the tip of the tongue are seen first and are commonly in an early stage, whereas lesions at the base and posterior one-third of the tongue that invade the floor of the mouth, the tonsils, or the muscles are advanced and have a higher incidence of nodal metastasis. Base of tongue cancer is highly infiltrative, and clinical understaging is common.[27] An early-stage lesion of the tongue can be cured with a local excision or hemiglossectomy (surgical removal of half the tongue). For the preservation of speech and swallowing functions, external beam treatment is the best choice for large T3 to T4 lesions. ^{192}Ir implants can external beam treatment. Brachytherapy requires a preprocedure tracheotomy because the tongue swells massively after the implant.

A study from the University of Iowa Healthcare[11] that focused on failure patterns after IMRT for oral cavity cases considered carcinomas of the oral tongue a high risk for contralateral lymph node involvement; therefore, bilateral neck is critical to include in the radiation field. The report explains that there is a much higher risk for contralateral regional failure in oral tongue cancer because oral tongue has multiple and rich lymphatic intercommunications compared with other regions of oral cavity. Some surgeons suggest performing continuous neck dissection for oral tongue cancer (i.e., en block resection of the primary tumor, the selective neck dissection, and the region between the primary tumor and regional lymph nodes). For anterior lateral oral tongue cancer, such surgery necessitates more extensive resection and potentially more complications. This area should be included

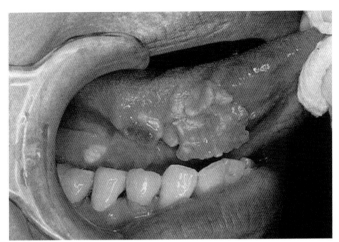

Fig. 29.20 Advanced exophytic carcinoma that had been noted for more than 6 months. (From Silverman S. *Oral Cancer.* 5th ed. Hamilton, Ontario, Canada: BC Decker; 2003. Reprinted by the permission of the American Cancer Society, Inc.)

as a high-dose radiation field during IMRT in postoperative RT. The report explains further that neck dissection may predispose aberrant migration of in-transit cancer cells to the opposite side of the neck. Therefore, contralateral neck should be included in the radiation field in postoperative IMRT for oral tongue cancer.[56] Treatment failures have included cases of regional metastasis traced to the multiple and rich lymphatic intercommunications of the oral tongue that crossed midline to the contralateral lymph node involvement.

The Oral Cavity: The Buccal Mucosa. The buccal mucosa is the mucous membrane that lines the inner surface of the cheeks and lips. Most lesions originate on the lateral walls, have a history of leukoplakia, and appear as a raised, exophytic growth. As it grows, the lesion invades the skin and bone. Usually, the patient notices a bump with the tip of the tongue. Pain is not associated with this lesion unless the nerves to the tongue or ear become involved. Advanced lesions bleed. Early lesions often appear as an inflammatory process, so care should be taken during a biopsy to obtain a differential diagnosis.

Stensen's duct can become obstructed. This enlarges the parotid gland, thereby necessitating surgical intervention. Small (1-cm) lesions can be excised, whereas larger lesions are treatable with combination surgery/RT, radical surgery, or aggressive RT alone.

If conventional RT is chosen as a treatment modality, a single photon or electron beam that spares contralateral tissues, especially the contralateral parotid, can be used. The submaxillary and subdigastric nodes are at risk. If positive, these nodes require a controlling dose. The classic large field technique usually consists of 5500 to 6000 cGy in 6 weeks, followed by a boost of 2000 cGy that spares the mandible.[20] In advanced tumors, RT is followed by surgical resection of the lesion and regional lymph nodes. Fibrosis of the cheek and trismus are not infrequent complications after radical RT. T1 lesions can be treated with oral cone alone, 6000 cGy in 15 fractions, or an implant to deliver 6000 cGy in 6 to 7 days.

Three-dimensional conformal therapy has been exclusively recommended to spare the contralateral parotid.[5] Large buccal mucosal tumors may be treated with 3D conformal therapy, with delivery of 7500 cGy with sparing of healthy structures.

The Oral Cavity: The Hard Palate. The hard palate is the semilunar area between the upper alveolar ridge and the mucous membrane that covers the palatine process of the maxillary palatine bones. It extends from the inner surface of the superior alveolar ridge to the posterior edge of the palatine bone. Hard palate carcinomas are quite rare and are mostly adenocarcinomas, adenoid cystic carcinomas known for a perineural (around nerves) pattern of spread. Most malignant tumors of the hard palate are of minor salivary gland origin. SCC is rare. They tend to spread to the bone and invade the maxillary antrum. Adenoid cystic types spread hematogenously to lungs and bone and along the second branch of the fifth cranial nerve to the middle fossa. These types of tumors seldom metastasize to lymph nodes. Surgical resection is the usual treatment, with postoperative RT given as needed in patients at high risk. Irradiation with surface molds can treat very superficial lesions.[5] Cancers in this area have been noted to be the result of secondary spread from the upper gum. A history of ill-fitting dentures or trauma is common. Postoperative RT is added in patients at high risk.

The Oral Cavity: The Retromolar Trigone. The retromolar trigone is the triangular space behind the last molar tooth. Carcinomas of this area are rare. Lesions can cause tongue pain, ear canal pain, or, if the muscles become involved, trismus. Indirect extension begins with early invasion of the anterior tonsillar pillar or the buccal mucosa. The retromolar trigone is included in the minimum target volume for the treatment of early tonsillar cancers.[27] Gomez and colleagues[5] indicate that they are indistinguishable from carcinomas that arise from the anterior tonsillar pillar. Most are moderately differentiated SCCs. CT scan and MRI in selected cases can show deep extension like bone invasion and positive neck nodes. Invasion of the pterygoid muscles that produce trismus is better imaged on MRI than on CT scan.[31] Lymphatic spread occurs to the submaxillary and subdigastric nodes. Mendenhall[31] report that local control rates for T1 and T2 lesions are similar with surgery or RT. Small lesions without bone invasion can be resected, but superficial T3 lesions can be treated with RT alone.[31] Gomez and associates[5] report that lesions of the retromolar trigone are treated in a highly selected manner. T1 and T2 tumors are treated with RT, but surgical resection is the preferred modality. More advanced tumors necessitate surgery and postoperative RT.

Early lesions may be treated with external RT alone with mixed beams. The large-field conventional treatment technique involves electrons and photons with single lateral fields or parallel opposing fields with 2:1 weighting that favors the diseased side. IMRT treatment doses for regions of the oral cavity have been provided previously; for conventional treatment, 6600 to 7400 cGy, 200 cGy/fraction is delivered. Lesions in this area have a high tendency for metastases to the neck; therefore, prophylactic neck treatment is critical.[5] An anterior field is included to treat the lower cervical nodes and bilateral supraclavicular fossa.

Surgery has been noted to be reserved for salvage of RT failures, but a recent report indicated that better locoregional control and disease-free survival were obtained with surgery and postoperative RT.[5]

> The subdivisions of the oral cavity include (1) the anterior two-thirds of the tongue, (2) the lip, (3) the buccal mucosa, (4) the retromolar trigone, (5) the floor of the mouth, and (6) the hard palate.

THE PHARYNX REGION

Anatomy

The pharynx is subdivided into three anatomic divisions: the oropharynx, the nasopharynx, and the hypopharynx, also referred to as the laryngopharynx (see Fig. 29.4). Attention should be provided to the distinct anatomic structures that define each subdivision: the

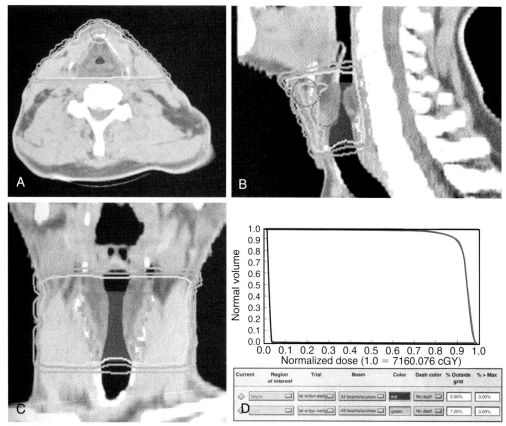

Fig. 29.21 (A) Three-dimensional treatment plan for laryngeal cancer, axial plane. (B) Three-dimensional plan, coronal plane. (C) Three-dimensional plan, sagittal view. (D) Dose-volume histogram. (From Hoppe RT, Phillips TL, Roach M. *Leibel and Phillips Textbook of Radiation Oncology.* 3rd ed. Philadelphia, PA: Saunders; 2010.)

nasopharynx, located behind the nose and extending from the posterior nares to the level of the soft palate; the oropharynx, located behind the mouth from the soft palate above to the level of the hyoid bone below; and the laryngopharynx or hypopharynx, extending from the hyoid bone to its termination in the esophagus.[34]

Clinical Presentation

The most common symptoms include persistent sore throat, painful swallowing, and referred otalgia. Often enlargement of cervical nodes is present. Halitosis, dyspnea, dysphasia, hoarseness, dysarthria, and hypersalivation may indicate advanced disease.[3]

Diagnostic Procedures and Staging

The patient history is part of a comprehensive evaluation. If the history includes strong tobacco and alcohol use, determination of habitual use is important, and intervention may be necessary to guide the patient toward cessation programs. Cessation is important for the patient to better tolerate the treatment and for better results. One recent study retrospectively evaluated the prognostic value of smoking and drinking status in patients with head and neck SCCs.[57] On the basis of data from 1,871 patients, evidence was observed that smoking and drinking were associated with inferior local control and survival. For survival, the results of former smokers and active smokers versus those who never smoked were also statistically significant. Adjusted 5-year local control and survival rates for those who never smoked and never drank were 87% and 77%, respectively, and for those who were both active smokers and active drinkers were 72% ($P = .007$) and 52% ($P = .0009$), respectively. The study provided conclusive data that showed that smoking and drinking were associated with poor outcomes in these patients.[57]

A finding of the study that may be of special interest regarding current smokers, because former smokers had a much better local control than did active smokers, was that it was more prudent to suggest that patients stop smoking (or minimize their smoking) as soon as the diagnosis was made to maximize the length of time without smoking before RT. Patients should not be told that they can wait until the first day of RT to change their smoking behavior because smoking at baseline is probably as deleterious as smoking during RT. Current smokers at baseline had a lower local control and slightly lower survival than former smokers.

Inspection includes indirect mirror examination (essential), palpation, biopsy (essential), fiberoptic endoscopy, and CT and MRI imaging to detect occult primaries and define anatomic extensions. In addition to the history, physical examination, CT or MRI of the head and neck, a chest radiograph, and routine blood cell counts and serum chemistries are part of the staging evaluation. Other pretreatment diagnostic evaluations, especially for nasopharyngeal tumors, include EBV-specific serologic tests and liver function tests. CT scan of the chest and a bone scan may be necessary for advanced nodal disease.[36,43] Pretreatment dental evaluation and initiation of dental prophylaxis are also recommended.

Histopathology

These tumors are predominantly SCCs (90%). Well-differentiated tumors are less common than in the oral cavity. Lymphoepithelioma may occur in the tonsil and the base of the tongue. Minor salivary gland carcinomas have been identified in this region. Non-Hodgkin lymphoma is seen in approximately 5% of tonsillar malignancies.

Staging

Refer to the *UICC TNM Classification of Malignant Tumors.*

Metastatic Behavior

Cervical lymph node involvement is common with OPC. Base-of-the-tongue tumors may have palpable nodes on presentation. The incidence rate of bilateral neck disease is up to 40%. Tonsillar lesions have palpable metastatic nodes at diagnosis in 60% to 70% of cases, pharyngeal wall lesions have involved nodes in 50% to 60% of cases, and soft palate carcinoma metastasizes about 40% to 50% of cases to the jugulodigastric nodes. Bilateral nodal disease is frequent, and retropharyngeal node involvement is common. Hematogenous metastasis is related to tonsillar and base of tongue primaries. Lung is the most common site.

RADIATION THERAPY FOR REGIONS OF THE PHARYNX

A report from the Stanford University Department of Radiation Oncology concludes that because of the morbidity associated with surgical resection of locally advanced SCC of the oropharynx and the similar survival rates between surgery and RT, RT has become the standard treatment for the oropharynx.[53]

Because cure rates are now relatively high, long-term morbidity ranging from xerostomia to mandibular necrosis has become an important issue. A number of studies have shown that with its irregular, often concave shapes and close proximity to critical healthy structures such as the parotid glands and mandible, IMRT appears to be the ideal treatment for carcinomas of the oropharynx and related sites. Advantages include not only excellent local regional control and overall survival but a decrease in late side effects compared with conventional RT techniques in the head and neck. The Sloan Kettering group confers with this view, citing xerostomia and hearing loss as the most common debilitating long-term side effects seen in patients with NPC.[51]

In a search for one standardized IMRT plan across current literature, discussions point out the rationale for developing the treatment plan. One study explains that clinically achievable dose-volume histogram (DVH) objectives and weights (optimization parameters used in planning) that account for the trade-offs between target coverage and organ-at-risk (OAR) sparing for a specific patient are unknown ahead of planning and are largely determined by the geometric relationship between OARs and targets.[59]

In creation of clinical plans, dosimetrists follow the physician's clinical requirements and in-house dosimetric guidelines that include dose limits to various anatomic structures of interest. It is now well-known that the use of IMRT makes possible the more effective sparing of healthy tissues such as the parotid gland. However, unless a structure is identified as important, contoured, and entered into the cost function, a significant dose may nonetheless be deposited. One study notes that after the larynx was included as an avoidance structure in an IMRT plan where disease extended inferiorly and close to the larynx, mean dose was reduced from 47.7 to 38.8 Gy.[60]

Findings of a search for one standard IMRT technique include variations based on the specific targeted site and patient conditions. Two views regarding such variation in the literature follow. From the international perspective, a study from Switzerland reports that the differences in IMRT dose-distribution definitions between institutions prevent meaningful DVH comparisons—a reminder of the fact that we still lack an international standardization of IMRT schedules, dose constraints, and contouring.[61] Among local institutions, Wu and colleagues[59] designed a multiinstitutional trial of IMRT for oropharyngeal cancer, in which they found high variations of target coverage and OAR sparing in a multicenter setting. Similarly, Wu and associates[59] distributed the CT scan of a patient with head and neck cancer to three institutions and found significant variation in the planning results.

Reports describing IMRT techniques for the pharynx region include various disease sites described further in this section of the chapter. Although studies group patient populations with diseases of the oropharynx, the hypopharynx, and the nasopharynx, the high level of beam sculpting with specific customized beam conformity is unique to each specific target. In general, the clinical planning goal in targeted RT such as IMRT is to deliver the prescribed dose to the mean volumes of specified anatomic structures, typically receiving 35 to 70 Gy while guided with thresholds from the literature.

The Sloan Kettering group recently reported on a study that tested the feasibility of hypofractionated "dose painting" IMRT with chemotherapy. Their goal was to determine rates of ototoxicity and xerostomia, regional control, distant metastasis, and overall survival. The treatment was designed as the hypofractionated regimen of 2.34 Gy/fx for a total of 70.2 Gy plus chemotherapy to treat nasopharyngeal carcinoma.[51]

The Oropharynx Region. The oropharynx consists of the base of the tongue, the tonsils (fossa and pillars), the soft palate, and the oropharyngeal walls. The oropharynx is situated between the axis and C3 vertebral bodies. The soft tissue regions include the anterior tonsillary pillars, the soft palate, the uvula, the base of the tongue, and the lateral-posterior pharyngeal walls (see Fig. 29.4 and 29.15).

Tumors in this region and treatment can have a profound effect on all of the basic aerodigestive functions. The tonsils are the most common site of disease. Clinically, a sore throat and pain during swallowing are the most common presenting symptoms. Upper spinal accessory nodes are involved bilaterally in 50% to 70% of patients. Early T1 to T2 lesions are treatable with external beam treatment alone. Large volumes are required for T3 to T4 lesions that encompass the cervical and supraclavicular neck nodes. Debate exists for the treatment of small and intermediate cancers, T1 to T3 tumors of the tonsillar fossa or soft palate. The issues are in regard to "the choice between conventional fractionated external beam treatment and accelerated fractionation, the optimal boost technique (external vs. interstitial RT), planned neck dissection after previous external beam treatment, and/or the use of adjuvant, neoadjuvant, or concomitant chemotherapy." A general trend is to aim for organ function preservation.

> The oropharynx is located posterior to the oral cavity from the soft palate above to the level of the hyoid bone below.

Fig. 29.22 shows a RapidArc treatment technique of the oropharynx. Despite the generally large tumors, RapidArc achieves conformal plans with an average confidence interval of 1.13. Coverage of both PTV$_{elect}$ and PTV$_{boost}$ is excellent, with an average of more than 99% of both PTVs receiving 95% of the prescription dose. Only 0.07% of PTV$_{boost}$ received more than 107%. For the boost volume, D99 was 66.9 Gy, and D95 was 68.3 Gy. For the elective volume, D99 was 55.0 Gy, and D95 was 56.9 Gy.[14] The maximum cord dose with the RapidArc was, on average, 45.7 Gy. The mean dose was 31.4 Gy to the ipsilateral parotid gland and 26.1 Gy to the contralateral gland. Stage III and IV cancers are treated with definitive RT and concurrent chemotherapy.[46]

The Hypopharynx Region. The hypopharynx (see Fig. 29.4) is composed of the pyriform sinuses, postcricoid, and lower posterior pharyngeal walls below the base of the tongue. It is anatomically situated between the vertebral bodies C3 and C6. The cricoid cartilage represents the inferior border, and the epiglottis is the superior border. The most common presenting symptoms include sore throat, odynophagia (painful swallowing), and a neck mass. Up to 25% of cases

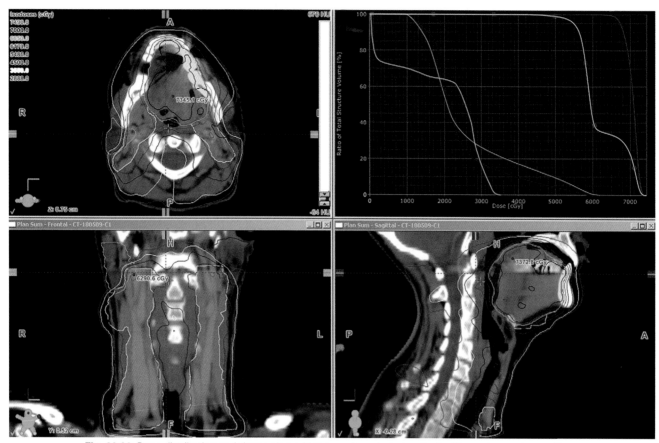

Fig. 29.22 Dose distribution and dose volume histogram for a typical patient with oropharynx tumor. (From Doornaert P, Verbakel WF, Bieker M, et al. Rapidarc planning and delivery in patients with locally advanced head and neck cancer undergoing chemoradiotherapy. *Int J Radiat Oncol Biol Phys.* 2011;79:429–435.)

present with a neck mass only; dysphagia and weight loss are common symptoms of locally advanced disease. More than 90% of cases present with dysphagia known as the hallmark of postcricoid carcinoma.[16]

Typically, disease of the hypopharynx is advanced. The pyriform sinus is the site of highest incidence of hypopharyngeal cancer. The male-to-female ratio ranges from 5:1 to 7:1 for pyriform sinus cancer and 3:1 to 4:1 for pharyngeal wall cancer. Postcricoid cancers occur predominantly in women.[16] A high rate (70%–75%) of nodal metastasis in pyriform sinus cancers is found, and the tumor is highly infiltrative. Treatment can also be debilitating. The rare T1 to T2 lesions are controllable through radiation or surgery, but most cases present as advanced T2 to T4 lesions and are not candidates for laryngeal preservation.[27] Most patients receive combined radical surgery and RT for curative purposes. Large radiation ports are common. A more conventional technique for the treatment of pyriform sinus, posterior pharyngeal wall, and postcricoid cancers was the classically defined beam arrangements. This include the opposed lateral photon fields, a low anterior neck photon field, and posterior cervical electron fields.[16]

Tumors of the posterior pharyngeal wall are considered unresectable. RT consists of large treatment volumes, including the entire pharynx and upper cervical esophagus and extending superiorly to include the nasopharynx vault; superior deep, middle, and low jugular; and Rouvière's (lateral retropharyngeal) lymph nodes at the base of the skull. Treatment planning can be complicated. Cases that involve tumor or lymphadenopathy that extends posterolaterally around the anterior aspect of the vertebral column to produce a horseshoe-shaped target volume have been reported. Rimmer, Lee, and Zelefsky[16] report that conformal RT with either an isocentric rotational technique with

MLC or a static five-field technique may effectively address the problem of a horseshoe-shaped target. Beitler, Amdur, and Mendenhall[27] describe this and any tumor that is wrapped around a vertebral body as a perfect case for IMRT.

> The laryngopharynx or hypopharynx extends from the hyoid bone to its termination in the esophagus.

The Nasopharynx Region. The nasopharynx includes the posterosuperior pharyngeal wall and lateral pharyngeal wall, the eustachian tube orifice, and the adenoids. The nasopharynx is a cuboidal structure that lies on a line from the zygomatic arch to the external auditory meatus, extending inferiorly to the mastoid tip. The nasopharynx lies behind the nasal cavities and above the level of the soft palate (see Fig. 29.4). The nasal cavity drains into the nasopharynx via the two posterior nares and also has on its lateral walls the two eustachian tubes, which connect to the middle ear. Disease in the nasopharynx can mimic an inflammatory process and cause considerable respiratory or auditory dysfunction.

Cranial nerve involvement occurs frequently. The 9th to the 12th cranial nerves can be affected by enlargement of the retropharyngeal nodes (see Fig. 29.10), as can the external carotid artery. Because of its proximity to the base of the brain, a lesion can directly invade the third nerve and most commonly involves the sixth nerve. Any cranial nerve involvement signifies advanced, widespread disease. The involvement of the trigeminal (V), the oculomotor nerves (III), and the trochlear (IV) nerves has been referred to as petrosphenoidal syndrome, with diplopia being the most common cranial nerve finding. The three branches of the trigeminal nerve, the ophthalmic, the maxillary, and the mandibular, are most frequently involved. See Table 29.3 for the cranial nerves and their related functions; Fig. 29.23 illustrates the ventral surface of the brain and shows attachment of the cranial nerves.

> The nasopharynx is located behind the nose and extends from the posterior nares to the level of the soft palate.

Staging for NPC differs from that for other head and neck cancers. The distribution and the prognostic impact of regional lymph node spread, particularly of the undifferentiated type, are different from those of other head and neck mucosal cancers and justify the use of a different N classification scheme. Lymphatic spread from a primary goes to the retropharyngeal, upper jugular, and spinal accessory nodes (level V). A solitary nodal mass in this level indicates examination of the nasopharynx.[21] Some 90% of these lesions are SCC or its variants. NPC has a tendency toward poor differentiation and unusual growth patterns. Pathologic types have been grouped by the World Health Organization. The following is a breakdown of types within North America. The figures are approximations that vary according to source.

Type 1: Keratinizing SCC (20% of cases)
Type 2: Nonkeratinizing carcinoma (10% of cases)
Type 3: Lymphoepithelioma (poorly differentiated carcinoma; 70% of cases)

Nonkeratinizing carcinoma and lymphoepithelioma are variants of SCC. Surgical intervention in the nasopharynx is extremely difficult. This disease is not associated with tobacco consumption. EBV is associated with NPC. The age distribution is bimodal, with a small peak in adolescence and young adulthood and a major peak between 50 and 70 years of age. The disease is uncommon in white populations; it comprises only 2% of all cases of head and neck cancer in the United States.[7] It has been noted to be rare among Japanese populations as well, although the literature makes reference to a study of an early-staged population from Hong Kong to the United States.[16]

A high incidence rate in southern Chinese (57% of all head and neck cancers) and Middle Eastern countries may be attributed to nitrosamines in salted fish among southern China. Eskimos and the mixed populations of Southeast Asia are included among the higher cases.

From 75% to 85% of patients with NPC have clinically positive cervical nodes, with about half of all cases having bilateral or contralateral disease. For conventional RT, radiation ports are quite large to encompass all the nodes and at-risk tissue. The lateral retropharyngeal node (node of Rouvière), which usually cannot be surgically removed,

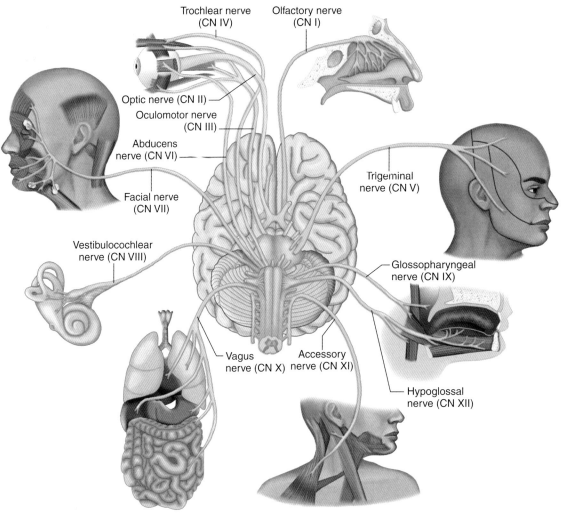

Fig. 29.23 Cranial nerves I through XII. (From Thibodeau GA, Patton KT. *The Human Body in Health and Disease.* 7th ed. St. Louis, MO: Mosby; 2018.)

and the jugulodigastric node are nearly always treated as tumor volume during any boost procedure.

NPC has an overall incidence rate of 25% of bloodborne metastasis. The nodal disease can be extensive; the primary lesion is often small. Patients with bilateral cervical nodes have up to a 40% to 70% likelihood of development of a distant metastasis, with bone, lung, and liver the most common sites. NPC disease spreads to adjacent subsites rather quickly and has a 30% to 40% local recurrence rate. For these reasons, aggressive, large-volume, radical RT is necessary.

Radiation treatment volumes are arranged to cover the possible pathways of spread (Fig. 29.24). The treatment portals are designed to deliver appropriate dose to gross disease (gross tumor volume) and areas at risk of microscopic extension (clinical target volume). This remains as the treatment objective regardless of treatment technique, in classically defined beam arrangements and in techniques with IMRT.

Treatment of NPC has seen dramatic changes in the past several years. Much of the early work on IMRT has centered on NPC because of accurate immobilization, the extent of critical structures in proximity to tumor, and the high incidence of morbidity with conventional treatment techniques. Although treatments with modified fractionation, such as hyperfractionation to 7440 cGy in twice-daily fractions,[27] are still being reported, IMRT is replacing conventional RT in the United States.[43] Several institutions have shown potential dosimetric improvement for IMRT over conventional techniques and 3D conformal techniques.[1] The preservation of salivary function with sparing of at least one parotid gland has been a primary objective of head and neck IMRT. Lee and colleagues[6] report that the ability to tailor dose to a desired distribution allows the simultaneous delivery of different fractionation schemes to different portions of the target. The primary target can be hypofractionated, and conventional fractionation can be delivered to subclinical neck disease, or conventional fractionation can be applied to the target with delivery of doses of less than 1.8 Gy to the secondary targets. Fusion of diagnostic MRI and treatment planning CT images provide accurate delineation of GTV and surrounding critical healthy structures. The CTV is defined as the GTV and areas with potential microscopic disease. The CTV should also include lymph node groups of high risk:

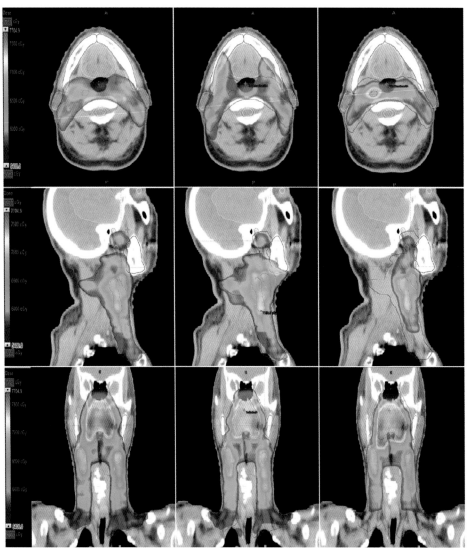

Fig. 29.24 Comparison of dose distributions between NPC standard plan and the individual plans delineated by two different physicians. The first column is the results of the standard plan. The second column represents the individual plan delineated by physician A, where the prescription dose distribution of planning tumor volume 2 is beyond the scope of the standard target. The third column is the individual plan delineated by physician B, where the prescription dose does not cover the entire standard target area. (From Peng, Y, Chen L, et al. Interobserver variations in the delineation of target volumes and organs at risk and their impact on dose distribution in intensity modulated radiation therapy for nasopharyngeal carcinoma. *Oral Oncol.* 2018;82:1–7.)

the upper deep jugular, submandibular, subdigastric, midjugular, posterior cervical, and retropharyngeal nodes. Also included as CTV are the lower neck and supraclavicular nodes, considered at lower risk for microscopic spread, along with margin for movement and setup error.[43] One prescribed treatment includes 7000 cGy delivered to the GTV and positive neck nodes. The high-risk CTV receives 5940 cGy, and the low-risk CTV receives 5000 to 5400 cGy (negative neck nodes). Also, 180 cGy/fraction per day for 5 days per week is delivered to the CTV for a total dose of 5940 cGy to the high-risk CTV. The low-risk CTV receives 5040 cGy, and the GTV receives a higher 212 cGy/fraction per day. Fig. 29.24 shows various treatment plans for NPC. Note the varying tumor volumes covering the target area.

Adjuvant chemotherapy seems to improve both local control and survival. Concomitant chemotherapy should be used along with radiation for stage III and IV (localized) tumors. Retreatment of local failures with a combination of external beam followed by an intracavitary brachytherapy boost is considered feasible. Overall, lymphoepithelioma and undifferentiated carcinomas have been reported to be more radiosensitive and have a better prognosis than SCC. Local control has improved along with advances in RT.[43]

THE LARYNX REGION

The larynx is contiguous with the lower portion of the pharynx above and is connected with the trachea below. It extends from the tip of the epiglottis at the level of the lower border of the C3 vertebra to the lower border of the cricoid cartilage at the level of the C6 vertebra. The larynx is subdivided into three sites (Fig. 29.25): the glottis, the supraglottis, and the subglottis region. Glottic cancer accounts for roughly 65% of larynx cancers, with a 30% site incidence rate in the supraglottic region. The remaining larynx cancers appear in the subglottic area.

Cahlon and colleagues[62] report that cancers of the larynx are the most common cancers of the upper aerodigestive tract. Cancer of the larynx has also been described as the most common head and neck cancer if one excludes skin malignancies.[63] The ratio of glottic to supraglottic carcinomas is about 3:1. Carcinomas of the glottis (true vocal cord) are not considered life-threatening, and the choice of therapy is based on the preservation of speech and maintenance of the airway. Historically, the treatment of larynx cancer focused on cure with aggressive surgery, which left the survivor with a difficult and challenged life from

the inability to communicate. The loss of vocalization has a profound psychologic and socioeconomic impact on quality of life.

Incidence characteristics are consistent, regardless of culture.[63] Laryngeal cancer is mostly a male-dominated disease (90%), with a peak incidence in the 50-year to 60-year age group. Laryngeal carcinomas display an extremely high etiology toward smoking. The use of black tobacco is associated with a higher risk than the use of blond tobacco. People who use their voices extensively in their work also appear to be at higher risk. The role of alcohol has been associated with the incidence of supraglottic cancer; the role related to glottic cancer is not clear. A synergistic role of alcohol with tobacco is favored instead of alcohol as an independent factor. Studies have involved the relation to gastroesophageal reflux. Chronic irritation from acid is believed to predispose patients to cancer.[17]

Studies involve the molecular basis for laryngeal cancer. Mutation of the *p53* gene is common and is seen in 47% of patients who are smokers but in only 14% of nonsmokers. This mutation has been identified in 55% of the tumors among drinkers and in 20% among nondrinkers. The transformation of this gene and antigen proliferation are suspected to be associated with HPV infection that may play a role in laryngeal cancer.[62] Garden, Morrison, and Ang[17] refer to this as a causal link that also affects the tonsil.

A persistent sore throat and hoarseness are classic presenting symptoms. Cervical lymph node involvement, if present, is seen in supraglottic lesions but not in glottic lesions. Tis (Tumor in situ) is rather common on the vocal cords. Glottic lesions are well to moderately differentiated, with supraglottic lesions being less differentiated and more aggressive. About 65% to 75% of glottic lesions appear on the anterior two-thirds of one cord. Cord mobility is a factor in the classification of the lesions. Early lesions are treated successfully with either surgery or RT; voice quality reportedly is better after RT alone.[62] Advanced lesions with fixed vocal cords as a result of extensive cartilage invasion are best treated with surgery and postoperative RT. Exophytic lesions are more responsive to RT than are infiltrative lesions. RT alone or concurrent with chemotherapy may be the preferred treatment for poorly differentiated carcinoma. Conservation surgery may be the preferred treatment for early verrucous carcinoma of the vocal cord.[62] Verrucous carcinoma is generally a well-differentiated, slow-growing, wartlike lesion that is relatively radioresistant. It has a tendency to convert to a highly anaplastic neoplasm after RT.[17]

Proper selection in treating Tis with transoral laser excision requires an experienced team. Laser excision performed to a narrow margin treats microinvasive cancer and spares the anterior commissure, allowing mucosal waves to travel across the glottis unimpeded. Voice problems worsen as the extent of resection increases. Generally, RT for Tis is based on anterior commissure involvement when the mucosal wave is impaired or when the patient is not in good medical condition. Limited risk of subclinical disease to the cervical lymphatics in the treatment of Tis and T1 lesions indicates a field that encompasses the primary lesion only.[13]

RADIATION THERAPY FOR REGIONS OF THE LARYNX

The University of Wisconsin reports treatment of primary carcinomas of the larynx and of the oral cavity, oropharynx, hypopharynx, and nasopharynx with definitive IMRT with or without concurrent chemotherapy as the standard of care.[15] Treatment delivery approaches have included either a moderate hypofractionation schedule of 6600 cGy at 220 cGy per fraction to the gross tumor (primary and nodal), with the standard dose fractionation of 5400 to 6000 cGy at 180 to 200 cGy per fraction to the elective neck lymphatics or a conventional dose and

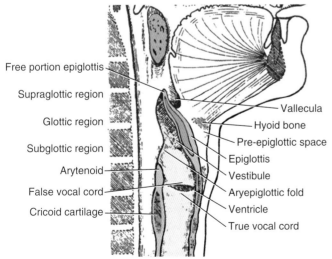

Free portion epiglottis

Supraglottic region

Glottic region

Subglottic region

Arytenoid

False vocal cord

Cricoid cartilage

Vallecula

Hyoid bone

Pre-epiglottic space

Epiglottis

Vestibule

Aryepiglottic fold

Ventricle

True vocal cord

Fig. 29.25 Anatomic regions and structures of the larynx. (From Lee NL, Phillips TL. Cancer of the larynx. In: Hoppe RT, Phillips TL, Roach M. *Leibel and Phillips Textbook of Radiation Oncology.* 3rd ed. Philadelphia, PA: Saunders; 2010.)

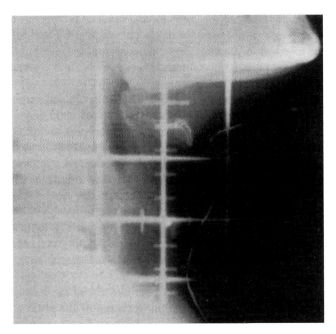

Fig. 29.26 Simulation image of a lateral port, T1N0 glottic cancer. (From Cox JD. *Moss' Radiation Oncology: Rationale, Technique, Results.* 7th ed. St. Louis, MO: Mosby; 1994.)

fractionation schedule of 7000 cGy at 200 cGy per fraction to the gross tumor (primary and nodal) with reduced dose to the elective neck lymphatics. The group reports similar treatment outcomes with either of the two treatment delivery schedules. Their study further concludes that a dose of 5000 cGy at 143 cGy per fraction may be sufficient to treat low-risk neck lymphatics.[15]

The accurate definition of gross tumor volume with CT treatment planning is reportedly correlated with effective local control. With conventional RT, glottic cancer is treated with opposing lateral fields angled to be parallel to the trachea, 5 × 5 cm (for T1 and early T2) to 6 × 6 cm. Wedges are indicated if the tissue inhomogeneities produce unacceptable hot spots in the posterior margins. Daily doses can be 200 to 220 cGy, up to a total dose of 6000 to 7000 cGy, depending on the size of the lesion and mobility of the cord. Multiple studies suggest that 120 cGy fractions of twice-daily treatments to 7440 to 7900 cGy are appropriate. If hyperfractionation is not feasible, daily fractions of greater than 200 cGy per day result in superior outcomes to smaller daily doses.[42] The treatment of small fields for early glottic cancers rarely results in severe complications. Large, fixed lesions need more aggressive therapy; T3 and T4 lesions of the glottis and subglottis are treated as supraglottic lesions.[62]

The radiation port borders can be clinically determined before simulation, but CT scans of the neck are used for computerized treatment planning. Fig. 29.26 depicts a typical conventional simulation lateral port, and Figs. 29.21 and 29.27 illustrates several planning techniques including IMRT, VMAT, HT, and 3D-CRT. Notice the corresponding dose histograms.

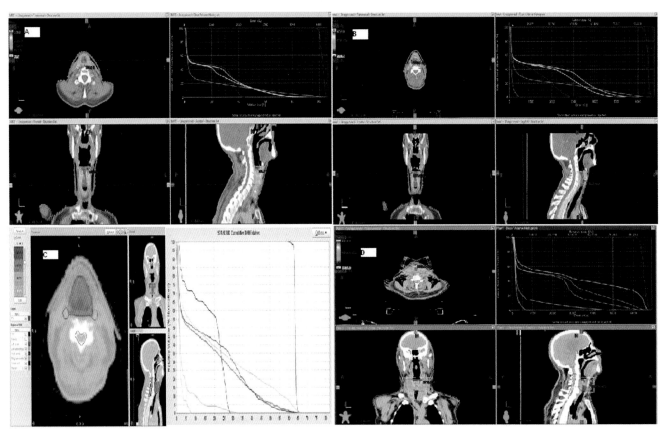

Fig. 29.27 Dose distributions and dose-volume histograms of four planning techniques for an early-stage (T1N0) glottis cancer: (A) intensity-modulated radiation therapy, (B) volumetric-modulated arc therapy, (C) Helical Tomotherapy (HT), and (D) three-dimensional conformal radiation therapy. (Reprinted by permission of Elsevier from Dosimetric comparison of helical tomotherapy, intensity-modulated radiation therapy, volumetric-modulated arc therapy, and 3-dimensional conformal therapy for the treatment of T1N0 glottic cancer, by Ekici K, Pepele E, Yaprak B, et al, Medical Dosimetry, 41, 329–333, 2016, by American Association of Medical Dosimetrists.)

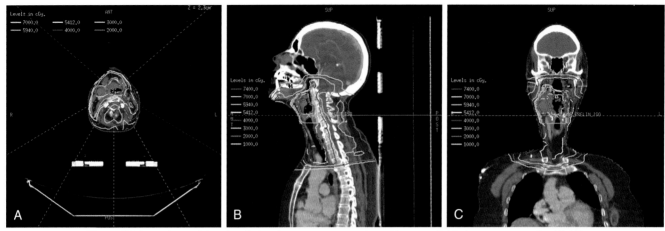

Fig. 29.28 Intensity-modulated radiation therapy treatment plan with seven fields for a postoperative T4 N1 M0 carcinoma of the larynx after total laryngectomy. (From Cahlon O, Lee N, Le Q, et al. Cancer of the larynx. In: Hoppe RT, Phillips TL, Roach M. *Leibel and Phillips Textbook of Radiation Oncology*. 3rd ed. Philadelphia, PA: Saunders; 2010.)

The typical radiation field borders are as follows:

Superior: upper thyroid notch

Inferior: cricoid cartilage (lower border of C6)

Anterior: 1-cm to 1.5-cm flash or shine over the skin surface at the level of the vocal cords

Posterior: just anterior to the vertebral body, including the anterior portion of the posterior pharyngeal wall

Large T3 to T4, transglottic lesions are treated with radiation alone. In the event of a recurrence, salvage surgery is an option. However, the voice is usually sacrificed. RT offers the best method of voice preservation.

Supraglottic lesions are frequently large and bulky but (despite appearances) do not usually invade the inferior false cord or the ventricles. These lesions tend to spread superiorly to the epiglottis. Lymph node metastasis is expected in 40% to 50% of patients. Therefore, the treatment volumes are much larger than the glottic ports.

Computer-optimized or inverse-planned IMRT has been described as an ideal treatment technique for a T3N1 supraglottic carcinoma. Although the expected benefits include voice preservation and less xerostomia than with conventional treatment, Fig. 29.28 illustrates an inverse-planned IMRT technique for T4N1 M0 SCC of the larynx.

Surgery can control 80% of supraglottic T1 to T2 lesions, whereas RT offers 75% local control. RT alone for T3 to T4 supraglottic lesions is contraindicated. Relapses are treated with surgery. The tumor dose needed to achieve control is 6600 to 7000 cGy. Subglottic cancers are treated with a total laryngectomy, with postoperative RT given for any residual disease.

Survival rates are good for glottic cancer: 80% to 90% without cord fixation, and 50% to 60% with fixation. Patients with supraglottic cancers have a 60% to 70% 5-year survival rate with negative nodes, but this rate drops to 30% to 50% if positive clinical nodes are present.[3] Garden and colleagues[17] note that because nearly all published series are retrospective single-institution studies, valid data on control rates remain a challenge to obtain. The management of early glottic carcinomas remains controversial and is often determined by the preference of the attending physician. Oncologists advocate either RT or voice-preserving partial laryngectomy. Equivalent control rates have been published with surgery (excision, cordectomy, or hemilaryngectomy) and RT.

THE SALIVARY GLANDS

The salivary glands consist of three large, paired major glands—the parotid, submandibular, and sublingual glands—and many smaller minor glands located throughout the upper aerodigestive tract. They play a role in digestion and tooth protection. The parotid gland is the largest of the three salivary glands; it is located superficial to and partly behind the ramus of the mandible and covers the masseter muscle. It fills the space between the ramus of the mandible and the anterior border of the SCM. The parotid contains an extensive lymphatic capillary plexus, many aggregates of lymphocytic cells, and numerous intraglandular lymph nodes in the superficial lobe. Lymphatics drain more laterally on the face, including parts of the eyelids, diagonally downward and posteriorly toward the parotid gland, as do the lymphatics from the frontal region of the scalp. Associated with the gland, both superficially and deeply, are parotid nodes that drain down along the retromandibular vein to empty into the superficial lymphatics and nodes along the outer surface of the SCM and into upper nodes of the deep cervical chain. Lymphatics from the parietal region of the scalp drain partly to the parotid nodes in front of the ear and partly to the retroauricular nodes in back of the ear, which, in turn, drain into upper deep cervical nodes.

Chong and Armstrong[13] report that tumors of the salivary gland are rare and constitute from 3% to 4% of all cancers of the head and neck region. Quon and associates[64] write that malignant tumors of the salivary glands account for 7% of head and neck cancers diagnosed in North America each year. The parotid is the site of the highest incidence rate of salivary gland tumors (80% to 90%). Of these tumors, more than two-thirds are benign, and between 15% and 31% are malignant. Tumors of the minor salivary glands account for 2% to 3% of all head and neck cancers; about 65% and 85% of these are malignant.[7,65] The submandibular gland is involved in about 10% of all instances. Although the causes of these glandular tumors are stated to be unknown, low-dose ionizing radiation in childhood may account for some cases of malignant salivary tumors. Radiation-induced malignancies have been associated with early radiation treatments for benign conditions such as acne, tinea capitis, and infected tonsils. These malignancies have also been associated with the atomic bomb survivors.

Female patients with a history of carcinoma of the major salivary glands have an incidence rate of breast cancer that is eight times higher than that of the healthy population.[65] Chong and Armstrong[13] report that firm epidemiologic data of this association are lacking. Most major and minor salivary cancers are of unknown origin, and etiologic factors are poorly understood. However, risk factors such as dental radiographs have been implicated for both benign and malignant salivary gland tumors. Parotid gland tumors in children are more likely to be malignant compared with the same tumors in adults.[65] Exposure to hardwood dust has been linked to the development of nasal cavity and paranasal sinus minor salivary gland adenocarcinomas.[63] Malignant neoplasms occur in patients with an average age of 55 years; benign tumors occur at around age 40 years. The incidence rates among genders are about equal, with a slight male predominance.

Histologically, the more common cell types for malignant tumors are adenoid cystic, mucoepidermoid, and adenocarcinoma. Most patients have development of an asymptomatic parotid mass that lasts, on average, from 4 to 8 months before presentation.[63] Presenting symptoms are localized swelling and pain, facial palsy, and rapid growth. Facial nerve involvement is highly suggestive of a malignancy. CT scan and MRI are not routinely used because they are ineffective in differentiating between benign and malignant salivary gland tumors. PET scans show an increased FDG uptake for both benign and malignant lesions as well. Although not useful in the evaluation of primary tumor, PET may play a role in the evaluation of distant metastasis.[16] FNAB is reported to be an accurate diagnostic technique, with overall sensitivities of greater than 90% and specificities of greater than 95%.[65] Controversy exists regarding diagnostic procedures that involve FNAB. A diagnosis via a lobectomy is done, and submandibular lesions are excised for a frozen section.[7] Some institutions reserve FNAB for inoperable and recurrent lesions. Incisional or excisional biopsies are never performed to establish a tissue diagnosis because such procedures increase the risk of recurrence, the risk of injury to the facial nerve, and subsequent surgical morbidity.[13]

The incidence of cervical node involvement varies according to the histologic subtype. High-grade mucoepidermoid tumors display a 44% metastatic behavior. The rate for this behavior is 5% in adenoid cystic tumors, 21% in malignant mixed tumors, 37% in SCC, and 13% in acinic cell carcinoma. Hematogenous metastases are common and range from about 13% for acinic cell carcinoma to 41% for adenoid cystic carcinoma. Lung metastases from adenoid cystic carcinomas may lie quiescent for years after presentation.[7]

Although tumors in this area are mostly benign, the risk of local recurrence is high. They are considered low-grade cancer and are optimally treated via total resection, with generous margins for sparing of facial nerves.

RADIATION THERAPY FOR REGIONS OF THE SALIVARY GLANDS

IMRT is effective in cases of perineural involvement of the facial, trigeminal, hypoglossal, and lingual nerves that necessitate treatment of the proximal nerve to the brainstem with sparing of the contralateral salivary gland, the eyes, the temporal lobes, and the brainstem itself. Subclinical intracranial disease in the cavernous sinus, adjacent to the brainstem, or within the petrous bone can be treated at 180 cGy/fraction; higher risk areas in the original tumor bed and high-risk lymph nodes in the neck can be treated at 200 cGy/fraction. Positive distal nerve margins may also be effectively treated with IMRT. The entire span of the nerve can be treated distally with sparing of critical healthy structures such as the lacrimal gland and eye.[65] Fig. 29.29 illustrates IMRT to a postoperative right submandibular salivary gland with perineural invasion. Fig. 29.30 shows the IMRT plan for a 46-year-old patient who underwent RT alone for a stage T2 N0 parotid gland tumor.

Improved results have also been reported with accelerated fractionation.[7] Accelerated fractionation techniques provide similar dose levels of RT in a shorter amount of overall time. This counteracts quick cellular proliferation of aggressive tumors by giving more dose in a shorter time. Treatment complications should be monitored.

THE PARANASAL SINUSES

Maxillary sinus

The maxillary sinus is a pyramid-shaped cavity lined by ciliated epithelium and bound by thin bone or membranous partitions. Carcinomas that arise from the ciliated epithelium or mucous glands perforate the bony walls almost from the start. The roof of the maxillary sinus is also the floor of the orbit. Tumors that involve the superior portion of the sinus readily extend into the orbit. The more posterior wall or infratemporal surface separates the sinus from the pterygopalatine fossa and the posterosuperior alveolar nerves. The nasal surface of the antrum is visible through the nostril, with the ostium of the sinus inferior to the middle turbinate. The alveolar process and the hard palate separate the maxillary sinus from the oral cavity.

Maxillary sinus disease accounts for 80% of all sinus cancers, with a 2:1 male prevalence. Most patients with carcinoma in the sinonasal region are older than 40 years. Adenocarcinoma of the nasal cavity and ethmoid sinus has been associated with wood dust exposure. SCCs of the maxillary sinus and nasal cavity are associated with chemical agents found in work related to nickel refinery and leather tanning. Thorotrast, an imaging contrast media used to image the maxillary sinus in the 1960s, includes radioactive thorium, which is now known to be a carcinogen. Chen, Ryu, and Donald[14] report that, unlike other respiratory tract carcinomas, cancers of the nasal cavity and paranasal sinus have no association with smoking. This is in contrast to Beitler and colleagues,[15] who write that "cigarette smoking is reported to increase the risk of nasal cancer, with a doubling of risk among heavy or long-term smokers and a reduction in risk after long-term cessation." Patients with this type of cancer have a history of long-standing sinusitis, nasal obstructions, and bloody discharge. Although chronic sinusitis is frequently a symptom with the malignant tumor, sinusitis is not a causative agent.[14] These cancers are mostly SCCs and tend to invade the floor of the orbit, ethmoid sinuses, hard palate, and zygomatic arch. Displacement of the eye is common. Physical examination should include inspection and bimanual palpation of the orbit, oral and nasal cavities, and nasopharynx and direct fiberoptic endoscopy. Neurologic examination should emphasize cranial nerve function because nasal cavity and paranasal sinus tumors are frequently associated with cranial nerve palsies, especially of the trigeminal branches. Cervical lymph nodes are palpated for adenopathy. Imaging has essentially replaced surgical exploration for staging and tumor mapping in this region. The most useful studies are CT scan and MRI. CT scan defines early cortical bone erosion more clearly, whereas MRI better delineates soft tissue and can differentiate among opacification of the sinuses from fluid, inflammation, or tumor. MRI may show subtle perineural spread and involvement of the cranial nerve foramen and canals. In addition, visualization of sagittal and coronal images with MRI advances visualization compared with CT scan in evaluation of intracranial or leptomeningeal spread.[14] Fusion of MRI with planning CT is useful in defining tumor not visible on CT scan alone. MRI or PET fusion with planning CT are also useful when induction chemotherapy is given where prechemotherapy images facilitate accurate mapping of the initial volume of gross tumor for precise target delineation.[66]

RADIATION THERAPY FOR REGIONS OF THE PARANASAL SINUSES

A study at Stanford University[42] reported that IMRT for patients with paranasal sinus and nasal cavity tumors has better outcomes compared with historical series and is well tolerated. The study notes that RT delivered via conventional techniques has been associated with significant complications. Severe visual toxicity has been observed, with

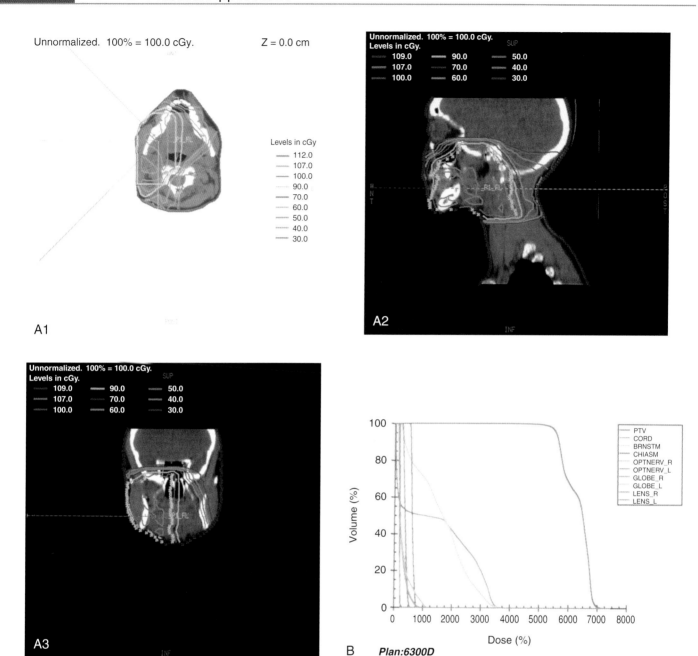

Fig. 29.29 T1N0M0 adenoid cystic carcinoma of the right submandibular salivary gland. Postoperative intensity-modulated radiation therapy to the right submandibular area and the pathways of the adjacent lingual nerve and the hypoglossal nerve to the base of skull to a dose of 5400 cGy; submandibular bed is boosted to 6300 cGy. (A) Isodose distributions: *A1,* Axial; *A2,* sagittal; *A3,* coronal. (B) Dose-volume histogram. (From Chong LM, Armstrong JG. Tumors of the salivary glands. In: Hoppe RT, Phillips TL, Roach M. *Leibel and Phillips Textbook of Radiation Oncology.* 3rd ed. Philadelphia, PA: Saunders; 2010.)

unilateral and bilateral blindness rates reported to be as high as 30% and 10%, respectively. Subsequent improvements in conventional and 3D-CRT techniques reduced the risk of blindness but did not eliminate it. IMRT planning for the department includes planning target volumes generated by adding a 3-mm to 5-mm margin to all clinical target volume structures. The surrounding OARs, including the optic nerves, optic chiasm, orbits, and brainstem, were contoured on the treatment planning CT. Elective nodal irradiation is routinely delivered to patients with T3 and T4 SCC of the maxillary sinus. For other histologies and subsites, elective nodal irradiation is given at the discretion of the treating oncologist. The Stanford study reports a good outcome with a clinical plan with the high-risk PTV dose of 6600 cGy in 220

cGy fractions, whereas the standard risk PTV dose is 5400 to 6000 cGy in 180 to 200 cGy fractions. Five patients who were undergoing postoperative RT were treated with a hyperfractionated RT course with the high-risk PTV receiving 7440 cGy in 120 cGy twice-daily fractions. Treatment plans were normalized to cover at least 95% of the PTV with the prescription isodose curve.[42] The plan included a stereotactic radiosurgical (SRS) boost to the site of gross residual disease or site of positive margin. The SRS boost prescription dose was 800 cGy in 1 fraction in 3 patients, which resulted in a total tumor biologic effective dose of 7910 cGy in 200 Gy fractions.

Cervical nodal spread is uncommon, but if it is present, the submandibular node is the first station involved and is treated. Surgery

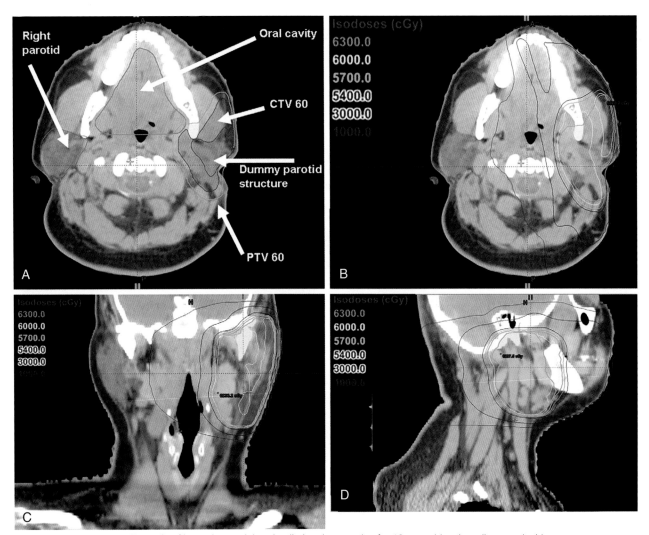

Fig. 29.30 Example of intensity-modulated radiation therapy plan for 46-year-old patient diagnosed with stage T2 N0, left, parotid, low-grade mucoepidermoid carcinoma. The planning tumor volume *(PTV)* was prescribed to 60 Gy in 30 fractions. Healthy tissues of concern included the oral cavity (mean dose, 26.8 Gy), contralateral parotid and submandibular glands (mean doses, 6.4 and 3.6 Gy, respectively), cochlea (mean and maximal dose, 20.6 and 30.5 Gy, respectively), and spinal cord (maximal dose, 14 Gy). The maximal hot spot was 105.3%, which was within the PTV. (From Schoenfeld JD, Sher DJ, Norris CM Jr, et al. Salivary gland tumors treatment with adjuvant intensity-modulated radiotherapy with or without concurrent chemotherapy. *Int J Radiat Oncol Biol Phys.* 2012;82:308–314.)

and RT are complicated because these tumors are often located close to multiple critical structures, including the eye, brain, optic nerves, brainstem, and cranial nerves. Adjuvant RT is favored based on aesthetic considerations as opposed to radical resections. Nevertheless, surgery is the principal treatment for control of small lesions of the nasal septum or those limited to the infrastructure of the maxillary sinus. Although primary RT for small lesions has a high cure rate, this approach has a significant chance of optic nerve injury from the high dose necessary to achieve good tumor control.[14]

Maxillary cancers are usually diagnosed at advanced stages. Most cases warrant treatment with combined surgery and postoperative RT. This is considered standard treatment. The results of radical surgical excisions such as craniofacial resection, total maxillectomy, or orbital exenteration have improved, especially with aggressive plastic reconstruction. However, these operations still produce significant morbidity.

Massive tumors with extensive involvement of the nasopharynx, base of skull, sphenoid sinuses, brain, or optic chiasm are considered

unresectable. Primary RT has been used with differing success depending on stage and extent of tumor. Treatment rationale for RT has incurred a change over the past decade from preoperative to postoperative treatment. Preoperative RT may obscure the initial extent of disease and erroneously lead to a more conservative resection, leaving microscopic disease behind. Preoperative RT also has been shown to increase infection rate and the risk of postoperative wound-healing complications. RT after surgery has the advantage of accurate pathologic review of all structures at risk. RT target volumes for the nasal cavity, ethmoid sinuses, and maxillary sinuses include both halves of the nasal cavity and the ipsilateral maxillary sinus in the typical postoperative setting. If tumor extends superiorly into the ethmoid air cells, the ethmoid sinuses and the ipsilateral medial orbital wall are included. A tongue depressor is used to displace the tongue from the field.

It is most advantageous to base the treatment volume on treatment planning CT, with MRI correlation. The complex anatomy of this region and the presence of numerous critical, dose-limiting structures (optic nerves, chiasm, eyes, lacrimal gland, pituitary, brainstem, etc.)

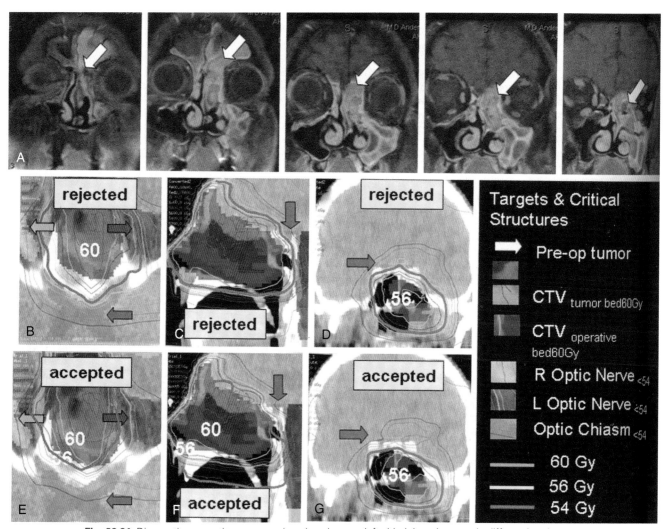

Fig. 29.31 Diagnostic magnetic resonance imaging shows a left-sided, invasive, poorly differentiated, naso-ethmoid carcinoma invading the bone. After resection, the goal was to deliver a dose of 60 Gy in 30 fractions to the tumor bed and 54 Gy to the operative bed with intensity-modulated radiation therapy (A). The plan was rejected because the 54-Gy isodose line *(light color)* was very close to the optic nerves and chiasm *(arrow;* B to D). The optimized plan was accepted (E to G). (From Beitler JJ, et al. Sinonasal cancer. In: Gunderson LL, Tepper JE, eds. *Clinical Radiation Oncology.* 3rd ed. Philadelphia, PA: Elsevier Saunders; 2012.)

render these tumors ideal candidates for a sophisticated treatment planning system.[14] A 3D system allows careful definition and comprehensive visualization of the tumor and normal anatomy through "beam's-eye view." The use of nonaxial and noncoplanar fields allows greater flexibility in treatment planning so that dose distribution conforms to tumor volume in 3D space, sparing the surrounding healthy tissue to a greater extent. This type of treatment planning has great potential for improving tumor control by allowing dose escalation. Compared with a classic treatment plan, which routinely includes one-half to one-third of the ipsilateral eye, greater sparing of the ipsilateral eye is possible without sacrificing tumor control with use of a 3D conformal plan. The presentation of inhomogeneity corrections for air cavities and dense bone is a significant advantage of this type of conformal planning system. Inverse-planned IMRT may render a greater therapeutic ratio for tumor of the paranasal sinuses compared with the more standard forward-planning 3D conformal therapy (Fig. 29.31). IMRT improves sparing of the optic critical structures, especially in unresectable, definitive cases where high doses are necessary for eradication of gross tumor. The SEER database shows an improving trend of overall survival rate for maxillary sinus. The overall survival rate for the

1980s, 39%; for the 1990s, 45% and between 2008 and 2014 was 58%. The overall treatment outcome is still poor, though, with less than 55% of patients surviving longer than 5 years. The most common patterns of treatment failure are local recurrence and distant metastasis.[66]

MANAGEMENT OF SYMPTOMS AND MORBIDITY

The incidence of morbidity is related to the treatment technique used, the size of the irradiated volume, the time/dose fractionation scheme used, the location and the extent of the disease, and the patient's age and nutritional status. The early- and late-responding tissues are affected differently by these factors. The interaction of radiation in cells is random and has no selectivity for any structure or site. This forms the basis of the great challenge in RT.

The amount of dose prescribed to eradicate a cancer ultimately is dependent on healthy tissue tolerance of that dose. Radiosensitivity is the innate sensitivity of cells, tissues, or tumors to radiation. Both healthy and cancer cells are affected by radiation. Cells vary in their expressed sensitivity to radiation. Generally, rapidly dividing cells are most sensitive (e.g., mucosa); nondividing or slowly dividing cells

TABLE. 29.6 Typical Curative Radiation Doses for Head and Neck Cancer

5000 cGy	Nodes
5000 cGy	Any subclinical disease
6000–6500 cGy	T1 lesions
6500–7000 cGy	T2 lesions
7000–7500 cGy	T3–T4 lesions

TABLE. 29.7 Approximate Dose-Tissue Response Schedule for Conventional Fractionation

Response	Dose (cGy)
Dry mouth	2000
Erythema	2000
Brachial plexus	5500
Spinal cord	4500–5000
Lhermitte's sign	2000–3000
Mandible, teeth, and gums	5000–6000
Mucositis	3000
Ears	4000
Cataracts	500–1000
Dry eye	4000
Optic nerve	5000
Retina	5000
Trismus	6000
Laryngitis	5000

generally are less radiosensitive, or radioresistant (e.g., muscle cells, neurons). Exceptions include small lymphocytes and salivary gland cells, which are nondividing but are radiosensitive. The incidence of morbidity is also higher when RT and surgery are combined. The difficulties consist of delayed wound healing from impaired blood supply and infection.[14] Specific curative doses for head and neck cancers are listed in Table 29.6. The tissue tolerance doses, the radiation doses to which healthy tissue can be irradiated and continue to function, are listed in Table 29.5. The radiation therapist should know the dose limitations to the specific tissues included in the typical head and neck volume. Table 29.7 provides an approximate dose-tissue response schedule for a conventional fractionation scheme. Studies report that treatment-related toxicities for head and neck cancer patients may include mucositis, pharyngitis, dysphagia, and skin toxicities, among other conditions. Despite IMRT's improvement of certain side effects. such as xerostomia, patients still experience dental caries, swallowing issues, osteoradionecrosis, and strictures leading to PEG tube placements.[67]

Contemporary issues include different response rates for HPV-positive oropharyngeal cancer, with overall survival rates near 90%. The good prognosis of the HPV-associated tumors as compared with regular cases of oropharyngeal cancer has raised concerns of over irradiation and needless aggressive treatment to these cases that show radiosensitivity. New protocols are exploring biomarkers, new PET protocols, dose-de-escalation concurrent with chemotherapy regimens for HPV-positive oropharyngeal cancer treatments.[67]

This brings focus to the very different characteristics of the HPV-positive cancer patient population observed in increasing numbers within the past decade. Of critical importance is the observance of a younger demographic reporting oropharyngeal cancers attributable to the HPV. As already expressed, this patient population has a better than normal prognosis and a longer life expectancy than the counterpart HPV-negative oropharyngeal cancer patient. The better prognosis warrants the need to examine methods to avoid toxicities and new strategies to mitigate common debilitating toxicities this population may have to live with.[68]

Dysphagia

Difficulty swallowing and issues regarding normal functioning of the throat is common among head and neck cancer patients as they undergo RT. Speech pathologists are instrumental in working with these patients to maintain or improve swallow physiology and function. However, it is not clear which interventions provide the greatest benefit or which exercise therapy on swallow physiology and function impact the overall quality of life for the patient.[68]

A recent metaanalysis study reveals that although the exact type or the timing of the interventions that are most effective is unclear, there is evidence that behavioral dysphagia intervention for jaw range-of-motion and swallow function shows benefit for the patient.[68]

Periodontal Disease and Caries

Because healing is poor after treatment, extractions of carious teeth after RT are not recommended. Aggressive extractions after high doses can lead to osteoradionecrosis. The teeth should be extracted before RT if the patient has carious teeth.

Nutrition

At the time of diagnosis, many patients have lost a significant amount of weight. Maintenance of adequate nutrition is a major problem for these patients; both the tumor and the treatment side effects, such as mucositis from both chemotherapy and RT (after 2000–3000 cGy), may contribute to this problem. Placement of a gastrostomy tube or nasogastric feeding may be necessary to maintain adequate nutrition. A PEG tube may be needed for patients who experience significant weight loss as a result of treatment side effects. Insertion of a PEG tube is a procedure (with use of a mild sedation) in which a tube is passed into the patient's stomach through the abdominal wall. The tube provides a means of nutrition for the patient who is unable to eat because of treatment side effects.

Mucositis/Stomatitis

The epithelial cells of the mucous membrane that line the oral cavity are extremely radiosensitive. Inflammation of the oral mucous membranes with edema and tenderness can occur. A pseudomembrane may form along the mucosal surface. This membrane can slough off and leave a friable, painful ulcerated surface. Areas that are adjacent to metallic tooth fillings within the treatment field may develop an increased reaction because of scatter radiation from the filling. Dental accessories may be available to eliminate scatter during treatment. Mouth care should involve avoidance of drying agents, such as alcohol- or glycerin-based products, and frequent brushing and rinsing of the oral cavity. An oral care regimen and the need for routine follow-up with a dentist should be part of the patient and family education (Box 29.6).

Xerostomia

Xerostomia occurs after 1000 cGy and diminished long-term salivary function at doses as low as 2000 cGy, posing a significant long-term side effect. The patient then becomes at risk for dental caries and oral infections. When the salivary glands are within the treatment field, the saliva may become scant and thick and ropy. In some patients, pilocarpine

---

BOX. 29.6 Recommended Oral Hygiene Program

- Clean teeth and brush gums after meals
- Use fluoride toothpaste or fluoride rinses daily
- Floss daily
- Rinse the mouth with salt and a baking soda solution (1 qt water, ½ tsp salt, ½ tsp baking soda)
- See a dentist regularly during treatment for a dental examination
- To reduce the severity of any head and neck complication, the patient should be encouraged to avoid the following:
  - Spicy hot foods, coarse or raw vegetables, dry crackers, chips, and nuts
  - Smoking, chewing tobacco, and alcohol
  - Sugary snacks
  - Commercial mouthwash that contains alcohol because it dries the mouth
  - Cold foods and drinks

BOX. 29.7 Recommended Skin Care Program

- Wash the skin with lukewarm water, pat dry.
- Use mild soaps (e.g., Basis, Neutrogena)
- Use water-based lotions or creams (e.g., Aquaphor, Eucerin)
- Avoid lotions with perfume and deodorants
- Avoid direct sunlight
- Do not use straight razors
- Avoid tight-fitting collars and hat brims
- Do not use aftershave lotions or perfumes
- Apply only nonadherent, hydrophilic dressings to wounds

---

hydrochloride (Salagen) has been useful in stimulating the production of saliva. The use of saliva substitutes is necessary along with other oral lubricants; XeroLube or vegetable oils help decrease the sensation of mouth dryness. The use of reinforced daily fluoride application to the teeth may strengthen the tooth enamel and minimize dental caries.

Cataract Formation

One of the most radiosensitive tissues in the head and neck area is the lens. Cataracts, which can be removed surgically, may develop after doses lower than 1000 cGy.[12]

Lacrimal Glands

Irradiation of the lacrimal gland may cause a dry, painful eye. Severe dry eye syndrome has been reported in 100% of patients receiving more than 5700 cGy. Obstruction to the tear duct, which is rare and usually associated with tumor involvement of the lacrimal duct, causes a constantly wet eye.[12]

Taste Changes

Treatment may affect the taste buds, which line the tongue and other parts of the oral cavity. Although the sensation affected (sweet, sour, salty, or bitter) varies, reports indicate that the sweet sensation is affected more than the salty sensation.[26] The incidence is dose dependent. The taste buds are radiosensitive, and atrophy and degeneration are noted at 1000 cGy. Although some recovery may occur within a few months after treatment, many patients continue to report persistent taste changes for several months after irradiation. The therapist should educate the patient and family regarding temporary or permanent effects and maintenance of nutritional status. One should encourage the patient to identify and consume foods that have or retain some taste (sweet and sour foods retain some taste). Patients should be encouraged to chew foods longer to allow more contact of the food with the taste buds. The sense of taste and smell are closely linked. Because the olfactory senses are not affected, the patient can smell the food before eating it to give the sense of some taste.[12]

Skin Reactions

Most patients experience some degree of acute skin effects. These effects vary depending on total dose, dose of daily fraction, type and energy of radiation used, the use of radiosensitizing/chemotherapy agents (methotrexate, 5-FU), the use of beam modifiers (bolus material), and individual differences among patients (complexity and nutrition). Reactions range from erythema or dryness to dry or moist desquamation. Adherence to principles of good wound care and maintenance of

a clean environment are recommended. Moisturizing lotions and gels can be applied to areas of dry desquamation; hydrocortisone cream can be applied to irritated, inflamed skin but should not be used on areas of moist skin reactions because it may enhance infection.[62] Box 29.7 lists elements of a recommended skin care program.

Repeat Treatment of Recurrent Disease

Studies and patient histories show that despite effective treatment of head and neck cancers such as SCC, 30% to 40% of patients will experience recurrence with isolated locoregional disease. Others will have a second primary cancer develop. Both cases will involve new growth in a previously irradiated area posing a great challenge for treatment. Historically, RT to a previously irradiated field was associated with significant acute and late morbidity with minimal control rates and poor patient outcomes. The risks of reirradiation have exceeded the benefits. Contemporary treatment techniques, such as conformal RT using IMRT and VMAT, are felt to have changed the therapeutic ratio for reirradiation cases. The modern treatment planning systems with better abilities to target gross tumor, with smaller fields, tighter margins, and targeted treatments are felt to be factors leading to a greater degree of sparing normal tissue and reducing collateral radiation dose. However, exact and specific details regarding the role of irradiation with contemporary treatment methods is still being studied.

Stereotactic body RT (SBRT) is now considered a viable modality for patients with unresectable, local recurrent, and previously irradiated head and neck cancers.[69]

A fatal complication of head and neck cancer reirradiation has been carotid blowout syndrome (CBOS). The response to the repeated radiation has been noted to include this complications where the carotid artery or one of its major branches ruptures. Early reports noted a higher rate of CBOS after SBRT as compared with conventional reirradiation techniques. Improved methods have been reported to reduce the risk of CBOS after SBRT. These include increasing the length of treatment delivery from daily to every other day and eliminating patients with skin invasion or tumor-related ulceration.[69] Repeat treatment with SBRT continues to be explored and analyzed to determine the best patient selection, fractionation, and dose constraints.

Despite modern conformal and targeted treatment techniques, morbidity still includes varying degrees of osteoradionecrosis, aspiration pneumonia, esophageal strictures, CBOS, and fistulas. A late toxicity also includes continued dependence on a feeding tube and tracheostomy.[70]

A 2018 study described the safety and efficacy of IMRT-based reirradiation of patients with a recurrent or second primary of a SCC of the head and neck referred to its findings as a favorable risk-to-benefit ratio. This study of 412 patients within 7 different medical facilities reported encouraging conclusions with guidelines for patient selection. Improved overall survival was reported among patients with nasopharynx and base-of-skull tumors. A factor for a good candidate was the lack of organ dysfunction before repeated treatment or after surgery. Also, the treatments implemented a longer time between courses of radiation treatments. Patients longer than 2 years from their previous treatment with resectable tumors often experience long-term survival. Recursive partitioning analysis (RPA), a method of identify patients with distinct, good survival patterns can identify patient candidates who will benefit from reirradiation treatments. Tumor location and degree of invasion appears to be more useful than general performance status such as a Karnofsky performance score for patient selection.[70]

Another study by Vargo, Caudell, and Dunlap[71] provides supportive findings that correspond with the previously mentioned factors reflecting favorable factors for reirradiation of recurrent or second primary head and neck cancers. A study of 414 patients with 9 US academic medical centers reported that IMRT and SBRT is better tolerated than historical accounts of repeat RT. Specific details of dose and fractionation were provided. Findings support RPA as an important prognostic tool to guide candidates. It is emphasized that supportive care is necessary for each patient. Further study is needed to optimize patient outcomes. [71]

ROLE OF THE RADIATION THERAPIST

The extent of RT side effects varies from patient to patient. During the initial consultation, the radiation oncologist should inform the patient of all possible complications that can arise from the treatment or disease process; this is usually accomplished during informed consent completion. The entire oncology team is responsible for assessing the efficiency of the treatment in terms of the health and well-being of the patient. The radiation therapist's role in patient assessment and as a gatekeeper to direct care or to avoid significant patient reactions (perhaps by interrupting treatment) is dependent on this knowledge.

Patients with head and neck cancer need to know that the side effects encountered are site specific and dose dependent. Patients also need to understand that communication of any discomfort they are experiencing to the radiation therapists or other team members is vital to good cancer treatment management of the head and neck region. Radiation therapists should encourage patients to express any fears they have about the side effects, disease outcomes, or procedures that can alter speech, food intake, or breathing. Patients should also be informed that follow-up after treatment is an important aspect of the management of head and neck cancer because they are at risk for a recurrence. Radiation therapists should give patients explicit instructions regarding physical changes to look for in tissue color, texture, new growths, or unexplained pain. Patients should be instructed to seek medical advice as soon as possible if they experience any of these changes.

Soreness of the throat and mouth is expected to appear in the second or third week of standard fractionated RT. Minor irritations often remain for about a month after treatment's end. Viscous lidocaine or dyclonine hydrochloride are good liquid pain relievers. Over-the-counter medication (approved by a physician) such as Orajel for babies and Ambersol can provide temporary relief.

Denture wearers may notice that the dentures no longer fit as a result of swelling of the gums. Loss of saliva is a common side effect of radiation to the oral cavity. Sipping of cool, carbonated drinks during the day may alleviate some of this. Lemon drops (sugar-free) help promote saliva production and taste. The radiation therapist should instruct the patient to choose foods that are easy to eat. As chewing and swallowing become more difficult, the therapist should recommend more liquid, semisolid meals moistened with sauces and gravies to make eating easier. Artificial saliva is a possible remedy; a physician should be consulted.

The cancer care team, including the therapist, should instruct the patient about wound care, cleaning of tracheostomies, and speech rehabilitation options. The therapist should be mindful of any weeping surgical sites or a change in the healing process that can indicate an infection. Proper skin care during treatment is an important aspect of patient care management. To better facilitate communication with a speech-impaired patient, the therapist should provide a pad and pencil. Hand signals should be arranged with the patient in the event something goes wrong in the treatment room during beam-on conditions. The radiation therapist must understand that the patient with head and neck cancer undergoes some structural and functional losses; the therapist should be ready to answer any questions and provide for the specific needs of the patient.

FUTURE DIRECTIONS

Greater results in RT may be achieved with the use of techniques such as 3D conformal therapy, proton beam therapy, or intracavitary boost delivery for limited tumors. A report on proton beam therapy for nasopharyngeal tumors has shown promising results. It suggests that the use of proton beams results in a significant increase in dose with increased sparing to healthy tissue. The high-cost and time-consuming planning is noted to be a disadvantage. Examples of the advantages of 3D conformal therapy and IMRT have been cited in several sections of this chapter. Computer-assisted multileaf collimators with a real-time portal imaging device allow the delivery of multiple beams with minimal human interventions. This development adds to available quality assurance, which is growing in importance as treatment volumes become more specific with escalating doses. Local control has been reported to be enhanced. Sparing of structures such as the unaffected parotid gland is achieved with IMRT, and tumor failure within the CTV has led to studies of radioresistant tumor subvolumes. These studies bring a new awareness for the selection of more aggressive treatment techniques where hypoxic regions are identified using modern imaging such as PET and biomarkers.

Recent studies that involve the treatment of patients with head and neck cancer with a helical tomotherapy unit focus on the elimination of systematic errors and random setup errors. Consideration of error includes the progressive deformation of the patient's soft tissue structures during the course of treatment. Protocols that use megavolt CT image guidance are now in practice. Variables under consideration include increased patient imaging dose and machine time in addition to precision.[66]

Publications describing candidates for repeated RT treatments because of recurrent disease or a second tumor indicate advances improving the therapeutic ratio. However, the literature includes recommendations for further studies to optimize treatment outcomes.

▎ SUMMARY

- The effective management of patients with head and neck cancer involves the close cooperation of radiation oncologists, medical oncologists, dentists, maxillofacial prosthodontists, nutritionists, head and neck surgeons, neurosurgeons, plastic surgeons, oral surgeons, pathologists, oncology nurses, radiologists, social workers, radiation therapists, speech therapists, pain service, neurology service, and of course, the patient.

- Integration of image guidance technology with IMRT and use of functional image information with PET fused with treatment planning have the potential to improve both tumor control and healthy tissue sparing.
- The lungs are the most common site of distant metastasis.
- The incidence of distant metastasis is greatest with tumors of the nasopharynx and hypopharynx.

- High-grade parotid tumors are known to involve the facial nerve and to cause paralysis.
- The preservation of salivary function with sparing of at least one parotid gland has been a primary objective of head and neck IMRT. A general benefit involves minimal side effects and morbidity from minimized exposure to healthy tissue.
- Thyroid cancer consistently shows the greatest positive trend in the SEER reports. It leads among all ages, races, and genders in trending incidence of primary cancers and is second only to liver cancer and inflammatory bowel disease in trending US cancer death rates for the time period reported.

- General etiologic risk factors for head and neck cancer include (1) tobacco and alcohol use, (2) UV light exposure, (3) viral infection, and (4) environmental exposures.
- Occupations associated with greater risk include (1) nickel refining, (2) furniture and woodworking (cancers of the larynx, nasal cavity, and paranasal sinuses), and (3) steel and textile work (oral cancer).
- EBV has been associated with nasopharyngeal carcinoma in all races.
- More than 80% of head and neck cancers arise from the surface epithelium of the mucosal linings of the upper digestive tract. These cancers are mostly SCCs.

REVIEW QUESTIONS

The answers to the Review Questions can be found by logging on to our website at: http://evolve.elsevier.com/Washington/principles

1. Multiple tumor types are included in the head and neck region. Which type of primary tumor is most common?
   a. Adenocarcinoma.
   b. Squamous cell carcinoma.
   c. Basal cell carcinoma.
   d. Fibrosarcoma.
2. The primary lymphatic drainage of the lower lip is to the:
   a. Submental nodes.
   b. Submaxillary nodes.
   c. Subdigastric node.
   d. Posterior cervical chain.
3. What healthy tissue is at most risk of radiation damage with treatment of the maxillary antrum?
   a. Brain.
   b. Eye.
   c. Skin.
   d. Pituitary.
4. The most common sign or symptom of oral cancer is:
   a. Ulceration.
   b. Hoarseness.
   c. Odynophagia.
   d. Xerostomia.
5. The most commonly involved group of nodes in oropharyngeal cancer is the:
   a. Submandibular nodes.
   b. Retropharyngeal nodes.
   c. Jugulodigastric nodes.
   d. Supraclavicular nodes.

6. A tumor confined to the larynx with cord fixation in glottic cancer is staged as a:
   a. T1.
   b. T2.
   c. T3.
   d. T4.
7. Palpation of the cricoid cartilage indicates the inferior border of the:
   a. Oral cavity.
   b. Oropharynx.
   c. Larynx.
   d. Hypopharynx.
8. For patients with carious teeth, when is dental work recommended when anticipating oral cavity irradiation?
   a. After treatment.
   b. Before treatment.
   c. Both a and b.
   d. Neither a nor b.
9. Postcricoid cancers occur predominantly in:
   a. Adult women.
   b. Adult men.
   c. Both women and men equally.
   d. Pediatric patients under 18 years.
10. Tumors of the head and neck may involve the cranial nerves that control the major senses. This involvement may lead to signs and symptoms that can point to a possible location of a tumor. Which cranial nerve may be involved in facial paralysis?
    a. XII.
    b. I.
    c. VIII.
    d. VII.

QUESTIONS TO PONDER

1. Most head and neck cancers are grouped together by anatomic site. Why then is there such diverse difference in biologic and clinical behavior between the same cell type and structures that are only a few millimeters apart?
2. What is the reason for the high incidence of a second primary for patients with early-stage squamous cell disease that was cured?

3. Can any biologic markers be identified early and decrease the toxicity and morbidity from treatments?
4. Do nonstandard RT fractionation schemes improve survivability at the expense of second malignancies?
5. Does chemotherapy have a role in the elective treatment of premalignant conditions seen in head and neck disease?

REFERENCES

1. Foote RL, Ang KK. Head and neck tumors; overview. In: Gunderson LL, Tepper JE, eds. *Clinical Radiation Oncology*. 3rd ed. Philadelphia, PA: Elsevier Saunders; 2012.
2. Noone AM, Howlader N, Krapcho M, et al, eds. SEER Cancer Statistics Review, 1975-2015, based on November 2017 SEER data submission, posted to the SEER website, April 2018. https://seer.cancer.gov/csr/1975_2015. Accessed July 17, 2018.
3. American Cancer Society. Cancer facts and figures 2018. Atlanta, GA: American Cancer Society. https://www.cancer.org/content/dam/cancer-org/research/cancer-facts-and-statistics/annual-cancer-facts-and-figures/2018/cancer-facts-and-figures-2018.pdf. Accessed July 17, 2018.
4. National Cancer Institute. *Surveillance, Epidemiology, and End Results Program*. Cancer stat facts: oral cavity and pharynx cancer; 2018. https://seer.cancer.gov/statfacts/html/oralcav.html. Accessed July 17, 2018.
5. Gomez DR, Kaplan MJ, Colevas AD, et al. Cancer of the oral cavity. In: Hoppe RT, Leibel SA, Phillips TL, eds. *Textbook of Radiation Oncology*. 3rd ed. Philadelphia, PA: Elsevier Saunders; 2010.
6. Lee N, Laufer M, Ove R, et al. Nasopharyngeal carcinoma. In: Gunderson LL, Tepper JE, eds. *Clinical Radiation Oncology*. 3rd ed. Philadelphia, PA: Elsevier Saunders; 2012.
7. Noone AM, Howlader N, Krapcho M, et al. (eds). SEER Cancer Statistics Review, 1975–2015, National Cancer Institute. Bethesda, MD, https://www.cancer.gov/types/head-and-neck/hp/oral-prevention-pdq/ based on November 2017 SEER data submission, posted to the SEER web site, April 2018. Accessed July 17, 2018.
8. National Cancer Institute. Oral Cavity, Pharyngeal, and Laryngeal Cancer Prevention (PDQ®)–Health Professional Version. https://www.cancer.gov/types/head-and-neck/hp/oral-prevention-pdq/#link/_122_toc. Updated June 28, 2018. Accessed July 17, 2018.
9. Blot WJ, McLaughlin JK, Winn DM, et al. Smoking and drinking in relation to oral and pharyngeal cancer. *Cancer Res*. 1988;48(11):3282–3287.
10. Talamini R, Bosetti C, La Vecchia C, et al. Combined effect of tobacco and alcohol on laryngeal cancer risk: a case-control study. *Cancer Causes Control*. 2002;13(10):957–964.
11. Pazdur R, Wagman LD, Camphausen KA. *Cancer Management: a Multidisciplinary Approach*. 13th ed. New York: UBM Medica; 2010.
12. Iwamoto RR, Haas ML, Gosselin KT. *Manual for Radiation Oncology Nursing Practice and Education*. 4th ed. Pittsburgh: Oncology Nursing Press; 2012.
13. Chong LM, Armstrong JG. Tumors of the salivary glands. In: Hoppe RT, Leibel SA, Phillips TL, eds. *Textbook of Radiation Oncology*. 3rd ed. Philadelphia, PA: Elsevier Saunders; 2010.
14. Chen AM, Ryu JK, Donald PJ. Cancer of the nasal cavity and paranasal sinuses. In: Hoppe RT, Leibel SA, Phillips TL, eds. Leibel and Phillips *Textbook of Radiation Oncology*. 3rd ed. Philadelphia, PA: Elsevier Saunders; 2010.
15. Beitler JJ, McDonald MW, Wadsworth JT, Hudgins PA. Sinonasal cancer. In: Gunderson LL, Tepper JE, eds. *Clinical Radiation Oncology*. 3rd ed. Philadelphia, PA: Elsevier; 2012.
16. Rimmer A, Lee N, Zelefsky M. Cancer of the hypopharynx. In: Hoppe RT, Leibel SA, Phillips TL, eds. Leibel and Phillips *Textbook of Radiation Oncology*. 3rd ed. Philadelphia, PA: Elsevier Saunders; 2010.
17. Garden AS, Morrison WH, Ang KK. Larynx and hypopharynx cancer. In: Gunderson LL, Tepper JE, eds. *Clinical Radiation Oncology*. 3rd ed. Philadelphia, PA: Churchill Livingstone; 2012.
18. American Joint Committee on Cancer. *Cancer Staging Manual*. 7th ed. New York, NY: Springer; 2010.
19. American Cancer Society. *Causes, Risk Factors, and Prevention: Risk Factors for Laryngeal and Hypopharyngeal Cancers*; 2017. https://www.cancer.org/cancer/laryngeal-and-hypopharyngeal-cancer/causes-risks-prevention/risk-factors.html#references. Accessed July 17, 2018.
20. Hoppe RT, Leibel SA, Phillips TL, eds. *Textbook of Radiation Oncology*. 3rd ed. Philadelphia, PA: Elsevier Saunders; 2010.
21. Kim S, Smith BD, Haffty BG. Prognostic factors in patients with head and neck cancer. In: Harrison LB, Sessions RB, Kies MS, eds. *Head and Neck Cancer: A Multidisciplinary Approach*. 4th ed. Philadelphia, PA: Lippincott Williams & Wilkins; 2013.
22. Gregoire V, et al. Management of the neck. In: Gunderson LL, Tepper JE, eds. *Clinical Radiation Oncology*. 3rd ed. Philadelphia, PA: Elsevier Saunders; 2012.
23. Hu KS, et al. Cancer of the oropharynx. In: Hoppe RT, Leibel SA, Phillips TL, eds. *Textbook of Radiation Oncology*. 3rd ed. Philadelphia, PA: Elsevier Saunders; 2010.
24. Wolfe MJ, Wilson K. Head and neck cancer. In: Sabel MS, Sondak VK, Sussman JJ, eds. *Surgical Foundations: Essentials of Surgical Oncology*. Philadelphia, PA: Mosby; 2007.
25. Chen RC, Khorsandi AS, Shatzkes DR, Holliday RA. The radiology of referred otalgia. *Am J Neuroradiol*. 2009;30(10):1817–1823. Accessed July 17, 2018.
26. Hornig JD, et al. Clinical evaluation of the head and neck. In: Harrison LB, Sessions RB, Kies MS, eds. *Head and Neck Cancer: A Multidisciplinary Approach*. 4th ed. Philadelphia, PA: Lippincott Williams & Wilkins; 2013.
27. Beitler JJ, Amdur RJ, Mendenhall WM. Cancers of the head and neck. In: Khan FM, Gerbi BJ, eds. *Treatment Planning in Radiation Oncology*. 3rd ed. Philadelphia, PA: Lippincott Williams & Wilkins; 2011.
28. Welz S, Monnich D, Pfannenberg C, et al. Prognostic value of dynamic hypoxia PET in head and neck cancer: results from a planned interim analysis of a randomized phase II hypoxia-image guided dose escalation trial. *Radiother Oncol*. 2017;124(3):526–532.
29. Marcu LG, Moghaddasi L, Bezak E. Imaging of tumor characteristics and molecular pathways with PET: developments over the last decade toward personalized cancer therapy. *Int J Radiat Oncol Biol Phys*. 2018;102(4):1165–1182.
30. Oosting SF, Brouwers AH, van Es SC, et al. 89Zr-bevacizumab PET visualizes heterogeneous tracer accumulation in tumor lesions of renal cell carcinoma patients and differential effects of anti-angiogenic treatment. *J Nucl Med*. 2015;56:63–69.
31. Mendenhall WM, et al. Oral cavity cancer. In: Gunderson LL, Tepper JE, eds. *Clinical Radiation Oncology*. 3rd ed. Philadelphia, PA: Elsevier Saunders; 2012.
32. Khandani AH, Sheikh A. Nuclear medicine. In: Gunderson LL, Tepper JE, eds. *Clinical Radiation Oncology*. 3rd ed. Philadelphia, PA: Elsevier Saunders; 2012.
33. Weng BM, Cohen JM. General principles of head and neck pathology. In: Harrison LB, Sessions RB, Kies MS, eds. *Head and Neck Cancer: A Multidisciplinary Approach*. 4th ed. Philadelphia, PA: Lippincott Williams & Wilkins; 2013.
34. Sabel M. Principles of surgical therapy. In: Sabel MS, Sondak VK, Sussman JJ, eds. *Surgical Foundations: Essentials of Surgical Oncology*. Philadelphia, PA: Mosby; 2007.
35. Fakhry C, Zevallos JP, Eisele DW. Imbalance between clinical and pathological staging in updated American Joint Commission on Cancer Staging System for human papillomavirus-positive oropharyngeal cancer. *J Clin Oncol*. 2018;36(3):217–219.
36. Cannon GM, et al. Oropharyngeal cancer. In: Gunderson LL, Tepper JE, eds. *Clinical Radiation Oncology*. 3rd ed. Philadelphia, PA: Elsevier Saunders; 2012.
37. Huang HS, O'Sullivan B. Overview of the 8th edition TNM classification for head and neck cancer. *Curr Treat Options Oncol*. 2017;18(7):40.
38. Brierley J, Gospodarowicz M, Wittekind C. *UICC TNM Classification of Malignant Tumors*. 8th ed. Chichester, UK: Wiley; 2017.
39. Amin M, Edge S, Greene F, et al. *AJCC Cancer Staging Manual*. 8th ed. New York, NY: Springer; 2017.
40. O'Sullivan B. Head and neck tumors. In: Brierley J, Gospodarowicz M, Wittekind C, eds. *UICC TNM Classification of Malignant Tumors*. 8th ed. Chichester, UK: Wiley; 2017.
41. O'Sullivan B, Lydiatt W, Haughey BH, et al. HPV- Mediated (p16+) Oropharyngeal Cancer. In: Amin M, Edge S, Greene F, et al. *AJCC Cancer Staging Manual*. 8th ed. New York, NY: Springer; 2017.
42. You YN, Donohue JH. Surgical principles. In: Gunderson LL, Tepper JE, eds. *Clinical Radiation Oncology*. 3rd ed. Philadelphia, PA: Elsevier Saunders; 2012.
43. Lee M, et al. Cancer of the nasopharynx. In: Hoppe RT, Leibel SA, Phillips TL, eds. *Textbook of Radiation Oncology*. 3rd ed. Philadelphia, PA: Elsevier Saunders; 2010.

44. Forastiere AA, Zhang Q, Weber RS, et al. Long-term results of RTOG 91-11: a comparison of three nonsurgical treatment strategies to preserve the larynx in patients with locally advanced larynx cancer. *J Clin Oncol.* 2013;31(7):845–852.

45. Sanguineti G. Oncology scan: rethinking treatment strategies for cancers of the larynx and pharynx. *Int J Radiat Oncol Biol Phys.* 2013;86(5): 805e–807e.

46. Doornaert P, Verbakel WF, Bieker M, et al. RapidArc planning and delivery in patients with locally advanced head and neck cancer undergoing chemoradiotherapy. *Int J Radiat Oncol Biol Phys.* 2011;79(2):429–435.

47. Romesser PB, Cahlon O, Scher ED, et al. Proton bean re-irradiation for recurrent head and neck cancer: multi-institutional report on feasibility and early outcomes. *Int J Radiat Oncol Biol Phys.* 2016;95(1):386–395.

48. Khan FM, Gerbi BJ, eds. *Treatment Planning in Radiation Oncology.* 3rd ed. Philadelphia, PA: Lippincott Williams & Wilkins; 2011.

49. Marks LB, Yorke ED, Jackson A, et al. Use of normal tissue complication probability models in the clinic. *Int J Radiat Oncol Biol Phys.* 2010;76(3):S10–S19.

50. Sher DJ, Thotakura V, Balboni T, et al. Treatment of oral cavity squamous cell carcinoma with adjuvant or definitive intensity modulated radiation therapy. *Int J Radiat Oncol Biol Phys.* 2011;81(4):e215–e222.

51. Bakst RL, Lee N, Pfister DG, et al. Hypofractionated dose painting intensity modulated radiation therapy with chemotherapy for nasopharyngeal carcinoma: a prospective trial. *Int J Radiat Oncol Biol Phys.* 2011;80(1):148–153.

52. Vann A, et al. *Portal Design in Radiation Therapy.* 3rd ed. DWV Enterprises. Columbia S.C.; 2013.

53. Daly ME, Le QT, Maxim PG, et al. Intensity-modulated radiotherapy in the treatment of oropharyngeal cancer: clinical outcomes and patterns of failure. *Int J Radiat Oncol Biol Phys.* 2010;76(5):1339–1346.

54. Beadle BM, Anderson CM. CTV guidance for head and neck cancers. *Int J Radiat Oncol Biol Phys.* 2018;100(4):903–905.

55. Khan FM. Introduction: process, equipment, and personnel. In: Khan FM, ed. *Treatment Planning in Radiation Oncology.* 2nd ed. Philadelphia, PA: Lippincott Williams & Wilkins; 2007.

56. Yao M, Chang K, Funk GF, et al. The failure patterns of oral cavity squamous cell carcinoma after intensity modulated radiotherapy: the University of Iowa experience. *Int J Radiat Oncol Biol Phys.* 2007;67(5):1332–1341.

57. Fortin A, Wang CS, Vigneault E. Influence of smoking and alcohol drinking behaviors on treatment outcomes of patients with squamous cell carcinomas of the head and neck. *Int J Radiat Oncol Biol Phys.* 2009;74(4):1062–1069.

58. Ghadjar P, Bojaxhiu B, Simcock M, et al. High dose-rate versus low dose rate brachytherapy for lip cancer. *Int J Radiat Oncol Biol Phys.* 2012;201283(4):1205–1212.

59. Wu B, McNutt T, Zahurak M, et al. Fully automated simultaneous integrated boosted: intensity modulated radiation therapy treatment planning is feasible for head and neck cancer: a prospective clinical study. *Int J Radiat Oncol Biol Phys.* 2012;84(5):e647–e653.

60. Caudell JJ, Burnett OL, Schaner PE, et al. Comparison of methods to reduce dose to swallowing-related structures in head and neck cancer. *Int J Radiat Oncol Biol Phys.* 2010;77(2):462–467.

61. Studer G, Peponi E, Kloeck S, et al. Surviving hypopharynx-larynx carcinoma in the era of IMRT. *Int J Radiat Oncol Biol Phys.* 2010;77(5):1391–1396.

62. Cahlon O, et al. Cancer of the larynx. In: Hoppe RT, Leibel SA, Phillips TL, eds. *Textbook of Radiation Oncology.* 3rd ed. Philadelphia, PA: Elsevier Saunders; 2010.

63. Schoenfeld JD, Sher DJ, Norris CM, et al. Salivary gland tumors treated with adjuvant intensity-modulated radiotherapy with or without concurrent chemotherapy. *Int J Radiat Oncol Biol Phys.* 2012;82(1):308–314.

64. Quon H, et al. Salivary gland malignancies. In: Gunderson LL, Tepper JE, eds. *Clinical Radiation Oncology.* 3rd ed. Philadelphia, PA: Elsevier Saunders; 2012.

65. Wiegner EA, Daly ME, Murphy JD, et al. Intensity-modulated radiotherapy for tumors of the nasal cavity and paranasal sinuses: clinical outcomes and patterns of failure. *Int J Radiat Oncol Biol Phys.* 2012;83(1):243–251.

66. Zeidan OA, Langen KM, Meeks SL, et al. Evaluation of image-guidance protocols in the treatment of head and neck cancers. *Int J Radiat Oncol Biol Phys.* 2007;67(3):670–677.

67. Lee N, Schoder H, Beattie B, et al. Strategy of using intra-treatment hypoxia imaging to selectively and safely guide radiation dose de-escalation concurrent with chemotherapy for locoregionally advanced human papillomavirus-related oropharyngeal carcinoma. *Int J Radiat Oncol Biol Phys.* 2016;96(1):9–17.

68. Greco E, Simic T, Ringash J, et al. Dysphagia treatment for patients with head and neck cancer undergoing radiation therapy: a meta-analysis review. *Int J Radiat Oncol Biol Phys.* 2018;101(2):421–444.

69. Gebhardt BJ, Vargo JA, Ling D, et al. Carotid dosimetry and the risk of carotid blowout syndrome after reirradiation with head and neck stereotactic body radiation therapy. *Int J Radiat Oncol Biol Phys.* 2018;101(1):195–200.

70. Ward MC, Caudell JJ, Isrow D, et al. Refining patient selection for reirradiation of head and neck squamous carcinoma in the IMRT era: a multi-institution cohort study by the MIRI collaborative. *Int J Radiat Oncol Biol Phys.* 2018;100(3):586–594.

71. Vargo JA, Caudell JJ, Dunlap NE, et al. A multi-institutional comparison of SBRT and IMRT for definitive reirradiation of recurrent or second primary head and neck cancer. *Int J Radiat Oncol Biol Phys.* 2018;100(3):595–605.

30

Central Nervous System Tumors

Megan Trad

OBJECTIVES

- Discuss epidemiologic factors of this tumor site.
- Identify, list, and discuss etiologic factors that may be responsible for inducing tumors in this anatomic site.
- Describe the symptoms produced by a malignant tumor in this region.
- Discuss the methods of detection and diagnosis for tumors in this anatomic region.
- List the varying histologic types of tumors specific to this region.
- Describe the diagnostic procedures used in the workup and staging for this site.
- Differentiate between histologic grading and staging.
- Describe in detail the anatomy and physiology of this anatomic region or organ.
- Identify the treatments of choice for this malignancy.
- Discuss the rationale for treatment with regard to treatment choice, histologic type, and stage of the disease.

- Describe in detail the treatment methods available for this diagnosis.
- Describe the differing types of radiation treatments that can be used for treatment of this tumor site.
- Identify the appropriate tumor lethal dose for various stages of this malignancy.
- Discuss the expected radiation reactions for the area based on time-dose-fractionation schemes.
- Discuss tolerance levels of the vital structures and organs at risk.
- Describe the instructions that should be given to a patient with regard to skin care, expected reactions, and dietary advice.
- Identify the psychologic problems associated with a malignancy in this site.
- Describe the various treatment planning techniques for this anatomic site.
- Discuss survival statistics and prognosis for various stages for this tumor site.

OUTLINE

KEY TERMS

Blood-brain barrier
Cerebellum
Cerebrospinal fluid
Cerebrum
Debulking
Edema
Gamma knife
Intracranial pressure
Karnofsky performance scale

Necrosis
Papilledema
Positron emission tomography
Radiation necrosis
Radiosensitizers
Regeneration
Tentorium
Ventricles

Central nervous system (CNS) tumors include brain and spinal cord tumors. As with most tumors, they can be classified as primary or secondary (metastatic) and benign or malignant; however, when tumors occur within the brain or spinal cord, both classifications are significant.[1] Radiation therapy is a vitally important primary and adjuvant treatment technique in the management of CNS tumors and provides a means of increasing survival time, minimizing neurologic deficits, and enhancing the quality of life of many patients with brain tumors.[2,3]

Although CNS tumors rarely metastasize, they are often locally invasive and create significant problems. Structures that become involved with these neoplasms are not capable of regeneration (repair or regrowth), so the damage done is most often permanent. Tumors of the CNS, even if benign histologically, are considered malignant in part because of their inaccessible location.[4] As shown in Table 30.1, many different cell types are believed to produce CNS and spinal axis tumors. Because CNS tumors arise in different areas of the cranium and spinal axis, the belief is that different molecular and genetic mechanisms are at work during various times of life.

CANCER OF THE CENTRAL NERVOUS SYSTEM

Epidemiology

According to the American Cancer Society, approximately 23,800 cases of primary brain tumors and other nervous system tumors are diagnosed annually in the United States.[5,6] Brain tumors account for 1.4% of all malignancies and so are considered relatively rare; however, 16,000 deaths are attributed to CNS tumors each year.[6] About 80% of CNS tumors involve the brain, whereas 20% involve the spinal cord. The incidence rate is 5 per 100,000 people and varies according to race, gender, and age. Brain tumors are the second leading cause of cancer death in children (behind leukemia).[5]

Age is a dominant variable, with the incidence of CNS tumors rising as a person ages. Nelson and colleagues[7] attribute this increase to three possible factors: (1) an increase in life expectancy, (2) the increasing availability and use of computed tomography (CT) and magnetic resonance imaging (MRI), and (3) an increased interest in geriatrics and an overall improvement in healthcare of the elderly. CNS tumors have a bimodal peak in incidence by age. The first peak is during childhood between the ages of 3 and 12 years, and the second is later in life in individuals between the ages of 50 and 80 years.[8] The adult incidence is highest between the age of 55 and 64 years, with a median age of diagnosis at 57 years.[6]

Many different tumor types are included in the CNS category, with a wide range in aggressiveness. Any of these tumors can occur at any location within the brain or spinal column. Approximately 16,400 of all CNS tumors occur in the cerebrum. Gliomas are the most common classification of brain tumors, with 30% of all CNS tumors and 80% of malignant brain cell tumors in this classification.[9] Approximately 45% of childhood tumors are gliomas, with most involving the cerebellum and, to a lesser degree, the brainstem.[9,10]

> Recent statistics regarding brain cancer incidence can be found at the American Cancer Society's website: www.cancer.org.

The function of the cerebrum includes interpretation of sensory impulses and voluntary muscular activities; it is the center for memory, learning, reasoning, judgment, intelligence, and emotions. The cerebellum is the part of the brain that plays a role in the coordination of voluntary muscular movement.

Although primary brain tumors are relatively uncommon, estimates are that 20% to 40% of patients with cancer eventually have brain metastasis develop throughout the course of the disease.[11] The most common primary site of disease responsible for brain metastases is the lung, which occurs in 30% to 60% of patients.[12] Most metastatic lesions occur in the cerebral hemispheres, with a single metastasis occurring 40% to 45% of the time. Brain metastases because of the conspicuous presenting symptoms may be the only indication of malignant disease. These metastases can occur early in the disease process or may not appear until years later. Factors such as the patient's age, Karnofsky performance scale (KPS) score, and neurologic signs and symptoms at the time of diagnosis are important variables in determination of a patient's prognosis.[1]

TABLE 30.1   Classification of Tumors of the Central Nervous System

Tumor Type	Normal Tissue Origin	General Function of Tissue
Glioma (includes glioblastoma, astrocytoma, glioblastoma multiforme, brainstem, and thalamus tumors)	Astrocytes	These star-shaped cells are commonly found between neurons and blood vessels that provide support and help regulate ions. They are an important part of the blood-brain barrier.
Medulloblastoma	Primitive neuroectodermal cells, or PNETs	These cells comprise a family of the small blue round cell mass and are the most common malignant nervous system tumors of childhood. These cells do not usually remain in the body after birth.
Oligodendroglioma	Oligodendrocyte	These smaller cells resemble an astrocyte. They produce a fatty insulating substance called myelin, which may be provided to many nearby axons.
Ependymoma	Ependyma	These cells line the ventricles and spinal cord. These cuboidal-shaped cells aid in the production and circulation of cerebrospinal fluid.
Meningioma	Meninges	These cells are comprised of three distinct coverings that protect the brain and spinal cord. CSF circulates within the meninges.
Lymphoma	Lymphocyte and microglia	Part of the immune system, these cells are the body's primary defense against infection and foreign substances. Microglial cells help support neurons and phagocytize bacteria and cellular debris.
Schwannoma	Schwann cell	These cells produce a fatty insulating substance called myelin, which insulates and protects nerves outside the CNS.

CNS, Central nervous system; *CSF,* cerebrospinal fluid; *PNETs,* primitive neuroectodermal tumors.

The Karnofsky performance scale (KPS) scores, which range from 0 to 100, are a clinical method of measuring the ability of patients with cancer to perform ordinary tasks. A higher score means the patient is better able to carry out daily activities. KPS may be used to determine a patient's prognosis, measure changes in a patient's ability to function, or decide whether a patient is available for inclusion in a clinical trial.

Etiology

The origin of primary CNS tumors is largely unknown. Brain tumor associations include occupational and environmental exposures, lifestyle and dietary factors, medical conditions, and genetic factors. Occupational and environmental factors include chemicals, synthetic rubber, pesticides, herbicides, ionizing radiation, and electromagnetic fields. The association between chemical exposure and brain tumors is limited to a few occupations. Workers in agriculture and healthcare delivery have shown higher incidence rates than normal. Lifestyle and dietary factors include cells phones, nitrates, hair dyes, and smoking. Medical conditions include drugs, viral infections, and acquired immunodeficiency syndrome (AIDS). Genetic factors, which include less than 5% of the etiology of brain tumors, include neurofibromatosis, tuberous sclerosis, Li-Fraumeni syndrome, and von Hippel-Lindau syndrome.[1,13] Some research indicates a twofold to threefold increase in incidence when a close relative is diagnosed with a glioma.[2]

Prognostic Indicators

The 5-year survival rates for patients with primary CNS tumors during the past four decades have ranged from 19% from 1960 to 1985 to an overall 35% during the past two decades.[3] Several factors have been identified as prognostic indicators for CNS tumors. The three most important factors are age, performance status, and tumor type. In numerous clinical trials with malignant gliomas, these prognostic factors had a greater influence on survival than the type or extent of the therapy evaluated. Unfortunately, one of the most common adult brain tumors, glioblastoma multiforme, is one of the most lethal, with only 2.2% of patients surviving 3 years.[14,15] The prognosis tends to be better in younger patients, with one exception; children younger than 4 years present a particular problem with respect to treatment regimen. Therapy must be modified because of their still developing brain, which is more sensitive to radiation; therefore, radiation treatment in children younger than 4 years old must be avoided if possible.

Late effects after CNS treatment in children are an area of concern. Radiation therapy to the brain has been linked to a significant decrease in IQ scores and to impaired mental functions such as processing speed, attention, and working memory.[16] Pediatric cancer long-term survivors also experience higher incidences of emotional distress such as anxiety and depression, which can diminish quality of life.[16]

The location of the tumor is of great importance and serves as a natural prognostic indicator for survival time and neurologic defects. In addition, the KPS measures the neurologic and functional status, which allows for measurements of the quantity and quality of neurologic defects. The KPS ranges from 0 to 100 and is measured in decades. Patients who are able to work or whose lifestyle is not affected significantly by the disease have scores in the 80 to 100 range. Patients who are unable to work but can still care for themselves have scores in the 50 to 70 range (Box 30.1). Patients who are chronically ill from the disease process have scores of 40 or below.

Tumor grade rather than size is the primary factor involved with prognosis. The tumors are normally grouped into benign, or low-grade,

---

BOX 30.1 Karnofsky Performance Scale

Performance Criteria

Able to carry on normal activity; no special care needed	100		Normal; no symptoms; no evidence of disease
	90		Ability to carry on normal activity; minor signs or symptoms of disease
	80		Normal activity with effort; some signs or symptoms of disease
Unable to work; able to live at home and care for most personal needs; a varying amount of assistance needed	70		Self-care; inability to carry on normal activity or do active work
	60		Occasional care for most needs required
	50		Considerable assistance and frequent medical care required
	40		Disabled; special care and assistance required
Unable to care for self; required equivalent of institutional or hospital care; disease may be progressing rapidly	30		Severely disabled; hospitalization indicated, although death not imminent
	20		Extremely sick; hospitalization necessary; active support treatment necessary
	10		Moribund; fatal processes progressing rapidly
	0		Dead

Performance Scale (Eastern Cooperative Oncology Group)

Grade

0	Fully active; able to carry on all predisease activities without restriction (Karnofsky score of 90 to 100)
1	Restricted in physically strenuous activity, but ambulatory and able to carry out work of a light or sedentary nature, such as light housework or office work (Karnofsky score of 70 to 80)
3	Capable of only limited self-care; confined to bed or chair 50% or more of waking hours (Karnofsky score of 30 to 40)
4	Completely disabled; unable to carry on any self-care; totally confined to bed or chair (Karnofsky score of 10 to 20)

Modified from Carter S, *Principles of Cancer Treatment* by New York, NY: McGraw-Hill; 1981.

---

and malignant, or high-grade, categories. The presence or absence of necrosis has prognostic significance. Necrosis is the death of a cell or cell group that results from disease or injury. The process is caused by the action of enzymes and can also affect part of a structure or an organ.

A pathologist examining a biopsy specimen under the microscope grades the specimen to describe its growth rate and prognosis. Because tumors of the CNS rarely spread to other parts of the body, no specific staging system is used. Instead, assessment of the type of tumor or grade, the tumor size and location, and the patient health and function level is used to estimate a prognosis. The tumor grading system classifies tumors from I to IV, with low-grade tumors (I and II) resembling the tissue of origin and growing at a slow pace and with high-grade tumors (III and IV) being poorly differentiated and growing rapidly (Box 30.2). As CNS tumors continue to grow, they can progress from a low-grade tumor to a high-grade tumor; however, this is more common in adult patients.

BOX 30.2 National Cancer Institute Tumor Grading

Grade	Tissue Description
I	The tissue is benign. The cells look nearly like healthy brain cells, and they grow slowly.
II	The tissue is malignant. The cells look less like healthy cells than do the cells in a grade I tumor.
III	The malignant tissue has cells that look very different from healthy cells. The abnormal cells are actively growing (anaplastic).
IV	The malignant tissue has cells that look most abnormal and tend to grow quickly.

From National Cancer Institute. *What You Need to Know About Brain Tumors.* Bethesda, MD: National Institutes of Health; 2009.

Low-grade tumors have cellularity patterns that look similar to those found in reactive hyperplasia, whereas marked cellularity has been recognized in high-grade tumors, with necrosis seen in the most aggressive tumors, typically, the higher the grade, the shorter the survival time. Almost all patients experience a recurrence (with high-grade tumors) after surgery, and 80% of all recurrences are within a 2-cm margin.[7]

Anatomy and Lymphatics

The brain is one of the most complex organs in the body (Fig. 30.1). It is composed of two cerebral hemispheres (right and left) and two cerebellar hemispheres. The cranial bones, meninges, and cerebrospinal fluid (CSF) provide an outer covering of protection for the brain.

The ventricles are cavities that form a communication network with each other, the center canal of the spinal cord, and the subarachnoid space. The ventricles, canals, and subarachnoid space are all filled with CSF, which provides buoyancy, protection, chemical stability, and prevention of brain ischemia. Ependymal cells, which line the choroid

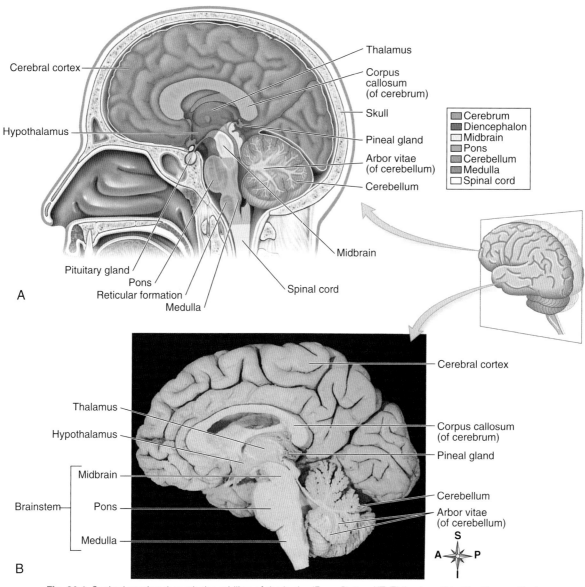

Fig. 30.1 Sagittal section through the midline of the brain. (From Patton KT, Thibodeau GA. *The Human Body in Health and Disease.* 7th ed. St. Louis, MO: Elsevier; 2018.)

plexuses, are responsible for secreting about 0.5 L of cerebral spinal fluid each day into the ventricles. These cavities are identified as the right and left lateral ventricles and the third and fourth ventricles. The lateral ventricles are located below the corpus callosum and extend from front to back. Each opens into the third ventricle. The lateral ventricles are able to communicate with the third ventricle via the interventricular foramen, which is a small oval opening. The third ventricle is connected to the fourth ventricle. The fourth ventricle lies between the cerebellum and inferior brainstem. Three small openings also allow the CSF to pass into the subarachnoid space. The openings also allow communication with the cord and subarachnoid space (see Fig. 30.1).

The supratentorial and infratentorial regions comprise the two major intracranial compartments, the cerebral and cerebellar hemispheres. The tentorium (a fold of dura mater, or the outer covering of the brain) separates these compartments. It passes transversely across the posterior cranial fossa in the transverse fissure and acts as a line of separation between the occipital lobe of the cerebrum and the upper cerebellum. The cerebral hemispheres and the sella, pineal, and upper brainstem regions are located in the supratentorial region. The infratentorial region, which leads to the upper spinal cord, houses the brainstem, pons, medulla, and cerebellum.

The CNS is composed of 40% gray matter and 60% white matter. The gray matter contains the supportive nerve cells and related processes. It forms the cortex, or outer part of the cerebrum, and surrounds the white matter. The white matter is composed of bundles of nerve fibers, axons that carry impulses away from the cell body, and dendrites that carry impulses toward the cell body. The nerve cells process and integrate nerve impulses from other neurons. The spinal cord is also composed of a gray substance that forms the inner core, which contains the nerve cells. The outer layer, or white substance, is the location of the nerve fibers. The gray matter varies at different levels of the spinal cord.

The blood supply for the brain comes from the internal carotid arteries and vertebral arteries via the circle of Willis. The blood that enters the brain contains oxygen, nutrients, and energy-rich glucose, which is the primary source of energy for the brain cells. If the blood supply to the brain is interrupted, dizziness, convulsions, or mental confusion may result.

The spinal cord is the continuation of the medulla oblongata and forms the inferior portion of the brainstem. The anterior and lateral portions contain motor neurons and tracts, whereas the posterior portions contain the sensory tracts. The motor neurons are nerve cells that convey impulses from the brain to the cord. This system allows communication between the spinal cord and various parts of the brain. The cord continues down to the level of the first and second lumbar vertebrae. This is an important anatomic reference point for the radiation therapy student. Many times, doses to the spinal cord must be calculated, and an understanding of where the spinal cord ends is important. From the spinal cord come 31 pairs of nerves referred to as the *cauda equina*. The spinal cord is surrounded by the same material that surrounds the brain, CSF, which flows between the arachnoid and pia arachnoid. Blood is supplied to the cord from the vertebral arteries and radicular branches of the cervical, intercostal, lumbar, and sacral arteries (Fig. 30.2). No lymphatic channels exist in the brain substance.

The blood-brain barrier (BBB), which hinders the penetration of some substances into the brain and CSF, exists between the vascular system and brain. Its purpose is to protect the brain from potentially toxic compounds. Substances that can pass through the BBB must be lipid soluble. Water-soluble substances need a carrier molecule to cross the barrier via active transport. Lipid-soluble substances include alcohol, nicotine, and heroin. Examples of water-soluble substances are glucose, some amino acids, and sodium. Various drugs pass the barrier with varying degrees of difficulty but never easily. Tumor cells that infiltrate healthy brain tissue cannot be reached by drugs that do not cross the BBB (Fig. 30.3).

Cerebrospinal fluid is a clear, colorless fluid that resembles water. The entire CNS contains 3 to 5 oz of this fluid, which is composed of proteins, glucose, urea (a compound formed in the liver and excreted by the kidney), and salts. The CSF performs several functional roles, including buoyancy to protect the brain, a link in the control of the chemical environment of the CNS, a means of exchanging nutrients and waste products with the CNS, and a channel for intracerebral transport. Blockage of CSF, because of tumor growth, may have disastrous effects on the patient. Interruption in the flow of CSF may contribute to increased intracranial pressure (ICP), which is pressure that occurs within the cranium. Increased ICP can cause headaches, vomiting, lethargy, seizures, and neurologic symptoms.

Natural History of Disease and Patterns of Spread

With few exceptions, most gliomas tend to spread invasively because they do not form a natural capsule that inhibits growth. These neoplasms are unique because they do not metastasize through a lymphatic drainage system and rarely metastasize outside the CNS; instead they expand through local invasion. Tumor cells may also break off and circulate within the CSF fluid, which allows tumors to spread to other parts of the CNS. The common route of spread for medulloblastomas and primitive neuroectodermal tumors, for example, is seeding via CSF into spinal and intracranial subarachnoid spaces.[17]

Local invasion and CSF seeding provide the major patterns of spread for CNS tumors. These tumors tend to have cells that can invade healthy brain tissue. Drop metastases occur via the CSF and can form secondary tumors. The confines of the brain itself limit the spread

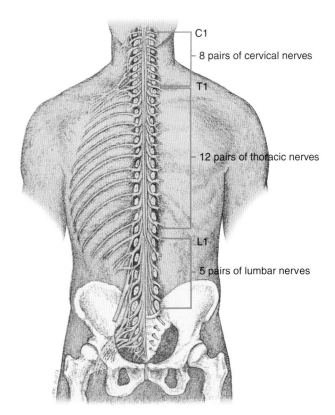

Fig. 30.2 Image depicts the spinal cords and associated nerves. Within the cervical spinal cord there are 8 associated nerves, 12 associated nerves within the thoracic vertebrae, and 5 lumbar nerves associated with the lumbar vertebrai.

C1
8 pairs of cervical nerves
T1
12 pairs of thoracic nerves
L1
5 pairs of lumbar nerves

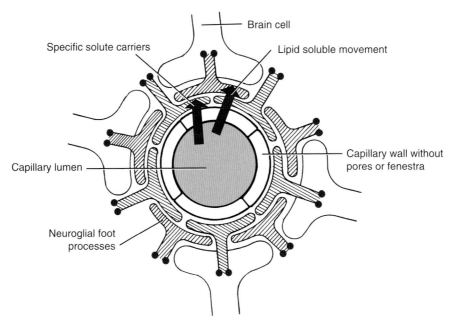

Fig. 30.3 Blood-brain barrier. (From Maisey M, Britton KE, Gilday DL. *Clinical Nuclear Medicine*, 2nd ed. New York: Chapman and Hall; 1992.)

of disease, but local recurrence is a major concern. Secondary seeding may grow along nerve roots, causing pain or cord compression. Although the lumbosacral area is the most frequent site of CSF seeding, any area along the spinal axis can become involved. Hematogenous spread is rare.

CNS tumors are characterized by their heterogeneity, which makes understanding their biology difficult. With an improved understanding of the reason and way that CNS tumors develop, grow, and progress, new treatment approaches can be developed and implemented.

Clinical Presentation

As stated, the location of the tumor correlates with the presenting symptoms. Table 30.2 provides an excellent correlation between common symptoms and tumor location. The initial symptom may be a headache, which is usually worse in the morning. This symptom results from the differences in the CSF drainage from the recumbent to upright positions. Seizures and difficulties with balance, gait, and ambulation are also common presenting signs. Focal signs are usually unilateral. Other neurologic symptoms can include aphasia, hemiplegia, and paresis. Ocular symptoms may result in decreased vision, oculomotor defects, proptosis, and ophthalmic defects. Other presenting signs may be expressive aphasia, sensory aphasia, mental and personality changes, short-term memory loss, hallucinations, and changes in intellectual functions. Increased ICP can result from the obstruction of CSF flow. The symptoms can result from direct invasion of the tissue by the tumor, destruction of brain tissue and bone, edema, and increased pressure.

Patients with spinal cord tumors have pain, weakness, loss of sensation, and bowel and bladder control problems. Although pain may be an early symptom, additional symptoms may signal a cord compression or vascular problems. Weakness usually occurs in the distal part of the extremity first and progresses proximally. Rapid deterioration of motor and sensory functions soon follows. Immediate treatment is necessary for patients who have a sudden onset of symptoms so that permanent paralysis may be prevented (Table 30.3). In contrast to brain lesions, the symptoms are more frequently bilateral.

Detection and Diagnosis

No screening tests are currently available to detect CNS tumors before they begin presenting symptoms. Because of this, diagnosis is usually made after a patient consults with a physician about physical symptoms. Most symptoms appear as the tumor creates increased ICP. ICP symptoms include headache, nausea, vomiting, blurred vision, trouble with balance, personality or behavioral changes, seizures, drowsiness, and in rare cases, coma.[1]

The initial workup is critical to a definitive diagnosis, and a complete history and physical examination are necessary. Because some CNS tumors are genetic or are associated with exposure to chemicals or related to infection, the medical, family, and social histories are extremely important. Information gathered from people other than the patient may also be beneficial in making a diagnosis. Mental changes, personality changes, and changes in behavior are not often noticed by the patient but are noticed by other individuals. Symptoms of long duration may indicate a slow-growing tumor, whereas the sudden onset of symptoms may point toward a tumor of higher grade and size.

A neurologic workup includes an evaluation in several key areas. The patient's mental status at the time of the diagnosis often reflects changes in behavior, mood, thought and speech patterns, and intelligence. Intellectual function is crucial, and the level of consciousness must be evaluated quickly. One test for intellectual function includes orientation to person, place, and time and the quickness of the responses to these questions. Further intellectual functions are determined with studying of speech, memory, and logical thought processes.

Coordination skills (including walking, balance, and gait), sensations, reflexes, and motor skills are also examined. Lesions that inhibit motor function tend to affect fine motor skills first and produce a spastic paralysis. Sensory functions can be tested with a pin, temperature, and vibrations. These functions can be affected before motor skills. Reflexes may be hyperactive with intracranial tumors early but may become hypoactive in later stages.

If spinal cord tumors are suspected, the evaluation of motor, sensory, and reflex functions is also important. Sensory testing is helpful in determination of the level of the lesion. Motor testing may reveal weakness.

TABLE 30.2	Symptoms, Signs, and Diagnostic Characteristics of Various Intracranial Tumors		
Tumor	**Common Symptoms**	**Common Signs**	**Diagnostic Characteristics**[a]
Primary			
Malignant astrocytoma	Headache, seizure, unilateral weakness, mental changes	Focal presentation related to tumor location	Enhancing CT lesion, tumor blush on angiography
Glioblastoma multiforme			CT lesion
Astrocytoma with anaplastic foci			No hypodense interior enhanced MRI or CT lesion
Brainstem or thalamus	Nausea, vomiting, ataxia	Increased intracranial pressure (papilledema) abducens and oculomotor nerve defects	May not enhance CT; biopsy may not be appropriate
Meningioma (B, M)	Localized headache, seizure	Focal presentation related to tumor location	Enhancing MRI or CT lesion associated with dura
Astrocytoma (B, M)	Headache, seizure, unilateral weakness, mental changes	Focal presentation related to tumor location	May not enhance on CT or MRI
Cerebral	Headache, seizure, unilateral weakness, mental changes	Focal presentation related to tumor location	
Cerebellar	Occipital headache	Increased intracranial pressure (papilledema), abducens and oculomotor nerve defects, coordination	
Brainstem or thalamus	Nausea, vomiting, ataxia	Increased intracranial pressure (papilledema), abducens and oculomotor nerve defects, coordination	May be seen only on MRI image; biopsy may not be appropriate
Optic nerve	Ocular symptoms	Ocular changes	Detailed MRI or CT scan
Pituitary (B, M)	Vertex headache, ocular changes	Ocular and endocrine abnormalities	Hormone analysis, resection histopathology
Medulloblastoma (M)	Morning headaches, nausea, vomiting	Coordination, increased intracranial pressure (papilledema), abducens and oculomotor nerve defects	MRI or CT scan, lumbar puncture recommended
Ependymoma (B, M)	Morning headaches, nausea vomiting	Coordination, increased intracranial pressure (papilledema), abducens and oculomotor nerve defects	MRI or CT scan, lumbar puncture recommended
Hemangioma, arteriovenous malformation (B, M)	"Migrainous" headache	Focal presentation related to tumor location	Angiography, biopsy may not be appropriate
Oligodendroglioma (B, M)	Insidious headache, mental changes	Focal presentation related to tumor location	Radiographic calcification
Sarcoma (M), neurofibroma (B)	Focal presentation related to tumor location	Focal presentation related to tumor location	
Pinealoma (B, M) germinoma	Various (ocular, vestibular endocrine)	Parinaud syndrome, endocrine changes, ocular changes, increased intracranial (papilledema), abducens and oculomotor nerve defects	Biopsy or resection may not be obtained; markers in CSF may be informative
Lymphoma (M), reticulum cell sarcoma, microglioma	Focal presentation related to tumor location	Focal presentation related to tumor location	"Soft" CT enhancement
Unspecified (B, M)	Focal presentation related to tumor location	Focal presentation related to tumor location	
Other			
Craniopharyngioma	Headache, mental changes hemiplegia, seizure, vomiting (and ocular changes)	Cranial nerve defects (II–VII)	Cystic/calcified lesion on MRI, bone erosion, mass effect from base of skull

[a]Unless noted, a biopsy is assumed.
B, Benign; CSF, cerebrospinal fluid; CT, computed tomography; M, malignant; MRI, magnetic resonance.
Modified from Gondi V, Vogelbaum MV, Grimm S, et al. Primary intracranial neoplasms. In: Halperin EC, Brady LW, Perez CA, et al, eds. *Perez and Brady's Principles and Practices of Radiation Oncology.* 6th ed. Philadelphia, PA: Lippincott Williams & Wilkins; 2013.

Ophthalmoscopy is a test designed to check for papilledema (edema of the optic disc), which results from increased ICP. Visual fields may decrease and blind spots increase as the disease progresses. An increase in ICP is usually the result of the flow of CSF becoming obstructed. This can indicate an increase in the tumor mass. If CSF flow is obstructed or production of the fluid is changed, hydrocephalus may

appear on CT scans. Infection, edema (swelling caused by the abnormal accumulation of fluid in interstitial spaces), or hemorrhage may also cause rising pressure.

Invasion, irritation, and compression of the brain by the tumor cause a variety of symptoms. Benign tumors generally cause symptoms produced by pressure, whereas malignant tumors can cause pressure

TABLE 30.3 Clinical Manifestations of Spinal Cord Tumors

Location	Findings
Foramen magnum	Eleventh and twelfth cranial nerve palsies; ipsilateral arm weakness early; cerebellar ataxia; neck pain
Cervical spine	Ipsilateral arm weakness with leg and opposite arm in time; wasting and fibrillation of ipsilateral neck, shoulder girdle, and arm; decreased pain and temperature sensation in upper cervical regions early; pain in cervical distribution
Thoracic spine	Weakness of abdominal muscles; sparing of arms; unilateral root pains; sensory level with ipsilateral changes early and bilateral with time
Lumbosacral spine	Root pain in groin region and sciatic distribution; weakened proximal pelvic muscles; impotence; bladder paralysis; decreased knee jerk and brisk ankle jerks
Cauda equina	Unilateral pain in back and leg, becoming bilateral when the tumor is large; bladder and bowel paralysis

Modified from Mehta M, Vogelbaum MA, Chang S, et al. Neoplasms of central nervous system. In: DeVita VT, Lawrence TS, Rosenberg SA, et al, eds. *DeVita, Hellman, and Rosenberg's Cancer: Principles and Practice of Oncology*. 9th ed. Philadelphia, PA: Lippincott Williams & Wilkins; 2011.

and destruction of CNS tissue. The initial presentation of symptoms depends on different anatomic locations. The involvement of specific regions of the brain generally produces symptoms specific to the areas controlled by those regions, thereby making tumor localization possible (Table 30.4).

Thus patients typically have symptoms that reflect the site of involvement. For example, if a tumor occurs in the frontal portion of the brain, symptoms likely to be identified include personality changes, memory defects, gait disorders, and speech difficulties. Lesions that occur in the parietal regions of the brain can produce symptoms such as loss of vision, spatial disorientation, and seizures.

Radiographs of the skull may show several changes that have occurred as a result of an ongoing tumor process. The pineal body may be calcified and deviated, increasing pressure may show erosion of the posterior clinoid process of the sphenoid bone, or calcification of certain tumors may be seen. Radiographs may show a hammered-metal appearance, which results from chronic pressure on the inner table of the skull. This condition is seen more often in radiographs of children. Erosive changes also may occur if the tumor invades the skull by eroding through the dura or outermost, toughest, and most fibrous membranes that cover the brain and spinal cord.

A CT scan can distinguish the CSF, blood, edema, and tumor from healthy brain tissue. The risks to the patient are minimal with CT scan. The use of iodine-based contrast to enhance the study increases the risk of an allergic reaction; however, this contrast is important for better visualization of the tumor's location, extent, and vascularization. Contrast-enhanced volume is indicative of a tumor. CT scans also provide information regarding the tumor growth patterns, and effects of the tumor on the skull. An area of higher or lower x-ray scattering power differentiates between necrosis or edema and calcification. CT scan used in conjunction with MRI can also confirm calcification or verify hemorrhage (Fig. 30.4).

Computed tomographic (CT) scanning for brain tumors can distinguish between soft tissue structures with CT numbers or Hounsfield units. Each pixel used to reconstruct a CT image is assigned a CT number from +1000 (bone) to −1000 (air) that corresponds to the density of the tissue within the pixel.

MRI is an important diagnostic tool in the diagnosis and grading of CNS tumors because of the superior image quality and the ability to show chemical changes that occur within the brain. For example, functional MRIs are currently being evaluated for their usefulness in radiation treatment planning and surgery. A functional MRI is a scan similar to a regular MRI except that the patient is asked a variety of questions or asked to perform specific tasks, such as wiggling toes, to identify which part of the brain controls that function. This information can be used to minimize damage to specific functions during surgery or to plan a radiation treatment around a specific function.

After radiation therapy or surgery, MRI also provides a method of evaluating tumor response or recurrence and is sensitive enough to detect tumors smaller than 1 cm. Another advantage MRI has over CT scan is that iodine contrast is not necessary to perform the procedure, which reduces the risk for a reaction. The contrast agent used in MRI is gadolinium, which is a noniodine-based intravenous (IV) contrast agent. Gadolinium helps differentiate between edema and the tumor and can detect surface seeding. With MRI, as with CT scan, three-dimensional imaging is possible; however, bone artifacts are absent, which makes it ineffective to use for radiation therapy treatment planning alone. MRI may also not be able to detect treatment-related changes from recurrent disease. CT scan is more cost effective, which allows for more economical use in follow-up after treatment (Fig. 30.5).

Positron Emission Tomography. Positron emission tomography (PET) is a beneficial diagnostic tool that may be useful in determination of differences between necrosis and malignancy, which are associated with areas of high metabolism. PET uses the radionuclide ^{18}F-fluorodeoxyglucose (FDG) to help detect lesions. PET incorporates the localizing ability of CT scanning with the ability of the FDG agent to concentrate lesions and help differentiate between various types of CNS lesions, infections, and degenerative processes.

A stereotactic biopsy (a procedure commonly performed during neurosurgery to guide the insertion of a needle into a specific area of the brain) allows all areas of the tumor and its borders to be studied before surgery causes changes in the appearance of the tumor. A biopsy is indicated if a lesion is deep-seated, is thought to be malignant, or occurs in older or debilitated patients who cannot tolerate a surgical procedure. The risks of a biopsy include an approximately 30% rate of inadequate diagnosis. Other risks include hemorrhage in the area of the biopsy and postoperative swelling.[18]

Debulking procedures are performed if the tumor location is accessible and the tumor volume is large. Debulking accomplishes a reduction in tumor size and the opportunity to obtain a pathologic diagnosis. A reduction in tumor size may sometimes make treatment with postoperative radiation therapy easier.

Cerebral angiography has value for planning surgical intervention as a means for surgeons to study the intrinsic vasculature (blood supply) of the tumor and surrounding blood vessels. However, this tool is of little value in establishing a definitive diagnosis.

Pathology

The most important prognostic factor for CNS tumors is the histopathologic diagnosis. Benign lesions are indicative of a better prognosis, and the potential for a cure with the use of surgery or radiation therapy exists. Intracranial tumors are considered locally malignant based on the limited space for expansion in the cranium. Treatment of the neural axis is indicated for some histopathologically malignant lesions such as medulloblastoma because of the risk of metastatic seeding.

Tumor growth is not hindered in most gliomas because CNS tumors do not form a natural capsule to contain them. Cellularity patterns differ according to the tumor grade. Low-grade tumors exhibit reactive

TABLE 30.4 Brain Tumor Localization Chart

	Frontal	Parietal	Temporal	Occipital
Symptoms	Often asymptomatic until late	Symptomatic earlier than frontal lobes	Speech disorders (left hemisphere dominant; not only for right-handed, but for most left-handed persons)	Seizures (relatively less common, but with auras, including flashing lights and unformed hallucinations)
	Symptoms of increased ICP	Symptoms of increased ICP		
	Bradyphrenia	Loss of vision	Loss of smell (superior lesion)	Loss of vision
	Personality changes	Spatial disorientation	Disturbance in hearing, tinnitus, etc.	Tingling (early)
	Libido changes	Tingling sensation	Speech disturbance	Weakness (late)
	Impetuous behavior	Dressing apraxia	Uncinate fits	
	Excessive jocularity	Loss of memory	Seizures with vocal phenomena in aura, including speech arrest	
	Defective memory	Seizures (focal sensory epilepsy)		
	Urinary incontinence	Weakness (anterior extension)	Hallucinations, dreams, déja vu	
	Seizures (generalized, becoming focal)		Space-perception disturbances	
	Gait disorders		Dysarthria	
	Weakness		Dysnomia	
	Loss of smell		Disturbance of comprehension	
	Speech disorder			
	Tonic spasms of fingers and toes			
Special Cerebral Functions	Behavioral problems (anterior location)	Anosognosia	Dysarthria	Visual agnosia
	Labile personality	Autotopagnosia	Sensory aphasia	Visual impulses
	Mental lethargy	Visual agnosia	Defective hearing	
	Defective memory	Graphesthesia (X)		
	Motor aphasia	Loss of memory		
		Proprioceptive agnosia		
Cranial Nerve Functions	Anosmia (inferior lesion)	Hemianopsia	Superior quadrantanopsia (X; could be homonymous hemianopsia with tumor extension)	Macular-sparing hemianopsia
	Nerve VI palsy with increased ICP	Papilledema (with increased ICP)		Horizontal nystagmus
	Papilledema with increased ICP		Central weakness of the cranial nerve VI	
	Foster Kennedy syndrome		Papilledema with increased ICP	
	Proptosis			
Motor System	Contralateral weakness (late)	Weakness	Dysdiadochokinesia (early)	Late appearance of motor signs, manifested by drift or dysdiadochokinesia
	Paresis (flaccid spastic)	Atrophy	Drift (secondary in later stages, involving arm more than leg)	
	Disturbed gait (midline lesion)	Clumsiness		
	Automatism	Dysdiadochokinesia		
	Persistence of induced movement (Kral's phenomenon)	Independent movements (unrecognized by patient)		
	Diagonal rigidity (arm [X]: leg [−])			
	Loss of skilled movement (X)			
	Urinary incontinence (super lesion)			
Sensory Functions	Rare involvement initially, unless invasion of sensory area (posterior lesion)	Dysesthesias (tingling; X)	Initially minimal	Somatosensory disturbances earlier than motor changes as adjacent structures are involved
		Pallesthesia (loss of vibratory sense; X)		
		Loss of touch, press and position sense (X), but pain and temperature usually unaffected		Visual phenomena, such as persisting images, unformed hallucinations, and aura
Reflex Changes	Tonic plantar reflex	Babinski's sign	May occur contralateral to tumor	No effect in early stages
	Hoffmann's sign	Hoffmann's sign		
	Grasp reflex			
	Babinski's sign			

ICP, Intracranial pressure; *X,* contralateral; −, ipsilateral.
Modified from Gondi V, Vogelbaum MV, Grimm S, et al. Primary intracranial neoplasms. In: Halperin EC, Brady LW, Perez CA, et al, eds. *Perez and Brady's Principles and Practices of Radiation Oncology.* 6th ed. Philadelphia, PA: Lippincott Williams & Wilkins; 2013.

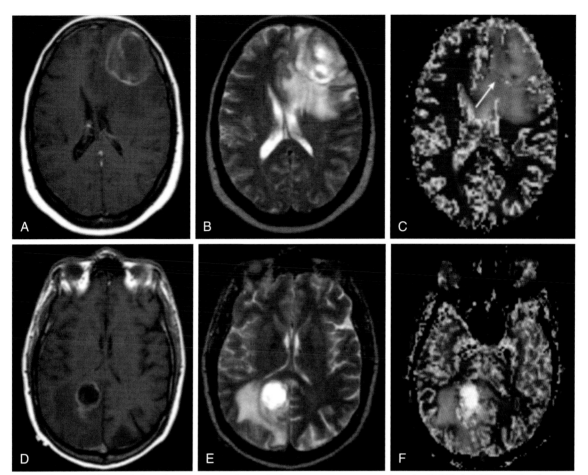

Fig. 30.4 Differentiation of tumor types using perfusion magnetic resonance imaging (MRI). Axial T1-weighted postgadolinium MRI demonstrating a metastasis from a lung carcinoma in one patient (A) and glioblastoma multiforme in another (D). Respective axial T2-weighted images demonstrate moderate edema with questionable involvement of the corpus callosum genu by the metastasis (B) and the corpus callosum by the glioblastoma (E). Perfusion MRI demonstrates hypovascularity in the peritumoral region, with only a minor increase in perfusion at the rim of enhancing tumor (C, *white arrow*), consistent with vasogenic edema without infiltrating tumor, compared with (F), which demonstrates increased perfusion in the peritumoral region, implying hypervascularity consistent with infiltrating high-grade glioma. (From Law M. Perfusion and MRS for brain tumor diagnosis. In: Edelman RR, Hesselink JR, Zlatkin MB, Crues JV, eds. *Clinical Magnetic Resonance Imaging*. 3rd ed, vol. 3. Philadelphia, PA: Saunders; 2006.)

hyperplasia with low cellularity, whereas marked cellularity is common in high-grade tumors. Necrosis is an important feature in high-grade tumors. Survival rates, with or without treatment, are clearly associated with tumor grade. Histopathology is more important than anatomic staging in determination of the clinical outcome and behavior of the tumor. In other words, the cell type associated with brain tumors is more important than the size of the tumor. Tissue diagnosis should be obtained in all patients with a brain tumor. The few exceptions include patients with diffuse intrinsic brainstem gliomas and optic nerve gliomas.[7]

Staging

No universal staging system is currently in use, and problems result because of the lack of a standardized method of staging. The American Joint Committee on Cancer uses a system based on the grade, tumor, metastasis (GTM) classification. Grade (G) has prognostic significance, with a range from well-differentiated to poorly differentiated (G1 to G3; https://www.cancer.org/cancer/brain-spinal-cord-tumors-adults/detection-diagnosis-staging/staging.html).

The Kernohan grading system has also been used. It is also a four-grade system, but it is difficult to use. The Kernohan system considers cellularity, anaplasia, mitotic figures, giant cells, necrosis, blood vessels, and proliferation.

Treatment Techniques

A multidisciplinary approach is necessary for the treatment of CNS tumors. A biopsy is extremely important for diagnostic purposes and essential for therapeutic decision-making.

Surgery. With the development of new surgical techniques, preoperative evaluation is even more important to further aid the surgeon. The tumor size and extent should be determined before surgery. The introduction of microsurgery, the ultrasonic aspirator, the laser, and perioperative sonography have made the surgeon's job easier. Computer-assisted stereotactic neuronavigation provides a new tool with the potential for great medical value.

When possible, surgery should be performed on tumors that are symptomatic and offer a chance for complete resection. Debulking is indicated with a large tumor volume and if a complete resection is not possible. Surgery can range from a debulking procedure to complete microsurgical removal. The primary goal for surgery is to remove the

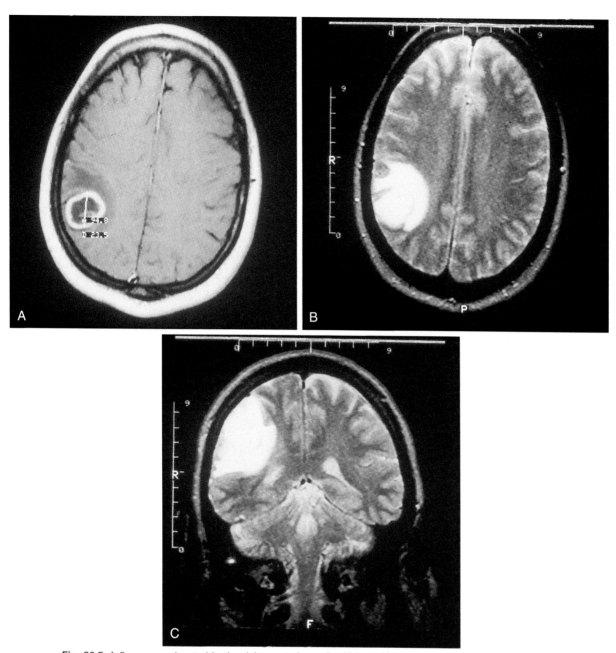

Fig. 30.5 A 3-cm mass located in the right posterior parietal lobe with surrounding edema. The peripheral aspect of the lesion exhibits gadolinium enhancement. (A) Axial magnetic resonance imaging cut shows a lesion with a necrotic center. (B) The mass is enhanced by gadolinium and shows surrounding edema. (C) Coronal image.

tumor and to obtain a histologic diagnosis. Surgery can be limited by the tumor location and extent, patient status, and risk of debilitating neurologic deficits. The patient's chances for survival are not enhanced with partial removal of the tumor. Tumor recurrence occurs from residual tumor that invades healthy brain tissue. Decreases in morbidity and mortality rates result from an earlier diagnosis, the use of steroid therapy, improvements in anesthetic techniques, and improved surgical methods. Surgical approaches to tumors depend on anatomic pathways, the tumor size, and the tumor location. General opinion in the surgical world is that early and radical excisions provide the best chance for a good outcome because of an accurate histologic diagnosis, control of a mass effect, and cytoreduction, which allow or enhance adjuvant therapy.[19]

Most patients with central nervous system tumors are prescribed steroids to reduce swelling and subside any symptoms that may exist. Steroids are naturally found within the body; however, pharmaceutical steroids increase the amount and work as a powerful antiinflammatory. Patients must take steroids exactly as prescribed by the doctor and be weaned off of the steroids gradually because the body stops producing natural steroids when an abundance is found in the bloodstream and needs to start producing them naturally again before being taken off the pharmaceutical steroid. Side effects of steroid use include weight gain, increased appetite, difficulty sleeping, increased risk of infection, and changes in mood, to name a few. Patients should be educated about side effects and that they should disappear after the steroid treatment has concluded.

Surgery also plays a crucial role in the management of some spinal cord tumors. Surgery can establish a diagnosis and make possible the removal of the tumor. Because of the location of the cord, a surgical resection is difficult at best to perform and impossible in some instances. Serious neurologic deficits are always a risk.

Radiation Therapy. Radiation therapy is indicated for malignant tumors that are incompletely excised, inaccessible from a surgical approach, and associated with metastatic lesions.

Several factors are considered in determination of the doses for treatment. Tumor type, tumor grade, and patterns of recurrence are particularly important. The radioresponsiveness of the tumor must also be considered.[20] The total dose must be limited by healthy tissue tolerance because radiation necrosis (tissue destruction) develops if tissue tolerance is exceeded. The risk of tumor progression must be balanced against the potential risk of necrosis when the dose is determined. In addition, consideration should be given to the side effects that may be induced. These side effects include acute reactions (or those encountered during the course of treatment), early-delayed reactions that occur from a few weeks until up to 3 months after treatment, and late-delayed reactions that occur months to years later. Threshold doses and the therapeutic ratio also must be considered.

Several approaches are available for treatment of tumors of the brain, depending on the type of disease, tumor location and extent, and whether the spinal axis requires treatment. Because brain malignancies can result from primary brain tumors, metastases from another site, or meningeal involvement, each type of malignancy must be handled appropriately.

The total surgical resection of a brain tumor for cure is an extremely difficult task to accomplish, partly because of the difficulty in obtaining generous enough resection margins in brain tissue. Radiation therapy usually follows surgery in an attempt to prevent tumor regrowth or recurrence. In the past, whole-brain irradiation has been used via lateral portals with a boost to the tumor bed after initial treatment. With the advent of CT scan and MRI, more accurate tumor localization allows smaller fields to be simulated and treated. Smaller field designs and unique configurations through the use of specialized multileaf collimation blocking make simulation and daily reproducibility of the setup an even more important part of the treatment process.

If brain metastases are present from another primary site of involvement, whole-brain irradiation in the past has been the preferred treatment. The belief being that even with a solitary mass, occult disease is often present, although undetected; therefore, the whole brain should be treated. Stereotactic radiosurgery (SRS), however, has emerged as an important treatment option for patients with isolated CNS tumors and solitary brain metastasis.[21] A common treatment technique for patients with a single unresectable brain metastasis currently is whole-brain radiation therapy (WBRT) with an SRS boost. New research, however, is indicating that eliminating the WBRT and delivering the entire dose via SRS provides more favorable cognitive outcomes, reduces late side effects, and has less of an impact on patient's quality of life.[22]

Simulation provides the foundation for all radiation treatment no matter the technique for delivery. The simulation procedure should be carefully explained to the patient before it begins. The complexity of the procedure and the necessity for daily reproducibility of the treatment setup should be stressed. Patients should be aware of the importance of their compliance and cooperation in relation to the outcome of the treatment. Accurate reproducibility is a must. Head rotation and tilting create the potential for difficulties in reproducibility. Immobilization is extremely important and can be achieved through the use of head-holding devices. The use of an immobilization system is beneficial for treating patients via lateral ports to a limited brain field with the

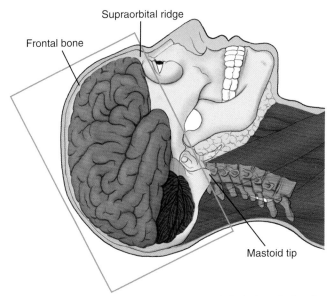

Supraorbital ridge

Frontal bone

Mastoid tip

Fig. 30.6 A lateral view of the skull shows a whole-brain radiation therapy field setup with the supraorbital ridge and mastoid tip as topographic bony reference marks. Note an equal amount of falloff or "flash" surrounding the cranium on the anterior, superior, and posterior margins.

patient in the supine position. The use of a thermoplastic mask greatly reduces errors in the reproducibility of the setup.

Lateral portal fields are used for treatment of the whole brain for palliative reasons. The inferior margin of the field may intersect the superior orbital ridge and external auditory meatus. In selection of the field size, 1 cm of flash or shine over should be seen at the anterior, posterior, and superior borders of the field (Fig. 30.6). The flash reduces the chances of clipping any of the anatomy as a result of the field size being too small. The fields may be treated isocentrically or with a fixed source-skin distance. The use of a thermoplastic mask greatly reduces errors in the reproducibility of the whole-brain setup for palliative reasons. The standard approach for palliative whole brain treatment involves 3000 to 3750 cGy in 10 to 15 fractions of 250 to 300 cGy per fraction.

One of the most complex CNS treatment targets is the craniospinal axis. Delivery of radiation needs to encompass the entire brain and spinal cord simultaneously. This is most common in the treatment of medulloblastoma. Other tumors such as intracranial germ cell tumor and ependymoma with evidence of distant CNS metastases may benefit from craniospinal axis treatment. Craniospinal cases are typically treated in the prone position, and treatment fields consist of two lateral whole brain fields and one or more posterior spinal fields. Care must be taken to match the beam divergence, with no overlap allowed. Hot or cold spots at the junction between the brain and spine fields can be avoided by feathering the gap. This can be accomplished by shifting the gap by 1 cm every 1000 cGy. This approach allows a 1-cm gap between fields daily. With this technique, the length of the brain and spine fields change daily. The central axis of the spine fields is shifted superiorly to accommodate the gap. The central axis of the brain field remains constant, whereas the field size changes to expand superiorly and inferiorly. Other methods of feathering the gap may also be used, such as using couch kicks to form a straight edge. In addition, craniospinal axis irradiation may be accomplished with tomotherapy or proton treatment. Each method has benefits over traditional linear accelerator treatment. (Chapters 15 and 16 provide more details on the treatment of adjacent fields with these treatment modalities.)

International Commission on Radiation Units 50 and 62. The International Commission on Radiation Units (ICRU) report numbers 50 and 62 are the international standards that determine the radiation tumor volumes. The gross tumor volume (GTV) is the gross tumor seen on the MRI, CT scan, or other imaging study. The clinical target volume (CTV) is the CNS tissue with suspected microscopic tumor; this usually extends 1 to 3 cm beyond the GTV. The planning target volume (PTV) is the margin beyond the GTV and CTV and accounts for factors such as internal organ motion, setup variation, and patient movement. This usually contains and extends 0.5 to 1 cm beyond the GTV and CTV. The treated volume (TV) is the volume enclosed by the desired prescription isodose line (usually greater than 95%); this contains the GTV, CTV, and PTV. The irradiated volume is the tissue volume that receives a significant dose of radiation and contains the GTV, CTV, and PTV.[23]

Organs at risk (OAR) and planning organ-at-risk volume should be delineated and the dose recorded based on the recommendations of ICRU reports. Depending on the tumor site, the OAR that may receive a radiation dose may include the lens of the eye, the optic nerve and chiasm, the brainstem, the parotid glands, and the spinal cord.

The treatment volume for gliomas is determined by the tumor's extent, which (as shown with CT scan and MRI) includes the GTV and related tumor edema. Fig. 30.7 shows an intensity-modulated radiation therapy (IMRT) plan for a patient with a high-grade glioma.

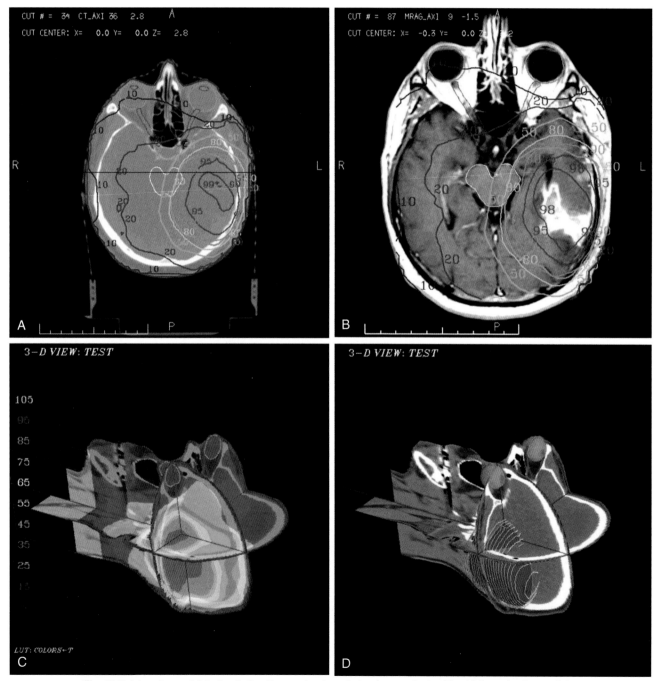

Fig. 30.7 Intensity-modulated radiation therapy treatment plan for a patient with a high-grade glioma of the right parietal region. (From Fraas BA, Eisbruch A, Feng M. Central nervous system tumors. In: Gunderson LL, Tepper JE, eds. *Clinical Radiation Oncology.* 4th ed. St. Louis, MO: Elsevier; 2016.)

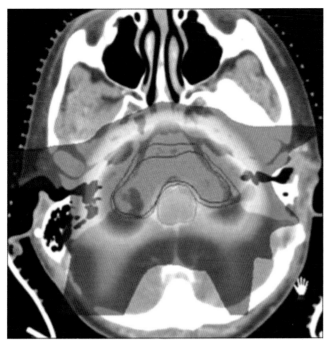

Fig. 30.8 Dose distribution on an MRI scan of a patient with an astrocytoma. Note the high dose region from this IMRT treatment plan (red) wraps around the brain stem. From Fraas BA, Eisbruch A and Feng M. Central Nervous System Tumors. In Gunderson LL, Tepper JE, eds. *Clinical Radiation Oncology*, 4th ed. St Louis, MO: Elsevier; 2016. Reprinted from The Lancet, Vol 13, Walcott BP, et al, Chordoma: current concepts, management, and future directions, e69-e76, 2012, with permission from Elsevier.

Because tumor cells have been found in edema of this patient, the area should be included in the treatment field with a 1-cm to 3-cm margin for malignant tumors.[24] Fig. 30.8 outlines the GTV on an MRI scan of a patient with an astrocytoma.

Conventional therapy has been enhanced through the use of three-dimensional treatment planning, IMRT, portal imaging, and multileaf collimators. Irregularly shaped fields can be created quickly through the use of these collimators, which eliminates the need to construct custom blocks. Three-dimensional treatment planning allows the use of multiple noncoplanar fields (Fig. 30.9) to a well-defined target volume. A frequently used noncoplanar field, called a *vertex field*, is best described with the patient in the supine field. The treatment, which requires a lateral treatment beam and a 90-degree couch kick, is directed superiorly from the top of the head and exits inferiorly through the neck region. Checking the accuracy of the patient's setup before treatment is recommended through the use of portal imaging and image-guided radiation therapy.

As a result of radiation treatments to the cranium, temporary hair loss occurs with doses ranging from 2000 to 4000 cGy. With doses of greater than 4000 cGy, hair loss may be permanent. Erythema, tanning, dry and moist desquamation, and edema are also side effects of the treatments. Early-delayed reactions include drowsiness, lethargy, a decreased mental status, and a worsening of symptoms. These reactions can occur up to 3 months after treatment, are usually temporary, and disappear without therapy. The occurrence of apparently new symptoms at this time is not necessarily indicative of treatment failure or the need for any change in therapy. Radiation necrosis is a complication that rarely occurs from 6 months to many years after irradiation. Late reactions are usually irreversible and progressive. Radiation cataracts can be avoided by shielding or keeping the eyes out of the field.

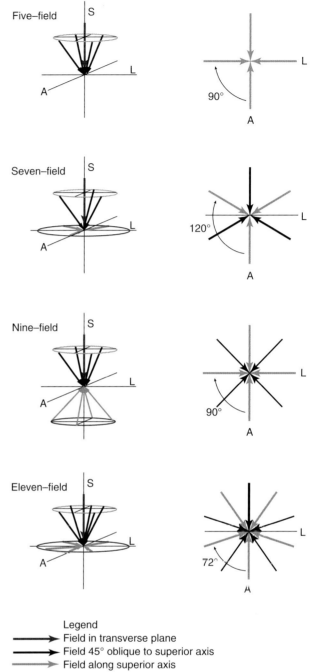

Legend
→ Field in transverse plane
→ Field 45° oblique to superior axis
→ Field along superior axis

Fig. 30.9 Comparison of various noncoplanar, three-dimensional treatment approaches with 5, 7, 9, and 11 static, noncoplanar treatment beams. Beam orientations are shown from a lateral prospective (*left*) and as viewed from above (*right*). (From Shaw EG, Debinski W, Robbins ME. Central nervous system tumors, overview. In: Gunderson LL, Tepper JE, eds. *Clinical Radiation Oncology*. 2nd ed. Philadelphia, PA: Churchill Livingstone; 2007.)

Radiation tolerance for healthy tissues within the CNS includes 4500 to 5000 cGy for whole brain, 6000 cGy for partial brain, and 4500 to 5000 cGy for the spinal cord. These tolerances are based on TD $_{5/5}$, which assumes a 5% incidence rate of complications at a 5-year period and QUANTEC (quantitative analysis of normal tissue effects in the clinic) data (Tables 30.5, 30.6, and 30.7).

TABLE 30.5 Predicted TD₅/₅ Tolerance Doses

Organ	Injury	One-Third	Two-Thirds	Whole Organ
Brain	Necrosis/infarction	6000	5000	4500
Brainstem	Necrosis/infarction	6000	5300	5000
Ear, mid/external	Acute serous otitis	3000	3000	3000[a]
Ear, mid/external	Chronic serous otitis	5500	5500	5500[a]
T-M joints mandible	Marked limitation of joint function	6500	6000	6000
Optic chiasma	Blindness	—	—	5000
Eye lens	Cataract	—	—	1000
Optic nerve	Blindness	—	—	5000
Retina	Blindness	—	—	4500
Parotid gland	Xerostomia	—	3200*	3200*
Skin	Necrosis/ulceration	7000	6000	5500 100 cm²
Spinal cord	Myelitis/necrosis	5000 5 cm²	5000 10 cm²	4700 20 cm²

*Qualitative Analysis of Normal Tissue Effects in the Clinic (QUANTEC) data indicate that the mean dose after conventional fractionation should not exceed 2000 cGy when sparing one parotid gland, and the mean dose should not exceed 2500 cGy when both parotid glands are spared when included in three-dimensional-conformal radiation therapy (3D-CRT) volume.

[a]Less than 50% of volume does not make a significant change.

$TD_{5/5}$, Tissue dose associated with a 5% injury rate within 5 years.

Modified from Emami B, Lyman J, Brown A, et al. Tolerance of normal tissue to therapeutic radiation. *Int J Radiat Oncol Biol Phys.* 1991;21:109–122.

TABLE 30.6 QUANTEC Summary Data: Approximate Dose/Volume/Outcome Data for Several Organs After Conventional Fractionation of 180 to 200 cGy per Fraction

Organ	Volume	Dose/Volume	Dose (Gy)	Toxicity Rate	Toxicity End Point
Brain			<60 Gy	<3%	Symptomatic necrosis
Brain			72 Gy	5%	Symptomatic necrosis
Brain			90 Gy	10%	Symptomatic necrosis
Brainstem			<54 Gy	<5%	Neuropathy or necrosis
Brainstem	D1–10 cc	≤59 Gy		<5%	Neuropathy or necrosis
Brainstem			<64 Gy	<5%	Neuropathy or necrosis
Optic nerve/chiasm			<55 Gy	<3%	Optic neuropathy
Optic nerve/chiasm			55–60 Gy	3%–7%	Optic neuropathy
Optic nerve/chiasm			>60 Gy	>7%–20%	Optic neuropathy
Spinal cord			50 Gy	0.2%	Myelopathy
Spinal cord			60 Gy	6%	Myelopathy
Spinal cord			69 Gy	50%	Myelopathy
Cochlea	Mean	≤45 Gy		<30%	Sensory-neural hearing loss

QUANTEC, Quantitative analysis of normal tissue effects in the clinic.

Modified from Marks LB, Yorke ED, Jackson A, et al. Use of normal tissue complication probability models in the clinic, *Int J Radiat Oncol Biol Phys.* 2010;76(3):S10–S19.

TABLE 30.7 QUANTEC Summary Data: Approximate Dose/Volume/Outcome Data for Several Organs Following Stereotactic Radiosurgery (Single Fraction) or Stereotactic Body Radiation Therapy (Multiple Fractions)

Organ	Volume	Dose/Volume	Dose (Gy)	Toxicity Rate	Toxicity End Point
Brain		V12 <5–10 cc		<20%	Symptomatic necrosis
Brainstem (acoustic tumors)			<12.5 Gy	<5%	Neuropathy or necrosis
Optic nerve/chiasm			<12 Gy	<10%	Optic neuropathy
Spinal cord (single-fx)			13 Gy	1%	Myelopathy
Spinal cord (hypo-fx)			20 Gy	1%	Myelopathy
Cochlea	Prescription dose	≤14 Gy		<25%	Sensory-neural hearing loss

QUANTEC, Quantitative analysis of normal tissue effects in the clinic.

Modified from Marks LB, Yorke ED, Jackson A, et al. Use of normal tissue complication probability models in the clinic, *Int J Radiat Oncol Biol Phys.* 2010;76(3):S10–S19.

Chemicals that enhance the lethal effects of radiation are known as *radiosensitizers*. Hypoxic cell sensitizers and halogenated pyrimidines are under investigation. Hypoxic cells are more radioresistant than are well-oxygenated cells. The use of sensitizers makes the cells more susceptible to the radiation without increasing the radiation effects to the healthy tissue, which is well oxygenated. Mitotically active tumor cells use these compounds more than replicating healthy glial cells and vascular cells.

Interstitial implants (brachytherapy) are done with the use of radioactive seeds (I-125) that are temporarily placed in tumors. Adjacent healthy tissue is spared from excessively high doses because of the rapid decrease of dose outside the high-dose volume. Conceptually healthy tissue can better tolerate the low-dose rate (given over a longer period as compared with external beam radiation therapy), so a higher dose can be delivered. Interstitial implants provide a less invasive treatment modality than surgery if recurrence occurs. Interstitial irradiation may provide an alternative in the treatment of infants and children. Brachytherapy may be beneficial to patients with recurrent disease, but it does not play a major role in the management of the disease.

SRS is an important treatment option for patients with isolated CNS tumors and solitary brain metastasis.[21] The process combines stereotactic localization techniques with a sharply collimated beam to direct the dose of radiation to a specific, well-defined lesion. The patient is positioned in a halo device that is used as an immobilization device to ensure the accuracy and reproducibility of the treatment setup. The target volume should be spherical and only up to 3 cm at its maximum dimension. Accuracy approaches 1 mm. A necrosing dose of radiation can be given in a single-fraction treatment or in multiple fractions. A local dose to the tumor can be increased with sparing of surrounding tissue. The process can be accomplished with the use of different sources of radiation. Heavy charged particles, a *Gamma knife* with multiple cobalt-60 sources (a type of radiosurgery with a sharply defined field, considered by some to be equivalent to resecting the irradiated region), and linear accelerator–based systems can be used with comparable results. The role of radiosurgery in the management of primary, metastatic, and recurrent disease is still under investigation; however, radiosurgery has showed promise in allowing patients to delay or avoid whole brain radiation treatment and its comorbidities.[21] (Chapter 15 provides more detailed information on SRS.)

> Radiosurgery with external beam treatment modalities includes linear accelerator–based and cobolt-60 accelerator–based treatments. More information is available at www.accuray.com, and www.gammaknife.org.

Chemotherapy. Progress has been slow in the area of chemotherapeutic drugs. Several reasons account for this. The presence of the BBB, the low number of effective drugs, lack of change in progression of disease with introduction of adjuvant therapy, and lack of adjuvant chemotherapy to increase the survival rate all have limited the use of chemotherapy in the treatment of CNS tumors.[25] Other reasons for the difficulty in finding useful drugs include the small number of patients with CNS tumors for use in clinical trials compared with more prevalent diseases, difficulties with measurement of the tumor response, and the fact that one measurement of response is survival time. Effective chemotherapy for CNS tumors is further hindered by the BBB, which impedes the penetration of the drugs into the brain. "The goal of blood-brain barrier disruption (BBBD) is maximizing delivery of agents to the brain while preserving neurocognitive function and quality of life, and minimizing systemic toxicity. BBBD is especially important in increasing the delivery of high molecular weight agents, such as proteins, antibodies, immunoconjugates, and viral vectors."[26]

Chemotherapeutic drugs can be administered orally, IV, directly into the tumor bed, and via direct carotid perfusion. Most chemotherapeutic drugs cause cytotoxic effects by disrupting DNA synthesis in rapidly dividing cells.

The designing of new drugs that allow better penetration of the BBB and can exhibit better distribution and lower toxicity has become extremely important. Limited studies suggest that the drug concentrations in the area around the tumor or in healthy brain tissue may be lower than those in the tumor itself, where the BBB is inefficient. The concentrations of drugs in the healthy brain tissue decrease as the distance from the tumor increases. Therefore, drug concentrations in the brain surrounding the tumor may be too low to eliminate infiltrating tumor cells. This can be a reason for therapeutic failures.[26] The nitrosourea drugs are lipid soluble, which allows them to cross the BBB. Because of this ability, these drugs can work against brain tumors.

Drugs of choice for CNS neoplasms include carmustine, procarbazine, vincristine, and lomustine. Temozolomide, also a lipid-soluble alkylating agent developed especially for the treatment of malignant gliomas, has been studied and showed some positive results, especially in patients with recurrent disease.[24] Multiagent chemotherapy plays a major role in the treatment of recurrent gliomas

Role of the Radiation Therapist

Patient education is a primary goal of the physician, radiation therapist, and oncology nurse. Although the physician and nurse initially discuss treatment procedures, side effects, skin care, nutrition, and psychosocial issues with the patient and family members, the emotional state of those persons at that time is generally not conducive to remembering and complying with all the information they are given. It becomes the responsibility of the therapist, who sees the patient daily, to reiterate and reinforce all these educational issues with the patient.

Daily contact allows the therapist to build a professional bond of trust, understanding, and communication with the patient. The therapist must be ready to step in and provide patients with emotional support, answers to questions and concerns, and referrals to persons they may need to see (e.g., social worker, pastor, nutritionist, office personnel, and support groups).

In addition, the therapist's daily contact also allows monitoring of the patient's mental and physical well-being. Some patients still feel overwhelmed, angry, and vulnerable and are in denial at the beginning of treatments.

A separate patient waiting area allows patients to talk and share their thoughts with other persons who have the same concerns. This area allows discussions regarding issues the patient may not be able to discuss with family members.

Patients undergoing treatment for CNS neoplasms can expect specific side effects. Most commonly, patients report fatigue. Reassuring patients that this is not unusual helps them a great deal to cope with the situation. Explaining to patients that the body requires plenty of rest while it tries to heal itself from the disease and the effects of daily treatment eliminates some concern, as does suggesting that patients pamper themselves and take a nap when they feel tired, rather than fight the fatigue.

A proper diet is a must for the healing process and well-being of the patient. If food becomes unappealing in looks, taste, and smell, the patient does not want to eat. The patient can try eating smaller portions several times a day rather than sitting down to a large meal. Large portions are sometimes discouraging to someone with no appetite. A change in the location of eating can sometimes help, as can having someone else cook. Nutritional supplements should be available to patients, including different kinds of supplements so patients can then purchase the brand that appeals to them most.

Frequent blood tests are not required, with the exception of patients receiving craniospinal irradiation. The white cell count and platelet counts may decrease in patients treated with craniospinal irradiation. These counts require close monitoring in the event the patient needs a break in treatment until the situation corrects itself.

Permanent hair loss with treatment for primary brain tumors does occur. A loan closet with wigs, turbans, and kerchiefs ranging in a wide variety of colors and styles should be available to patients. Shops specializing in these items should also be suggested. Therapists should caution patients to use a mild shampoo to prevent skin irritation. Moisturizing creams can be prescribed for dry desquamation and other products for moist desquamation. Therapists can also recommend skin conditioners if erythema tanning occurs.

The patient should be cautioned against exposing to direct sunlight areas of the body being treated. The radiation from the sun in combination with the radiation from treatment enhances the adverse side effects.

Most patients begin to feel a sense of security that develops over the course of treatment from the daily contact with the therapy team. When treatment ends, patients feel a sense of loss and abandonment after weeks of daily attention being focused on them and their needs. In some facilities, patients can be called 1 week to 10 days after the completion of treatment (before the first follow-up visit) just to check on them and evaluate their physical and mental condition. This may provide the patient with a sense of ongoing care.

The therapist must also be watchful for signs of medical complications that may arise as a result of the treatment. Early intervention of potential problems can prevent unnecessary suffering later in the course of treatment. Attention to detail regarding treatment setups and parameters is a must, and providing professional, competent, efficient, and accurate treatment in a relaxed and friendly atmosphere completes the role of the therapist.

Case I. A 62-year-old Asian female was treated for moderately well-differentiated invasive ductal carcinoma in her left breast. She had detected a lump in her breast approximately 1 month before surgery, which included a lumpectomy and a sentinel node biopsy. No lymph nodes were detected. She was diagnosed with T2 N0 M0, stage IIA breast cancer. She received adjuvant chemotherapy and radiation therapy that consisted of 5000 cGy in 25 fractions to the left breast with opposed tangents and a boost to 6500 cGy with 9-MeV electrons.

Twenty-four months after the completion of the initial treatment, she was diagnosed with a solitary bone metastases to L4 and received a dose of 3000 cGy in 10 fractions to the spine. The patient had a Karnofsky performance status of 70 at the time of her spinal irradiation. During the workup for the lumbar spine metastases, several small foci of brain metastases were revealed on a MRI scan.

WBRT was initiated (3000 cGy in 10 fractions), with left and right laterals, together with a decreasing doses of corticosteroids. Acute side effects were limited to mild skin toxicity, hair loss, and considerable fatigue. Evaluation after six cycles of additional chemotherapy showed no evidence of disease. The patient continues to be monitored and is now 28 months out since her initial diagnosis.

SUMMARY

- Approximately 24,000 cases of primary brain tumors and other nervous system tumors are diagnosed annually in the United States. The tumors account for 1.4% of all malignancies. About 80% of CNS tumors involve the brain, whereas 20% involve the spinal cord.
- CNS tumors can be primary or secondary (metastatic) and benign or malignant.
- In recent years, radiation therapy has played a significant role in the treatment of CNS tumors, providing a means of increased survival time and enhancing the quality of life of many patients with brain tumors.
- The three most important as prognostic indicators for CNS tumors are age, performance status, and tumor type.
- Tumors are normally grouped into benign, or low-grade, and malignant, or high-grade, categories, with grade rather than size as the primary prognostic factor.

- The BBB, which hinders the penetration of some substances into the brain and CSF, exists between the vascular system and brain. Its purpose is to protect the brain from potentially toxic compounds.
- PET is a beneficial diagnostic tool that may be useful in determination of differences between necrosis and malignancy, which are associated with areas of high metabolism.
- A multidisciplinary approach is necessary for the treatment of CNS tumors, as a biopsy is extremely important for diagnostic purposes and essential for therapeutic decision-making.
- Radiation therapy is indicated for malignant tumors that are incompletely excised, inaccessible from a surgical approach, and associated with metastatic lesions.
- Daily contact allows the therapist to build a professional bond of trust, understanding, and communication with the patient. The therapist must be ready to step in and provide patients with emotional support, answers to their questions and concerns, and referrals.

REVIEW QUESTIONS

The answers to the Review Questions can be found by logging on to our website at: http://evolve.elsevier.com/Washington/principles

1. Karnofsky performance status (KPS) is:
   a. A measure of the biologic grade of the tumor.
   b. A measure of the neurologic and functional status of the patient.
   c. Measured in cGy.
   d. Direct measurement of the chance of 5-year survival.
2. The purpose of the BBB is to:
   I. Hinder the penetration of some substances into the brain and CSF.
   II. Protect the brain from potentially toxic substances.
   III. Protect the brain from radiation.

IV. Prevent the passage of lipid-soluble or water-soluble substances into the brain.
   a. I and III.
   b. II and III.
   c. I and II.
   d. II and IV.
3. Which of the following are important factors to consider in the initial workup for a definitive diagnosis of CNS neoplasms?
   a. Family and social histories.
   b. Changes in behavior or personality.
   c. Difficulties with speech, memory, or logical thought processes.
   d. All of the above.

4. What does *not* belong in this group?
   a. High dose fractionation.
   b. Increased ICP.
   c. Edema.
   d. Papilledema.
5. Surgery for CNS neoplasms can be limited by:
   a. Tumor location and extent.
   b. Patient status.
   c. Risk of causing neurologic deficits.
   d. All of the above.
6. The most common brain lesion is:
   a. Astrocytoma.
   b. Glioma.
   c. Metastatic.
   d. Medulloblastoma.
7. Little is known concerning the _____, development, and growth mechanisms of CNS tumors.
   a. Etiology.
   b. Dose response.
   c. Effects of alcohol.
   d. BBB.
8. Which of the following does *not* provide protection for the brain?
   a. Cerebellum.
   b. Cranial bones.
   c. Meninges.
   d. CSF.
9. The most important prognostic factor for CNS tumors is the histopathologic diagnosis.
   a. True.
   b. False.
10. Cells are more radiosensitive when they are
    a. Slow growing.
    b. Anoxic.
    c. Well oxygenated.
    d. Homogeneous.

QUESTIONS TO PONDER

1. Explain the benefits and risks involved in treatment of patients who have CNS neoplasms with surgery, radiation therapy, and chemotherapy.
2. What are the presenting signs and symptoms anticipated with patients who have CNS tumors?
3. Explain the purpose of the feathered-gap technique for treatment to the craniospinal axis.
4. Analyze the expected side effects from radiation therapy to the CNS.
5. Differentiate between SRS and Gamma knife treatment.
6. Explain the use and effect of steroids in treatment of patients with CNS neoplasms.
7. Discuss the clinical application of two-dimensional and three-dimensional treatment approaches to CNS tumors.

REFERENCES

1. American Cancer Society. Brain cancer. http://www.cancer.org/cancer/braincnstumorsinadults/index. Accessed February 16, 2018.
2. Chang SM, Mehta MP. *Principles and Practice of Neuro-Oncology: A Multidisciplinary Approach.* New York, NY: Demos Medical; 2011.
3. Deorah S, Lynch CF, Sibenaller ZA, Ryken TC. Trends in brain cancer incidence and survival in the United States: surveillance, epidemiology, and end results program, 1973 to 2001. *Neurosurg Focus.* 2006;20(4):E1.
4. Ohgahi H, Kleinhues P. Epidemiology and etiology gliomas. *Acta Neuropathol.* 2005;109:93–108.
5. American Cancer Society. *Cancer Facts and Figures 2018.* Atlanta, GA: American Cancer Society.
6. National Cancer Institute. SEER stat fact sheets: brain and other nervous system cancer. http://seer.cancer.gov/statfacts/html/brain.html. Accessed February 16, 2018.
7. Nelson DF, Jenkins RB, Scheithauer BW, et al. Central nervous system tumors. In: Rubin P, ed. *Clinical Oncology: A Multidisciplinary Approach for Physicians and Students.* 8th ed. Philadelphia, PA: Saunders; 2001:789–822.
8. Ostrom QT, Gittleman H, Liao P, et al. CBTRUS statistical report: primary brain and other central nervous system tumors diagnosed in the United States in 2010–2014. *Neuro Oncol.* 2017;19(suppl 5):v1–v88.
9. Goodenberger ML, Jenkins RB. Genetics of adult glioma. *Cancer Genet.* 2012;205(12):613–621.
10. Smith M, Hare ML. An overview of progress in childhood cancer survival. *J Pediatr Oncol Nurs.* 2014;10:160–164.
11. Merrick J, Chow E, Sahgal A. *Bone and Brain Metastases: Advances in Research and Treatment.* New York, NY: Nova Science; 2011.
12. Stelzer KJ Epidemiology and prognosis of brain metastases. *Surg Neurol Int.* 2013;4(suppl 4):192–202.
13. Ramis R, Tamayo-Uria I, Gómez-Barroso D, et al. Risk factors for central nervous system tumors in children: new findings from a case-control study. *PLoS One.* 2017;12(2):1–14.
14. Cheo ST, Lim GH, Lim KHC. Glioblastoma multiforme outcomes of 107 patients treated in two Singapore Institutions. *Singapore Med J.* 2017;58(1):41–45.
15. Smoll NR, Schaller K, Gautschi OP. Long-term survival of patients with glioblastoma multiforme (GBM). *J Clin Neurosci.* 2013;20(5):670–675.
16. Rodgers SP, Trevino M, Zawaski JA, Gaber MW, Leasure JL. Neurogenesis, exercise, and cognitive late effects of pediatric radiotherapy. *Neural Plast.* 2013:(3);455–461.
17. Phi SH, Choi SA, Lim SH, et al. ID3 contributes to cerebrospinal fluid seeding and poor prognosis in medulloblastoma. *BMC Cancer.* 2013;13(1):1–16.
18. Heper AO, Erden E, Savas A, et al. An analysis of stereotactic biopsy of brain tumors and nonneoplastic lesions: a prospective clinicopathologic study. *Surg Oncol.* 2005;64:82–88.
19. Johns Hopkins Medicine. Neurology and neurosurgery. https://www.hopkinsmedicine.org/neurology_neurosurgery/centers_clinics/brain_tumor/about-brain-tumors/. Accessed February 16, 2018.
20. Hall EJ, Giaccia AJ. *Radiobiology for the Radiologist.* 8th ed. Alphen aan den Rijn, South Holland, Netherlands: Wolters Kluwer; 2018.
21. Halasz LM, Rockhill JK. Stereotactic radiosurgery and stereotactic radiotherapy for brain metastases. *Surg Neurol.* 2013;4:S185–S191. Int.
22. Tsao M, Xu W, Sahgal A. A meta-analysis evaluating stereotactic radiosurgery, whole brain radiotherapy, or both for patients presenting with a limited number of brain metastases. *Cancer.* 2012;118(9):2486–2493.
23. International Commission on Radiation Units and Measurements (ICRU). *Prescribing, Recording, and Reporting, Photon Beam Therapy: Report 50.* Washington, DC: ICRU; 2001.
24. Lassman AB, Matceyevsky D, Corn BW. High grade gliomas. In: Gunderson LL, Tepper JE, eds. *Clinical Radiation Oncology.* 4th ed. Philadelphia, PA: Elsevier; 2015:469–482.
25. Wijaya J, Fukuda Y, Schuetz JD. Obstacles to brain tumor therapy: key ABC transporters. *Int J Mol Sci.* 2017;18(12):1–35.
26. Doolittle ND, Murillo TP, Neuwelt EA. Blood–brain barrier disruption chemotherapy. In: Newton HB, ed. *Handbook of Brain Tumor Chemotherapy.* San Diego, CA: Academic Press; 2006:262–273.

31

Digestive System Tumors

Leila Bussman-Yeakel

OBJECTIVES

- Identify, list, and discuss epidemiologic and etiologic factors that may be responsible for induction of tumors in the colon, rectum, anus, esophagus, and pancreas.
- Describe the symptoms produced by malignant tumors that arise in the colon, rectum, anus, esophagus, and pancreas.
- Discuss the methods of detection and diagnosis for tumors in the colon, rectum, anus, esophagus, and pancreas.
- List the varying histologic types of tumors that occur in the colon, rectum, anus, esophagus, and pancreas.
- Describe the diagnostic procedures used in the workup and staging of these sites.
- Describe in detail the most common routes of tumor spread for these digestive system sites.
- Describe and diagram the lymphatic routes of spread for tumors of the colon, rectum, anus, esophagus, and pancreas.
- Differentiate between histologic grading and staging.
- Describe in detail the anatomy and physiology of the colon, rectum, anus, esophagus, and pancreas.

- Identify and discuss the rationale for treatment with regard to treatment choice, histologic type, and stage of the disease.
- Describe the differing types of radiation treatment techniques that can be used for tumors of the rectum, anus, esophagus, and pancreas.
- Identify the appropriate tumor lethal dose or prescribed dose for each site.
- Discuss the expected radiation reactions for the area based on time-dose-fractionation schemes.
- Discuss tolerance levels of the vital structures and organs at risk.
- Describe the instructions that should be given to a patient with regard to skin care, expected reactions, and dietary advice.
- Discuss the rationale for use of multimodality treatments for each diagnosis.
- Describe the various treatment planning techniques.
- Discuss survival statistics and prognosis for various stages of each cancer listed: rectum, anus, esophagus, and pancreas.

OUTLINE

KEY TERMS

Abdominoperineal resection
Achalasia
Anterior resection
Barrett esophagus
Carcinoembryonic antigen
Chemoradiation
Chronic ulcerative colitis
Endocavitary radiation therapy
Endoscopic retrograde cholangiopancreatography
Endoscopic ultrasound scan
Familial adenomatous polyposis
Gardner syndrome
Hematochezia

Hereditary nonpolyposis colorectal syndrome
Intensity-modulated radiation therapy
Intraoperative radiation therapy
Leukopenia
Low anterior resection
Neoadjuvant
Odynophagia
Peritoneal seeding
Tenesmus
Three-point setup
Thrombocytopenia
Tylosis
Volume-modulated arc therapy

This chapter discusses the three major malignant diseases of the gastrointestinal (GI) system that are managed with radiation therapy (i.e., cancers of the rectum, esophagus, and pancreas). Colorectal cancer is the most common GI malignancy; it is the second leading cause of death from cancer among men and women combined, but it is associated with the best prognosis of all GI malignancies.[1] Cancers of the esophagus and pancreas are usually diagnosed at an advanced stage and do not have many long-term survivors.

COLORECTAL CANCER

Epidemiology and Etiology

The incidence rate of colorectal cancer has been steadily declining since 1980 in men and women older than 50 years. However, the incidence rate is rising in those younger than 50 years. Colon cancer diagnosed in those younger than 50 years increased from 6% in 1990 to 11% in 2013, with most cases occurring in people in their 40s.[2] About 101,420 cases of colon cancer and 44,180 cases of rectal cancer are projected to occur each year.[1] The disease affects men more commonly than women. Cancer of the colon is ranked third in incidence when men and women are compared separately. The risk of development of cancer of the large bowel increases with age, with more than 90% of cases occurring in people older than 55 years of age.[1,2] Colorectal cancer is the second leading cause of cancer death in the United States; it accounts for approximately 50,000 deaths annually. Death rates from colorectal cancer have been declining as a result of early detection and better treatment.[1,2]

The cause of colorectal cancer has largely been attributed to a diet high in animal fat and low in fiber. The excess fat in a person's diet may act as a promoter of the development of colon cancer. A diet high in processed and red meats and low in fruit and vegetables has been associated with an increased risk of colorectal cancer. The intake of fiber in diets may act as an inhibitor, diluting fecal contents and increasing fecal bulk, resulting in quicker elimination, and therefore minimizing the exposure of the bowel epithelial lining to the carcinogens. Other risk factors for the development of colorectal cancer include obesity,

smoking, type 2 diabetes, excessive alcohol consumption (more than two drinks/day in men or one drink/day in women), and minimal physical activity. There has been a steady increase in the obesity rates among adults age 20 to 74. Men who are obese have a 50% higher increased risk of developing colon cancer compared with those who are of normal weight. Women who are obese have a 20% increased risk of developing colon cancer.[1,2]

Recent studies have shown that the risk of colorectal cancer may be decreased with the regular use of nonsteroidal antiinflammatory drugs and postmenopausal hormone therapy. However, the use of these drugs as a preventive measure is not recommended.[1,2]

Other principal factors in the development of colon cancer include chronic ulcerative colitis, carcinomas that arise in preexisting adenomatous polyps, and the hereditary cancer syndromes. These syndromes are familial adenomatous polyposis (FAP) and hereditary nonpolyposis colorectal syndrome (HNPCC), or Lynch syndrome.[1-5] Individuals also at an increased risk for the development of colorectal cancer are those with a first-degree relative with colorectal cancer or adenomatous polyps before age 60 years. An increased risk also exists if two or more first-degree relatives at any age had colorectal cancer or adenomatous polyps in the absence of a hereditary syndrome.[1-5]

Chronic ulcerative colitis usually occurs in the rectum and sigmoid area of the bowel but may spread to the rest of the colon. This condition is characterized by extensive inflammation of the bowel wall and ulceration. A patient experiences attacks of bloody mucoid diarrhea up to 20 times a day. These attacks persist for days or weeks and then subside, only to recur. The risk of development of colon cancer depends on the extent of bowel involvement, age of onset, and severity and duration of the active disease. The earlier the age at onset and the longer the duration of the active disease, the higher the risk of cancer. Studies have shown the risk to be 3% at 15 years' duration, with an increase to 5% at 20 years.[4,5] Only 1% of patients with a diagnosis of colorectal cancer have a history of chronic ulcerative colitis.

Adenomatous polyps are growths that arise from the mucosal lining and protrude into the lumen of the bowel. They are classified as tubular or villous, based on their growth pattern and microscopic

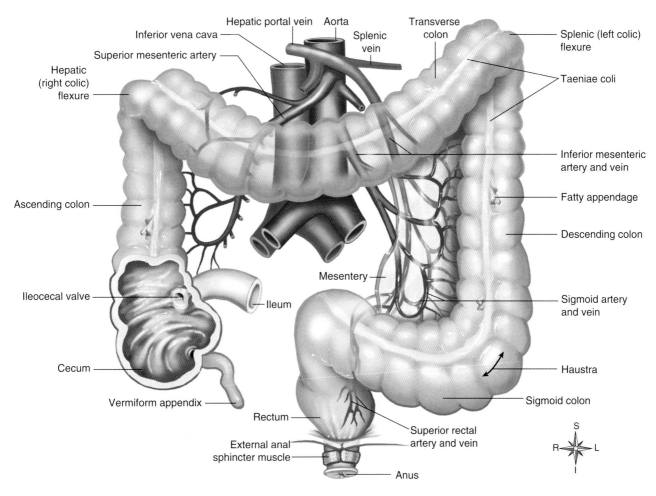

Fig. 31.1 Anatomy of the large bowel. (From Thibodeau GA, Patton KT. *The Human Body in Health and Disease.* 7th ed. St. Louis, MO: Mosby; 2018.)

characteristics. Polyps are considered a precursor to the development of a malignancy. The larger the polyp, the greater the risk of malignant transformation. Villous adenomas are 8 to 10 times more likely than tubular adenomas to be malignant.[6]

Virtually all patients with the hereditary condition FAP, if left untreated, have colon cancer develop.[4] FAP is characterized by the studding of the entire large bowel wall by thousands of polyps. Persons affected with this disease do not have polyps at birth. Progression to extensive involvement of the colon usually occurs by late adolescence. The cause of FAP is associated with a mutation on the adenomatous polyposis coli gene on chromosome 5.[7,8] FAP is treated with the complete removal of the colon and rectum. Gardner syndrome is another inherited disorder similar to FAP. Patients with Gardner syndrome have adenomatous polyposis of the large bowel and other abnormal growths, such as upper GI polyps, periampullary tumors, lipomas, and fibromas.[4,5]

The frequent occurrence of colorectal cancer in families without polyposis has been termed Lynch syndrome, **formerly known as HNPCC.**[1,4,5] This is the most common form of hereditary colorectal cancer syndrome.[1] The cause of Lynch syndrome (HNPCC) has been attributed to mutations in repair genes located on chromosome 2, 3, or 7. Lynch syndrome has classically been defined as colorectal cancer that develops in three or more family members, with at least two first-degree relatives and involving people in at least two generations with

one family member with a diagnosis before the age of 50 years.[2,7,8] Patients with this family history of colon cancer usually have right-sided colon cancers develop at a much younger age than in the general population. These patients are also at an increased risk for the development of a second cancer of the colon and adenocarcinomas of the breast, ovary, endometrium, and pancreas. Individuals with this family history should undergo physical examinations regularly and consider genetic testing.

Anatomy and Lymphatics

Cancer of the large bowel is usually divided into cancer of the colon or rectum because the symptoms, diagnosis, and treatment are different based on the anatomic area involved. A major factor that determines the treatment and prognosis is whether a lesion occurs in a segment of bowel that is located retroperitoneally or intraperitoneally. This is discussed further in the section on the anatomy and lymphatic drainage of these areas.

The colon is divided into eight regions: the cecum, ascending colon, descending colon, splenic flexure, hepatic flexure, transverse colon, sigmoid, and rectum. Located intraperitoneally, the cecum, transverse colon, and sigmoid have a complete mesentery and serosa and are freely mobile (Fig. 31.1). Lesions that occur in these regions can usually be surgically removed with an adequate margin unless the tumor is adherent or invades adjacent structures. Treatment failure or recurrence is most likely attributed to peritoneal seeding.

Located retroperitoneally, the ascending and descending colon and the hepatic and splenic flexures are considered immobile. They lack a true mesentery and a serosal covering on the posterior and lateral aspect. Because of the retroperitoneal location and lack of a mesentery for these regions, early spread outside the bowel wall and invasion of the adjacent soft tissues, kidney, and pancreas are common.

The rectum is continuous with the sigmoid and begins at the level of the third sacral vertebra. Like the sigmoid, the upper rectum is covered by the peritoneum, but only on its lateral and anterior surfaces. The peritoneum is then reflected over the anterior wall of the rectum onto the seminal vesicles and bladder in males or the vagina and uterus in females, forming a cul-de-sac termed the *rectovesical pouch* or *rectouterine pouch,* respectively. The lower half to two-thirds of the rectum is located retroperitoneally. Three transverse folds divide the rectum into areas known as the upper valve, middle valve, and lower valve, or ampulla (Fig. 31.2). The middle valve is located 11 cm superior from the anal verge and represents the approximate location of the peritoneal reflection.[9] Because of the retroperitoneal location, tumors of the rectum can invade adjacent structures of the pelvis, such as the prostate, bladder, vagina, and sacrum. Treatment options depend on the location of the lesion.

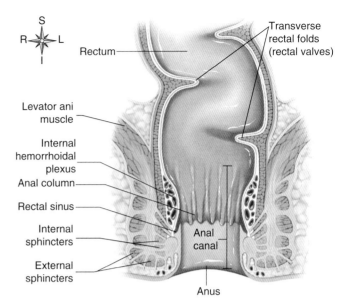

Fig. 31.2 A coronal section through the rectum. (From Patton KT. *Anatomy and Physiology.* 10th ed. St. Louis, MO: Elsevier; 2019.)

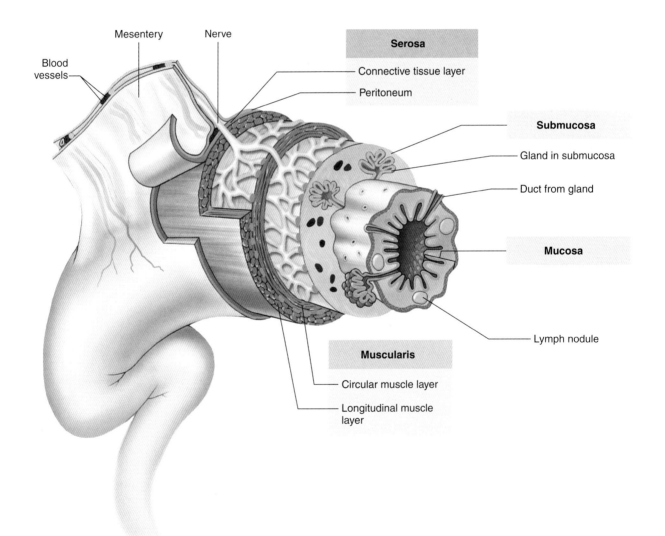

Fig. 31.3 A cross section of the bowel wall. (From Thibodeau GA, Patton KT: The human body in health & disease, ed 7, St. Louis, 2018, Mosby, Copyright Elsevier (2018).)

A cross section through a segment of large bowel reveals four main layers: the mucosa, submucosa, muscularis propria, and serosa (Fig. 31.3).[10,11] These layers are used in the staging system to define the amount of involvement through the bowel wall. The mucosa, or innermost layer, forms the lumen of the bowel and consists of two supporting layers: the lamina propria and the muscularis mucosa. The next layer, the submucosa, is rich in blood vessels and lymphatics. The muscularis propria contains two muscle layers, one circular and one longitudinal, which are responsible for peristalsis. Beneath the muscularis layer is a lining of fat termed the *subserosal layer*. The outermost layer is the serosa. Not all segments of the colon have a serosal layer. This layer is provided by the visceral peritoneum.

The lymphatic drainage of the colon follows the mesenteric vessels. The right colon follows the superior mesenteric vessels and includes the ileocolic and right colic nodes (see Fig. 31.1). The left colon follows the inferior mesenteric vessels and includes the regional nodes termed the midcolic, inferior mesenteric, and left colic. The sigmoid region drains into the inferior mesenteric system but also includes the nodes along the superior rectal, sigmoidal, and sigmoidal mesenteric vessels.[10] Lymphatic drainage of the upper rectum follows the superior rectal vessels into the inferior mesenteric system. Middle and lower rectum lymphatic drainage is along the middle rectal vessels, with the principal nodal group that comprises the internal iliac nodes.[12,13] Other nodal groups at risk for involvement with rectal cancer are the perirectal, lateral sacral, and presacral nodes.[10,14] Low rectal lesions that extend into the anal canal can drain to the inguinal nodes (Fig. 31.4).

With any of these regions, other nodal groups may be involved or at risk for involvement if the tumor has invaded an adjacent structure. For example, if a rectal cancer has invaded the vagina or prostate, the external iliac nodes may be involved with disease.

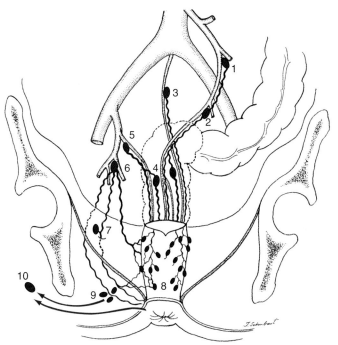

Fig. 31.4 Lymphatic drainage of the rectum: *1* and *2,* Nodes at the origin of the inferior mesenteric artery and origin of the sigmoid vessels; *3,* nodes of the sacral promontory; *4,* sacral nodes; *5* and *6,* internal iliac nodes, hypogastric; *7,* external iliac nodes that may be involved in low rectal lesions; *8,* nodes located at the rectal wall; *9,* ischiorectal nodes; and *10,* inguinal nodes. (From del Regato JA, Spjut HJ, Cox JD. *Ackerman and del Regato's Cancer: Diagnosis, Treatment, and Prognosis.* 6th ed. St Louis, MO: Mosby; 1985.)

Clinical Presentation

Patients with rectal cancer usually have rectal bleeding, which may be bright red blood in the toilet or may be mixed in or on the stool.[1,2] This bleeding is termed hematochezia. Other symptoms include a change in bowel habits, diarrhea versus constipation, or a change in the stool caliber.[1,9,14] Pencil-thin stools, constipation, or diarrhea may be indicative of a tumor that fills the rectal valve area and causes an obstructive-type process. Dark or black-colored stools may also be a symptom of cancer in the colon. This symptom results from a chemical reaction of hemoglobin and the intestinal enzymes and bacteria that gives stool a dark color. Tenesmus (spasms of the rectum accompanied by a desire to empty the bowel) may be a patient's report with locally advanced rectal cancer. Pain in the buttock or perineal area may occur from tumor extension posteriorly.[4,9]

Presenting symptoms of patients with lesions in the left colon are similar to those of rectal cancer. Blood in the stool, a change in stool caliber, obstructive symptoms, and abdominal pain are the most common reports.[2,4,5] In contrast, patients with right-sided colon lesions usually have abdominal pain, which is often accompanied by an abdominal mass. Nausea and vomiting are other possible symptoms. Occult blood in the stool and microcytic anemia are two other symptoms of colon cancer.[4,5]

Detection and Diagnosis

In general, cancer in the large bowel is diagnosed via findings of physical examination and radiographic and endoscopic studies. Together, these findings provide crucial information in the detection and extent of the disease process. In 2019, the American Cancer Society (ACS) changed the screening guidelines for the early detection of colorectal cancer, lowering the age recommendations from 50 to 45 years of age for a person at average risk.[1,15] Screening tests include a fecal occult blood test or fecal immunochemical test annually, fecal immunochemical test-DNA exam every 3 years, flexible sigmoidoscopy, double-contrast barium enema, or computed tomographic colonography (CTC) every 5 years. A colonoscopy should follow any positive test results. A colonoscopy, the preferred screening test, examines the entire colon and can visualize polyps and allow them to be removed for examination. Colonoscopy is done every 10 years.[1,2,7,15] Another technique for evaluation of the colon, CTC, uses a CT scanner and three-dimensional (3D) software to examine the inside the large intestine without insertion of the lengthy scope through the rectum. The examination requires less bowel preparation than a conventional colonoscopy and results in a radiation dose that is equivalent to a barium enema. The procedure can be used for patients who refuse colonoscopy or who are unable to complete a regular colonoscopy procedure because of a combination of technical factors. The fecal immunochemical test-DNA or Cologuard is a new type of stool test that detects mutations in the DNA of cells found in the stool that have been shed by a colorectal cancer or large adenoma. This test also detects blood in the stool.[2,15]

Individuals at high risk, those with a family history of FAP or Lynch syndrome, should undergo colonoscopies before age 45 years and should determine a plan for screening with their healthcare providers.[2,4] These persons also benefit from counseling to consider genetic testing.

The initial procedure for any patient with a malignancy is a thorough history and physical examination. For all patients with colorectal cancer, a digital rectal examination should be performed, and attention should be given to the approximate size of the lesion, the mobility, the location from the anal verge, and the rectal wall involved.[14] Enlarged perirectal nodes may also be detected during the digital examination.

A proctosigmoidoscopy is performed as a complementary procedure and allows a more accurate depiction of the size and location of the lesion. This procedure also determines whether the mass is exophytic or ulcerative. A tissue diagnosis is obtained from a biopsy during the endoscopic procedure. A pelvic examination should be performed for colon or rectal cancer to rule out any other pelvic masses. An anterior extrarectal mass (a lesion in the cul-de-sac) may be indicative of peritoneal seeding. In women, an anterior rectal mass may invade the vaginal wall and put the external iliac nodes at risk for involvement. The left supraclavicular and inguinal lymph nodes should also be palpated, especially in patients with low rectal lesions nearing the dentate line.[12,13] Supraclavicular lymph node involvement indicates extensive incurable disease and generally occurs as a result of spread from metastatically involved paraaortic nodes via the thoracic duct. The physical examination should also assess potential sites of distant spread. Palpation of the abdomen should be performed to check for masses in the abdomen, liver, and ascites.

Endoscopic procedures, colonoscopies, and proctosigmoidoscopies can assess the size, location of lesion, and circumferential extent and provide the distance of the lesion from the anal verge. They are also used for obtaining biopsies of lesions or removing polyps for histologic confirmation of malignancy.

After a diagnosis is established, a patient undergoes a staging workup for determination of the extent or amount of spread of the disease. A chest radiograph is usually obtained for detection of metastasis to the lungs. CT scan or magnetic resonance imaging (MRI) of the pelvis is done for evaluation of whether the tumor has extended into other pelvic organs or structures and for determination of pelvic lymph node involvement. An abdominal CT scan may also be obtained for detection of metastasis to the liver or other abdominal structures.[14]

Positron emission tomography (PET) has been used as part of the staging workup for location of areas of uptake in the primary tumor, lymph nodes, or distant metastasis. PET scans have shown uptake in lymph nodes that was not seen on initial CT scan. A combined PET-CT scan examination provides better anatomic correlation of areas of involvement than PET alone. PET-CT scan is becoming a commonly used examination for cancer staging and radiation treatment planning.[16]

Laboratory studies used in the diagnosis and workup of colon cancer include a complete blood count (CBC) and blood chemistry profile. Elevated liver function test results indicate the need for imaging of the liver with CT scan or with sonography. The tumor specimen may also be evaluated for changes in the KRAS gene in the cancer cells. If this mutation is found, the patient does not benefit from treatment with monoclonal antibodies such as cetuximab or panitumumab. Carcinoembryonic antigen (CEA) is a type of protein molecule that may be associated with certain malignant tumors, such as colon and ovarian cancer. It is sometimes used as a tumor marker for colon cancers. If the protein marker levels are above normal before treatment, they are expected to fall to normal levels after treatment. Levels of more than 20 ng/mL before therapy may be associated with widespread metastatic disease. A rising CEA level usually indicates a recurrence of the cancer. For this reason, the protein molecule serves as indicator for disease. The higher the level, the more disease may be present.

Pathology and Staging

Adenocarcinoma is the most common malignancy of the large bowel; it accounts for 90% to 95% of all tumors.[4,17] Other histologic types include mucinous adenocarcinoma, signet-ring cell carcinoma, and squamous cell carcinoma.[12,13]

The American Joint Committee on Cancer (AJCC) tumor, node, metastasis (TNM) system may be used clinically (before surgery) or

after surgery. The TNM system is the more commonly used system. (For more information on staging colorectal cancer, see: https://www.cancer.org/cancer/colon-rectal-cancer/detection-diagnosis-staging/staged.html.)

The TNM system has incorporated changes from previous staging systems into the current system. The revisions in the staging systems reflect the two most important prognostic indicators of survival: the number of nodes positive for tumor and the depth of penetration through the bowel wall.[4,5,10,12]

The staging system devised by Dukes in the 1930s was the first useful system.[10] Tumors were classified according to the level of invasion into the bowel wall and the absence or presence of nodes positive for tumor. The tumors were given a letter designation from A to C. Dukes's A designation indicates a lesion that has not penetrated through the bowel wall. The B designation indicates a lesion that has penetrated the bowel wall with nodes negative for tumor, and the C designation indicates a lesion with nodes positive for tumor. The TNM system is the more commonly used system.

More than 95% of colon and rectal cancers are adenocarcinomas. These are cancers of the cells that line the inside of the colon and rectum. There are some other, rarer types of tumors of the colon and rectum.[2,7]

Routes of Spread

As implied in the staging system, malignancies of the large bowel usually spread via direct extension, lymphatics, and hematogenous spread. Direct extension of the tumor is typically in a radial fashion, with penetration into the bowel wall rather than longitudinally.[5]

Lymphatic spread occurs if the tumor has invaded the submucosal layer of the bowel. The initial lymphatic and venous channels of the bowel wall are found in the submucosal layer. Lymphatic spread is orderly. The initial nodes involved for rectal cancer are the perirectal nodes. Approximately 50% of patients have nodes positive for tumor at the time of diagnosis.[5]

Blood-borne spread to the liver is the most common type of distant metastasis. The mechanism of spread involves the venous drainage of the GI system (the portal circulation). The second most common site of distant spread is the lung. This spread results from tumor embolus into the inferior vena cava (IVC).[5]

Lesions may also spread within the peritoneal cavity. The growth of a tumor through the bowel wall onto the peritoneal surface of the colon can result in tumor cells shedding into the abdominal cavity. These shed cells then take up residence on another surface (i.e., peritoneal lining, cul-de-sac) and begin to grow. This process is called peritoneal seeding. The implantation of tumor cells onto a surface at the time of surgery is another mechanism of spread.

Treatment Techniques

Surgery is considered the treatment of choice. The tumor, an adequate margin, and the draining lymphatics are removed. The type of procedure depends on the location of the tumor. For colon tumors, the removal of a large segment of bowel, the adjacent lymph nodes, and the immediate vascular supply is common with procedures such as a right hemicolectomy or left hemicolectomy. Some colon surgeries are done laparoscopically instead of with the traditional open procedure. Patients who undergo laparoscopic colectomy recover from the procedure sooner and have a shorter hospital stay than patients who undergo an open procedure. For rectal cancer, the two most common procedures are the low anterior resection (LAR) and the abdominoperineal resection (APR). The use of a laparoscopic surgical procedure for rectal cancer is more difficult to perform.

The **LAR** involves the removal of the tumor plus a margin (an en bloc excision) and the immediately adjacent lymph nodes. The bowel is then reanastomosed. Therefore a colostomy is not necessary. This procedure is used in the treatment of colon cancers and select rectal cancers.

An APR is used in patients with rectal cancer in the lower third (distal 5 cm) of the rectum. An anterior incision is made into the abdominal wall to construct a colostomy. Then, a perineal incision is made to resect the rectum, anus, and draining lymphatics, with the entire en bloc specimen pulled out through the perineal opening. The final phase of the procedure involves the reconstruction or reperitonealization of the pelvic floor through the use of an absorbable mesh, omentum, or peritoneum. This is extremely important for the patient who needs postoperative radiation therapy. Reperitonealization allows the small bowel to be displaced superiorly, reducing the amount of small bowel in the treatment field and minimizing the treatment toxicity from radiation therapy.[9]

Radiation Therapy

Radiation therapy is most commonly used as an adjuvant treatment for rectal cancer. This treatment is done either before or after surgery and in conjunction with chemotherapy.

Postoperative adjuvant radiation therapy with concurrent chemotherapy is advocated based on the high local failure rate of surgery alone in patients with rectal cancer who have nodes positive for tumor or tumor extension beyond the wall. Postoperative radiation therapy and chemotherapy consistently have been shown to improve local control and survival rates in patients with rectal cancer. A major advantage of postoperative adjuvant treatment is that the physician has pathologic confirmation of the extent of the tumor spread through the wall to nodes or distant sites. This information is critical in determining whether adjuvant treatment is necessary.[12]

Preoperative radiation therapy is another commonly used technique for patients who have large rectal cancers that have invaded through the muscle layer (T3) or who have imaging studies (MRI) that show enlarged lymph nodes that indicate N1 or N2 disease. The goal of this treatment is sphincter preservation. Radiation therapy combined with chemotherapy is done before surgery to shrink the tumor so that a LAR can be done, rather than an APR, to spare the patient a colostomy. The potential advantages of preoperative radiation therapy are downstaging of the primary tumor, which decreases the chance of tumor spillage or seeding at the time of surgery; increased radiosensitivity because of well-oxygenated cells in the nonoperative pelvis; increase in local control of the disease; and less acute side effects.[12,18-20] A disadvantage to preoperative radiation therapy is the lack of pathologic tumor (T) staging that results in the irradiation of a patient with a T1 or T2 tumor. Preoperative or neoadjuvant chemoradiation is the most common treatment used today for locally advanced rectal cancer.[18,19,21,22]

Radiation alone has also been used in patients who have conditions that are medically inoperable or who have locally advanced rectal cancer that is deemed unresectable.[12,13] In this setting, radiation provides palliation and is rarely curative. Radiation combined with chemotherapy (5-fluorouracil [5-FU]) has proved more effective than radiation alone in relieving symptoms, decreasing tumor progression, and increasing overall survival.

Chemotherapy. The addition of adjuvant chemotherapy combined with radiation therapy in the preoperative or postoperative setting in high-risk rectal and colon cancer cases (T3 or N1, N2) has shown an increase in overall survival rates (Fig. 31.5).[12,18,19,23] Many studies have shown decreased disease recurrence and improved survival rates with a combination of 5-FU and pelvic radiation therapy. The National

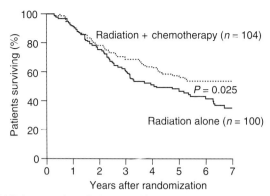

Fig. 31.5 Improved survival rates with postoperative radiation and chemotherapy versus radiation alone. (Modified from Krook JE, Moertel CG, Gunderson LL, et al. Effective surgical adjuvant therapy for high-risk rectal carcinoma. *N Engl J Med.* 1991;324:709–715.)

Comprehensive Cancer Network (NCCN) has established treatment guidelines for patients with colon and rectal cancer. The current recommendations for T3 rectal cancer are for continuous venous infusion 5-FU or oral capecitabine during radiation therapy in the preoperative or neoadjuvant setting.[18,19] In the neoadjuvant setting, the chemoradiation is followed by curative resection and then additional 5-FU with or without leucovorin, FOLFOX (5-FU, leucovorin, oxaliplatin) regimen, or capecitabine with or without oxaliplatin. In the postoperative setting, 5-FU with or without leucovorin or FOLFOX is done first followed by radiation therapy with continuous 5-FU. Once the radiation therapy is completed, additional chemotherapy with 5-FU with or without leucovorin or FOLFOX is done. In the case of recurrent or metastatic rectal cancer, the same drugs can be used or a regimen called FOLFIRI may be used. FOLFIRI consists of 5-FU, leucovorin, and irinotecan.[5,14] Two monoclonal antibodies, bevacizumab and cetuximab, are being studied in the use of advanced or metastatic colon or rectal cancer. Bevacizumab (Avastin, Genentech, San Francisco, CA) is a drug that blocks the growth of new blood vessels to the tumor and hinders the supply of oxygen and nutrients necessary for continued growth of the tumor. This drug is used in combination with FOLFOX or FOLFIRI. Cetuximab (Erbitux, Bristol-Myers Squibb, NY) blocks the effects of hormone-like factors that promote cancer cell growth and thus cause cell death. Cetuximab may be used alone or in combination with other chemotherapy drugs in patients who do not respond to the chemotherapy agent irinotecan.[7,14]

Field Design and Critical Structures. Patients who undergo preoperative or postoperative adjuvant radiation therapy for rectal cancer are at a high risk for local recurrence. These patients include those with extension beyond the bowel wall, tumor adherence (T3, T4), or lymph nodes positive for tumor (N1, N2). The treatment fields are typically designed to encompass the primary tumor volume and pelvic lymph nodes, which shrinks the field to treat the primary target volume to a higher dose. Anatomic boundaries of the portals depend on whether the patient underwent an anterior resection or anteroposterior (AP) resection directly related to the areas at risk for recurrence. For patients with rectal cancer, most recurrences occur in the posterior aspect of the pelvis, including metastasis to the internal iliac and presacral lymph nodes.[12,13] These two nodal groups are not included in a standard surgical resection for rectal cancer and need to be encompassed in radiation portals.[12,13] For irradiation of the pelvis, the dose-limiting structure or organ at risk (OAR) is the small bowel. The small bowel dose should be less than 45 Gy. Radiation treatment techniques and the field design must take into consideration the amount of small bowel in the field to minimize treatment-related toxicities. The reduction of the small bowel dose is achieved through patient positioning and positioning devices, bladder distention, multiple-shaped fields, and dosimetric weighting.[4,5,12] The dose to the small bowel is more easily reduced during preoperative radiation therapy than during postoperative radiation because with postoperative radiation, the rectum and peritoneum have been removed, which allows the small bowel to be displaced more inferiorly in the pelvis and results in more small bowel within the radiation field. The dose delivered to the large volume (tumor plus regional nodes) is 4500 cGy, with the coned-down volume (primary tumor bed) receiving 5000 to 5500 cGy in 6 to 6.5 weeks. Doses in excess of 5000 cGy are not advisable unless the small bowel can be excluded from the field.[4,5,12,24] In the neoadjuvant treatment setting, a newer short-course radiation therapy regimen has been used. The NCCN states that 2500 cGy in 5 fractions may be given as an alternative for T3 N0 patients followed by surgery within 1 week. This approach is more commonly performed in Europe but is in use in the United States. Short-course radiation therapy may be an option for patients who live farther from a cancer center, whose health is declining or are unable to receive chemotherapy.[21–24]

Traditionally, a three-field technique in which the patient is positioned prone (posteroanterior [PA] and opposed laterals wedged) is used, which allows a homogenous dose to the tumor bed with sparing of anterior structures, such as the small bowel. A four-field PA/AP and opposed laterals technique may be used when the anterior structures such as the prostate or vagina are at risk for involvement or are involved. For patients who have undergone an anterior resection, the superior extent of the field is placed 1.5 cm superior to the sacral promontory, which correlates to L5 to S1 innerspace.[4,9] Depending on the superior extent of the lesion and clinical indications, the field may need to be placed at the L4 to L5 interspace or extend superiorly to include the paraaortic lymph node chain. The more superiorly the field extends, the more precautions are necessary to avoid small bowel injury and complications. The width of the PA/AP field is designed to provide adequate coverage of the iliac lymph nodes. This border is placed 2 cm lateral to the pelvic brim and inlet. The inferior border generally includes the entire obturator foramina, although this may vary depending on the location of the lesion. The recommended inferior margin is 3 to 5 cm beyond the gross tumor before surgery or below the most distal extent of dissection after surgery (Fig. 31.6). A rectal tube is inserted at the time of simulation. Contrast (30 to 40 cm^2) is injected into the rectum to facilitate the localization of critical structures and design of treatment fields. A radiopaque marker or BB is placed on the anal verge to reference the perineal surface on digitally reconstructed simulation radiographs (DRRs).

Lateral treatment portals and prone positioning with full bladder distention allow the small bowel to be excluded from the treatment volume. This position also assists in the localization of critical posterior structures. Anatomically, the rectum and perirectal tissues are extremely close to the sacrum and coccyx. In locally advanced disease, the tumor may spread along the sacral nerve roots and result in tumor recurrence in the sacrum. Therefore the posterior field edge is placed 1.5 to 2.0 cm behind the anterior bony sacral margin. In advanced situations, the entire sacral canal plus a 1.5-cm margin is recommended.[4,12] This margin allows day-to-day variances in the patient setup caused by movement. Anteriorly, the field border is placed at the anterior edge of the femoral heads to ensure coverage of the internal iliac nodes. The lower third of the rectum lies immediately posterior to the vaginal wall and prostate, which places these organs and their draining lymphatics at risk for involvement. If the rectal lesion has invaded anterior structures (prostate or vagina), the anterior border is placed on pubic symphysis for inclusion of the external iliac nodes (Fig. 31.6B).[4,5,12]

The use of a CT simulator allows the physician to more accurately localize and outline the pertinent anatomic structures described previously. The CT simulator software enables physicians to digitize in different colors the target volume and critical healthy structures, such as the rectum, bladder, and lymph nodes on each CT slice. The intimate relationships of target versus healthy tissues are available at the time of simulation and with the patient in treatment position. This assists the physician and the dosimetrist in the accurate placement of the isocenter and in the design of the fields. A DRR is produced to show the radiation field outline, the treatment isocenter, and the pertinent anatomic structures (Fig. 31.7). The CT images can be sent electronically directly to dosimetry for treatment planning.

The CT simulation procedure requires the radiation therapist to position patients prone on a positioning device, such as a belly board, with the elbows "in" so that they do not hit the sides of the CT gantry during the scan. Patients may also be positioned supine if treated using volume-modulated arc therapy (VMAT) or intensity-modulated radiation therapy (IMRT). The supine position is a more stable and comfortable for the patient than prone. A vacuum bag immobilization device under the legs provides a reproducible setup. It is extremely important that patients be as straight as possible before the scan because they cannot be repositioned once the scan is complete. Patients may be given oral contrast to drink 45 minutes before the CT simulation to allow the small bowel to be localized on the CT scans. Additional contrast is typically placed in the rectum at the time of simulation, and the tube is removed before scanning. IV contrast may also be used at the time of simulation. The contrast allows blood vessels to be highlighted and assists in the outlining of lymph node groups at risk.

Initially, patients should be straightened with the external laser system and any useful topographic anatomy. With the lasers, temporary reference marks can be drawn on the patient and marked with small radiopaque BBs. These marks may be used later in the simulation process as a reference to check patient positioning or to help place fiducial marks after topograms are acquired (if fiducial marks are necessary with the virtual simulation software). The reference isocenter is used to ensure that the patient did not move during the scan. The reference isocenter is also used as the zero coordinates from which the treatment isocenter is marked. A typical topogram may extend from the level of the second lumbar vertebrae to below the lesser trochanters. After the CT scan, the physician determines the treatment isocenter while the patient is still on the CT couch; images are reviewed by the physician, and the treatment isocenter is determined based on the areas contoured on the CT images. The isocenter coordinates are then programmed into the movable lasers in the scanner room, and the patient is marked accordingly. The patient then goes home with marks that will actually be used for treatment delivery.

IMRT and **VMAT** are more recent techniques that are used in the treatment of rectal cancer. VMAT combines IMRT with arc therapy. The multileaf collimator leaves move while the treatment unit rotates 360 degrees around the patient to provide a highly conformal dose. IMRT and VMAT use inverse forward planning to place dose limits on OARs such as the small bowel, colon, bladder, and femoral heads. VMAT allows more dose conformity to the planning target volume and spares the small bowel more than conventional methods. IMRT and VMAT are more costly than 3D conformal methods, and although more tissues are exposed to low doses of irradiation with VMAT, the benefit of sparing more healthy tissues is considered a greater advantage. Treatment of rectal cancer with VMAT consisting of two full arcs is becoming a more commonly used approach than 3D conformal prone treatment fields.

Dose-limiting structures for treatment of ascending or descending colon cancer include the kidney and the small bowel. Contrast studies

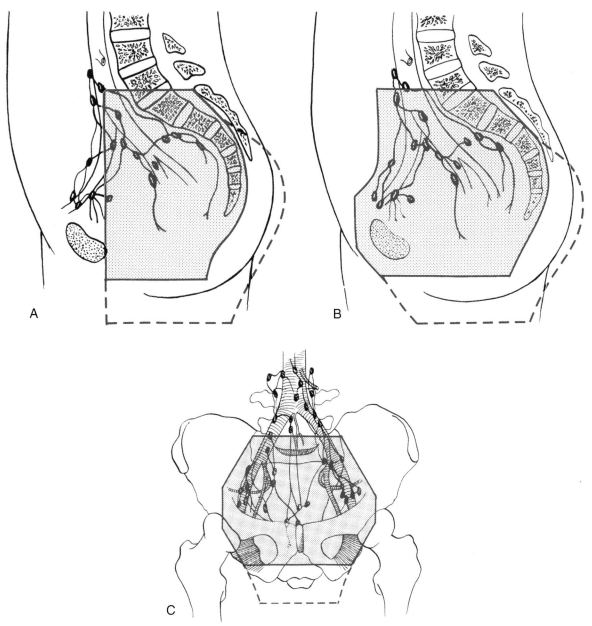

Fig. 31.6 Radiation treatment fields. In all figures, the *dotted line* indicates the field extension to be used after an abdominal-perineal resection. (A) A standard lateral field. (B) A lateral field to include external iliacs in patients who have involvement of structures with external iliac lymph node drainage. (C) A standard anteroposterior/posteroanterior field.

for assessment of renal function and kidney localization should be performed before treatment or at the time of simulation to ensure the adequate sparing of at least one kidney. For example, with treatment of a right-sided colon lesion, 50% or more of the right kidney may be in the field; therefore the left kidney must be spared.[12,13] Three-dimensional conformal radiation therapy techniques and IMRT may be used. IMRT allows more sparing of the kidneys, liver, and small bowel and is more commonly used.

In patients with locally advanced colorectal cancer or recurrent disease, local control is difficult to achieve because of limited surgical options that result from fixation of the tumor to pelvic organs (prostate, uterus) or unresectable structures, such as the presacrum or pelvic sidewall. If microscopic residual disease exists, an external beam dose of 6000 cGy or greater is necessary to provide a reasonable chance for control. This dose is even higher (>7000 cGy) if gross residual disease

exists. These doses exceed the healthy tissue tolerance dose of abdominal or pelvic structures and cannot be safely delivered with conventional external beam.

The radiation therapist is also responsible for ensuring the accurate delivery of the radiation treatments. Today, image-guided radiation therapy (IGRT) is used to ensure radiation fields are correctly aligned before initiation of treatment. Many different types of image guidance technologies exist. One type is the linear accelerator equipped with a kV imager along with electronic portal imaging device (EPID). The kV imager produces an image of greater contrast and detail than the equivalent EPID image taken with 6-MV photons. Radiation therapists have the responsibility of taking the pretreatment port of the treatment field or orthogonal pair and then matching the bony anatomy on the kV image with the DRR from simulation and applying any shifts (i.e., anterior, posterior, superior) in treatment position before turning on

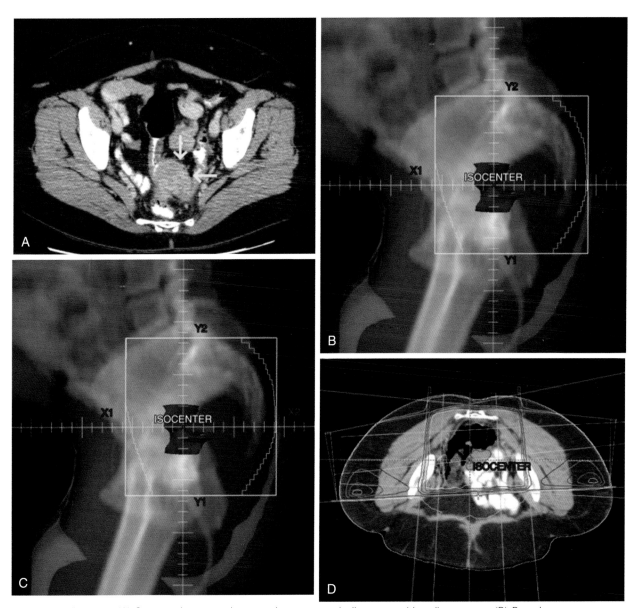

Fig. 31.7 (A) Computed tomography scan shows tumor *(yellow arrows)* invading rectum. (B) Beam's-eye lateral view. (D) Isodose distribution of primary fields. (From Czito BG, Hsu D, Palta M, et al. Colon cancer. In Clinical Oncology: Gunderson L, Tepper JE, eds. 4th ed. Philadelphia, PA: Elsevier; 2016.)

the beam. Another IGRT system is cone-beam CT (CBCT). The resultant scan is used to compare cone-beam scan with the simulation CT scan. The simulation CT scan is registered to allow the CBCT to be compared with it. Bony anatomy, soft tissues, or fiducial marks, are matched to determine whether any shifts in isocenter are necessary.

Recall the dose limits of radiation for the kidneys, liver, and small bowel. What is the healthy tissue tolerance for each of these OARs? Which of the three organs is most sensitive to radiation damage? IMRT may help reduce the dose to OARs.

Intraoperative Radiation Therapy. Intraoperative radiation therapy (IORT) is a mechanism for supplementing the external beam dose to assist in obtaining local control of the tumor while sparing dose-limiting healthy structures.[14] IORT is a specialized boost technique similar to brachytherapy. IORT is also used when cancer recurs in the pelvis. As the name implies, IORT involves an operative

procedure that requires general anesthesia. The radiation oncologist and surgeon must work closely with one another to determine whether IORT is appropriate and which diagnostic tests are helpful in planning the IORT and external beam radiation treatments. A contraindication for IORT is the presence of distant metastasis. The surgeon and radiation oncologist also determine the optimal sequence of surgery and external radiation by discussing the benefits and side effects of each.[9,14]

Patients who undergo an IORT procedure may receive a dose of 1000 to 2000 cGy of electrons in a single fraction directly to the tumor bed. Critical dose-limiting structures (i.e., kidney, bowel) are shielded or surgically displaced out of the radiation portal so that these healthy tissues receive little or no radiation. This dose, delivered in a single fraction, is two to three times the dose if delivered at conventional fractionation of 180 to 200 cGy/fraction. For example, an IORT single dose of 1500 cGy equals 3000 to 4500 cGy fractionated external radiation. With the effective IORT dose added to the 4500 to 5000 cGy,

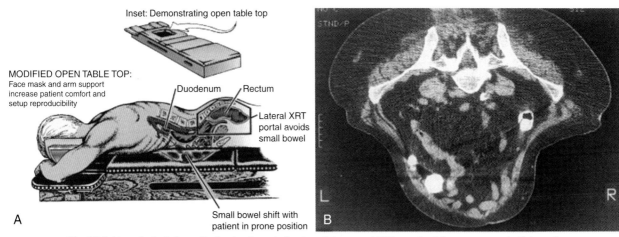

Inset: Demonstrating open table top

MODIFIED OPEN TABLE TOP:
Face mask and arm support
increase patient comfort and
setup reproducibility

Duodenum

Rectum

Lateral XRT
portal avoids
small bowel

A

Small bowel shift with
patient in prone position

B

Fig. 31.8 Use of a belly board in the treatment of colorectal cancer. (A) The patient lies prone on a belly board, allowing the small bowel to be displaced anteriorly. (B) Computed tomography scan confirms displacement of the small bowel. (A, From Rich T, Ajani JA, Morrison WH, et al. Chemoradiation therapy for anal cancer. Radiation plus continuous infusion of 5-fluorouracil with or without cisplatin. *Radiother Oncol.* 1993;27:209-215.) B, From Janjan NA, Delclos ME, Crane CH. Colon and rectum. In: Cox JD, Ang KK eds. *Radiation Oncology: Rationale, Techniques, Results.* 9th ed. St. Louis, MO: Mosby; 2010.)

delivered with conventional external beam radiation, the total effective dose equals 7500 to 9500 cGy. A dose this high cannot be safely given with standard external irradiation.[17,25]

The IORT dose is calculated at the 90% isodose line, with the energy and dose delivered depending on the depth or amount of residual disease. Electron energies of 9 to 12 MeV are used after a gross total resection, or minimal residual and high energies of 15 to 18 MeV are used for patients who have recurrent disease with gross residual or unresectable disease. Some newer portable equipment is now available for use in the operating room.

The precise role of IORT in the treatment of large bowel cancer is still being studied. IORT continues to be used in locally advanced and recurrent colorectal cancer. This treatment in addition to combined modality therapy is associated with better local control and survival rates.[25] Moreover, toxicity can be significant. Further study is needed before IORT becomes a widely accepted tool in the treatment of colorectal cancer.

Side Effects. The acute and chronic side effects of irradiation to the pelvis or abdomen are directly related to the dose, volume, and type of tissue irradiated. The larger the area treated, the greater are the associated toxicities. The toxicities of treatment increase with escalating doses and depend on the healthy tissue tolerances of the structures in the irradiated volume. For patients with colorectal cancer, the main dose-limiting structure for acute and chronic side effects is the small bowel. Acute toxicities of treatment include diarrhea, abdominal cramps and bloating, proctitis, bloody or mucus discharge, and dysuria. Patients may also experience leukopenia (an abnormal decrease in the white blood cell count) and thrombocytopenia (an abnormal decrease in the platelet count). GI and hematologic toxicities are increased when chemotherapy is used with radiation therapy.[12,13] In patients who have their perineum treated, a brisk skin reaction (moist desquamation) may result, which sometimes necessitates a treatment break.

Chronic effects occur less often than acute side effects but are more serious. Persistent diarrhea, increased bowel frequency, proctitis, fistula, urinary incontinence, and bladder atrophy have occurred in patients after radiation therapy. The most common long-term complication is damage to the small bowel that results in enteritis, adhesions, and obstruction.[9,14] The incidence of small bowel obstruction that necessitates surgery may be decreased by radiation oncologists and

surgeons working together to determine methods for minimizing the amount of small bowel in the radiation field.

As mentioned previously, treatment techniques and fields are designed to limit the dose to the small bowel. These include surgical and radiation therapy interventions. For example, the surgeon can reconstruct the pelvis to minimize the amount of small bowel in the pelvis after an AP resection. The surgeon can help limit the volume of tissue irradiated by placing clips to demarcate the tumor bed, which allows the radiation oncologist to more precisely outline the area at risk instead of requiring a more generous treatment volume.[9,14]

Radiation therapy techniques for limiting the small bowel dose are numerous and involve the efforts of the radiation oncologist, radiation therapists, and dosimetrists. Before CT simulation, the patient drinks oral contrast to highlight the small bowel on the CT simulation scan. Because the patient is scanned in treatment position, the physician can use this information along with previous imaging studies, such as CT scan and barium studies, to determine the tumor–small bowel relationship and design the radiation field. Treatment with the patient in a prone position with a full bladder causes the small bowel to shift superiorly out of the treatment field and further reduces the dose to the small bowel (Fig. 31.8). VMAT or IMRT reduces the dose to the small bowel and allows the patient to be treated in a supine position. The patient must be in a stable and reproducible position with use of IMRT or VMAT.

The radiation oncologist and dosimetrist work together to further reduce the small bowel dose by carefully planning the initial and boost-field volumes with the use of 3D conformal treatment planning with multileaf collimation (MLC). High-energy beams (≥6 MV) are preferable with 3D conformal treatment planning because of the depth-dose characteristics that deliver a homogeneous dose to the target volume while allowing the more anterior healthy structures to be spared. A multiple-field approach (three or four fields) coupled with weighting of the fields to the posterior in patients with rectal cancer further reduces the dose to the anteriorly located small bowel (Fig. 31.9). The use of IMRT and VMAT is another method of reducing dose to small bowel and other healthy tissues.

Role of the Radiation Therapist

The radiation therapist plays a major role in the education of patients and their families. Communication is the key factor in making a

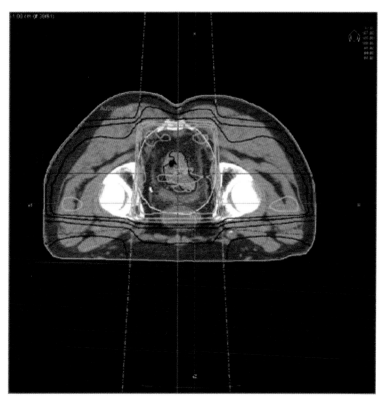

Fig. 31.9 Isodose distribution of a three-field plan for the treatment of rectal cancer. (From Minsky BD, Rödel CM, Valentini V. Rectal cancer. In: Gunderson L, Tepper JE, eds. *Clinical Oncology*. 4th ed. Philadelphia, PA: Elsevier; 2016.)

patient's experience with a cancer diagnosis and treatment less traumatic and anxiety ridden. The therapist's first major role with the patient is in simulation. The therapist should inform the patient that the simulation is not a treatment but a planning session to locate and outline the area that needs treatment. The therapist should describe the procedure to the patient, indicating the length of time it will take and pointing out that the treatments do not require the same amount of time. The patient's position during the treatment should also be discussed. The therapist should inform the patient about the contrast materials that are used during the procedure, the skin marks to be used to align the patient, and the importance of maintaining those marks. If tattoos are used to indicate treatment isocenter or positioning marks, the patient should be told about the process of a needle stick and the permanency of these marks before the simulation to obtain consent. If the patient is treated in the prone position, the therapist should explain the procedure before the patient is positioned. After the simulation begins, the therapist should continually update the patient on what is happening throughout the procedure. Keeping patients informed reduces the anxiety that they may experience. Instrumental music played during the simulation or treatment can calm and further reduce a patient's anxieties and fears.

At the time of the first treatment, therapists should familiarize patients with the treatment room and the location of the camera and audio equipment and explain what patients should do if they need something (e.g., raising their right hand). A common fear of patients is being alone in the room. Therapists should discuss the actual length of time that the machine is on per treatment. Therapists should also inform the patients about the types of noises that are heard as the machine is programmed and treatment is initiated. If the patient's family members are also present, the therapist may offer to show them the treatment room and control area so that they may see the video camera; however, the family should not be in the control area during

the initiation of treatment so that the therapist's performance is not hindered.

The therapist should assess the information given to the patient regarding treatment instructions (e.g., full bladder) and potential side effects. Written materials regarding bladder distention, a low-residue diet, and available support services should be distributed during the first week of treatment.

As treatments progress, the therapist is responsible for inquiring about how the patient is feeling, monitoring any treatment-related side effects, and checking on the patient's emotional well-being. If the patient reports abdominal cramping and diarrhea, the therapist should determine whether the patient is following a low-residue diet or has a prescription for an antidiarrheal agent, such as diphenoxylate (Lomotil, Pfizer, NY) or loperamide (Imodium, Janssen Pharmaceuticals, Beerse, Belgium). The therapist should ask the patient about the physician's instructions regarding the prescription. In some instances, the patient may not be taking the medication correctly. Dietary suggestions regarding which foods to avoid or recommendations for a low-residue diet are the therapist's responsibility. If the patient is experiencing diarrhea, instructions to avoid whole-grain breads or cereals, fresh fruits, raw vegetables, fried or fatty foods, milk, and milk products may be helpful. Recommended foods include white bread; meats that are baked, broiled, or roasted until tender; peeled apples; bananas; macaroni and noodles; and cooked vegetables (Table 31.1).[7] If the patient still reports diarrhea after diet and medications have been discussed, the patient may need to be referred back to the physician or dietitian for further evaluation.

Skin reactions on the perineum or in the region of the gluteal cleft may occur with the three-field technique. Skin reactions range from brisk erythema (treated with topical steroid creams) to moist desquamation (requiring sitz baths, Domeboro solution). Therapists play an important role in monitoring the perineal area, which the patient

TABLE 31.1 Dietary Guidelines for Patients Receiving Pelvic Irradiation

Recommended Foods	Foods to Avoid
White bread	Whole-grain breads or cereals
Meat baked, broiled, or roasted until tender	Fried or fatty foods
Macaroni	Milk and milk products
Cooked vegetables	Raw vegetables
Peeled apples and bananas	Fresh fruit

cannot easily see. The therapist meets with the patient daily and can assess whether the reaction has intensified. The therapist can question patients to determine the way in which they are caring for their skin. If the patient has a moist desquamation, recommendations include taking sitz baths in tepid water, wearing loose undergarments or none at all, and allowing the area to be exposed to air and kept dry after the bath. These suggestions keep the area clean, dry, and less irritated.

The physical side effects of treatment are often the most visible and easiest to address; however, the therapist must be alert to the emotional needs of the patient and family. The psychosocial aspect of a cancer diagnosis and treatment can be just as painful as the treatment or cancer itself. Therapists are not expected to diagnose but should listen to what the patient is saying and be available to offer suggestions and support. Sometimes, all the patient needs is for someone to listen and know someone cares. The therapist should provide the patient with information about community or hospital services, such as the ACS, the hospital oncology social worker or chaplain, and other support groups in the area. Patients with a colostomy may be having difficulty adjusting to their appliance, so the therapist can refer them to an endostomal therapist, (a healthcare professional trained to care for individuals with stomas) for assistance. The therapist should listen to patients and determine the way their diagnosis and treatment has affected their self-image and self-esteem. The ACS's written materials about specific types of cancer or other publications for patients with cancer should be handed out or made available to the patient. These documents can be used by patients as references and shared with families and friends because patients may have trouble remembering much of this information when given verbally by the physician.

Many patients today access much of the information about their cancer and its treatment on the internet (for instance, much useful information is posted on the ACS website, www.cancer.org).

Case I

Preoperative Radiation for Rectal Cancer. A 70-year-old woman presented to her primary care physician with a reported change in bowel habits, blood in the stool, and weight loss. A colonoscopy was obtained that revealed a rectal mass starting at 5 cm from the anal verge. Biopsies were positive for invasive adenocarcinoma. As part of the patient's staging workup, a CT of the chest, abdomen, and pelvis was obtained. An MRI of the pelvis was also completed. The CT of the pelvis confirmed the presence of a large rectal mass with involvement of the internal sphincter. The MRI of the pelvis showed a low rectal mass with extension into the mesorectal space and enlargement of multiple pelvic lymph nodes. The rest of the imaging studies were negative for any distant metastasis.

Based on the imaging studies, the patient was staged as T3d, N2a, and M0 or Stage III B. Because the tumor had spread beyond the bowel wall into the mesorectal space, surgery to obtain negative margins would be difficult. Therefore a course of neoadjuvant chemoradiation was recommended. An APR was planned after the completion of chemoradiation.

The patient received oral capecitabine chemotherapy and 5040cGy in 28 fractions to the primary tumor. The radiation treatment technique used was VMAT with four full 360-degree arcs to the pelvis with IMRT planning minimizing the dose to OARs: small bowel, colon, bladder, and femoral heads. Therapists would perform daily onboard imaging and match to bony anatomy (pelvic bones).

Case II

A 51-year-old man presented to his primary care physician with a 1-year history of intermittent hematochezia and mucus. He recently had development of rectal discomfort. Physical examination results revealed a mass that was freely mobile and exophytic on the left rectal wall beginning about 4 to 5 cm above the anal verge. A colonoscopy was done and showed a 2-cm to 3-cm polypoid mass in the lower rectum. The mass was biopsied and found to be a moderately differentiated adenocarcinoma. A CT scan of the chest, abdomen, and pelvis was performed, and results were negative for metastatic disease. An MRI of the pelvis was also completed. This showed a 3.8-cm-long mass in the rectum that did not involve the sphincter but was close to the mid- and caudal left levator ani muscle. The muscularis propria was involved without any extension to the perirectal fat. One 6-mm perirectal lymph node and two sacral lymph nodes were suspicious for cancer. Endoscopic ultrasound scan (EUS) could have been performed but was not believed necessary as it would not have changed the management of the case. The patient was given a stage of IIIA T2 N1 M0 based on imaging studies.

Because the tumor was located close to the sphincter, the patient was recommended to undergo **neoadjuvant chemoradiation** to shrink the tumor to facilitate a better surgery with negative margins. The patient's chemotherapy consisted of infusion 5-FU and capecitabine.

A radiation dose of 5040 cGy to the pelvis was prescribed and delivered with a three-field approach, with posterior and right and left lateral IMRT fields. The patient was treated prone with full bladder distension to minimize the amount of small bowel in the treatment field. Daily IGRT, with an OBI kV imager, was useful in matching the boney landmarks in the and sacrum.

ANAL CANCER

Epidemiology and Etiology

Cancers of the anus occur more often in women than in men and constitute approximately 1% to 2% of all large bowel malignancies.[3] The ACS predicts that about 8300 new cases of anal cancer will occur each year: 5530 in women and 2770 in men.[1] The median age at the time of diagnosis is 60 years.[1] A general age distribution of 30 to 90 years is reported. The human papilloma virus infection (HPV) is considered the causative factor in 90% of anal cancers.[3,26] Other etiologic factors for the development of anal cancer are associated with genital warts, genital infections, anal intercourse, intercourse before age 30 years, human immunodeficiency virus infection, and immunosuppression.[26-29] HPV-16 is the type of virus found in squamous cell cancers of the anus. It is also found in some genital and anal warts. HPV has been found to make two proteins, E6 and E7, which are able to shut down two tumor suppressor proteins, p53 and Rb, in healthy cells. When these tumor suppressors are rendered inactive, cells can become cancerous.[27,30] Cigarette smoking has also been associated with the development of anal cancer.[27]

Anatomy and Lymphatics

The anal canal is 3 to 4 cm long and extends from the anal verge to the anorectal ring at the junction of the anus and rectum. The anal canal is lined with a hairless, stratified squamous epithelium up to the dentate or pectinate line. At this line, the mucosa becomes cuboidal in transition to the columnar epithelium found in the rectum (Fig. 31.2).[11,14]

Lymphatic spread occurs initially to the perirectal and anorectal lymph nodes. If the tumor extends above the dentate line, the nodal groups at risk are the internal iliac and lateral sacral nodes; this is similar to rectal cancer. With involvement below the dentate line, inguinal lymph nodes may be involved. Inguinal lymph node involvement is found in approximately 10% to 30% of patients.[14,30]

Clinical Presentation

The most common presenting symptom is rectal bleeding (bright red). Other symptoms are pain, change in bowel habits, and the sensation of a mass. Pruritus or itching has been reported less often and is associated with a perianal lesion.[26,27,30]

Detection and Diagnosis

A thorough physical examination should be performed that includes a digital anorectal examination (with notation of anal sphincter tone and direct extension to other organs) and palpation of the inguinal lymph nodes. Anoscopy or proctoscopic examination and biopsy should be obtained. A further workup includes a CT scan of the abdomen and pelvis to evaluate the liver and perirectal, inguinal, pelvic, and paraaortic nodes. A PET scan for further assessment of spread of tumor to lymph nodes or liver or an MRI has been advocated. Transrectal sonography may also be done to determine depth of invasion into the bowel wall.[27,30] A chest radiograph, a CBC, and liver function tests also are performed.

Pathology, Staging, and Routes of Spread

Squamous cell carcinoma is the most common histology of anal cancer; it comprises approximately 80% of cases.[26,30] The next most frequent type is basaloid, or cloacogenic, cancer. These tumors occur in the region of the dentate line where the epithelium is in transition. Also found in this region are adenocarcinoma (arising from the anal glands), mucoepidermoid tumors, and melanoma. Cancers that occur in the perianal region are typically squamous or basal cell carcinomas consistent with skin cancers.

The most commonly used staging system is the AJCC system. In this clinical system, tumors are staged according to their size and extent. (For more information about staging anal cancer, see https://www.cancer.org/cancer/anal-cancer/detection-diagnosis-staging/staging.html)

Tumors of the anal canal spread most frequently via direct extension into the adjacent soft tissues. Lymphatic spread occurs relatively early to pelvic nodes but more commonly to inguinal lymph nodes, whereas hematogenous spread to the liver or lungs is less common. The incidence rate of inguinal node involvement may be as high as 20% for tumors more than 4 cm in diameter and as high as 60% with direct invasion of adjacent pelvis structures.[30]

Treatment Techniques

Combination radiation therapy and chemotherapy (5-FU and mitomycin C [MMC]) is advocated as the preferred method of treatment and is considered the standard of care for most patients. Cisplatin in combination with 5-FU has also been used. Cisplatin is associated with fewer side effects and is more easily tolerated by the patient.[7,26,27,30] Radiation alone may be advocated for patients who cannot tolerate chemoradiation. Studies have shown that the multimodality (radiation and chemotherapy) approach provides good local control and colostomy-free survival. Most series report survival rates from 65% to 80% at 5 years, with a local control rate of 60% to 89%.[7,27,30] An AP resection with a wide perineal dissection is the most common surgical procedure for anal cancer. This procedure is no longer done as the initial treatment, but it is done in the case of local recurrence after conventional chemoradiation.[7,27,30]

A variety of radiation techniques exist for the treatment of anal cancer. Current radiation treatment techniques today includes VMAT fields. Traditionally, a four-field or AP/PA pelvic field with electron fields to the inguinal nodes, including a boost to the tumor bed with a perineal electron field or another multifield technique, has been used. The pelvic field extends from the lumbosacral-sacroiliac region to 3 cm distal to the lowest extent of the tumor (noted by a radiopaque marker at the time of simulation). The inferior border typically flashes the perineum, which results in brisk erythema and moist desquamation of the perineal tissues. The lateral border may extend to include treatment of the inguinal lymph nodes on the AP field only, placing that field edge at the midlateral aspect of the femoral heads. The PA field is kept narrower because the anteriorly located inguinal nodes do not receive much contribution from the posterior field. This also avoids an excessive dose to the femoral heads and yet encompasses the tumor bed and deep pelvic nodes. Anterior electron fields centered over each inguinal region and abutting the PA lateral border are used to further supplement the dose to the inguinal lymph nodes. These fields require careful matching to avoid overlap into the pelvic fields from the inguinal electron fields.

Many structures are identified as OARs in treatment of anal cancer, such as the femoral head and necks, genitalia/perineum, small bowel, and bladder. For this reason, VMAT is the standard treatment of anal cancer. The inverse planning of IMRT allows doses to be conformed to the primary tumor and has shown improved dosimetric coverage of inguinal lymph nodes. The use of VMAT greatly reduces the doses to healthy tissues (OARs) compared with the conventional 3D conformal AP/PA technique and reduces the side effects patients experience.[21,23,26,30–32]

A variety of radiation dose schemes have been used. The NCCN recommendations for T2 to T4 anal cancer is a dose of 4500 cGy to the pelvis and inguinal nodes followed by a shrinking field boost to reduce small bowel toxicity with an additional 900 to 1400 cGy delivered to the primary tumor.[33] A higher total dose is advocated for T3 or T4 disease.[19,34] Total radiation doses range from 5400 to 5900 cGy.[29,32,35]

Chemoradiation, although a very effective treatment, is associated with much acute toxicity. Almost all patients treated with AP/PA fields experience a perineal skin reaction, with about half of the patients encountering moist desquamation. IMRT has reduced the type and severity of skin reactions patients experience. Nausea, vomiting, and mild to moderate diarrhea are also reported. The most severe and life-threatening complication is bone marrow suppression from the irradiation to the pelvis and the 5-FU and mitomycin regimen.[7,26,29,30] Radiation therapists are responsible for monitoring a patient's blood counts and reporting any low counts, including the absolute neutrophil count, to the radiation oncologist. The radiation therapist sees the patient daily and should keep a watchful eye on the perineal skin and advise patient on proper skin care. The radiation therapist should also refer patients to the oncology nurse or radiation oncologist for further advisement on skin care in case a break in treatment is warranted.

In conclusion, radiation therapy in combination with chemotherapy is considered the standard of care for the treatment of anal cancer and provides sphincter preservation and satisfactory cure rates.

Case III

Anal Cancer. A 53-year-old woman presented with noticeable bleeding in her stool and anal pain. A physical examination was performed, and a mass was palpated. The patient then underwent a sigmoidoscopy, which showed a 6-mm mass extending into the anal canal. The lesion was an ulcerating fissure with raised edges located on the right lateral aspect of the canal. A biopsy obtained demonstrated a well-differentiated squamous cell carcinoma. Staging workup procedure included a PET-CT of the pelvis that confirmed the mass in the anal canal and showed no evidence of disease in inguinal lymph nodes or distant spread. The patient was stage II T2 N0 M0.

To maintain continuity of the GI tract, chemoradiation was the recommended course of treatment. Chemotherapy consisting of 5-FU and MMC was given during the first and fifth weeks of radiation treatment. The patient was prescribed 5040 cGy in 28 treatments to the anal mass plus margin, and 4200 cGy was delivered to the elective nodal regions, including the inguinal and pelvic nodes. The treatment technique used VMAT with four full 360-degree arcs.

ESOPHAGEAL CANCER

Epidemiology and Etiology

Cancer of the esophagus accounts for 1% of all cancers in the United States, with approximately 17,650 cases reported each year.[1] Men are three to four times more commonly affected than are women (13,750 vs. 3,900, respectively).[1,5] Most cancers of the esophagus are diagnosed in patients between 55 and 85 years of age.[36] Esophageal cancer is usually diagnosed at an advanced stage and is nearly a uniformly fatal disease. Each year, the ACS estimates about 16,080 esophageal cancer–related deaths will occur in the United States.[1] Survival rates have been improving, with a current 21% overall survival rate at 5 years compared with only 9% 5-year survival in 1989.[1] Cancer of the esophagus occurs with the greatest frequency in northern China, northern Iran, and South Africa.[36-38] This has been attributed to environmental and nutritional factors.

Many risk factors or etiologic factors contribute to the development of esophageal cancer. Certain risk factors increase one's chance of development of a squamous cell carcinoma or adenocarcinoma of the esophagus. For example, the most common and important etiologic factors in the development of squamous cell cancer of the esophagus in western countries are excessive alcohol and tobacco use. The combination of these two factors has a synergistic effect on the mucosal surfaces, which increases the risk of esophageal cancer and other aerodigestive malignancies.[34,39,40] Excessive alcohol use has been an implicated risk factor for the development of squamous cell carcinomas. The use of tobacco products has been shown to cause squamous cell carcinomas. Tobacco use has also been shown to increase an individual's chance of development of adenocarcinoma of the esophagus.[36-38] The risk of development of esophageal cancer increases with the number of packs of cigarettes smoked per day and the amount of alcohol consumed.

Barrett esophagus is a condition in which the distal esophagus is lined with a columnar epithelium rather than a stratified squamous epithelium. This mucosal change usually occurs with gastroesophageal (GE) reflux. One theory to explain this phenomenon is that chronic chemical trauma that results from reflux causes the mucosa to undergo metaplasia, leading to various degrees of dysplasia that are precancerous.[36-38] Adenocarcinoma of the esophagus occurs in patients with a history of Barrett esophagus. Longstanding GE reflux disease (GERD) is associated with the development of adenocarcinomas of the distal esophagus. Approximately 30% of esophageal cancers are associated with GERD.[36,41] Patients with GERD may or may not have development of Barrett esophagus.

Dietary factors have also been implicated in the development of cancer of the esophagus. Diets low in fresh fruits and vegetables and high in nitrates (i.e., cured meats and fish, pickled vegetables) have been cited as risk factors for persons from Iran, China, and South Africa. A diet high in fruits and vegetables is considered a preventive measure against the development of esophageal and other cancers. Overweight and obesity have been linked to the development of adenocarcinomas.[36,40,41]

Other conditions predispose individuals to the development of esophageal cancer. They include achalasia, Plummer-Vinson syndrome, caustic injury, and tylosis.

Achalasia is a disorder in which the lower two-thirds of the esophagus loses its normal peristaltic activity. The esophagus becomes dilated (termed *megaesophagus*), and the esophagogastric junction sphincter also fails to relax, which prohibits the passage of food into the stomach. Clinical symptoms include progressive dysphagia and regurgitation of ingested food. Patients with achalasia have a 5% to 20% risk of development of squamous cell cancer of the esophagus.[36]

Tylosis is a rare inherited disorder that causes excessive skin growth on the palms of the hands and soles of the feet. Individuals with this condition are at significant risk of about 40% of development of a squamous cell carcinoma. A mutation on chromosome 17 is thought to cause tylosis and the associated squamous cell carcinoma.[36]

Many believe that some risk factors, such as use of tobacco or alcohol abuse, cause esophageal cancer by damaging the DNA of cells that line the inside of the esophagus. The DNA of esophageal cancer cells microscopically often shows many abnormalities; however, no special changes have been described that are typical of this cancer. Long-term irritation of the lining of the esophagus, as with GERD, Barrett esophagus, achalasia, esophageal webs, or scarring from swallowing lye, can promote the formation of cancers.[36]

Prognostic Indicators

Tumor size is an important prognostic tool. According to a series by Hussey and colleagues,[39] patients with tumors less than 5 cm in length had a better 2-year survival rate (19.2%) than did patients with lesions larger than 9 cm (1.9%). Tumors 5 cm or less in length were more often localized (40% to 60%), whereas tumors larger than 5 cm had distant metastasis 75% of the time.[39] Other factors that indicate a poor prognosis are weight loss of 10%, a poor performance status, and age greater than 65 years.

Anatomy and Lymphatics

The esophagus is a thin-walled 25-cm-long tube lined with stratified squamous epithelium. The esophagus begins at the level of C6 and traverses through the thoracic cage to terminate in the abdomen at the esophageal gastric junction (T10 to T11).

For accurate classification, staging, and recording of tumors in the esophagus, the AJCC has divided the esophagus into three regions: upper thoracic, middle thoracic, and lower thoracic or GE junction. The staging system is also subdivided based on pathology: squamous cell carcinoma or adenocarcinoma. Because lesions are localized with an endoscopy, reference is made to the distance of the lesion from the upper incisors (front teeth). This distance is also used in defining each region (Fig. 31.10).[10]

The cervical esophagus extends from the cricoid cartilage to the thoracic inlet (suprasternal notch [SSN]), corresponding to vertebral levels C6 to T2 to T3 and measuring about 18 cm from the upper incisors. The thoracic inlet (SSN) to the level of the tracheal bifurcation (carina)—24 cm from the incisors—defines the upper thoracic portion. The middle thoracic esophagus begins at the carina and extends proximally to the esophageal gastric junction, or 32 cm from the incisors. The lower thoracic portion includes the abdominal esophagus and is approximately 8 cm long at a level of 40 cm from the incisors.[10]

The esophagus lies directly posterior to the trachea and is anterior to the vertebral column. Located laterally and to the left of the esophagus is the aortic arch. The descending aorta is situated lateral and posterior to the esophagus (see Fig. 31.10). During an endoscopy, an indentation is visible where the aorta and left mainstem bronchus are in contact with the esophagus. Because of the

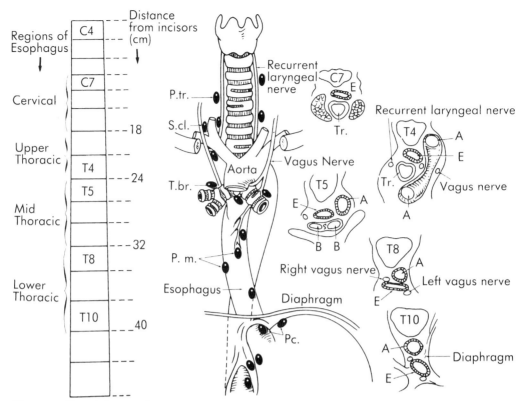

Fig. 31.10 The relationship of the esophagus with surrounding anatomic structures, including divisions of the esophagus and their location from the upper central incisors. (From Cox JD, Ang KK, eds. *Radiation Oncology: Rationale, Techniques, Results.* 9th ed. St. Louis, MO: Mosby; 2010.)

esophagus's intimate relationship with these structures, tumors are often locally advanced, fistulas may occur, and surgery is often not feasible.[34,39,40]

Histologically, the esophagus consists of the usual layers of the bowel common to the GI tract (i.e., the mucosa, submucosa, and muscular layers). However, the esophagus lacks a serosal layer. The outermost layer, the adventitia, consists of a thin, loose connective tissue. This is another factor that contributes to the early spread of these tumors to adjacent structures.[39]

The esophagus has numerous small lymphatic vessels in the mucosa and submucosal layers. These vessels drain outward into larger vessels located in the muscular layers (Fig. 31.11). Lymph fluid can travel the entire length of the esophagus and drain into any adjacent draining nodal bed, which places the entire esophagus at risk for skip metastasis and nodal involvement.

Although the entire length of the esophagus is at risk for lymphatic metastasis, each region still has primary or regional nodes that specifically drain the area. For example, the upper third (cervical area) of the esophagus drains into the internal jugular, cervical, paraesophageal, and supraclavicular lymph nodes. The upper and middle thoracic portion has drainage to the paratracheal, hilar, subcarinal, paraesophageal, and paracardial lymph nodes. Finally, the principal draining lymphatics for the distal or lower third of the esophagus include the celiac axis, left gastric nodes, and nodes of the lesser curvature of the stomach (Fig. 31.12). Lymphatic spread is unpredictable and may occur at a significant distance from the tumor. Nodes positive for tumor outside a defined region represent distant metastasis rather than regional spread. For example, supraclavicular nodal involvement in a primary tumor located in the cervical esophagus is considered regional lymph node involvement, but this is a distant metastasis for tumors that arise in the thoracic esophagus.[10]

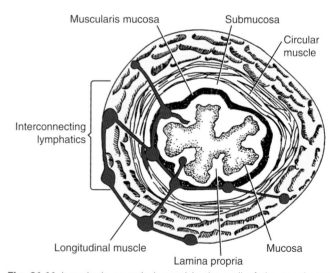

Fig. 31.11 Lymphatic vessels located in the wall of the esophagus. (From Cox JD, Ang KK, eds. *Radiation Oncology: Rationale, Techniques, Results.* 9th ed. St. Louis, MO: Mosby; 2010.)

Clinical Presentation

The most common presenting symptoms are dysphagia and weight loss, which occur in 90% of patients. Patients report food sticking in their throat or chest and may point to the location of this sensation. Initially, patients have difficulty with bulky foods, then with soft foods, and finally even with liquids. Patients may recall having this difficulty in swallowing for 3 to 6 months before the diagnosis. Regurgitation of undigested food and aspiration pneumonia may also occur. Odynophagia (painful swallowing) is reported in approximately 50% of

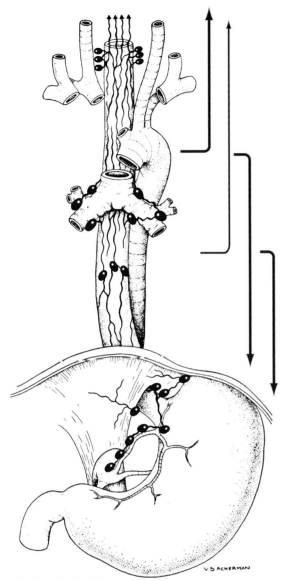

Fig. 31.12 Lymphatic drainage of the esophagus. The *arrows* represent potential spread to cervical, mediastinal, and subdiaphragmatic lymph nodes, based on the location of the esophageal lesion. Subdiaphragmatic involvement is unusual in the upper-third tumors. (From del Regato JA, Spjut HJ, Cox JD. *Ackerman and del Regato's Cancer: Diagnosis, Treatment, and Prognosis.* 6th ed. St Louis, MO: Mosby; 1985.)

patients. Patients may report pressure or a burning sensation similar to heartburn. Weight loss, as a result of the difficulty in swallowing food, is a common finding. Symptoms of a locally advanced tumor include the following: hematemesis (vomiting blood), coughing (caused by a tracheoesophageal fistula), hemoptysis, Horner syndrome, and hoarseness, as a result of nerve involvement.[34,39]

Detection and Diagnosis

A thorough history and physical examination should be performed. Information should be obtained regarding weight loss and the use of alcohol and tobacco. The physical examination should include palpation of the cervical and supraclavicular lymph nodes and abdomen for assessment of potential spread to the nodes or liver. A chest radiograph and barium swallow are necessary for localizing the lesions causing the dysphagia. A barium swallow depicts characteristic features of esophageal cancers. The reported incidence of tumors

located in each third of the esophagus varies in the literature. Lesions in the upper third of the esophagus occur with the least frequency. The most common site of occurrence in the United States is in the lower one-third of the esophagus and the GE junction. A CT scan of the chest and upper abdomen should be obtained. This scan may show extramucosal spread and invasion of adjacent structures such as the trachea or aorta. Spread to lymph nodes in the thorax and abdomen can be also assessed. Blood-borne metastases to the liver and adrenals may be imaged via CT scan, although small lesions may not be detectable.[34,36]

A histologic confirmation is obtained during an esophagoscopy. A rigid or flexible endoscope can be used to examine the entire esophagus, with brushings and biopsies of all suspicious lesions obtained. **EUS** is also helpful for visualizing the tumor, its depth of invasion, and lymph node status.[40] A bronchoscopy should also be performed for all upper-third or middle-third lesions to detect any possible communication or fistula of the tumor with the tracheobronchial tree.[10,34,39]

The PET scan has become a standard test for the staging workup of patients with esophageal cancer. Fluorodeoxyglucose (FDG), a sugar, is taken up by cancer cells because of their high mitotic activity. Recent studies have shown the effectiveness of PET in the staging of esophageal cancer. A PET scan demonstrates involvement of lymph nodes and liver, as well as the primary tumor. Metastatic disease was detected in 15% to 20% of patients with PET after the original workup with endoscopy and CT scan.[41]

Pathology and Staging

The most common pathologic types of esophageal cancer are squamous cell carcinoma and adenocarcinoma. Squamous cell carcinomas are found most frequently in the upper and middle thoracic esophagus.[34] Adenocarcinoma typically occurs in the distal esophagus and GE junction; however, it can occur in other regions of the esophagus. In the United States, the most common pathologic type and site that occurs is adenocarcinomas of the distal esophagus and GE junction.[37,41,42] A variety of other epithelial tumors arise in the esophagus but are rare. These include adenoid cystic carcinoma, mucoepidermoid carcinoma, adenosquamous carcinoma, and undifferentiated carcinoma.[39,40]

Nonepithelial tumors also arise in the esophagus, although these are rare. Leiomyosarcoma (a tumor of the smooth muscle) is the most common nonepithelial tumor. Leiomyosarcomas yield a more favorable prognosis than do squamous cell carcinomas. Malignant melanoma, lymphoma, and rhabdomyosarcoma are other nonepithelial tumors that can occur in the esophagus.[39]

The tumor specimen may be examined for a specific gene or protein called *HER2*. Some patients with cancer of the esophagus have an excess of this protein on the surface of the cancer cells. This protein allows the cancer cells to grow. In addition, if the *HER2/neu* oncogene is overexpressed in adenocarcinoma of the esophagus, the disease may carry a poorer prognosis. Patients whose cancer is found to have excess *HER2* may benefit from targeted therapy with a monoclonal antibody called trastuzumab.[34]

The AJCC staging system for esophageal cancer is available more information about staging esophageal cancer. See: https://www.cancer.org/cancer/esophagus-cancer/detection-diagnosis-staging/staging.html

Squamous cell carcinoma and adenocarcinoma of the esophagus have separate staging systems. The staging for squamous cell carcinoma includes tumor location relative to the pulmonary vein and histologic grade. The staging for adenocarcinoma of the esophagus includes tumor grade but does not include location.[10]

Routes of Spread

Because the esophagus is distensible, lesions are large before they cause obstructive symptoms. Spread is usually longitudinal. Occasionally, skip lesions may be present at a significant distance from the primary lesion. This is principally the result of submucosal spread of the tumor through interconnecting lymph channels. Locally advanced disease, invasion into adjacent structures, and early spread to draining lymphatics are common in esophageal cancer. Because the esophagus lacks a serosa layer, tracheoesophageal fistulas or bronchoesophageal fistulas may easily occur.[34] Distant metastasis can occur in many different organs, with the liver and lung being the most common.

Treatment Techniques

The treatment of esophageal cancer is highly complex and technically difficult. Most patients have locally advanced or metastatic disease at the time of diagnosis and need multimodality treatment. Treatment is usually categorized as curative or palliative and may be given with surgery or radiation for the locoregional problem and chemotherapy for distant spread of disease. Patients who receive either modality (surgery or radiation) alone have a significant risk of local recurrence and distant metastasis. The primary goal of either treatment is to provide relief of the dysphagia and a chance for cure. Many different combined modality treatment regimens are being studied to determine whether one approach provides a better local control and survival outcome than others. The two most commonly used combined modality techniques are definitive chemoradiation therapy and neoadjuvant chemoradiotherapy followed by surgery.[26,43,44] Definitive chemoradiation therapy has been the current nonsurgical standard for the treatment of esophageal cancer. Current studies are evaluating preoperative chemoradiotherapy with different chemotherapeutic agents and definitive chemoradiotherapy for locoregional cancers of the esophagus. Current studies are being done to review biomarkers on DNA repair protein that might predict a patient's response to chemotherapy or radiation.[39]

A variety of surgical techniques exist for the resection of esophageal cancer. In many centers, surgical resection is limited to the middle and lower thirds of the esophagus. The cervical esophagus is not considered a surgically accessible site in many institutions and is often managed with radiation therapy and chemotherapy. Curative surgery usually involves a subtotal or total esophagectomy. The type of procedure chosen depends on the location of the lesion and extent of involvement. Typically, the entire esophagus is removed. The continuity of the GI system is maintained by placing either the stomach or left colon in the thoracic cavity. Complications from surgery include anastomotic leaks (which can be life-threatening), respiratory failure, pulmonary embolus, and myocardial infarctions. Strictures, difficulty in gastric emptying, and GE reflux are mechanical side effects that result from surgery. Even after a curative resection, most patients have distant failure with blood-borne spread to the lungs, liver, or bone.

Radiation Therapy. Neoadjuvant chemoradiation followed by curative surgery remains the treatment standard.[45–47] Radiation therapy with chemotherapy is considered the current nonsurgical treatment of choice for esophageal cancer. Studies have showed a clear advantage for radiation therapy and chemotherapy compared with radiation therapy alone.[34,39,40] Radiation therapy alone might be used in patients who are medically unable to undergo combined modality treatment.

Chemotherapy. The poor survival rates of esophageal cancer are associated with the high percentage of patients with local failure and with distant metastases after curative treatment. The addition of combination chemotherapy has resulted in a decrease in local and distant failures and an increase in the overall survival rate compared with radiation alone (Figs. 31.13 and 31.14).[34,39,40,48]

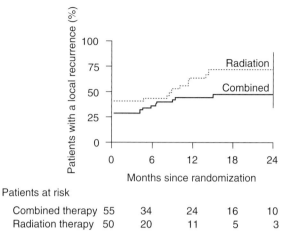

Fig. 31.13 A comparison of radiation alone with combined radiation and chemotherapy regarding the time to a local recurrence in patients with esophageal cancer. (From Herskovic A, Martz K, al-Sarraf M, et al. Combined chemotherapy and radiotherapy compared with radiotherapy alone in patients with cancer of the esophagus. *N Engl J Med.* 1992;326:1596.)

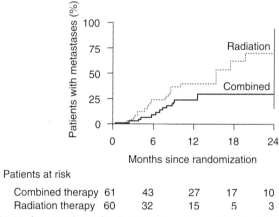

Fig. 31.14 A comparison of radiation alone with combined radiation and chemotherapy regarding the time to a distant metastasis in patients with esophageal cancer. (Modified from Herskovic A, Martz K, al-Sarraf M, et al. Combined chemotherapy and radiotherapy compared with radiotherapy alone in patients with cancer of the esophagus. *N Engl J Med.* 1992;326:1595.)

Carboplatin and paclitaxel have replaced continuous-infusion 5-FU and cisplatin as the standard drugs used in the treatment of esophageal cancer. These two drugs have less toxicity and are better tolerated by the patient than 5-FU and cisplatin. Combined-modality therapy has definite local control and survival benefits. Many drug combinations are being studied and are in use.[47]

Field Design and Critical Structures. Esophageal cancer spreads longitudinally, with skip lesions up to 5 cm from the primary lesion. Regional spread to draining lymphatics is a common early presentation and must be taken into consideration in the design of the radiation field. The cervical, supraclavicular, mediastinal, paraesophageal, and subdiaphragmatic (celiac axis) lymph node regions are at risk. The degree to which these nodal groups are at risk depends on the location of the primary tumor. Supraclavicular nodes are involved more often with a proximal lesion than a distal lesion. However, neck or abdominal nodal disease involvement can occur with any esophageal primary site.[34,39,40]

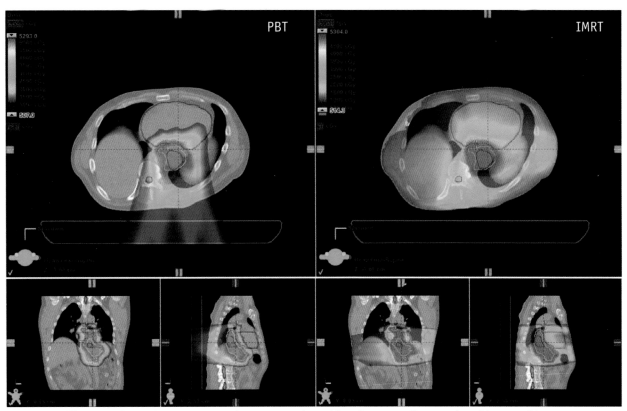

Fig. 31.15 Proton beam treatment for gastroesophageal junction tumor. Note sparing of heart and lungs. (From Chuong, MD, Hallemeier, CL, Jabbour, SK, et al. Improving outcomes for esophageal cancer using proton beam therapy. *Int J Radiation Oncol Bio Phys.* 2016;95[1]:488–497.)

The clinical treatment volume includes the regional lymphatics and encompasses the primary tumor with a 3-cm to 4-cm margin above and below the gross tumor volume and a 1-cm radial margin.[34] The margin on the lymph nodes should be expanded 0.5 to 1.5 cm from the gross tumor volume. The planning target volume is also expanded an additional 0.5 to 1 cm for radial or lateral margins.[34,47] Lesions of the upper third of the esophagus are treated with a field that begins at the level of the thyroid cartilage and ends at the level of the carina to include supraclavicular, low anterior cervical, and mediastinal lymph nodes.[34] In patients with tumors of the distal third of the esophagus, the inferior margin must include the celiac axis lymph nodes, which are located at the T12 to L1 vertebral level. The superior extent of the treatment field should include the paraesophageal nodes and mediastinal nodes and may not include the supraclavicular nodes because they are at a low risk of being involved.[34,39,40] For tumors of the midthoracic esophagus, the anatomic borders included in the treatment field include the periesophageal lymph nodes and mediastinal nodes but may not include the supraclavicular fossa or the esophagogastric junction.[34,48]

A variety of radiation techniques are used in the treatment of esophageal cancer. This includes 3D conformal fields (AP/PA, laterals, or obliques), IMRT fields, and VMAT. The technique chosen is dependent on the location of the esophageal cancer, proximal versus distal, and which technique minimizes the dose to OARs. Many critical structures need to be considered, such as the lung, heart, spinal cord, kidneys, and liver. Many studies have been done to determine which technique provides adequate coverage of the target volume with minimal dose to healthy tissues. IMRT and VMAT result in radiation dose distributions that are highly conformal to the target volume and have shown better sparing of healthy tissues, such as lung, heart, and spinal cord than 3D conformal fields.[39,49–55]

The use of proton beam therapy for the treatment of esophageal cancer is also being evaluated. The characteristic properties of a proton beam result in no exit dose, thus sparing the anatomic structures beyond the target. The use of intensity-modulated proton therapy (IMPT) or pencil beam scanning paints the dose to the target level resulting in a highly conformal dose distribution. Preliminary studies show that proton therapy significantly reduces the dose to the lung, heart, liver, and spinal cord more than traditional IMRT with photons or 3D conformal techniques.[15,45,51,52] Treatment field arrangements that have been used include two posterior oblique fields or AP and two posterior oblique fields, which allows sparing of anterior structures such as the heart and lungs[14,21] (see Fig. 31.15).

For treatment of the esophagus with radiation alone, the prescribed dose is 60 to 65 Gy. With preoperative combined radiation and chemotherapy, the total dose is 41.4 to 50.4 Gy to minimize healthy tissue toxicity. The dose for definitive chemoradiation is 50 to 50.4 cGy.[50] Both of these doses exceed the radiation tolerance dose of the spinal cord, which is 45 to 50 Gy. Careful dosimetry planning for VMAT or static IMRT is necessary to ensure the dose constraints for lung, heart, spinal cord, kidney, and liver doses are met.

Patients are typically placed in the standard supine position for simulation. Because lateral treatment field arrangements or rotational arcs may be used, the patient's arms are often positioned above the head, with the patient clasping the elbows or wrists. This position can be difficult for the patient to hold and maintain, which can cause reproducibility problems later during treatment. Custom-made immobilization devices such as body casts, foaming cradles, and vacuum bag devices greatly assist the daily reproducibility of the setup. Care should be taken when making the immobilization device to ensure it fits within the bore of the CT scanner. With or without a custom-made device, measurements of the elbow-to-elbow separation and a photograph of the patient arm position assist in the consistency of the daily setup.

For the simulation of patients with their arms along their sides for cancers of the upper esophagus, the elbows should be bent slightly out from the body so that a set of marks can be placed on the thoracic cage for a three-point setup. The arms are mobile and are not reliable for positioning and maintaining the established isocenter daily. A thermoplastic mask that fits over the shoulders may be used to maintain shoulder and head position. Marks may be placed on midline at the inferior field edge of patient in addition to the isocenter mark for alignment and straightening purposes. A set of three reference points are placed lower on the thoracic cage and are used to establish the isocenter. The AP source-skin distance, or setup distance, is double-checked and maintained, especially with oblique treatment fields.

A liquid or pudding-type contrast may be given at the time of the CT simulation to visualize the esophagus. Patients with severe dysphagia may not tolerate this, especially in the supine position. Oral contrast may not be used at all for simulation or treatment to maintain consistency in daily treatment setup. The patient is instructed not to eat 2 to 3 hours before the simulation or for treatment. Intravenous contrast may be used to assist in definition of target volume for treatment. The simulation may also include a four-dimensional (4D) CT scan to assess the amount of respiratory motion that occurs and how this affects internal target volumes. Margins for clinical treatment volumes may need to be adjusted based on the 4D CT data. Respiratory gating may be beneficial for the treatment of some patients.[45,42,49,47]

The radiation therapist ensures that the patient is straight and places reference marks on the thoracic cage and radiopaque markers on these marks for visualization on the scan. The coordinates of these reference marks, pilot, or scout length may be recorded. A scan from above the mandible to the iliac crest to include the entire esophagus and stomach may be obtained. After the scan, the physician digitizes in different colors the target volume and critical anatomy as listed previously. The treatment isocenter also is identified. After the CT scan, the physician determines the treatment isocenter while the patient is still on the CT couch. Images are reviewed by the physician, and the treatment isocenter is determined based on the areas contoured on the CT images. The isocenter coordinates are then programmed into the movable lasers in the scanner room, and the patient is marked accordingly. The patient then goes home with marks that will actually be used for treatment delivery. Patient setup information, such as positioning and immobilization devices, is recorded at the time of simulation. Field size parameters and gantry or couch angles are recorded once treatment planning is complete. Axial (transverse) and sagittal treatment planning images are seen in Fig. 31.16, which represent the dose distribution for a patient with a distal esophageal tumor.

Side Effects

After 2 weeks of radiation treatment, patients begin to experience esophagitis. They report substernal pain during swallowing and the sensation of food sticking in their esophagus. Patients may be unable to eat solid foods and may need a diet of bland, soft, or pureed foods. In addition, patients should eat small, frequent meals that are high in calories and protein (Table 31.2). High-calorie liquid supplements such as Carnation Instant Breakfast and Ensure are good alternatives for a high-calorie snack during the day or at bedtime.

To ease the pain of swallowing, the physician may suggest that the patient take liquid analgesics or viscous lidocaine before meals. These drugs provide local and systemic pain relief. Esophagitis can become severe by the end of the treatment and may even necessitate the placement of a nasogastric tube.

Concomitant chemotherapy increases the sensitivity of the esophageal mucosa to radiation. Therefore more severe esophagitis and possibly ulceration may occur. The radiation tolerance of the esophagus is 65 Gy delivered with 1.8-Gy to 2.0-Gy fractions. When concurrent chemotherapy is administered, the total radiation dose safely delivered is 50

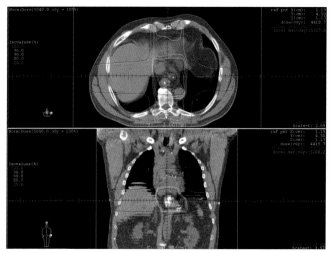

Fig. 31.16 Three-dimensional treatment planning for a patient with distal gastroesophageal junction cancer. Axial and sagittal representations illustrate the dose distribution. (From Blackstock AW, Russo S. Cancer of the esophagus. In: Gunderson L, Tepper JE, eds. *Clinical Oncology.* 4th ed. Philadelphia, PA: Elsevier; 2016.)

TABLE 31.2 Dietary Guidelines for Patients Receiving Thoracic Irradiation	
Recommended Foods	**Foods to Avoid**
Cottage cheese, yogurt, and milkshakes	Hot and spicy foods
Puddings	Dry to coarse foods
Smoothies	Crackers, nuts, and potato
Casseroles	chips
Skinless poultry	Raw vegetables, citrus fruits,
Scrambled eggs	and juices
Meats and vegetables in sauces or gravies	Alcoholic beverages
Low-fat tofu	Tobacco
	Acidic foods

Gy, based on the increased treatment-related toxicities associated with combined-modality treatment. Decreased blood counts, nausea, and vomiting also occur with chemotherapy. A break in a patient's treatment may be necessary if the leukocyte or platelet count becomes too low.

Radiation pneumonitis or pericarditis may occur if a large volume of lung or heart is in the radiation field. Proper field shaping and careful treatment planning greatly reduce the likelihood of severe complications. Perforation and fistula formation can result from rapid shrinkage of a tumor that was adherent to the esophageal-tracheal wall.

Long-term side effects from irradiation of the esophagus include stenosis or stricture as a result of scar formation. Dilations of the esophagus can be performed to relieve the obstructive symptoms and restore the patient's ability to swallow. Transverse myelitis is a late complication that should not occur if the radiation treatments are delivered and planned precisely and accurately.

Recall the dose limits of radiation for the lung, heart, and spinal cord. What is the healthy tissue toxicity for each of these OARs? Which of the three organs is most sensitive to radiation damage? Careful planning with IMRT or VMAT may help reduce the dose to OARs.

Role of the Radiation Therapist

Patients who undergo radiation therapy for esophageal cancer need a lot of supportive care. They usually experience substantial weight loss as a result of the tumor's obstructive process and are nutritionally compromised. Esophagitis, as a result of the treatment, can cause more weight loss and further debilitate the health of the patient. The therapist should question patients about the way they are feeling, their appetite, and their food intake. Dietary suggestions regarding recommended foods or those to avoid should be made available to the patient. Some radiation therapy centers have printed sheets for the therapist or nurse to give to the patient. Many centers also have a dietitian to whom the patient may be referred for meal planning and dietary supplements.

Esophagitis can be emotionally and physically draining for these patients. The therapist should try to monitor the patient's emotional well-being as much as the physical aspects. The therapist should inform the patient about local cancer support groups that assist in coping with side effects of radiation treatments and disease.

Case IV: Midesophagus

A 64-year-old man presented to his local physician with a 1-month history of dysphagia and painful swallowing. This was especially noticeable when eating hot foods and foods with a scratchy texture such as chips or crackers. The patient had an upper GI barium swallow study that revealed a midesophageal lesion that was several centimeters in length and extended 30 to 34 cm from the incisors. The lesion did not appear to be completely circumferential. Biopsies of the lesion were taken and found to be poorly differentiated high grade invasive squamous cell carcinoma.

A PET-CT scan was done to assist in the staging workup. The PET scan showed increased FDG uptake in the known area of the lesion and in a right azygous lymph node. No other sites of distant metastasis were noted. An EUS of the esophagus was discussed but not ordered because the outcome would not change the plan for treatment. The patient was at stage IIB T2 N1 M0 of the middle third of the esophagus. The thoracic surgery team saw the patient and believed he was not a surgical candidate based on the patient's poor performance on recent pulmonary function tests and his history of chronic obstructive pulmonary disease and cardiac issues. The patient was then seen for definitive chemoradiation therapy. The patient was to receive carboplatin and paclitaxel administered on a weekly basis as a radiation sensitizer. Radiation consisted of a total dose of 5040 cGy delivered in 28 fractions. The initial larger treatment fields were treated to 4500 cGy in 25 fractions with a four-field technique (anterior, posterior, right, and left laterals) with IMRT static fields. A shrinking field boost for an additional three treatments with the same beam arrangement and IMRT technique brought the total dose to 5040 cGy.

Case V: Lower Third of Esophagus

A healthy 75 year old man presented with an increase in reflux symptoms with central chest burning and bitterness in his mouth which he had experienced over the last year. Over the last 2 months, he began to have a sensation of solid food sticking at the level of the lower aspect of the sternum. He did not take any regular medications for this. At times, this would lead to spontaneous regurgitation. His weight has fallen approximately 6 pounds. He was seen by a local endoscopist who proceeded with an esophagogastroduodenoscopy (EGD) revealing a medium-size hiatal hernia and a nodular mass at the level of the GE junctions. Biopsies of the area revealed adenocarcinoma. The patient denies any chest of other abdominal symptoms. He denies any pain. The patient is a nonsmoker and drinks alcoholic beverages very minimally.

The patient underwent a staging workup that included CT of the chest, abdomen, and pelvis to check for metastatic spread. Pending the results of the CT scan, the patient will have a PET scan to further check for spread of the disease regionally and distantly. If no metastatic spread is noted, an EGD, an endoscopic ultrasound, will be completed to locally stage the tumor.

The CT of the chest, abdomen, and pelvis showed a moderate esophageal hiatal hernia with irregular mural thickening at the GE junction at the region of the known biopsy-proven cancer. The scan also showed a mildly enlarged distal right paraesophageal lymph node, suspicious for metastasis. In addition, there were opacities in the right lung that may be infectious or inflammatory in nature. There is evidence of diffuse, mild cylindrical bronchiectasis in the lower lungs, which may be secondary to recurrent microaspiration. There was no evidence of hepatic metastasis or abdominal or pelvic lymphadenopathy. A PET scan was then obtained. The PET demonstrated uptake at the site of the GE cancer and in the right paraesophageal metastatic lymph node.

Next, the patient underwent an EGD and EUS. The malignancy was found 41 cm from the incisors. The endoscope was able to get past the stenosis, and on EUS, the mass was found spanning from 39 to 41 cm from the incisors. Suspicious subcarinal nodes were identified in the mediastinum. A fine-needle aspiration (FNA) was done and came back positive for malignancy. The patient was staged as a T3 N1 M 0 stage III.

Based on the findings, the patient was referred to radiation oncology and medical oncology to discuss treatment options. The treatment recommendation is for trimodality therapy consisting of neoadjuvant (preoperative) chemoradiation followed by surgery. An Ivor Lewis esophagectomy was planned following completion of the chemoradiation therapy.

The patient was unable to receive the usual chemotherapy regimen of carboplatin and paclitaxel because of an elevated bilirubin. Instead he was prescribed FOLFOX (5-FU, oxaliplatin, leucovorin) every 2 weeks for 3 cycles. The side effects from this course of chemotherapy was discussed with the patient. This includes fatigue, cytopenia, diarrhea, nausea, vomiting, mouth sores, rash joint pain, and hair thinning. Radiation would be delivered concurrently with the chemotherapy.

Treatment with proton therapy was recommended with a dose of 5000 cGy prescribed to the gross disease plus margin and 4500 cGy to elective nodes and esophageal margin. The treatment field arrangement consists of two posterior oblique fields delivered with IMPT. The patient was instructed to eat nothing through the mouth (NPO) 2 hours before treatment to ensure an empty stomach. A light snack such as toast or crackers may be consumed, but no heavy or large meals. Liquid intake should be limited to less than 3 oz of noncarbonated beverage. Side effects, including fatigue, nausea, esophagitis, and radiation dermatitis, were discussed with the patient.

PANCREATIC CANCER

Epidemiology and Etiology

Cancers of the pancreas account for approximately 2% of all cancers diagnosed annually in the United States. Each year, the ACS estimates that about 56,770 new cases of pancreatic cancer will occur. The incidence rate of pancreatic cancer has been increasing for the past 10 years.[5,43] Pancreatic cancer is the fourth leading cause of cancer-related deaths in the United States, with an estimated 45,750 deaths expected to occur each year.[1,5,43,53] Pancreatic cancer has a high mortality rate and is considered one of the deadliest malignancies. It occurs more commonly

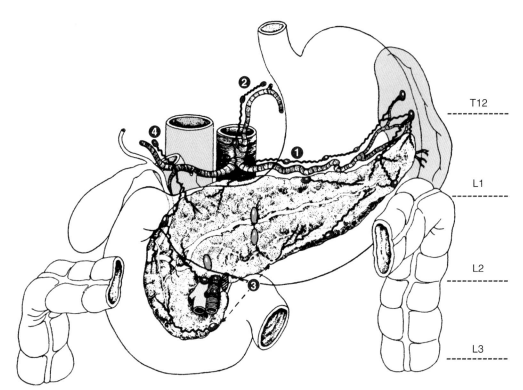

Fig. 31.17 Anatomy and lymphatic drainage of the pancreas. Note the intimate relationship of the pancreas with the duodenum, stomach, transverse colon, spleen, and common bile duct. The four main trunks of lymphatic drainage: *1,* Left side drains along the tail into splenic hilar nodes; *2,* superior pancreatic lymph nodes and the celiac axis; *3,* inferior pancreatic, mesenteric, and left paraaortic nodes; *4,* right-side drainage to anterior and posterior pancreaticoduodenal nodes and right paraaortic nodes. (From del Regato JA, Spjut HJ, Cox JD. *Ackerman and del Regato's Cancer: Diagnosis, Treatment, and Prognosis.* 6th ed. St. Louis, MO: Mosby; 1985.)

in men than in women, with incidence and mortality rates greater in black persons than in white persons. The disease rarely occurs in persons younger than 45 years, with most patients in the 50- to 80-year age group.

No known cause exists for the development of pancreatic cancer, although smokers have a two times higher risk of development of pancreatic cancer.[1] Cigarette smoking is thought to cause about 20% of pancreatic cancers.[5,43,53] Lynch syndrome H, familial breast cancer associated with the *BRCA2* mutation, *p16* gene mutations in familial pancreatic cancer, and hereditary pancreatitis have been implicated as risk factors for the development of pancreatic cancer.[43,53] Exposure to industrial chemicals such as benzidine and beta-naphthylamine over an extended period is related to an increased incidence of pancreatic cancer. Obesity, lack of physical activity, and diets high in fats, red meat, and processed meat (bacon, sausage) are thought to increase one's risk of development of pancreatic cancer. Conversely, diets high in vegetables and fruits lower one's risk for pancreas cancer. More studies are being conducted to determine whether a high-fat diet does indeed cause pancreatic cancer. Pancreatic cancer is also more common in people with type 2 (adult-onset) diabetes.[1,53]

Anatomy and Lymphatics

The pancreas is located retroperitoneally at the T12 to L2 level and lies transversely in the upper abdomen. The pancreas is divided into three anatomic regions: the head, body, and tail. The head of the pancreas is located in the C-loop of the duodenum. The body lies just posterior to the stomach near the midline and is anterior to the IVC. Extending laterally to the left, the tail terminates in the splenic hilum. The pancreas is in direct contact with the duodenum, jejunum, stomach, major vessels (IVC), spleen, and

kidney. Tumors of the pancreas commonly invade these structures and are therefore usually unresectable at the time of diagnosis.

Numerous lymph node channels drain the pancreas and its surrounding structures. The main lymph node groups include the superior and inferior pancreaticoduodenal nodes, porta hepatis, suprapancreatic nodes, and paraaortic nodes. Tumors that arise in the tail of the pancreas drain to the splenic hilar nodes (Fig. 31.17). Most patients have advanced local or metastatic disease at the time of diagnosis.[6]

Clinical Presentation

The four most common presenting symptoms of pancreatic cancer are jaundice, abdominal pain, anorexia, and weight loss. Tumors that arise in the head of the pancreas may obstruct the biliary system and result in jaundice. An obstruction of the biliary system results in excess bilirubin to be excreted in urine and less bilirubin to enter the bowel, which results in dark urine and light-colored stools. Patients who are jaundiced also report pruritus or itching.[1] Tumors that occur in the body or tail of the pancreas are not associated with obstruction of the biliary system and commonly involve severe back pain and weight loss. Pancreatic cancers occur most frequently in the head and neck of the pancreas.[53]

Detection and Diagnosis

A thorough history and physical examination are extremely important. The abdomen should be assessed for palpable masses. The tumor's obstruction of the biliary system can result in an enlarged pancreas, gallbladder, or liver. Palpable supraclavicular nodes or rectal masses discovered during a digital rectal examination indicate peritoneal spread. All of these signs suggest an advanced stage disease. The presence or absence of jaundice is assessed by paying particular attention to the sclera, skin, and oral cavity mucosa.[53]

The most valuable and important diagnostic test is a CT scan of the abdomen. This scan provides a complete view of the abdominal structures most likely involved with the tumor. This image localizes the mass in the pancreas and depicts whether it is a head, body, or tail primary. The scan also shows whether the tumor has invaded surrounding structures, such as the duodenum, superior mesenteric vessels, or celiac axis vessels. Spread to the regional lymph nodes, peritoneal implants, and distant metastasis to the liver can also be assessed.

The resectability of the tumor can be determined with the information found on the CT scan. Liver metastasis and the involvement of the superior mesenteric artery or other major vessels are two contraindications to surgery. A CT-guided fine-needle biopsy of the primary tumor or metastatic lesions may be performed to establish the diagnosis.

MRI may also be used to evaluate local extension of the tumor into adjacent structures. The MRI may provide better soft tissue delineation than CT scan and can provide information related to respectability of pancreatic tumor.[53,54]

A PET scan is an additional test that may be done. PET scans are useful for showing spread of the cancer outside of the pancreas to lymph nodes or liver or into adjacent tissues. This information is used in conjunction with the CT scan findings.[8,53-55]

Endoscopic retrograde cholangiopancreatography (ERCP) is used in evaluation of the obstruction and potential involvement of the biliary system. A biopsy of the ampulla or duodenum may be obtained at the time of the ERCP. This procedure is even more beneficial for the diagnosis of a primary tumor of the biliary system. Ultrasound scan has also been used to assess ductal obstruction, blood vessel invasion, and liver metastasis.

With EUS, a transducer is passed down the esophagus to the duodenum adjacent to the pancreas. This examination is more useful than CT scan for visualization of small lesions in the head of the pancreas and evaluation of the potential involvement of lymph nodes and vasculature.[8] EUS, along with FNA, is used as a tool to obtain tissue for diagnosis with less chance of tumor seeding as compared with a percutaneous approach.

A laparoscopy to obtain a biopsy is commonly performed before any surgical intervention and may rule out small liver metastases (1 to 2 mm) that were undetectable on a CT scan.[53] A laparoscopic procedure does not require a big incision and is much easier on the patient.[53] According to a study done by Warshaw and colleagues,[56] laparotomy results indicated that 40% of patients had small metastases in the liver or on parietal peritoneal surfaces. These patients were spared the morbidity of unnecessary abdominal surgery. If the patient's tumor appears to be resectable, based on the diagnostic workup, exploratory surgery and a biopsy are performed to determine the histology of the pancreatic mass.

Carbohydrate antigen-19 (CA-19) or serum carbohydrate antigen is a tumor marker that is often elevated in pancreatic cancer. It is not considered effective as a screening tool because it can be elevated in other cancers, such as ovarian, GI, and hepatocellular carcinoma, and inflammatory conditions of the pancreas or liver. A blood value is obtained before and after surgery. If the CA-19 level remains elevated after treatment, residual disease or metastasis is present.

Pathology and Staging

Adenocarcinomas comprise 80% of pancreatic cancers. Other histologic types include islet cell tumors, acinar cell carcinomas, and cystadenocarcinomas.[5,33]

A formal TNM staging system for pancreatic cancer is available at https://www.cancer.org/cancer/pancreatic-cancer/detection-diagnosis-staging/staging.html.

Cases with disease confined to the pancreas, T1 to T3, are generally considered resectable.[43] More than 50% of patients who are

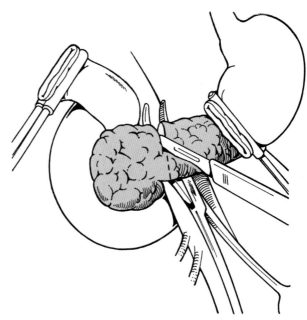

Fig. 31.18 Pancreaticoduodenectomy (Whipple procedure); resection of the head of the pancreas, duodenum, distal stomach, gallbladder, and common bile duct. (From Beazley RM, Cohn I Jr: Tumors of the pancreas, gallbladder, and extrahepatic ducts. In Murphy G, Lawrence W, Lenhard R, ed: American Cancer Society textbook of clinical oncology, Atlanta, 1995, American Cancer Society.)

diagnosed with pancreatic cancer have distant metastasis at the time of diagnosis.[8,53,54]

Routes of Spread

Cancers of the pancreas are locally invasive. Lymph node involvement or direct extension into the duodenum, common bile duct, stomach, and colon is not uncommon at the time of diagnosis. The tumor often encases or invades the superior mesenteric artery, portal vein, and celiac axis artery, rendering the tumor unresectable. Hematogenous spread to the liver via the portal vein is another common pathway of spread.

Treatment Techniques

Surgery is the treatment of choice. Most tumors, however, are unresectable. Pancreas tumors are categorized into resectable, borderline resectable, or locally advanced unresectable based on the extent of disease and likelihood of resectability. Borderline resectable means the cancer is localized but the tumor abuts major vessels in the abdomen such as the superior mesenteric vein (SMV) or portal vein, making it difficult to resect the tumor and have negative margins. Locally advanced pancreatic cancer that is unresectable is when the tumor mass encases the major abdominal vessels such as the SMV, portal vein, or the superior mesenteric artery and surgery is not recommended.[48, 82] Contraindications for a curative surgical procedure are liver metastasis, extrapancreatic serosal implantation, and invasion or encasement of major vessels.[55,57]

The most common potentially curative surgical procedure is a pancreaticoduodenectomy (Whipple procedure), which involves a resection of the head of the pancreas, entire duodenum, distal stomach, gallbladder, and common bile duct (Fig. 31.18). Reconstruction is done to maintain the continuity of the biliary-GI system. The remaining pancreas, bile ducts, and stomach are anastomosed onto various sites of the jejunum (Fig. 31.19). The operative mortality rate from this procedure has greatly improved in recent years; it has been as high as 30%, but it is now less than 5%. The surgeon should place clips to outline

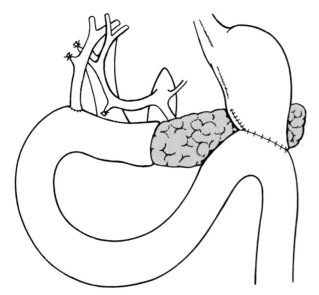

Fig. 31.19 Reconstruction of the biliary and gastrointestinal system. The remaining pancreas, stomach, and bile ducts are anastomosed to the jejunum. (From Beazley RM, Cohn I Jr: Tumors of the pancreas, gallbladder, and extrahepatic ducts. In Murphy G, Lawrence W, Lenhard R, ed: American Cancer Society textbook of clinical oncology, Atlanta, 1995, American Cancer Society.)

the extent of the tumor to assist the radiation oncologist in planning adjuvant radiation therapy fields.[53]

Because pancreatic cancers are often locally advanced at the time of diagnosis, neoadjuvant chemotherapy with or without radiation is considered standard of care. Induction chemotherapy plus chemoradiation therapy has been effective in downstaging the tumor and making resection possible in borderline resectable or locally advanced-unresectable pancreatic cancer.[54,57] Palliative biliary bypass procedures are often performed for unresectable tumors to redirect the flow of bile from obstructed ducts back into the GI system. Typically, this is done by anastomosing the uninvolved bile ducts into the jejunum. Resolving the obstruction provides patients with relief of jaundice.

The two general types of surgery used to treat cancer of the pancreas are as follows[8]:

- Potentially curative surgery is used when imaging tests suggest that removal of all the cancer is possible.
- Palliative surgery may be done if imaging tests show that the tumor is too widespread to be completely removed. This is done to relieve symptoms or to prevent certain complications such as blockage of the bile ducts or the intestine by the cancer.

Pancreatic cancer surgery is one of the most difficult operations a surgeon can do. It is also one of hardest for patients to undergo. Multiple complications may occur, and several weeks may be necessary for patients to recover.

Radiation Therapy. Because of the high rate of distant metastasis and locoregional failure rate after surgery alone, combined-modality therapy versus observation was investigated in a randomized trial of patients with resected tumors. Adjuvant combined-modality treatment after surgery resulted in a significant improvement in the overall survival rate of 18 to 29 months compared with no further treatment.

Radiation therapy and chemotherapy are considered the preferred treatments for borderline resectable, and locally advanced, unresectable pancreatic cancers. Studies that compared radiation alone with radiation and chemotherapy alone have shown that the combined-modality treatment provides modestly improved survival rates.[5,58,59]

Chemotherapy. As mentioned, chemotherapy is used with radiation therapy as an adjuvant treatment in resected pancreatic tumors and as

TABLE 31.3	Approximate Tissue Tolerance Dose for Specific Dose Limiting Structures Related to the Treatment of Pancreatic Cancer	
Kidneys	1500–1800 cGy
Liver	3000–3200 cGy
Small bowel	4500 cGy
Spinal cord	5000 cGy
Stomach	4500 cGy

QUANTEC, Quantitative Analysis of Normal Tissue Effects in the Clinic. Modified from Marks LB, Yorke ED, Jackson A, et al. Use of normal tissue complication probability models in the clinic. *Int J Radiat Oncol Biol Phys.* 2010;76(3):S10–S19; and from Emami B, Lyman J, Brown A, et al. Tolerance of normal tissue to therapeutic irradiation. *Int J Radiat Oncol Biol Phys.* 1991;21:109–122.

neoadjuvant treatment with or without radiation for borderline resectable and locally advanced unresectable disease.[54,55,57] Gemcitabine is the most common drug used in the treatment of pancreatic cancer and was found to result in better survival rates than with 5-FU.[60] Different drug combinations and sequences are being investigated for improving survival rates. Gemcitabine has been paired with various drugs such as capecitabine, paclitaxel or oxaliplatin to see if these combinations results in better survival.[57] FOLFIRINOX, a four-drug regimen consisting of leucovorin, 5-FU, irinotecan, and oxaliplatin, is another drug combination being explored for borderline resectable or locally advanced pancreatic cancer.[54,57] More research is needed to determine what drugs and in what combinations provide the best outcome for patients with pancreatic cancer.[54,55,57] Even with combined-modality treatment, the overall survival rate of patients with pancreatic cancer is extremely poor.

Field Design and Critical Structures. The primary tumor bed and draining lymphatics, as defined by surgical clips in the adjuvant setting or on CT scan in the neoadjuvant setting, are the key target volumes. The typical treatment field arrangement used is VMAT with two to three full 360-degree arcs. IMRT static fields may also be used. A dose of 45 to 54 Gy is delivered in 1.8Gy fractions with a reduction in the field volume after 45 Gy.[33] The upper abdomen contains many dose-limiting structures that must be considered for the designing and planning of radiation treatments. These structures include the kidneys, liver, stomach, small bowel, and spinal cord. Table 31.3 contains the tolerated dose (TD) 5/5 and tissue tolerance data of these structures. Conformal 3D treatment planning and IMRT or VMAT systems may allow higher doses of radiation to be delivered while keeping the dose-limiting structures within tolerance. Three-dimensional treatment planning permits the design of coplanar and noncoplanar beams that use a couch rotation to enter at unique angles to avoid critical structures and allow a higher dose to be achieved. Intensity-modulated systems use unique beam directions; however, they also vary the beam intensity and shape of the field with the use of MLCs. Studies that compare IMRT with 3D conformal have shown that IMRT and VMAT further reduce the dose to the liver, kidneys, stomach, and small bowel than 3D conformal.[56,61,62] Ongoing research studies are being conducted to see whether dose escalation is possible with IMRT techniques as a result of the improved dose conformality to the tumor volume and sparing of critical structures.[63] Stereotactic body radiotherapy (SBRT) alone and in combination with chemotherapy is one option of the NCCN recommendations for locally advanced pancreatic cancer. Additional studies are ongoing for the use of SBRT in locally advanced unresectable pancreas cancers.[62–66] Preliminary studies have shown that treatment with SBRT has similar or better local control rate as conventional external beam. In some studies, SBRT resulted in the tumor shrinking enough that allowed resection of the tumor to be done.[66] Treatment-related GI toxicities, duodenal bleeding, and ulcers have been a concern, especially in early studies when higher total doses were delivered.[65] Dose fraction schemes vary from 25 to 33 Gy in three to five fractions to 45 Gy in three fractions.[23,58,67] These lower total doses were applied to reduce toxicity to OARs such as the duodenum, small bowel, and stomach.[62,65,68] The SBRT short treatment time has been viewed as a benefit for the patient's quality of life when compared with 5 to 6 weeks of conventional radiotherapy.[64] The short treatment course of SBRT may also be more cost-effective when compared with the standard course of external beam treatments.[66] SBRT is a complex treatment that may include respiratory gating, breath hold, and IGRT. IGRT is of extreme importance in treatment of patients with SBRT. The therapist is responsible for obtaining CBCT and kV images before treatment.[64,65] Proton beam therapy may provide another future treatment option for patients with locally advanced and unresectable pancreas cancer. The characteristic finite depth in tissue that protons travel may provide an advantage of sparing more healthy tissue. This is critically important in treatment of the upper abdomen because of the kidneys, liver, small bowel, and stomach being in such close proximity to the target volume. Some studies have shown that proton beam therapy results in less dose delivered to the kidneys, liver, and small intestine when compared with IMRT or VMAT. For CT simulation, the patient is placed in the supine position with the arms above the head for easier placement of the lateral isocenter marks. A vacuum device or foaming cradle immobilization device is made before the simulation. The therapist should make sure the patient is straight on the table before the immobilization device is made. This can be accomplished by using the sagittal laser and lining up midline structures such as SSN, xiphoid, and pubic bone. The device is measured to ensure that it fits inside the scanner, and an image of patient setup is taken. With simulation of a patient for SBRT, a full-body vacuum device for immobilization is made that might include abdominal compression.[62] The pancreas is an area associated with a large amount of movement. The simulation should include a 4D CT scan to determine the amount of respiratory-related motion.[11] The CT simulation also requires that contrast be administered. With this simulation, the patient is instructed to drink contrast 30 minutes to 1 hour before the scan. If oral contrast is used, the NCCN guidelines suggest giving the patient the same amount of water before treatment each day to reproduce the same amount of stomach distention. Conversely, no oral contrast may be used, and the patient is instructed to be NPO before simulation and treatment, ensuring an empty stomach to maintain similar internal anatomy for each treatment.[33] Some centers may inject IV contrast for kidney localization or blood vessels to assist in determining nodal volumes. Fiducial markers may be inserted into the pancreas before CT simulation for patients treated with SBRT.[62,66]

The radiation therapist places reference marks on the patient's abdomen before scanning. A scan from above the diaphragm to below the iliac crest is obtained. The physician can digitize in the location of the target volume, lymph nodes, porta hepatis, and superior mesenteric artery to ensure coverage of these structures in the treatment field. The OARs, kidneys, liver, stomach, small bowel, and spinal cord, may be outlined as well.

Once the treatment isocenter has been identified, the radiation therapist makes the appropriate shifts from the reference isocenter and marks the final three points to be used for treatment. The CT images are then sent to the dosimetrist for 3D conformal planning or IMRT or VMAT planning. IMRT or VMAT highly conformal dose distributions and treatment planning dose constraints allows dose to kidneys, liver, stomach and spinal cord to be minimized[11,60,33] (Fig. 31.20).

Side Effects. The most common reports of patients receiving radiation for pancreatic cancer are nausea and vomiting. Antiemetics

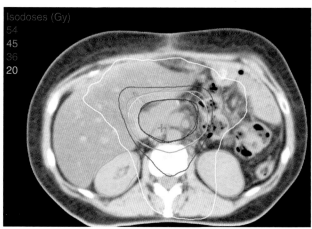

Fig. 31.20 Dose distribution obtained with VMAT treatment for pancreatic tumor. Note the kidneys and spinal cord are outlined in blue and tan, respectively. (From Avanzo M, Chiovati P, Boz G. Image-guided volumetric arc radiotherapy of pancreatic cancer with simultaneous integrated boost: optimization strategies and dosimetric results. *Physica Medica* 32(1):169–175.)

may be given to mitigate these adverse effects. Other potential acute side effects include leukopenia, thrombocytopenia, diarrhea, and stomatitis. Long-term side effects such as renal failure are rare and suggest the possibility of the kidney receiving a higher dose of radiation.

Case VI: Locally Advanced Pancreatic Cancer, Potentially Resectable

A 64-year-woman presented to her physician with a 27-lb unintentional weight loss over 3 months, lower abdominal bloating, and pressure. CT scan of the abdomen/pelvis showed a 2.6 × 3.6-cm pancreatic head mass with massive cystic enlargement of the pancreatic duct through the pancreatic neck, body, and tail with atrophy of the associated pancreatic parenchyma. The common bile duct was also enlarged and measured up to 1.5 cm in caliber. Intrahepatic biliary ductal dilation was observed. The area of ill-defined abnormality in the pancreatic head bordered the SMV abutting approximately 40% of the wall, which also appeared to abut the superior mesenteric artery, although to a lesser extent. A CT scan of the chest was done and was negative for metastasis. EUS was done and showed a 3.7 × 3.5-cm mass in the pancreatic head, which was biopsied. The pathology report came back as adenocarcinoma, moderately differentiated. An ERCP was done to place a stent to relieve obstruction of bile duct.

The patient was referred to radiation oncology for neoadjuvant radiation therapy and chemotherapy for her borderline resectable pancreatic cancer. She enrolled in a clinical trial that began with neoadjuvant FOLFIRINOX for four cycles and then began chemoradiation after a 2- to 6-week break. The chemoradiation with Xeloda was followed by a break before surgery. More chemotherapy with gemcitabine was given adjuvantly after surgery.

The patient had a 4D CT scan simulation to determine tumor movement with breathing. Oral contrast was administered. A dose of 5040 cGy at 180 cGy per 28 fractions was delivered via VMAT with two 360-degree arcs. Daily IGRT with kV imaging was performed with the therapists matching the spine from T-10 to L-4.

Case VII: Pancreatic Cancer

A 69-year-old woman in her usual state of health began to notice dark urine in June. She also noticed she was losing weight. In addition to this, she later developed jaundice. She then went to see her primary care provider in August for a routine medical exam. Blood tests were ordered, and she was found to have elevated liver function tests. This prompted an ultrasound of liver and pancreas to be ordered. This showed narrowed bile ducts. Next, a CT scan of the abdomen and pelvis was obtained. The CT showed narrowed bile ducts at the head of the pancreas and soft tissue mass. Because of findings on the CT scan, an ERCP was ordered. This demonstrated a stricture in the lower third of the main bile duct. A biopsy and brushings of the common bile duct were done that were suspicious for adenocarcinoma. A stent was placed in the bile duct to alleviate the obstruction. Following her stent placement, her symptoms of jaundice and dark urine resolved. During his time, the patient continued to lose weight, nearly 10% of her body weight.

A PET MRI scan was ordered that showed increased metabolic activity in the pancreatic head and tail. A mass in the head of pancreas was visualized measuring 2.4 × 2.8. × 3.2 cm. There was also a suspicious lymph node. The head of pancreas mass had less than 180-degree contact with the SMV. No evidence of distant metastasis was seen. The patient was referred to the gastroenterology department. An endoscopic ultrasound was ordered and performed that identified a 3.4-cm mass in the head of the pancreas with invasion into the SMV and splenoportal confluence. A FNA biopsy of the pancreas head showed adenocarcinoma. Because of the less than 180-degree of invasion of the SMV, the tumor is considered a borderline resectable pancreatic cancer. She was referred to medical and radiation oncology for the consideration of neoadjuvant treatment.

The plan of treatment is 4 months of induction chemotherapy followed by chemoradiation. The patient received FOLRINOX that resulted in a decrease in the size of pancreas lesions and no distant metastasis.

She began chemoradiation, receiving capecitabine as a radiosensitizer. The radiation oncologist prescribed a course of 5000 cGy in 25 fractions to the GTV with a dose of 4500 cGy delivered to elective lymph nodes. The patient was treated with VMAT with three full 360-degree arcs and instructed to be NPO 3 hours before treatment, the same as for simulation.

▮ SUMMARY

Colorectal Cancer

- The risk of development of cancer of the large bowel increases with age, with more than 90% of cases in people over 50 years of age. Cancer of the large bowel more commonly affects the rectum or distal colon. Colorectal cancer is the second leading cause of cancer death in the United States; it accounts for approximately 51,000 deaths annually.
- The colon is divided into eight regions: cecum, ascending colon, descending colon, splenic flexure, hepatic flexure, transverse colon, sigmoid, and rectum.
- Patients with rectal cancer usually have rectal bleeding. Other symptoms include a change in bowel habits, diarrhea versus constipation, and a change in the stool caliber.
- Cancers in the large bowel are diagnosed via findings of the physical examination and radiographic and endoscopic studies.
- Adenocarcinoma is the most common malignancy of the large bowel; it accounts for 90% to 95% of all tumors. Other histologic types include mucinous adenocarcinoma, signet-ring cell carcinoma, and squamous cell carcinoma.
- Surgery is considered the treatment of choice for rectal cancer. Radiation therapy is most commonly used as an adjuvant treatment for rectal cancer, either done before or after surgery and in conjunction with chemotherapy.

Anal Cancer

- The etiologic factors for the development of anal cancer are associated with human papillomaviruses, genital warts, genital infections, anal intercourse in men or women before age 30, and immunosuppression.
- The most common presenting symptom is rectal bleeding. Other symptoms are pain, change in bowel habits, and the sensation of a mass.
- Squamous cell carcinoma is the most common histology of anal cancer; it comprises approximately 80% of cases.
- Combination radiation therapy and chemotherapy is advocated as the preferred method of treatment and is considered the standard of care for most patients. A variety of radiation techniques exist for the treatment of anal cancer. VMAT and IMRT techniques are more commonly done than a four-field or AP/PA pelvic field with matching electron fields to the inguinal nodes.

Esophageal Cancer

- Risk factors such as use of tobacco or alcohol abuse cause esophageal cancer. Long-term irritation of the lining of the esophagus, as with GERD, Barrett esophagus, achalasia, esophageal webs, or scarring from swallowing lye, can cause esophageal cancers.
- The esophagus is a 25-cm-long tube lined with stratified squamous epithelium. The esophagus begins at the level of C6 and traverses through the thoracic cage to terminate in the abdomen at the esophageal gastric junction (T10 to T11).
- The most common presenting symptoms are dysphagia and weight loss, which occur in 90% of patients.
- The most common pathologic types of esophageal cancer are squamous cell carcinoma and adenocarcinoma. Squamous cell carcinomas are found most frequently in the upper and middle thoracic esophagus. Adenocarcinoma typically occurs in the distal esophagus and GE junction. Adenocarcinoma is the most commonly occurring type in the United States.
- Because the esophagus is distensible, lesions are large before causing obstructive symptoms. Spread is usually longitudinal. Occasionally, skip lesions may be present at a significant distance from the primary lesion.
- The treatment of esophageal cancer is highly complex and technically difficult. Radiation therapy with concurrent chemotherapy is considered the current nonsurgical treatment of choice for esophageal cancer. Trimodality therapy may be done for cancers in the lower one-third of the esophagus. Chemoradiation is done first, followed by resection if feasible and if no distant metastasis is present.

Pancreatic Cancer

- Cancers of the pancreas account for approximately 2% of all cancers diagnosed annually in the United States and have a high mortality rate. No known cause exists for the development of pancreatic cancer, although smokers have a two to three times higher risk of development of pancreatic cancer.
- The pancreas is located retroperitoneally at the L1 to L2 level, lies transversely in the upper abdomen, and is divided into three anatomic regions: the head, body, and tail.

- The four most common presenting symptoms of pancreatic cancer are jaundice, abdominal pain, anorexia, and weight loss.
- The most valuable and important diagnostic test is a CT scan of the abdomen, which provides a complete view of the abdominal structures most likely involved with the pancreatic tumor.
- Adenocarcinomas comprise 80% of pancreatic cancers.
- Surgery is the treatment of choice. Most tumors, however, are unresectable.
- Radiation therapy and chemotherapy are considered the preferred treatments for locally advanced, unresectable pancreatic cancers.

■ REVIEW QUESTIONS

The answers to the Review Questions can be found by logging on to our website at: http://evolve.elsevier.com/Washington/principles

1. Which of the following methods may reduce dose to the small bowel during pelvic radiation therapy?
   a. Supine position.
   b. Prone position.
   c. Treatment with a full bladder.
   d. Both b and c.
2. The principal advantage of IMRT or VMAT over conventional 3D conformal in the treatment of rectal, anal, or pancreatic cancer is:
   a. Fewer long-term radiation side effects.
   b. Better dose conformity to target volumes.
   c. More sparing of healthy structures (OARs).
   d. All of the above.
3. The principal lymph node group involved in patients with rectal cancer is the:
   a. Common iliac nodes.
   b. Hepatic nodes.
   c. Paraaortic nodes.
   d. Internal iliac nodes.
4. The principal etiologic factor(s) in the development of adenocarcinomas of the esophagus in North America is (are):
   a. A diet high in fat and high in nitrate content.
   b. A diet low in fat and high in vegetables and fruits.
   c. GERD.
   d. Barrett's esophagus.
5. A common site of blood-borne metastasis from rectal, pancreatic, or esophageal malignancies is the:
   a. Brain.
   b. Bone.
   c. Adrenal gland.
   d. Liver.
6. For radiation treatment to the thorax for esophageal cancer, the dose-limiting structure of most concern is the:

   a. Spinal cord.
   b. Heart.
   c. Esophagus.
   d. Trachea.
7. The radiation-field design most commonly used to avoid the critical structure in Question 6 is:
   a. Lateral-opposed fields.
   b. AP/PA fields.
   c. Conformal 3D VMAT or IMRT.
   d. Wedge pair.
8. Which of the following are common presenting symptoms of pancreatic cancer?
   I. Jaundice.
   II. Nausea and vomiting.
   III. 10% weight loss.
   IV. Anorexia.
      a. I and II.
      b. II and III.
      c. I, II, and IV.
      d. I, III, and IV.
      e. I, II, III, and IV.
9. Which of the following statements regarding pancreatic cancer is *not* correct?
   a. It is locally invasive into surrounding structures.
   b. Hematogenous spread to the liver at the time of diagnosis is common.
   c. The 5-year survival rate is 50%.
   d. Most tumors are unresectable.
10. For irradiation of the upper abdomen for pancreatic cancer, the most radiosensitive dose-limiting structure is the:
    a. Kidney.
    b. Liver.
    c. Small bowel.
    d. Spinal cord.

■ QUESTIONS TO PONDER

1. Describe the rationale for the use of neoadjuvant preoperative radiation therapy and adjuvant postoperative radiation therapy for rectal cancer.
2. What is the rationale for a 4D CT scan and respiratory gating when simulating patients with cancer of the esophagus or pancreas?
3. What are the theoretic advantages and disadvantages of proton therapy for the treatment of esophageal cancer?
4. What techniques are used to decrease or limit the radiation dose to the small bowel? Why are these important?

5. In treatment of the thorax for esophageal cancer, the arms and shoulders can create problems with the reproducibility of the setup. What can be done to ensure consistency in the daily setup of the treatment fields?
6. What is the main advantage of CT simulation and 3D conformal irradiation techniques?
7. What is the purpose of chemoradiation?
8. Barrett's esophagus and GERD are factors that are associated with the development of what histologic type of esophageal cancer?

REFERENCES

1. American Cancer Society. *Cancer Facts & Figures 2019*. Atlanta, GA: American Cancer Society; 2019.
2. American Cancer Society. *Colorectal Cancer Facts and Figures, 2017–2019*. Atlanta, GA: American Cancer Society; 2019.
3. American Cancer Society. *Cancer Facts & Figures 2017*. Atlanta, GA: American Cancer Society; 2017.
4. Czito C, Willet CG. Colon cancer. In: Gunderson LL, Tepper JE, eds. *Clinical Radiation Oncology*. 3rd ed. St. Louis, MO: Elsevier Saunders; 2012.
5. Minsky BD, Welton ML, Pineda CE. Cancer of the colon. In: Hoppe RT, Phillips TL, Roach M, eds. *Leibel and Phillips Textbook of Radiation Oncology*. 3rd ed. Philadelphia, PA: Saunders; 2010.
6. O'Kane GM, Knox JJ. Locally advanced pancreatic cancer: an emerging entity. *Curr Probl Cancer*. 2018;42:12–25.
7. American Cancer Society. Colorectal cancer. http://www.cancer.org/cancer/colonandrectumcancer/index. Accessed March 11, 2019.
8. American Cancer Society. *Colorectal Cancer Facts and Figures, Special Edition*; 2014. http://www.cancer.org/research/cancerfactsfigures/colorectalcancerfactsfigures/colorectal-cancer-facts-figures-2011-2013-page. Accessed March 19, 2019.
9. Minsky BD, Welton ML, Venook AP. Cancer of the rectum. In: Hoppe RT, Phillips TL, Roach M, eds. *Leibel and Phillips Textbook of Radiation Oncology*. 3rd ed. Philadelphia, PA: Saunders; 2010.
10. Amin MB, ed. *AJCC Cancer Staging Manual*. 8th ed. New York, NY: Springer; 2017.
11. Reese AS, Lu W, Regine WF. Utilization of intensity-modulated radiation therapy and image guided radiation therapy in pancreatic cancer: is it beneficial? *Semin Radiat Oncol*. 2014;24:132–139.
12. Palta M, Willett G, Czito BR. Pancreatic cancer. In: Halperin EC, Brady LW, Perez CA, et al., eds. *Perez and Brady's Principles and Practices of Radiation Oncology*. 6th ed. Philadelphia, PA: Lippincott Williams & Wilkins; 2013.
13. Li CC, Chen CY, Chien CR. Comparison of intensity modulated radiotherapy vs 3Dimensional conformal radiotherapy for patients with non-metastatic esophageal squamous cell carcinoma receiving definitive concurrent chemoradiotherapy: a population based propensity score matched analysis. *Medicine (Baltimore)*. 2018;97(22):e10928.
14. Minsky BD, Rodel C, Valentini V. Rectal cancer. In: Gunderson LL, Tepper JE, eds. *Clinical Radiation Oncology*. 3rd ed. St. Louis, MO: Elsevier Saunders; 2012.
15. Wolf AM, Fontham ET, Church TR, et al. Colorectal cancer screening for average-risk adults: 2018 guideline update from the American Cancer Society. *CA Cancer J Clin*. 2018;68:250–281.
16. Anderson C, Koshy M, Staley C, et al. PET-CT fusion in radiation management of patients with anorectal tumors. *Int J Radiat Oncol Biol Phys*. 2007;69:155–162.
17. Gunderson LL, Dozois RR. Intraoperative irradiation for locally advanced colorectal carcinomas. *Perspect Colon Rectal Surg*. 1992;5:1–23.
18. Franke AJ, Parekh H, Starr JS, et al. Total neoadjuvant therapy: a shifting paradigm in locally advanced rectal cancer management. *Clin Colorectal Cancer*. 2018;17(1):1–12.
19. Sao Julioa GP, Habr-Gama A, Vailati BB, et al. New strategies in rectal cancer. *Surg Clin N Am*. 2017;97:587–604.
20. Wang J, Wei C, Tucker SL, et al. Predictors of postoperative complications after trimodality therapy for esophageal cancer. *Int J Radiation Oncol Biol Phys*. 2013;86:885–891.
21. Grass F, Mathis K. *Novelties in Treatment of Locally Advanced Rectal Cancer. F1000Res*. 2018;7:F1000 Faculty Rev-1868.
22. Mowery YM, Salama JK, Yousuf Z, et al. Neoadjuvant long-course chemoradiation remains strongly favored over short-course radiotherapy by radiation oncologists in the United States. *Cancer*. 2017;123:1434–1441.
23. Cummings BJ, Brierley JD. Anal cancer. In: Halperin EC, Brady LW, Perez CA, et al., eds. *Perez and Brady's Principles and Practices of Radiation Oncology*. 6th ed. Philadelphia, PA: Lippincott Williams & Wilkins; 2013.
24. National Comprehensive Cancer Network. *NCCN Radiation Therapy Compendium, Rectal Cancer Guidelines*. Version 3. NCCN; 2018. https://www.nccn.org/professionals/radiation/default.aspx. Accessed November 6, 2019.
25. Holman FA, Bosmans SJ, Haddock MG, et al. Results of a pooled analysis of IOERT containing multimodality treatment for locally recurrent rectal cancer: results of 565 patients of two major treatment centres. *Eur J Surg Oncol*. 2017;43:107–117.
26. Ghosn M, Kourie HR, Abdayem P, et al. Anal cancer treatment: current status and future perspectives. *World J Gastroenterol*. 2015;21(8):2294–2302.
27. American Cancer Society. Anal cancer. http://www.cancer.org/cancer/analcancer/index. Accessed March 11, 2019.
28. Chuong MD, Hallemeir CL, Jabbour SK, et al. Improving outcomes for esophageal cancer using proton beam therapy. *Int J Radiation Biol Phys*. 2015;95(1):488–497.
29. Julie D, Goodman KA. Advances in the management of anal cancer. *Curr Oncol Rep*. 2016;18:20.
30. Callister MD, Haddock MG, Martenson JA. Anal carcinoma. In: Gunderson LL, Tepper JE, eds. *Clinical Radiation Oncology*. 3rd ed. St. Louis, MO: Elsevier Saunders; 2012.
31. Elson JK, Kachnic LA. Intensity-modulated radiotherapy improves survival and reduces treatment time in squamous cell carcinoma of the anus: a National Cancer Data Base study. 124(22):4383–4439.
32. Minsky BD, Welton ML, Pineda CE. Cancer of the anal canal. In: Hoppe RT, Phillips TL, Roach M, eds. *Leibel and Phillips Textbook of Radiation Oncology*. 3rd ed. Philadelphia, PA: Saunders; 2010.
33. National Comprehensive Cancer Network. *NCCN Radiation Therapy Compendium, Pancreatic Adenocarcinoma Guidelines*. NCCN. Version 1. 2019. https://www.nccn.org/professionals/radiation/default.aspx. Accessed November 6, 2019.
34. Blackstock AW, Russa S. Cancer of the esophagus. In: Gunderson LL, Tepper JE, eds. *Clinical Radiation Oncology*. 3rd ed. St. Louis, MO: Elsevier Saunders; 2012.
35. National Comprehensive Cancer Network. NCCN Radiation Therapy Compendium. *Anal Cancer Guidelines*. Version. 1. 2018. https://www.nccn.org/professionals/radiation/default.aspx. Accessed November 6, 2019.
36. American Cancer Society. Esophageal cancer. http://www.cancer.org/cancer/esophaguscancer/index. Accessed March 11, 2019.
37. Miao Y, Lui R, Pu Y, Yun L. Trends in esophageal and esophagogastric junction cancer research from 2007 to 2016: a bibliometric analysis. *Medicine*. 2017;96(20):e6924.
38. Regine WF, Winter K, Abrams RA, et al. Postresection CA 19-9 and margin status as predictors of recurrence after adjuvant treatment for pancreatic carcinoma: analysis of NRG oncology RTOG trial 9704. *Adv Rad Oncol*. 2018;3:154–162.
39. Czito BG, DeNittis AS, Palta M, et al. Esophageal cancer. In: Halperin EC, Brady LW, Perez CA, et al., eds. *Perez and Brady's Principles and Practices of Radiation Oncology*. 6th ed. Philadelphia, PA: Lippincott Williams & Wilkins; 2013.
40. Minsky BD, Goodman K, Warren R. Cancer of the esophagus. In: Hoppe RT, Phillips TL, Roach M, eds. *Leibel and Phillips Textbook of Radiation Oncology*. 3rd ed. Philadelphia, PA: Saunders; 2010.
41. Wang A, Chengpei Z, Fu L, et al. Citrus fruit intake substantially reduces the risk of esophageal cancer: a meta-analysis of epidemiologic studies. *Medicine*. 2015;94(39):e1390.
42. Lin JC, Tsai JT, Chang CC, et al. Comparing treatment plan in all locations of esophageal cancer volumetric modulated arc therapy versus intensity-modulated radiotherapy. *Medicine*. 2015;94(17):1–9.
43. Ajani JA, Walsh G, Komaki R, et al. Preoperative induction of CPT-11 and cisplatin chemo-therapy followed by chemoradiation therapy in patients with locoregional carcinoma of the esophagus or gastroesophageal junction. *Cancer*. 2004;100(11):2347–2354.
44. Crane CH, O'Reilly EM. Ablative radiotherapy doses for locally advanced pancreatic cancer. *Cancer J*. 2017;23(6):350–354.
45. Badiyan SN, Hallemeier CL, Lin SH, et al. Proton beam therapy for esophageal cancers: past, present, and future. *J Gastrointest Oncol*. 2017;9(5):692–971.
46. Fleshman J, Sargent DJ, Green E, et al. Laparoscopic colectomy for cancer is not inferior to open surgery based on 5-year data from the COST Study Group Trial. *Ann Surg*. 2007;246(4):655–664.

47. National Comprehensive Cancer Network. *NCCN Radiation Therapy Compendium, Esophagus and Esophgastric Junction Guidelines.* NCCN. Org. Version 1. 2018. https://www.nccn.org/patients/guidelines/esophageal/4/index.html. Accessed November 6, 2019.

48. Shah AP, Abrams RA. Pancreatic cancer. In: Gunderson LL, Tepper JE, eds. *Clinical Radiation Oncology.* 3rd ed. St. Louis, MO: Elsevier Saunders; 2012.

49. Hafeez S, Bedford JL, Tait DM, et al. Normal tissue sparing with respiratory adapted volumetric modulated arc therapy for distal oesophageal and gastro-oesophageal tumours. *Acta Oncologica.* 2014;53(1):149–154.

50. Kole TP, Aghayere O, Kwah J, Yorke ED, Goodman KA. Comparison of heart and coronary artery doses associated with intensity-modulated radiotherapy versus three-dimensional conformal radiotherapy for distal esophageal cancer. *Int J Radiation Oncol Biol Phys.* 2012;83:1580–1586.

51. Lin SH, Komaki R, Liao Z, et al. Proton beam therapy and concurrent chemotherapy for esophageal cancer. *Int J Radiation Oncol Biol Phys.* 2012;83:345–351.

52. Stauder MC, Miller RC. Stereotactic body radiation therapy (SBRT) for unresectable pancreatic carcinoma. *Cancer.* 2010;2:1565–1575.

53. American Cancer Society. Pancreatic cancer. http://www.cancer.org/cancer/pancreaticcancer/index. Accessed March 11, 2019.

54. Palta M, Willett CG, Czita BR. Cancer of the colon and rectum. In: Halperin EC, Brady LW, Perez CA, et al., eds. *Perez and Brady's Principles and Practices of Radiation Oncology.* 6th ed. Philadelphia, PA: Lippincott Williams & Wilkins; 2013.

55. Lopez NE, Prendergast C, Lowy AM. Borderline resectable pancreatic cancer: definitions and management. *World J Gastrointerol.* 2014;20(31):10740–10751.

56. Warshaw AL, Swanson RS. What's new in general surgery: pancreatic cancer in 1988, possibilities and probabilities. *Ann Surg.* 1988;208:541.

57. Wolff RA. Adjuvant or neoadjuvant therapy in the treatment in pancreatic malignancies. Where are we? *Surg Clin N Am.* 2018;90:95–111.

58. Bilimoria KY, Bentrem DJ, Ko CY, et al. Multimodality therapy for pancreatic cancer in the U.S. *Cancer.* 2007;110(6):1227–1234.

59. Bodner WR, Hilaris BS, Mastoras DA. Radiation therapy in pancreatic cancer: current practices and future trends. *J Clin Gastroenterol.* 2000;30:230–233.

60. Goodman KA, Regine WF, Dawson LA, et al. Radiation therapy oncology group consensus panel guidelines for the delineation of the clinical target volume in the postoperative treatment of pancreatic head cancer. *Int J Radiation Oncol Biol Phys.* 2012;83:901–908.

61. Brown MW, Ning H, Arora B, et al. A dosimetric analysis of dose escalation using two intensity-modulated radiation therapy techniques in locally advanced pancreatic carcinoma. *Int J Radiat Oncol Biol Phys.* 2006;65(1):274–283.

62. Chuong MD, Springett GM, Freilich JM, et al. Stereotactic body radiation therapy for locally advanced and borderline resectable pancreatic cancer is effective and well tolerated. *Int J Radiation Oncol Biol Phys.* 2013;86:516–522.

63. Ben-Josef E, Shields AF, Vaishampayan U, et al. Intensity-modulated radiotherapy (IMRT) and concurrent capecitabine for pancreatic cancer. *Int J Radiat Oncol Biol Phys.* 2004;59(2):454–459.

64. Petrelli F, Comito T, Ghidini A. Stereotactic body radiation therapy for locally advanced pancreatic cancer: a systematic review and pooled analysis of 19 trials. *Int J Radiation Oncol Biol Phys.* 2017;97(2):331e322.

65. Shier D, Butler J, Lewis R. *Hole's Human Anatomy and Physiology.* 13th ed. New York, NY: McGraw-Hill; 2013.

66. Shridhar R, Almhanna K, Meredith KL, et al. Radiation therapy for esophageal cancer. *Cancer Control.* 2013;20:97–110.

67. Perez K, Safran H, Sikov W, et al. Complete neoadjuvant treatment for rectal cancer: the Brown University oncology group CONTRE study. *Am J Clin Oncol.* 2017;40(3):283–287.

68. Nichols RC Jr , Huh SN, Prado KL, et al. Protons offer reduced normal-tissue exposure for patients receiving post-operative radiotherapy for resected pancreatic head cancer. *Int J Radiation Oncol Biol Phys.* 2012;83:158–163.

32

Gynecological Tumors

Kameka Rideaux

OBJECTIVES

- Discuss the etiology and epidemiologic data for gynecologic tumors.
- Discuss common presenting symptoms related to malignant gynecologic tumors and treatments.
- List the histopathology of tumors categorized in the gynecologic region.
- Discuss the latest screening methods and diagnostic procedures used in the diagnosis and staging of gynecologic tumors.
- List and classify the lymphatic chains, and illustrate the most common routes of spread.
- Discuss the pathologic appearance and staging of gynecologic tumors.
- Describe the anatomy and physiologic components of the female reproductive system.
- Formulate treatment rationales based on the information obtained from staging, histology, and patient assessment.

- Identify the tumor lethal dose based on the disease staging.
- Discuss the tolerance doses for the organs at risk.
- Differentiate between the various treatment practices as related to the gynecologic tumor.
- Describe patient instructions that should be given in regard to expected side effects, skin care, and dietary concerns.
- Discuss the range of psychologic issue associated with gynecologic malignancies and radiation treatments.
- Compare and contrast the medical, surgical, and radiation management options for gynecologic tumors.
- Discuss the reasoning for a multimodal approach to gynecologic tumors.
- Discuss the possible fractionation schemes that can be used in the treatment of gynecologic cancers and the side effects related to each.

OUTLINE

KEY TERMS

In the management of gynecologic malignancies, clinicians must have a comprehensive understanding that extends beyond the disease itself to the complex psychologic and physical impacts to patients. This chapter provides radiation therapists with information regarding gynecologic malignancies that can be applicable to the work environment. The objective of this chapter is to facilitate a clear understanding of anatomy and radiation therapy standard practices that enable the radiation therapist to provide optimal services to patients with gynecologic tumors. Gynecologic cancers are tumors that originate in the female reproductive system and can be divided into carcinomas of the cervix, uterus, ovaries, vulva, and vagina. A sagittal view of the female pelvis can be seen in Fig. 32.1. Each section of this chapter is separated into individual cancers to emphasize that although the cancers have similarities, the origins, behaviors, and treatments are very different. The main function of the radiation therapist during a course of treatment is to focus attention on the interpretation and implementation of complex treatments, patient assessment, and patient safety and monitoring.

ANATOMY

Vulva

The vulva is the outermost portion of the female genitalia. The major parts include the labia majora and labia minora, the clitoris, and the area bound by these three, which is called the vestibule. The vestibule is the triangular space that is located anterior to the vaginal opening and contains the opening of the female urethra. The perineum refers to the area between the change to vagina and anus in females and the scrotum and anus in males.

Vagina

The vagina is a muscular tube that extends 6 to 8 inches from the cervix of the uterus to the vulva. It is surrounded by the rectum, urethra, and bladder, specifically anterior to the rectum and posterior to the bladder. Superiorly, the cervix projects through the vaginal wall and creates a circular sulcus called the vaginal fornices. The fornices serve as an anatomic landmark that surrounds the superior portion of the vagina. The vaginal canal is composed of smooth muscle and lined with a layer of stratified squamous epithelium formed by epithelial cells. The vaginal wall or mucosa is of great importance in the discussion of brachytherapy treatments. The vaginal wall has three layers: the mucosa, muscularis, and adventitia.

Cervix and Uterus

The uterus is a hollow, pear-shaped structure that is divided into three main parts: the cervix, the body, and the fundus. The cavity of the uterus is small because of the thickness of the uterine walls. The three layers of the wall of the uterus are the inner endometrium (mucous membrane), the middle myometrium (smooth muscles), and the outer perimetrium (parietal peritoneum). The thickness of the endometrial layer varies with estrogen changes in the body. The fallopian tubes extend laterally from the superior uterus. These hollow structures transfer the ova from the ovaries to the uterus. The parametrium refers to the connective tissue that is immediately lateral to the uterine cervix.

The cervix (the part of the uterus that extends into the superior vaginal wall) is a firm, rounded structure from 1.5 to 3 cm in diameter. The cervix is the lowest part of the uterus where it connects with the superior portion of the vagina. The part of the cervix closest to the body of the uterus is the endocervix, and the part closest to the vagina is the exocervix. The cervical os is the opening of the cervix (vaginal end) and is lined with squamous cell epithelium. Squamous cell epithelium of the cervix connects with the columnar epithelium of the endocervix, which is called the squamocolumnar junction, or transformation zone. Squamous cell carcinoma of the cervix usually originates at this junction.

CERVICAL CANCER

Epidemiology

Cervical cancer remains a considerable burden worldwide and is reported to be the third most common malignancy in women. According to the National Institutes of Health, the incidence rates in the United States are much lower than in other countries, with a rank of 14th in incidence.[1] The American Cancer Society (ACS) estimates that about 13,250 women in the United States will be diagnosed with cervical cancer, and about 4,170 will die of this disease each year.[2] Historically, mortality rates flourished because precancerous conditions of the cervix are asymptomatic and were not detectable. However, the mortality rate of cervical cancer has progressively declined because of effective screening methods and advances in treatments.[17] The most effective and widely accepted cervical screening examination is the Papanicolaou's smear (Pap smear), which detects early dysplasia and has increased the diagnosis of preinvasive cancers. Despite this discovery, the incidence and mortality rates of cervical cancer remain high in developing countries where women have limited access to screening.[1] Presently, in the United States, a high incidence rate of cervical cancer is found among Hispanic and black women. Cancers of the cervix are astonishingly low among Jewish women. Most cases of cervical cancers have been found in women younger than the age of 50 years, but the disease is rare under the age of 20 years.[17] Women with lower socioeconomic status may not have access to cervical screenings, which places them at a higher risk for the development of cervical cancer.[2-4]

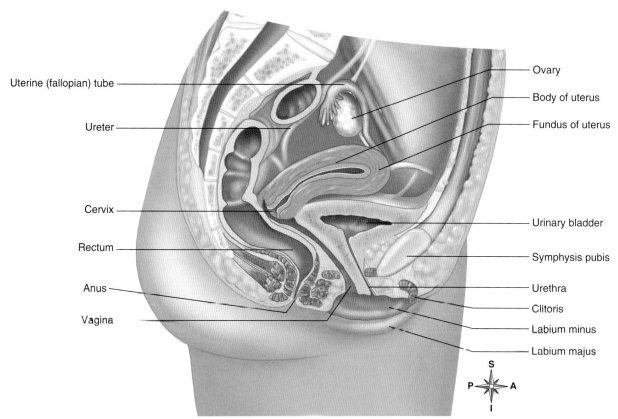

Fig. 32.1 A sagittal view of the female pelvis. (From Thibodeau GA, Patton KT: *The human body in health & disease*, ed 7, St. Louis, 2018, Mosby, Copyright Elsevier (2018).)

Cervical cancers are histologically classified by their tissue of origin. The two primary types of cervical carcinomas are squamous carcinoma and adenocarcinoma. Squamous cell carcinoma is the most common and accounts for 80% to 90% of cervical cancers.[11] These cancers originate in the squamous cells of the exocervix. The second most common type, adenocarcinoma, accounts for 10% to 20% of cervical cancers and typically carries a worse prognosis. These tumors arise inside the endocervical mucus-producing gland cells and can become bulky. This cancer has a high rate of distant metastasis and is difficult to detect. About 3% to 5% of cervical cancers are composed of both squamous carcinoma and adenocarcinoma and are called adenosquamous carcinomas. Other rare histologies include melanoma, clear cell, and neuroendocrine.[3]

Etiology

The World Health Organization defines *risk factor* as "any attribute, characteristic or exposure of an individual that increases the likelihood of developing a disease or injury."[5] Identification of the risk factors for cervical cancer provides valuable information that allows clinicians to advise and accurately screen patients at high risk. Epidemiologic studies have revealed a strong correlation between sexual behaviors and the risk of cervical cancer. Multiple sexual partners and sexual intercourse at an early age are some behaviors that increase the risk of cervical and other gynecologic cancers. Research has also revealed a strong correlation between sexually transmitted diseases and cervical cancer, specifically herpes simplex type 2 and the human papilloma virus (HPV).[11] HPV is the most common sexually transmitted infection in the United States and is responsible for more than 90% of cervical cancers.[2,6] HPV has a high prevalence among adolescent girls. Only certain subtypes of HPV, specifically 16 and 18, are responsible for most cervical cancers. Studies of HPV and cervical cancer reveal that HPV needs 10 to 20 years to progress into cervical cancer. An important highlight is that

most HPV infections clear within 2 years without progressing into cancer.[3] Additional risk factors associated with cervical cancer are oral contraceptives with estrogen alone (without progesterone), smoking, hormonal factors, obesity, low socioeconomic status, nulliparity, and immunosuppression.

Clinical Presentation

Cervical cancers are characteristically slow growing and develop over decades before becoming clinically evident; therefore, the early stages of cervical cancers are asymptomatic. As cervical cancers progress into more advanced stages, more recognizable symptoms begin to manifest, such as abnormal vaginal discharge, pelvic or back pain, painful urination, and hematuria or hematochezia (the passage of bright red, bloody stools).[2,3] The most common presenting symptom for cervical cancer is abnormal vaginal bleeding. Patients with more advanced disease may present with bowel symptoms, which suggest tumor invasion into the rectum. Edema in lower extremities or pelvic pain may indicate lymphatic obstruction or nerve involvement.

Screening

The prevention of cervical cancer largely depends on public education about regular screenings. Screenings are pivotal to prevention and early diagnosis. Currently, vaccines are available to prevent the transmission of some subtype of the HPV. In asymptomatic women, a thorough history and physical examination, including a pelvic examination, are performed to detect cervical cancer.[20] Clinical examinations are performed to visualize the cervix, obtain a Pap smear, conduct a colposcopy examination, and palpate the cervix and lymph nodes. The primary screening test for cervical cancer is a Pap smear, which is sensitive, specific, and cost effective.[2] Pap smears identify abnormal cells that may develop into cancer.

During a Pap examination, a healthcare provider inserts a speculum into the vagina to reveal the cervix. The cells of the cervix are collected with a cervical brush and then prepared for analysis underneath a microscope. Current guidelines recommend that women have a Pap smear every 3 years beginning at the age of 21 years old. Women aged 30 to 65 years should have an HPV and Pap cotesting every 5 years or a Pap test alone every 3 years.[20] Women with certain risk factors may need more frequent screening or continued screening over the age of 65 years. Continued screening after a total hysterectomy is not recommended. One-half of women diagnosed with cervical cancer in the United States were never screened, and 10% were not screened in the past 5 years.[2,3]

Detection and Diagnosis

A colposcopy is performed on women who have abnormal Pap smear results or who are at a high risk for the development of cervical cancer. This test uses a magnifying microscope to examine the cervix for visible abnormalities. Cervical intraepithelial neoplasm is a precancerous condition in which squamous cells that line the cervix become dysplastic. This condition is not cancer and usually lasts years before development into invasive cervical cancer. During a colposcopy, abnormal areas can be excised with a punch biopsy method. In this type of biopsy the clinician removes a small piece of tissue from the cervix with forceps. In cases in which the transformative zone cannot be seen under colposcopy, endocervical curettage removes tissue from the endocervical canal. Another option is the cone biopsy (conization), whereby a cone-shaped piece of tissue is removed from the cervix (exocervix and endocervix) and examined by a pathologist. Conization is performed when no tumor is visible on the cervix but the clinician suspects an endocervical tumor. Cone biopsies offer two approaches for abnormal cell removal: the loop electrosurgical excision procedure (LEEP) and the cold knife cone biopsy. The LEEP removes abnormal cells from the cervix with a thin wire loop heated with electric current. The cold knife biopsy method uses a scalpel or laser for the removal of tissue.

Imaging Studies

For accurate staging of patients, a clinician may perform any of the following diagnostic examinations: a chest x-ray, magnetic resonance imaging (MRI), computed tomographic (CT) scan, positron emission tomography (PET)-CT scan, cystoscopy, or proctoscopy. A CT scan and MRI are both equally effective in assisting clinicians to detect the extent of lymph nodes involvement. A PET-CT scan is more sensitive than an MRI or a CT scan in the detection of lymph nodes and therefore has become the most widely used type of imaging test in the staging of cervical cancer. Besides detection of lymph nodes, a PET/CT scan is useful for the detection of distant metastasis, such as disease in the lung, liver, and bone. MRI has exceptional soft tissue resolution and is used to evaluate parametrial and vaginal extension. A notable contraindication of MRI is that it excludes patients with pacemakers or any type of internal metallic objects, including some prosthetics. Cystoscopy and proctoscopy is indicated only if imaging examination results reveal possible bladder or rectum invasion or if patients have symptoms suggestive of bladder or rectal invasion.[3]

Staging

After a patient is diagnosed with cancer, medical oncologists should construct a treatment plan and determine a prognosis. Before staging, clinicians must know the extent of the disease. The most commonly used staging systems for cervical cancer are the International Federation of Gynecology and Obstetrics (FIGO) and the American Joint Commission on Cancer (AJCC) tumor node metastasis (TNM)

TABLE 32.1	FIGO Staging for Cervical Cancer
FIGO Stage	**Surgical-Pathologic Findings**
I	Cervical carcinoma confined to the uterus (disregard extension to the corpus)
IA	Invasive carcinoma diagnosed only with microscopy; stromal invasion with a maximum depth of 5.0 mm measured from the base of the epithelium and a horizontal spread of 7.0 mm or less; vascular space involvement, venous or lymphatic, does not affect classification
IA1	Measured stromal invasion ≤3.0 mm in depth and ≤7.0 mm in horizontal spread
IA2	Measured stromal invasion >3.0 mm and ≤5.0 mm with a horizontal spread ≤7.0 mm
IB	Clinically visible lesion confined to the cervix or microscopic lesion >T1a/IA2
IB1	Clinically visible lesion ≤4.0 cm in greatest dimension
IB2	Clinically visible lesion > 4.0 cm in greatest dimension
II	Cervical carcinoma invades beyond uterus but not to pelvic wall or to lower third of vagina
IIA	Tumor without parametrial invasion
IIA1	Clinically visible lesion ≤4.0 cm in greatest dimension
IIA2	Clinically visible lesion >4.0 cm in greatest dimension
IIB	Tumor with parametrial invasion
III	Tumor extends to pelvic wall or involves lower third of vagina or causes hydronephrosis or nonfunctional kidney
IIIA	Tumor involves lower third of vagina, no extension to pelvic wall
IIIB	Tumor extends to pelvic wall or causes hydronephrosis or nonfunctional kidney
IV	Tumor invades mucosa of bladder or rectum or extends beyond true pelvis (bullous edema is not sufficient to classify a tumor as T4)
IVA	Tumor invades mucosa of bladder or rectum (bullous edema is not sufficient to classify a tumor as T4)
IVB	Tumor extends beyond true pelvis or invading the mucosa of the bladder or rectum

Based on Federation of Gynecology and Obstetrics treatment of cervical cancer. *FIGO*, International Federation of Gynecology and Obstetrics.

staging systems (Table 32.1). The FIGO system is widely used by gynecologists and gynecologic oncologists. These two staging systems are very similar, with the only difference being that the FIGO system excludes stage 0. Both staging systems classify cervical cancers based on the extent of the tumor (T), cancer spread to lymph nodes (N), and spread to distant sites (M). For more information on AJCC staging for cervix cancer see https://www.cancer.org/cancer/cervical-cancer/detection-diagnosis-staging/staged.html. Accessed November 19,2019.

The most significant prognostic factor in patients with invasive carcinoma of the cervix is staging. Other determining factors of survival include age, race, socioeconomic status, tumor size, location, and lymph node involvement. Patients without lymph node involvement show improved 5-year survival rates compared with those with paraaortic or pelvic lymph node metastasis.

The incidence rate of pelvic and paraaortic nodal involvement is local-stage dependent, with less than 5% and less than 1% for stage I,

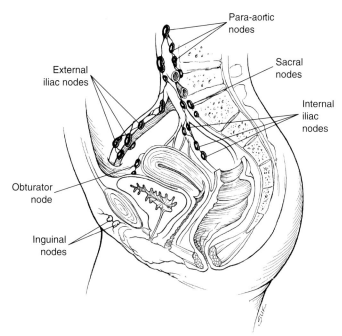

Fig. 32.2 Lymph node drainage of the pelvis.

TABLE 32.2	**Treatment Considerations**
Pretreatment Evaluation	**Key Factors for Radiation**

I. Treatment selection
  A. Sites of possible
    regional involvement
     1. Guide operative
      procedures
     2. Guide external beam
      planning
  B. Extent of primary disease
    1. Selection of local
     treatment
I. Assign FIGO stage
II. Predict prognosis
	Primary radiation therapy should be
	  considered in cases where:
	The tumor is still confined to the cervix
	  but surgical removal is not possible.
	Surgery will cause damage to the bladder
	  and rectum
	Surgery alone (>stage Ib2) is not ade-
	  quate.
	Patient is unable to undergo surgery.
	There is nodal involvement.

	Radiation is usually administered with a
	  combination of external beam therapy
	  and brachytherapy implants.
	Postoperative radiation is normally deliv-
	  ered to patients who have pelvic node
	  involvement, positive tumor margins
	  or a combination of high risk factors
	  including size greater than 4 cm, deep
	  stromal invasion, and LVSI.[9]

FIGO, International Federation of Gynecology and Obstetrics; *LVSI,* lymphovascular space involvement.

15% and 5% for stage Ib, 30% and 15% for stage II, and 50% and 30% for stage III, respectively. For stages IB and IIA, the involvement of lymph nodes results in approximately a 50% reduction in survival rates.[3,7]

Cervical cancers are slow-growing tumors that directly invade adjacent tissues. Metastasis includes direct extension into the uterus, the vagina, the parametrium, the abdomen, the pelvis, the rectum, and the bladder. Cervical cancer may also spread via hematogenous routes. The most common distant sites involved are the lungs, the liver, and bone. Lymphatic involvement is usually orderly, involving parametrial nodes, followed by pelvic (Fig. 32.2), common iliac, periaortic, and even supraclavicular nodes. With paraaortic nodal involvement, a 35% risk exists for supraclavicular spread.[3]

Treatment Modalities and Considerations

The treatment selected for a patient is based on a number of different factors, including extension of primary disease, sites of possible regional involvement, the performance status of the patient, and preservation of childbearing function (Table 32.2). Women with pre-invasive cancers can be treated with cryotherapy or laser therapy to eliminate abnormal cells; other techniques have been described in the detection and diagnosis section. Cryotherapy uses liquid nitrogen to freeze the cervix, and laser therapy uses laser beams to target abnormal cells.

Localized cervical carcinoma may be treated with surgery, radiation, or a combination of both radiation and surgery. For early-stage 0 (carcinoma in situ) and stage IA1 invasive cancers, the typical treatment is a total abdominal hysterectomy (TAH) with or without a small amount of vaginal tissue, referred to as the vaginal cuff. After this surgical procedure, women can no longer conceive children, and menstruation ceases. These patients may undergo brachytherapy treatment alone because the risk of nodal metastasis is very low. The other option in this group of patients is radical trachelectomy, in which the cervix is removed and the uterus remains in place. The advantage of this procedure is that patients maintain their fertility. The survival outcomes of these three modalities are similar. Radiation may play a role for patients with medically inoperative conditions.

Primary radiation therapy should be considered if the tumor is still confined to the cervix but surgical removal is not possible, surgery would cause damage to the bladder and rectum, surgery alone (more that stage IB2) is not adequate, or the patient is not physically able to undergo surgery. The treatments selected for stages IB1 and IIA are controversial because surgery and radiation therapy yield similar control and survival data. Because of the preservation of vaginal pliability and ovarian function, surgery is often used for younger women, whereas radiation is used for women who have a higher risk for surgical complications. Postoperative irradiation is given to patients with pelvic nodes positive for tumor, with surgical margins positive for tumor, and with disease that is an incidental finding in a less-than-definitive surgical procedure, as for benign disease. Some patients with negative nodes may benefit from postoperative radiation therapy. Patients with a combination of deep stromal invasion (invasion of more than one-third to two-thirds of the stroma), lymphovascular space involvement (LVSI), or large tumor diameter (≥4–5 cm) may benefit from the addition of postoperative radiation therapy.[8] If radiation is selected, then it is usually a combination of external beam therapy and brachytherapy implants. Combined modalities should be considered if there is a high risk of reoccurrence or if neither treatment alone would control the disease.

Patients with advanced-stage disease are treated with radiation with or without chemotherapy. Radiation treatments consist of a combination of external beam therapy and brachytherapy implants. Total tumor doses are increased from 70 Gy for low-volume disease to 85 Gy for advanced or bulky disease. Some patients with stage IVa disease can be treated with a high dose of whole pelvis radiation, intracavitary radiation, and parametrial radiation or pelvic exenteration, combined with chemotherapy. When clinicians use brachytherapy, they must be careful not to deliver excessive dose to the vaginal mucosa, which could result in fibrosis, vaginal stenosis, and atrophy.

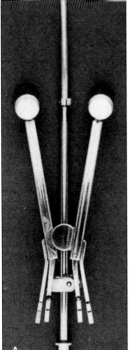
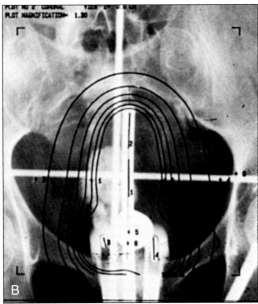
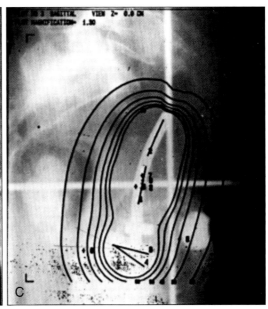

Fig. 32.3 (A) Intracavitary device for brachytherapy. (B and C) Treatment plan for cervical carcinoma showing a radiograph of the intracavitary irradiation in situ with its dose distribution in cGy/h. (A From Niederhuber JE, Armitage JO, Doroshow JH, et al. *Abeloff's Clinical Oncology*. 6th ed. Philadelphia, PA: Elsevier; 2020; B and C From Shingleton SM, Kim RY. Treatment of cancer of the cervix. In: Gusberg SB, Shingleton HM, Neppe G, eds. *Female Genital Cancer*. New York, NY: Churchill Livingstone; 1988:297.)

Because of the thickness of the pelvic area, high-energy photon beams are necessary for external beam treatment. Low-energy photons lead to higher doses to achieve the same tumor dose as higher-energy photons with minimized dose to the bladder and rectum.[3] Shrinkage of bulky tumor during the external beam portion of the treatment results in better geometry for the brachytherapy implant. A standard intrauterine tandem (a small, hollow, curved cylinder that fits through the cervical os and into the uterus) and vaginal colpostats (two golf club–shaped, hollow tubes) are placed laterally to the tandem into the vaginal fornices (see Fig. 32.3). However, some patients may not have the anatomy to accommodate ovoids, and a tandem and ring or cylinder may be used or interstitial implants may be necessary to supplement disease as the bulk increases. Brachytherapy can be delivered either as inpatient with low dose rate or as outpatient with high dose rate. With high dose rate, the fractionation of brachytherapy is increased from one to two implants to five to six implants.

Numerous dose, field, and sequencing arrangements are possible for external beam radiation therapy (EBRT) and brachytherapy. The actual protocol used is based on the radiation oncologist's clinical experience. Examples of doses and configurations include the following: a 70-Gy tumor dose via an implant alone for stage IA disease, 75 to 85 Gy via 45-Gy pelvic radiation therapy, plus a 35-Gy to 40-Gy tumor dose from brachytherapy for stages IB2-IVA. Some centers give a greater percentage of the dose with midline blocking to allow higher implant doses, and some give higher pelvic radiation therapy doses without midline blocking to cover the volume more evenly and sacrifice the amount of the brachytherapy dose. Low-dose-rate implants are usually paired (i.e., two are given approximately 2 weeks apart to achieve higher tolerated doses and allow further tumor regression). The goal is to deliver 50 to 60 Gy to microscopic disease, 60 to 70 Gy to small macroscopic

disease, and 70 to 90 Gy to large macroscopic disease (or its high-dose-rate equivalent) while limiting the volume and dose to the bladder, colorectal tissues, and small intestine. Central doses are traditionally prescribed to the Point A prescription point, usually defined as 2 cm superior to the cervical os and 2 cm lateral to the endocervical canal where the uterine artery crosses the ureter. Point B is 3 cm lateral to point A. Increasingly, with image-guided brachytherapy, the doses to tumor and tissues at risk for disease involvement are described by the isodose line that adequately covers the volume to be treated once the plan is generated.[3]

Treatment

Radiation therapy may be used to treat all stages of cervical cancer. Surgery is reserved for patients with medically operable conditions in early stages (in situ, IA, IB1, and IIA) for whom cure rates are similar and morbidity may be less. Surgery may be followed by radiation therapy if pelvic nodes are positive for tumor, surgical margins are positive for tumor, and simple hysterectomy was performed, and more radical surgery is indicated because the disease is more advanced. Patients with stages IB2, IIB, III, and IVa are usually treated with irradiation alone or in combination with chemotherapy.

The whole pelvis is initially treated with a four-field (minimum, 16-MV photons) technique. The lower border generally falls at the inferior aspect of the obturator foramen unless the vagina is involved, in which case the lower extent of the border is at least 4 cm below the most inferior extent of the disease (and may include the entire vaginal length). The upper border is usually at the top or bottom of L5 or may be extended upward to L4 for a portion of the treatment, depending on the suspected level of potential nodal involvement. The lateral borders are 1.5 to 2.0 cm lateral to the pelvic sidewall in the anteroposterior/posteroanterior (AP/PA) plane. Laterally, the anterior border is at or anterior to the pubic symphysis, with a block designed to include the external iliac nodes; the posterior border includes S3. In patients with anterior or posterior extension, AP/PA fields alone or widening of the laterals is necessary to extend anterior to the pubis or posterior to include S4 and S5. The actual field borders are best finalized with incorporation of a CT scan or MRI in the treatment planning and localization of the lymph nodal areas of involvement (or those at risk) and the cervical disease. AP/PA fields allow midline blocking early if a greater percentage of the dose is to be administered with brachytherapy and, therefore, possibly decrease the dose given to the entire rectum and bladder. The four-field technique allows exclusion of the anterior bladder and posterior rectum in patients for whom the external beam dose is to be taken to 45 to 50 Gy. In patients with a high risk for paraaortic nodes to be treated, extended AP lateral fields are delineated.[3]

Anal markers, rectal barium, vaginal markers, and bladder contrast may be helpful for delineation of critical structures during the simulation process. Prone positioning with a belly board or full bladder may allow the exclusion of the small bowel without jeopardizing the tumor coverage. Small bowel contrast can allow minor field reductions that prevent complications while allowing higher tumor or nodal doses.

Patients with FIGO stage IB2-IIA disease have 5-year survival rates that range from 70% to 90%, depending on the size of the disease. There are reported 5-year disease-specific survival rates of 90%, 86%, and 67% in patients with stage IB tumors with cervical diameters of less than 4 cm, 4 to 4.9 cm, and greater than 5 cm, respectively. Five-year survival rates of 65% to 75%, 35% to 50%, and 15% to 20% have been reported in patients with stage IIB, IIIB, and IV tumors, respectively, treated with radiation therapy alone. The addition of platinum-containing regimens may further improve local control and survival. However, both local control and distant disease recurrence remain a common problem in patients with stage IIIB and IVA disease.

ENDOMETRIAL CANCERS

Epidemiology

Endometrial cancers are the most common gynecologic malignancy and the fourth most common cancer in women in the United States. The ACS estimates that about 60,250 new cases of cancers of the body of the uterus will be diagnosed each year. Most endometrial cancers are adenocarcinomas.[2] Endometrial cancers usually arise in the lining of the uterus and begin to grow and invade the uterine wall. The uterus is located in the pelvis between the bladder and rectum. It is divided into three parts: the body, cervix, and fundus. The three inner layers of the uterus are divided into the serosa (parietal peritoneum), myometrium (smooth muscle), and endometrium (mucous membrane). Endometrial cancers originate from the endometrium layer of the uterus. This layer is greatly affected by fluctuations in estrogen levels. Most cases of endometrial cancer affect postmenopausal women at the age of 55 years and older. Incidence rates of endometrial cancers are higher among white women, but black women have a higher mortality rate.[3]

Most endometrial cancers are adenocarcinomas, which account for more than 80%. Less frequently seen endometrial cancers include clear cell, papillary serous, mucinous, and squamous cell. Uterine sarcomas are rare but are the most malignant. Papillary serous adenocarcinoma is also an extremely malignant form of endometrial carcinoma that tends to spread rapidly and widely throughout the abdominal cavity and is usually associated with a poor survival outcome. Clear cell adenocarcinoma has similar characteristics.

Etiology

Endometrial cancers are hormone-related cancers, so risk factors result from the female hormone estrogen. The major risk factor for endometrial cancers is a high cumulative exposure to estrogen that is not hindered by progesterone.[21] Because of this risk factor, standard practice is to prescribe estrogen with progesterone. Estrogen replacement therapy and obesity are two important factors that increase estrogen exposure. Obese women have a threefold to fivefold higher risk of developing endometrial cancer. Other risk factors include estrogen replacement without progesterone, never giving birth (nulliparity), late menopause, early menarche, irregular menstruation, diabetes, and a history of infertility. Women taking tamoxifen are at a higher risk for endometrial cancers, as are those with hereditary colon cancer.[21]

Clinical Presentation

Endometrial adenocarcinoma most commonly presents with postmenopausal bleeding. Approximately one-third of postmenopausal bleeding is cancer related, specifically cervical or endometrial. Most endometrial cancers are diagnosed in stage I (Table 32.3); more advanced disease presents with hematuria, hematochezia, constipation, lower extremity edema, pain, and abdominal distention. Recent studies have highlighted the increased risk of endometrial cancer in women who take the drug tamoxifen, which has led some to suggest that surveillance of this subset of patients is warranted.[3] Most endometrial cancers are early stage; 80% of patients present with stage I disease. Poor prognostic factors include higher grade, increased depth of invasion into the myometrial muscle, lymph node involvement, and lymphovascular space invasion (LVSI) and size of tumor. LVSI occurs when cancer cells invade blood vessels or lymph channels.

Screening

Currently, no screening test for endometrial cancer is recommended for asymptomatic women. Endometrial biopsy is 90% accurate in the detection of cancer but is not recommended for screening. A physical examination is important to inspect and palpate the vulva, the vagina, and the cervix to rule out metastatic disease. Pap smears may raise some suspicion of endometrial cancers but do not diagnose this type of cancer. Women with high risk factors should be placed under close surveillance by their physicians. The ACS recommends that at the time of menopause, physicians educate women about the risks and symptoms of endometrial cancers. Women should be counseled to report unexpected bleeding or spotting. For women who are at high risk, an annual biopsy may be done starting at the age of 35 years.

Detection and Diagnosis

The gold standard method for the evaluation of symptomatic women is fractional dilation and curettage. However, endometrial biopsy and aspiration curettage can be a less invasive option. Pathologic examination is essential for a definitive diagnosis of endometrial cancer. A thorough history is taken, and a physical examination is performed. An ultrasound scan can be used in some cases to evaluate the thickness of the endometrial cavity.

Imaging Studies

After the diagnosis of endometrial cancer is confirmed, imaging studies are ordered to determine staging and the extent of disease. These diagnostic studies may consist of an ultrasound scan, a chest x-ray, PET, a CT scan, MRI, a cancer antigen 125 (CA-125) blood test, cystoscopy, proctoscopy, or surgical staging. A chest x-ray is ordered if metastatic spread to the lungs is suspected. A transvaginal ultrasound scan evaluates the thickness of the endometrium, which may indicate cancer invasion into the myometrial layer of the uterus. PET and CT scans are useful in the accurate determination of the locations of metastatic spread. CA-125 levels are used to predict which patients are predisposed to invasive or extrauterine disease. Cystoscopy and proctoscopy examinations are used to determine any cancer spread to the bladder or rectum.

Staging

Adenocarcinoma is the most common type of endometrial cancer. Papillary serous adenocarcinoma is a highly malignant form of endometrial cancer that spreads rapidly throughout the abdominal cavity. This type of cancer yields a very poor prognosis. Uterine sarcomas are a rare type of endometrium carcinoma, and prognosis is correlated with the extent of disease at diagnosis (Table 32.3). Histologic grade is a good predictor of tumor spread and survival rates. For information on AJCC staging for endometrial cancer see https://www.cancer.org/cancer/endometrial-cancer/detection-diagnosis-staging/staging.html. Accessed November 19, 2019

Metastasis

Spread to pelvic and paraaortic nodes is common in endometrial carcinomas. Lymphatic spread occurs initially to the internal and external iliac pelvic nodes. For stage I disease, about 10% of patients have nodes positive for tumor. This increases to between 25% and 35% for stage II disease, a poorly differentiated histology, or a deep myometrial invasion. About 20% can have positive paraaortic nodes and lymphovascular invasion without pelvic involvement. If pelvic nodes are involved, the chance of paraaortic node involvement is 60%.

Treatment Modalities and Consideration

The most important prognostic factors at diagnosis are stage, grade, depth of invasive disease, LVSI, and histologic subtype. LVSI is a predictor of nodal disease and a prognostic indicator for disease recurrence in all stages of endometrial cancers. Treatment can involve surgery or radiation therapy, depending on the stage, grade, and medical condition of the patient. In early-stage cancers, surgery alone or in combination with adjuvant therapies can yield definitive results.

Surgical management of endometrial cancers includes a total hysterectomy and bilateral salpingo-oophorectomy with or without lymphadenectomy. Salpinges-oophorectomy is the surgical removal of the fallopian tubes and ovaries. Widespread debate still exists about the benefits of lymphadenectomy in terms of overall survival. Adjuvant therapies, such as postoperative radiation and chemotherapy, are considered for high-grade tumors. Clinical trials show an improvement in local control with postoperative radiation but not overall survival. The radiation modality used is external beam radiation or intracavitary brachytherapy.

Irradiation alone may be used for patients with medically inoperable conditions. Preoperative EBRT is not commonly used but may be beneficial in patients with extensive disease of the cervix and vagina.[3]

Simulation and Treatment

Most endometrial cancers are seen after surgery. For stage IB, grades 1 and 2, and sometimes stage IA, grade 2, a vaginal cylinder or colpostats alone are used to treat the vaginal cuff. Typical low-dose-rate brachytherapy doses, a 60-Gy to 70-Gy surface dose in two treatment sessions, or high-dose-rate brachytherapy dose fractions of 7 Gy to a 0.5-cm depth are prescribed for three treatment sessions (Table 32.4). For stage IB or higher or for grade 3 disease, an increased risk of pelvic nodal involvement exists and pelvic radiation therapy is given (see Table 32.4). Fields are similar to cervical fields. Heyman capsule techniques or an intrauterine tandem are used if the uterus is still present for implantation. For postoperative treatment, a domed cylinder or vaginal colpostats are used if brachytherapy is necessary. Pelvic nodal doses of 40 to 50 Gy are recommended, with boosting up to 65 Gy for gross involvement. The endometrial cavity can be taken to 75 to 90 Gy with combined external beam therapy and low-dose-rate brachytherapy, but the bladder and rectum must be kept to about 65 to 75 Gy or less, and the small bowel must be kept at or below 45 to 50 Gy if treatment is with radiation therapy alone. High-dose-rate brachytherapy may also be used with equivalent doses. Simulation with CT guidance is needed for the pelvic external beam treatment and possibly also for the brachytherapy portion, but image-guided treatment planning is increasingly used.

OVARIAN CANCER

Epidemiology

Ovarian cancer is the fifth most common cancer among women in the United States and the leading cause of death from gynecologic cancers. The ACS estimates about 22,250 new cases and 14,100 deaths from ovarian cancer are expected each year.[2] Ovarian cancer primarily presents in older women, with roughly half in women 63 years old or older. Most patients with ovarian cancers present with advanced disease, which is attributed to nonspecific symptoms. White women have ovarian cancer more frequently than do black women. Ovarian cancer originates in the tissue of the ovaries, which produces an ovum each month. There is an ovary located several centimeters to the left and right of midline within the pelvis. Most ovarian cancers are either epithelial carcinoma or malignant germ cell tumors, which are more prevalent in younger women.

Etiology

The etiology of ovarian cancer is not well understood. Many theories have been postulated about the causation of ovarian cancer; however, none have been validated. Ovarian cancer risk factors include: nulliparity, early menarche, smoking, immunosuppression, family history of breast or ovarian cancer, pelvic inflammatory disease, first childbirth after age 35 years, late menopause, and Jewish descent. Specifically, Ashkenazi Jewish women have a higher risk of ovarian cancer than the general population because of hereditary mutations of the BRACA1 and BRACA2 genes. Women with mutations of these genes are more predisposed to the development of ovarian cancer. However, the most significant risk factor is advancing age, followed by family history. Women at high risk for ovarian cancers should consider risk-reducing methods. Oral contraceptives (combined with progesterone), hysterectomy, and prophylactic oophorectomy have been noted in a number of studies to reduce the risk of ovarian cancer.

Clinical Presentation

Most women are not diagnosed until symptoms develop as the disease progresses, which is most commonly in stage IIIC. The most common presenting symptoms are abdominal or pelvic pain, abdominal distension caused by ascites, and vague gastrointestinal symptoms. Symptoms are usually a result of the mass itself or ascites. Early-stage cancers can be discovered during routine examinations as a palpable mass in asymptomatic women. Ovarian cancer is most common in women between the ages of 50 and 70 years. CA-125 is a poor screening tool for early-stage ovarian cancers but extremely useful as a prognostic indicator to monitor the effectiveness of chemotherapy in ovarian cancers.

Screening

The high mortality rate of ovarian cancer is associated with the fact that more than 70% of ovarian cancers are advanced stage at diagnosis. A strong correlation is found between the stage of cancer and survival outcome. Five-year survival rates for women with late-stage ovarian cancer range from 20% to 30%; conversely, women diagnosed with earlier-stage disease have cure rates that range from 70% to 90%.[14] Currently, no recommended screening exists for the general population. Transvaginal ultrasound scan and CA-125 blood tests are most often

TABLE 32.3	**FIGO Staging for Endometrial Cancer**
FIGO Stage	**Definition**
I	Tumor confined to the corpus uteri, including the endocervical glandular involvement
IA	Tumor confined to the endometrium or invading less than half of the myometrium
IB	Tumor confined to uterus, ≥50% myometrial invasion
II	Cervical stromal invasion but not extending beyond the uterus
III	Tumor invasion into serosa, adnexa, vagina, or parametrium
IIIA	Tumor involving the serosa and or the adnexa (direct extension or metastasis)
IIIB	Vaginal or parametrial involvement
IIIC1	Pelvic node involvement
IIIC2	Paraaortic node involvement
IVA	Tumor invasion into bladder or bowel mucosa
IVB	Distant metastases (including abdominal metastases) or inguinal lymph node involvement

FIGO, International Federation of Gynecology and Obstetrics.
Based on International Federation of Gynecology and Obstetrics treatment of carcinoma of the corpus uteri.[9,15]

TABLE 32.4	**Postoperative Treatment**		
	G1	**G2**	**G3**
None		± Brachytherapy	Brachytherapy
<50%	± Brachytherapy	Brachytherapy	Brachytherapy ± External beam radiotherapy: whole pelvis irradiation
≥50%	Brachytherapy ± External beam radiotherapy: whole pelvis irradiation	Brachytherapy ± External beam radiotherapy: whole pelvis irradiation	Brachytherapy + External beam radiotherapy: whole pelvis irradiation

used to screen women with high risk factors for ovarian cancer. These tests are inadequate for detection of early-stage ovarian cancer; they lack sensitivity and specificity.[14] Studies show that CA-125 is elevated in 75% to 90% of patients with advanced disease but in only 50% of patients with stage I disease. For ovarian cancers, no improved survival benefit is seen with undergoing screenings.[3,18]

Detection and Diagnosis

Patients suspected of ovarian cancer should undergo a physical examination, including a pelvic examination, complete blood count, CA-125 blood test, and diagnostic imaging studies.[18] CT scan, MRI, ultrasound, and chest x-rays can be ordered to evaluate metastatic disease. Clinicians must acquire a detailed history to identify women at high risk for ovarian cancers. Ovarian cancer is a surgically staged disease. Biopsies can be obtained through a laparotomy, which provides a thorough evaluation of the ovaries and surrounding anatomy. During exploratory laparotomy, debulking can be performed in cases of advanced disease to remove the tumor and areas of involvement. After surgery, a definitive diagnosis can be ascertained and adjuvant therapies planned.

Staging

Staging is based on the FIGO and the AJCC methods of TNM staging. Poor survival rates are associated with increased staging[16,19] (Tables 32.5). For more information on the AJCC staging system for ovarian cancer see https://www.cancer.org/cancer/ovarian-cancer/detection-diagnosis-staging/staging.html. Accessed November 19, 2019

Metastasis

Advanced disease typically spreads through direct extension of adjacent organs, peritoneal fluid, or lymph nodes. Hematogenous spread is rare. About 80% of patients with ovarian cancers present with abdominal cavity involvement. Ovarian cancer cells exfoliate into fluid in the peritoneal cavity, which is called peritoneal seeding. Pelvic or paraaortic lymph nodes are frequently involved in lymphatic spread. Ovarian

cancers can metastasize via direct spread to the neighboring uterus, ovaries, and fallopian tubes and colon. Distant metastasis can occur with spread to the liver, lung, diaphragm, bladder, or colon.

Treatment Modalities and Consideration

Surgery plays a vital role in the management of ovarian cancers. Surgery and adjuvant chemotherapy are most commonly used as treatment options. The primary treatment for early-stage ovarian cancer is a TAH and bilateral salpingo-oophorectomy with surgical evaluation for staging. In some cases, one ovary can be spared to preserve fertility. Chemotherapy is administered after surgery. The role of radiation therapy in early-stage ovarian cancer is controversial. Radiation therapy has not been proven to improve survival outcomes or recurrence rates. Traditionally, whole abdominal radiation or radioisotope P-32 were used as adjuvant postoperative treatments. Today, adjuvant chemotherapy has replaced whole abdominal radiation and radioisotopes for ovarian cancers. Radiation therapy, however, may have a role in isolated nodal recurrence of ovarian cancer after chemotherapy. Palliative radiation may be a useful therapy for recurrent or metastatic disease. It can be used to alleviate symptoms such as bleeding, pain, or obstructions.

Simulation and Treatment

Ovarian fields are also treated after surgery after staging and optimal debulking by the gynecologic oncologist. The entire peritoneal cavity must be covered with an open-field technique that extends from the diaphragm to the pelvic floor. When no liver shielding is used, the upper abdominal dose is limited to 25 to 28 Gy in 1.0-Gy to 1.2-Gy fractions. Partial renal blocking is used to limit the dose to a total of 18 to 20 Gy. The pelvis is then boosted up to a total dose of 50 Gy at 1.8 Gy/fraction. Higher-energy photons are recommended with AP/PA fields to limit the dosage variation to less than or equal to 5%. This is rarely done today because of high toxicities to critical organs in the abdominal region.

VULVAR CANCERS

Epidemiology

Approximately 6,200 women in the United States are expected to be diagnosed with cancer of the vulva each year, and an estimated 1200 will die of this disease.[2] Vulva cancers are uncommon malignancies that account for 4% of all gynecologic cancers and less than 1% of all cancers in women. This is primarily a disease of elderly women, with more than half of the cases occurring in women over the age of 70 years.[2] It is worth noting another age group is composed of patients under the age of 40 years. The vast majority of vulvar tumors are squamous

TABLE 32.5 International Federation of Gynecology and Obstetrics Staging and Survival Rates for Ovarian Cancer

FIGO Staging	5-Year Survival Rates
STAGE I	
Tumor confined to ovaries	
IA: Involves one ovary (capsule intact); no tumor on ovarian surface; no malignant cells in ascites or peritoneal washings	90%
IB: Involves both ovaries (capsule intact); no tumor on ovarian surface; no malignant cells in the ascites or peritoneal washings	86%
IC: Tumor limited to one or both ovaries with any of the following: capsule ruptured, tumor on ovarian surface, malignant cells in ascites or peritoneal washings	83%
STAGE II	
Tumor involves one or both ovaries with pelvic extension	
IIA: Extension or implants on uterus or fallopian tubes or ovaries	71%
IIB: Extension or implants onto other pelvic structures	66%
STAGE III	
Tumor involves one or both ovaries with spread to the peritoneum or metastasis to retroperitoneal lymph nodes	
IIIA: Microscopic peritoneal metastases beyond the pelvis or limited to the pelvis with extension to the small bowel or omentum	47%
IIIB: Macroscopic peritoneal metastases beyond the pelvis less than 2 cm in size	42%
IIIC: Macroscopic peritoneal metastases beyond pelvis greater than 2 cm or lymph node metastases	33%
STAGE IV	19%
Distant metastases excluding peritoneal metastasis	

Based on the International Federation of Gynecology and Obstetrics for treatment of carcinoma of the ovary.[15]

TABLE 32.6 International Federation of Gynecology and Obstetrics Staging for Vulvar Cancer

FIGO Staging

STAGE I

IA: Tumor confined to the vulva or perineum, ≤2 cm in size with stromal invasion ≤1 mm, negative nodes

IB: Tumor confined to the vulva or perineum, >2 cm in size or with stromal invasion >1 mm, negative nodes

STAGE II

Tumor of any size with adjacent spread (one-third lower urethra, one-third lower vagina, anus), negative nodes

STAGE III

IIIA: Tumor of any size with positive inguinofemoral lymph nodes, 1 lymph node metastasis greater than or equal to 5 mm, 1 to 2 lymph node metastasis(es) of less than 5 mm

IIIB: 2 or more lymph nodes metastases greater than or equal to 5 mm, 3 or more lymph nodes metastases less than 5 mm

IIIC: Positive node(s) with extracapsular spread

STAGE IV

IVA: Tumor invades other regional structures (two-thirds upper urethra, two-thirds upper vagina), bladder mucosa, rectal mucosa, or fixed to pelvic bone

IVB: Any distant metastasis including pelvic lymph nodes

Based on International Federation of Gynecology and Obstetrics for treatment of vulvar cancer.
FIGO, International Federation of Gynecology and Obstetrics.

cell carcinomas that grow slowly. Generally, these cancers remain in a precancerous state referred to as vulvar intraepithelial neoplasm (VIN) for years before progressing to squamous cell carcinoma. Squamous cell carcinomas represent the majority of vulvar cancers. The most common site for these carcinomas is the labia minora and majora, but they can also be found on the clitoris and perineum. Vulvar cancers are palpable and should be diagnosed at an early stage; however, quite the opposite occurs, with 39% of patients diagnosed in an advanced stage. This may be attributed to the embarrassment that patients feel or misdiagnosis by clinicians.

Etiology

The cause of vulvar cancers is not clear, especially in older women. Recent research studies postulate that vulvar cancers can be categorized into two types of diseases.[13] The first type affects younger patients and is caused by HPV; the second type affects older women with a history of vulvar inflammation or lichen sclerosis. HPV 16 and 18 have been identified in the development of both vulvar and cervical cancers. Other risk factors include smoking, a history of genital warts, leukoplakia, immune system deficiency, multiple sexual partners, and sexual intercourse at a young age.

Clinical Presentation

Most women with precancerous conditions do not experience any symptoms. As vulva cancer progresses from VIN to more invasive stages, symptoms become more demonstrable. Women with vulvar cancers typically present with a history of pruritus, a palpable mass on the vulva, painful urination, and vaginal bleeding.[13] The disease is usually unifocal, with the labia as the most common location.

Detection and Diagnosis

Clinicians must acquire a detailed history and conduct a thorough pelvic examination. Annual gynecologic examinations can help detect tumors at an early stage. Tumors of the vulva usually appear raised, ulcerated, and wartlike or leukoplakic. A suspicious mass in the vulva region should be biopsied to make a definitive diagnosis.

Staging

According to the American Society of Clinical Oncology, squamous cell cancers of the vulva have a 5-year survival rate of 93% for early-stage disease. Conversely, most advanced-stage diseases have a modest 5-year survival rate of 29%. Adenocarcinomas have an extraordinary 5-year survival rate of 100% for early-stage disease; advanced disease yields a 74% survival rate. Prognosis is mainly determined by tumor staging at diagnosis.[22]

Vulva cancers can spread via direct extension to adjacent structures, regional lymph nodes, or hematogenous routes. As the depth of tumor invasion increases, the risk of metastasis to lymph nodes is more probable. Lymphatic node status is the most important prognostic factor for vulva cancers. The most common routes of spread of vulva cancers are through direct extension to adjacent organs or lymphatics. Vulvar cancers spread in a very orderly pattern from inguinal lymph nodes to pelvic lymph nodes. Hematogenous spread is rare.[22] (Table 32.6). For more information on AJCC staging for vulvar cancer see https://www.cancer.org/cancer/vulvar-cancer/detection-diagnosis-staging/staging.html. Accessed November 19, 2019

Treatment Modality and Consideration

The choice of treatment is dependent on the size, depth, and location of the tumor. Historically, radical vulvectomy was the standard of treatment for all vulva cancers. Although surgery is still the most common treatment for these cancers, more conservative approaches are being used. Most early-stage disease can be treated with a wide local excision, as opposed to the radical vulvectomies performed in the past. More invasive disease with positive inguinal lymph nodes is treated with a wide local incision and an inguinofemoral lymphadenectomy (nodal dissection) or postoperative radiation. Radiation has shown a clear benefit as an adjuvant therapy in patients with two or more nodal metastases.[13]

The role of radiation therapy in the treatment of vulva cancer is expanding. Preoperative radiation can be an option for patients with tumors close to critical structures (i.e., clitoris, rectum, urethra). In these cases, radiation can shrink tumors and salvage structures that would otherwise be injured or removed during surgery. Definitive radiation can be used to treat very large tumors, where surgery may not be possible. Postoperative radiation can be used for patients with positive nodes in the pelvic or groin region.

Simulation and Fields

Patients with vulvar cancers are usually simulated in the supine position with their legs in frog-leg position. Placing the legs in frog-leg position helps decrease dose to the soft tissues of the thighs. Bolus is used on the vulva to eliminate cold spots within the treatment area.

A wide anterior field may be used to treat the nodes, including the inguinal nodes, and a narrow posterior field used to protect the femoral

necks. The inguinal nodes are supplemented with electron fields anteriorly to make up for the dose that was missed by narrowing the posterior field. Intensity-modulated radiation therapy (IMRT) may also be used, as it can spare healthy tissues further, particularly skin, femoral necks, and bowel, and therefore reduce long-term complications associated with standard field radiation therapy for vulvar carcinoma. This is a difficult cancer to treat effectively.

VAGINAL CANCER

Etiology

The etiology of vaginal cancer is not well understood. A strong correlation exists between HPV and the development of vaginal cancer. Other risk factors include smoking, multiple sexual partners, sexual intercourse at an early age, sexually transmitted diseases, diethylstilbestrol exposure, immunosuppression, and a history of vaginal irritation.[10]

Epidemiology

Primary vaginal cancers are extremely rare malignancies. In the United States, approximately 5,200 women will be diagnosed, and about 1,350 will die of vaginal cancers each year.[2] Most vaginal cancers are the result of direct extension from other adjacent sites located in the pelvis. Most primary vaginal cancers are squamous cell carcinomas and occur primarily in women aged 70 years or older. Hispanic women are most at risk for this malignancy, followed by black women. Vaginal carcinomas most commonly appear in the upper one-third of the vagina.

Clinical Presentation

Most patients who present with vaginal intraepithelial neoplasms are asymptomatic at the time of diagnosis. Abnormal Pap smear results typically prompt a diagnosis. Invasive vaginal cancers most commonly cause abnormal bleeding or vaginal discharge after coitus or after menopause. Other symptoms include a painless mass, constipation, painful urination, and hematochezia.

Detection and Diagnosis

Clinicians must acquire a detailed history and conduct a thorough pelvic examination. Annual gynecologic examinations can help detect tumors at an early stage. Currently, no recommended screening exists for vaginal cancers. Vaginal cancers are surgically staged.

Treatment Modalities and Consideration

Early-stage vaginal cancers that are limited to the vagina can be effectively treated with radiation alone or with surgery. The most common strategy for delivery of radiation is through EBRT and brachytherapy (intracavitary). Patients with small stage IA tumors (<2 cm) can be effectively treated with brachytherapy alone. The entire vaginal wall is treated with a dose of 60 to 70 Gy. Larger tumors (>2 cm) are treated with a combination of EBRT and brachytherapy. Studies reveal improved tumor control with combined radiation therapy treatments than with brachytherapy or external radiation alone. The whole pelvis receives a dose of 40 to 50 Gy with a conventional technique followed by brachytherapy. Great consideration is given to boost the parametrium in cases of extensive disease. For patients with more advanced disease, EBRT and brachytherapy are recommended to a dose of 70 to 80 Gy.[3]

Intracavitary brachytherapy is performed with the use of a vaginal cylinder loaded with cesium or iridium radioactive sources. These cylinders are inserted into the vagina.

Methods of Delivering Radiation and Concurrent Chemotherapy. IMRT provides a means to deliver external beam radiation while modulating the dose and sparing more healthy tissue. IMRT allows for dose escalation to the gross disease, which consequently improves the probability of tumor control. IMRT is used for all types of gynecologic cancers, particularly in the postoperative setting, in patients who need extended field radiation because of positive nodes and in patients with vulvar carcinoma. However, one has to be careful with the use of IMRT; because of the tight margins, there is a higher potential to miss the target. Organ motion and setup discrepancies need to be accounted for when planning margins for target volumes for IMRT.

In 1999, five studies showed that concurrent chemotherapy with radiation therapy was better than radiation alone in patients with cervical carcinoma. Soon after the results were published, the National Cancer Institute published guidelines recommending the use of concurrent cisplatin with radiation therapy in the treatment of cervical carcinoma. Therefore, standard treatment in the United States for patients with locally advanced cervical cancer is concurrent weekly cisplatin and pelvic or extended field radiation therapy. These results have been extrapolated for other cancers, including vulva and vagina cancers. For endometrial carcinoma, the sequencing of chemotherapy and radiation therapy is controversial. Some centers give concurrent chemotherapy and radiation followed by more chemotherapy; others use a "sandwich" approach, where the patient receives chemotherapy for three courses followed by radiation therapy and then three more courses of chemotherapy; and other centers give six courses of chemotherapy followed by radiation therapy.

Treatment Side Effects

Radiation therapy treatment requires a unique understanding of the radiosensitivity of the various gynecologic structures and their lymphatic drainage. The vulva and perineum usually show the most acute side effects, partially because of the radiosensitivity of these structures and the quality of the treatment beams used for treatment. Treatment doses near 70 Gy can cause considerable fibrosis. The response of an organ to radiation depends on dose, type of tissue, and volume of tissue exposed to radiation. The dose response of organs depends on the dose and volume of tissue exposed to radiation. The dose tolerance of the vagina is high, reaching doses of 100 Gy before extensive fibrosis is caused. The uterus and cervix can also tolerate high doses of radiation, which facilitates the effective delivery of brachytherapy to these organs. The ovaries are the most radiosensitive structures. Age appears to be a significant factor in the dose response of radiation to the ovaries. For example, a dose of 4 to 5 Gy produces permanent cessation of menstruation or menopause in about 65% of women younger than 40 years, in 90% of women 40 to 44 years, and in 100% of women older than 50 years. Many other critical structures that surround the gynecologic region should be considered when delivering radiation. The bladder is located anterior to the vagina and cervix and inferior to the uterus; it expands forward and away from these structures when filled. A dose of 30 Gy to the whole bladder or 75 to 80 Gy to a part of the bladder causes acute cystitis. This acute condition results in bladder irritation with dysuria, frequency, and urgency. Chronic cystitis can occur with doses above 50 to 60 Gy. The rectum is located posterior to the vagina and cervix, with a whole organ dose tolerance of 60 Gy. Acute symptoms such as diarrhea, bleeding, urgency, and pain begin at 30 to 40 Gy. Stricture, bleeding, and perforation are late effects that occur when dose exceeds tolerance levels. The small bowel may sometimes drop down into the pelvis and lie on top of the uterus and bladder. The tolerance dose of the small bowel is 45 Gy.

Management of Symptoms

Acute side effects of pelvic radiation therapy include fatigue, diarrhea, dermatitis, and dysuria. Fatigue may develop as early as the first week of treatment, and it could be exacerbated or complicated by anemia and depression as the patient continues to come to terms with the disease. Rest, reassurance, adequate nutrition, and antidepressants may make the course of treatment more tolerable. Anemia, as a result of blood loss or from disease treatment, should be corrected, especially if the patient is symptomatic, to a hemoglobin level above 10 g/dL and ideally above 11 g/dL. Diarrhea usually occurs the second or third week of treatment and is related to large and small bowel treatment. The addition of chemotherapy can significantly worsen this problem. Low-fiber diets, sucralfate (Carafate Axcan Pharma, Birmingham, AL) as a small bowel–coating agent, diphenoxylate (Lomotil, Pfizer, New York, NY), and loperamide are useful in alleviating this problem. Exclusion of as much bowel as possible from the radiation therapy fields also helps. This is done with the use of belly boards, the prone position with a full bladder on smaller fields, MLC shielding, serial field size reduction, and increasingly, IMRT.

> Reducing the dose to the small bowel is important in reducing side effects to the gastrointestinal tract. The use of belly boards, positioning the patient prone to displace the small bowel, and treating with a full bladder all help to reduce the dose to normal tissues in the pelvis.

Other acute effects of treatment of pelvic fields include nausea and upper gastrointestinal bleeding. Nausea can be treated prophylactically with agents such as prochlorperazine (Compazine, GlaxoSmithKline, Philadelphia, PA) or granisetron (Kytril, Roche Pharmaceuticals, Nutley, NJ), and gastritis can be treated with H_2 blockers (e.g., Tagamet, Zantac, Pepcid, and Axid), sucralfate, or other acid inhibitors. Dermatitis is more common with treatment with low-energy beams, with AP/PA only fields, with perineal flash, or with use of bolus when indicated, and with concomitant chemotherapy. Domeboro soaks, Aquaphor ointment, and natural care gels can lessen the severity and speed healing. The prevention and early treatment of local infection and correction of anemia and nutritional problems may also speed skin healing.

Dysuria usually occurs during the third or fourth week of treatment and can be lessened by treatment with a full bladder, partial bladder exclusion, and maintenance of a partially full bladder during brachytherapy. Medications such as phenazopyridine (Pyridium, Pfizer, New York, NY) and Urised can be used to anesthetize the bladder, or oxybutynin (Ditropan, ALZA Corporation, Vacaville, CA), hyoscyamine (Levsin), and terazosin (Hytrin) can be used to relax the bladder and relieve urinary frequency. Infections should be treated early and completely. Bleeding may also complicate the treatment as a result of anal irritation, bladder irritation, and hemorrhagic tumor. Rectal irritation can be treated with hemorrhoidal preparations, steroids, topical anesthetic agents, and sitz baths.

Late side effects can include menopause, vaginal dryness/narrowing/shortening, chronic cystitis, proctosigmoiditis, enteritis, and bowel obstruction. Use of replacement hormonal therapy may be considered, vaginal dryness can be treated with moisturizing agents such as Replens or hormonal creams, and shrinkage can be prevented with vaginal dilators or regular sexual activity. Chronic tissue inflammation or ulceration is treated with local medications, pentoxifylline (Trental, Sanofi, Paris), nutritional support, antiinflammatory agents, and pain medications. Bowel obstruction is treated surgically.

ROLE OF THE RADIATION THERAPIST

Treatment Delivery

The primary role of the radiation therapist in the control of these diseases is to perform the simulation and treatment delivery with precision and accuracy. Patient positioning is an important component. Radiation therapists must often rely on their own experience regarding the way to position a particular patient for optimal comfort and stability. The pelvis can present considerable difficulty for simulation and treatment reproducibility. Reminding the patient to maintain a full bladder when it is used to exclude the small bowel, encouraging the patient to remain on a low-residue diet when diarrhea is a problem, and remaining open and responsive to patient concerns helps to get the patient through treatment with positive outcomes (optimal cure) and minimal discomfort.

Patient Assessment

The radiation therapist is a critical link in patient assessment. The radiation therapist is in daily contact with the patient (more so than the physician or nurse), which allows monitoring of early changes in the patient's physical status. In addition, closer communication often exists between the patient and the radiation therapist compared with the physician or nurse. Concerns and observations should be communicated to the medical staff members initially for more in-depth assessment. In some institutions, standing orders are written with specific expectations for suggestions to the patient and communications with medical staff members. Knowledge of institutional policy is important.

The skin should be carefully assessed, especially beginning in the third week of radiation therapy. The infraabdominal, gluteal, and

inguinal folds are the earliest to show a skin reaction. The vulvar folds also exhibit an early skin reaction. Pelvic irradiation may cause diarrhea, with consequent weight loss and electrolyte imbalance. Loose or soft stools are common, but the primary concern is watery diarrhea, which should be communicated immediately to medical staff members.

Skin irritation and bowel irregularities are common outcomes of pelvic irradiation. Close monitoring of symptoms is necessary, and specific medical attention may need to be initiated in the event of increasing severity.

Reassurance

The radiation therapist has a responsibility to maintain a caring, professional atmosphere. Questions should be answered as much as knowledge permits, and medical staff should be kept aware of patient concerns and questions. Chart rounds are an excellent forum for this communication, but otherwise, the radiation therapist should communicate with the nurse, physician assistant, or physician.

SUMMARY

Gynecologic malignancies are common and may account for a significant proportion of the routine patient load at a radiation oncology facility. The basic knowledge presented here should enhance the radiation therapist's role in managing these cases while enabling a deeper understanding of the treatment rationale and potential outcome.

- The most common gynecologic cancer is endometrial, followed by ovarian, cervical, and other gynecologic cancers.
- Treatment options for gynecologic malignancies are the most diverse in the field of radiation therapy.
- The treatment design of gynecologic cancers must consider the extent of the primary lesion and the probability of metastases to the draining lymph nodes. Lymphatic drainage is adjoining, so if there is nodal involvement at one level, inclusion of the next higher nodal group in the treatment field may be reasonable.
- Lymphatic drainage includes the inguinal lymph nodes, pelvic nodes (the internal and external iliac chain), and periaortic nodes.
- The deep inguinal nodes drain into the external iliac chain, and the internal and external iliac chains join and then drain into the periaortic nodes.
- Ovarian and endometrial lymphatics run along the ovarian artery to the periaortic lymph nodes at the level of the kidneys and then progress to involve the inguinal lymphatics.
- The primary lymphatic drainage route of the cervix and some additional routes of the ovary and uterus are the external iliac, obturator, and hypogastric (internal iliac) lymphatic chains.

- The upper portion of the vagina follows the same lymphatic route as the cervix. The lower vagina follows the lymphatic drainage of the vulvar into inguinal nodes.
- The radiation therapist has three main functions during the course of therapy: treatment delivery, ongoing patient assessment, and patient reassurance.
- The radiation therapist is often more involved in the physical assessment of the patient than the physician is. Concerns and observations should be reported to the appropriate medical staff.
- Positioning a patient for treatment with regard for comfort and stability is dependent on the radiation therapist's own experience with that patient.
- Gynecologic radiation therapy treatment requires an understanding of the radiosensitivity of the various gynecologic structures. For instance, the most radiotolerant structure is the uteral canal, whereas the most radiosensitive is the ovary.
- Gynecologic radiation therapy planning requires consideration of lymphatic drainage patterns to ensure appropriate field coverage. Treatment design must also consider the extent of the primary lesion and probability of metastases to draining lymph nodes.
- Anemia is among the most common side effects of treatment, especially for cervical cancer. Hemoglobin restoration to optimal levels greatly increases treatment tolerability for the patient.
- Rest, reassurance, adequate nutrition, and antidepressants may help make treatment more tolerable for patients.

REVIEW QUESTIONS

The answers to the Review Questions can be found by logging on to our website at: http://evolve.elsevier.com/Washington/principles

1. Which of the following risk factors are associated with cervical cancer?
   I. HPV.
   II. Low socioeconomic status.
   III. Multiple sexual partners.
      a. I only.
      b. I and III.
      c. II and III.
      d. I, II, and III.
2. A rectal examination can often be used to determine local invasion of_____ cancer.
   a. Endometrial.
   b. Cervical.

   c. Ovarian.
   d. None of the above.
3. What is the most common gynecologic malignancy in the United States?
   a. Endometrial cancer.
   b. Vaginal cancer.
   c. Ovarian cancer.
   d. Cervical cancer.
4. What is the most common cause of gynecologic cancer deaths?
   a. Endometrial cancer.
   b. Vaginal cancer.
   c. Ovarian cancer.
   d. Cervical cancer.

5. A history of breast or colon cancer is a risk factor for development of which gynecologic cancer?
   a. Ovarian.
   b. Vulvar.
   c. Vaginal.
   d. Endometrial.

6. Which screening tool is responsible for the decreased incidence rate of cervical cancer?
   a. Mammogram.
   b. Pap smear screenings.
   c. Colposcopy.
   d. CA-125 screenings.

7. What is the most common presenting symptom in cervical cancer?
   a. Abnormal vaginal bleeding.
   b. Increased abdominal girth.
   c. Ascites.
   d. Satiety.

8. What are the risk factors associated with endometrial cancer?
   I. Obesity.
   II. Estrogen replacement therapy.
   III. Nulliparity.
   a. I only.
   b. I and II.
   c. II and III.
   d. I, II, and III.

9. The most common treatment for endometrial cancers is _____.
   a. Radiation.
   b. Chemotherapy.
   c. Surgery.
   d. Both a and c.

10. What is the rounded superior portion of the body of the uterus?
    a. Cervix.
    b. Fundus.
    c. Internal Os.
    d. Both a and c.

11. Cervical cancer that has spread outside the cervix and not to the upper third of the vagina and not to the pelvic sidewall is which stage?
    a. I.
    b. II.
    c. III.
    d. IV.

12. Which is true of a cervical cancer with a stage III classification?
    I. The cancer invades beyond the uterus but not to the pelvic sidewalls.
    II. The cancer involves the lower third of the vagina.
    III. Bladder or rectum involvement is possible.
    a. I.
    b. II.
    c. III.
    d. I, II, and III.

13. What is the most common histologic form of endometrial cancer?
    a. Squamous cell.
    b. Adenocarcinoma.
    c. Epithelial.
    d. Germ cell

REFERENCES

1. Corpus uteri. In: Edge SB, ed., et al. *American Joint Committee (AJCC) Cancer Staging Manual.* 7th ed. New York, NY: Springer; 2010: 406-407.
2. American Cancer Society. *Cancer Facts and Figures: 2018.* Atlanta, GA: American Cancer Society; 2018.
3. Halperin E, Wazer D, Perez C, et al. *Perez and Brady's Principles and Practice of Radiation Oncology.* Philadelphia, PA; Wolters Kluwer Health/ Lippincott Williams & Wilkins; 2013.
4. National Cancer Institute. *NIH fact sheet;* 2018. http://www.cancer. gov/types/uterine/hp/endometrial-treatment-pdq. Accessed November 5, 2018.
5. Mitrović-Jovanović A, Stanimirović B, Nikolić B, et al. Cervical, vaginal and vulvar intraepithelial neoplasms. *Vojnosanit Pregl.* 2011;68(12):1051–1056.
6. Centers for Disease Control. HPV-associated cancer statistics: 2011-2015. http://www.cdc.gov/cancer/hpv/statistics. Accessed November 5, 2018.
7. American Joint Committee on Cancer. *AJCC Cancer Staging Manual.* 8th ed. Chicago, IL Springer; 2017.
8. Sedlis A, Bundy BN, Rotman MZ, et al. A randomized trial of pelvic radiation therapy versus no further therapy in selected patients with stage IB carcinoma of the cervix after radical hysterectomy and pelvic lymphadenectomy: a *Gynecologic Oncology Group study. Gynecol Oncol.* 1999;73:177–183.
9. Colombo N, Preti E, Landoni F, et al. Endometrial cancer: ESMO clinical practice guidelines for diagnosis, treatment and follow-up. *Ann Oncol.* 2011;22(suppl 6):vi35–vi39.
10. Di Donato V, Bellati F, Fischetti M, et al. Vaginal cancer. *Crit Rev Oncol Hematol.* 2012;81(3):286–295.
11. Center for Disease Control. Cervical cancer. http://www.cdc.gov/cancer/cervical/. Accessed November 5, 2018.
12. Hacker N, Eifel P, van der Velden J. Cancer of the vulva. *Int J Gynaecol Obstet.* 2012;J119(suppl 2):S90–S96.
13. Rauh-Hain JA, Krivak TC, del Carmen MG, et al. Ovarian cancer screening and early detection in the general population. *Rev Obstet Gynecol.* 2011;4(1):15–21.
14. Lengyel E. Ovarian cancer development and metastasis. *Am J Pathol.* 2010;177(3):1053–1064.
15. Nezhat F, DeNoble S, Saharia P, et al. The safety and efficacy of laparoscopic surgical staging and debulking of apparent advanced stage ovarian, fallopian tube. primary peritoneal cancers. *JSLS.* 2010;14(2):155–168.
16. Pierce Campbell CM, Menezes LJ, Paskett E, et al. Prevention of invasive cervical cancer in the United States: past, present, and future. *Cancer Epidemiol Biomarkers Prev.* 2012;21(9):1402–1408.
17. Pignata S, Cannella L, Leopardo D, et al. Follow-up with CA125 after primary therapy of advanced ovarian cancer: in favor of continuing to prescribe CA125 during follow-up. *Ann Oncol.* 2011;22(suppl 8):viii40–viii44 .
18. Prat J. Staging classification for cancer of the ovary, fallopian tube. and peritoneum. *Int J Gynaecol Obstet.* 2014;124(1):1–5.
19. Saslow D, Solomon D, Lawson HW, et al. ACS-ASCCP-ASCP Cervical Cancer Guideline Committee: American Cancer Society, American Society for Colposcopy and Cervical Pathology, and American Society for Clinical Pathology screening guidelines for the prevention and early detection of cervical cancer. *CA Cancer J Clin.* 2012;62:147–172.
20. Trabert B, Wentzensen N, Brinton L, et al. Is estrogen plus progestin menopausal hormone therapy safe with respect to endometrial cancer risk? *Int J Cancer.* 2013;132(2):417–426.
21. Woelber L, Trillsch F, Mahner S, et al. Management of patients with vulvar cancer: a perspective review according to tumour stage. *Ther Adv Med Oncol.* 2013;5(3):183–192.

33

Male Reproductive and Genitourinary Tumors

Megan Trad

OBJECTIVES

- Recognize the route of lymphatic spread from the prostate.
- Compare and contrast the treatment techniques and modalities for prostate carcinoma along with associated pros and cons.
- Describe how computed tomographic scanning and improvements in treatment planning have enabled physicians to increase the dose delivered to the prostate.
- Recognize the importance of rectal and bladder filling in the treatment of prostate cancer and the need for daily prostate targeting.

- Discuss the treatment methods and techniques for patients with seminoma.
- List the routes of spread for renal cell carcinoma.
- Outline the principles of bladder-sparing radiation for bladder carcinoma.

OUTLINE

KEY TERMS

Bowen disease	Morphology
Bulbous urethra	Penile urethra
Corpora cavernosa	Prostate gland
Corpus spongiosum	Prostatic hypertrophy
Cryptorchidism	Smegma
Impotence	Trigone

PROSTATE

Epidemiology

Carcinoma of the prostate is the most common malignancy in males in the United States with approximately one in nine men having prostate cancer in their lifetime.[1] An estimated 164,700 new cases are diagnosed each year, and approximately 29,450 men die of the disease each year, making it the second leading cause of cancer-related deaths among men in America.[1] The incidence rate increases with each decade of life; more than 60% of prostate carcinomas occur in men 65 years and older, with an average age of diagnosis of 66 years.[1] Black men in the United States have one of the highest incidence rates of prostate cancer in the world, significantly higher than that of white men of comparable age.[1]

Prognostic Indicators

Tumor Stage and Histologic Differentiation. Strong prognostic indicators in prostate carcinoma are the clinical stage and pathologic grade of tumor differentiation. Larger and less-differentiated tumors are more aggressive and have a greater incidence of lymphatic and distant metastases.

Age. Conflicting reports have been published on age as a prognostic factor. Some reports indicate that men older than 70 years are most often diagnosed with a higher grade and stage of disease.[2] Other reports indicate that age does not determine the aggressiveness of the disease, and prognosis should be based on whether the risk category is low, intermediate, high, or very high for that particular patient.[3] It is known that men are at an increased risk as they get older and that it is rare for a man to be diagnosed with prostate cancer before the age of 40.[1]

Race. Black males have the highest incidence rate of prostate cancer. Black men are also more likely to be diagnosed at an advanced stage and also have the highest mortality rates.[1] For reasons unknown, Asian and Hispanic/Latino men have the lowest incidence rate of prostate cancer.[1]

Prostate-Specific Antigen Level. Several reports strongly suggest a close correlation between pretreatment and posttreatment prostate-specific antigen (PSA) levels and the incidence of failure-free survival.[4] PSA levels should be recorded over a length of time after treatment to gain a true picture of the success of the treatment. In the past, postradiation therapy nadir has been thought to be the main indicator of treatment success. The American Society for Radiation Oncology (ASTRO) has determined, however, that postradiation nadir cannot be a sole determinant in deeming treatment a success, a more accurate predictor also includes looking at Gleason score and staging in addition to the posttreatment PSA.[5] It can be inferred, however, that lower the posttreatment nadir, the lower the likelihood of PSA rising posttreatment.[5]

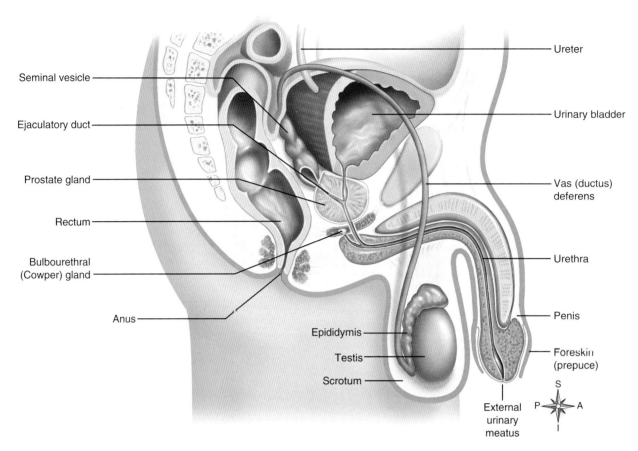

Fig. 33.1 Anatomy of the prostate in relationship to the bladder, rectum, and other surrounding structures. (From Thibodeau GA, Patton KT, eds. *The Human Body in Health and Disease.* 7th ed. St. Louis, MO: Mosby; 2018.)

Lymph Node Status. With the increased use of PSA, the need for lymph node dissection as a staging tool for prostate cancer has diminished. It has been found that for patients with favorable risk factors, the likelihood of regional lymph node involvement is less than 5%.[5] Patients who present with intermediate risk features have a 10% to 15% chance of having positive lymph node involvement, and likelihood increases to 40% to 50% for those patients who present with high-risk features.[5]

Anatomy. The prostate gland surrounds the male urethra between the base of the bladder and the urogenital diaphragm. The prostate is a walnut-shaped, solid organ that consists of fibrous, glandular, and muscular elements. It is attached anteriorly to the pubic symphysis by the puboprostatic ligament and separated posteriorly from the rectum by Denonvilliers' fascia (retrovesical septum), which attaches above to the peritoneum and below to the urogenital diaphragm. The seminal vesicles and vas deferens pierce the posterosuperior aspect of the gland and enter the urethra at the verumontanum (Fig. 33.1).

Natural History of Disease

Local Growth Patterns. Most prostate carcinomas are multifocal and develop in the peripheral glands of the prostate, whereas benign prostatic hyperplasia arises from the central (periurethral) portion. As the tumor grows, it may extend into and through the capsule of the gland, invade periprostatic tissues prand seminal vesicles, and if untreated, involve the bladder neck or rectum. The incidence rate of microscopic

tumor extension beyond the capsule of the gland, at the time of radical prostatectomy, in patients with clinical stages T1b/c or T2 disease, ranges from 10% to 50% and is also very much dependent on tumor grade and PSA. If allowed to progress, prostate cancer has been seen to invade the perineural spaces and regional and distant lymphatics, and metastasize to the bone or other organs.

Regional Lymph Node Involvement and Distant Metastases. The tumor size and degree of differentiation affect the tendency of prostatic carcinoma to metastasize to regional lymphatics.

As smaller, nonpalpable tumors are diagnosed with the use of PSA screening, the incidence of metastatic pelvic lymph nodes decreases. Lymphatic spread from the prostate is orderly, first involving the periprostatic and obturator nodes, followed by external iliac, hypogastric, common iliac, and paraaortic nodes (Fig. 33.2). Approximately 7% of patients have involvement of the presacral lymph nodes, including the promontorial and middle hemorrhoidal group, without evidence of metastases in the external iliac or hypogastric lymph nodes. Metastases to the paraaortic nodes occur in 5% to 25% of patients. Patients with pelvic lymph node metastases are more likely to have development of distant metastases than those with nodes negative for tumor. The incidence rate of distant metastases ranges from 20% in stage T1b to 90% in stage N1 to N3.

Clinical Presentation

Patients with prostate carcinoma may report decreased urinary stream, frequency, difficulty in starting urination, dysuria, and infrequently

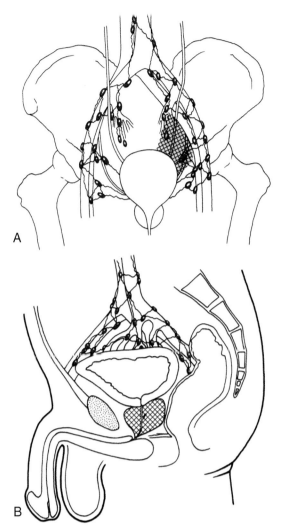

Fig. 33.2 (A) Location of lymph nodes most frequently involved in carcinoma of the prostate. The hatched area outlines the zone usually dissected in a limited staging lymphadenectomy. **(B)** Sagittal view. (A, From Perez CA. Prostate. In: Perez CA, Brady LW, eds. *Principles and Practice of Radiation Oncology*. 3rd ed. Philadelphia, PA: Lippincott-Raven; 1998.)

even hematuria. All of these symptoms can also be caused by conditions other than cancer, such as benign prostatic hypertrophy (enlargement of the prostate gland, which leads to narrowing of the urethra) and infection. Some tumors are diagnosed at the time of a transurethral resection (a surgical procedure of the prostate performed for lower urinary tract obstructive symptoms), although this procedure is performed much less often because of the efficiency of current medications. Bone pain or other symptoms associated with distant metastasis are seen less frequently at the time of the initial diagnosis.

More than 20 years ago, almost 40% of patients diagnosed with carcinoma of the prostate had M1 disease (distant metastasis). This number has been reduced to less than 5% through the increased awareness by the public and physicians of the disease and the growing use of PSA testing. The American Cancer Society suggests that men without a family history of prostate cancer begin screening at age 50 years. Earlier screening, around age 40 to 45 years, is suggested for men with a higher propensity for development of the disease.[3]

Detection and Diagnosis

Complete physical and rectal examinations are mandatory. A rectal examination is used to palpate the prostate and feel for any abnormalities or enlargements. It is also important in the evaluation of seminal vesicles. Although in most patients, the seminal vesicles cannot be palpated, a firm area that extends above the prostate suggests that the seminal vesicles are involved by malignancy. Approximately 50% of prostatic nodules found during rectal examination are confirmed to be malignant at the time of a biopsy.

The diagnosis of prostatic carcinoma can be obtained only through histologic confirmation. A transrectal ultrasound-guided needle biopsy is the standard method of diagnosis in the United States. This may also be done with blending or fusing of an MRI, where 12 or more core biopsies are taken. Generally the MRI scan is obtained before the biopsy (Box 33.1).

Much research has been done to determine whether diagnosis through transrectal ultrasound scan yields accurate results to eliminate the need for biopsy. In one long-term study on the evaluation of accuracy of ultrasound scan versus biopsy, research showed that 30% of cases showed some overlap of benign and malignant lesions.[6] Most believe that this level of inaccuracy is too high, and therefore, a biopsy is always necessary.[7] Also, with ultrasound scan, tumors less than 1 cm are difficult to detect.[8] Transrectal magnetic resonance imaging (MRI) is increasingly used in the evaluation of these patients.[9]

Screening. Carcinoma of the prostate can be asymptomatic until it reaches a significant size. An annual digital rectal examination of the prostate should be performed in all men older than 50 years. A digital rectal examination has a 70% sensitivity rate and 50% specificity rate in detection of prostate cancer. Radioimmunoassays for prostatic acid phosphatase, which have a sensitivity rate of only 10% and a specificity rate of 90% for malignant tumors, have been largely replaced by PSA testing.

Prostate-Specific Antigen Testing. PSA tests measure the amount of PSA, a specific protein in the blood that is produced by the prostate. PSA blood levels are routinely obtained in men older than 50 years. Tracking of PSA levels over time allows physicians to monitor rising levels and indicate a problem even before a tumor is detectable. PSA is not a tool to specifically identify cancer because it is present in healthy prostatic tissue, benign hyperplasia, malignant tumors, and seminal fluid. Although a normal PSA value, in general, is said to be 4 ng/mL or less, PSA level must be adjusted for age. However, more recent studies have shown that some men with PSA levels below 4.0 ng/mL have prostate cancer and that many men with higher levels do not have prostate cancer.

For a 49-year-old man, a normal PSA is 2.5 ng/mL or less, whereas a 70-year-old man has a low risk of prostate cancer with a PSA of 6.5 ng/mL. This is because as men age, prostate size increases, with higher PSA levels as a result of benign hypertrophy. An elevated PSA value with no palpable disease of the prostate (stage T1c) is now the most common presentation for this disease because of increased screening and awareness.

Prostate-Specific Antigen in the Selection of Patients for Therapy and Post-treatment Evaluation. Several studies have shown a close correlation between PSA levels and clinical and pathologic tumor stage and lymph node status, especially in conjunction with Gleason score and histologic tumor grade. A group of patients with PSA levels below 2.8 ng/mL and Gleason scores below 4 had an incidence rate of nodal disease or seminal vesicle involvement of approximately 1% at the time of prostatectomy, but 60% of patients with a PSA level above 40 ng/mL and a Gleason score above 8 had these findings (Fig. 33.3).[10] PSA is also of great value in the follow-up of patients treated with radical prostatectomy or radiation therapy.[13] In the months after a radical prostatectomy, for example, PSA levels should be undetectable.

Pathology and Staging

Most malignant tumors of the prostate are adenocarcinomas. Gleason devised a quantitative histologic grading system based on the morphologic tumor characteristics.[11] The pathologist evaluates the predominant degree of differentiation of the tumor (primary pattern) and the less frequent component (secondary pattern) based on the morphology of the lesion (e.g., glandular pattern, distribution of glands, stromal invasion; Fig. 33.4A). The primary and secondary tumor grades are each labeled from 1 to 5. The two grades are added for a Gleason score of 2 to 10. The Gleason score correlates closely with prognosis, with lower scores representing more slowly growing, nonaggressive tumors and higher scores their more invasive, metastatic counterparts (Fig. 33.4B). Perez and colleagues[15] found that the histologic differentiation of the tumor was strongly correlated with the incidence of distant metastases and survival but not as closely with locoregional failure.

Findings from the digital examination of the prostate and imaging studies determine the stage of the disease, which is classified according to the American Joint Committee on Cancer (AJCC).[13] (For more information on prostate cancer staging, see: https://www.cancer.org/cancer/prostate-cancer/detection-diagnosis-staging/staging.html.)

Stage T1 lesions are not detectable on digital rectal examination. T1a lesions are well-differentiated adenocarcinomas that are incidentally found during a transurethral resection of the prostate. They involve 5% or less of resected tissue. Stage T1b tumors are also subclinical, but they are more diffuse or have a larger volume, frequently with multifocal involvement of the prostate (>5% of tissue resected). T1c tumors are identified with a needle biopsy (e.g., because of elevated PSA levels).

Stage T2 tumors are palpable and confined within the capsule of the prostate gland. T2a tumors involve one lobe; T2b involve both lobes.

Stage T3 lesions are more locally extensive, beyond the edges of the prostate or into the seminal vesicles. T3a denotes extracapsular extension, either unilateral or bilateral. T3b indicates seminal vesicle invasion.

Stage T4 tumors are fixed to the pelvic sidewall or invade adjacent structures such as rectum or bladder. Regional nodal status is described

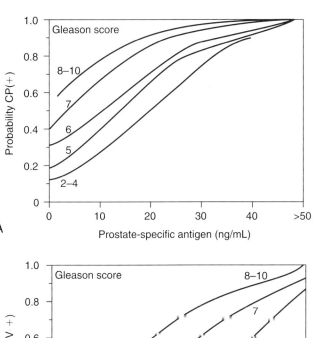

A

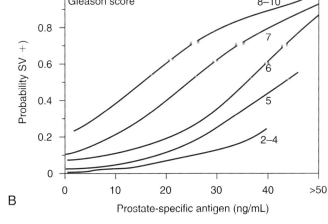

B

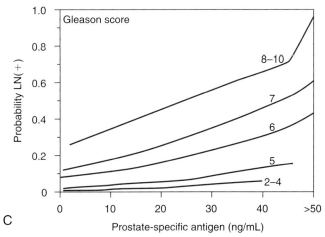

C

Fig. 33.3 (A) Probability of capsular penetration *(CP+)* as a function of the serum prostate-specific antigen (PSA) and preoperative Gleason score. (B) Probability of seminal vesicle involvement *(SV+)* as a function of the serum PSA and preoperative Gleason score. (C) Probability of lymph node involvement *(LN+)* as a function of the serum PSA and preoperative Gleason score. (From Partin AW, Yoo J, Carter HB, et al. The use of prostate specific antigen, clinical stage and Gleason score to predict pathological stage in men with localized prostate cancer. *J Urol.* 1993;150:110-114.)

as negative (N0) or positive (N1). Distant disease is designated M1a: nonregional nodes, M1b: bone, and M1c: other sites.

Whether prostate cancer is localized (T1 and T2), is more extensive (T3 and T4), or has metastasized to lymph nodes (N1) or distantly (M1) has great bearing on subsegment survival (Fig. 33.5).

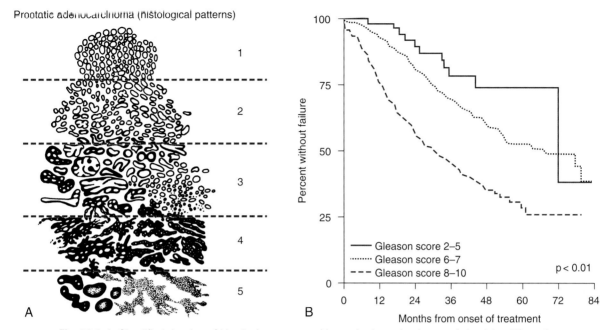

Prostatic adenocarcinoma (histological patterns)

Fig. 33.4 A. Simplified drawing of histologic patterns, with emphasis on the degree of glandular differentiation and relation to stroma. The all black area in the drawing represents the tumor tissue and glands with all cytologic detail obscured, except in the right side of pattern. B. Survival correlated with the Gleason score (N-566). (A. From Gleason DF, et al: Histologic grading and clinical staging of prostatic carcinoma. In Tannenbaum M, editor: Urologic pathology: the prostate, Philadelphia, 1977, Lea and Fabiger. B. From Pilepich MV, Krall JM, Sause WT, et al: Prognostic factors in carcinoma of the prostae. analysis of RTOG Study 75-06, Int J Radiat Oncol Biol Phys 13:339–349, 1987.)

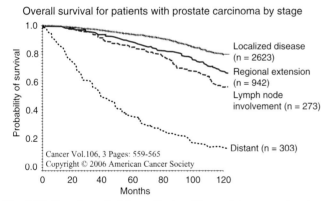

Fig. 33.5 Overall survival for patients with prostate cancer by stage. (From Taylor SH, et al. Inadequacies of the current American joint committee on cancer staging system for prostate cancer. https://www.ncbi.nlm.nih.gov/pubmed/16369982. Accessed November 5, 2019.)

Treatment Techniques

Many valid treatment options are available for patients with prostate cancer; these options span all treatment modalities, and all have an excellent prognosis if the cancer is caught early. Patients must be made aware of all of their treatment options and the long-term risks associated with each because the different forms of therapy can affect the quality of life and sexual function to varying degrees.

In general, localized carcinoma of the prostate has a fairly slow clinical course. The National Cancer Institute Consensus Development Conference on Management of Localized Prostate Cancer has concluded that radical prostatectomy and radiation therapy are equally effective treatments in appropriately selected patients for tumors limited to the prostate. However, based on patient and tumor characteristics, other valid options may be available.

Observation. Because in many cases, prostate cancer is such a slow-growing disease, watchful waiting (active surveillance) is a viable treatment option in some patients with specific staged disease or age. Several studies have reported on patients who, after a histologic diagnosis of prostatic carcinoma, were managed conservatively and monitored without specific anticancer treatment until symptoms developed.[14,15] The literature indicates that the tumors that are not poorly differentiated can have a protracted course associated with significant competing mortality and marginal benefit from therapy at 10 years.[14,15] Observation is a reasonable management for patients older than 75 years. It can also be offered to younger patients, 65 to 75 years old, with small, well-differentiated tumors. However, in today's health environment in the United States, most patients do not readily accept delaying definitive therapy unless they are very elderly with indolent-behaving disease or in very poor general health from other comorbidities.

According to many urologists, stage T1a disease, which is found incidentally, necessitates no treatment because it may take many years before the disease becomes a clinical problem. One recent study, however, documented that 34% or 110 of 324 patients who initially were managed with observation eventually underwent a second form of treatment.[3] According to the National Comprehensive Cancer Network, observation is a valid treatment option for patients who have a T1 to T2 staged tumor, Gleason score of 2 to 6, a PSA less than 10 ng/mL, and a life expectancy of more than 10 years.[15] Observation is also thought to be a valid treatment option if the patient presents with any stage disease but has a life expectancy of less than 5 years.[18]

Prostatectomy. Patients with resectable stage T1 or T2 prostate cancer who are in good general medical condition and have a life expectancy of at least 10 years are candidates for radical prostatectomy. Impetus has been given to the use of bilateral nerve-sparing surgery because an increasing number of tumors are diagnosed at earlier stages, and a lower incidence rate of sexual impotence (the inability to obtain an erection) has been reported with this surgery (15% to 80%, depending on the patient's age and tumor extent) compared with classic radical prostatectomy (close to 100%).[16] The most recent advancement in prostate surgery is the robotic-assisted laparoscopic prostatectomy. This procedure uses advanced cameras and robotic arms to perform the surgery through small incisions to minimize erectile and bladder side effects.

Patients diagnosed at stage T3 disease, or high-risk prostate cancer, have an increased risk of disease progression and cancer-related death. Because of this, radical prostatectomy alone is not efficient for disease control, and a secondary form of treatment including radiation therapy and hormone therapy is necessary.[17] PSA progression–free survival rate was 76% and overall survival rate was 78% at 5 years after treatment for patients treated with the combination therapy (radiation therapy plus hormonal therapy) versus 45% and 60%, respectively, for patients treated with radiation alone.[18]

Hormonal Therapy.
Although considered an ineffective form of treatment alone, hormone therapy plays a large role in halting the proliferation of prostate cancer cells by cutting off the supply of testosterone.[19] In 1941, Huggins, Stevens, and Hodges[20] reported prostate tumor regression and diminished serum acid phosphatase levels after orchiectomy or estrogen administration. Orchiectomy removes 95% of circulating testosterone and is followed by a prompt, long-lasting decline in serum testosterone levels. The introduction of drugs that mimic the removal of the testosterone source has since replaced this invasive and irreversible surgery.[19]

A prescription known as a maximal androgen blockade (MAB) is currently the mainstay of hormonal therapy and mimics the results of a bilateral orchiectomy. A MAB consists of an injection of luteinizing-releasing hormone (LHRH) and gonadotropin-releasing hormone receptor blockers given once monthly or every 3 months.[19] Some examples of LHRH drugs include leuprolide, goserelin, and triptorelin. These injections stop the production of testosterone. Antiandrogens are also given to block testosterone from reaching the prostate and are taken daily in the form of a pill. After patients' PSA levels have dropped to sufficiently low levels, patients may be allowed to discontinue hormone therapy as long as they continue to be evaluated.[19]

Hormonal therapy has long been used to reduce metastatic tumor burden and palliate symptoms; however, more recently, hormonal therapy has been added to radiation in locally advanced and high-grade tumors. The Radiation Therapy Oncology Group 86-10 and 92-02 studies have shown an advantage in disease control and survival with short-term hormonal administration (2 months before and during radiation) in bulky Gleason score 2 to 6 tumors and with long-term hormonal therapy (2 years) in Gleason score 8 to 10 tumors. Testosterone ablation appears to help by reducing tumor bulk locally while also controlling microscopic, clinically undetected metastatic disease.[21,22]

Chemotherapy.
Chemotherapy is limited in its use for prostate cancer to patients whose cancer has spread outside of the prostate or whose disease does not respond to hormone therapy. In 2011, the US Food and Drug Administration (FDA) approved the use of abiraterone acetate in the treatment of metastatic progressive prostate cancer. Abiraterone acetate was approved for use after clinical trials showed a medium overall survival of 14.8 months compared with 10.9 months in the placebo arm.[23] Following progression of disease during or after the use of abiraterone acetate, docetaxel plus prednisone has shown a response in PSA and pain relief and a small survival advantage in patients with metastatic disease.[23,24] Effective cytotoxic systemic treatment is thought to be necessary to truly eradicate the occult metastatic disease, which is prevalent in patients with locally advanced, poorly differentiated tumors.

External Radiation.
The treatment of prostate cancer with radiation therapy has progressed significantly over the years with the greater utilization of intensity-modulated radiation therapy (IMRT) and conformal beam therapy, which has increased survival rates to more than 90% in patients with low-stage disease and also minimized treatment-related side effects.[25] In planning for a course of radiation, a decision must first be made regarding treatment volume and whether the patient is at low risk or high risk for recurrence. A patient is considered high risk if the PSA concentration is greater than 20 ng/mL and has a Gleason score of 8 or higher and a tumor staging of T2c or greater according to the AJCC.[26] For patients with a good prognosis or low risk of recurrence (initial PSA, ≤10 ng/mL; Gleason, ≤6), 78% of patients with irradiation and 80% of patients with prostatectomy at 5 years after treatment were disease free with PSA criteria, which is the strictest and most objective measure. Recent studies have also found no significant difference in survival rates of high-risk patients who choose radiation therapy in conjunction with hormonal therapy over radical prostatectomy.[26]

Historical Use of Radiation Therapy in the Treatment of Prostate Cancer.
In the past, before extensive prostate cancer screening, the irradiation of pelvic lymph nodes was thought to be necessary to reduce the risk of metastasis. The inclusion of pelvic lymph nodes greatly increased the treatment portal size and minimized the dose able to be delivered to the prostate because of the side effects to the bladder and rectum.[27,28] A treatment technique known as a four-field box technique with lateral portals was commonplace and was used to treat pelvic lymph nodes along with the prostate gland and seminal vesicles. With this four-field box technique, the upper border was set at the midsacral level, and the lower border was determined by the inferiormost aspect of the prostate. The lateral margins of the anterior field were 1.5 to 2 cm from the lateral pelvic brim (Fig. 33.6A). For the lateral field, the anterior margin was 1 cm posterior to the projection of the anterior cortex of the pubic symphysis (Fig. 33.6B). The small bowel was spared anteriorly at the upper aspect of the field, mindful of the location of the external iliac nodes. The posterior border was generally at the posterior ischium, with shielding of the posterior rectal wall as appropriate. Barium or a plastic catheter with radiopaque markers was used to define the rectum if computed tomographic (CT) planning was not available. The position of the seminal vesicles was verified with CT scan, and the posterior field margin had to allow for coverage of these structures with adequate margin. Typical simulation films for a pelvic nodal field are shown in Fig. 33.7A and B. Field dimensions and blocking were then defined with CT scan contours and planning.

With this technique, field size was typically 15 × 15 cm at the patient surface (16.5 cm at the isocenter; see Fig. 33.6A). The reduced field for treatment of the prostate and seminal vesicles only was determined with CT scan, and therefore, size varied according to prostate and seminal vesicle size, usually in the range of 8 to 10 cm, including margins. A final cone down was also used to encompass only the prostate and minimize the dose to surrounding structures. The location varied as well but was generally related to the pubic symphysis. The inferior margin was determined with retrograde urethrogram, implanted marker, or CT scan.

The introduction of three-dimensional (3D) imaging has allowed for the escalation of dose to the prostate gland with minimization of the dose to the bladder and rectum. Three-dimensional conformal radiation therapy, IMRT, and image-guided radiation therapy (IGRT) are now the standards of treatment, which dramatically change the way patients are both treated and simulated.[29]

Simulation.
CT simulation is necessary in the creation of a 3D or IMRT treatment plan, which is currently the gold standard in prostate external beam irradiation. Before patients come into the simulator, they

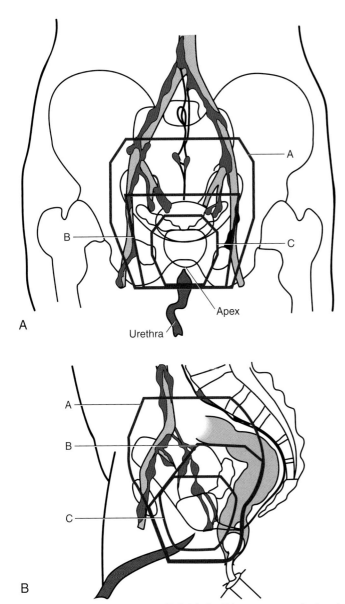

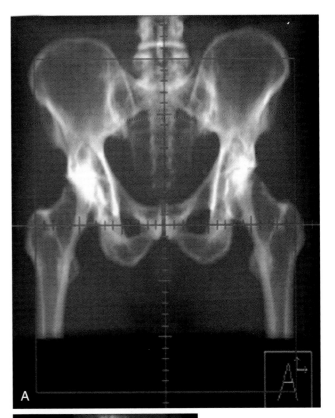

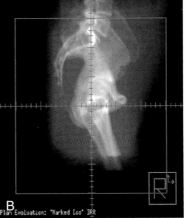

Fig. 33.6 **(A)** Anteroposterior (AP) fields for (A) prostate, seminal vesicles, and pelvic nodes; (B) prostate and seminal vesicles; and (C) prostate only. **(B)** Lateral fields for same regions. (From Kuban DA, El-Mahdi AM: Cancers of the genitourinary tract. In: Khan FM, Potish RA, eds. *Treatment Planning in Radiation Oncology.* Baltimore, MD: Lippincott Williams & Wilkins; 1998.)

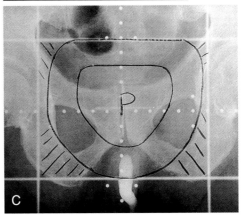

Fig. 33.7 (A) Anteroposterior (AP) projection and isocenter placement simulation films for computed tomographic scan planning. (B) Lateral simulation field. (C) AP urethrogram shows inferior field margin. (C, From Kuban DA, El-Mahdi AM. Cancers of the genitourinary tract. In: Khan FM, Potish RA, eds. *Treatment Planning in Radiation Oncology.* Baltimore, MD: Lippincott Williams & Wilkins; 1998.)

are asked to have an empty rectum and a full bladder. Some clinics, to better immobilize the bladder, insert a rectal balloon on a daily basis for treatment. If this is the case, the rectal balloon needs to be inserted during simulation as well. Patients are simulated in the supine position, and the construction of a leg immobilization device is carried out with a foaming cradle or a vacuum bag. CT images of the pelvis are taken in 3–5-mm thicknesses, with scanning superiorly below the diagram and inferiorly to midfemur. An isocenter is set within the prostate with the CT images. It is marked anteriorly and laterally, both right and left, with radiographic markers or BB's. The patient is then scanned every 3 mm with the same superior and inferior margins with care to scan through the plane of the BBs. The isocenter is tattooed on the patient at the three points (see Fig. 33.7A and B). Scans are then transferred to the treatment planning computer. Some facilities use bladder and urethral contrast to better visualize and avoid these structures in treatment planning.

Conformal Three-Dimensional and Intensity-Modulated Radiation Therapy Treatment Planning and Delivery. The development of sophisticated radiation treatment planning computers has allowed the planning CT scan to be reconstructed in three dimensions. The target (prostate or prostate and seminal vesicles) and the surrounding healthy structures can be anatomically defined. These organs are outlined on each CT slice. Margins are generally dependent on intended dose, setup error, and internal organ motion. The latter two may vary depending on external immobilization and techniques for correcting for internal prostate movement such as fiducial markers, rectal balloon, or transabdominal ultrasound scan (B-mode acquisition technology). In general, required margins on the clinical target volume (CTV) to achieve the planning target volume are usually in the range of 0.5 to 1.0 cm for conformal and IMRT techniques when daily preprostate localization is carried out. Treatment plans are constructed to deliver 76 Gy to 95% of the PTV volume.[25]

Because the prostate is located interior to the bladder and just anterior to the rectum, the prostate location should be verified daily before treatment. Bladder and rectal filling and slight differences in patient positioning on the treatment table can change the prostate position from day to day. Verification of the prostate location can be done in many ways. Some institutions use ultrasound imaging (B-mode acquisition technology [BAT]), as prostate, bladder, and rectum can all be seen on ultrasound scan. Patients are treated with a full bladder, which helps in visualizing the bladder-prostate interface and in moving the bladder out of the field. With proper alignment of the prostate within the radiation field, not only is the proper dose delivered, with marginal misses avoided, but also, the bladder and rectum are maximally spared. Another technique is the injection of a material into the peritoneum that will increase the space between the rectum and the prostate.[30] SpaceOAR Hydrogel is a substance that is injected in between the prostate and the rectum, increasing the space between them. The hydrogel remains in the body for 3 months and then is absorbed into the body and excreted during urination. Studies have identified that the use of SpaceOAR Hydrogel is associated with significantly less rectal pain during treatment as well as less long-term rectal complications.[30] Studies have also shown that patients using the gel were 78% more likely to retain sexual function and had less long-term urinary and bowel complications, which increased quality of life.[30]

Image-guided radiation therapy (IGRT) has become the most widely used treatment technique for the localization and treatment of the prostate with radiation therapy. With IGRT, therapists image daily before treatment and make small adjustments to the patient's setup to ensure that the patient is aligned identical to the treatment planning images. Exact daily alignment is more important than ever, as treatment planning has allowed for dose escalation and tighter margins around the prostate.[31]

Beam design may vary but typically uses five or six oblique treatment angles. A common technique is five fields that consist of right and left posterior oblique fields, right and left anterior oblique fields, and a posterior-anterior field. Treatment fields are shaped or conformed to the prostate with multileaf collimators (MLCs) designed by the computer plan (Fig. 33.8(B)). Volumetric-modulated arc therapy and tomotherapy have also been used to further spare healthy tissue. In these treatment techniques, gantry and collimator movement happen simultaneously so that treatment is delivered through a single or multiple arcs.

The introduction of CT has led to the ubiquitous use of IMRT, which is a more advanced technique that specifies the chosen dose to the tumor volume and acceptable dose levels for surrounding healthy structures such as bladder, rectum, and femoral heads. Although five to eight different beam angles are typically used, MLC settings change while each field is being treated, shielding the critical structures a

portion of the time and thus treating the tumor volume to a higher dose than the organs of lesser tolerance. Although this technique tends to produce extremely conformal fields with tight margins, inhomogeneity of dose tends to be greater, with differentials in the 5% to 15% range. Care must be taken that the highest doses are within the tumor volume and not in healthy structures where tolerance is exceeded. It is with this technique that doses of 80 Gy or more can be delivered to the prostate (Fig. 33.9). Dose-volume histograms (DVHs) must be constructed to determine the volume of the critical organs (rectum, bladder, and femur) receiving high doses (see Fig. 33.9E).

A word should be said about dose prescription. Care should be taken to define the prescription point. Up to a 5% difference can be found with standard conformal techniques and more for IMRT, depending on whether the total dose is prescribed to isocenter, the CTV, or the PTV. Although doses prescribed to isocenter may appear higher on paper, the dose to the CTV and PTV is actually considerably lower. For definitions of tumor and planning volumes, see Table 33.1. Conventional doses consist of 76 Gy in 38 fractions with 2.0 Gy per fraction. Clinical trials are investigating the use of hypofractionation with delivery of 70.2 Gy in 26 fractions at 2.7 Gy per fraction. With this hypofractionation scheme, the lower dose is estimated to be actually equivalent to delivery of 84.4 Gy in 2.0-Gy fractions. Although whether hypofractionation has any clinical benefit is still undetermined, it does shorten the treatment time by 2.5 weeks.[32] Further efforts have been made to increase the dose delivered to the prostate. The use of IGRT in combination with the modulated fields has allowed doses greater than 78 Gy to be successfully delivered.[31] Please refer to the IGRT section of Chapter 15 in this textbook for more information on this treatment technique.

Proton Therapy. Proton therapy is a form of external beam radiation therapy in the treatment of many cancers, including the prostate, that has grown in popularity over the last several years. Protons are positively charged particles and deposit their radiation differently than x-rays, which many argue offer considerable advantages over photon treatment.[33] Compared with an x-ray beam, a proton beam has a low "entrance dose" (the dose delivered between the surface and the tumor), a high dose designed to cover the entire tumor, and no "exit dose" beyond the tumor (Fig. 33.10A and B).[34] This unique characteristic gives proton therapy the ability to deposit a radiation dose in a precise manner and a specific location within the body, thus minimizing damage to the surrounding healthy tissue. This may lead to better cancer control with fewer side effects and long-term complications.

For this type of treatment, patients are treated from right and left lateral fields up to a dose of 76 to 82 Gy. Brass apertures are placed in the beams path to shape the beam to the desired field size. Because proton beams are sensitive to the amount and density of tissue traversed, lateral beams provide the most accurate, reproducible arrangement for prostate cancer therapy. Lateral beams are not always well suited to treatment of seminal vesicles, however. When seminal vesicles are involved, the beam arrangement needed to cover them treats far too much rectum because seminal vesicles wrap around the bladder posteriorly. Therefore, some patients with more extensive tumors, which necessitate seminal vesicle irradiation, may not be good candidates for proton therapy.

Much research in the recent years has compared the use of IMRT and proton therapy in the treatment of prostate cancer. Some studies identify as much as a 26% to 39% reduction in the risk of secondary malignant neoplasms in patients treated with protons versus IMRT treatment.[33] Other studies indicate a lack of beneficial findings in research of the two treatment modalities and even report that patients with IMRT had 34% fewer gastrointestinal (GI) problems.[35] Long-term follow-up of patients and more research are needed to better

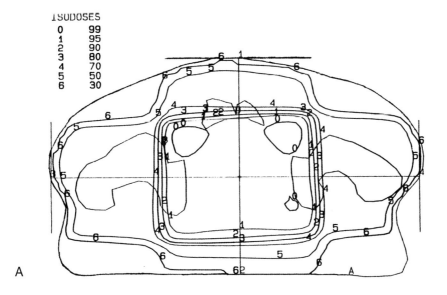

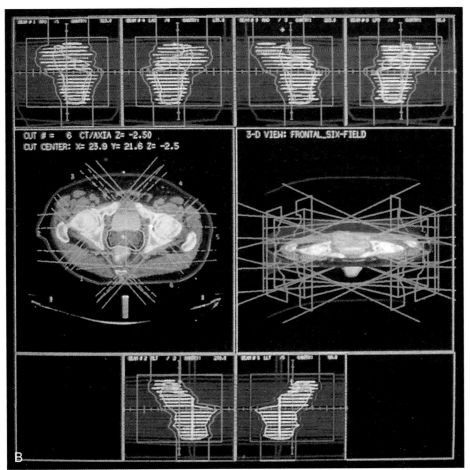

Fig. 33.8 (A) Historic four-field pelvic plan to include lymph nodes. **(B)** Dosimetry for a patient with favorable-risk prostate cancer generated by six contemporary conformal-based planning methods. Top row: left, four-field plan with lateral field reduction posteriorly at 46 Gy; right, 10-field conformal boost plan (as used in the MD Anderson dose-escalation trial). Middle row: left, seven-field conformal plan with 40% weighting of lateral fields, right, plan using the Peacock multileaf intensity-modulating collimator (MIMiC) to deliver intensity-modulated radiation therapy. Bottom: left, a seven-field conformal plan with 50% weighting of lateral fields; right, plan using multileaf collimation (MLC) for intensity-modulated radiation therapy. The prescribed dose was 75.6 Gy to the planning target volume, except in the 10-field conformal boost plan, in which the dose was prescribed to the isocenter. (From Lee AK, Pollac A. The prostate. In: Cox JD, Ang KK, eds. *Radiation Oncology: Rationale, Technique, Results.* St. Louis, MO: Mosby Elsevier; 2010:676-729.)

understand risks and benefits of each form of treatment, but currently, the standard treatment technique is IMRT. Please refer to Chapter 15 and 16 for more information on proton therapy.

Interstitial Brachytherapy. The introduction of the transrectal ultrasound scan in the late 1980s elevated low-dose-rate brachytherapy, and it now has been documented to have similar survival outcomes to radical prostatectomy and external beam therapy.[36] This procedure is done with either spinal or general anesthesia and uses a grid or template against the perineum with the patient in the dorsal lithotomy position. Transrectal ultrasound scan is used to direct the needles, which are either preloaded or attached to the Mick applicator that deposits the permanently placed radioactive seeds. Dosimetric

planning may be done in advance by taking ultrasound images every 5 mm from the base of the prostate through the apex and then loading these into the treatment planning computer. Seeds are then distributed throughout the prostate 1 cm apart. Isodoses are then computed (Fig. 33.11A and B).

Alternatively, this planning can be done in the operating room just before the procedure. In general, for the average gland, approximately 25 needles and 100 or so seeds are used. The commonly used permanent isotopes are I-125 (half-life, 60 days), Pd-103 (half-life, 17 days) and Cs-131 (half-life, 9.7 days). The usual dose for implant alone with ^{125}I is 160 Gy to the prostate plus margin.[36]

After implantation, patients return for a CT scan after a month and then every 3 months for the first year. PSA levels are also recorded

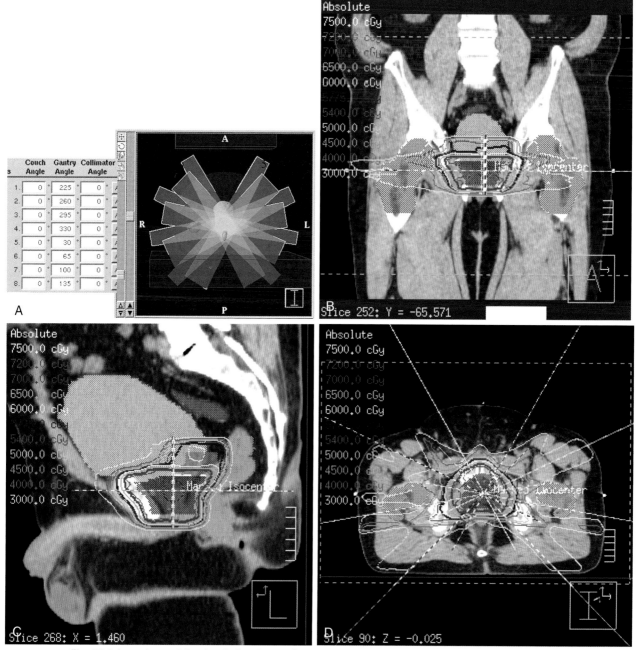

Fig. 33.9 Intensity-modulated radiation therapy for prostate cancer. (A) Beam angles (8). (B) Coronal dose distribution. (C) Sagittal dose distribution. (D) Axial dose distribution.

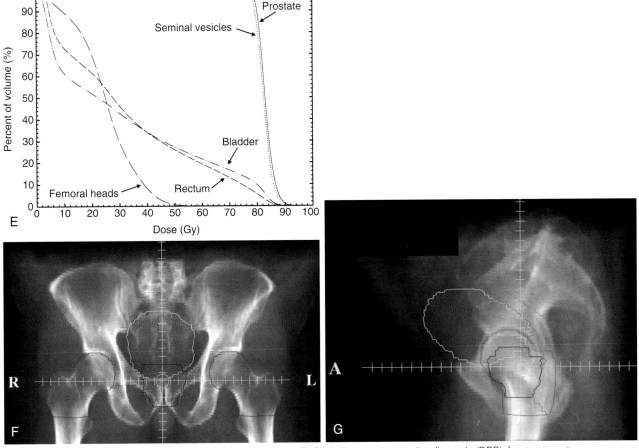

Fig. 33.9, cont'd (E) Dose-volume histogram. (F) Digitally reconstructed radiograph (DRR) for treatment setup, anterior view. (G) DRR, lateral view.

TABLE 33.1 Volume Definitions for Treatment Planning

Volume	Definition
GTV	Palpable or visible extent of tumor
CTV	GTV plus margin for subclinical disease extension
PTV	CTV plus margin for treatment reproducibility (patient/organ movement, daily setup error)
Treatment volume	Volume enclosed by appropriate isodose in achieving the treatment purpose

CTV, Clinical target volume; *GTV*, gross tumor volume; *PTV*, planning target volume.

and evaluated. A study by Dallas and associates[36] documented a PSA relapse-free survival rate at 98.8% for patients at intermediate risk and at 100% survival for patients at low risk.

Interstitial implant can also be used as a boost after moderate-dose external beam radiation. Patients chosen for this procedure are those with significant risk of tumor extension outside the prostate capsule. Typically, a dose of 45 Gy to the prostate, seminal vesicles, and possibly pelvic nodes is delivered with external beam. This is then followed 2 to 4 weeks later by an implant, as a boost, to the prostate. The implant dose is decreased to 110 Gy with I-125 and 90 Gy with Pd-103.

High-dose-rate iridium is another way to deliver a boost after a moderate-dose external beam. The isotope used for this type of treatment is typically iridium-192 (Ir-192).[37] Compared with I-125 and Pd-103, which are permanent implants, this is a temporary implant technique. Similar to permanent isotopes, a perineal template is used to introduce needles and catheters into the prostate. The catheters are left in place, and the patient is hospitalized. A common dosage scheme is 7 fractions of 6.5 Gy over 3.5 days for a total dose of 45.5 Gy.[37]

Radiation After Prostatectomy. Three situations arise in the post-prostatectomy setting: (1) PSA does not decrease to the undetectable range immediately after prostatectomy, signaling that all of the tumor has not been removed; (2) PSA is undetectable after surgery, but tumor margins contain tumor or seminal vesicles are involved; and (3) PSA is undetectable immediately after surgery but, after a period, begins to rise. In the latter two circumstances, radiation to the prostate fossa is commonly applied. In the first situation, the PSA may still be detectable because of metastatic disease, and therefore, local radiation is not beneficial. Care must be taken to prove that the only disease remaining is in the surgical bed before local therapy is applied.

CT scan planning can be used similar to the procedure for an intact prostate. The surgical bed, or area where the prostate and seminal vesicles are normally found, is contoured as the target volume. Care is taken to include any site found worrisome by the surgeon or noted as being involved by the pathology report. Four-field or six-field conformal techniques were commonplace in the past, with field sizes in the 10 × 8 cm range. Currently, IMRT treatment techniques are used to further customize the dose to the prostate bed. Doses for microscopic disease immediately after surgery with undetectable PSA are generally at the 64 to 66 Gy level, with higher doses, in the 70-Gy range, for rising

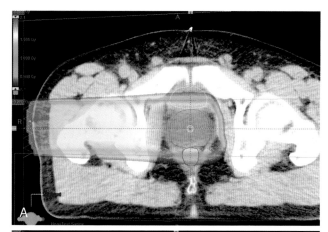

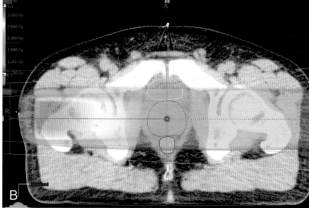

Fig. 33.10 (A) Lateral proton beam. (B) Lateral photon beams. Both images are a single right lateral beam. Notice the lack of exit dose on the proton beam.

PSA. Care must be taken to evaluate rectal and bladder DVHs. After surgical removal of the prostate, the bladder and rectum tend to move into the prostatic space, necessitating inclusion of a significant portion of these organs if the area at risk is to be adequately treated. It is not unusual that desired dose levels are compromised by critical organ (rectum and bladder) tolerance.

Results of Treatment

Surgery. Overall, survival is a poor measure of treatment outcome for prostate cancer therapy because this is a slowly progressive disease that many men die with but not of. Many other medical conditions in elderly men affect the death rate. Therefore, cause-specific survival based on death from cancer per se is a better measure. For evaluation of a particular therapy and its efficacy in eradicating the disease, PSA disease-free survival is generally used in the case of prostate cancer. Because a rising PSA after treatment signals disease recurrence, it is an objective and early measure of disease status. The outcome is also very much dependent on prognostic factors, such as tumor stage, histologic grade (Gleason score), and pretreatment PSA. Patients who have had prostatectomy can be additionally classified according to pathologic features: extracapsular tumor extension, seminal vesicle involvement, and lymph node status.

For prostatectomy, overall PSA progression-free survival rates range from 70% to 85% at 5 years and 45% to 75% at 10 years. For those patients with the best prognosis, T1 to T2, PSA of 10 ng/mL or less, Gleason of 6 or less, the PSA progression-free rate is 80% to 85% at 10 years.[38,39] On the contrary, however, the PSA progression-free rate at 10 years is only 50% for pretreatment PSA greater than 10 ng/mL, 70% with extracapsular extension, 40% with seminal vesicle involvement, and 10% with lymph nodes positive for tumor.[38,39] Clinical disease usually becomes detectable long after the PSA rises. In the Johns Hopkins surgical series, only 4% of men had local recurrence, and 8% had distant disease 10 years after prostatectomy.[39]

Radiation. Both external beam radiation and radioisotopic implant treatment yield similar results to surgery if like groups are compared. With treatment of patients with radiation, we do not, of course, have the pathologic factors such as extracapsular extension, seminal vesicle involvement, and lymph node status by which to group patients into prognostic categories. Tumor stage, grade, and PSA, however, provide substantial information for comparison. With external beam therapy, the best prognostic group (T1–T2, PSA ≤10 ng/mL, Gleason ≤6) has a PSA disease-free survival rate of 80% at 10 years, just as for surgery,[40] and newer techniques (IMRT) with higher doses provide even better results.[41] Similar patients show PSA disease-free survival rates of 80% to 90% of the time with implants.[42,43] The patients with implants tend to be a more highly select group with smaller amounts of disease, which may account for slightly better outcome statistics. Patients with more advanced disease, T3 or PSA greater than 10 ng/mL or Gleason 7 to 10, tend to have more guarded prognosis—again, similar to those surgically treated.[17,44]

As radiation techniques become more highly conformal and doses are increased, early reports on outcome appear promising. The randomized study from the University of Texas MD Anderson Cancer Center that compared 70 Gy with 78 Gy reported a 39% absolute gain in PSA disease-free survival rate at 8 years for patients with pretreatment PSA greater than 10 ng/mL treated to 78 Gy[45,46] (Fig. 33.12). No advantage was found for higher doses in patients with pretreatment PSA of 10 ng/mL or less. Other investigators have seen improved outcomes with higher doses as well (Table 33.2). A randomized study has shown improvement in 5-year PSA progression–free survival rates for patients with both low and intermediate/high risk treated with 79.2 Gy compared with 70 Gy.[47] Because serum PSA is a good marker for recurrent disease and has been shown to highly correlate with prostate biopsy results, routine postradiation biopsies are no longer done, except in randomized trials. Biopsies become important, however, when local treatment for prostate recurrence is planned. Because these therapies, such as prostatectomy and repeat irradiation, usually carry significant complication rates, it is essential to ensure that local disease is, in fact, present, because a PSA rise could also be caused by nodal or distant disease.

Palliative radiation. Irradiation doses of 50 to 60 Gy may be effective in the treatment of massive, locally extensive prostatic carcinoma or significant-size pelvic lymph node disease, which may produce pain, hematuria, urethral obstruction, or leg edema.

Radiation is frequently used in the treatment of distant metastases from carcinoma of the prostate. Marked symptomatic relief is noted in more than 80% of patients treated with doses of 30 Gy in 2 weeks. Most commonly, osseous sites are treated with localized fields. Although unusual, brain metastases may be successfully treated with doses of 30 Gy in 10 fractions to the entire cranial contents, just as for other primary sites. For palliation of pain, larger doses per day are also effective and may be especially prudent in patients in poor general condition and with very limited life spans.

If multiple skeletal sites are involved by the tumor and produce symptoms, radioactive strontium-89 or radium-226 can be administered intravenously, with some degree of pain relief occurring in 80% of patients.[48] Samarium-153 is a newer isotope that is also used for this purpose.[49]

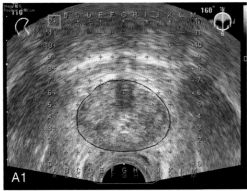

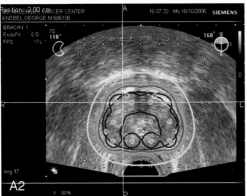

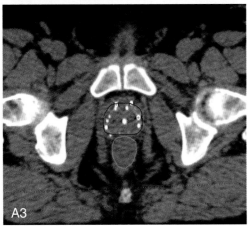

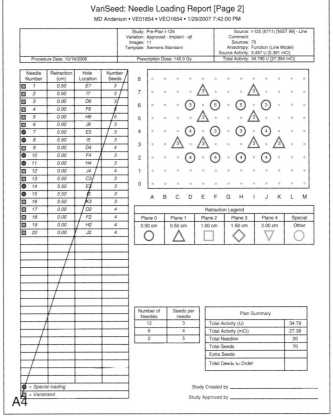

VariSeed: Needle Loading Report [Page 2]

MD Anderson • VE01654 • VEO1654 • 1/29/2007 7:42:00 PM

	Study: Pre-Plan I-125	Source: I-125 (6711) [NIST 99] - Line
	Variation: Approved - Implant - sjf	Comment:
	Images: 11	Sources: 70
	Template: Siemens Standard	Anisotropy: Function (Line Model)
		Source Activity: 0.497 U [0.391 mCi]
Procedure Date: 10/16/2006	Prescription Dose: 145.0 Gy	Total Activity: 34.790 U [27.394 mCi]

Needle Number	Retraction (cm)	Hole Location	Number Seeds
1	0.50	E7	3
2	0.50	I7	3
3	0.00	D6	3
4	0.00	F6	3
5	0.00	H6	5
6	0.00	J6	3
7	0.50	E5	3
8	0.50	I5	3
9	0.00	D4	4
10	0.00	F4	3
11	0.00	H4	3
12	0.00	J4	4
13	0.50	C3	3
14	0.50	E3	3
15	0.50	G3	3
16	0.50	K3	3
17	0.00	D2	4
18	0.00	F2	4
19	0.00	H2	4
20	0.00	J2	4

● = Special loading
■ = Varistrand

Retraction Legend

Plane 0	Plane 1	Plane 2	Plane 3	Plane 4	Special
0.00 cm	0.50 cm	1.00 cm	1.50 cm	2.00 cm	Other
○	△	□	◇	▽	○

Number of Needles	Seeds per needle
12	3
6	4
2	5

Plan Summary	
Total Activity (U)	34.79
Total Activity (mCi)	27.39
Total Needles	20
Total Seeds	70
Extra Seeds	
Total Seeds to Order	

Study Created by _____

Study Approved by _____

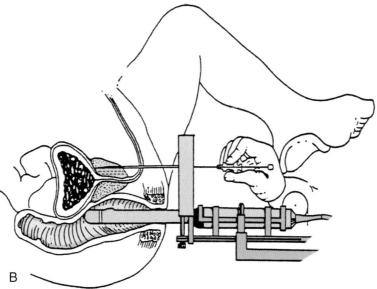

Fig. 33.11 (A 1–3) Prostate implant treatment planning. (B) Ultrasound-guided transperineal template implant technique. (From Kuban DA, El-Mahdi AM. Cancers of the genitourinary tract. In: Khan FM, Potish RA, eds. *Treatment Planning in Radiation Oncology*. Baltimore, MD: Lippincott Williams & Wilkins; 1998.)

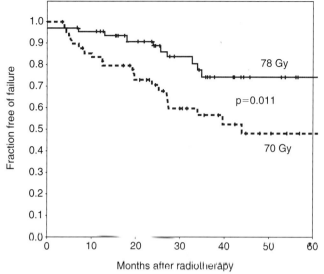

Months	0	10	20	30	40	50	60
70 Gy	53	43	33	20	13	9	5
78 Gy	53	50	40	29	18	12	8

Fig. 33.12 Kaplan-Meier freedom from failure (FFF) curves for patients with prostate-specific antigen (PSA) levels of more than 10 ng/mL with dose randomization (70 Gy vs. 78 Gy). The numbers of patients at risk at 10-month intervals are shown above the graphs. (From Kuban DA, Tucker SL, Dong L, et al. Long term results of the MD Anderson randomized dose-escalation trial for prostate cancer, *Int J Radiat Oncol Biol Phys.* 2008;70:67–74.)

TABLE 33.2 Five-Year Prostate-Specific Antigen Disease-Free Survival Rate With Higher Versus Lower Dose Irradiation

Study	Total No. of Patients	Dose (GY)	% 5-YEAR PSA-DFS (ng/ml) ≤10	10-20	>20
Hanks	232	<71.5	ND	29	8
		71.5–75.7	ND	57	28
		≥75.7	ND	73	30
			≤10	>10	
Kuban	301	70	85	61	
		78	87	81	
			Favorable	Unfavorable	
Lyons	738	<72	81	41	
		≥72	98	75	
			Favorable	Intermediate	High
Zelefsky	1100	64.8–70.2	79	49	21
		75.6–86.4	90	67	50

Favorable, PSA ≤10 ng/mL, Gleason ≤6, T1-T2; *intermediate,* one factor worse; *ND,* no difference based on dose; *PSA-DFS,* prostate-specific antigen disease-free survival; *unfavorable or high,* ≥2 factors worse. Data from Hanks G, Hanlon AL, Schultheiss TE, et al. Dose escalation with 3D conformal treatment: five year outcomes, treatment optimization, and future directions. *Int J Radiat Oncol Biol Phys.* 1998;41:501–510; Kuban D, Tucker SL, Dong L, et al. Long-term results of the M. D. Anderson randomized dose-escalation trial for prostate cancer. *Int J Radiat Oncol Biol Phys.* 70:67–74, 2008; Lyons JA, Kupelian PA, Mohan DS, et al. Importance of high radiation doses (72 Gy or greater) in the treatment of stage T1–T3 adenocarcinoma of the prostate. *Urology* 2000;55:85–90; and Zelefsky MJ, Fuks Z, Hunt M, et al. High dose radiation delivered by intensity modulated conformal radiotherapy improves the outcome of localized prostate cancer. *J Urol.* 2001;166:876–881.

Side Effects and Complications

Surgery. The most significant morbidity is incontinence and sexual impotence, which is related to the type of radical prostatectomy. Moderate stress incontinence requiring pads is reported to be 5% to 8% by major university centers.[50] Surveys of patients, however, show this rate to be considerably higher, at 25% to 30%.[38] The preservation of potency is related to the tumor stage, unilateral or bilateral resection of the neurovascular bundle, and patient age. With a bilateral nerve-sparing procedure, potency rates range from 76% in men younger than 60 years to 49% for those older than 65 years. Potency rates are less, of course, if nerves can only be spared unilaterally because of close proximity to tumor or if the patient did not have full erectile function before surgery.[38]

Radiation Therapy. Acute GI side effects of radiation include diarrhea, abdominal cramping, rectal discomfort, and occasionally rectal bleeding, which may be caused by transient proctitis. Patients with hemorrhoids may have discomfort develop earlier than other patients, and aggressive symptomatic treatment should be instituted promptly. A higher incidence of both acute and late GI effects occurs when larger volumes of the pelvis are irradiated.

Severe late sequelae of treatment include persistent proctitis, rectal bleeding, and ulceration. Although the incidence rate of grade 2 (moderate) GI complications is low (5%) with doses in the 64 to 70 Gy range, this rate can more than double (14%) when higher doses of 75 to 81 Gy are used.[51] Storey and colleagues[52] have shown that the rectal complication rate is related to the amount of rectum treated to doses of 70 Gy or higher. Therefore, attention to DVHs is imperative when dose escalating. When the amount of treated rectum is kept to a minimum, grade 2 complication rates can be reduced to 5% or less.[41,51] Fortunately, severe grade 3 and 4 GI complications occur infrequently, in less than 2% of patients. To date, no strong relationship to irradiated bladder volume has been shown for urinary complications. Urinary toxicity is thought to perhaps be related to the urethra, which is contained within the prostate and cannot be spared. Moderate (grade 2) urinary complications occur in 10% to 15% of patients and mainly necessitate medication for urgency or frequency. More severe (grade 3) urinary complications such as urethral strictures occur in only 1% to 3% of patients.[41,51,52] Late GI and urinary complication rates for patients with implant are similar to those for patients treated with external beam therapy.[42]

Sexual impotence (erectile dysfunction) has been observed in 30% to 60% of formerly potent patients treated with external irradiation and in 20% to 30% of those treated with interstitial implant.[38,53] These percentages are, of course, dependent on patient age, definition of potency, and degree of potency pretreatment. Data are also greatly influenced by physician versus patient reporting via survey. The latter tends to produce higher rates of dysfunction and complications.

PENIS AND MALE URETHRA

Epidemiology

Carcinoma of the penis is relatively rare in the United States; the estimated incidence is 1 per 100,000 each year, which accounts for less than 1% of cancers in men.[54] This tumor is extremely rare in circumcised Jewish men; circumcision performed early in life protects against carcinoma of the penis, but this is not true if the operation is done in adult life. The higher incidence in some areas of South America, Africa, and Asia, and in black men seems to be related to the absence of the practice of neonatal circumcision. Phimosis (narrowing of the opening of the prepuce) is common in men with penile carcinoma. Smegma (a white secretion that collects under the prepuce of the foreskin) is carcinogenic in animals, although the component of smegma responsible for its carcinogenic effect has not been identified.[55]

Carcinoma of the male urethra is also rare. No racial or geographic predisposing factors are recognized. Although the cause remains unknown, some correlation exists between the incidence of carcinoma of the urethra and chronic irritation and infections, venereal diseases, and strictures. The average age at the time of presentation is 58 to 60 years, although 10% of these tumors occur in men younger than 40 years.[55] The human papilloma virus (HPV) has been identified in about half of all diagnosed penile cancers and is believed to be the cause for the recent rise in incidence of penile cancer in many developing countries.[54,55]

Prognostic Indicators

The principal prognostic factors in carcinoma of the penis are the extent of the primary lesion and the status of the lymph nodes. The incidence of nodal involvement is related to the extent and location of the primary lesion. Tumor-free regional nodes imply an excellent long-term disease-free survival rate, 85% to 90%.[56,57] Patients with involvement of the inguinal nodes do considerably worse, and only 40% to 65% experience long-term survival. Pelvic lymph node involvement implies an even worse prognosis; less than 35% of these patients survive. Tumor differentiation is another important prognostic factor.[58]

The overall prognosis for carcinoma of the urethra in males varies considerably with the location of the primary lesion. The prognosis for distal lesions is generally similar to that for carcinoma of the penis. Lesions of the bulbomembranous urethra are usually extensive and associated with a dismal prognosis. Tumors of the prostatic urethra have prognostic features similar to those of bladder carcinoma. Superficial lesions have a good prognosis and may be managed with a transurethral resection, whereas deeply invasive tumors have a greater tendency to develop inguinal or pelvic lymph node and distant metastases.

Anatomy and Lymphatics

The basic structural components of the penis include two corpora cavernosa and the corpus spongiosum (Fig. 33.13A). These are encased in a dense fascia (Buck fascia), which is separated from the skin by a layer of loose connective tissue. Distally, the corpus spongiosum expands into the glans penis, which is covered by a skin fold known as the *prepuce*.

Composed of a mucous membrane and the submucosa, the male urethra extends from the bladder neck to the external urethral meatus (Fig. 33.13B). The posterior urethra is subdivided into the membranous urethra, the portion that passes through the urogenital diaphragm, and the prostatic urethra, which passes through the prostate. The anterior urethra passes through the corpus spongiosum and is subdivided into *fossa navicularis* (a widening within the glans), the penile urethra (which passes through the pendulous part of the penis), and the bulbous urethra (the dilated proximal portion of the anterior urethra).

The lymphatic channels of the prepuce and the skin of the shaft drain into the superficial inguinal nodes located above the fascia lata. For practical purposes, lymphatic drainage may be considered bilateral. Some disagreement exists regarding whether the glands and deep penile structures drain into the superficial or deep inguinal lymph nodes. The lymphatics of the fossa navicularis and penile urethra follow the lymphatics of the penis to the superficial and deep inguinal lymph nodes. The lymphatics of the bulbomembranous and prostatic urethra may follow three routes: external iliac, obturator and internal iliac, and presacral lymph nodes. The pelvic (iliac) lymph nodes are rarely involved in the absence of inguinal lymph node involvement.

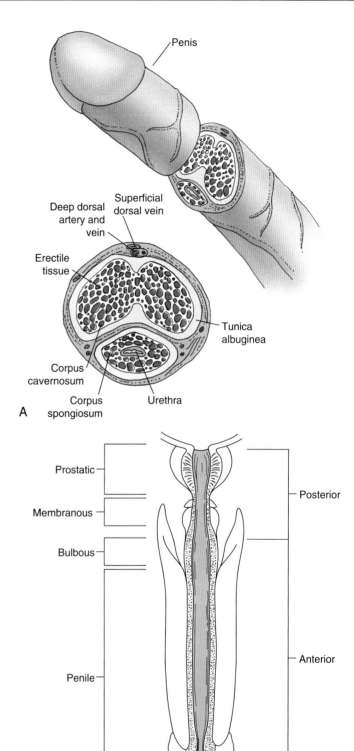

Fig. 33.13 (A) Cross section of the penis shaft. (B) Anatomic subdivisions of the male urethra. (A, From Gartner L. *Color Textbook of Histology*. 3rd ed. St. Louis, MO: Saunders Elsevier, 2006. Fig 21.21. B, From Perez CA, Pilepich MV. Penis and male urethra. In: Perez CA, Brady LW, eds. *Principles and Practice of Radiation Oncology*. 2nd ed. Philadelphia, PA: JB Lippincott; 1992.)

Clinical Presentation

The presence of phimosis may obscure the primary lesion. Secondary infection and an associated foul smell are common, whereas urethral obstruction is unusual. Inguinal lymph nodes are palpable at the time of presentation in 30% to 45% of patients.[56] However, the lymph nodes contain tumor in only half the patients; enlargement of the lymph nodes is often related to inflammatory (infectious) processes. Conversely, 20% of patients with clinically normal inguinal lymph nodes have occult metastases.

Patients with urethral carcinoma may exhibit obstructive symptoms, tenderness, dysuria, urethral discharge, and occasionally initial hematuria (blood in the urine). Lesions of the distal urethra are often associated with palpable inguinal lymph nodes at the time of presentation.

Detection and Diagnosis

Penile lesions can be seen on examination and documented with biopsy. Urethral lesions are evaluated with urethroscopy and cystoscopy. Inguinal lymph nodes should be thoroughly evaluated. Radiographic assessment of the regional lymphatics is of questionable value because of the extensive inflammatory changes often present in the lymph nodes. CT scan is useful in the identification of enlarged pelvic and paraaortic lymph nodes in patients with involved inguinal lymph nodes. Nodal involvement can be confirmed with biopsy or dissection.

Pathology and Staging

Most malignant penile tumors are well-differentiated squamous cell carcinomas. No significant correlation between the histologic grade and survival time has been found. Bowen disease is squamous cell carcinoma in situ that may involve the shaft of the penis and hairy skin of the inguinal and suprapubic areas. Erythroplasia of Queyrat is an epidermoid carcinoma in situ that involves the mucosal or mucocutaneous areas of the prepuce or glans. This carcinoma appears as a red, elevated, or ulcerated lesion. Some patients with erythroplasia of Queyrat have invasive squamous cell carcinoma at the time of the diagnosis. Extramammary Paget disease is a rare intraepithelial apocrine carcinoma. The most common sites are the scrotum, inguinal folds, and perineal region. Primary lymphoma of the penis is extremely rare as well.

Cancers metastatic to the penis are also rare. The most common neoplasms that metastasize to the penis are carcinomas from the genitourinary organs, followed by carcinomas from the GI and respiratory systems. Priapism as an initial presenting feature or later development occurs in 20% to 50% of these patients.[59] Approximately 80% of urethral carcinomas in males are well-differentiated or moderately differentiated squamous cell carcinomas.[60] Others include transitional cell carcinomas (15%), adenocarcinomas (5%), and undifferentiated or mixed carcinomas (1%). More than 90% of carcinomas of the prostatic urethra are of the transitional cell type. Adenocarcinomas occur only in the bulbomembranous urethra. The AJCC staging systems for carcinoma of the penis and male urethra are used to stage cancers of the penis and male ureathra.[13] (For more information on the staging for cancer of the penis, see: https://www.cancer.org/cancer/penile-cancer/detection-diagnosis-staging/staging.html.)

Routes of Spread

Most carcinomas of the penis start in the preputial area and arise in the glands, the coronal sulcus, or the prepuce. Extensive primary lesions may involve the corpora cavernosa or even the abdominal wall. The inguinal lymph nodes are the most common site of metastatic spread. About 20% of patients with clinically nonpalpable inguinal nodes have micrometastases. Pathologic evidence of nodal metastases is reported in about 35% of all patients and in approximately 50% of those with palpable lymph nodes.[60] Distant metastases are uncommon (about 10%), even in patients with advanced locoregional disease, and usually occur in patients who have inguinal lymph node involvement.

The natural history of carcinoma of the male anterior urethra is similar to that of carcinoma of the penis. Most tumors are low grade and progress slowly at primary and regional sites rather than spread to distant areas. Tumors of the penile urethra spread to the inguinal lymph nodes, and tumors of the bulbomembranous and prostatic urethra metastasize first to the pelvic lymph nodes.[60]

Treatment Techniques

Carcinoma of the Penis. Therapy is usually performed in two phases: initial management of the primary tumor and later treatment of the regional lymphatics. Surgery for the primary tumor ranges from local excision or chemosurgery in a small group of highly selected patients, particularly those with small lesions of the prepuce, to a partial or total penectomy. Although surgical resection is usually a highly effective and expedient treatment modality, it may not be acceptable to sexually active patients.

Bowen disease and erythroplasia of Queyrat can be treated with topical 5-fluorouracil (5-FU; 5% cream), a local excision, or superficial x-rays (4500 to 5000 cGy in 4 to 5 weeks). The principal advantage of radiotherapeutic management of the primary lesion in penile carcinoma is organ preservation. Many different techniques, doses, and fractionation schemes have been used.[61] Interstitial implants have been found to be an organ-preserving alternative with similar prognostic outcomes in early-stage disease. Most patients who experience local failure after radiation therapy can have surgical salvage.

Nodal management with observation and delayed intervention when signs of nodal involvement appear has replaced elective nodal dissection for the following reasons: (1) the 1% to 3% surgical mortality rate, (2) the morbidity associated with lymphadenectomy, and (3) the relatively low incidence rate of nodal metastasis (10% to 20%) in patients with clinically normal lymph nodes. Survival rates are high with this treatment.[57] Patients with lymph nodes clinically negative for tumor who are at risk for microscopic nodal metastases because of a primary tumor more advanced than stage I or a moderately to poorly differentiated histology can receive elective radiation to the inguinal lymph nodes (5000 cGy in 5 weeks) with a high probability of tumor control and low morbidity. Generally, clinically involved and resectable regional lymph nodes are managed with radical lymphadenectomy. Some patients can be treated with combined radiation and lymphadenectomy and, if necessary, pelvic lymph node dissection.

Chemotherapy. The use of chemotherapy for carcinoma of the penis is limited. Some degree of tumor regression has been described with systemic agents, such as bleomycin, 5-FU, and methotrexate. A response to cisplatin has also been reported.[62] Systemic therapy is usually reserved for metastatic and recurrent disease or those lesions so advanced as to be incurable with surgery and radiation.

Carcinoma of the Male Urethra. Noninvasive carcinoma of the proximal urethra can be treated with a transurethral resection. For lesions of the distal urethra, results with penectomy or radiation therapy are similar to those for carcinoma of the penis, and the 5-year survival rates of 50% to 60% are comparable.[63] Involved regional lymph nodes are treated with lymphadenectomy. Most patients, however, have advanced invasive lesions, which are difficult to manage with radical surgery or radiation therapy.

Radiation Therapy Techniques. If indicated, circumcision must be performed before the start of radiation therapy to minimize radiation therapy–associated morbidity.

External irradiation. External beam therapy requires specially designed accessories, including bolus, to achieve a homogeneous dose distribution to the entire organ involved. One device consists of a plastic box with a central circular opening that can be fitted over the penis. The space between the skin and box must be filled with

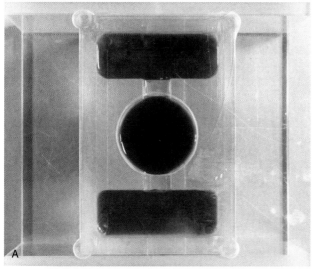

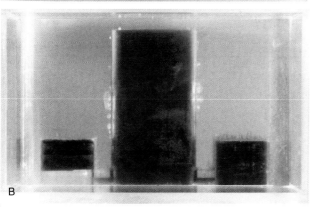

A

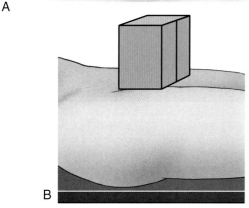

B

Fig. 33.14 (A) View from above of a plastic box with a central cylinder for external irradiation of the penis. The patient is treated in the prone position. The penis is placed in the central cylinder, and water is used to fill the surrounding volume in the box. The depth dose is calculated at the central point of the box. (B) Lateral view. (From Levy L. *Mosby's Radiation Therapy Study Guide.* St. Louis, MO: Mosby; 2011:Fig. 9.18.)

tissue-equivalent material (Fig. 33.14). This box can be treated with parallel-opposed megavoltage beams. An ingenious alternative to the box technique is the use of a water-filled container to envelop the penis while the patient is in a prone position.

A more complex device consists of a Perspex tube (plexiglass) attached to a base plate that rests on the skin. This device is placed as close as possible to the base of the penis, and a flexible tube is connected to a vacuum pump. The suction effect keeps the penis in a fixed position during treatment. Appropriate bolus is placed outside the

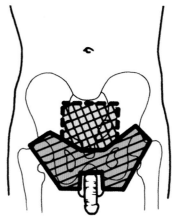

Fig. 33.15 Portals encompassing the inguinal and pelvic lymph nodes. (From Perez CA, Pilepich MV. Penis and male urethra. In: Perez CA, Brady LW, eds. *Principles and Practice of Radiation Oncology.* 2nd ed. Philadelphia, PA: JB Lippincott; 1992.)

tube. The patient can also be treated in the prone position, with the penis hanging through a small hole placed in the Perspex's cylinder.

A well-established association exists between large fraction size and late tissue damage. The daily fraction in most reported series is 250 to 350 cGy for a total dose of 5000 to 5500 cGy, although a smaller daily fraction size, 180 to 200 cGy, and a higher total dose are preferable. A total dose of 6500 to 7000 cGy, with the last 500 to 1000 cGy delivered to a reduced portal, should result in reduced incidence of late fibrosis.

Regional lymphatics can be treated with external beam megavoltage radiation. The fields should include bilateral inguinal and pelvic (external iliac and hypogastric) lymph nodes (Fig. 33.15). The posterior pelvis may be partially spared with anterior loading of the beams. Depending on the extent of nodal disease and the proximity of the detectable tumor to the skin surface or the presence of skin invasion, the application of a bolus to the inguinal area should be considered. If clinical and radiographic evaluations show no gross enlargement of the pelvic lymph nodes, the dose to these nodes may be limited to 5000 cGy. In patients with palpable lymph nodes, doses of 6500 to 7000 cGy in 7 to 8 weeks, 180 to 200 cGy per day, with reduced fields after 5000 cGy are required. If grossly involved nodes are respectable, this is typically the preferred treatment. Radiation can be applied after surgery for extracapsular extension or microscopic residual disease.

Brachytherapy. A mold is usually built in the form of a box or cylinder with a central opening and channels for the placement of radioactive sources (needles or wires) in the periphery of the device. The cylinder and sources should be long enough to prevent underdosage at the tip of the penis. A dose of 6000 to 6500 cGy at the surface and approximately 5000 cGy at the center of the organ is delivered in 6 to 7 days. The mold can be applied continuously, in which case an indwelling catheter or intermittent catheterization is used. Single-plane or double-plane implants can also be used to deliver 6000 to 7000 cGy in 5 to 7 days.[61] In extensive lesions that involve the shaft of the penis (stage III), obtaining an adequate margin with brachytherapy procedures is difficult, similar to the situation seen in attempting a partial penectomy.

Results of Treatment

Carcinoma of the Penis. Because of the rarity of this type of cancer, reports of treatment results are scarce. A significant proportion of patients have been treated surgically, with 5-year survival rates that range from 25% to 80%, depending on the stage of the primary tumor and inguinal lymph node involvement.[62,63]

In patients 41 to 57 years old treated with various radiation techniques (mold, interstitial, and external beam), 5-year survival rates range from 45% to 68%. A 5-year survival rate of 66% and a tumor control rate of 86% have been reported in patients with stage I carcinoma of the penis treated with radiation, compared with a 5-year survival rate of 70% and a tumor control rate of 81% in patients treated with surgery.[60] Survival and local control rates were only slightly affected by the treatment modality in stage II disease but were lower in stage III disease treated surgically. If radiation did not control the primary lesion after 6 months, the penis was amputated and a significant number of cases were salvaged. Of patients initially treated surgically or with radiation, 8% and 20%, respectively, had development of inguinal lymph node metastases. Overall, 8% of patients treated surgically and 10% of those irradiated died of inguinal lymph node metastases and tumor spread.

In one study, 80% of patients treated with radiation therapy had tumor control and conservation of the penis.[64] Although irradiation alone or combined with lymph node dissection controlled lymph node metastases smaller than 2 cm in four patients, radiation therapy was successful in controlling lymph node metastases in only one of seven patients who had N2 or N3 disease.

Carcinoma of the Male Urethra. Most patients with male urethral carcinoma are treated surgically. Partial or total penectomy is performed for distal urethral lesions, depending on the tumor location and extent. The associated 5-year disease control rate is in the 50% range in the absence of lymph node involvement. Tumors of the proximal urethra require total penectomy, and those located even more proximally at the prostatic urethra require prostatectomy and often cystectomy as well. The prognosis for these patients is not nearly as good.[63]

Side Effects and Complications

Irradiation of the penis produces brisk erythema, dry or moist desquamation, and swelling of the subcutaneous tissue of the shaft in almost all patients. Although they are uncomfortable, these reversible reactions subside within a few weeks with conservative treatment. Telangiectasia and fibrosis are usually asymptomatic, common, late consequences of radiation therapy.

Most strictures after radiation therapy are at the meatus. Meatal-urethral strictures occur with a frequency of up to 40%.[64,61] This incidence rate compares with that of urethral strictures after penectomy.

Ulceration, necrosis of the glans, and necrosis of the skin of the shaft are rare complications. Lymphedema of the legs has occurred after inguinal and pelvic radiation therapy and is related to field size, dose, and whether lymph node dissection preceded radiation.

URINARY BLADDER

Epidemiology

Approximately 81,190 new cases and 17,240 deaths from bladder cancer are reported in the United States annually.[65] The incidence peaks in the seventh decade, with the average age of diagnosis at 73 years.[65] In men, this cancer is the fourth most prevalent malignant disease. It occurs about four times more often in men than in women.

Prognostic Indicators

The tumor extent and the depth of muscle invasion are important factors that affect the tumor's behavior and the outcome of therapy. Tumor **morphology** is also important because papillary tumors are usually low grade and superficial with a favorable prognosis. Infiltrating

lesions tend to be higher grade, sessile, and nodular; they invade muscle, vascular, and lymphatic spaces and generally have a worse prognosis. The degree of histologic differentiation must also be considered because well-differentiated tumors are less aggressive and have a better prognosis than poorly differentiated tumors, which are usually more invasive.[65]

Anatomy and Lymphatics

The urinary bladder, when empty, lies entirely within the true pelvis. The empty bladder is roughly tetrahedral; each of its four surfaces is shaped like an equilateral triangle. The base of the superior surface (the only surface covered with peritoneum) is behind, and the apex is in front. The apex of the bladder is directed toward the upper part of the pubic symphysis and is joined to the umbilicus by the middle umbilical ligament, the urachal remnant. The sigmoid colon and the small intestine rest on the superior surface.

In the male, the rectovesical pouch separates the upper part of the bladder base from the rectum. The seminal vesicles and deferent duct separate the lower part of the base from the rectum.

The parietal peritoneum of the suprapubic region of the abdominal wall is displaced so that the bladder lies directly against the anterior abdominal wall without any intervening peritoneum.

The ureters pierce the wall of the bladder base obliquely. During the contraction of the muscular bladder wall, the ureters are compressed, which prevents reflux. The orifices of the ureters are posterolateral to the internal urethral orifice, and with the urethral orifice, they define the trigone (the triangular portion of the bladder formed by the openings of the ureters and urethra orifice). The sides of the trigone are approximately 2.5 cm in length in the contracted state and up to 5 cm in the distended state (Fig. 33.16). In the male, the bladder neck rests on the prostate.

The epithelium, or urothelium, is transitional. The mucous membrane is only loosely attached to the subjacent muscle layer by a delicate vascular submucosa (lamina propria), except over the trigone, where the mucosa is firmly attached.

The lymphatics of the bladder form two plexuses, one in the submucosa and one in the muscular layer. They accompany the blood vessels into the perivesical space and ultimately terminate in the internal iliac lymph nodes. Some lymphatics may find their way into the external iliac nodes. From these nodes, the lymphatics progress to the common iliac and paraaortic lymph nodes.

Clinical Presentation

Most patients with bladder cancer, 75% to 80%, present with gross painless hematuria. Clotting and urinary retention may occur. Approximately 25% of patients have symptoms of vesical irritability, although almost all patients with carcinoma in situ experience frequency, urgency, dysuria, and hematuria.

Detection and Diagnosis

In addition to a complete history and physical examination, including rectal and pelvic examination, each patient should have a chest x-ray examination, urinalysis, complete blood cell count, liver function tests, cystoscopic evaluation, and bimanual examination performed with anesthesia. Biopsy is done for diagnosis. An abdominal CT scan with contrast should be obtained before cystoscopy, so that the upper tracts can be evaluated. Retrograde pyelogram, ureteroscopy, brush biopsy, and cytology can then be done, if necessary. CT scan or MRI is used to evaluate bladder wall thickening and to detect extravesical extension and lymph node metastases. Bone scans are obtained for patients with T3 and T4 disease and those with bone pain.

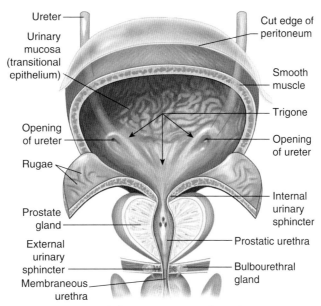

Fig. 33.16 A ventral view of the urinary bladder and prostate, illustrating the location of the trigone of the bladder. (From Huether SE, McCance KL: *Understanding pathophysiology,* ed 7, St. Louis, 2020, Elsevier.)

Pathology and Staging

Most bladder cancers (98%) are epithelial in origin. In the Western hemisphere, approximately 92% of epithelial tumors are transitional cell carcinomas, 6% to 7% are squamous cell carcinomas, and 1% to 2% are adenocarcinomas. Squamous or glandular differentiation can be seen in 20% to 30% of transitional cell carcinomas. Patients whose bladders are chronically irritated by long-term catheter drainage (e.g., paraplegics) or bladder calculi are at risk of development of squamous cell carcinoma.

Morphologically, bladder cancers can be separated into the following four categories: (1) papillary, (2) papillary infiltrating, (3) solid infiltrating, and (4) nonpapillary, noninfiltrating, or carcinoma in situ. At the time of diagnosis, 70% of these cancers are papillary, 25% show papillary or solid infiltration, and 3% to 5% indicate carcinoma in situ. The tumor node metastasis (TNM) AJCC staging system is used to evaluate bladder cancers.[13] (For more information on staging bladder cancer, see: https://www.cancer.org/cancer/bladder-cancer/detection-diagnosis-staging/staging.html.)

This system combines histologic findings from transurethral resection specimens and clinical findings from bimanual examination with anesthesia. Pathologic staging is based on histologic examination of cystectomy specimens. In the AJCC system, these stages are preceded by the prefix p (e.g., pT3).

The presence of muscle invasion categorizes the lesion as T2 to T4b. Although a bimanual examination of the patient with anesthesia and radiographic studies are helpful in further evaluating the various stages, understaging is common.

Routes of Spread

Bladder cancer spreads via direct extension into or through the wall of the bladder. In a small proportion of cases, the tumor spreads submucosally under intact, normal-appearing mucosa. Intraepithelial involvement of the distal ureters, prostatic urethra, and periurethral prostatic ducts is frequently found with multifocal or diffuse carcinoma in situ. Approximately 75% to 85% of new bladder cancers are superficial (Tis, Ta, or T1), and about 15% to 25% of patients have evidence of muscle invasion at the time of the diagnosis. Those with superficial disease can have development of muscle invasion when tumors recur

after conservative therapy. Of all patients with muscle-invasive bladder cancer, approximately 50% have evidence of muscle invasion at the time of the initial diagnosis, and the remaining 40% initially exhibit more superficial disease that later progresses. Perineural invasion and lymphatic or blood vessel invasion are common after the tumor has invaded muscle.

Lymphatic drainage occurs via the external iliac, internal iliac, and presacral lymph nodes. Published data correlate the incidence of pelvic lymph node metastases with the depth of tumor invasion in the bladder wall (Table 33.3).[66] The most common sites of distant metastasis are the lung, bone, and liver.

Treatment Techniques

For carcinoma in situ, a radical cystectomy is usually curative. However, most patients and urologists prefer more conservative initial management. For lesions that are smaller than 5 cm, reasonably well delineated, and without involvement of the bladder neck, prostatic urethra, or ureters, treatment consists of electrofulguration followed by intravesical chemotherapy or Bacillus Calmette-Guérin (BCG).

Ta and T1 disease is usually treated with a transurethral resection and fulguration. Patients with diffuse grade 3, T1 disease, or involvement of the prostatic urethra or ducts are difficult to treat locally and may be initially treated with a cystectomy.

Intravesical immunotherapy chemotherapy is often administered after a transurethral resection for T1, grade 2 or 3 lesions. Most physicians withhold intravesical treatment for patients with T1, grade 1 tumors. The most commonly used agents are BCG, mitomycin-C, and interferon. Patients require close follow-up with cystoscopy, cytology, and resection as indicated.

Definitive treatment with transurethral resection is not applicable to most patients with muscle-invasive disease. Failure to completely eradicate high-grade disease, progression to muscle invasion, or involvement of the prostatic urethra or prostatic periurethral ducts usually signals the need for radical cystectomy.

Partial Cystectomy. Carefully chosen patients with relatively small, solitary, well-defined lesions with muscle invasion or superficial disease

TABLE 33.3   Incidence of Histologically Positive Lymph Nodes Correlated With Pathologic Stage in Bladder Cancer

Pathologic Stage	No. of Patients	Positive Lymph Nodes (%)
pT1	41	5
pT2	20	30
pT3a	13	31
pT3b	28	64
pT4	8	50

Modified from Skinner DG, Tift JP, Kaufman JJ. High dose, short course preoperative radiation therapy and immediate single stage radical cystectomy with pelvic node dissection in the management of bladder cancer. *J Urol.* 1982;127:671–674.

not suitable for transurethral resection of bladder tumor (TURBT) may be treated with segmental resection. However, recurrence rates can be as high as 50% to 70%, and the primary lesion must be located at the bladder dome, right or left bladder wall, and well removed from the ureteral orifices and trigone area such that partial cystectomy is technically feasible. Many patients who are disease free 5 years after partial cystectomy owe their survival to salvage treatment with total cystectomy or radiation. In the Stanford series, radical cystectomy was the most successful salvage treatment.[65]

Radical Cystectomy With or Without Preoperative Radiation. Radical cystectomy is recommended for superficial disease (Tis, Ta, T1) in which all attempts at conservative management have proven unsuccessful. Patients are included who experience recurrence after transurethral resection or intravesical chemotherapy, or cancer has progressed to now invade musculature. Cystectomy is also indicated for patients with recurrent tumors in whom bladder capacity has been so reduced by repeated transurethral resections and intravesical chemotherapy treatments that the successful eradication of the tumor by these conservative means would produce an unsatisfactory functional result.

For clinical stage T2, T3, and resectable T4a disease, radical cystectomy is commonly used. Preoperative radiation was recommended in years past for large tumors with deep muscle invasion because the risk of understaging was high and local recurrence rates were substantial. More recently, however, staging evaluation and surgical technique has improved such that local recurrence rates are in the 7% to 15% range.[67,68] Little research is available evaluating the effectiveness of preoperative and postoperative radiation in the treatment of bladder cancer. One study, however, of patients with T3-T4 bladder cancer demonstrated higher 5-year local control rates (87%–93%) using postoperative radiation therapy versus cystectomy alone (50%). These patients also had improved disease-free survival (44%–49% vs. 25%).[69]

Trimodality Bladder Preservation Therapy. Because removal of the bladder has a significant impact on the patient's quality of life, much research has been devoted to finding a viable alternative.[69] Trimodal bladder preservation therapy consists of a TURBT. A TURBT consists of a scope being placed into the bladder via the urethra. Tumors within the bladder wall can then be removed and examined, leaving the bladder intact.[70] Following the TURBT is a course of concurrent chemoradiation therapy.[69] Radiation courses primarily

consist of a radiation dose of approximately 40 Gy, which allows for a quick determination of effectiveness. Patients who have an incomplete response and are suitable for surgery proceed to immediate cystectomy, whereas the remainder receive additional chemoradiation with a total radiation dose of 64 to 65 Gy.[69] Patients who undergo trimodal bladder preservation therapy must continue with long-term cystoscopic surveillance, with salvage cystectomy performed for invasive recurrences.[69]

Research indicates that trimodal bladder preservation therapy has achieved a complete response of more than 70% at cystoscopic evaluation; therefore, only 30% of patients who attempted trimodality therapy ultimately underwent cystectomy.[69] In addition, 5-year overall survival rates range from 48% to 65%.[69]

Interstitial Implants. Interstitial radiation therapy for bladder cancer is used more commonly in Europe than in the United States. This technique may be used alone, with external beam radiation, or after partial cystectomy. Suitable patients are those with solitary high-grade T1 to T3a lesions that measure less than 5 cm and whose general medical condition permits a surgical procedure. In experienced hands, selected patients can achieve excellent local control and survival. Overall, however, results appear similar to external beam approaches, and no comparative trials have been attempted.

Radiation Therapy
Initial Target Volume. Portals should include the total bladder and tumor volume, prostate and prostatic urethra, and pelvic lymph nodes. Similar to the prostate, in the past, a four-field (anteroposterior/posteroanterior [AP/PA], laterals) pelvic technique was used. Fields extend 1 cm inferiorly to the caudal border of the obturator foramen and superiorly to just below the sacral promontory or just below the S1 to L5 disc interspace on the AP projection. These fields include the perivesical, obturator, external iliac, and internal iliac lymph nodes but clearly not the common iliac nodes. The field widths extended 1.5 cm laterally to the bony margin of the pelvis at its widest point. The irradiation portals are usually at least 12 × 12 cm to include the empty bladder.[71] The anterior boundary of the lateral fields should be at least 1 cm anterior to the most anterior portion of the bladder mucosa seen on an air contrast cystogram or CT scan or 1 cm anterior to the anterior tip of the symphysis, whichever is more anterior. Posteriorly, the fields extend at least 2 cm posterior to the most posterior portion of the bladder or 2 cm posterior to the tumor mass if it is present on a pelvic CT scan. The lateral fields should be shaped with MLCs inferiorly to shield the tissues outside the symphysis anteriorly and to block the entire anal canal and as much of the posterior rectal wall as possible (Fig. 33.17). High-energy photons (10–20 MV) are most suitable.

Because of the high degree of movement and placement uncertainty on a daily basis of the bladder, oncologists have struggled to limit the exposure to surrounding structures with the use of IMRT. Studies are now taking place to evaluate the use of adaptive radiation therapy or IGRT. With use of daily CT images, oncologists can reduce the field size from 2 to 3 cm down to 1 to 1.6 cm and significantly reduce radiation-induced complications.[72]

Boost Target Volume. The contour of the primary bladder tumor volume is obtained from findings gathered via a bimanual examination, cystoscopy, and CT scan. If the radiation oncologist is satisfied that all initial sites of the tumor are limited to one section of the bladder, the high dose volume should exclude the uninvolved areas of the bladder (see Fig. 33.17). Treatment of the bladder while full can help in

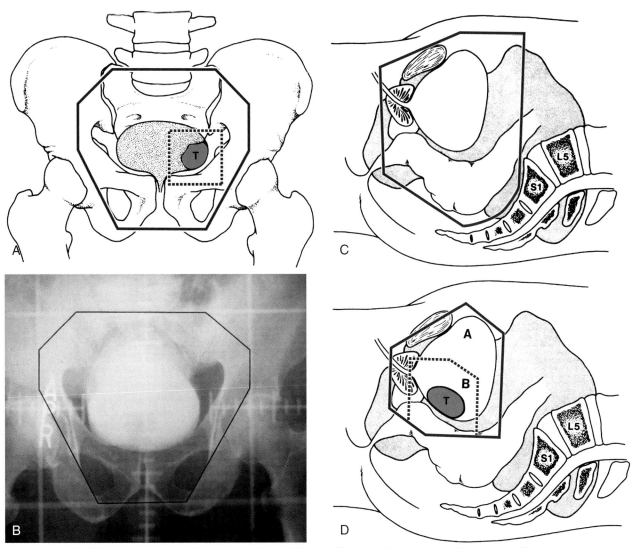

Fig. 33.17 (A) Diagram of the anteroposterior (AP) pelvic field used for carcinoma of the bladder. The boost volume is outlined with dashed lines. *T*, Residual primary tumor. (B) Conventional simulation film of the AP portal. (C) Diagram of the lateral pelvic field encompassing the bladder and pelvic lymph nodes. (D) Reduced portals after 4500 to 5000 cGy (A) and 6500 or 7000 cGy (B).

this regard. Lateral or oblique beams, arcs, or other field combinations can be used.

Simulation is performed with the patient in the supine position. A Foley catheter is inserted into the bladder through the use of sterile technique, and 150 to 250 mL of iodinated contrast material (20% concentration) is injected to outline the posterior portion of the bladder. For visualization of the anterior wall of the bladder on lateral (cross-table) radiographs, 100 to 150 mL of air is injected. Currently, CT scan planning is preferred and is helpful for large tumor masses with extravesical extension.

Doses. The larger pelvic field to include the bladder and pelvic lymph nodes is generally treated to a dose of 45 to 50 Gy at 180 cGy/day, which requires 5 to 5.5 weeks of treatment. With chemotherapy, the nodal dose is usually kept at 45 Gy. A smaller boost volume, as previously described, is taken to 65 Gy, or possibly 70 Gy, if radiation alone is used.

TESTIS

Epidemiology

The American Cancer Society estimates that 9,310 new cases of testicular cancer and 400 deaths from the disease occur each year in the United States.[73] The incidence of this tumor is rare, with an estimated 1 in every 250 men; however, with treatment, the mortality rate of this cancer is reported to be just 1 in 5000.[73] Although testicular tumors are relatively rare, they are the most common malignancy in men between 15 and 35 years of age, with an average age of 33 years.[73,74] The incidence is lowest in Asian, African, Puerto Rican, and North American black men. Higher rates are reported among white men in the United States, United Kingdom, and Denmark. The origin of testicular tumors may be related to gonadal dysgenesis, as strongly suggested by a higher incidence in men with undescended testes. Cryptorchidism (undescended testes) also increases the risk of intraabdominal testicular tumors. Patients with one testicular tumor are at increased risk for development of a contralateral malignancy; 2% to 4% may have a contralateral lesion within 5 years.[74] Although cryptorchidism is a risk factor, 90% of patients will not have a history of cryptorchidism.[74]

The greatest incidence rates of testicular carcinomas are found in men ranging in age from 20 to 34 years. Many individuals in this age range have not even begun to have or are not finished having children. Because treatment techniques for these types of cancers include chemotherapy and often radiation therapy, the option of sperm banking must be presented to the patient. Chemotherapy commonly causes infertility during treatment and for an undetermined amount of time afterwards. Radiation therapy is thought to not affect the patient's fertility, but a small dose does reach the opposite testicle. For this reason, it is often necessary to deposit sperm in a sperm bank before any treatment has started to plan for the future.

Prognostic Indicators

In seminoma, the tumor stage is a significant prognostic factor. The histologic subtype and mild elevation of serum beta human chorionic gonadotropin (hCG) likely have no prognostic implications. In stages II and III, the outcome is related to the bulk of the retroperitoneal disease, which is associated with an increased propensity for distant metastasis. Patients with stage III or IV disease have a worse prognosis because of the possibility of mediastinal and supraclavicular lymph node involvement or distant metastasis.

The prognosis of nonseminomatous tumors is related to the stage of the disease as well. Most patients with stage I or II disease survive with modern multiagent chemotherapy. In these patients, the levels of tumor markers and the volume of metastasis do have prognostic value. Patients with choriocarcinoma have a poor prognoses.

Anatomy and Lymphatics

The testes are contained in the scrotum and suspended by the spermatic cords. The left testis is usually longer than the right. The testis is invested by the tunica vaginalis, tunica albuginea, and tunica vasculosa. The functioning testis houses the spermatozoa in different stages of development and is responsible for testosterone production.

A close network of anastomosing tubes in a fibrous stroma at the upper end of the testis constitutes the rete testis and vasa efferentia. These small tubes converge in the vas deferens, a continuation of the epididymis, which is a hard, cordlike structure about 60 cm in length and 5 mm in diameter. The vas deferens enters the pelvis along the spermatic cord and empties into the seminal vesicles (two lobulated membranous pouches located on top of the prostate). The ejaculatory ducts, one on each side, begin at the base of the prostate, run forward and downward between its middle and lateral lobes, and end in the verumontanum after entering the prostate.

The lymphatics from the hilum of the testes accompany the spermatic cord up to the internal inguinal ring along the cords of the testicular-spermatic veins. These lymphatics drain into the retroperitoneal lymph nodes between the level of T11 and L4 but are concentrated at the level of the L1 through L3 vertebrae. They drain to the left renal hilum on the left side and to the pericaval lymph nodes on the right. Crossover from the right to the left side is common, but crossover in the opposite direction is rare. From the retroperitoneal lumbar nodes, drainage occurs through the thoracic duct to lymph nodes in the mediastinum and supraclavicular fossa and occasionally to the axillary nodes.

Clinical Presentation

Usually, a testicular tumor appears as a painless swelling or nodular mass in the scrotum and is sometimes noted incidentally by the

patient or a sexual partner.[75] Occasionally, patients report a dull ache, heaviness, or pulling sensation in the scrotum or an aching sensation in the lower abdomen. Approximately 10% of patients have acute and severe pain, which may be related to torsion of the spermatic cord. Frequently, patients relate the appearance of the mass to a previous trauma, although this is coincidental rather than etiologic. Rarely, patients exhibit symptoms of metastatic disease, such as a neck mass, respiratory symptoms, or low back pain. Gynecomastia occurs in approximately 10% of patients with testicular germ cell tumors producing hCG such as choriocarcinoma.[74]

Detection and Diagnosis

A complete history and physical examination are mandatory. If a testicular tumor is suspected, a testicular ultrasound scan should be performed.[74] The appropriate surgical procedure to make the diagnosis and remove the primary tumor is radical orchiectomy through an inguinal incision instead of a biopsy. A biopsy of the mass is not possible because seeding into the scrotum could occur and spread the disease. Although beta hCG levels are slightly elevated in 17% of patients with pure seminoma, any elevation of alpha-fetoprotein (AFP) signals nonseminomatous disease. Beta hCG or AFP levels are elevated in more than 80% of patients with disseminated nonseminomatous disease.[74] Serum markers (beta hCG, AFP) are assayed before and after orchiectomy because they can be used to document persistent or recurrent cancer and may predict the responsiveness of nonseminomas to surgery or chemotherapy.

A CT scan of the chest, abdomen, and pelvis forms the basis of the staging process for evaluation of pelvic, abdominal, mediastinal, and supraclavicular lymph nodes and the pulmonary parenchyma. A semen analysis and sperm banking should be considered for patients in whom treatment is likely to compromise fertility and who intend to have children in the future. Note that viable sperm in patients with testicular cancer may be limited, and so sperm banking does not guarantee a possible reproductive future.

Pathology and Staging

A representation of the dual origin of testicular tumors is shown in Fig. 33.18. About 95% of testicular neoplasms originate in germinal elements. The most common type of testicular tumor is seminoma, which has three histologic subtypes: classic, anaplastic, and spermatocytic. The prognoses are not significantly different for the various subtypes.[73,74] The nonseminomatous tumors include embryonal carcinoma, teratoma, choriocarcinoma, and yolk sac tumor (embryonal adenocarcinoma in the prepubertal testis). The most common single-cell type is embryonal carcinoma. Yolk sac tumors are the most common in children. Choriocarcinoma accounts for about 1% of these tumors. It is not uncommon for more than one cell type to be found in the same patient.

The European Organization for Research on Treatment of Cancer (EORTC)/International Union Against Cancer (UICC) and the AJCC staging systems are used to stage testicular cancers. The EORTC/UICC system or some modification is perhaps the most widely used. (For more information of staging testicular cancer, see: https://www.cancer.org/cancer/testicular-cancer/detection-diagnosis-staging/staging.html and

Routes of Spread

Although the routes of dissemination are similar for seminoma and nonseminoma, the propensity for involvement of various sites differs. Pure seminoma has a much greater tendency to remain localized or involve only lymph nodes, whereas nonseminomatous germ cell tumors of the testes may spread via lymphatic or hematogenous routes.

Seminoma spreads in an orderly manner, initially to the lymph nodes in the retroperitoneum. From the retroperitoneal nodes, the seminoma spreads to the next echelon of draining lymphatics in the

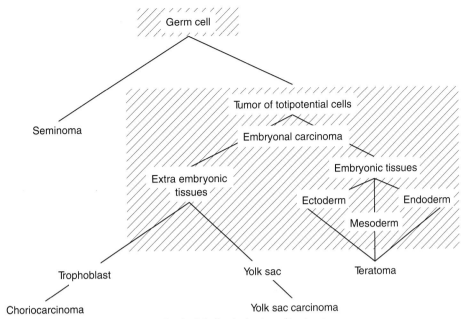

Fig. 33.18 Dual origin for derivation of testes tumors.

mediastinum and supraclavicular fossa (stage III disease).[74] Only rarely and late does pure seminoma spread hematogenously to involve the lung parenchyma, bone, liver, or brain (stage IV disease). Less than 5% of patients have stage III or IV disease at the time of presentation. The orderly route of spread for pure seminoma has been confirmed with surveillance studies. In one study of 255 patients, of 33 patients with relapses, 29 had disease in the retroperitoneal lymph nodes. The site of the second relapse when infradiaphragmatic irradiation was used for the first relapse was the supradiaphragmatic nodes.[76]

Nonseminomatous tumors that metastasize outside the lymph nodes usually involve the lungs and liver.

Treatment Techniques

The initial management goal for a suspected malignant germ cell tumor of the testis is to obtain serum AFP and beta hCG measurements and then perform a radical inguinal orchiectomy with high ligation of the spermatic cord. Further management depends on the pathologic diagnosis of the stage and extent of the disease.

Seminoma. The most commonly applied treatment for patients with stage I seminoma is radical orchiectomy and postoperative irradiation of the paraaortic or paraaortic and ipsilateral pelvic nodes. Because of the low incidence rate of pelvic nodal involvement (0.5% to 3%, as shown by the Leeds Conference and surveillance studies), paraaortic radiation alone has been suggested to be adequate.[77-79] In addition, a randomized trial has shown equally good results with paraaortic radiation alone.[80] Although for years, the standard radiation dose for seminoma has been 2500 cGy/fraction, a randomized trial showed that 2000 cGy in 10 fractions produced the same low relapse rate as 3000 cGy in 15 fractions.[81] Therefore, some are moving to the shorter fractionation scheme. Surveillance studies performed in Canada and the United Kingdom with patients receiving no further treatment after orchiectomy have indicated recurrence rates of approximately 20%.[78,79] Of patients in whom the tumor recurred, 99.5% had salvage with subsequent radiation or chemotherapy. If surveillance is chosen over radiation, consistent follow-up is mandatory. The use of chemotherapy in stage 1 disease has increased as the result of a clinical study that identified the use of one dose of carboplatin as an alternative to radiation therapy.[99] This study found that patients with stage 1 seminoma showed the same tumor response as with radiation therapy with just one dose of carboplatin, which markedly reduced the risk of contralateral cancer and reduced the frequency of follow-up that surveillance alone requires.[82]

For patients with stage IIA disease (<2-cm-diameter mass), the radiation dose and portals for the paraaortic and ipsilateral pelvic lymph nodes are similar to those used for stage I disease, including adequate margin to cover the enlarged nodes. For stage IIB disease (<5-cm-diameter mass), the paraaortic and ipsilateral pelvic lymph nodes should be irradiated with appropriate modification of the treatment field to encompass the larger mass. The dose to the entire nodal volume is 2500 cGy in 160-cGy to 180-cGy fractions or 2000 cGy in 10 fractions, with an additional boost of 500 to 1000 cGy in 180-cGy to 200-cGy fractions with reduced fields to cover the gross tumor. At some institutions, the preferred primary treatment modality for stage IIB disease is chemotherapy.

The optimal therapy for patients with stage IIC retroperitoneal disease (5 to 10 cm in transverse diameter) must be individualized. If the mass is centrally located and does not overlap most of one kidney or significantly overlap the liver, primary radiation therapy can be applied, with chemotherapy reserved for relapse. However, if the location of the mass is such that the radiation volume covers most of one kidney or a significant volume of the liver, the potential morbidity of radiation therapy can be avoided with the use of primary cisplatin-containing combination chemotherapy.

Stage IID is rare. Patients in this stage should be treated with primary cisplatin-containing combination chemotherapy.

The current standard therapy for stages III and IV disease is four courses of cisplatin-containing combination chemotherapy. Often, residual masses may exist in the abdominal or mediastinal area after four cycles of chemotherapy. The 1989 Germ Cell Consensus Conference in Leeds, England, concluded from the available data that patients should be observed after appropriate chemotherapy and that further exploratory surgery or consolidative irradiation should be given only for overt disease progression.[78] This, however, is a controversial issue.

Nonseminoma. The initial treatment for nonseminoma is radical inguinal orchiectomy, followed by cisplatin-based chemotherapy. The most commonly accepted standard regimens include four courses of either cisplatin, vinblastine, and bleomycin or bleomycin, VP-16, cisplatin. Several investigators are exploring the use of fewer courses of cisplatin-containing combination chemotherapy and the use of single-agent cisplatin, carboplatin, or ifosfamide. One-third of patients treated with chemotherapy have a radiographically apparent residual mass or masses after chemotherapy. In general, these masses should be excised because approximately 40% are teratomas and another 10% to 15% are carcinomas. Presumptive evidence exists to indicate that unresected teratomas may give rise to later relapse and that patients have a lower risk of recurrence after surgical excision. Patients with persistent carcinoma need additional chemotherapy but generally do well after treatment.

Irradiation has little role in the management of patients with disseminated nonseminoma, except in the palliation of brain and other metastatic sites. Chemotherapy is the mainstay of treatment in this advanced state.[75]

Radiation Therapy. Patients with stage I testicular seminoma should receive megavoltage irradiation to the paraaortic or paraaortic and ipsilateral pelvic lymph nodes. The top of the portal should be at the T10 to T12 level to ensure treatment of nodes at the level of the renal hilum. The inferior border should be at the bottom of L5 or at the top of the obturator foramen, depending on whether pelvic nodes are treated. The lateral border must include the paraaortic lymph nodes and ipsilateral renal hilum (usually 10–12 cm wide). A shaped field with 2-cm margins is designed to encompass the ipsilateral pelvic lymph nodes (Fig. 33.19). CT planning, to be sure that nodal areas are included and the kidneys are avoided, is now commonly done. Previously, renal contrast was given so that the kidneys could be seen on plain x-rays. Testicular shielding for decreasing primary and, to a lesser degree, scattered irradiation should be applied if the patient wants to preserve fertility.[83]

The recommended dose to retroperitoneal and pelvic lymphatics for stages I and IIA disease is 25 to 35 Gy in 15 to 20 fractions for 3 to 4 weeks.[75] For IIA disease, a boost of 500 to 600 cGy to the known nodal involvement is often delivered. For stage IIB and IIC tumors, the portals are the same as those in stages I and IIA, except that the fields should be modified to cover the palpable or radiographic mass with an adequate margin. The first 2000 to 2500 cGy is delivered to the entire nodal volume, followed by a boost of 500 to 1000 cGy in 180-cGy to 200-cGy fractions to a reduced field to encompass the mass with an adequate margin of at least 2 cm.

If the primary radiation therapy field encompasses most of one kidney, care must be taken to protect at least two-thirds of the contralateral kidney from receiving doses higher than 1800 cGy. Care should also be taken to limit the radiation dose to a significant volume of the liver to less than 3000 cGy. If these parameters cannot be met, chemotherapy typically becomes the treatment of choice.

Mediastinal Irradiation. In the 1960s and early 1970s, the use of prophylactic mediastinal irradiation to treat patients who had stage I or II testicular seminoma was common. Compiled data from six series suggest that supradiaphragmatic relapse is extremely rare, even for patients with relatively poor staging with stage IIA or IIB disease, if prophylactic mediastinal irradiation is withheld. Mediastinal relapse occurred in only 8 of 250 patients, and 7 of 8 patients had salvage with radiation. Because the possible survival benefit of elective mediastinal irradiation is only 0.4%, most radiation oncologists have abandoned its use for stage IIA and IIB disease.[84]

Paraaortic Versus Ipsilateral Iliac and Paraaortic Irradiation. There is growing interest in Europe and the United Kingdom

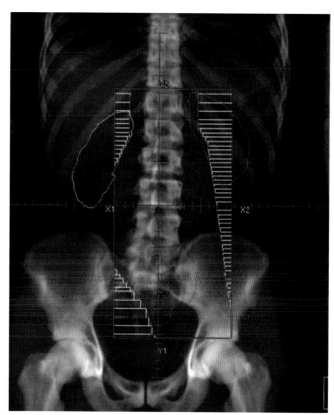

Fig. 33.19 Contoured anterior and posterior radiation treatment fields for clinical stage I or IIA left testicular cancer. (From Kubo H, Shipley WU. Reduction of the scatter dose to the testicle outside the radiation treatment fields, *Int J Radiat Oncol Biol Phys.* 1982;8:1741–1745.)

in reducing the radiation volumes for the treatment of stage I disease by omitting irradiation of the pelvic lymph nodes.[80] Less than 3% of patients have involved pelvic nodes, and the reduction of the irradiated volume is unlikely to cause a significant increase in relapse rate. Furthermore, salvage chemotherapy is very effective. The most commonly used field in the United States, however, still encompasses both paraaortic and ipsilateral pelvic nodes (see Fig. 33.19).

Results of Treatment

Rates of disease-free survival for stage I testicular seminoma approaches 99% at 5 years.[73] Corresponding cause-specific survival rate is 100%.

For patients with stage IIA and IIB disease, rates of disease-free and cause-specific survival are 90% and 95%, respectively.[84–86]

Survival for patients with stage IIC, IID, and III disease depends on the initial bulk of the tumor and the therapeutic approach. With radiation alone, tumor-free survival rates range from 30% to 50%, and primary chemotherapy yields a progression-free survival rate of 91%.[86] Chemotherapy is highly effective as a salvage treatment for failure after radiation as well.

Side Effects and Complications. In general, paraaortic and pelvic radiation is well tolerated. Patients often have nausea and occasionally diarrhea during the treatment course, which is usually controlled with appropriate medication. Severe dyspepsia or a peptic ulcer occurs in only 3% to 5% of patients who undergo irradiation.[87]

Patterns of case studies have shown that a significant increase in late complications occurred with wide-field irradiation for seminoma and Hodgkin disease with doses greater than 2500 cGy. However, no late complications were reported with lower doses.[88] The complication rate increased to 2% with 3500 cGy and to 6% with 4000 to 4500 cGy. Reports have also suggested an increased risk of cardiovascular disease after mediastinal radiation, which is no longer routinely prescribed.[88]

Approximately 50% of patients with seminoma have a decreased sperm count at the time of diagnosis. Further decreases are noted after pelvic and paraaortic irradiation, even if gonadal shielding is used. Typically, the uninvolved testicle receives 1% to 2% of the prescription dose because of scattered radiation through the body tissues.[83] Spermatogenesis may be affected by doses as low as 50 cGy, and cumulative doses above 200 cGy are likely to induce permanent sterility.[89]

Second Primary Malignancy. A 5% to 10% incidence rate of second malignancy has been reported in patients treated with radiation therapy for testicular seminoma. These second malignancies arise from inside and outside the radiation treatment portal. Whether they result from radiation treatment, the predisposition of patients with testicular seminoma to development of a second primary, or a combination of both is not clear. Among 10-year survivors diagnosed with testicular cancer, the overall risk of development of a second solid tumor is approximately twice that of the general population. The risk of development of tumors of the bladder, pancreas, and stomach, organs typically at least partially within the treatment portal, is as high as three to four times that of the general population, according to a large study in which patients had long-term follow-up.[90] Risk appears to be similar with either radiation or chemotherapy but is highest when the two are combined: three times that of the population.

KIDNEY

Epidemiology

Renal Cell Carcinoma. The estimated number of new cases of kidney and renal pelvis cancers reported each year in the United States is 63,340; these cancers result in approximately 14,970 deaths, representing 2% of all new cancers and cancer deaths annually.[91] The average age at the time of diagnosis is 55 to 60 years, with a male-to-female ratio of 2:1.[91]

Several environmental, occupational, hormonal, cellular, and genetic factors are associated with the development of renal cell carcinoma (RCC).[91] Cigarette and tobacco use, obesity, and analgesic abuse (i.e., phenacetin-containing analgesics, which were widely used between their introduction in 1887 and 1983 before a ban was imposed by the FDA) have been correlated with an increased risk and incidence of kidney cancer. A higher incidence of RCC has also been reported among leather tanners, shoe workers, and asbestos workers. Exposure to cadmium, petroleum products, and thorium dioxide (a radioactive contrast agent used in the 1920s) may cause RCC in humans.

The association of renal cell cancer and von Hippel-Lindau disease, a genetic disorder characterized by the formation of tumors and fluid-filled sacs in many parts of the body, has long been established. Various tumor-produced growth factors have been described in the initiation or progression of RCC.[92,93]

Renal Pelvic and Ureteral Carcinoma. About 7% of all renal neoplasms and less than 1% of all genitourinary tumors are transitional cell carcinomas of the upper urinary tract.[91] For renal pelvic tumors, the incidence in men versus women is 3:1, and the peak incidence is in the fifth and sixth decades of life. About one-third of patients with upper urinary tract tumors have development of bladder carcinoma. Etiologic factors for renal pelvic and ureteral cancer are similar to those for tumors of the urinary bladder. Urban residency, cigarette and tobacco use, aminophenol exposure (e.g., benzidine, β-naphthylamine), renal stones, and analgesics (e.g., chronic phenacetin abuse)

have been associated with an increased risk of development of upper urinary tract tumors.[93]

Prognostic Indicators

Renal Cell Carcinoma. The major prognostic factors for survival in patients with RCC are the stage and histologic grade of the tumor. Reported 5-year survival rates are 81% for stage I, 74% for stage II, 53% for stage III, and 8% for stage IV disease.[112] Renal vein or vena cava involvement, without corresponding regional lymph node metastasis, is not a poor prognostic sign if the entire tumor thrombus is removed. The mean survival time for patients with metastasis at the time of diagnosis is approximately 4 months, and only about 10% of patients survive 1 year.[91]

Renal Pelvic and Ureteral Carcinoma. Stage and grade are important prognostic factors in carcinoma of the renal pelvis and ureter. One report noted that 54 patients with transitional cell carcinoma of the renal pelvis and ureter had a median survival time of 91.1 months for early-stage tumors and 12.9 months for more advanced tumors.[94] When patients were stratified according to low or high tumor grade, the median survival time was 66.8 months versus 14.1 months, respectively.

Anatomy and Lymphatics

The kidneys and ureters and their vascular supply and lymphatics are located in the retroperitoneal space between the parietal peritoneum and the posterior abdominal wall. The kidneys are located at a level between the 11th rib and the transverse process of the third lumbar vertebra. The renal axis is parallel to the lateral margin of the psoas muscle. Each kidney is about 11 to 12 cm in length, with the right kidney usually 1 to 2 cm lower than the left. Gerota fascia envelops the kidney in its fibrous capsule and the perinephric fat.

The collecting system lies on the anteromedial surface of the kidney and forms a funnel-shaped apparatus that is continuous with the ureter. The ureters course posteriorly, parallel to the lateral border of the psoas muscle, until they curve anteriorly in the pelvis to join the base of the bladder posteriorly.

The lymphatic drainage of the kidney and renal pelvis occurs along the vessels in the renal hilum to the paraaortic and paracaval nodes. The lymphatic drainage of the ureter is segmented and diffuse and involves any of the following: renal hilar, abdominal paraaortic, paracaval, common iliac, internal iliac, or external iliac nodes.

The topographic relationship of the kidneys, renal pelvis, and ureters to other abdominal organs is illustrated in Fig. 33.20.

Clinical Presentation

Renal Cell Carcinoma. RCC may appear as an occult primary tumor or with signs and symptoms. In one report, the classic triad of gross hematuria, a palpable abdominal mass, and pain occurred in only 9% of patients. Two of three components of the triad occurred in 36% of patients, whereas hematuria, gross or microscopic, was noted in 59% of patients.[95] Several paraneoplastic syndromes or systemic symptoms of RCC have been described, and the tumor may masquerade behind a variety of symptom patterns.

Renal Pelvic and Ureteral Carcinoma. Gross or microscopic hematuria is the most common sign in patients who have a renal pelvic or ureteral tumor; it occurs in 70% to 95% of cases.[93] The other less common symptoms include pain (8% to 40%), bladder irritation (5% to 10%), and other constitutional symptoms (5%). Approximately 10% to 20% of patients have a flank mass from the tumor or associated hydronephrosis. Otherwise, physical findings are unremarkable.

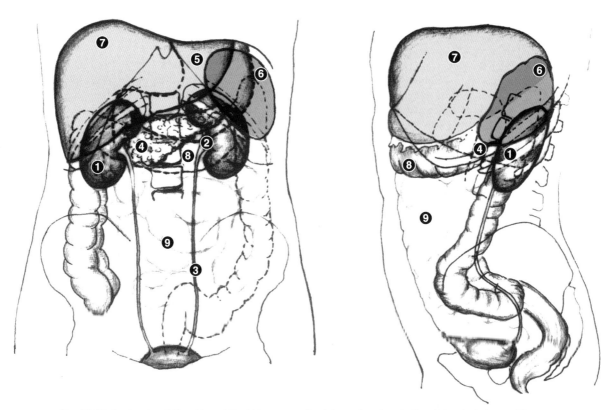

Fig. 33.20 Anatomic relationships of the kidneys, renal pelvis, and ureters to the abdominal viscera. The surrounding structures as numbered (*1*, right kidney; *2*, left renal pelvis; *3*, left ureter; *4*, pancreas; *5*, stomach; *6*, spleen; *7*, liver; *8*, transverse colon; *9*, small bowel) become dose-limiting factors in the planning of abdominal or retroperitoneal irradiation. (A) Anteroposterior view. (B) Lateral view. (Courtesy Peter P. Lai, MD.)

Detection and Diagnosis

Renal Cell Carcinoma. The diagnosis of RCC is established clinically and radiographically in most patients. After a radiographic diagnosis is made, a thorough staging workup is performed to determine resectability. A metastatic workup that includes a bone scan, chest radiograph, and CT or MRI scan of the abdomen and pelvis should be performed before surgery. If metastatic lesions are detected, a histologic confirmation of the most easily accessible lesion should be obtained.

An intravenous pyelogram can identify the tumor, determine its location, and show the function of the contralateral kidney when surgery is contemplated. However, an intravenous pyelogram is not sensitive or specific for small to medium-sized tumors. Ultrasound scan provides accurate anatomic detail of extrarenal extension of the tumor. In addition, it differentiates solid from cystic renal lesions. Renal arteriography detects neovascularity, arteriovenous fistula, and pooling of contrast medium, and it accentuates capsular vessels. Contrast-enhanced or dynamic CT scan provides extremely accurate information about the location and size of the tumor and lymph node enlargement. A CT scan plus digital subtraction angiography provides adequate diagnostic and anatomic details with much less morbidity than arteriography. Inferior venacavography is sometimes used to detect the extent of the tumor thrombus involvement within the vena cava.

Renal Pelvic and Ureteral Carcinoma. Excretory urography is frequently used in evaluation of patients with renal pelvic carcinoma. The most common finding is a filling defect in the renal pelvis or collecting system. Retrograde pyelography accurately delineates upper-tract filling defects and defines the lower margin of the ureteral lesion. CT scan or MRI of the abdomen and pelvis before and after contrast gives useful information regarding tumor extension. Angiography is not often used. Endoscopic ureteroscopy with percutaneous nephroscopy is a recently developed technique. A brush cytology or biopsy from such an endoscopic retrograde procedure has a diagnostic accuracy of 80% to 90%.[92]

Pathology and Staging

The proximal tubular epithelium is the tissue of origin for RCC. Clear cell carcinoma is the predominant subtype. Some reports indicate that spindle cell (sarcomatoid variant) carcinoma is associated with a poor prognosis. A tumor's high nuclear grade is associated with an increased incidence of lymph node involvement and a short survival time.[95]

Transitional cell carcinoma accounts for more than 90% of malignant tumors of the renal pelvis and ureter, and squamous cell carcinoma accounts for 7% to 8%.[92] Adenocarcinoma of the upper urothelial tract is rare. Squamous cell carcinoma of the renal pelvis is often deeply invasive and is associated with a worse prognosis than transitional cell carcinoma. High-grade renal pelvic or ureteral tumors are associated with poor survival rates.[94]

The AJCC system for the classification of kidney cancers is available at https://www.cancer.org/cancer/kidney-cancer/detection-diagnosis-staging/staging.html.

Routes of Spread

Renal Cell Carcinoma. Progression of kidney cancer may occur in the following ways: (1) via local infiltration through the renal capsule to involve the perinephric fat and Gerota fascia; (2) via direct extension in the venous channels to the renal vein or inferior vena cava; (3) via rctrograde venous drainage to the testis; (4) via lymphatic drainage to the renal hilar, paraaortic, and paracaval nodes; and (5) via hematogenous route to any part of the body, including the lung, liver, central nervous system, skeleton, and other organs. The incidence rate of lymph node metastasis is 12% to 23%.[93]

Approximately 18% of patients with RCC have metastasis at diagnosis.[96] It has also been found that more than 50% of RCC patients will develop metastatic disease within 3 years after nephrectomy.[96] Common metastatic sites include the lung (45%), lymph nodes (22%), bone (30%), liver (22%), adrenal glands (9%), and central nervous system (8%).[96]

Spontaneous regression of metastatic RCC after nephrectomy has been reported but is extremely rare.

Renal Pelvic and Ureteral Carcinoma.
Upper urinary tract carcinoma is a multifocal process; patients with cancer at one site in the upper urinary tract are at greater risk of development of tumors elsewhere in the urinary tract.

Transitional cell carcinoma of the upper urothelial tract may spread via direct extension, blood, or lymphatics. The implantation of tumor cells in the bladder has been demonstrated, especially in previously traumatized areas.

Treatment Techniques

Renal Cell Carcinoma.
Standard treatment for patients with localized RCC T1 and T2 is radical nephrectomy, which consists of the complete removal of the intact Gerota fascia and its contents, including the kidney, adrenal gland, and perinephric fat. Regional lymphadenectomy is often performed at the time of radical nephrectomy.

The role of preoperative radiation therapy before nephrectomy has not been defined. Tumor shrinkage and increased resectability have been reported in patients who received preoperative irradiation, but no survival benefit has been noted.[97]

Definitive radiation treatment may be indicated if the patient is not a candidate for surgical resection. It is limited, of course, by the inability to deliver high doses of radiation to the upper abdomen, where most surrounding structures, including the kidney, have low tolerance. Therefore, the intent typically becomes palliative.

Because of the impact to quality of life that a radical nephrectomy poses to patients, urologists have begun investigating partial nephrectomy specifically for cases in which a radical nephrectomy would leave the patient in need of immediate dialysis (bilateral RCC, a horseshoe kidney, or a solitary kidney).[97] Partial nephrectomy is also necessary for patients with unilateral RCC with a contralateral kidney at risk for compromised function, for example, in patients with diabetes or hypertension.[97] After favorable initial outcomes, patient selection expanded to include localized primary tumors with diameter of 4 cm or less and exophytic location, regardless of renal function.[97] Partial nephrectomy does pose a higher risk of local recurrence; however, cancer-specific mortality appears similar to a radical approach.[97]

Renal Pelvic and Ureteral Carcinoma.
Management of renal pelvic and ureteral carcinoma consists of nephroureterectomy with the excision of a cuff of bladder and bladder mucosa. Less aggressive surgery, such as nephrectomy and partial ureterectomy, is accompanied by a ureteral stump recurrence rate of 30%. More conservative surgical excision has been advocated for patients with low-stage, low-grade, and solitary lesions. The survival rate for patients with solitary, well-differentiated tumors after surgical resection is greater than 90%.[98]

Combination chemotherapy consisting of methotrexate, vinblastine, doxorubicin (Adriamycin), and cisplatin produces an objective response of more than 70% in limited groups of patients who have metastatic transitional cell carcinoma of the bladder, ureter, or renal pelvis.[99] For patients who have high-stage and high-grade tumors with local extension or patients with regional lymph node metastases, combination chemotherapy and radiation offer the best chance of disease control.

Radiation Therapy Techniques

Renal Cell Carcinoma.
Radiation is most commonly delivered in the postoperative setting for a tumor left behind or for recurrence after surgery. The treatment volume includes the renal fossa and site of gross recurrence, if present, along with the paraaortic nodal drainage sites in the adjuvant setting.

Postoperative radiation doses range from 4500 to 5500 cGy; the usual recommended dose that can be safely given to the upper abdomen with an acceptable complication rate is 5040 cGy at 180 cGy/fraction over 5 to 6 weeks. A boost of 540 cGy in three fractions to a smaller volume may be added, with special care, to bring the total tumor dose to 5580 cGy. The remaining kidney should not receive doses above 1800 cGy. For a right-sided tumor, a field reduction may be needed at 3600 to 4000 cGy to ensure that no more than 30% of the liver parenchyma is irradiated to a higher dose. The nominal dose for the spinal cord should be limited to 4500 cGy with 180-cGy fractions. No attempt is made to include the entire surgical incision in the treatment field for patients who receive postnephrectomy irradiation, unless specific knowledge exists of significant wound contamination by tumor spillage.[100]

The patient is usually treated via isocentric, parallel-opposed AP/PA-shaped fields. CT planning is used to define the area at risk and healthy structures. Treatment plans include (1) equal weighting of parallel-opposed AP/PA fields, (2) bias loading (i.e., 3:1 or 2:1 posterior loading), and (3) other wedge pair techniques. A shrinking-field technique should be used to reduce exposure to dose-limiting adjacent structures. High-energy photons, 10 MV or higher, should be used. An example of a typical postoperative treatment field and technique is shown in Fig. 33.21. Although the kidney is shown, this does, of course, represent the renal bed after surgical removal.

Radiation can also be used for palliation of a symptomatic renal mass that is unresectable or for the patient who is inoperable. Depending on the patient's symptoms and longevity, a shorter treatment scheme can be used. Similar treatment plans encompassing the kidney are applied.

Renal Pelvic and Ureteral Carcinoma.
Postoperative radiation has been applied to patients with renal pelvic and ureteral carcinoma. The treatment portal usually includes the entire renal fossa, ureteral bed, and ipsilateral bladder trigone area. The extent is dictated by clinical information obtained at the time of surgery and a pathologic analysis of the resected specimen (Fig. 33.22). Because of the high incidence of lymph node involvement, the treatment portal should also include the paraaortic and paracaval areas. As in RCC of the kidney, the postoperative radiation dose is limited by the tolerance of healthy tissues in the treatment field. The usual dose is 5040 cGy in 180-cGy fractions, with a possible boost of an additional 540 cGy in three fractions to a reduced volume. The technique is generally AP/PA parallel opposed for the large field with the same technique or oblique beams for the boost.

Results of Treatment

Results of studies of postoperative radiation therapy for RCC have varied, which makes conclusions regarding efficacy difficult to draw (Table 33.4). Survival benefit remains questionable. Of note is that loco-regional failure is rarely reported and compared. Older treatment

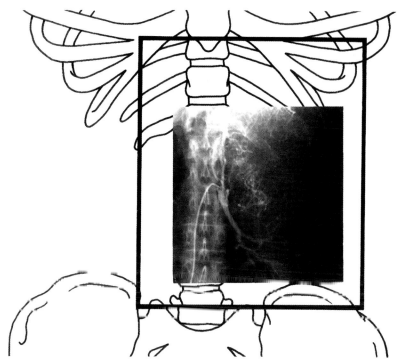

Fig. 33.21 Radiation dose distribution corresponding to the treatment portal in Figure 35.22. Note that a combination of anteroposterior/posteroanterior (AP/PA) plus oblique portals with wedges are used to encompass the entire lesion with an isodose curve of 5400 cGy. The spinal cord dose is less than 4150 cGy. (From Lai PP. Kidney, renal pelvis, and ureter. In: Perez CA, Brady LW, eds. *Principles and Practice of Radiation Oncology*. 2nd ed. Philadelphia, PA: JB Lippincott; 1992.)

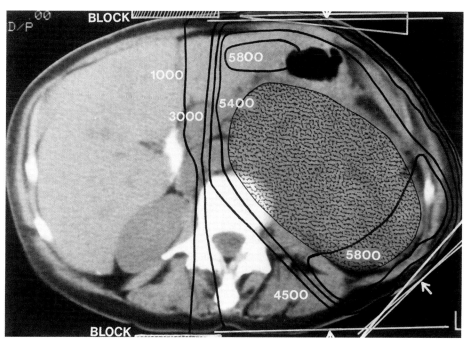

Fig. 33.22 A postoperative radiation portal for cancer of the renal pelvis and ureter. Usually, the entire renal fossa, urethral bed, and ipsilateral area are included; the exact extent is determined with pathologic information. (From Lai PP. Kidney, renal pelvis, and ureter. In: Perez CA, Brady LW, eds. *Principles and Practice of Radiation Oncology*. 2nd ed. Philadelphia, PA: JB Lippincott; 1992.)

techniques without CT planning were used, often, with severe or even fatal complications. Therefore, postoperative radiation is not widely applied for renal, renal pelvis, or ureteral malignancies. Sufficient evidence of residual disease from evaluation of surgical findings and specimens must be present to warrant postoperative radiation. Similarly,

preoperative radiation has shown questionable benefit in past studies and is generally no longer applied.

Side Effects. The side effects and complications from radiation treatment of cancer of the kidney, renal pelvis, and ureters are

TABLE 33.4 Renal Cell Carcinoma: 5-Year Survival Rates After Nephrectomy or Postoperative Irradiation and Nephrectomy

Author	Stage	No. of Patients	Radiation Dose/ Fraction Size (cGY)	Treatment	5-Year Survival Rate	Local Recurrence (%)
Peeling et al. (1969)[a]		96		N	52% (50/96)	
		68		N + RT	25% (17/68)	
Rafla (1970)[b]	All	96		N	37% (35/94)	
		94		N + RT	57% (46/81)	
	Renal vein	36		N	30% (11/36)	
	± Others	40		N + RT	40% (14/35)	
	Renal pelvis	50		N	32% (16/49)	
	± Others	60		N + RT	60% (30/50)	
	Renal capsule	52		N	28% (15.52)	
	± Others	69		N + RT	57% (34/59)	
Rafla and Parikh (1984)[c]		135		N	18% (24/135)	
		105	4500	N + RT	38% (40/105)	
Finney (1973)[d]		48		N	47% (17/35)	7
		52	5500/204	N + RT	36% (14/39)	7
Kjaer et al. (1987)[e]		33		N	63%[§]	1
		32	5000/250	N + RT	38%[¶]	0

[a]This retrospective study has incomplete staging information and no description of the radiation dose or technique. The end point was 5-year survival, with no mention of local recurrence.

[b]This is the only report that described the benefits of irradiation with survival *and* local recurrence as end points. Unfortunately, there was no description of the radiation dose or technique. The study was performed in the era before computed tomography; therefore, local recurrence is an underestimate. Subgroup analysis (involvement of renal vein, renal pelvis, renal capsule + others) indicated an effect of radiation therapy on survival.

[c]The authors also showed some data that attested to the benefits of radiation therapy in patients with renal capsular, renal vein, and regional lymphatic involvement.

[d]This is a randomized study, but no staging information is available. The incidences of local recurrence and distant metastasis are similar. However, there are four fatal liver complications among the patients who received radiation therapy.

[e]In this randomized study, 27 or 32 patients assigned to the irradiation arm completed treatment; 12 of 27 (44%) reported significant complications, with five fatal complications related to irradiation.

N, Nephrectomy; *RT,* postoperative radiation therapy.

Modified from Lai PP: Kidney, renal pelvis, and ureter. In: Perez CA, Brady LW, eds. *Principles and Practice of Radiation Oncology.* 2nd ed. Philadelphia, PA: JB Lippincott; 1992.

similar to those expected from irradiation of the abdomen and pelvis. Acute side effects include nausea, vomiting, diarrhea, and abdominal cramping, which usually respond to conservative medical management.[100] The complication rate is related to the total dose and fraction size. With careful attention given to the treatment technique and dose-volume distribution, many complications can be eliminated.

SUMMARY

- Male reproductive and genitourinary tumors range from the most common form of cancers found in men, such as prostate cancer, to the relatively rare, such as penile and urethral carcinomas.
- Testicular cancer, although relatively rare, is the most common malignancy found in men between the ages of 20 and 34 years.
- As with all other types of cancers, early detection is the most important factor in gaining control over the disease.
- A clear understanding of lymphatic drainage and surrounding anatomy is vital to gaining a better understanding of the treatment rational and dose limitations.
- Several areas of controversy surround the many treatment options available to patients with prostate cancer. Different forms of treatment can affect quality of life and sexual function to varying degrees.

- Ever-evolving technologies, such as CT simulation and IMRT, with associated increases in radiation dose, have improved disease control rates and decreased the side effects related to radiation therapy.
- The potential side effects of treatment to the abdomen and pelvis are similar to those of other sites treated with radiation, including skin reaction, fatigue, weight loss, nausea and vomiting, diarrhea, and hair loss in the area being irradiated.
- Genitourinary cancer management has proven to be a fruitful proving ground in the development of dose escalation treatment regimens and conformal treatment delivery. The treatment of these cancers with today's technology has led to the refinement of IMRT treatment delivery, IGRT, and, to a degree, particulate therapies.

REVIEW QUESTIONS

The answers to the Review Questions can be found by logging on to our website at: http://evolve.elsevier.com/Washington/principles

1. The most common pathology of malignant tumors of the prostate is:
   a. Squamous cell carcinoma.
   b. Adenocarcinoma.
   c. Transitional cell carcinoma.
   d. Burkitt cell carcinoma.
2. The most common type of kidney tumor is:
   a. Transitional cell lymphoma.
   b. Choriocarcinoma.
   c. Adenocarcinoma.
   d. Seminoma.
3. The cancer with the highest incidence rate for males is:
   a. Prostate cancer.
   b. Penile cancer.
   c. Kidney and ureteral cancer.
   d. Lung cancer.
4. For patients with bladder cancer, the bladder should be _____ during whole-bladder radiation.
   a. Empty
   b. Partially full
   c. Full
   d. Localized with contrast material
5. A side effect associated with the treatment of prostate cancer, in which the adult male is unable to obtain an erection, is:
   a. Benign prostatic hypertrophy.
   b. Transurethral resection of the prostate.
   c. Impotence.
   d. None of the above.

6. The prostate gland is located _____ to the rectum.
   a. Posterior.
   b. Anterior.
   c. Superior.
   d. Both b and c.
7. The tumor of the male reproductive and genitourinary system that requires the lowest dose to control the disease is:
   a. Prostate.
   b. Kidney.
   c. Seminoma.
   d. Bladder.
8. The tumor of the male reproductive and genitourinary system for which a brachytherapy implant is most likely used to control the disease is:
   a. Prostate.
   b. Kidney.
   c. Testis.
   d. Bladder.
9. The most common testicular tumor pathology is:
   a. Seminoma.
   b. Choriocarcinoma.
   c. Teratoma.
   d. Embryonal carcinoma.
10. The increased incidence of what sexually transmitted disease has raised the number of penile cancer diagnosis over the last few years?
   a. AIDS.
   b. HPV.
   c. Chlamydia.
   d. Herpes.

QUESTIONS TO PONDER

1. Discuss the role of a digital rectal examination and PSA in the screening of the prostate cancer.
2. Compare and contrast the following prognostic indicators related to carcinoma of the prostate: tumor stage, grade, PSA level, and race.
3. Examine the following specific treatment options for carcinoma of the prostate: surgery, external beam radiation therapy, brachytherapy, hormonal therapy, and chemotherapy.
4. Discuss the general management of cancer of the urinary bladder and surgery versus radiation.
5. Compare the treatments for testicular seminoma and nonseminoma.
6. Discuss the role of the radiation therapist in the treatment of patients with genitourinary tumors.

REFERENCES

1. American Cancer Society. *Cancer Facts and Figures: 2018*. Atlanta, GA: American Cancer Society, 2018.
2. Brassell SA, Rice KR, Parker PM, et al. Prostate cancer in men 70 years or older, indolent or aggressive: clinicopathological analysis and outcomes. *J Urol*. 2011;185(1):132–137.
3. Rice KR, Colombo ML, Wingate J, et al. Low risk prostate cancer in men less than 70 years old: to treat or not to treat. *Urol Oncol*. 2013;30:755–760.
4. Shekarriz B, Upadhyay J, Bianco FJ, et al. Impact of preoperative serum PSA level from 0 to 10 ng/ml on pathological findings and disease-free survival after radical prostatectomy. *The Prostate*. 2001;48(3):136–143.
5. Lee AK, Pollac A. The prostate. In: Cox JD, Ang KK, eds. *Radiation Oncology: Rationale, Technique, Results*. St. Louis, MO: Mosby Elsevier; 2010:676–729.
6. Maricic A, Valencic M, Sotosek S, et al. Transrectal sonography in prostate cancer detection- our 25 years experience of implementation. *Coll Antropol*. 2010;34(2):239–242.
7. Rifkin MD, Zerhouni EA, Gatsonis CA, et al. Comparison of magnetic resonance imaging and ultrasonography in staging early prostate cancer: results of a multi-institutional cooperative trial. *N Engl J Med*. 1990;323:621–626.
8. Chodak GW, Wald V, Parmer E, et al. Comparison of digital examination and transrectal ultrasonography for the diagnosis of prostate cancer. *J Urol*. 1986;135:951–954.
9. Schnall MD, Imai Y, Tomaszewski J, et al. Prostate Cancer: local staging with endorectal surface coil MR imaging. *Radiology*. 1991;178:797–802.
10. Partin AW, Kattan MW, Subong EN, et al. Combination of prostate specific antigen, clinical stage and Gleason score to predict pathological stage in men with localized prostate cancer. *J Am Med Assoc*. 1997;277:1445–1451.

11. Gleason D, Veterans Administration Cooperative Urological Research Group. Histologic grading and clinical staging of prostatic carcinoma. In: Tannenbaum M, ed. *Urologic Pathology: The Prostate*. Philadelphia, PA: Lea and Febiger; 1977.

12. Perez CA, Garcia D, Simpson JR, et al. Factors influencing outcome of definitive radio-therapy for localized carcinoma of the prostate. *Radiother Oncol*. 1989;16:1–21.

13. Amin MB. American Joint Committee on Cancer, *AJCC Cancer Staging Manual*. 8th ed. New York, NY: Springer-Verlag; 2017.

14. Herden J, Heidenreich A, Weissbach L. Risk stratification: a tool to predict the course of active surveillance for localized prostate cancer? *BJU Int*. 2017;120(2):212–218.

15. Klotz L, Vesprini D, Sethukavalan P, et al. Long-term follow-up of a large active surveillance cohort of patients with prostate cancer. *J Clin Oncol*. 2015;33:272–272.

16. Wang X, Wang X, Liu T, He Q, Wang Y, Zhang X. Systematic review and meta-analysis of the use of phosphodiesterase type 5 inhibitors for treatment of erectile dysfunction following bilateral nerve-sparing radical prostatectomy. *PLoS One*. 2014;9(3):1–10.

17. Nagao K, Matsuyama H, Matsumoto H, et al. Identification of curable high-risk prostate cancer using radical prostatectomy alone: who are the good candidates for undergoing radical prostatectomy among patients with high-risk prostate cancer? *Int J Clin Oncol*. 2018;23(4):757–764.

18. Bolla M, Collette L, Blank L, et al. Long-term results with immediate androgen suppression and external irradiation in patients with locally advanced prostate cancer (an EORTC study): a phase III randomized trial. *Lancet*. 2002;360:103–106.

19. Malik S. Using hormone therapy for the management of prostate cancer. *Nurs Residential Care*. 2014;16(2):75–77.

20. Huggins C, Stevens RE, Hodges CV. Studies on prostatic cancer II: the effects of castration on advanced carcinoma of the prostate gland. *Arch Surg*. 1941;43:209–223.

21. Hanks GE, Pajak TF, Porter A, et al. RTOG Protocol 92-02: a phase III trial of the use of long term total androgen suppression following neoadjuvant hormonal cytoreduction and radiotherapy in locally advanced carcinoma of the prostate. *Int J Radiat Oncol Biol Phys Suppl*. 2000;48(3):112.

22. Pilepich MV, Krall JM, al-Sarraf M, et al. Androgen deprivation with radiation therapy compared with radiation therapy alone for locally advanced prostatic carcinoma: a randomized comparative trial of the Radiation Therapy Oncology Group. *Urology*. 1995;45:616–623.

23. Roviello G, Francini E, Petrioli R, et al. Role of chemotherapy in the treatment of metastatic castration-resistant prostate cancer patients who have progressed after abiraterone acetate. *Cancer Chemother Pharmacol*. 2015;76(3):439–445.

24. Eisenberger MA, De Witt R, Berry W, et al. A multicenter phase III comparison of docetaxel (D) + prednisone (P) and mioxantone (MTZ) + P in patients with hormone-refractory prostate cancer (HRPC). *J Clin Oncol*. 2004;22(suppl):4.

25. Good D, Lo J, Lee WR, et al. A knowledge-based approach to improving and homogenizing intensity modulated radiation therapy planning quality among treatment centers: an example application to prostate cancer planning. *Int J Radiat Oncol Biol Phys*. 2013;87(1):176–181.

26. Kenneth W, Ming-Hui C, Judd M, et al. Radical prostatectomy vs radiation therapy and androgen-suppression therapy in high-risk prostate cancer. *BJU Int*. 2012;8:1116.

27. Lawton CA, DeSilvio M, Roach M III, et al. An update of the phase III trial comparing whole pelvic to prostate only radiotherapy and neoadjuvant to adjuvant total androgen suppression: updated analysis of RTOG 94-13, with emphasis on unexpected hormone/radiation interactions. *Int J Radiat Oncol Biol Phys*. 2007;69:646–655.

28. Roach M III, DeSilvia M, Lawton C, et al. Phase III trial comparing whole-pelvic versus prostate-only radiotherapy and neoadjuvant versus adjuvant combined androgen suppression: radiation Therapy Oncology Group 9413. *J Clin Oncol*. 2003;21(10):1904–1911.

29. Reddy NMS, Nori D, Chang H, et al. Prostate and seminal vesicle volume based consideration of prostate cancer patients for treatment with 3D-conformal or intensity-modulated radiation therapy. *Med Phys*. 2010;37(7):3791–3801.

30. Hamstra D, Mariados N, Sylvester J, et al. Continued benefit to rectal separation for prostate RT: final results of a phase III trial. *Int J Radiat Oncol Biol Phys*. 2017;97(5):976–985.

31. Eade TN, Guo LX, Forde E, et al. Image-guided dose-escalated intensity-modulated radiation therapy for prostate cancer: treating to doses beyond 78 gy. *BJU Int*. 2012;109(11):1655–1660.

32. Pollack A, Walker G, Horwitz EM, et al. Randomized trial of hypofractionated external-beam radiotherapy for prostate cancer. *J Clin Oncol*. 2013;31(31):3860–3868.

33. Fontenot JD, Lee AK, Newhauser WD. Risk of secondary malignant neoplasms from proton therapy and intensity-modulated x-ray therapy for early-stage prostate cancer. *Int J Radiation Oncology Biol Phys*. 2009;74(2):616–622.

34. University of Texas MD Anderson Cancer Center. Proton therapy center. https://www.mdanderson.org/patients-family/diagnosis-treatment/care-centers-clinics.html. Accessed November 5, 2019.

35. Sheets NC, Goldin GH, Meyer AM, et al. Intensity-modulated radiation therapy, proton therapy, or conformal radiation therapy and morbidity and disease control in localized prostate cancer. *J Am Med Assoc*. 2012;307(15):1611–1620.

36. Dallas NL, Malone PR, Jones A, et al. The results of real-time brachytherapy for the management of low- and intermediate-risk prostate cancer in patients with prostate volumes up to 100 mL. *BJU Int*. 2012;110(3):383–390.

37. Komiya A, Fujiuchi Y, Ito T, et al. Early quality of life outcomes in patients with prostate cancer managed by high-dose-rate brachytherapy as monotherapy. *Int J Urol*. 2013;20(2):185–192.

38. Eastham JA, Scardino PT. Radical prostatectomy for clinical stage and T2 prostate cancer. In: Volgelzang NJ, et al, ed. *Comprehensive Textbook of Genitourinary Oncology*. 2nd ed. Philadelphia, PA: Lippincott Williams & Wilkins; 2000.

39. Partin AW, Walsh PC. Management of stage B (T1c–T2) prostate cancer. Surgical management of localized prostate cancer In: Radhavan D, et al, eds. *Principles and Practice of Genitourinary Oncology*. Philadelphia, PA: Lippincott-Raven; 1997.

40. Kupelian P, Katcher J, Levin H, et al. External beam radiotherapy versus radical prostatectomy for clinical stage T1–2 prostate cancer: therapeutic implications of stratification by pretreatment PSA levels and biopsy Gleason scores. *Cancer J Sci Am*. 1997;3:78–87.

41. Zelefsky MJ, Fuks Z, Hunt M, et al. High dose radiation delivered by intensity modulated conformal radiotherapy improves the outcome of localized prostate cancer. *J Urol*. 2006;176:1415–1419.

42. Blasko JC, Wallner K, Grimm PD, Ragde H. Prostate specific antigen based disease control following ultrasound guided 125 iodine implantation for stage T1/T2 prostatic carcinoma. *J Urol*. 1995;154:1096–1099.

43. Blasko JC, Grimm PD, Sylvester JE, et al. Palladium-103 brachytherapy for prostate carcinoma. *Int J Radiat Oncol Biol Phys*. 2000;46:839–850.

44. Bolla M, Collette L, Blank L, et al. Long-term results with immediate androgen suppression and external irradiation in patients with locally advanced prostate cancer (an EORTC study): a phase III randomized trial. *Lancet*. 2002;360:103–106.

45. Kuban DA, Tucker SL, Dong L, et al. Long term results of the MD Anderson randomized dose-escalation trial for prostate cancer. *Int J Radiat Oncol Biol Phys*. 2008;70:67–74.

46. Pollack A, Zagars GK, Starkschall G, et al. Prostate cancer radiation dose response: results of the M.D. Anderson phase III randomized trial. *Int J Radiat Oncol Biol Phys*. 2002;53:1097–1105.

47. Al Z, DeSilvio ML, Slater JD, et al. Comparison of conventional-dose vs high-dose conformal radiation therapy in clinically localized adenocarcinoma of the prostate: a randomized controlled trial. *J Am Med Assoc*. 2005;294:1233–1239.

48. Porter AT, McEwan AJ, Powe JE, et al. Results of randomized phase III trial to evaluate the efficacy of strontium-89 adjuvant to local external beam irradiation in the management of endocrine metastatic prostate cancer. *Int J Radiat Oncol Biol Phys*. 1993;25:805–813.

49. Anderson PM, Wiseman GA, Dispenzieri A, et al. High-dose samarium-153 ethylene diamine tetramethylene phosphonate: low toxicity of skeletal irradiation in patients with osteosarcoma and bone metastases. *J Clin Oncol*. 2002;20:189–196.

50. Catalona WJ, Bigg SW. Nerve-sparing radical prostatectomy: evaluation of results after 250 patients. *J Urol.* 1990;143:538–544.

51. Litwin MS, Hays RD, Fink A, et al. Quality of life outcomes in men treated for localized prostate cancer. *J Am Med Assoc.* 1995;273:129–135.

52. Zelefsky MJ, Fuks Z, Hunt M, et al. High dose radiation delivered by intensity modulated conformal radiotherapy improves the outcome of localized prostate cancer. *J Urol.* 2001;166:876–881.

53. Storey MR, Pollack A, Zagars G, et al. Complications from dose escalation in prostate cancer: preliminary results of a randomized trial. *Int J Radiat Oncol Biol Phys.* 2000;48:635–642.

54. American Cancer Society. Penile cancer. http://www.cancer.org/cancer/penilecancer/detailedguide/penile-cancer-key-statistics. Accessed June 11, 2018.

55. Chipollini J, Chaing S, Peyton CC, et al. Original study: national trends and predictors of locally advanced penile cancer in the United States (1998–2012). *Clin Genitourin Cancer.* 2018;16:e121–e127.

56. DeKernion JB, Tynberg P, Persky L, et al. Carcinoma of the Penis. *Cancer.* 1973;32:1256–1262.

57. Stadler WM, et al. In: Volgelzang NJ, et al, ed. *Comprehensive Textbook of Genitourinary Oncology.* 2nd ed. Philadelphia, PA: Lippincott Williams & Wilkins; 2000.

58. Li Z, Yao K, Chen P, et al. Modification of N staging systems for penile cancer: a more precise prediction of prognosis. *Br J Cancer.* 2015;112(11):1766–1771.

59. Kamaleshwaran KK, BKP B, Jose R, Shinto AS. Penile metastasis from prostate cancer presenting as malignant priapism detected using gallium-68 prostate-specific membrane antigen positron emission tomography/computed tomography. *Indian J Nucl Med.* 2018;33(1):57–58.

60. Gupta R, Gupta S, Basu S, Dey P, Khan IA. Primary adenocarcinoma of the bulbomembranous urethra in a 33-year-old male patient. *J Clin Diagn Res.* 2017;11(9):PD07–PD08.

61. Elwell CM, Jones WG. *Comprehensive Textbook of Genitourinary Oncology.* 2nd ed. Philadelphia; Lippincott Williams & Wilkins; 2000.

62. Eisenberger MA, De Witt R, Berry W, et al. A multicenter phase III comparison of docetaxel (D) + prednisone (P) and mioxantone (MTZ) + P in patients with hormone-refractory prostate cancer (HRPC). *J Clin Oncol.* 2004;22(suppl):4.

63. Rabbani F. Prognostic factors in male urethral cancer. *Cancer.* 2011; 117(11):2426–2434.

64. Salaverria JE, Hope-Stone HF, Paris AM, et al. Conservative treatment of carcinoma of the penis. *Br J Urol.* 1979;51:32–37.

65. American Cancer Society. Bladder cancer. http://www.cancer.org/cancer/bladdercancer/detailedguide/bladder-cancer-key-statistics. Accessed June 11, 2018.

66. Skinner DG, Tift JP, Kaufman JJ. High dose, short course preoperative radiation therapy and immediate single stage radical cystectomy with pelvic node dissection in the management of bladder cancer. *J Urol.* 1982;127:671–674.

67. Montie JE, Straffon RA, Stewart RH. Radical cystectomy in men treated for localized prostate cancer. *J Am Med Assoc.* 1995;273:129–135.

68. Skinner DG, Liekovsky G. Management of invasive and high grade bladder cancer. In: Skinner DG, Liekovsky G, eds. *Diagnosis and Management of Genitourinary Cancer.* Philadelphia, PA: WB Saunders; 1988.

69. Smith A, Baler AV, Milowsky M., Chen RC. Bladder cancer. In: Neiderhuber JE, et al, eds. *Abeloff's Clinical Oncology.* 5th ed. Philadelphia, PA: Saunders; 2014:1445–1462.

70. Kansas City Urology Care. Transurethal resection of bladder tumor. http://www.kcurology.com/treatments/transurethral-resection-of-bladder-tumor-turbt.html. Accessed November 5, 2019.

71. Sternberg CN, Donat SM, Bellmunt J, et al. Chemotherapy for bladder cancer: treatment guidelines for neoadjuvant chemotherapy, bladder preservation, adjuvant chemotherapy, and metastatic cancer. *Urology.* 2007;69:62–79.

72. Pos F, Remeijer P. Adaptive management of bladder cancer radiotherapy. *Semin Radiat Oncol.* 2010;20(2):116–120.

73. American Cancer Society. Testicular cancer. http://www.cancer.org/cancer/testicularcancer/detailedguide/testicular-cancer-key-statistics. Accessed July11, 2018.

74. Friedlander TW, Ryan CJ, Small EJ, Torti F. Testicular cancer. In: Neiderhuber JE, et al., ed. *Abeloff's Clinical Oncology.* 5th ed. Philadelphia, PA: Saunders; 2014.

75. Adra N, Einhorn LH. Testicular cancer update. *Clin Adv Hematol Oncol.* 2017;15(5):386–396.

76. Duchesne GM, Horwich A, Dearnaley DP, et al. Orchidectomy alone for stage I seminoma of the testis. *Cancer.* 1990;65:1115–1118.

77. Logue JP, Harris MA, Livsey JE, Swindell R, Mobarek N, Read G. Para-aortic radiation for stage I seminoma of the testis. *Int J Radiat Oncol Biol Phys.* 2000;48(suppl):208.

78. Thomas G, James W, Van Oosterom A, Kawai T. Consensus statement on the investigation and management of testicular seminoma 1989. *EORTC Genitourinary Group Monogr.* 1990;7:285–294.

79. Warde P, Gospodarowicz MK, Panzarella T, et al. Stage I testicular seminoma: results of adjuvant irradiation and surveillance. *J Clin Oncol.* 1995;13:2255–2262.

80. Fossa SD, Horwich A, Russell JM, et al. Optimal planning target volume for stage I testicular seminoma: a medical research council randomized trial: medical research council testicular tumor working group. *J Clin Oncol.* 1999;17(4):1146.

81. Jones WG, Fossa SD, Mead GM, et al. Randomized trial of 30 versus 20 Gy in the adjuvant treatment of stage I Testicular Seminoma: a report on medical research council trial TE188, European Organization for research and treatment of cancer trial 30942. *J Clin Oncol.* 2005;23(6):1200–1208.

82. Timothy R, Oliver D, Graham M, et al. Randomize trial of carboplatin versus radiotherapy for stage I seminoma: mature results on relapse and contralateral testis cancer rates in MRC TE19/EORTC 30982 study. *J Clin Oncol.* 2011;29(8):957–962.

83. Lieng H, Chung P, Lam T, Warde P, Craig T. Basic original report: testicular seminoma: scattered radiation dose to the contralateral testis in the modern era. *Pract Radiat Oncol.* 2018;8:e57–e62.

84. Sagerman RH, Kotlove DJ, Regine WF, et al. Stage II seminoma: results of postorchiectomy irradiation. *Radiology.* 1989;172:565–568.

85. Lai PP, Bernstein MJ, Kim H, et al. Radiation therapy for stage I and IIA testicular seminoma. *Int J Radiat Oncol Biol Phys.* 1993;28:373–379.

86. Zagars GK, Babaian RJ. The role of radiation in stage II testicular seminoma. *Int J Radiat Oncol Biol Phys.* 1987;13:163–170.

87. Fossa SD, Aass N, Kaalhus O. Radiotherapy for testicular seminoma stage I: treatment results and long-term post-irradiation morbidity in 365 patients. *Int J Radiat Oncol Biol Phys.* 1989;16.383–388.

88. Coia LR, Hanks GE. Complications from large field intermediate dose infradiaphragmatic radiation: an analysis of the Patterns of Care Outcome Studies for Hodgkin's disease and seminoma. *Int J Radiat Oncol Biol Phys.* 1988;15:29–35.

89. Shapiro E, Kinsella TJ, Makuch RW, et al. Effects of fractionated irradiation on endocrine aspects to testicular function. *J Clin Oncol.* 1985;3: 1232–1239.

90. Travis LB, Fosså SD, Schonfeld SJ, et al. Second cancers among 40,576 testicular cancer patients: focus on long-term survivors. *J Natl Cancer Inst.* 2005;97(18):1354–1365.

91. American Cancer Society. Kidney cancer. http://www.cancer.org/cancer/kidneycancer/detailedguide/kidney-cancer-adult-key-statistics; 2018.

92. Emily K, Stefan Z. Renal Cell Carcinoma in von Hippel–Lindau Disease—from tumor genetics to novel therapeutic strategies. *Front Pediatr.* 2018;6:16.

93. Linehan WM, WU S, Longo DL. Cancer of the kidney and ureter. In: DeVita VT, Hellman S, Rosenbers GA, eds. *Cancer: Principles and Practice of Oncology.* 10th ed. Philadelphia, PA: Wolters Kluwer Health; 2015.

94. Ridge CA, Pua BB, Madoff DC. Epidemiology and staging of renal cell carcinoma. *Semin Intervent Radiol.* 2014;3(1):3–8.

95. Pritchett TR, Lieskovsky G, Skinner DG. Clinical manifestations and treatment of renal parenchymal tumors. In: Skinner DG, Liekovsky G, eds. *Diagnosis and Management of Genitourinary Cancer.* Philadelphia, PA: WB Saunders; 1988.

96. Brafau BP, Cerqueda CS, Villalba LB, Izquierdo RS, Gonzalez BM, Molina CN. Metastatic renal cell carcinoma: radiologic findings and assessment of response to targeted antiangiogenic therapy busing multidetector CT. *RadioGraphics.* 2013;33(6):1691–1716.

97. Pili R, Kauffman E, Rodriguez R. Cancer of the kidney. In: Neiderhuber JE, et al., ed. *Abeloff's Clinical Oncology*. 5th ed. Philadelphia, PA: Saunders; 2014.

98. Mufti GR, Gove JR, Badenoch DF, et al. Transitional cell carcinoma of the renal pelvis and ureter. *Br J Urol*. 1989;63:135–140.

99. Richie JP. Carcinoma of the renal pelvis and ureter. In: Skinner DG, Liekovsky G, eds. *Diagnosis and Management of Genitourinary Cancer*. Philadelphia, PA: WB Saunders, 1988.

100. Lai PP. Kidney, renal pelvis, and ureter. In: Perez CA, Brady LW, eds. *Principles and Practice of Radiation Oncology*. 2nd ed. Philadelphia, PA: JB Lippincott; 1992.

34

Breast Cancer

Erin F. Gillespie, T. Jonathan Yang, Simon N. Powell, Lior Z. Braunstein

OBJECTIVES

- Discuss the changing epidemiology and risk factors for development of breast cancer.
- Describe the anatomy of the breast and regional nodal basins (axillary, supraclavicular, and internal mammary) and important considerations in relation to the anatomy.
- Appreciate the diversity of clinical presentations of breast cancer.
- Discuss the methods of breast cancer detection.
- Describe varying histologic types of breast cancer.
- Discuss breast cancer staging.

- Discuss the prognostic factors associated with breast cancer outcomes.
- Compare and contrast the rationale and treatment selection for various definitive breast cancer regimens.
- Compare the different radiation therapy approaches that are available for breast cancer.
- Create radiation treatment fields and understand planning considerations for different breast cancer treatments.
- Discuss radiation toxicity and long-term risks encountered during and after breast radiotherapy.

OUTLINE

KEY TERMS

Axillary lymph nodes

Breast-conserving therapy

Ductal carcinoma in situ

Internal mammary lymph nodes

Lymphovascular invasion

Mammographically occult breast cancer

Mastectomy

Partial breast irradiation

Supraclavicular fossa

Triple negative breast cancers

EPIDEMIOLOGY AND RISK FACTORS

Incidence

Breast cancer is the most common noncutaneous malignancy in the United States and the second most common cause of cancer death. Estimates predict over 250,000 new diagnoses and that it is responsible for more than 40,000 deaths in the United States each year.[1] Approximately one in eight women will develop breast cancer by the age of 70 years.[2] Of note, the incidence of breast cancer in the United States declined by approximately 2% per year from 1999 to 2007, presumably due to the discontinuation of long-term hormone replacement therapy in postmenopausal women, which has been associated with an increased risk in development of breast cancer.[3,4] However, since then, rates have steadily increased again 0.4% per year as of 2013.[1]

Risk Factors

Gender. Breast cancer occurs 100 times more frequently in women than in men. It is the most common malignancy in women yet represents less than 1% of malignancies in men. Treatment paradigms typically mirror those of their female counterparts.[5] The median age of detection of breast cancer in men is 65 to 67 years, approximately 5 to 10 years later than the median age in women.[6,7]

Age. Breast cancer risk increases with age.[8] Between 2012 and 2014, the probability of breast cancer development in American women at the age of 40 was 1 in 68, at the age of 50 was 1 in 43, at the age of 60 was 1 in 29, at the age of 70 was 1 in 25. Lifetime risk is 1 in 8.[2] Despite increasing prevalence with age, outcomes tend to be more favorable for patients diagnosed at older age, typically as a result of more indolent tumor biology, in contrast to younger patients, who are more likely to present with aggressive biology, such as triple-negative tumors.[9,10]

Race. Although breast cancer is the most common malignancy among all women regardless of ethnicity, the incidence of breast cancer in the United States is slightly higher in white versus black women (122/100,000 women vs. 117/100,000 women, respectively).[11] Despite this, black women tend to present with more advanced disease and have a higher mortality rate (see "Prognostic Factors" section). Furthermore, there is a growing body of evidence to suggest different causes of carcinogenesis between patients of different genetic backgrounds.[12]

Weight. Among postmenopausal women, those with a body mass index (BMI) of more than 33 kg/m^2 are at 1.3 times higher risk for development of breast cancer compared with women with a BMI of less than 21 kg/m^2.[13] One hypothesis for the association between increased BMI and breast cancer is based on putatively higher levels of estrogen in obese women resulting from the peripheral conversion of estrogenic precursors by aromatase in adipose tissues.[14]

Hormonal and Reproductive Factors. Breast cancer risk rises with prolonged estrogen exposure. Early menarche and late menopause are hypothesized to increase breast cancer risk because of endogenous estrogen exposure. Nulliparous women are at increased risk for breast cancer compared with parous women who have the protective effect of pregnancy seen even 10 years after delivery.[15] Women whose first pregnancy is at a later age have an increased risk of breast cancer. As an example, lifetime breast cancer risk for a woman with a first full-term birth at age 35 is similar to that of a nulliparous woman.[16]

The risk of breast cancer in the setting of exogenous endocrine therapy, such as estrogenic hormone replacement therapy, depends on the type and duration of the therapy. Women who have prolonged use of hormone replacement therapy are at an increased risk of development of breast cancer.[17] Epidemiologic studies generally have not supported an association between oral contraceptive use and lifetime risk of breast cancer.[18,19]

Breast Pathology. Proliferative benign breast lesions are associated with an increased risk of breast cancer. Atypical ductal hyperplasia (ADH) and atypical lobular hyperplasia (ALH) represent abnormal noninvasive proliferations and are considered pathologic diagnoses. Most of these have cellular features of ductal carcinoma in situ (DCIS) or lobular carcinoma in situ (LCIS). Atypical hyperplasia leads to a substantial increase in the risk (4 to 5 times) of subsequent breast cancer.[20,21] Fig. 34.1 shows ADH, ALH, and LCIS as seen with histopathology.

Similarly, breast density reflects the ratio of glandular to adipose tissue as measured on mammography, and it is also associated with increased breast cancer risk. Women with mammographically dense breast tissue are four to five times more likely to develop subsequent breast cancer.[22]

History of Breast Cancer. Women with a personal history of noninvasive (DCIS) or invasive breast cancer exhibit an increased risk of contralateral breast cancer.[23] This risk increases for those treated curatively for breast cancer at a young age. Consequently, patients with a history of breast cancer must be closely monitored for the development of a contralateral breast malignancy, in addition to monitoring of the treated breast.

Genetics. As with nearly all other cancers, family history of breast cancer strongly influences personal risk. A woman with a first-degree relative with breast cancer has a twofold risk of development of breast cancer. A woman with two first-degree relatives with breast cancer has a threefold risk of development of breast cancer compared with a woman with no affected first-degree relatives. In addition, the age at diagnosis of the affected first-degree relative also influences a woman's breast cancer risk: a first-degree relative diagnosed before age 30 years confers a threefold risk of developing breast cancer, whereas if diagnosed after age 60 years, risk increases only 1.5-fold.[24]

Only 5% to 6% of all breast cancers are directly attributable to mutations in the breast cancer–susceptibility genes *BRCA1* or *BRCA2*.

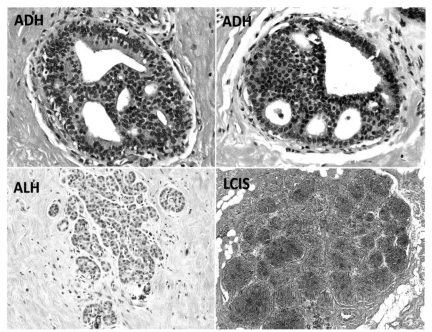

Fig. 34.1 Histopathologic features of cancer precursor lesions: atypical ductal hyperplasia *(ADH)*, atypical lobular hyperplasia *(ALH)*, and lobular carcinoma in situ *(LCIS)*.

Women with these mutations face a high risk of development of breast cancer. The cumulative breast cancer risk by age 70 years among women who are *BRCA1* carriers ranges above 60% and, in women who are *BRCA2* carriers, ranges up to 55%.[25] *BRCA1/2* mutations also increase breast cancer risk in men. For example, in men with *BRCA2* mutation, the lifetime breast cancer risk is approximately 6%, compared with 0.1% among men overall.[26]

Lifestyle. Several lifestyle parameters have been studied for their association with breast cancer risk. A metaanalysis that compared 92,000 light drinkers and 60,000 nondrinkers showed a small (5%) but significant association between breast cancer risk and light alcohol intake in women.[27] Tobacco use, a risk factor among many cancers, has also been found to be associated with increased risk of breast cancer, more so in current than past tobacco users, yet with an elevated risk among both.[28] Night shift work is also recognized by the World Health Organization as a probable carcinogen. A recent study on nurses reported that working after midnight was associated with elevated risk of breast cancer.[29] The elevated cancer risk has been proposed to be the result of nocturnal light exposure and suppression of nocturnal melatonin production by the pineal gland.[30]

Radiation Exposure. Radiation exposure at a young age has been associated with increased breast cancer risk.[31] This has been demonstrated most convincingly among patients treated for Hodgkin lymphoma at a young age who underwent mantle-field irradiation and subsequently developed secondary cancers. The risk of breast cancer is inversely related to age at treatment and declines steeply. Women who received radiation before the age of 20 years have a 34% predictive risk of development of breast cancer 25 years after treatment, and those who received radiation after the age of 29 years have a predicted risk of 3.5%.[32] The risk of breast cancer is dose dependent, with a dose greater than 4 Gy to the breast associated with a 3.2 times increased risk of breast cancer compared with a dose less than 4 Gy. Breast cancer risk increased eightfold with a prior breast dose of more than 40 Gy.[33]

ANATOMY

General Introduction

The mammary glands are composed of glandular tissue, subcutaneous fat, and fibrous connective tissue. The glands are rudimentary in men, consisting of only a few small ducts, and well developed in women, as they are the most prominent superficial structure of the anterior thoracic wall. The glands are supported by deep fascia overlying the pectoral muscles (pectoralis major and minor) posteriorly and are attached to the dermis with superficial fascia anteriorly. Fig. 34.2 illustrates the anatomy of the breast.

The adult breast is located between the second and sixth ribs in the sagittal plane and extends from the sternochondral junctions to the midaxillary line in the axial plane. Breast tissue is also located in the axilla, extending along the inferolateral edge of the pectoralis major and forming the axillary tail of Spence. Two-thirds of the breast rest on the deep pectoral fascia that overlies the pectoralis major, and one-third of the breast rests on the fascia that covers the serratus anterior. The retromammary bursa, which contains adipose tissue, is a loose connective tissue plane between the breast and deep pectoral fascia that allows breast movements. The suspensory ligaments of Cooper run from pectoral fascia and branch out through and around breast tissue to connect to the skin overlying the breast, supporting the breast in its normal position and maintaining its shape.

Breast Structure

The breast parenchyma consists of 15 to 20 sections or lobes that are embedded in adipose tissue. Each lobe is drained by a lactiferous duct that opens at the nipple. Ductal carcinoma is a type of breast cancer that originates from the lactiferous ducts. In each lobe are numerous lobules that contain the milk-producing alveoli arranged in grapelike clusters. Lobular carcinoma is a type of breast cancer that originates from the lobules of the breast. The nipple is a conical prominence in the center of the areola that is composed mostly of smooth muscle fibers that compress the lactiferous ducts. It contains no fat, hair, or sweat glands. In young, nulliparous women, the nipples are usually at the

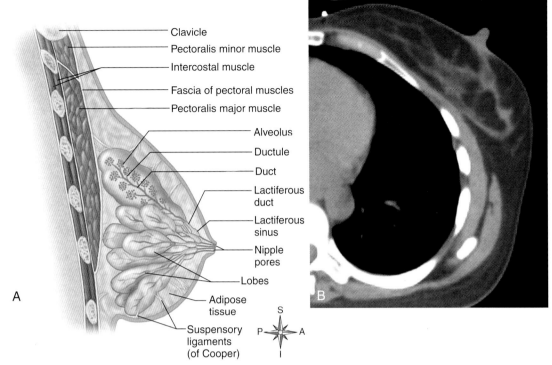

Fig. 34.2 (A) Sagittal section of the breast. (B) Axial section of the breast with computed tomographic scanning: the breast tissue is shown with variable density, and the muscles, ribs, and lung are visualized. (A, From Thibodeau GA, Patton KT: *The Human Body in Health and Disease*. 7th ed. St. Louis, MO: Mosby; 2018.)

level of the fourth intercostal spaces. However, the position of the nipples can vary considerably in women. The circular, pigmented area that surrounds the nipple is the areola. It contains numerous nerve endings and sebaceous glands.

Blood Supply and Lymphatics

Arteries, Veins, and Nerves. The arterial supply of the breast is derived from the medial mammary branches and anterior intercostal branches of the internal mammary artery medially, and the lateral thoracic and thoracoacromial artery branches of the axillary artery and the posterior intercostal arteries laterally.

The venous drainage of the breast is mainly to the axillary vein through the lateral thoracic and lateral mammary veins. Medially, the internal mammary vein is responsible for venous drainage through its perforating branches. In addition, the intercostal veins communicate with the vertebral plexus of Batson, a system of small veins that runs vertically through and around the vertebral column. This system drains the proximal humeri, shoulders, skull, vertebral bodies, bony pelvis, and proximal femurs. Venous blood can flow in both directions in this system because of the absence of valves and low pressure in the channels. Malignant cells in the blood that drain through the intercostal veins from the breast can therefore enter the axial skeleton, resulting in metastatic disease.

The nerves of the breast derive from anterior and lateral cutaneous branches of the fourth through sixth intercostal nerves. Branches of the intercostal nerves pass through the deep fascia that covers the pectoralis major, the breast parenchyma, and subcutaneous tissue and finally convey sensory fibers to the skin of the breast.

Lymphatic Drainage. The lymphatic channels follow the duct and lobular complexes and drain into lymph nodes. *Intra*mammary lymph nodes are located within the breast parenchyma. Although they can be involved with a metastatic tumor from the primary cancer within the breast, *intra*mammary involvement is part of the nodal staging. In describing the extent of lymph node metastasis, the number and

location (intramammary, axillary, supraclavicular/infraclavicular, internal mammary) of regional lymph nodes involved are considered.

Axillary lymph nodes. Primary deep lymphatic drainage of the breast occurs to the ipsilateral axilla. Between 10 and 50 lymph nodes are scattered throughout each axilla. These can be divided into three major sections (levels I, II, and III) based on location in relation with the pectoralis minor muscle and the sequential drainage patterns. Level I lymph nodes are located lateral of the pectoralis minor and are the most superficial lymph nodes in the axilla. They often represent the first station of drainage from the breast. Level II lymph nodes are located beneath the muscle. Level III lymph nodes, or the infraclavicular lymph nodes, are located cranial and medial to the pectoralis minor. Orderly spread of tumor cells from level I to II to III lymph nodes is most common, but skip metastasis can also occur. Surgically, the most common axillary lymph node dissection requires retrieval of level I and II lymph nodes. In a large lymphoscintigraphy study conducted at the Netherlands Cancer Institute, level I to II axillary lymph nodes were the most common location for sentinel lymph nodes regardless of the tumor location.[35] Fig. 34.3 shows the location of axillary level I to III lymph nodes.

Internal mammary lymph nodes. The internal mammary lymph nodes are located in the parasternal space, embedded in fat in the intercostal spaces, and they run alongside the corresponding artery and vein. Most internal mammary nodal recurrences in breast cancer are seen in the first, second, and third intercostal spaces.[34] Innerquadrant tumors have a higher risks of internal mammary lymph node involvement, with approximately 30% of patients with drainage localized to these lymph nodes.[35] Fig. 34.4 shows the location of the internal mammary node (IMN); see Fig. 34.4A–C) and radiographic features of IMN recurrence (see Fig. 34.4D).

Supraclavicular lymph nodes. The supraclavicular lymph nodes are located within the supraclavicular fossa, a space defined by the omohyoid muscle and tendon laterally and superiorly, the internal jugular vein medially, and the clavicle and subclavian vein inferiorly. The supraclavicular lymph nodes not only provide drainage for the internal mammary lymph node and

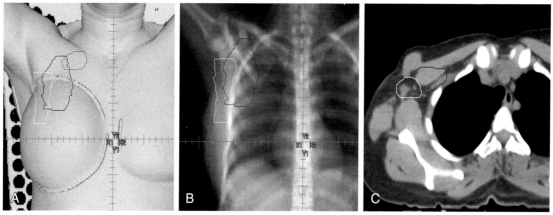

Fig. 34.3 Locations of level I, II, and III axillary lymph nodes on: (A) skin rendering; (B) anterior-posterior digitally reconstructed radiograph; and (C) axial section of computed tomographic scan. The anatomy of the axilla is defined by the position of the pectoralis minor muscle (circled in C), which attaches to the coracoid process (shown in B).

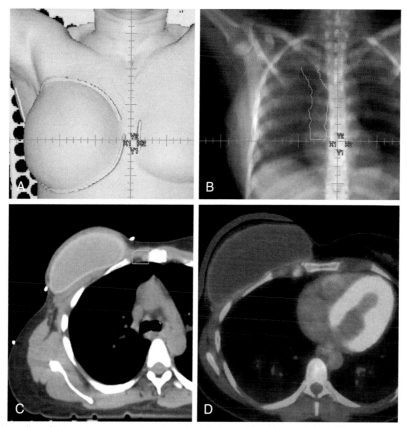

Fig. 34.4 Location of internal mammary lymph nodes chain on: (A) skin rendering, (B) anterior-posterior digitally reconstructed radiograph, and (C) axial section of computed tomographic scan. (D) A metabolically active internal mammary lymph node from recurrent breast cancer on positron emission tomographic scan.

axillary lymph node chains, but a small number of breast tumors, especially centrally located tumors, have direct drainage to the supraclavicular nodes. Fig. 34.5 shows the location of supraclavicular lymph nodes.

CLINICAL PRESENTATION

Mammographic Signs

The most frequent presentation of early-stage breast cancer is an asymptomatic, nonpalpable mass detected as an abnormality on a screening mammogram. On mammogram, two primary findings can be detected: a mass with ill-defined or speculated edges or irregular, pleomorphic calcifications. Further diagnostic studies, such as a diagnostic mammography and ultrasound scan, can help better determine the etiologies of these findings. Biopsy confirms breast cancer suspicion

pathologically. These procedures are detailed later in this chapter within the "Detection and Diagnosis" section. An example of an abnormal mammogram, highly suspicious for breast cancer, is seen in Fig. 34.6.

Physical Signs

The most common physical sign of early stage breast cancer is a painless mobile mass. When a patient presents with a breast mass, a detailed physical examination, including evaluation of the contralateral breast and bilateral regional lymph nodes (axilla, supraclavicular, infraclavicular, neck), is indicated. Because the treatment approach for breast cancer can vary by clinical presentation, such as tumor size, location, and skin involvement, detailed documentation of a patient's initial physical findings is essential. Physical signs of a locally advanced breast cancer include enlarged or matted axillary or supraclavicular lymph nodes, abnormal breast contours, nipple discharge

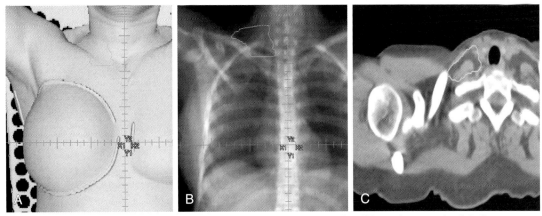

Fig. 34.5 Locations of supraclavicular lymph nodes on: (A) skin rendering, (B) anterior-posterior digitally reconstructed radiograph, and (C) axial section of computed tomographic scan.

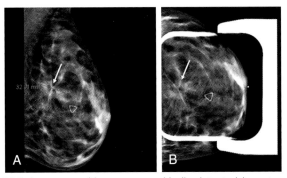

Fig. 34.6 A woman with mammographically detected breast cancer *(arrow)* on: (A) mediolateral oblique view of mammogram, and (B) craniocaudal compression view.

or retraction, and a palpable mass with or without fixation to the chest wall or involvement of the skin. Skin findings, such as erythema, thickening, peau d'orange, and ulcerations, are also indications of advanced disease. Inflammatory breast cancer (IBC), an aggressive form of breast cancer, presents with rapid onset, skin erythema and induration, and asymmetric enlargement and often is generally not associated with a palpable mass.

DETECTION AND DIAGNOSIS

Detection

Most breast cancers in the United States are diagnosed as a result of an abnormal screening imaging study, with a smaller proportion presenting clinically because of symptoms (breast pain, palpable lump, nipple discharge, etc.). Breast cancer incidence appeared to rise between 1994 and 1999, remaining stable after 2000.[36] This increased rate of breast cancer diagnosis in the 1990s was attributed to increased detection of early-stage and in situ disease, representing the prevalence of disease as screening began, rather than truly new cases. Conversely, the mortality rate of breast cancer began to steadily decline in 1990, with the recent age-adjusted mortality rate reaching 22.8 per 100,000, the lowest level since 1969.[37] This decreasing risk of breast cancer death can be partially attributed to early detection and highlights the importance of routine screening.

Imaging Studies. Several imaging technologies have been developed for breast cancer screening. The most established screening modalities include mammography, ultrasound, and magnetic resonance imaging (MRI). Breast self-examination is of varying efficacy in terms of early detection and has fallen out of favor among national screening guidelines.[7]

Mammography. Annual mammography is the mainstay of breast cancer screening in the United States. US surveillance data indicated that 78% of the invasive breast cancers detected on mammograms had no lymph node involvement.[38] Multiple studies also demonstrate a reduction in breast cancer mortality following the routine use of screening mammogram. A large international meta-analysis published in 2012 reviewed 11 randomized studies that included more than 670,000 women, showing a 20% relative risk reduction in breast cancer death among women who underwent mammogram screening compared with those who did not.[39] The benefit of decreased breast cancer mortality was found in women from age 40 to 69 years.[40] In addition to improved breast cancer–specific survival, mammographic screening was also shown to improve overall survival in an analysis of 240,000 women who were followed for over 15 years in Sweden.[41]

Routine mammographic imaging includes two views of each breast: craniocaudal (CC) and mediolateral oblique (MLO). The breast is lifted, positioned on the imaging plate, and compressed from above to generate the CC view. For the MLO view, which is used to maximize the coverage of the breast tissue, the breast is compressed from the side, obliquely angled down medial to lateral by 30 degrees. The radiation dose absorbed by the breast during screening mammogram depends on the breast thickness. The American College of Radiology recommends that the mean glandular dose exposure for a breast that is 4.2 cm thick should not exceed 3 mGy per image. There is no evidence that routine screening in women starting at age 40 years is associated with an elevated breast cancer risk from radiation exposure.[42]

It is important to distinguish screening and diagnostic mammography. A screening mammogram is performed in a patient with no clinical symptoms of breast cancer; a diagnostic mammogram is performed in a patient who presents with clinical suspicion, such as abnormal clinical examination or abnormal screening mammogram results. The diagnostic mammogram is performed with a radiologist's supervision, and views obtained are tailored to the clinically suspicious abnormality. Some of the diagnostic mammogram views include magnification (of calcifications) and spot compression (of architectural asymmetry) to further delineate the morphology or shape of suspicious disease; true lateral view, along with CC view, to triangulate suspicious disease; and rolled view to confirm that a finding seen only on one of the screening mammogram views is a three-dimensional (3D) lesion.

Mammography can miss 10% to 15% of breast cancers (mammographically occult), which is particularly so for lobular carcinomas. This is often a result of radiographic overlap between glandular tissue and tumor, which renders the tumor difficult to discern, or there may be a radiolucent growth pattern. Women with dense breasts have higher rates of mammographically occult breast cancers as a result of mammography's reduced sensitivity in this population. Because increased breast density is an independent risk factor for breast cancer,[43] other strategies have been used for screening, such as the addition of ultrasound.

More recently, breast tomosynthesis, also known as 3D mammography, has been incorporated frequently as an adjunct to standard mammography. Tomosynthesis uses a moving x-ray source and digital detector to generate 3D data of the breast architecture. This modality adds 3D thin slice reconstruction to standard mammography to provide better visualization by excluding overlapping structures seen on a two-dimensional view. This improvement in lesion delineation decreases the false-positive rate, prompting fewer biopsies.[44,45]

Ultrasound. Ultrasound is used in conjunction with mammography for screening in women who have dense breast tissue that is not adequately evaluated by mammogram alone. Ultrasound is not appropriate as a single screening modality because it is unable to detect calcifications and is not sensitive enough to detect small lesions. When used as an adjunct to mammogram, ultrasound increases the sensitivity in detection of early-stage breast cancer but decreases specificity. A large trial conducted through the American College of Radiology Imaging Network showed that ultrasound in combination with mammography for screening in women at high risk with dense breasts yields an additional 1.1 to 7.2 cancers per 1000 women screened compared with mammogram alone. However, an increased number of false positives was also demonstrated (i.e., a reduction in specificity).[46] Diagnostically, ultrasound is used to further evaluate abnormalities detected on screening mammogram. It is useful in evaluation of the extent of disease, and it can also be used in evaluation of the axilla for suspicious lymph nodes. Ultrasound is also the preferred imaging modality for biopsy guidance among lesions that are sonographically detectable.

Magnetic resonance imaging. MRI is more sensitive, but less specific, than mammography in the detection of breast cancer, with sensitivity reported between 88% and 100%[47,48] and specificity reaching as low as 72%,[49] as shown in a meta-analysis study by Peters et al., pooling 44 different studies. An MRI of the breast covers more tissue than observed with mammography alone and also includes visualization of the chest wall (Fig. 34.7). No data yet show a benefit for MRI screening in women with an average risk for breast cancer. In women with higher breast cancer risk, MRI results in higher rates of detection that can potentially translate into a survival benefit.[50] Among these patients, MRI also performs with similar specificity. Based on data from multiple MRI-based breast cancer screening trials, in 2007, the American Cancer Society published that screening MRI in combination with mammogram is recommended for women with 20% or greater lifetime risk of breast cancer, including women with a strong family history of breast or ovarian cancer and women who were treated for Hodgkin disease. Table 34.1 details the results of several large prospective studies in assessing the role of MRI in breast cancer screening for women with a high lifetime risk. In addition to screening, MRI is also useful in providing imaging guidance for biopsy of lesions that are better visualized on MRI than other imaging modalities.

Breast Palpation. Clinical breast examination is an important aspect of breast cancer detection. The skin over the breast is evaluated for color and textural changes. With the patient in the sitting and supine positions, the breast is examined visually and with palpation for mobility and the presence of a mass. The presence of chest wall fixation is assessed through a series of muscle-tensing maneuvers by the patient. Dimpling of the skin, nipple retraction, nipple discharge, and axillary lymph node enlargement are evaluated during the clinical examination. Although studies have shown that clinical breast examination in addition to mammography results in greater sensitivity in breast cancer detection compared with mammography alone, it also results in a higher false-positive rate.[51]

Diagnosis

The diagnosis of breast cancer is a pathologic one, dependent on the microscopic evaluation of breast tissue that exhibits distinct cellular features. The requisite tissue can be obtained via several complementary modalities.

Fine-Needle Biopsy. Fine-needle aspiration (FNA) involves the guided placement of a relatively small-gauge needle into the suspicious tissue in the breast. Sonographically detectable tumors are typically biopsied under ultrasound guidance. Sonographically occult tumors that harbor calcifications can be biopsied under stereotactic mammographic guidance. Lesions that neither harbor calcifications, nor can be seen on ultrasound, may be detectable by MRI, prompting MRI-guided biopsy. In any FNA modality, the needle is attached to a syringe in which the evacuated blood or tissue is collected. This material is prepared on slides for cytologic evaluation. FNA of the axillary lymph nodes can also be performed under imaging guidance to establish the axillary disease status.

Core Needle Biopsy. Core needle biopsy is similar to fine-needle biopsy in that a syringe and a larger-gauge needle are used to aspirate

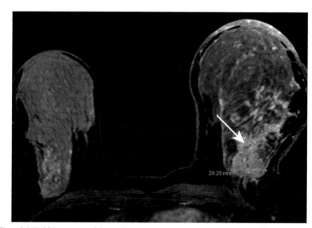

Fig. 34.7 Woman with a 3-cm tumor seen on magnetic resonance imaging (MRI; *arrow*). In addition to imaging of the breasts, an MRI can also delineate the chest wall anatomy with high resolution, which is a benefit over mammogram.

TABLE 34.1 Breast Magnetic Resonance Imaging Screening Study Results for Women With High Lifetime Risk for Development of Breast Cancer

	No. of Women	Age Range (Years)	MAMMOGRAM Sensitivity (%)	MAMMOGRAM Specificity (%)	MRI Sensitivity (%)	MRI Specificity (%)
The Netherlands[122]	1909	25–70	33	95	80	90
United Kingdom[123]	649	35–49	40	93	77	81
Germany[124]	529	≥30	33	97	91	97
United States[125]	390	≥25	25	98	100	95
Canada[126]	236	25–65	36	>99	77	95

MRI, Magnetic resonance imaging.

a core of tissue from the breast mass. Pathologic review can then offer robust architectural information about the growth pattern within the lesion. This approach offers a more definitive histologic diagnosis compared with FNA, mitigates inadequate sampling, and allows for distinction between invasive versus in situ cancer.

Excisional Biopsy. If a core needle biopsy is nondiagnostic, conflicts with imaging results or clinical suspicion, or has high risk features such as atypical hyperplasia, radial scar, papilloma, or LCIS, excisional biopsy is recommended.[52] Excisional biopsy involves surgical removal of the entire lesion in question.

In addition to determination of the histology of invasive or in situ breast cancer with biopsy of the lesion, assessment for expression of estrogen, progesterone, and human epidermal growth factor-2 (HER2) receptors status on the biopsy specimen is also important for a comprehensive assessment of treatment strategies. The prognostic implication of receptor status is discussed below.

PATHOLOGY

In Situ Cancers

The American Joint Committee on Cancer (AJCC) classifies breast cancers into in situ cancers and invasive cancers. The in situ cancers include DCIS and LCIS. DCIS is carcinoma confined to the preexisting duct system of the breast without penetration of the basement membrane and invasion of surrounding tissues on microscopic examination. DCIS can be characterized by its architectural patterns and nuclear grade. It represents approximately one-quarter of all breast cancers. DCIS is associated with a very low risk for axillary metastasis and breast cancer mortality. It is detected as a mammographic abnormality in 80% to 90% of women. Therefore the incidence of DCIS has increased dramatically in the era of routine screening mammography.

The five major subtypes of DCIS based on pathologic examination of architectural features are as follows: comedo type, which is characterized by prominent necrosis in the center of the involved spaces; cribriform type, which is characterized by the formation of back-to-back glands without intervening stroma; micropapillary type and papillary type, which show projection of tumor cells into the lumen; and solid type, which shows no

significant necrosis, gland formation, or projections of tumor cells. Although architectural classification of DCIS is descriptive, classification of DCIS based on nuclear grade (low, intermediate, and high) can affect clinical management. Low-grade lesions have a low proliferative rate and are typically estrogen and progesterone receptor (PR) positive. High-grade lesions have a high proliferative rate and tend to be associated with overexpression of HER2. Estrogen receptor positivity is associated with 90% low-grade DCIS and 25% high-grade DCIS. Low-grade and high-grade DCIS also have different patterns of growth within the breast. Low-grade lesions tend to have more diffuse and discontinuous pattern of spread, sometimes with distances of 1 cm between two involved areas, and high-grade DCIS tends to spread continuously.[53]

LCIS is similar to DCIS in that it has not demonstrated the ability to invade the basement membrane and spread. However, it is important to clarify that LCIS is considered a marker for increased risk of development of breast cancer rather that a disease that requires treatment. It is characterized by discohesive epithelial cells that fill the acinar spaces. Mastectomy studies have shown that LCIS is multicentric in 90% of patients and bilateral in up to 50% of patients.[54] The treatment for LCIS is usually excision alone with close follow-up, but prophylactic bilateral mastectomies have also been used to reduce risk.

Invasive Cancers

Invasive ductal carcinoma is the most common invasive cancer of the breast; it accounts for 70% to 80% of invasive lesions, and approximately 50% of invasive ductal carcinomas include a DCIS component. It originates in the ductal component of the breast, penetrates the basement membrane, and invades surrounding glands and adipose tissue. On pathologic examination, these lesions invade the surrounding tissues haphazardly and create irregular, stellar shapes. Under the microscope, nests and cords of tumor cells are seen that induce fibrosis as they infiltrate the breast tissue, which allows for the mass to be palpable and to present as a solid, dense structure on imaging. Invasive ductal carcinoma (often abbreviated IDC) is also subdivided into grades based on histology, with well-differentiated tumors with gland formation having a lower grade and poorly differentiated tumors without gland formation having a higher grade. Higher-grade lesions are associated with higher risk of recurrence, which is discussed in the "Prognostic Factors" section. Fig. 34.8 shows

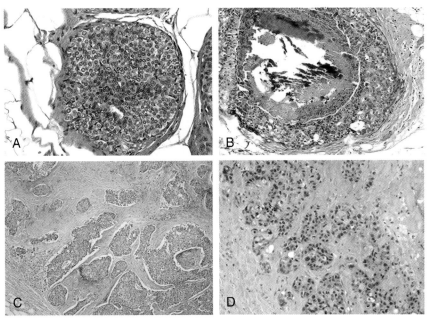

Fig. 34.8 Histopathologic features of: (A and B) ductal carcinoma in situ, and (C and D) invasive ductal carcinoma.

histopathologic features of DCIS (see Fig. 34.8A and B, precursor of invasive breast cancer) and invasive ductal carcinoma (see Fig. 34.8C and D).

Given that invasive ductal carcinoma is frequently associated with DCIS, the term *extensive intraductal component* (EIC) is used to describe DCIS that comprises 25% or more of the primary tumor and its presence in the healthy surrounding breast tissue. The definition also includes DCIS with focal areas of invasion. The presence of EIC is associated with high risk of local recurrence after lumpectomy with or without radiation therapy.[55,56] This high risk was thought to be because EIC-positive tumors were significantly more likely to have residual cancer (predominantly DCIS) at greater distances from the primary invasive ductal carcinoma than EIC-negative tumors.[57]

Invasive lobular carcinoma is the second most common type of invasive breast cancer; it accounts for 5% to 10% of all invasive lesions. It originates from the glands, or lobules, of the breast. Under the microscope, these tumors are characterized by small cells that infiltrate the surrounding tissues in a single-file pattern, often growing in a target-like configuration around the healthy breast ducts. Unlike invasive ductal carcinoma, it is not commonly associated with fibrosis formation. Invasive lobular carcinomas (often abbreviated ILC) have a higher frequency of bilateral breast involvement than invasive ductal carcinomas. They are more common in older women and, in general, are more well differentiated.[58] Invasive lobular carcinomas are usually estrogen receptor (ER) positive.

Other invasive cancers of the breast are less common, including tubular carcinoma, mucinous carcinoma, medullary carcinoma, tubulolobular carcinoma, metaplastic carcinoma, micropapillary carcinoma, and adenoid cystic carcinoma. Each carcinoma is characterized by its unique pathologic features, and the prognosis of most of them is more favorable than ductal carcinoma.

STAGING

The AAJCC tumor node metastasis (TNM) staging system for breast cancer is an internationally accepted system for determination of disease stage. More information about breast cancer staging can be found at: https://www.cancer.org/cancer/breast-cancer/understanding-a-breast-cancer-diagnosis/stages-of-breast-cancer.html. It is based on analyses of survival in diverse patients who represent all stages of disease. A unified staging system is important because it facilitates discussion of treatment options, prognosis, and outcomes between providers around the globe. Routine updates of the staging system are performed to reflect outcomes of current practice trends. The current staging system is more complex than prior versions, as it now includes an anatomic stage as well as a prognostic stage, and incorporates hormonal status, HER2 status, and grade into the stage grouping.

Clinical Stage

The clinical stage (cTNM) is based on findings from physical examination and imaging studies (mammography, ultrasound scan, MRI, computed tomographic [CT] scan). The size of the tumor and lymph node involvement can be derived from physical examinations and further aided with imaging. The presence of distant metastasis is hard to conclude from physical examination and necessitates information from imaging for clinical suspicion. Extensive imaging is not necessary to designate a patient to have M0 disease if the clinical history and examination do not suggest the presence of distant metastasis, particularly in early-stage disease. Accurate clinical staging is important, especially in patients who have locally advanced breast cancer and are undergoing neoadjuvant chemotherapy (chemotherapy before surgery). The clinical staging for these patients can influence postsurgical treatment decisions, such as whether the patient should receive adjuvant radiation therapy.

For clinical T stage, the larger the tumor is, the higher its T stage. Tumor with extension to the chest wall or skin (ulceration or skin nodules) is classified as stage T4. IBC has the highest T stage classification of T4d. Clinical N stage is based on the location and extent of regional lymph nodes involvement, with involvement of the typical first drainage station lymph nodes being lower N stage (e.g., axillary lymph nodes involvement is N1) and more extensive lymph nodes involvement being higher N stage (supraclavicular lymph nodes, internal mammary lymph nodes, and axillary lymph nodes involvement).

Pathologic Stage

The pathologic stage (pTNM) is based on detailed pathologic examination of the primary tumor from the lumpectomy or mastectomy and review of the regional lymph nodes from the sentinel lymph node biopsy or axillary lymph node dissection. For invasive cancer, the T stage is based on the size of the invasive component of the tumor, with larger tumors having higher pathologic T stages. For multiple primary tumors, the size of the largest tumor determines the pathologic T stage. The number of positive lymph nodes and their locations define the N stage. A woman with one to three axillary lymph nodes involved is classified to have N1 disease, with four to nine axillary lymph nodes involved is N2 disease, and with 10 or more axillary lymph nodes involved is N3 disease. Pathologic staging is generally considered to be more accurate than clinical staging in determination of the extent of patient's disease and the prognosis of the patient. The prognostic implication of patient's stage is discussed subsequently.

PROGNOSTIC AND PREDICTIVE FACTORS

A host of clinical and pathologic features are associated with breast cancer recurrence and survival outcomes. Some of these associations, like tumor size or nodal status, have a clear causal link to subsequent disease events, whereas others, such as age or race, are hypothesized to drive adverse biology but have yet to be fully revealed with regard to the mechanism that drives future risk. This section will review prognostic and predictive factors that are relevant for patients with nonmetastatic breast cancer. The reader should also appreciate the difference between prognostic factors, which indicate an outcome driven by inherent tumor biology regardless of therapeutic intervention, and predictive factors, which determine the extent to which a tumor will respond to (or resist) a given treatment.

Although many risk factors are reported to be independently prognostic and predictive of outcome, some exhibit robust interactions that change their significance within a given context. These "synergies" are difficult to parse in small studies but have been demonstrated in larger population level analyses. As an example, the adverse nature of young age at diagnosis was discussed above; however, among patients with HER2-amplified breast cancer who receive HER2-targeted therapy, age seems to have little correlation with outcome.

Clinical Characteristics

Clinical features have historically been the mainstay of risk prediction because these were the most readily apparent parameters with which to classify patients. Age and race, for example, two clear identifiers, have, for decades, been employed for risk stratification. Younger age at diagnosis is associated with worse survival among those with breast cancer. It is unclear, however, if age is merely a proxy for other adverse biologic features, because young women typically present with larger tumors that are estrogen receptor (ER) negative, both of which indicate adverse outcomes. When adjusting for these factors using multivariate regression methods, younger age remains an adverse feature, with worse survival outcomes and more aggressive biology.[59] With regard to race, black women are at higher risk of developing triple-negative breast cancer (TNBC) that is ER negative, PR negative, and HER2 negative. This entity is a biologically more aggressive subtype for which neither endocrine therapy nor HER2-directed therapies are effective.[60] Aside from biology, however, several studies have demonstrated that black women undergo less breast cancer screening (24% vs. 35%) and less treatment after diagnosis (87% vs. 92%). In addition, black women wait longer from diagnosis to treatment (29 vs. 22 days) and undergo breast-conserving surgery without adjuvant therapy more frequently (8% vs. 7%), all of which further contributes to adverse outcomes.[61] Although black women have a lower incidence of breast cancer compared with white women in the United States, these factors may contribute to the higher mortality rate in this population (28 vs 20 per 100,000 in 2015).[37]

Pathologic Characteristics

Stage. Pathologic stage is prognostic for outcomes in women with breast cancer. Breast cancer staging is based on the TNM system and is discussed in the previous section. AJCC stage groupings have seen increasingly detailed subgroupings in recent years with the aim of stratifying breast cancer risk and incorporating biologic factors in addition to anatomic features.

Tumor. T stage is dependent on the tumor size and status of skin or chest wall involvement at the time of presentation. Tumor size is measured as the largest diameter of the primary breast cancer or the size of the largest lesion when multiple foci exist. Larger tumors are associated with worse outcomes. A large study that involved 24,740 patients showed that for tumors less than 2 cm, the 5-year breast cancer survival rate was 91%, compared with 63% for tumors greater than 5 cm, independent of nodal involvement.[62] Although tumor location by quadrant influences the pattern of lymph node spread, no evidence indicates that the location of the primary tumor directly affects prognosis. Fixation of a mass to the chest wall (T4a) is a notably adverse feature, as is skin involvement (T4b), which suggests lymphovascular compromise. IBC (stage T4d) is an uncommon but highly aggressive presentation. Women with IBC present with symptoms that can include rapid swelling, erythema, skin induration, warmth, pain, and texture changes (reddened area with texture resembling the peel of an orange, "peau d'orange"). Although breast cancer must still be diagnosed by biopsy, the IBC subset is further established by the clinical presence of rapid-onset erythema occupying at least one-third of the breast and lasting no longer than 6 months. Biopsy of evidence of dermal lymphatic invasion is not sufficient to make the diagnosis of IBC in the absence of these clinical findings.

Lymph nodes. The number of axillary lymph nodes involved by tumor is a strong prognostic indicator. An increasing number of involved lymph nodes, regardless of other risk factors, signifies an increasing probability of future disease events.[3] Even among small tumors (<2 cm), one study showed that the 5-year survival rate for patients with no lymph node involvement was 96%, compared with 86% in patients with one to three involved nodes and 66% in patients with more than three involved nodes.[62]

Pathologic review of resected lymph nodes may identify macrometastases (>2 mm), micrometastases (≤2 mm and >0. 2 mm), or isolated tumor cells (<0.2 mm), Lymph node macrometastasis is a well-established prognostic factor, whereas the prognostic significance for micrometastasis or isolated tumor cells remains under study. The ability to detect smaller tumor deposits is a more recent phenomenon, driven largely by refined immunohistochemical techniques. Nevertheless, evidence suggests that patients with micrometastases have a worse outcome in certain settings. In the Swedish Sentinel Node Multicenter Cohort Study, which included more than 3000 patients, patients with nodal micrometastases were found to have lower breast cancer–specific survival rates compared with patients with no nodal involvement at 5 years (94% vs. 97%). These patients also had higher rates of recurrence (event-free survival rate, 80% vs. 87% in node-negative cases). However, no difference in survival was found between patients with isolated tumor cells and those with no nodal involvement.[63]

Grade. As with most malignancies, invasive breast cancer can present in a variety of histologic grades. One system used in classification of tumor grade is the modified Scharf Richardson Bloom system. Here, the overall tumor grade is based on the addition of the individual scores for differentiation, mitosis, and nuclear morphism, each having a score of 1 to 3 for a total score of 3 to 9. Low-grade tumors have scores of 3 to 5, intermediate grade tumors have scores 6 to 7, and high-grade tumors have scores 8 to 9. Higher-grade tumors are associated with high risks for local recurrence and worse breast cancer survival.[64,116]

Lymphovascular Invasion. Lymphovascular invasion (LVI) refers to the invasion of lymphatic spaces and/or blood vessels by tumor emboli. The negative prognostic value of LVI was first described in the 1960s and has been maintained through multiple studies that show clear correlation between LVI and poor outcomes. In a recent study of more than 3000 patients, LVI was found to be associated with higher risks of recurrence and worse breast cancer–specific survival at 5 years (81% vs. 92%) and 10 years (66% vs. 85%) compared with patients with no LVI, independent of lymph node involvement status, tumor grade, and ER status.[65] In addition, LVI has been associated with a higher risk of chest wall and regional failure,[66] but not in-breast recurrence.

Receptor Status. Tumor samples are analyzed to determine the level of expression of ERs and PRs, along with HER2/neu expression (HER2) and gene amplification in breast cancer cells. As discussed above, a vast body of literature has established the therapeutic benefit of endocrine therapy in the setting of ER-positive tumors, which also exhibit a 5% to 10% lower risk of recurrence compared with patients with ER-negative cancer.[67] Similarly, higher PR expression has also been correlated with better response to endocrine therapy, longer time to recurrence, and better overall survival.[68,69]

Overexpression of HER2 (or gene amplification) is found in 15% to 20% of breast cancers and has historically indicated an adverse prognosis. However, in the modern era of HER2-directed therapies, this subtype of breast cancer now fares more favorably with several ongoing trials seeking to de-escalate aggressive regimens for these patients.[70] Overexpression of HER2 tends to be associated with poorly differentiated, aggressively behaving tumors. Nevertheless, with the integration of anti-HER2 therapy as part of the systemic regimen for patients with HER2-amplified breast cancers, survival of this patient population is greatly improved,[71] and HER2 overexpression status has evolved into a predictive tool in identifying patients who should receive HER2-directed therapy.

Patients with TNBCs, defined as breast cancers with absent expression of ER, PR, and HER2, have poorer prognosis compared with patients with other breast cancer subtypes with receptor expressions. TNBC behaves more aggressively than other types of breast cancer, and lacks targeted approaches (endocrine therapy, HER2-directed therapy). A 2012 study of more than 12,000 women showed that women with TNBC experienced adverse survival, independent of age, stage, race, and tumor grade.[72] In this study, patients with TNBC were three times more likely to succumb to breast cancer compared with women with other subtypes. In addition, numerous reports have suggested that local failure within the breast is increased in women with TNBC.

A woman with triple-negative breast cancer does not have the three most common types of cell membrane receptors–estrogen, progesterone, and the HER-2/neu gene. These receptors are important for passing signals to cancer cells. This means that the cancer cells have tested negative for estrogen receptors (ERs), progesterone receptors (PRs), and epidermal growth factor receptor 2 (HER2). Some of the most effective breast cancer treatments work by targeting one or more of these receptors. For example, the drug trastuzumab is targeted to the HER2 receptor, whereas tamoxifen is effective in blocking the ER and preventing the hormone from stimulating breast cancer cells.

Gene Expression Profiles

Gene expression profiling is a rapidly emerging field whereby measurement of transcriptional activity is used to classify cancers based on therapeutic response and risk assessment. Profiles may range from measuring the activity of just a few genes (e.g., 21 genes measured in the OncotypeDX score) to measuring the entire tumor transcriptome for more detailed investigative analysis. Gene expression studies have identified several distinct breast cancer subtypes that differ in prognosis and treatment response[73] and can be broadly separated into four groups: luminal A, luminal B, HER2-amplified, and basal like. Luminal breast cancers are the most common and comprise the ER-positive subset that tends to respond to endocrine therapy and exhibit more indolent biology, with luminal A exhibiting more favorable outcomes than luminal B. HER2-amplified tumors, as discussed above, respond to anti-HER2 agents and were previously among the least favorable with regard to outcome. Basal-like tumors are typically approximated by the absence of ER, PR, or HER2 overexpression and overlap significantly with the triple-negative subtype described above.[74,75]

Beyond these subgroups, a number of transcriptional profiles are in use for risk stratification and treatment decision-making. For example, assays, such as Oncotype Dx (Genomic Health, Redwood City, CA) MAammaPrint (Agendia, Amsterdam, Netherlands), and Prosigna (Nanostring Technologies, Seattle, WA) have been validated on cohorts with known recurrence outcomes. These assays yield scores that serve as a proxy for tumor biology, response to therapy, and risk of local or distance recurrence, and can inform physician decision-making with regard to which therapies are most likely (or not) to benefit a given patient.

TREATMENT MANAGEMENT

A multidisciplinary approach that includes input regarding surgery, radiation therapy, and systemic therapy is necessary for optimal breast cancer treatment. Historically, breast cancer was treated aggressively via radical mastectomy, often without radiation therapy or chemotherapy. Advancements in the management of breast cancer came from randomized controlled trials conducted by large national cooperative groups, such as the National Surgical Adjuvant Breast and Bowel Project (NSABP), the Radiation Therapy Oncology Group, and many others. Collectively, these have shown the value of adjuvant systemic therapy among appropriately selected patients to reduce the risk of distant metastasis, and adjuvant radiation therapy to reduce the risk of locoregional failure. The precise indications for the use of each treatment modality continue to evolve, with improved definition of risk factors. Box 34.1 shows how local and regional treatment has evolved over the past 100 years. Locoregional therapies maximize local control and improve long-term survival. Patients with high risk of distant metastasis typically receive systemic therapy to prevent metastatic disease. The National Comprehensive Cancer Network guidelines provide clinicians guidance in selection of appropriate treatment regimens for patients.[76]

BOX 34.1 Evolution of the Treatment of Early-Stage Breast Cancer

- 1894: Halstead developed the radical mastectomy.
- 1926: Keynes began to use radium brachytherapy as the sole treatment for women with operable breast cancer.
- 1948: Patey developed modified radical mastectomy with resection of pectoralis minor.
- 1965: Madden developed modified radical mastectomy with preservation of pectoralis minor.
- 1960s: Early trials of breast-conserving surgery followed by radiation therapy (Guy's Hospital) were shown to be inferior for women with T2 tumors compared with mastectomy.
- 1970s: Milan initial study for women with T1N0 breast cancer showed equivalence of breast-conserving surgery followed by radiation therapy when compared with mastectomy. The breast-conserving surgery was quadrantectomy.
- 1980s: Hellman became the leading American proponent, in speeches and debates, for the conservative management of women who had breast cancer. At the time, he was the chairman at Harvard and was the one who fought the surgeons and brought breast-conserving surgery to people's attention.
- 1980s: National Surgical Adjuvant Breast and Bowel Project B6 and other randomized clinical trials conclusively showed equivalence for breast-conserving surgery (wide local excision) followed by radiation therapy for women with T1 and T2 breast cancer when compared with mastectomy.
- 1990s: Do all patients need radiation therapy? Wide local excision alone without radiation therapy was shown to be inferior.
- 2000s: Development of new radiation therapy regimens after wide local excision, including hypofractionated whole breast irradiation and partial breast irradiation.
- 2010s: Development of new radiation therapy techniques for simulation and treatment, including, magnetic resonance imaging (MRI)/computed tomography (CT) simulation, partial breast irradiation (PBI), intensity-modulated radiation therapy (IMRT), and volumetric modulated arc therapy (VMAT) options.

Surgery

Breast-Conserving Surgery. For patients with early stage breast cancer, breast-conserving therapy followed by adjuvant radiation therapy has been shown to provide the survival equivalent of mastectomy, with a low rate of recurrence in the treated breast in multiple randomized studies with long-term follow-up.[77–80] The selection of patients for appropriate breast-conserving surgery, often described as lumpectomy or wide location excision or partial mastectomy, which involves removal of the primary tumor with a healthy tissue margin, is crucial for its success. Decisions regarding treatment are influenced by the extent of the primary tumor, the pattern of tumor growth within the breast, and the patient's personal preference. Although breast-conserving surgery is the preferred treatment when possible, it is not appropriate for all patients. For very large tumors or tumors that involve multiple quadrants of the breast (multicentric), a mastectomy may be the best treatment choice. However, lumpectomy can become an option for patients with larger tumors that had a good response to neoadjuvant (preoperative) chemotherapy such that the tumor volume is reduced.[81]

Some patients with a history of connective tissue disease, especially those with scleroderma, are at higher risk of development of acute and late radiation related toxicities.[82] Given that radiation therapy is to follow breast-conserving surgery, special considerations must be given to these patients regarding the suitability of breast-conserving therapy. Some of the contraindications to breast-conserving surgery include:

1. Multicentric disease with two or more primary tumors in separate quadrants of the breast such that they cannot be encompassed in a single excision.
2. Diffuse malignant microcalcifications on mammography.
3. Persistent positive resection margins after multiple attempts of re-excision.
4. Pregnancy.

Mastectomy. Mastectomy is the complete surgical resection of breast tissue. It is indicated for patients who are not candidates for breast-conserving therapy, patients who prefer mastectomy, and for prophylactic purposes in extremely high-risk populations. Some patients choose to have mastectomy rather than breast-conserving therapy for various reasons, including a desire to avoid postlumpectomy radiation therapy, although this practice is discouraged for patients with access to radiation therapy, as mastectomy can result in high incidence of chronic pain and morbidity and is considered overtreatment. In patients with *BRCA1* and *BRCA2* mutations, prophylactic mastectomy reduces the risk of development of breast cancer by more than 90% and has been associated with improved overall survival. Outside of these patients with high risk for development of breast cancer, women with breast cancer who undergo prophylactic contralateral mastectomy do not benefit from improved oncologic outcomes compared with women who had unilateral mastectomy.[83]

Multiple types of mastectomy for oncologic purposes have evolved over the years and range from the most invasive (radical mastectomy) to the least invasive and frequently practiced today (total mastectomy). New modifications to mastectomy continue to evolve, including skin-sparing and even nipple-sparing approaches.

Radical mastectomy (halsted mastectomy). This mastectomy involves the removal of the breast with overlying skin, the pectoralis muscles, and all the axillary lymph nodes. Although this approach improves local control, it does not lead to improved long-term survival. The complication rate from radical mastectomy is high, and complications can be severe, often leaving the patient with a concave chest wall, arm weakness, shoulder stiffness, and lymphedema. This technique is rarely used today.

Modified radical mastectomy. The practice of modified radical mastectomy today usually includes removal of the breast and the underlying fascia together with removal of the level I and II axillary lymph nodes. Equivalent outcomes with less toxicity have been shown through multiple studies that compare modified radical mastectomy with radical mastectomy.[84,85] The original modification (Patey) was to spare the pectoralis major muscle but to remove the pectoralis minor muscle and dissect the level I, II, and III axillary lymph nodes. With further development, both the pectoralis minor and level III lymph nodes were spared to reduce the risk of complications, primarily lymphedema.

Total mastectomy. A total mastectomy removes the entire breast; however, removal of level I and II lymph nodes is not performed. With the common practice of sentinel lymph node biopsy (discussed subsequently), total mastectomy is now performed frequently. In Fig. 34.9, the difference between a wide local excision and mastectomy is shown. The average volume of resection in wide local excision is about 100 mL, whereas a mastectomy can resect from 500 to 2000 mL, depending on the size of the breast.

Nipple-sparing mastectomy. This surgery originated for the purposes of prophylactic mastectomy and has become increasingly common for early-stage breast cancer. Outcomes show higher rates of recurrence, likely because of variable amounts of residual breast tissue remaining.[86] This procedure should be performed by a high-volume breast surgeon and only for well-selected patients.

Axillary Staging. The axillary lymph nodes receive 85% of the lymphatic drainage from the breast. The likelihood of axillary lymph node involvement is related to tumor size, location, grade, and presence of lymphovascular invasion. Physical examination is not a reliable method in determination of axillary lymph node involvement, and pathologic staging of the axilla is an important part of breast cancer management. In the past, removal of all level I and level II axillary lymph nodes was the standard practice to stage the axilla. However, recent randomized controlled trials have shown that sentinel lymph node biopsy is equivalent to axillary dissection for the clinically negative axilla.

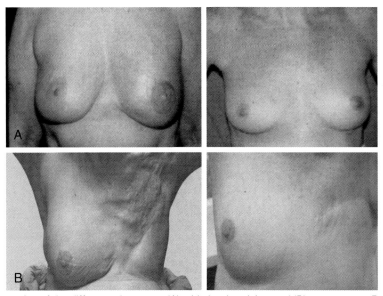

Fig. 34.9 Illustration of the difference between: (A) wide local excision, and (B) mastectomy. For breast-conserving surgery, the incision can be circumareolar *(left)* or over the lesion *(right)*. In (B), the left panel shows a radical mastectomy, but the right panel shows preservation of the pectoralis major muscle.

Sentinel lymph node biopsy. In patients with clinical node negative breast cancer (cN0), a negative sentinel lymph node biopsy accurately identifies patients without axillary lymph node involvement and therefore prevents the use of more extensive surgery. This procedure involves injection of radioactive colloid or blue dye into the breast tissue in the vicinity of the tumor. The tracer enters the lymphatic channels and flows to the lymph nodes that are first in line to receive the drainage from the tumor. These lymph nodes are then identified by localizing the tracers either visually (blue dye) or by using a Geiger counter (radioactive colloid) See Fig. 5.3. The lymph nodes are then removed for pathologic determination.

For patients with metastasis involving one to two positive sentinel lymph nodes, randomized data shows no differences in recurrence or survival rates were found whether a subsequent axillary dissection was performed or not.[87] Of note, all patients were treated with lumpectomy and underwent adjuvant whole breast radiation, which suggests that radiation is able to control microscopic disease in residual involved low axillary (level 1) lymph nodes. For patients with three or more sentinel lymph nodes, axillary dissection is generally recommended. The use of sentinel node biopsy alone in the setting of neoadjuvant chemotherapy is being investigated in an ongoing trial by the ALLIANCE cooperative group.

Axillary dissection. Axillary lymph node dissection today usually involves the removal of level I and level II lymph nodes. It was a routine component of staging and management of breast cancer until the emergence of sentinel lymph node biopsy. Therefore use of axillary dissection in patients with no clinically apparent axillary lymph nodes (cN0 stage) is now rarely used. Axillary lymph node dissection is still indicated for most patients with clinically positive axillary lymph node involvement. Patients who undergo axillary dissection have a threefold risk of development of chronic lymphedema of the ipsilateral arm.[88]

Breast Reconstruction

Breast reconstruction has been shown to improve psychologic status and quality-of-life in women who undergo mastectomy,[89] and the practice has been increasing in the United States, involving 61% in 2009 and 71% in 2014. Breast reconstruction can either be carried out at the time of mastectomy (immediate reconstruction) or after the completion of adjuvant therapies (delayed reconstruction). An advantage of immediate reconstruction is the streamlining of surgical procedures, which decreases the overall surgical time and also provides benefits in preserving body image in women. The two general types of reconstructive options are implant-based reconstruction (saline solution or silicone implants, preceded by the use of a tissue expander to create the correct size of a "pocket" to accommodate the implant) and autologous tissue reconstructions with tissues that are transferred from a donor site, such as the rectus abdominus muscle or latissimus dorsi muscle. Implant-based reconstructions are often done in two stages, with the expander placed at the time of initial mastectomy and exchanged for a permanent implant after several weeks of expansion. In the setting of postmastectomy radiation, the implant exchange can occur before radiation or after, at which time, a waiting period of 4 to 6 months is recommended. There is very little difference in outcome based on the timing of implant exchange and therefore is left to the surgeon's discretion.[90] In the setting of postmastectomy radiation, implant-based reconstruction carries a much higher risk of surgical complications than autologous reconstruction.[91] Nonetheless, there has been an increase in the practice of implant-based reconstruction and a decrease in autologous reconstruction in the United States.[92]

Systemic Therapy

Despite early diagnosis, complete staging, and the improvement in locoregional treatment techniques for breast cancer, some patients will relapse distantly. Distant metastases are likely the result of clinically occult micrometastases at the time of diagnosis. Systemic therapies, including chemotherapy, endocrine therapy, and targeted biological therapy, play an important role in eradicating this disease.

Adjuvant Therapy. Adjuvant systemic therapy selection is based on tumor characteristics and patient risk. In those with breast cancer, risk stratification for adjuvant cytotoxic chemotherapy is being increasingly employed to enhance the precision with which these aggressive therapies are used. Factors such as tumor size, grade, lymph node involvement, and molecular profiling/subtyping assay results (Oncotype DX; Mammaprint; Prosigna; see "Prognostic Factors" section) are taken into consideration in the decision of whether a patient should receive chemotherapy. Patient factors, such as age and comorbidities, are important considerations as well. A long and distinguished history of clinical trials and meta-analyses has shown that among appropriately selected patients, adjuvant chemotherapy can improve long-term overall survival.[93,94]

Patients with HER2-amplified breast cancer typically receive a combination of chemotherapy with HER2-directed therapies, such as trastuzumab. Trastuzumab is an anti-HER2 monoclonal antibody that targets HER2 activity, inhibits proliferation, and induces cell death. Large randomized trials have shown that trastuzumab with chemotherapy significantly improves disease-free survival by 30% to 50% and overall survival by 30% to 40%.[95] More recent studies have shown that the combination of dual HER2-directed therapy is superior to trastuzumab alone in women with metastatic breast cancer.[96]

Patients with ER-positive breast cancer typically also receive adjuvant endocrine therapy.[16–18] In premenopausal women, tamoxifen for at least 5 years improves both disease-free and overall survival rates.[97] Tamoxifen is a selective ER modulator that inhibits the growth of breast cancer cells by competitive antagonism of the ER. Aromatase inhibitors suppress plasma estrogen levels by inhibiting or inactivating aromatase, an enzyme responsible for converting estrogenic precursors to estrogens peripherally. Aromatase inhibitors have been shown to improve outcomes for postmenopausal women with hormone receptor–positive disease compared with tamoxifen.[98]

Neoadjuvant Therapy. Neoadjuvant systemic therapy is that which is administered before surgery. Aims of neoadjuvant therapy include tumor downstaging the disease to enable breast conservation, axillary node resolution to mitigate the need for axillary dissection, and response assessment to evaluate the activity of a given regimen on the gross tumor burden. When compared with adjuvant systemic therapy, neoadjuvant therapy results in long-term disease outcomes that are comparable.[11,19,20] Neoadjuvant therapy may include cytotoxic chemotherapy, HER2-directed therapy, and/or endocrine therapy. If a patient cannot receive systemic therapy (i.e., because of significant medical comorbidities) and has ER-positive disease, endocrine therapy is then given in the neoadjuvant setting in lieu of chemotherapy. Neoadjuvant systemic therapy is the standard approach in the treatment of inflammatory breast cancer. In rare cases, radiation is administered neoadjuvantly for nonresponsive inflammatory breast cancers.

RADIATION THERAPY

Why Is Radiation Therapy Important?

Radiation therapy plays an essential role in the management of breast cancer by eradicating subclinical disease after surgical removal of tumor. For patients with DCIS, radiation therapy after lumpectomy reduces the risk of local recurrence, but confers no survival benefit.[99–101] In a large metaanalysis of 3000 women with DCIS, radiation therapy reduced the rate of local recurrence by 54%, regardless of patient's age, surgical margin status, and tumor characteristics.[102] In women with early-stage breast cancer, breast-conserving therapy (lumpectomy followed by adjuvant radiation) and mastectomy yield similar long-term outcomes,[78,79] with multiple trials showing that the addition of whole breast radiation after lumpectomy for invasive cancer significantly reduces local relapse.[103] Individual series of breast-conserving surgery followed by radiation therapy yield recurrence rates that are frequently less than 5% to 10% with excellent outcomes.[104–107] For many years, it was unclear whether this improvement in local control conferred a survival benefit, but a landmark meta-analysis conducted by the Early Breast Cancer Trialists' Collaborative Group (EBCTCG) included more than 10,000 women and demonstrated that adjuvant whole breast radiation reduces disease recurrence at 10 years from 35% to 19%, with a concomitant reduction in 15-year mortality from 25% to 21%.[21] These rates have been further improved with advances in surgical techniques and systemic therapies; significantly lower rates are seen using contemporary approaches.

In women who undergo mastectomy for locally advanced disease, postmastectomy radiation therapy (PMRT) is used to treat the areas at risk for recurrence, often including the chest wall and regional lymphatics (axilla, supraclavicular fossa, and internal mammary lymph nodes). The benefits of PMRT in improving oncologic outcomes have been well documented in multiple studies, culminating in a large meta-analysis conducted by the EBCTCG, which included more than 9000 women. In this report, PMRT was found to significantly reduce the relative risk of local recurrence by 73%. Again, more importantly, this translated into improvement for both breast cancer–specific survival and overall survival at 15 years.[77] A subsequent trial, known as EORTC 22922, randomized node positive or high-risk node negative patients to regional nodal irradiation. This study again demonstrated a significant benefit to PMRT with regard to disease-free survival, but notably showed no overall survival benefit because of limited follow-up among other possible reasons.

In summary, breast irradiation for appropriately selected patients after lumpectomy or mastectomy improves locoregional disease control and can confer a survival benefit.

Breast irradiation is among the most technically challenging procedures performed in a radiation oncology department. Given that treatment volumes can often be visualized on setup, radiation oncologists routinely rely on therapists to ensure interfractional reproducibility and to visually confirm appropriate treatment fields on a daily basis. Tasked with accurate clinical setup, radiation therapists are required to have an exceptional clinical understanding of the desired target volumes and critical healthy structures to avoid. Furthermore, because breast anatomy varies widely among patients, radiation oncologists often rely on the therapist to have input on the most appropriate immobilization and setup to ensure optimal reproducibility. Breast irradiation, from the simulator to the linear accelerator, demands that the therapist be thorough, alert, precise, and often creative.

Simulation. Breast irradiation is very much dependent on accurate positioning and immobilization techniques—these are the first steps to development of an effective and safe treatment plan. Discussion with the radiation oncologist regarding optimal positioning for appropriate target coverage is essential, especially when regional lymph nodes are to be included in the target volumes. Many commercially available devices assist in patient positioning for treatment of breast cancer. These range from custom-molded foam casts to prone boards to supine boards with adjustable head and arm supports. An important element of reproducibility in immobilization is the ability to index the patient to the immobilization device comfortably and reproducibly.

Supine positioning and immobilization. The patient is asked to disrobe above the waist, and jewelry is removed. The patient lies supine in the selected immobilization device on the simulator table. When lying supine, patients with large or pendulous breasts often have breast tissue that is displaced upward by gravity into the infraclavicular area. These patients can be positioned on an immobilization device with an adjustable incline so that the head and thorax are slightly elevated. This brings the breast tissue inferiorly, which is necessary to adequately irradiate the breast and avoid treating the upper arm when tangential beams are used. This approach can also reduce skin folds in the supraclavicular area. Care must be taken, however, to avoid overelevating the patient and causing folding of the skin in the inframammary area. Furthermore, overelevating the patient can also increase lung volume in the supraclavicular field and potentially compromise lymph nodes' coverage. Discussion with the radiation oncologist on the appropriate treatment position is necessary.

Both arms are preferably abducted, externally rotated, and supported over the head in a reproducible manner, although modifications can be made for patients with limited upper extremity range of motion. Elevation of the ipsilateral arm above the head has been shown to decrease the volume of the heart in the tangential fields when compared with the 90-degree position.[108] It also allows tangential radiation beams to treat the breast or chest wall while avoiding the patient's upper arm. Adjustment of the ipsilateral arm position can help reduce skin folds in the axilla and supraclavicular areas to reduce skin side effects. If the patient is unable to elevate the contralateral arm above the head, the arm should rest on the tabletop with the hand palm down. Patients should not place the contralateral hand on the abdomen or grasp the belt or waistband of their clothing. Such a position of the contralateral hand and arm is poorly reproducible and can result in distortion of the thoracic anatomy, including rotation and displacement of the uninvolved breast into the treatment field.

The patient's head should be midline, with the neck neutral to slightly extended if treatment is limited to the breast or chest wall. If the regional lymphatics also require irradiation, then the head should be turned slightly to the contralateral side. If the head is rotated too far, then the spinal cord is moved closer to the supraclavicular field edge because it is behind the axis of rotation. The patient's chin should be slightly extended to minimize neck skin folds. The patient's body should be straight (in the sagittal plane) and level from side to side. A visual confirmation with use of the lasers in the simulation suite should be performed before a CT scout image is obtained if a CT simulator is used, or a fluoroscopic image if a conventional simulator is used.

Identical daily positioning of the patient's arm and head is extremely important for the accuracy of the treatment process. The feet can be held together to reduce lower body rotation and to enhance setup reproducibility. A triangular sponge or bolster may be placed under the patient's knees for comfort. The same immobilization devices must be used each time the patient is treated. The patient position should be well documented and explained in the setup instructions. Photographs or digital images of the patient in the treatment position are extremely helpful, especially for patients with unusual setup positions that need further clarification.

Prone positioning and immobilization. Prone breast positioning provides the benefit of minimizing lung or heart tissue in the treatment fields as the breast falls away from the chest wall. It requires the patient to climb onto a prone board and lie on the stomach with the ipsilateral arm over the head. The ipsilateral breast gravitationally falls through an opening in the breast board, and the contralateral breast is displaced away from the field on an angled platform to avoid dose from tangential beams entering or exiting. Prone positioning is better suited for women with larger breasts that pull away from the chest wall when laying facedown. Women with small breasts or

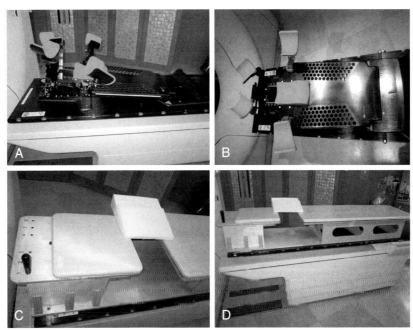

Fig. 34.10 (A and B) Supine, and (C and D) prone breast boards for radiation therapy.

with breast implants derive little benefit from the prone position. If the chest wall needs to be included in the target volume, the heart can also fall forward, so in some circumstances, the prone position is disadvantageous. The prone position may compromise the ability to match fields and therefore should not be used if treatment of regional lymph nodes is necessary, although ongoing trials are exploring regional nodal irradiation in the prone position. Thus it is an important decision to ascertain which position is the most favorable for each individual patient. Examples of both supine and prone breast boards are shown in Fig. 34.10.

Treatment Design. With treatment of the whole breast or chest wall, radiopaque markers or wires are placed on the patient to delineate the region of interest at the time of simulation. Some radiation oncologists prefer to wire the visible or palpable breast tissue (because it may be more accurate for distinguishing breast tissue from adipose tissue). Others prefer to place wires at the borders of the possible treatment fields, for intact breast or chest wall treatment, to get an idea of the extent of exposure to the lung or heart and determine whether any repositioning may be needed. In the latter scenario, wires are placed medially at the midsternum, laterally at the level of midaxilla, superiorly at the bottom of the clavicular head, and inferiorly approximately 2 cm below the inframammary fold. For postmastectomy patients, the position of the inframammary fold is estimated from the contralateral breast or from adjacent anatomic landmarks. Radio-opaque wires provide guidance in defining the posterior edge of the medial and lateral tangent. In cases in which patients are treated to the chest wall with electrons, the desired target to be covered is defined by the wires for en face beam design and treatment planning. Therefore skin markings of any sort placed at the time of simulation are to help guide the design of the treatment planning process. As shown in Fig. 34.11, supine tangential fields to cover the right breast are seen to include a small amount of chest wall and lung, which should be within safe tolerance. Assessment of whether prone coverage is able to further reduce the lung in the treatment beam and maintain breast tissue coverage can only be done at simulation (Fig. 34.12 is an example of prone whole breast irradiation fields).

Recently, external beam partial breast irradiation (PBI) has become more widely used for the treatment of early-stage breast cancer in select women. The precise indications for the use of PBI are evolving, although it is most widely employed for favorable early-stage patients without lymph node involvement. For PBI, field and plan design requires visualization of the lumpectomy cavity and the surgically placed localization clips. Typically, however, the radiation oncologist will still require wire placement for entire breast fields, as above, in the event that PBI dosimetry is suboptimal and the treatment has to be converted to whole breast irradiation. In addition, the ratio of the partial breast target volume to whole breast volume is generally kept to less than 25% to achieve the required dose constraints. Fig. 34.13 provides an example of the PBI treatment plan.

In designing breast radiation treatments, the lung and heart are two critical structures that are carefully mapped. Irradiated lung and heart volumes should be minimized without compromising target coverage. Consequently, several techniques have been developed, especially for left-sided treatments, in an effort to decrease heart volume within the treatment fields, including deep inspiratory breath hold (DIBH). Cardiac volumes that receive more than 50% of the prescribed dose have been shown to decrease significantly with this technique.[109-112] Successful simulation with DIBH necessitates input from the radiation oncologist, physicists, therapists, and patient because some patients may not be able to tolerate breath holding.

Intact breast treatment fields. Whole breast irradiation is typically administered with tangential fields. The purpose of this field arrangement is to maximize coverage of breast tissue and minimize radiation dose to underlying structures, primarily the lung and heart. Field borders for tangential beams are as follows, but they may be modified by physical examination and clinical judgment.

- Superiorly, at the following points:
  - Superior extent of the palpable breast tissue
  - Edge of the head of the clavicle
- Inferior
  - 2 cm below the inframammary fold or 2 cm below lowest edge of the breast

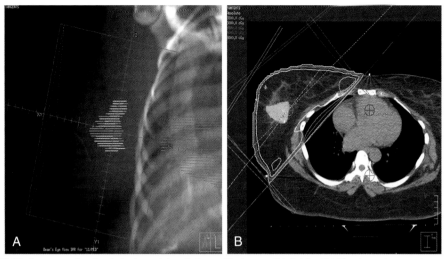

Fig. 34.11 An example of whole breast irradiation with tangential fields. (A) The beam's-eye view on the digitally reconstructed radiograph. (B) An axial section of the treating planning computed tomographic scan at the level of the lumpectomy cavity.

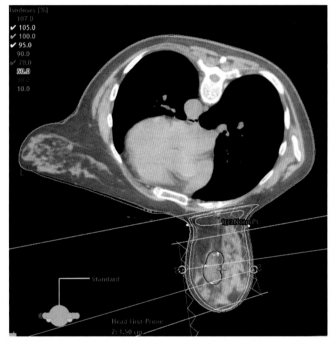

Fig. 34.12 An example of whole breast irradiation with prone tangential fields. Prone technique, when suitable, can lead to a reduction in lung volume included in the irradiation fields compared with the supine technique.

- Medial
  - At midline of patient, as determined with palpation of suprasternal notch and xiphoid process
  - Exclusion of contralateral breast in the treatment fields is important
- Lateral
  - Midaxillary line or 2 cm beyond breast tissue laterally
- Anterior
  - Flash approximately 2 to 3 cm to include the entire breast and allow for the possibility of edema that may occur during treatment
- Posterior
  - Include the chest wall; often includes up to 3 cm of lung

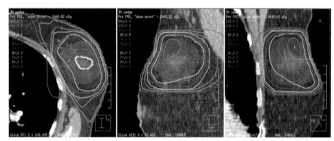

Fig. 34.13 An example of the dose distribution for partial breast irradiation. The prescribed dose is confined to the lumpectomy cavity with a defined healthy tissue margin.

Most contemporary approaches use an isocentric method of tangential field irradiation. In these techniques, the isocenter is placed at a specified depth in the patient's breast or near the chest wall. At many institutions, the isocenter is placed approximately halfway between the ribs and skin, at a point approximately midway between the medial and lateral entrance points of the beam. With this technique, the gantry angles are adjusted to create a nondivergent (straight) deep border. Other techniques place the isocenter at the deep edge of the tangential field and split the radiation beam in half (beam-split/half-beam block technique), blocking the deep half of the beam and allowing 180-degree opposed beams to be used.

With both techniques, the tangential field arrangement produces a single-plane deep (or posterior) margin in the beam's-eye view. The deep border of the medial tangent and the deep border of the lateral tangent form a single plane, ensuring a tight dose edge to the treatment plan.

The steps for simulation and field design for tangential beams for intact breast radiation therapy are presented. Breast simulation is important to approach on a case-by-case basis because of diverse clinical scenarios in breast cancer treatments and should be discussed with the treating oncologist.

1. Set the patient on the breast board. Be sure the patient is centered and leveled.
2. Mark superior, inferior, medial, and lateral borders on the patient with radiopaque wires.
3. Place the isocenter midway between superior-inferior borders and medial-lateral borders. Depth of the isocenter can either be in the breast or on the chest wall (posterior edge of tangential fields) and should be discussed with the treating oncologist.

4. Rotate the gantry to the desired angle for the medial tangent field. Adjust the angle as needed to align the wires from the medial and lateral margins. Adjust the collimator angle as needed such that the medial field edge is parallel to the chest wall. Be sure the skin flash is adequate.

5. Set up the lateral tangent field by rotating the gantry to the desired angle. Adjust the angle to make sure the medial and lateral wires are aligned and form a coplanar plane with the medial tangent field. Rotate the collimator the same number of degrees in the opposite direction of that used for the medial tangent field. Be sure the skin flash is adequate.

6. The amount of lung included in the tangential fields should be carefully considered and should be discussed with the treating radiation oncologist. If necessary, some of the breast tissue farthest away from the tumor bed may be omitted to provide an adequate balance of breast coverage without covering excessive amounts of lung and heart.

Computerized treatment planning of the tangential field pair is necessary to visualize the dose distribution throughout the treatment volume and surrounding organs at risk. Wedges or a custom compensator may be needed to improve dose homogeneity. Multileaf collimators provide the dose homogeneity compensation function, used either statically (segmentation) or dynamically. Skin doses are often adequate because of tangentially configured radiation beams. Bolus can be used to increase skin dose, if clinically warranted. Whole breast irradiation is typically prescribed to 4500 to 5000 cGy over 4.5 to 5 weeks or with a hypofractionated approach of 3990 to 4240 cGy over 15 or 16 fractions, sometimes followed by a boost, as clinically warranted.[22,23,113-115]

For prone intact breast irradiation, the breast falls away from the chest wall through an opening in the prone breast board. Visual inspection of the patient is important to ensure the entire breast tissue is included in the opening; this inspection is performed before the CT simulation scan. The tangential fields are designed to include the entire breast, similar to supine position, with the exception that usually minimal or no lung tissue is included in the fields. Tattoos are placed medially and laterally at the same horizontal level in the central axis of the breast. Additional tattoos are placed for longitudinal alignment. The treatment is delivered with isocenters on the skin medially and laterally at the same anterior shift from the central axis tattoos (source-to-skin distance [SSD] 100 cm technique). Prone positioning is best suited for women with larger breasts and mobile breast tissue.

Boost irradiation depends on the clinical context but is often used in the setting of younger patients with higher-grade tumors or concern about adequacy of the surgical margins.[117,118] An en face electron beam is the technique of choice at most institutions, although a deep-seated tumor may require the use of "mini-tangents" if the tumor bed is beyond the electron range. In planning the electron boost, care must be taken to ensure that the treatment volume adequately encompasses the tumor bed. The boost irradiation field is often designed during CT simulation, and the electron energy is modulated to ensure adequate coverage of the visualized tumor bed. Dose is prescribed to the 80 or 90% isodose line of the given electron beam.

Patients with extremely large or pendulous breasts are particularly challenging to treat. Numerous devices and techniques have been developed to stabilize the breast and permit a reasonably reproducible setup. Elastic netting can be placed over the breasts; however, this works best on smaller breasts because the material is not dense enough to support a larger breast on the chest wall. Systems that use thermoplastic materials to mold the breast into an appropriate position are available commercially. Thermoplastic sheets may also be molded to the patient and fastened around the patient's back with bandage material. A simple ring can be placed around the breast to immobilize and retain the breast in position on the anterior chest.[4] A foam wedge can also be fashioned and positioned to support pendulous breast tissue located far to the patient's lateral chest. Prone position with a commercially available board may also be advantageous to give a homogeneous dose to the breast. Care must be taken not to underdose the chest wall.

Accelerated PBI has gained popularity as an adjuvant therapy for those with favorable risk profiles. This technique delivers hypofractionated doses of daily or twice-daily radiation with a 1 cm to 2 cm margin to the postsurgical bed over 1 to 2 weeks. The rationale behind PBI is that most recurrences for breast cancer occur in the immediate vicinity of the original tumor.[84,106] Because radiation therapy is effective at reducing local recurrences, PBI delivers radiation to only the areas at risk of local recurrence and spares surrounding tissues (the rest of the breast, lung, and heart). PBI can be delivered in many ways, including balloon-based brachytherapy, interstitial brachytherapy, and external beam radiation therapy (EBRT), with EBRT being the most common form used. Short-term outcomes have shown good local control with EBRT PBI.[118]

The isocenter for EBRT PBI is most typically placed in the center of the lumpectomy cavity, and the treatment fields are designed to deliver homogeneous dose to the cavity plus a margin. Several beam arrangements for PBI have been used. An arrangement of two photon beams and an en face electron beam can be used to achieve dose homogeneity and limit dose to the lung.[119] The electron energy is determined based on the depth of the tumor bed. Other beam arrangements, including four noncoplanar photon beams and noncoplanar photon beams with en face electrons, have all been employed with varying degrees of success in different settings. Many clinical factors, such as location of lumpectomy cavity, patient breast size, and patient arm mobility, are taken into consideration in the design of EBRT PBI treatment fields.

Postmastectomy treatment fields. Women with lymph node involvement who undergo mastectomy may benefit from PMRT to the chest wall and regional lymph nodes as described above. One critical aspect of comprehensive irradiation for breast cancer is the avoidance of junctional inconsistency between the treatment fields (i.e., internal mammary, supraclavicular, and tangential fields). Both hot (overdosing) and cold (underdosing) spots can result from a combination of divergence and geometric distortion of the radiation beams. Excess dose can lead to match-line fibrosis and a poor cosmetic result. Conversely, underdosed regions raise the potential for tumor recurrence. For chest wall and regional lymph node irradiation, patients are treated in the supine position. Below are the general field designs for chest wall and regional lymph node irradiation, but individual anatomy must be considered on a per-patient basis.

Chest wall tangents: Standard tangential fields may cover some but not all of the level I and level II (lower) axillary lymph nodes. If the dual isocenter technique is used, the couch is kicked with the patient's feet away from the gantry for each tangent to prevent superior divergence of the tangents into the supraclavicular field.

- Superior, at the following points:
  - Inferior edge of the head of the clavicle/inferior border of the supraclavicular field; a "match-line" plane is created, with blocking required if collimation is used for the tangential fields
- Inferior
  - 2 cm below the inframammary fold or 2 cm below lowest edge of the breast; use the contralateral breast for reference
- Medial
  - At midline of patient, as determined by palpation of suprasternal notch and xiphoid process
  - If the ipsilateral internal mammary lymph nodes are to be treated, the medial border should extend to the contralateral side sufficiently to cover the IMN nodes
  - Include the mastectomy scar

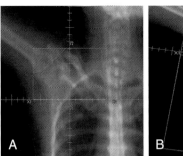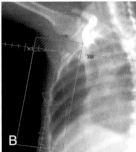

Fig. 34.14 A patient receiving postmastectomy radiation therapy. (A) The beam's-eye view of the supraclavicular field. (B) The medial tangential field covering the chest wall. The deep border of a chest wall field is deeper than in a breast-only treatment.

- Lateral
  - Midaxillary line
  - Include the mastectomy scar
- Anterior
  - Flash to include the chest wall plus about 2 to 3 cm beyond the skin
- Posterior
  - Include the chest wall; this often may include 2 to 3 cm posterior to the edge of the ribs

Supraclavicular and axillary fields: The field includes level II axillary lymph nodes not included in the tangent fields with level III and supraclavicular nodes. This is typically an anterior 6-MV photon field, beam split inferiorly at the match line (to prevent inferior divergence into the tangents) and angled 10 to 15 degrees away from the cervical spine, with dose prescribed to 3 cm. With CT-based planning, customized target coverage can be achieved by altering the energy of the photon beam. See Fig. 34.14 for an example of tangential photon fields matching a supraclavicular field.

- Superior
  - Generally, to encompass the superior extent of the supraclavicular lymph nodes. This is often above the acromioclavicular joint and below the cricoid cartilage, although individual patient anatomy will differ; the superior border needs to encompass the target volume, which is the supraclavicular fossa
  - Superior skin flash is avoided if possible, but target coverage is the primary consideration.
- Medial
  - The insertion of the sternomastoid muscle onto manubrium; posteriorly, the beam avoids the spinal cord and runs along the edge of vertebral laminae and pedicles.
- Lateral
  - Approximately 2 to 3 cm lateral of the humeral head if covering the full axilla; the coracoid process if covering level III axilla and avoiding the dissected axilla
- Inferior
  - Inferior edge of the clavicular head, which is the superior border of the tangent fields (i.e., the match line)
  - The inferior half of the beam is blocked at the supraclavicular field isocenter, creating a vertical straight edge at the inferior border and preventing divergence of dose into the tangent fields

Posterior axillary boost (PAB) field: A PAB field is sometimes used to increase the midaxillary dose to the prescribed level. This is done because the lymph nodes lateral to the coracoid become progressively deeper from the anterior surface as compared with the supraclavicular nodes, and the dose from an anterior supraclavicular field alone may be insufficient. The PAB field uses the identical inferior border as the supraclavicular field, preserving the vertical straight edge. The borders are typically as follows:

- Superior
  - Follows the clavicle (blocking is used above the clavicle)

- Medial
  - Midclavicular line (often where the first rib and clavicle cross)
- Lateral
  - Same as the supraclavicular field
- Inferior
  - Same as the supraclavicular field

Internal mammary lymph node field: among patients who require IMN radiation, a number of options exist. Elective treatment of the IMNs usually targets the first three ipsilateral intercostal spaces (from the top of the first rib to the top of the fourth rib), often 2.5 to 4 cm from the midline of the sternum. One method of irradiating the IMNs is the extended, partially wide, or deep tangential field configuration. Rather than placing the edge of the medial tangential field at the patient's midline, the field is extended beyond the midline to the contralateral side by approximately 3 cm. Although this arrangement is usually successful in encompassing the ipsilateral IMNs, it results in a significant increase in the volume of lung irradiated (Fig. 34.15). The extended tangential field also encroaches on the contralateral breast tissue, which causes an increase in scattered dose to the breast. Furthermore, in the treatment of left-sided lesions, a fairly large portion of the heart can be included in the extended tangential field.

An alternative method of irradiating the IMNs involves the use of an electron field. This field arrangement is subject to the difficulties of matching photon and electron fields, which may result in a hot or cold spot at the junctional regions. Given that the superior IMNs are anatomically deeper, a mixed-beam approach (photon and electron) has been used with the photon field also encompassing the medial supraclavicular nodes.[120] With CT simulation, different techniques can be evaluated for the best dose distribution and nodal coverage. The general borders for IMN fields of differing techniques are:

- Superior
  - Inferior border of the supraclavicular field
- Medial
  - About 1 cm contralateral of midline for the partially wide tangent technique, or about 4 cm ipsilateral of midline if planning a matching electron field to cover the IMNs
- Lateral
  - In the midaxillary line as per the usual tangent approach
- Inferior
  - 2 cm below the estimated breast tissue
- Electron strip IMN field: if an electron technique is used, a rectangular electron field is matched to the tangents medially, covering the first three intercostal interspaces and about 4 cm wide

The chest wall and regional lymph nodes are typically treated to 4500 to 5000 cGy over 4.5 to 5.0 weeks. An electron boost is sometimes employed based on clinical considerations. The steps for simulation and fields design for PMRT are presented. Breast simulation is important to approach on a case-by-case basis.

1. Set the patient on the breast board. Ensure the patient is centered and leveled.
2. Mark superior, inferior, medial, and lateral borders on the patient with radiopaque wires.
3. With CT simulation, take a scout image to visualize the superior border marker. If a fluoroscopic simulation is used, take fluoroscopic images of the area with the superior marker. The superior marker indicates the superior border of the tangential fields and the inferior border of the supraclavicular field and should be at the caudal edge of the clavicular head. If excessive lung tissue is in the supraclavicular field superior to the marker, adjustment to patient's position (if patient is on an incline, flatten the patient) or the marker (move the marker superior) may

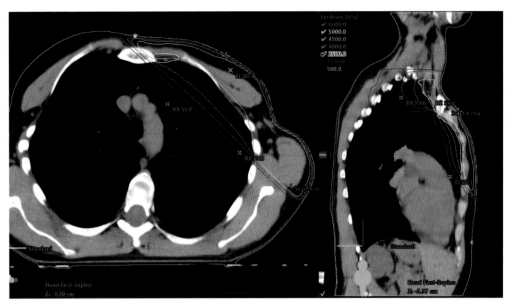

Fig. 34.15 An example of the "partially wide tangents" technique to treat the ipsilateral internal mammary node (IMN) and the chest wall. The superior portions of the photon tangential fields are wider to cover the IMN, which results in an increase in the lung volume irradiated. The patient is immobilized with slight rotation to the right to improve the position of the heart in relation to the chest wall.

be necessary. Discussion with the treating radiation oncologist is warranted.

4. Rotate the gantry 10 to 15 degrees away from the cervical spine. Design the supraclavicular field as indicated previously. Place the isocenter in the center of the field, then move it inferiorly to the inferior border of the field (on the marker or the superior border of the tangents). Place blocks to avoid treating the vertebral body, acromioclavicular joint, and part of humeral head. If PAB is needed, use the same isocenter as supraclavicular field to design the PAB. For the PAB field, place the block above the clavicle to avoid treating the supraclavicular lymph nodes, acromioclavicular joint, and part of the humeral head.

5. For chest wall tangential fields, place the isocenter midway between the superior-inferior borders and the medial-lateral borders. The depth of the isocenter should be in the chest wall.

6. Rotate the gantry to the desired angle for medial tangent field. Adjust the angle as needed to align the wires from the medial and lateral margins. Adjust the collimator angle as needed such that the medial field edge is parallel to the chest wall. Be sure the skin flash is adequate. A superior block is then placed by following the superior marker match line.

7. Set up the lateral tangent field by rotating the gantry to the desired angle. Adjust the angle to ensure the medial and lateral wires are aligned and form a coplanar plane with the medial tangent field. Rotate the collimator the same number of degrees in the opposite direction of that used for the medial tangent field. Be sure the skin flash is adequate. A superior block is then placed by following the superior marker match line.

8. The amount of lung included in the tangential fields should be carefully considered and should be discussed with the treating radiation oncologist.

9. For IMN fields with an en face electron beam, the electron beam angle should be 4 to 7 degrees toward the 0-degree gantry when compared with the medial photon tangent beam. This is to avoid a hotspot inside the breast tissue where electrons diverge to overlap with photons.

The single isocenter technique is another method for matching the tangents and supraclavicular fields if the tangent field length is less than 20 cm. Here, the isocenter is set at the match line between the supraclavicular and tangent fields. The supraclavicular field has an inferior half-beam block that prevents inferior divergence, whereas the tangents have a superior half-beam block to prevent superior divergence, thereby limiting field overlap. This method simplifies daily setup and eliminates the need for couch rotation.

Another method of treating the nonreconstructed chest wall is to use an en face electron beam. This method has been validated in prospective studies, yet typically results in a significant skin reaction.[121,122] The target area (ipsilateral chest wall) should be wired. A large electron cone (25 cm × 25 cm) is often needed to encompass the entire target. The gantry generally is rotated 30 degrees away from the 0-degree gantry, and the SSD is usually set up to be more than 105 cm to achieve target coverage and allow clearance of the electron cone over the patient. The simulation and field design for regional lymph node irradiation are the same as previously mentioned.

Static field intensity-modulated radiation therapy (IMRT) or volumetric modulated arc therapy (VMAT) are additional techniques used for comprehensive breast/chest wall and regional nodal irradiation. These are currently being studied but are more widely adopted as safety data emerge. While particular planning considerations are optimized, a number of reports have begun to disseminate safe and effective approaches.[123,124] VMAT provides the advantage of excellent target coverage of chest wall and regional lymph nodes with minimization of high doses to critical structures, such as the heart and lung. The dose homogeneity is much greater with IMRT or VMAT compared with four-field 3D radiotherapy. However, as with many IMRT techniques, the low-dose exposure is more extensive, raising concern for uncertain and uncommon long-term toxicities.

With CT-based treatment planning techniques utilizing static or dynamic multileaf collimation, excellent dose homogeneity can be achieved. Doses are generally prescribed to a point or to a volume defined by an isodose line generated from the 3D-based treatment plan. In patients receiving whole breast irradiation, the target isodose line should not be more than 5 mm from the skin surface. For patients receiving PMRT with or without breast reconstruction, bolus is typically necessary to adequately dose the skin. The thickness of the bolus

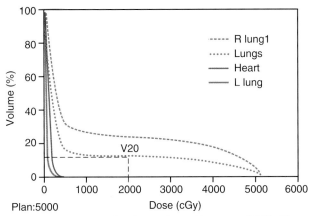

Fig. 34.16 An example of a dose-volume histogram (DVH). The percentage of the organ is plotted on the y-axis, with the dose to the organ on the x-axis. In this DVH, the patient is receiving minimal dose to her heart and the opposite left lung (yellow), and the ipsilateral right lung is receiving 10 to 40 Gy to 20% to 30% of the volume of the right lung. The average total lung dose is indicated.

used depends on the beam energy. For 6-MV photons, 0.3 to 0.5 cm of bolus is recommended, and for higher-energy photons, 1 cm of bolus is recommended. Evaluation of the dose-volume histogram (DVH) is also important to ensure appropriate target volume coverage by the dose desired and also to ensure all healthy tissue dose constraints are met, as excess dose to healthy tissue can potentially lead to significant toxicities. On the x-axis of the DVH is typically a scale of radiation dose, and the y-axis can vary between different parameters and commonly is a scale of percentage of the target volume (Fig. 34.16). A plot of the dose-volume relationship of a target can then be generated, with each x-y cross point representing the dose received (x-axis) by a portion target volume (V) (y-axis). A healthy tissue dose constraint commonly used is to limit the volume of ipsilateral lung to be equal to or less than 30% of the prescribed dose (V 20 Gy ≤30%) and to limit the volume of heart to 5% or less of the prescribed dose (V 40 Gy ≤5%).

Treatment Complications. Although radiation is effective in providing locoregional disease control, some patients may experience radiation-related side effects. Patients undergoing radiation are assessed weekly by the treating physician for acute toxicity (appointments often referred to as "status checks" or "on-treatment visits") and are reassessed typically at 4 to 8 weeks after completion of therapy and routinely thereafter for intermediate and late toxicity evaluations. Toxicities are graded by nurses and physicians with a standardized scoring system, one of which is the Common Terminology Criteria for Adverse Events (CTCAE) by the National Cancer Institute. There is increasing interest in collecting patient-reported outcomes (PROs) in which the patient directly completes surveys written in layperson terms regarding side effects. The PRO-CTCAE is one example, with recent piloting performed to modify the questions for radiation side effects.[125]

Acute skin changes. Skin and subcutaneous tissue changes are expected in the irradiated treatment volume. The skin dose depends on the exact treatment technique used for each patient. Variables in the treatment plan that affect the skin dose include the type of radiation (photons or electrons), beam energy, boost technique (external beam or brachytherapy), wedge, bolus, fraction size, total dose, number of treatment fields and physical conformation of the patient.

Special consideration must be given to the physical conformation of the patient. Skin folds tend to intensify skin reactions as a result of bolus effect and are therefore the most sensitive areas. Proper positioning is necessary to help minimize folds in potential problem areas. Axillary folds may be minimized by adjusting arm abduction. Skin folds in the inframammary, supraclavicular, and neck areas may be altered or eliminated by increasing or decreasing the superior-inferior incline of the patient. Obese patients or those with large, pendulous breasts may need netting or thermoplastic material for the immobilization and reduction of skin folds. Regardless of immobilization, however, radiation dermatitis has been found in multiple studies to be more severe in obese patients.

During a standard (or conventionally fractionated) radiation treatment schedule, skin reaction intensifies according to the escalating dose. Dryness and redness (erythema) of the skin are common after a skin dose of about 30 Gy. Dry desquamation, which involves the flaking of superficial layers of the epidermis, may appear after the delivery of about 40 Gy to the skin. Moist desquamation, which involves the loss of superficial and deep epidermal layers, occurs when doses to the skin exceed 50 Gy. Moist desquamation may arise earlier in treatment in areas where skin folds or bolus reduce the skin-sparing properties of megavoltage beams. The treatment of the large breast is more difficult because of these acute effects and can result in a less acceptable cosmetic outcome. In the era of more hypofractionated regimens, the peak dermatitis reaction often occurs within 1 to 2 weeks after the completion of radiation.

Care of irradiated skin varies according to the type and severity of the reaction. Patients should be advised regarding measures that protect the skin from further irritation and damage. The treatment area must be kept clean through normal gentle cleansing, sun exposure should be avoided, and lotion without irritants should be applied. Patients experiencing moist desquamation may need daily skin care to help prevent infection and minimize fluid loss. Wound dressings with nonstick bandaging techniques are essential; care must be taken to avoid placing adhesives or tape in the treatment area. Cornstarch should be avoided in areas of moist desquamation because it cakes. Moist areas may promote fungal growth and increase the risk of wound infection. Silvadene cream is often prescribed to promote healing and avoid infection.

Severe acute reactions may result in a longer healing time and higher incidence of chronic skin changes. The only treatment shown to reduce the peak skin reaction has been topical steroids, most commonly mometasone, with data strongest among patients undergoing postmastectomy radiation.[126] Most chronic skin changes are cosmetic and rarely problematic, including hyperpigmentation, hair loss, telangiectasia, and subcutaneous fibrosis. The grading for some of the radiation-induced skin side effects can be found in Table 34.2.

Fibrosis. Significant radiation-induced fibrosis is a rare, late event but can impact cosmesis after treatments. The rate of significant fibrosis is directly related to radiation dose, with the EORTC boost trial showing a doubling of moderate to severe fibrosis (15%–30%) with the addition of a 16-Gy tumor bed boost.[127] Patients with collagen vascular disease, especially lupus and scleroderma, have been shown to have an increased risk of radiation-induced fibrosis.[128]

Fatigue. Patients receiving radiation therapy may report generalized fatigue. The incidence appears to be related to the radiation dose, treatment volume, and site of involvement. Breast cancer patients not undergoing chemotherapy tend to experience a very minor degree of fatigue. Other factors (such as a history of recent surgery or chemotherapy, the patient's general medical and psychological condition, current medications, pain, or anemia) may contribute to fatigue.

TABLE 34.2	**Common Terminology Criteria for Adverse Events**				
Adverse Event	**1**	**2**	**3**	**4**	**5**
Radiation dermatitis	Faint erythema or dry desquamation	Moderate to brisk erythema; patchy, moist desquamation, most confined to skin folds and creases; moderate edema	Moist desquamation in areas other than skin folds and creases; bleeding induced by minor trauma or abrasion	Life-threatening consequences; skin necrosis or ulceration of full-thickness dermis; spontaneous bleeding from involved site; skin graft indicated	Death
Skin (pain)	Mild pain	Moderate pain; limiting instrumental ADL	Severe pain; limiting self-care ADL		
Pruritus	Mild or localized; topical intervention indicated	Intense or widespread; intermittent; skin changes from scratching; limiting instrumental ADL	Intense or widespread; constant; limiting self-care ADL or sleep; oral corticosteroid or immunosuppressive therapy indicated		
Skin hyperpigmentation	Hyperpigmentation covering <10% BSA; no psychosocial impact	Hyperpigmentation covering >10% BSA; associated with psychosocial impact			
Skin hypopigmentation	Hypopigmentation covering <10% BSA; no psychosocial impact	Hypopigmentation covering >10% BSA; associated with psychosocial impact			
Telangiectasia	Telangiectasias covering <10% BSA	Telangiectasias covering >10% BSA; associated with psychosocial impact			
Superficial soft tissue fibrosis	Mild induration, able to move skin parallel to plane (sliding) and perpendicular to skin (pinching up)	Moderate induration, able to slide skin, unable to pinch skin; limiting instrumental ADL	Severe induration; unable to slide or pinch skin; limiting joint or orifice movements; limiting self-care ADL	Generalized; associated with signs or symptoms of impaired breathing or feeding	Death

ADL, Activities of daily living; *BSA,* body surface area.

Lymphedema. Impairment of lymph flow can result from sentinel node biopsy, axillary dissection, or radiation therapy, and this can result in lymphedema. The risk of lymphedema increases most dramatically with the extent of axillary surgery (up to 25%), although the severity and risk of lymphedema may be further increased by radiation therapy. Clinically significant lymphedema was noted on the AMAROS trial to be 23% among patients undergoing axillary lymph node dissection compared with 11% among patients with a sentinel lymph node biopsy and nodal radiation.[129]

Cardiac effects. Cardiotoxicity, such as coronary artery disease and cardiomyopathy, is related to both the volume of heart irradiated and the dose the heart received. Older radiation treatment techniques for the breast delivered a significant dose of radiation to the heart, resulting in a higher incidence of cardiovascular disease.[77] A population-based case-control study in Sweden and Denmark involving more than 2000 women showed that the rates of major coronary events increased with mean dose to the heart by approximately 7% per Gy and that the effect began a few years after exposure and continued into the third decade after radiation therapy.[130] However, this study included women treated for breast cancer starting in 1958 with now outdated techniques.

Contemporary techniques include heart avoidance, which reduces incidental cardiac irradiation and appear to reduce cardiotoxicity. With the National Cancer Institute's Surveillance, Epidemiology, and End Results program, investigators found that women diagnosed with left breast cancer in 1973 to 1979, and who were treated with adjuvant radiation therapy, had significant higher rates of ischemic heart disease compared with women who were treated between 1980 and 1984, and 1985 and 1989 (10.2% vs. 9.4% vs. 5.8%, respectively).[131] With continuous improvement in breast cancer radiation treatment delivery,

modern techniques, such as DIBH, prone breast irradiation, PBI, and IMRT, can deliver a full dose to the intended treatment area and keep the heart dose to a minimum.

Pneumonitis. Symptomatic pneumonitis is an uncommon side effect of breast irradiation that can occur 1 to 3 months after radiation treatment. Patients with radiation-induced pneumonitis present with dry cough, dyspnea, and pulmonary infiltrate radiographically within the treatment volume. The symptoms respond to corticosteroids, and in most cases, the symptoms resolve. On the MA20 randomized trial (2015), symptomatic pneumonitis occurred in only 0.2% of patients who received whole breast tangent irradiation, compared with 1.2% of patients treated with regional nodal radiation.[132]

Secondary cancers. Radiation therapy for breast cancer can cause secondary cancers either within the treatment fields or from scattered radiation. In a recent analysis, the overall relative risk for development of cancer after breast irradiation is, on average, 1.2 times higher than in the general population. At 15 years, the risk of contralateral breast cancer in women who received radiation is 9.3% compared with 7.5% in those who did not.[77] More recent studies suggest that the effect of contralateral breast cancer is increased in women younger than 45 years of age. In a study conducted in the Netherlands, women younger than 45 years old who were treated with postlumpectomy radiation therapy had a 1.5-fold increased risk of contralateral breast cancer.[133] Furthermore, a strong dose-response relationship with the risk of contralateral breast cancer is found between the dose received by the medial breast and medial contralateral breast. Other nonbreast cancer malignancies have also been associated with breast irradiation, such as esophageal cancer and lung cancer, especially in smokers.[134]

REVIEW QUESTIONS

The answers to the Review Questions can be found by logging on to our website at: http://evolve.elsevier.com/Washington/principles

1. The pathologic staging system for breast cancer incorporates:
   - I. Lymph node status.
   - II. Tumor extent.
   - III. Distant metastasis.
   - IV. Hormonal status.
     - a. I and II.
     - b. II and III.
     - c. I, II, III.
     - d. I, II, III, and IV.
2. The most common presentation of early-stage breast cancer is:
   - a. Nipple discharge.
   - b. Pain.
   - c. Palpable mass.
   - d. Asymptomatic, nonpalpable mass detected as an abnormality on screening mammogram.
3. Which is an indication for the use of breast-conserving surgery?
   - a. Multicentric disease with two or more primary tumors in separate quadrants of the breast such that they cannot be encompassed in a single excision.
   - b. Diffuse malignant microcalcifications on mammography.
   - c. A small, well-localized tumor.
   - d. Persistent positive resection margins after multiple attempts of re-excision.
4. Why does adjuvant postmastectomy radiation therapy play an important role in women with breast cancer?
   - I. It improves locoregional control.
   - II. It improves breast cancer–specific survival.
   - III. It improves cosmesis.
     - a. I only.
     - b. II only.
     - c. I and II.
     - d. I, II and III.
5. Which radiation treatment technique is not used after breast-conserving surgery?
   - a. Radiation with wide-field electrons.
   - b. Supine whole breast irradiation.
   - c. Prone whole breast irradiation.
   - d. PBI to the lumpectomy cavity.

6. What is not a target of regional lymph node irradiation?
   - a. Cervical lymph nodes.
   - b. Supraclavicular lymph nodes.
   - c. Axillary lymph nodes.
   - d. Internal mammary lymph nodes.
7. The skin usually reacts in a pattern that is dose dependent. Which of the following do you expect to see first for radiation administered with a standard fraction schedule?
   - a. Dry desquamation.
   - b. Erythema.
   - c. Moist desquamation.
   - d. Radiation pneumonitis.
8. The sentinel lymph node biopsy uses _____ in an effort to identify the flow of lymphatic fluid.
   - a. Iodinated contrast material.
   - b. Barium contrast material.
   - c. Blue dye or radioactive material.
   - d. A mixture of oxygen and carbon dioxide.
9. Which of the following is not commonly used in the early detection of breast cancer?
   - a. Bone scan.
   - b. MRI.
   - c. Mammogram.
   - d. Ultrasound.
10. Which of the following normal tissues is of most concern in the treatment of breast cancer using tangential fields?
    - I. Spinal cord.
    - II. Liver.
    - III. Lung.
    - IV. Heart.
      - a. 1 and 2 only.
      - b. 2 and 3 only.
      - c. 3 and 4 only.
      - d. 1, 2, 3, and 4.

QUESTIONS TO PONDER

1. Discuss the significant prognostic factors for breast cancer.
2. Compare and contrast the lymph node drainage of breast cancer.
3. Describe the methods for detection and diagnosis of breast cancer.
4. Discuss important considerations for positioning the patient in breast (both supine and prone) and chest wall irradiation.
5. Describe the acute effects experienced by patients undergoing radiation treatments to the breast and chest wall.

REFERENCES

1. Siegel RL, Miller KD, Jemal A. Cancer statistics, 2017. *CA Cancer J Clin.* 2017;67(1):7–30.
2. DeSantis CE, Ma J, Sauer AJ, et al. Breast cancer statistics, 2017, racial disparity in mortality by state. *CA Cancer J Clin.* 2017;67(6):439–448.
3. Marshall SF, Clarke CA, Deapen D, et al. Recent breast cancer incidence trends according to hormone therapy use: the California Teachers Study cohort. *Breast Cancer Res.* 2010;12(1):R4.
4. Chlebowski RT, Kuller LH, Prentice RL, et al. Breast cancer after use of estrogen plus progestin in postmenopausal women. *N Engl J Med.* 2009;360(6):573–587.
5. DeSantis C, Siegel R, Bandi P, et al. Breast cancer statistics. *CA Cancer J Clin.* 2011;61(6):409–418.
6. Nahleh ZA, Srikantiah R, Safa M, et al. Male breast cancer in the veterans affairs population: a comparative analysis. *Cancer.* 2007;109(8):1471–1477.
7. Anderson WF, Althuis MD, Brinton LA, et al. Is male breast cancer similar or different than female breast cancer? *Breast Cancer Res Treat.* 2004;83(1):77–86.
8. Siegel RL, Miller KD, Jemal A. Cancer statistics, 2019. *CA Cancer J Clin.* 2019;69(1):7–34.
9. Arvold ND, Taghian AG, Niemierko A, et al. Age, breast cancer subtype approximation, and local recurrence after breast-conserving therapy. *J Clin Oncol.* 2011;29:3885–3891.

10. Braunstein LZ, et al. Breast-cancer subtype, age, and lymph node status as predictors of local recurrence following breast-conserving therapy. *Breast Cancer Res Treat*. 2017;161:173–179.

11. Centers for Disease Control and Prevention. Vital signs: racial disparities in breast cancer severity: United States, 2005–2009. *MMWR*. 2012;61(45):922–926.

12. Polak P, et al. A mutational signature reveals alterations underlying deficient homologous recombination repair in breast cancer. *Nat Genet*. 2017;49:1476–1486.

13. van den Brandt PA, Spiegelman D, Yaun SS, et al. Pooled analysis of prospective cohort studies on height, weight, and breast cancer risk. *Am J Epidemiol*. 2000;152(6):514–527.

14. Key TJ, Appleby PN, Reeves GK, et al. Body mass index, serum sex hormones, and breast cancer risk in postmenopausal women. *J Natl Cancer Inst*. 2003;95(16):1218–1226.

15. Bruzzi P, Negri E, La Vecchia C, et al. Short term increase in risk of breast cancer after full term pregnancy. *BMJ*. 1988;297(6656):1096–1098.

16. Colditz GA, Rosner B. Cumulative risk of breast cancer to age 70 years according to risk factor status: data from the Nurses' Health Study. *Am J Epidemiol*. 2000;152(10):950–964.

17. Collaborative Group on Hormonal Factors in Breast Cancer. Breast cancer and hormone: replacement therapy: collaborative reanalysis of data from 51 epidemiological studies of 52,705 women with breast cancer and 108,411 women without breast cancer. *Lancet*. 1997;350(9084):1047–1059.

18. Vessey M, Painter R. Oral contraceptive use and cancer: findings in a large cohort study, 1968-2004. *Br J Cancer*. 2006;95(3):385–389.

19. Marchbanks PA, McDonald JA, Wilson HG, et al. Oral contraceptives and the risk of breast cancer. *N Engl J Med*. 2002;346(26):2025–2032.

20. Hartmann LC, Sellers TA, Frost MH, et al. Benign breast disease and the risk of breast cancer. *N Engl J Med*. 2005;353(3):229–237.

21. Cote ML, Ruterbusch JJ, Alosh B, et al. Benign breast disease and the risk of subsequent breast cancer in African American women. *Cancer Prev Res*. 2012;5(12):1375–1380.

22. McCormack VA, dos Santos Silva I. Breast density and parenchymal patterns as markers of breast cancer risk: a meta-analysis. *Cancer Epidemiol Biomarkers Prev*. 2006;15(6):1159–1169.

23. Nichols HB, Berrington de Gonzalez A, Lacey Jr JV, et al. Declining incidence of contralateral breast cancer in the United States from 1975 to 2006. *J Clin Oncol*. 2011;29(12):1564–1569.

24. Collaborative Group on Hormonal Factors in Breast Cancer. Familial breast cancer: collaborative reanalysis of individual data from 52 epidemiological studies including 58,209 women with breast cancer and 101,986 women without the disease. *Lancet*. 2001;358(9291):1389–1399.

25. Mavaddat N, Peock S, Frost D, et al. Cancer risks for BRCA1 and BRCA2 mutation carriers: results from prospective analysis of EMBRACE. *J Natl Cancer Inst*. 2013;105(11):812–822.

26. Liede A, Karlan BY, Narod SA. Cancer risks for male carriers of germline mutations in BRCA1 or BRCA2: a review of the literature. *J Clin Oncol*. 2004;22(4):735–742.

27. Bagnardi V, Rota M, Botteri E, et al. Light alcohol drinking and cancer: a meta-analysis. *Ann Oncol*. 2013;24(2):301–308.

28. Gaudet MM, Gapstur SM, Sun J, et al. Active smoking and breast cancer risk: original cohort data and meta-analysis. *J Natl Cancer Inst*. 2013;105(8):515–525.

29. Hansen J, Stevens RG. Case-control study of shift-work and breast cancer risk in Danish nurses: impact of shift systems. *Eur J Cancer*. 2012;48(11):1722–1729.

30. Schernhammer ES, Hankinson SE. Urinary melatonin levels and breast cancer risk. *J Natl Cancer Inst*. 2005;97(14):1084–1087.

31. El-Din MAA, et al. Breast cancer after treatment of Hodgkin's lymphoma: risk factors that really matter. *Int J Radiat Oncol Biol Phys*. 2009;73:69–74.

32. Aisenberg AC, Finkelstein DM, Doppke KP, et al. High risk of breast carcinoma after irradiation of young women with Hodgkin's disease. *Cancer*. 1997;79(6):1203–1210.

33. van Leeuwen FE, Klokman WJ, Stovall M, et al. Roles of radiation dose, chemotherapy, and hormonal factors in breast cancer following Hodgkin's disease. *J Natl Cancer Inst*. 2003;95(13):971–980.

34. DeSelm C, et al. A 3-dimensional mapping analysis of regional nodal recurrences in breast cancer. *Int J Radiat Oncol Biol Phys*. 2019;103:583–591.

35. Estourgie SH, Nieweg OE, Olmos RA, et al. Lymphatic drainage patterns from the breast. *Ann Surg*. 2004;239(2):232–237.

36. Jemal A, Simard EP, Dorell C, et al. Annual Report to the Nation on the Status of Cancer, 1975-2009, featuring the burden and trends in human papillomavirus(HPV)-associated cancers and HPV vaccination coverage levels. *J Natl Cancer Inst*. 2013;105(3):175–201.

37. American Cancer Society Facts & Figures 2017-2018, Atlanta: American Cancer Society, Inc., 2017

38. Weaver DL, Rosenberg RD, Barlow WE, et al. Pathologic findings from the Breast Cancer Surveillance Consortium: population-based outcomes in women undergoing biopsy after screening mammography. *Cancer*. 2006;106(4):732–742.

39. Independent UK Panel on Breast Cancer Screening. The benefits and harms of breast cancer screening: an independent review. *Lancet*. 2012;380(9855):1778–1786.

40. Nelson HD, Tyne K, Naik A, et al. Screening for breast cancer: an update for the U.S. Preventive Services Task Force. *Ann Internal Med*. 2009;151(10):727–737, W237–W742.

41. Nystrom L, Andersson I, Bjurstam N, et al. Long-term effects of mammography screening: updated overview of the Swedish randomised trials. *Lancet*. 2002;359(9310):909–919.

42. Mettler FA, Upton AC, Kelsey CA, et al. Benefits versus risks from mammography: a critical reassessment. *Cancer*. 1996;77(5):903–909.

43. Vachon CM, van Gils CH, Sellers TA, et al. Mammographic density, breast cancer risk and risk prediction. *Breast Cancer Res*. 2007;9(6):217.

44. Gennaro G, Toledano A, di Maggio C, et al. Digital breast tomosynthesis versus digital mammography: a clinical performance study. *Eur Radiol*. 2010;20(7):1545–1553.

45. Andersson I, Ikeda DM, Zackrisson S, et al. Breast tomosynthesis and digital mammography: a comparison of breast cancer visibility and BI-RADS classification in a population of cancers with subtle mammographic findings. *Eur Radiol*. 2008;18(12):2817–2825.

46. Berg WA, Blume JD, Cormack JB, et al. Combined screening with ultrasound and mammography vs mammography alone in women at elevated risk of breast cancer. *J Am Med Assoc*. 2008;299(18):2151–2163.

47. Bluemke DA, Gatsonis CA, Chen MH, et al. Magnetic resonance imaging of the breast prior to biopsy. *J Am Med Assoc*. 2004;292(22):2735–2742.

48. Esserman L, Hylton N, Yassa L, et al. Utility of magnetic resonance imaging in the management of breast cancer: evidence for improved preoperative staging. *J Clin Oncol*. 1999;17(1):110–119.

49. Peters NH, Borel Rinkes IH, Zuithoff NP, et al. Meta-analysis of MR imaging in the diagnosis of breast lesions. *Radiology*. 2008;246(1):116–124.

50. Rijnsburger AJ, Obdeijn IM, Kaas R, et al. BRCA1-associated breast cancers present differently from BRCA2-associated and familial cases: long-term follow-up of the Dutch MRISC Screening Study. *J Clin Oncol*. 2010;28(36):5265–5273.

51. Chiarelli AM, Majpruz V, Brown P, et al. The contribution of clinical breast examination to the accuracy of breast screening. *J Natl Cancer Inst*. 2009;101(18):1236–1243.

52. Svane G, Silfversward C. Stereotaxic needle biopsy of non-palpable breast lesions: cytologic and histopathologic findings. *Acta Radiol Diagn*. 1983;24(4):283–288.

53. Holland R, Hendriks JH, Vebeek AL, et al. Extent, distribution, and mammographic/histological correlations of breast ductal carcinoma in situ. *Lancet*. 1990;335(8688):519–522.

54. Schnitt SJ, Morrow M. Lobular carcinoma in situ: current concepts and controversies. *Semin Diagnostic Pathol*. 1999;16(3):209–223.

55. Kreike B, Hart AA, van de Velde T, et al. Continuing risk of ipsilateral breast relapse after breast-conserving therapy at long-term follow-up. *Int J Radiat Oncol Biol Phys*. 2008;71(4):1014–1021.

56. Jacquemier J, Kurtz JM, Amalric R, et al. An assessment of extensive intraductal component as a risk factor for local recurrence after breast-conserving therapy. *Br J Cancer*. 1990;61(6):873–876.

57. Holland R, Connolly JL, Gelman R, et al. The presence of an extensive intraductal component following a limited excision correlates with prominent residual disease in the remainder of the breast. *J Clin Oncol*. 1990;8(1):113–118.

58. Orvieto E, Maiorano E, Bottiglieri L, et al. Clinicopathologic characteristics of invasive lobular carcinoma of the breast: results of an analysis of 530 cases from a single institution. *Cancer*. 2008;113(7):1511–1520.

59. Fredholm H, Eaker S, Frisell J, et al. Breast cancer in young women: poor survival despite intensive treatment. *PLoS One*. 2009;4(11):e7695.

60. Carey LA, Perou CM, Livasy CA, et al. Race, breast cancer subtypes, and survival in the Carolina breast cancer study. *J Am Med Assoc*. 2006;295(21):2492–2502.

61. Silber JH, Rosenbaum PR, Clark AS, et al. Characteristics associated with differences in survival among black and white women with breast cancer. *J Am Med Assoc*. 2013;310(4):389–397.

62. Carter CL, Allen C, Henson DE. Relation of tumor size, lymph node status, and survival in 24,740 breast cancer cases. *Cancer*. 1989;63(1):181–187.

63. Andersson Y, Frisell J, Sylvan M, et al. Breast cancer survival in relation to the metastatic tumor burden in axillary lymph nodes. *J Clin Oncol*. 2010;28(17):2868–2873.

64. Rakha EA, El-Sayed ME, Lee AH, et al. Prognostic significance of Nottingham histologic grade in invasive breast carcinoma. *J Clin Oncol*. 2008;26(19):3153–3158.

65. Rakha EA, Martin S, Lee AH, et al. The prognostic significance of lymphovascular invasion in invasive breast carcinoma. *Cancer*. 2012;118(15):3670–3680.

66. Freedman GM, Fowble BL. Local recurrence after mastectomy or breast-conserving surgery and radiation. *Oncology*. 2000;14(11):1561.

67. Grann VR, Troxel AB, Zojwalla NJ, et al. Hormone receptor status and survival in a population-based cohort of patients with breast carcinoma. *Cancer*. 2005;103(11):2241–2251.

68. Harvey JM, Clark GM, Osborne CK, et al. Estrogen receptor status by immunohistochemistry is superior to the ligand-binding assay for predicting response to adjuvant endocrine therapy in breast cancer. *J Clin Oncol*. 1999;17(5):1474–1481.

69. Bartlett JM, Brookes CL, Robson T, et al. Estrogen receptor and progesterone receptor as predictive biomarkers of response to endocrine therapy: a prospectively powered pathology study in the Tamoxifen and Exemestane Adjuvant Multinational trial. *J Clin Oncol*. 2011;29(12):1531–1538.

70. Ross JS, Fletcher JA. The HER-2/neu oncogene in breast cancer: prognostic factor, predictive factor, and target for therapy. *The Oncologist*. 1998;3(4):237–252.

71. Harris L, Fritsche H, Mennel R, et al. American Society of Clinical Oncology 2007 update of recommendations for the use of tumor markers in breast cancer. *J Clin Oncol*. 2007;25(33):5287–5312.

72. Lin NU, Vanderplas A, Hughes ME, et al. Clinicopathologic features, patterns of recurrence, and survival among women with triple-negative breast cancer in the National Comprehensive Cancer Network. *Cancer*. 2012;118(22):5463–5472.

73. Cancer Genome Atlas N. Comprehensive molecular portraits of human breast tumours. *Nature*. 2012;490(7418):61–70.

74. Loi S, Haibe-Kains B, Desmedt C, et al. Definition of clinically distinct molecular subtypes in estrogen receptor-positive breast carcinomas through genomic grade. *J Clin Oncol*. 2007;25(10):1239–1246.

75. Fan C, Oh DS, Wessels L, et al. Concordance among gene-expression-based predictors for breast cancer. *N Engl J Med*. 2006;355(6):560–569.

76. Gradishar WJ, Anderson BO, Blair SL, et al. Breast cancer version 3.2014. *J Natl Compr Canc Netw*. 2014;12(4):542–590.

77. Clarke M, Collins R, Darby S, et al. Effects of radiotherapy and of differences in the extent of surgery for early breast cancer on local recurrence and 15-year survival: an overview of the randomised trials. *Lancet*. 2005;366(9503):2087–2106.

78. Fisher B, Anderson S, Bryant J, et al. Twenty-year follow-up of a randomized trial comparing total mastectomy, lumpectomy, and lumpectomy plus irradiation for the treatment of invasive breast cancer. *N Engl J Med*. 2002;347(16):1233–1241.

79. Veronesi U, Cascinelli N, Mariani L, et al. Twenty-year follow-up of a randomized study comparing breast-conserving surgery with radical mastectomy for early breast cancer. *N Engl J Med*. 2002;347(16):1227–1232.

80. van Dongen JA, Voogd AC, Fentiman IS, et al. Long-term results of a randomized trial comparing breast-conserving therapy with mastectomy: European Organization for Research and Treatment of Cancer 10801 trial. *J Natl Cancer Inst*. 2000;92(14):1143–1150.

81. Fisher B, et al. Effect of preoperative chemotherapy on local-regional disease in women with operable breast cancer: findings from National Surgical Adjuvant Breast and Bowel Project B-18. *J Clin Oncol*. 1997;15:2483–2493.

82. Wo J, Taghian A. Radiotherapy in setting of collagen vascular disease. *Int J Radiat Oncol Biol Phys*. 2007;69(5):1347–1353.

83. Chung A, Huynh K, Lawrence C, et al. Comparison of patient characteristics and outcomes of contralateral prophylactic mastectomy and unilateral total mastectomy in breast cancer patients. *Ann Surg Oncol*. 2012;19(8):2600–2606.

84. Fisher B, Jeong JH, Anderson S, et al. Twenty-five-year follow-up of a randomized trial comparing radical mastectomy, total mastectomy, and total mastectomy followed by irradiation. *N Engl J Med*. 2002;347(8):567–575.

85. Cuzick J, Stewart H, Rutqvist L, et al. Cause-specific mortality in long-term survivors of breast cancer who participated in trials of radiotherapy. *J Clin Oncol*. 1994;12(3):447–453.

86. Galimberti V, et al. Nipple-sparing and skin-sparing mastectomy: review of aims, oncological safety and contraindications. *Breast*. 2017;34:S82–S84.

87. Giuliano AE, et al. Effect of axillary dissection vs no axillary dissection on 10-year overall survival among women with invasive breast cancer and sentinel node metastasis. *J Am Med Assoc*. 2017;318(10):918–926.

88. Kwan W, Jackson J, Weir LM, et al. Chronic arm morbidity after curative breast cancer treatment: prevalence and impact on quality of life. *J Clin Oncol*. 2002;20(20):4242–4248.

89. Atisha D, Alderman AK, Lowery JC, et al. Prospective analysis of long-term psychosocial outcomes in breast reconstruction: two-year postoperative results from the Michigan Breast Reconstruction Outcomes Study. *Ann Surg*. 2008;247(6):1019–1028.

90. Cordeiro PG, et al. What is the optimum timing of post-mastectomy radiotherapy in two-stage Prosthetic Reconstruction: radiation to the tissue expander or permanent implant? 135:1509.

91. Pusic AL, et al. Patient-reported outcomes 1 year after immediate breast reconstruction: results of the mastectomy reconstruction outcomes consortium study. *J Clin Oncol*. 2017;35:2499.

92. Jagsi R, Jiang J, Momoh AO, et al. Trends and variation in use of breast reconstruction in patients with breast cancer undergoing mastectomy in the United States. *J Clin Oncol*. 2014;32(9):919–926.

93. Early Breast Cancer Trialists' Collaborative Group (EBCTCG). Effects of chemotherapy and hormonal therapy for early breast cancer on recurrence and 15-year survival: an overview of the randomised trials. *Lancet*. 2005;365:1687–1717.

94. Early Breast Cancer Trialists' Collaborative Group (EBCTCG), Peto R, Davies C, et al. Comparisons between different polychemotherapy regimens for early breast cancer: meta-analyses of long-term outcome among 100,000 women in 123 randomised trials. *Lancet*. 2012;379(9814):432–444.

95. Romond EH, Perez EA, Bryant J, et al. Trastuzumab plus adjuvant chemotherapy for operable HER2-positive breast cancer. *N Engl J Med*. 2005;353(16):1673–1684.

96. Swain SM, Kim SB, Cortes J, et al. Pertuzumab, trastuzumab, and docetaxel for HER2-positive metastatic breast cancer (CLEOPATRA study): overall survival results from a randomised, double-blind, placebo-controlled, phase 3 study. *Lancet Oncol*. 2013;14(6):461–471.

97. Early Breast Cancer Trialists' Collaborative Group (EBCTCG), Davies C, Godwin J, et al. Relevance of breast cancer hormone receptors and other factors to the efficacy of adjuvant tamoxifen: patient-level meta-analysis of randomised trials. *Lancet*. 2011;378(9793):771–784.

98. Dowsett M, Cuzick J, Ingle J, et al. Meta-analysis of breast cancer outcomes in adjuvant trials of aromatase inhibitors versus tamoxifen. *J Clin Oncol*. 2010;28(3):509–518.

99. Wapnir IL, Dignam JJ, Fisher B, et al. Long-term outcomes of invasive ipsilateral breast tumor recurrences after lumpectomy in NSABP B-17 and B-24 randomized clinical trials for DCIS. *J Natl Cancer Inst*. 2011;103(6):478–488.

100. EORTC Breast Cancer Cooperative Group, EORTC Radiotherapy Group, Bijker N, et al. Breast-conserving treatment with or without radiotherapy in ductal carcinoma-in-situ: ten-year results of European Organisation for Research and treatment of cancer randomized phase III trial 10853: a study by the EORTC breast cancer cooperative group and EORTC radiotherapy group. *J Clin Oncol*. 2006;24(21):3381–3387.

101. Holmberg L, Garmo H, Granstrand B, et al. Absolute risk reductions for local recurrence after postoperative radiotherapy after sector resection for ductal carcinoma in situ of the breast. *J Clin Oncol.* 2008;26(8):1247–1252.

102. Early Breast Cancer Trialists' Collaborative Group (EBCTCG), Correa C, McGale P, et al. Overview of the randomized trials of radiotherapy in ductal carcinoma in situ of the breast. *J Natl Cancer Inst Monogr.* 2010;2010(41):162–177.

103. Clark RM, Whelan T, Levine M, et al. Randomized clinical trial of breast irradiation following lumpectomy and axillary dissection for node-negative breast cancer: an update. Ontario Clinical Oncology Group. *J Natl Cancer Inst.* 1996;88(22):1659–1664.

104. Liljegren G, Holmberg L, Adami HO, et al. Sector Resection with or without postoperative radiotherapy for stage-I breast-cancer: 5-year results of a randomized trial. *J Natl Cancer Inst.* 1994;86(9):717–722.

105. Forrest AP, Stewart HJ, Everington D, et al. Randomised controlled trial of conservation therapy for breast cancer: 6-year analysis of the Scottish trial. Scottish Cancer Trials Breast Group. *Lancet.* 1996;348(9029):708–713.

106. Veronesi U, Marubini E, Mariani L, et al. Radiotherapy after breast-conserving surgery in small breast carcinoma: long-term results of a randomized trial. *Ann Oncol.* 2001;12(7):997–1003.

107. Fisher B, Bryant J, Dignam JJ, et al. Tamoxifen, radiation therapy, or both for prevention of ipsilateral breast tumor recurrence after lumpectomy in women with invasive breast cancers of one centimeter or less. *J Clin Oncol.* 2002;20(20):4141–4149.

108. Hurkmans CW, Borger JH, v Giersbergen A, et al. Implementation of a forearm support to reduce the amount of irradiated lung and heart in radiation therapy of the breast. *Radiother Oncol.* 2001;61(2):193–196.

109. Remouchamps VM, Letts N, Vicini FA, et al. Initial clinical experience with moderate deep-inspiration breath hold using an active breathing control device in the treatment of patients with left-sided breast cancer using external beam radiation therapy. *Int J Radiat Oncol Biol Phys.* 2003;56(3):704–715.

110. Korreman SS, Pedersen AN, Aarup LR, et al. Reduction of cardiac and pulmonary complication probabilities after breathing adapted radiotherapy for breast cancer. *Int J Radiat Oncol Biol Phys.* 2006;65(5):1375–1380.

111. Korreman SS, Pedersen AN, Nottrup TJ, et al. Breathing adapted radiotherapy for breast cancer: comparison of free breathing gating with the breath-hold technique. *Radiother Oncol.* 2005;76(3):311–318.

112. Lu HM, Cash E, Chen MH, et al. Reduction of cardiac volume in left-breast treatment fields by respiratory maneuvers: a CT study. *Int J Radiat Oncol Biol Phys.* 2000;47(4):895–904.

113. Whelan T, MacKenzie R, Julian J, et al. Randomized trial of breast irradiation schedules after lumpectomy for women with lymph node-negative breast cancer. *J Natl Cancer Inst.* 2002;94(15):1143–1150.

114. Whelan TJ, et al. Long-term results of hypofractionated radiation therapy for breast cancer. *N Engl J Med.* 2010;362:513–520.

115. Bentzen S, et al. The UK Standardisation of Breast Radiotherapy (START) Trial B of radiotherapy hypofractionation for treatment of early breast cancer: a randomised trial. *Lancet.* 2008;371:1098–1107.

116. Bartelink H, Horiot JC, Poortmans P, et al. Recurrence rates after treatment of breast cancer with standard radiotherapy with or without additional radiation. *N Engl J Med.* 2001;345(19):1378–1387.

117. Bartelink H, Horiot JC, Poortmans PM, et al. Impact of a higher radiation dose on local control and survival in breast-conserving therapy of early breast cancer: 10-year results of the randomized boost versus no boost EORTC 22881-10882 trial. *J Clin Oncol.* 2007;25(22):3259–3265.

118. Chen PY, Wallace M, Mitchell C, et al. Four-year efficacy, cosmesis, and toxicity using three-dimensional conformal external beam radiation therapy to deliver accelerated partial breast irradiation. *Int J Radiat Oncol Biol Phys.* 2010;76(4):991–997.

119. Taghian AG, Kozak KR, Doppke KP, et al. Initial dosimetric experience using simple three-dimensional conformal external-beam accelerated partial-breast irradiation. *Int J Radiat Oncol Biol Phys.* 2006l64(4):1092-1099.

120. Lievens Y, Poortmans P, Van den Bogaert W. A glance on quality assurance in EORTC study 22922 evaluating techniques for internal mammary and medial supraclavicular lymph node chain irradiation in breast cancer. *Radiother Oncol.* 2001;60(3):257–265.

121. Overgaard M, Hansen PS, Overgaard J, et al. Postoperative radiotherapy in high-risk premenopausal women with breast cancer who receive adjuvant chemotherapy: Danish Breast Cancer Cooperative Group 82b Trial. *N Engl J Med.* 1997;337(14):949–955.

122. Overgaard M, Jensen MB, Overgaard J, et al. Postoperative radiotherapy in high-risk postmenopausal breast-cancer patients given adjuvant tamoxifen: Danish Breast Cancer Cooperative Group DBCG 82c randomised trial. *Lancet.* 1999;353(9165):1641–1648.

123. Ho AY, et al. Long-term pulmonary outcomes of a feasibility study of inverse-planned, multibeam intensity modulated radiation therapy in node-positive breast cancer patients receiving regional nodal irradiation. *Int J Radiat Oncol Biol Phys.* 2019;103(5):1100–1108.

124. Dumane VA, et al. Reduction in low-dose to normal tissue with the addition of deep inspiration breath hold (DIBH) to volumetric modulated arc therapy (VMAT) in breast cancer patients with implant reconstruction receiving regional nodal irradiation. *Radiat Oncol.* 2018;24;13(1):187.

125. Sandler KA, et al. Content validity of anatomic site-specific Patient-Reported Outcomes Version of the Common Terminology Criteria for Adverse Events (PRO-CTCAE) item sets for assessment of acute symptomatic toxicities in radiation oncology. *Int J Radiat Oncol Biol Phys.* 2018;102(1):44–52.

126. Ho AY, et al. A randomized trial of mometasone furoate 0.1% to reduce high-grade acute radiation dermatitis in breast cancer patients receiving postmastectomy radiation. *Int J Radiat Oncol Biol Phys.* 2018;101(2):325–333.

127. Bartelink H, et al. Whole-breast irradiation with or without a boost for patients treated with breast-conserving surgery for early breast cancer: 20-year follow-up of a randomised phase 3 trial. *Lancet Oncol.* 2015;16:47–56.

128. Morris MM, Powell SN. Irradiation in the setting of collagen vascular disease: acute and late complications. *J Clin Oncol.* 1997;15(7):2728–2735.

129. Donker M, et al. Radiotherapy or surgery of the axilla after a positive sentinel node in breast cancer (EORTC 10981-22023 AMAROS): a randomised, multicentre, open-label, phase 3 non-inferiority trial. *Lancet Oncol.* 2014;15:1303–1310.

130. Darby SC, Ewertz M, McGale P, et al. Risk of ischemic heart disease in women after radiotherapy for breast cancer. *N Engl J Med.* 2013;368(11):987–998.

131. Giordano SH, Kuo YF, Freeman JL, et al. Risk of cardiac death after adjuvant radiotherapy for breast cancer. *J Natl Cancer Inst.* 2005;97(6):419–424.

132. Whelan TJ, Olivotto IA, Parulekar WR, et al. Regional nodal irradiation in early-stage breast cancer. *N Engl J Med.* 2015;373(4):307–316.

133. Hooning MJ, Aleman BM, Hauptmann M, et al. Roles of radiotherapy and chemotherapy in the development of contralateral breast cancer. *J Clin Oncol.* 2008;26(34):5561–5568.

134. Taylor C, et al. Estimating the risks of breast cancer radiotherapy: evidence from modern radiation doses to the lungs and heart and from previous randomized trials. *J Clin Oncol.* 2017;35(15):1641–1649.

35

Pediatric Solid Tumors

Heather Mallett

OUTLINE

Although rare, pediatric cancers present a great challenge in the radiation oncology community. The implications of managing childhood cancers with surgery, radiation, and chemotherapy are often far-reaching, and there is a persistent need to mitigate long-term, treatment-related toxicities. Treatment often requires a collaborative approach among many disciplines. Care must be highly coordinated between medical, surgical, and radiation oncology with support from social services, physical therapists, nutritionists, educators, and others. In addition to treatment of each patient's malignancy, consideration and care must be given to the emotional, logistical, family, cultural, and other factors that affect each child's life. The resources required in managing the care of a child are immense and typically necessitate referral to a specialized children's cancer program.

Although cancer is largely considered a disease of older age groups, the incidence of childhood cancers (ages 0 to 19 years) is on the rise. An estimated 15,270 new cancer cases are expected to occur each year, accounting for less than 1% of all cancers diagnosed. An estimated 1,790 deaths are expected annually.[1] Although incidence rates have been slowly increasing since 1975, the childhood cancer death rate has declined by more than two-thirds since 1969, which may be attributed to improvements in the management of leukemia and high rates of participation in clinical trials. Although the overall outlook for children with cancer has improved significantly over the last 50 years, cancer remains the second leading cause of death among children past infancy (age 1 to 14 years), preceded only by accidents, accounting for 13% of deaths in 2015.[2] The most common childhood cancers in children aged 0 to 14 years are leukemia and central nervous system (CNS) tumors, which together account for 50% of all cancers in this age group. Other frequently encountered cancers in this age group are neuroblastoma, Wilms tumor, and malignant lymphomas. For adolescents (age 15 to 19 years), common cancers include Hodgkin lymphoma, germ cell tumors, and CNS tumors.[3] Table 35.1 outlines common childhood cancers and the role of radiation therapy.

There are very few etiologic agents associated with childhood cancers. In adults, a variety of lifestyle-related risk factors play a role in many types of cancer; however, these factors typically take many years to influence cancer risk. As such, they are not thought to play much of a role in childhood cancers.[2] Although a few environmental factors, such as radiation exposure, have been linked with some types of childhood cancers, most cancers of this age group have not been shown to have environmental causes.[2] Pediatric cancers are more frequently associated with genetic conditions including xeroderma pigmentosa; ataxia telangiectasia; Bloom, Faconi, and Down syndromes; neurofibromatosis (NF); Li-Fraumeni syndrome; and others. However, it is now known that genetically defined cancer susceptibility accounts for less than 10% of pediatric cancers. Cytogenetic and molecular markers that correlate with prognosis are being increasingly identified, which allows treatment to be tailored accordingly. Although treatment paradigms for many childhood cancers have shifted in recent years, radiation continues to play a central role in the management of CNS tumors, soft tissue sarcomas, Ewing sarcoma, Wilms tumor, Hodgkin lymphoma, and a variety of other benign and malignant conditions.

Because of the complicated nature of childhood cancers and the endless pursuit of better treatment strategies, a concerted effort is made to enroll as many pediatric patients as possible in clinical trials. Approximately two-thirds of children with cancer in North America are treated on clinical protocols.[3] More than 50% of patients are involved in clinical trial investigations led by the Children's Oncology Group (COG) in the United States and by similar international groups. Because many radiation therapists rarely encounter pediatric patients, the remainder of this chapter highlights selected childhood cancers, their unique treatments, and important age-specific considerations.

BRAIN TUMORS

Overview/Epidemiology

CNS cancers are the second most common cancers in children (after leukemia) and encompass a wide spectrum of lesions histologically and anatomically. Pediatric CNS tumors comprise about 20% of all childhood cancers and remain a leading cause of death in children despite improvements in 5-year survival from 62.9% for patients diagnosed in 1980 to 1989 to 75.3% for those diagnosed in 2000 to 2006.[4] Within the CNS, the brain is the most common site of disease. The World Health Organization (WHO) anatomic classification of CNS tumors is given in Table 35.2. Within the brain, common sites of disease include the cerebellum and brainstem.

There are important differences between brain tumors seen in childhood and those occurring in adulthood. Children are more frequently diagnosed with low-grade, infratentorial lesions when

TABLE 35.1 Common Neoplasms That Occur in Children and Adolescents

Disease Type	Percentage of Childhood Cancers	Role for Radiation Therapy
Acute leukemias	24	
ALL	18	1. Limited amount of benefit from preventive cranial irradiation (high-risk) T-cell tumors, <5% of ALL cases
	4	2. Therapeutic CNS RT for CNS relapse
		3. TBI in BMT for recurrent/high-risk ALL
Acute myeloblastic leukemia		1. TBI in BMT
Central nervous system tumors	18	
Glial tumors	12	1. Local RT for many low-grade histotypes; often at progression for <5–10 years of age
		2. Local RT for all high-grade tumors
Ependymomas	1	1. Local RT for virtually all presentations
Craniopharyngiomas	1	1. Local RT for biopsied, incompletely resected, or progressive/recurrent tumors
Medulloblastomas and other embryonal CNS tumors	3	1. Systematic craniospinal irradiation plus local boost for children ≥3–4 years of age
		2. Local RT in children <3–4 years of age (investigational)
Malignant lymphomas	15	
Hodgkin disease	9	1. Local (involved field) in combined-modality therapy
Malignant lymphoid tumors	6	2. TBI in transplantation settings for recurrent disease
		1. Limited local or TBI (BMT) indications
Neuroblastoma	5	1. Locoregional RT for regionally advanced disease
		2. Locoregional consolidation in metastatic presentations
		3. Palliative RT (bone, soft tissue)
Wilms tumor	4	1. Locoregional RT in advanced disease or unfavorable histologic findings
		2. Visceral RT in metastatic disease
Retinoblastoma	4	1. Focal RT in conjunction with systemic chemotherapy
		2. Ocular RT in consolidative or progressive/recurrent settings
Soft tissue sarcomas	7	
Rhabdomyosarcomas	4	1. Locoregional RT for most presentations (intermediate/advanced or alveolar histologic types)
Other soft tissue tumors	3	1. Locoregional RT based on histologic findings, site and size of tumor, and patient age
Bone sarcomas	6	
Osteosarcoma	3	1. Limited postoperative or primary use in central sites
Ewing sarcoma	2	1. Local RT for "nondispensable" primary site
		2. Local postoperative RT following marginal resection
		3. Visceral and bone RT in metastatic disease
Hepatic tumors	1	1. Limited postoperative or palliative RT
Germ cell tumors	5	1. Limited locoregional RT

ALL, Acute lymphoblastic leukemia; *BMT,* bone marrow transplantation; *CNS,* central nervous system; *RT,* radiation therapy; *TBI,* total body irradiation.
From Kun LE. Childhood cancers overview: In: Gunderson LL, Tepper JE, eds. *Clinical Radiation Oncology.* 3rd ed. Philadelphia, PA: Elsevier; 2012; Modified from SEER Cancer Statistics. www.seer.cancer.gov; and Li J, Thompson TD, Miller JW, et al. Cancer incidence among children and adolescents in the United States, 2001–2003. *Pediatrics* 2008;121(6):e1470–e1477. Accessed November 6, 2019.

TABLE 35.2 Distribution of Primary Brain and Central Nervous System Tumors

Type of Tumor	Percentage
Brain tumors	68.9
Pituitary tumors	12.2
Cranial nerve tumors	6.3
Spinal cord and cauda equina tumors	5.1
Meninges tumors	2.9
Pineal gland tumors	2.9
Other CNS tumors	1.8

CNS, Central nervous system.
Modified from Halperin EC, Wazer DE, Perez CA, Brady LW, eds. *Perez and Brady's Principles and Practice of Radiation Oncology.* 6th ed. Philadelphia, PA: Lippincott Williams & Wilkins; 2013 accessed November 6, 2019.

TABLE 35.3 Relative Incidence of Brain Tumors

Type of Tumor	Percentage of Total
Supratentorial (50%–55%)	
Low-grade astrocytoma	23
Anaplastic astrocytoma, glioblastoma, and PNET	10
Ependymoma	3
Pineal and germ cell tumors	4
Pituitary and craniopharyngioma	5
Other	4
Infratentorial (45%–50%)	
Medulloblastoma	15
Low-grade astrocytoma	15
Ependymoma	5
Brainstem glioma	10

PNET, Primitive neuroectodermal tumor.
Data from Duffner PK, Cohen ME, Myers MH, et al. Survival of children with brain tumors: SEER program, 1973–1980. *Neurology* 1986;36:597–601; and from Surveillance, epidemiology, and end results program. National Cancer Institute website. SEER.cancer.gov. Accessed November 6, 2019.

compared with their adult counterparts. Primitive neuroectodermal tumor (PNET) lesions, like medulloblastoma, also tend toward younger ages. Table 35.3 illustrates relative incidences from a combination of patient series. Most tumors occur sporadically; however, some congenital disorders and genetic defects predispose toward development of brain tumors. Examples include NF, Li-Fraumeni syndrome, and defects in the retinoblastoma tumor suppressor gene. For long-term survivors, late effects of treatment are a major concern, as neurocognitive effects of CNS irradiation have been well described and correlated with radiation dose, volume, and patient age.[3] Because the disease and its treatment can result in significant morbidity for children, individualized multidisciplinary care that involves neurosurgery, endocrinology, pediatric and radiation oncology, neuropsychology, rehabilitation, social work, and other services is a necessity.

> Astrocytes are star-shaped glial cells within the central nervous system (CNS) that perform a variety of support tasks, including synaptic support between blood vessels and brain tissue and control of the blood-brain barrier, and they have an important role in maintaining homeostasis at the synapse.

Low-Grade Astrocytoma

Astrocytomas are tumors that arise from the supporting cells of the brain and are typically classified as either low grade (WHO grade I and II) or high grade (WHO grade III or IV).

Low-grade astrocytomas tend to exhibit continued slow, relentless growth and occur with equal frequency in the cerebrum and posterior fossa. Pilocytic astrocytomas are the most common low-grade lesions in the pediatric group. Patients with low-grade astrocytomas typically present with a long history of nonspecific and nonlocalizing symptoms. Headaches, degenerating coordination, visual impairment, or poor school performance can subtly worsen for months or years, and seizures can eventually develop in those with hemispheric lesions. On imaging, low-grade astrocytomas are well circumscribed and solid, often with a cystic component. Typically, less surrounding edema or mass effect is found than with high-grade lesions (Fig. 35.1A). In general, these lesions follow an indolent clinical course, with overall survival rates at 10 and 15 years as high as 80% to 100%.

Surgery is the mainstay of treatment for low-grade astrocytomas. Complete resection is most likely to be accomplished in patients with small tumors and those arising in noneloquent parts of the brain, as well as in patients with generally well-circumscribed pilocytic tumors.[4] If discovered in an extremely young child without major neurologic deficits, a low-grade brain tumor requires no immediate treatment; however, the patient should be monitored closely. This strategy may effectively delay therapy in this group of patients who are most susceptible to treatment effects. Ideally, after the child reaches an age at which the brain is more mature and less susceptible to injury (usually 3 to 5 years of age), resection can be performed. The extent of resection is a significant prognostic indicator; if the lesion is completely removed, long-term prognosis is excellent. Incomplete resection is associated with lesser control. Chemotherapy has been increasingly used in low-grade gliomas and may allow delay and possible avoidance of radiation.

Radiation therapy is typically reserved for unresectable or recurrent lesions and those with postsurgical residual tumor in locations where further growth could lead to significant neurologic problems. A dose of 5000 to 5400 cGy in 180 cGy fractions is commonly used. Because infiltration of surrounding brain tissues is usually limited with low-grade gliomas, a 1.5-cm clinical target volume (CTV) beyond the lesion plus an additional 0.5 cm for the planning target volume is generally an adequate margin with three-dimensional (3D) treatment planning and intensity-modulated radiation therapy (IMRT) technique. Fusion of magnetic resonance (MR) images with computed tomography (CT) images is helpful in delineating volumes and designing precise fields to better spare critical healthy tissues. Radiation therapy has enhanced the long-term control of residual tumors in most series, but progression may occur years later. Long-term follow-up with imaging and neurologic evaluation is necessary.

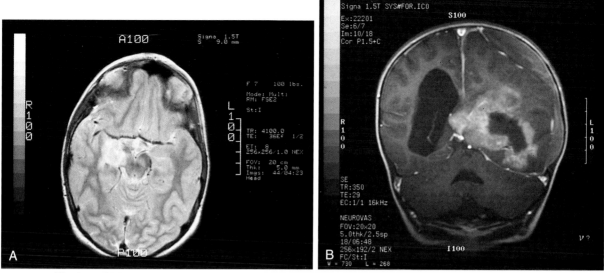

Fig. 35.1 (A) Low-grade astrocytoma. Note the regular border and minimal edema. (B) Glioblastoma multiforme. Note the invasive borders, edema, and midline shift of normal structures.

High-Grade Astrocytoma

In contrast to their low-grade counterparts, high-grade astrocytomas (anaplastic astrocytoma and glioblastoma multiforme) are highly malignant and tend to behave aggressively. They grow rapidly, invade and destroy adjacent brain tissue, and can occasionally spread through the CNS or to distant sites. High-grade gliomas are typically supratentorial and are associated with rapidly progressing neurologic symptoms including headaches, lethargy, motor or sensory loss, seizures, and altered mental status. On imaging, these lesions enhance with contrast because of their disruption of the blood-brain barrier, have irregular borders, and contain areas of necrosis and surrounding edema (Fig. 35.1B). Steroids are frequently prescribed to reduce edema and related symptoms. MRI imaging using T1 and T2/FLAIR sequences (Fig. 35.2) is important in high-grade gliomas for definition of tumor boundaries and determination of extent of edema.[36]

The management of high-grade astrocytomas requires multiple modalities, with neurosurgery being the first step. The goal of surgery is complete resection, although clear margins are difficult to achieve. Surgical resection also yields the histologic diagnosis and decompresses adjacent structures. As such, surgery often provides immediate symptomatic relief, but residual tumor (gross or microscopic) almost always remains. Because it is widely accepted that complete resection is rare in cases of high-grade gliomas, many neurosurgeons operate with the goal of a maximum safe resection compatible with a good neurologic outcome. The extent of resection is an important prognostic indicator with better outcomes for those with complete resection than for those without complete resection. Radiation therapy is routinely used after surgery, usually in combination with chemotherapy (typically temozolomide). Radiation treatment volumes for high-grade gliomas are typically large because of the infiltrating nature of these tumors. The CTV includes any gross residual tumor that remains after surgery, the surgical bed, and surrounding edema. A 3-cm margin is typically placed around the CTV because autopsy studies in adults have shown that tumor infiltrates microscopically beyond the gross tumor for up to 2 cm. A dose of 45 to 50 Gy is

typically delivered to this volume, with a "boost" delivered to a smaller volume to bring the cumulative dose to 54 to 60 Gy. Many studies have investigated dose escalation (>70 Gy), hyperfractionated treatment courses, and stem cell transplant in attempts to improve survival; however, little progress has been made, and overall prognosis remains poor.

In adult high-grade gliomas, studies have shown improved survival for those who received surgery and adjuvant radiation therapy plus temozolomide followed by temozolomide alone, which is the current standard of care. This approach is being investigated in younger patients, although the benefit and optimal sequencing of chemotherapy are still uncertain. CNS tumor research groups have shown improvement in survival rates with some combinations of chemotherapy.[5] Chemotherapy is particularly useful in infants to delay the need for radiation therapy while the brain matures, thus hopefully reducing the late effects of radiation.

Optic Glioma

Optic tract and hypothalamic gliomas are typically considered one entity and collectively account for approximately 5% of all CNS tumors in the pediatric age group.[4] These tumors tend to be low grade and behave indolently; as such, they are typically classified as grade 1 astrocytomas. Visual disturbance is the most common presenting symptom. NF is a significant risk factor, with 10% to 38% of patients having NF.[3] For asymptomatic or indolently behaving tumors, observation may be the initial strategy. Because visual and hormonal functions can be impaired with disease progression, these tumors frequently necessitate treatment. For unilateral optic nerve tumors, surgery can be considered. Primary chemotherapy may be delivered in young children in an effort to delay radiation therapy.[6,7] Indications for radiation therapy include progressive disease on chemotherapy for children younger than 10 and progressive disease at diagnosis or after surgery for older patients.[4] MRI is vital for treatment planning, as it can effectively characterize the intraorbital lesion and its intracranial extent. Tumors can be bilateral or track along the optic nerves, chiasm, and optic tracts.

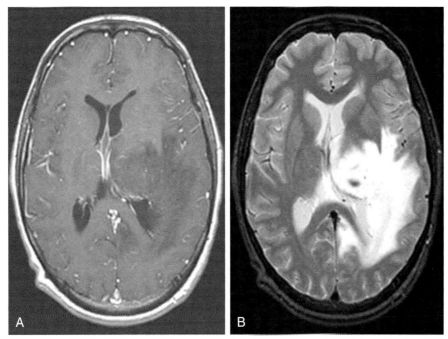

Fig. 35.2 T1 (A) and T2/FLAIR (B) magnetic resonance imaging sequences for a high-grade glioma. Note the contrast enhancing edema and midline shift on both images. (From Gunderson LL, Tepper JE. *Clinical Radiation Oncology.* 4th ed. Philadelphia, PA: Elsevier; 2016.)

Target volumes must take into account potential spread of these tumors. Doses of 45 to 50 Gy for younger children and 50 to 54 Gy for those older than 5 years are commonly delivered with 3D conformal therapy, IMRT, or proton therapy. This yields long-term survival in the 50% to 80% range, although many patients are left with significant neuroendocrine and neuropsychologic sequelae.[4] Given the indolent nature of this disease, long-term follow-up is necessary.

Ependymoma

Ependymoma is the third most common CNS tumor in children, affecting approximately 236 children (mostly younger than 4 years of age) annually in the United States. Ependymomas arise from cells that line the ventricles, and may occur anywhere within the CNS but have the highest prevalence within the posterior fossa, arising from the floor or roof of the fourth ventricle.[3] The presenting symptoms and preoperative imaging results often mimic medulloblastoma and are typically the result of increased intracranial pressure. Cerebrospinal fluid (CSF) metastatic seeding is unusual, occurring in 5% to 10% of patients, but far more likely in infratentorial and anaplastic ependymomas.[4] Because there is a risk of dissemination, evaluation of the entire brain and spinal canal is necessary. Although debate exists about the clinical significance of histologic grade of ependymomas, a correlation does seem to exist between higher grade and poorer outcome.[8] The standard of care for a child with localized ependymoma is gross total resection and postoperative radiation therapy. The extent of surgical resection is the most important prognostic factor.[4] The radiation therapy treatment volume includes the surgical bed and any gross residual tumor, as defined by MRI, with a 1-cm CTV margin. The recommended total dose is 59.4 Gy using conventional fractionation.[3] With contemporary surgery and radiation therapy, event-free survival at 3 years is approximately 75%.[3] If CSF seeding is noted, then **craniospinal irradiation** (CSI) with techniques similar to those used for medulloblastoma is needed.

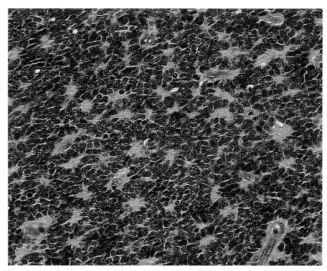

Fig. 35.3 Histologic appearance of medulloblastoma revealing pseudorosette consisting of tumor cells that form a pattern with radial arrangement of cells like that of rose petals (From Phillips J, Tihan T, Fuller G. Practical molecular pathology and histopathology of embryonal tumors. *Surgical Pathology Clinics* 8(1):73–88, 2015.)

Chemotherapy has been used adjuvantly or even before surgery, especially for the youngest patients, or to improve resectability, but the value has yet to be established.

Medulloblastoma

Medulloblastoma is the prototype posterior fossa malignancy and constitutes about 20% of all childhood brain tumors. Medulloblastoma is a type of PNET believed to arise from cerebellar stem cells. The histologic appearance is a classic "small, round blue cell" tumor that forms pseudorosettes.[9] Fig. 35.3 illustrates the microscopic appearance of this histology.

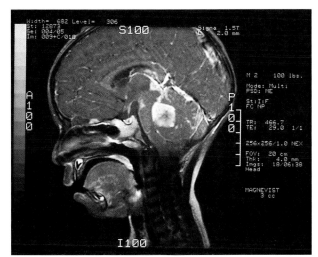

Fig. 35.4 Magnetic resonance imaging scan of medulloblastoma. Pressure on the brainstem and cerebrospinal fluid (CSF) obstruction are evident. Diffuse CFS seeding can be present.

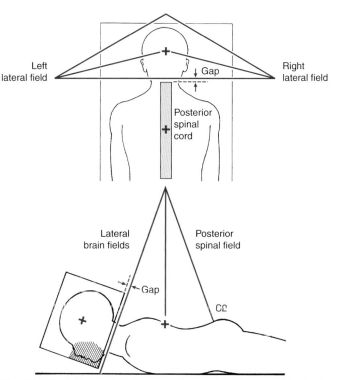

Fig. 35.5 Radiation portal alignment for medulloblastoma. The brain portal collimator angle is adjusted for spinal field divergence. The junction gap is moved 1 cm daily or weekly.

The tumor usually arises in the midline of the cerebellum (cerebellar vermis) and projects into the fourth ventricle and brainstem. These tumors have an inherent tendency to metastasize via cerebrospinal pathways, and approximately 30% to 35% of patients present with CSF seeding.[4] Among the varying histologies of medulloblastoma, anaplastic medulloblastoma has the greatest propensity for dissemination through the CSF.[3]

The presenting symptoms of medulloblastoma usually occur over a period of weeks to a few months. Several symptoms can develop as a result of the invasion and compression of the fourth ventricle, which may stop or decrease the inferior flow of CSF with resultant hydrocephalus. Headaches and early-morning vomiting can occur. Other symptoms include ataxia and cranial nerve abnormalities from invasion of the brainstem. CT and MRI imaging usually show a round, central cerebellar, enhancing mass (Fig. 35.4), and hydrocephalus is often noted. Steroids and a ventriculostomy can be used to reduce pressure in the acute situation. Because of the propensity for CSF seeding, imaging the entire CNS via MRI is critical, and a lumbar puncture is often done to look for tumor cells in the CSF.

Chang, Housepian, and Herbert[10] initially developed a staging system at Columbia University that related to tumor size, invasion of the fourth ventricle and brainstem, and amount of CSF spread. With the known importance of surgical debulking, therapy is now based on residual tumor of greater than 1.5 cm^2 and the extent of CSF or gross neuroaxis **metastases**. Medulloblastoma is one CNS tumor that can develop extracranial metastases, usually in bone. The intense, technical multidisciplinary therapy necessary for medulloblastomas must be performed in a center with pediatric cancer expertise.

Maximal tumor resection is vital to good outcomes. Gross total resection and residual tumor less than 1.5 cm^2 result in superior outcomes to lesser resection. A posterior occipital craniotomy is used. The often purple, friable, bulging tumor is usually quickly evident. Although the central mass is removed easily, the tumor can infiltrate into the brainstem or laterally into the cerebellar peduncles. Despite the importance of resection, surgery alone is rarely curative, and maximal resection can lead to a higher risk of complications, such as posterior fossa syndrome. Routine use of ventriculoperitoneal shunts is discouraged because of the risk of tumor seeding into the peritoneal cavity and a higher complication rate.

CSI is required adjuvantly because the entire subarachnoid space is at risk for disease dissemination. The benefit of postoperative radiation therapy was documented by Patterson and Farr[11] as early as 1953 and became part of the standard of care. CSI is technically challenging, and several methods may be used, depending on the institution.

The most common technique uses lateral-opposed fields for the brain and intracranial CSF spaces from the posterior orbits down through the upper cervical spine. Careful shielding must be designed for the anterior globe, pharynx, and neck. The treatment couch is angled a few degrees to compensate for divergence of the beam inferiorly into the spinal cord. The collimator is angled on the brain fields to match the divergence of the superior margin of the posteroanterior spinal radiation field. Depending on the height of the child, one or two posterior fields are used to encompass the spine down to the level of the S2/S3, where the thecal sac terminates on MRI. The lower spine field widens to cover the sacral nerve roots. This technique is illustrated in Fig. 35.5. Some centers have used electrons or protons in treatment of the spinal CSF space to avoid radiation exposure to healthy tissues anterior to the spine. However, this requires precise physics and extensive tissue compensators and is not available at most centers. Often 6 MV x-rays are commonly used for each field. Customarily, a gap is used between the spinal fields and the lateral brain fields to account for beam divergence. Usually, the junction between the brain and superior spine field and the junction between the superior and inferior spine fields (in taller children) are moved superiorly and inferiorly 0.5 to 1 cm daily or weekly (a term called *feathering the gap*). This technique prevents excessive dose gradients at the match lines and eliminates the potential for a spinal cord overdose or a low-dose area that can allow tumor cells to survive. Optimally, these children should be immobilized in a prone position, unless doing so is deemed unsafe, with the chin extended to avoid dose from the posterior/anterior (PA) spine field from exiting the oral cavity. Some centers use a similar CSI technique with the patient in the supine position. Custom head holders, body cradles, or a rigid commercial vacuum bag system are helpful. Because of the critical importance of field junctions, reproducible positioning of the head and careful marking of treatment portal edges are paramount. If sedation is needed, the anesthesia staff members may need some modifications of the previous technique to ensure airway safety and the accomodation of monitoring equipment monitoring equipment.

CSI is typically prescribed at 150 to 180 cGy/day. Antiemetics are often needed because the gastrointestinal tract receives significant dose from the exiting spine fields. Because of late sequelae, an attempt has been made to reduce the CSI dose or use chemotherapy as a substitute. Some now prescribe 2340 cGy CSI, with higher doses if CSF metastases are seen.[12] Chemotherapy is used during and after radiation. Because the most frequent site of recurrence is the posterior fossa, that region is boosted with 3D or IMRT fields after CSI. Some studies have treated only the decompressed tumor bed with a 1.5-cm margin rather than the entire posterior fossa. State-of-the-art treatment planning and delivery can avoid excessive doses to the cochlea and ear canals, improving long-term hearing. The daily fraction is usually 180 cGy/day up to a total of 5400 cGy.[12] For average-risk patients, a combined approach of 2340 cGy to the CSI and 5400 cGy to the posterior fossa, followed by chemotherapy, has resulted in 5-year survival of 80% or better.[13]However, a dose of 36 Gy to the CSI is required for high-risk patients.[3]

The entire radiation treatment course for medulloblastoma is 6 to 7 weeks, excluding any potential treatment breaks that may occur as a result of surgical complications, low blood counts and infection, or gastrointestinal toxicity. Despite the rigors of treatment, the addition of radiation and chemotherapy has increased survival rates to more than 80%.[14]

Brainstem Glioma

Brainstem gliomas represent approximately 10% of all pediatric CNS tumors and are a particularly devastating disease, with more than 90% of patients dying within 2 years of diagnosis.[15] Because the brainstem serves as a conduit from the brain to the cranial nerves, lesions of the area commonly cause cranial nerve deficits that affect vision, facial function, and swallowing. These cranial nerve defects may develop over the course of weeks to months. Most of these lesions are diffuse and located in the pons, yielding a diagnosis of diffuse infiltrating pontine glioma (DIPG). Because they are diffuse in nature and located in an elegant area of the brain, these lesions are entirely unresectable. These tumors have a characteristic appearance on MRI and do not typically necessitate a biopsy. However, if biopsied, most of these diffuse tumors are found to be high-grade astrocytomas.

The mainstay of treatment is radiation therapy. The radiation therapy volume should cover the entire MRI abnormality with an additional 1-cm to 2-cm margin. Doses of 180 cGy/fraction are delivered with 3D conformal radiation therapy (CRT) or IMRT to a total dose of about 5400 cGy. Historically, survival is poor, and DIPG is considered uniformly fatal despite excellent initial response to radiation therapy and corticosteroids.[3] The use of hyperfractionated radiation therapy, dose escalation, and the addition of concurrent chemotherapy have not yielded much improvement. Local progression and worsening neurologic function typically occur within a few months and necessitate prolonged supportive care.

Rarely, the brainstem glioma is an exophytic lesion that extends from the posterior aspect of the brainstem. These lesions tend to have a low-grade histology and are amenable to surgical resection by select pediatric neurosurgeons.

Brain tumors are the most common solid tumor in children and adolescents. They are often treated with surgery and adjuvant radiation therapy. Each type and location of brain tumor necessitates individualized multidisciplinary treatment. Three-dimensional treatment planning and delivery or intensity-modulated radiation therapy (IMRT) are used to spare healthy tissues and reduce late effects, which are more severe the younger the patient's age when irradiated. Craniospinal radiation is among the most technically challenging and high-risk procedures for therapists, and careful attention must be given to field matching. More information is available via the Children's Oncology Group and Childhood Brain Tumor Foundation (www.cbtf.org).

Central Nervous System Germ Cell Tumors

CNS germ cell tumors develop from embryologic nests of tissue in the midline brain, usually in the suprasellar or pineal region. Before neurosurgical biopsy became safe, empiric treatment of the tumor mass with radiation was common. In most instances, a biopsy can now be performed to guide the treatment. Germinoma is the most common histology and is quite radiosensitive. It can be treated with low-dose CSI followed by a primary tumor boost to 5000 cGy, or with cisplatin-based chemotherapy, followed by local field irradiation.[16] In non-CSI cases, whole ventricular radiation to the primary mass and the supratentorial CSF ventricle spaces to a dose of 3000 to 4500 cGy, depending on the response to chemotherapy, may be used.[17] Nongerminomatous germ cell tumors often require chemotherapy, CSI, and primary tumor boost.

Benign Tumors of the Central Nervous System

Pituitary adenomas usually occur in adolescents and adults but can also be seen in young children. These patients can have excessive hormone production, visual disturbance from pressure on the optic chiasm, or diabetes insipidus (DI). Transsphenoidal hypophysectomy or medical management to counteract hormone production usually supplants radiation in the treatment of children. Localized radiation therapy with multiple fields with a dose of 4500 to 5040 cGy or stereotactic radiation therapy can be given to control these tumors (see Chapter 27).

Craniopharyngiomas arise from embryologic remnants of pharyngeal pouch tissues. These tumors eventually enlarge (usually with a prominent cystic component) and disrupt the hypothalamic pituitary axis (which may cause DI or precocious puberty), impair vision, or induce seizures. Surgery and radiation therapy can be effective, with the goal of reducing visual or late side effects. Today, these tumors are usually treated with 3D CRT or IMRT with narrow margins from 5000 to 5400 cGy. Because panhypopituitarism almost always develops, a pediatric endocrinologist must be included on the management team for these patients.

Meningiomas and acoustic neuromas are histologically benign lesions that occur far more often in patients who have NF. These lesions are treated with observation, or surgery if they progress and cause neurologic symptoms. Radiation may be necessary for unresectable lesions. Arteriovenous malformations (AVMs) in less surgically accessible locations can be treated with stereotactic radiosurgery. Usually 1500 to 2000 cGy is delivered in a single fraction, with control of potentially deadly rebleeding in 80% of patients.[18] Doses and control rates depend on the size of the AVM.

Late Effects of Treatment

The treatment of large areas of the brain and spinal cord in pediatric patients can have a variety of devastating late sequelae. Because survival rates for children with CNS tumors were so poor for many decades, only now, as survival outcomes are improving, are these late effects being adequately addressed. The late effects of radiation are typically worse the younger the child's age at the time of treatment, and as such, every effort should be made to delay radiation in very young children when possible.

Radiation therapy is known to affect the microvasculature of the brain, as well as the cells that produce myelin, which disrupts neurogenesis and causes cortical atrophy. Because of this, patients may fail to acquire new knowledge and skills at an age-appropriate rate and show a progressive decline in IQ over time. The magnitude of the deficit depends mostly on age at treatment; however, neurocognitive effects are also correlated with tumor location, dose, volume irradiated, and other treatment factors.[4] In addition to the aforementioned cognitive effects, the development of behavioral difficulties may also occur. The end result for many patients is impaired school and social performance that deteriorates over time.[4] Endocrine deficits, particularly growth hormone deficiency, are common and correlate with the dose of radiation to the hypothalamic-pituitary axis.[4] Patients may also find the acute hair loss to be psychologically traumatic, especially when the high doses of radiation used results in permanent hair loss. In pediatric radiation therapy, it is important to consider the issue of secondary malignancies; overall risk is approximately 5% to 10% over 3 decades of follow-up.[3]

CSI can decrease the height of vertebral bodies and lead to a short-waisted adult. Secondary malignancies may develop many years later in the CNS, bones and soft tissues, or bone marrow as a result of radiation and chemotherapy.[19]

Because of the toxicities mentioned above, the following strategies may be used to avoid or minimize the long-term effects of treatment for pediatric brain tumors[4]:

- Avoidance of radiation therapy altogether (for low-grade astrocytomas for whom surgery alone may be a good option)
- Delay of radiation therapy using chemotherapy
- Daily use of anesthesia and rigid immobilization to allow reduced margins
- Use of CT/MRI for better treatment planning and delivery
- Use of new radiation modalities (proton therapy)
- Reduced target volumes
- Reduction of cumulative dose
- Use of smaller fraction sizes where appropriate

In addition to the radiation-induced toxicities mentioned, the post-surgical deficits of motor sensory loss, poor coordination, or cranial nerve dysfunction can last a lifetime. For all patients, careful follow-up and early intervention, both medically and educationally, are required and can lessen many of the late effects. Although parents may be frightened, the risks for late effects must be discussed when informed consent for a child's radiation treatment is obtained. Despite these risks, parents are almost always ecstatic that even an impaired child has survived a life-threatening brain tumor.

RETINOBLASTOMA

Epidemiology

Retinoblastoma is a PNET that develops in the retina, which is the specialized light-sensitive tissue at the back of the eye that detects light and color. Although retinoblastoma is the most common intraocular tumor in young children, only about 300 cases are diagnosed annually in the United States.[20] Retinoblastoma is a disease of the very young; two-thirds of all cases are diagnosed before 2 years of age, and 95% of cases are diagnosed before 5 years of age.[3] A well-documented hereditary pattern exists, with 25% to 35% of patients presenting with a germline mutation. The retinoblastoma gene (*RB1*) is a well-studied tumor suppressor gene located on chromosome 13 that inhibits cell cycle progression past the G1-S restriction point.[21,22] When mutated, the *RB1* gene fails to make functional proteins, and cells are unable to regulate cell division. Retinoblastoma is a recessive genetic defect (13q-14 deletion); as such, both alleles of the *RB1* gene must be mutated for the disease to occur. Individuals who inherit one defective copy of the gene are more likely to develop retinoblastoma, as a defect in the other copy of the gene may be acquired over time. Patients with an inherited defect in one copy of the gene account for most cases of bilateral retinoblastoma and have a significant risk of developing other types of tumors. However, at least 65% of retinoblastomas are unilateral and without evidence of inheritance.[23]

Diagnosis and Staging

Retinoblastoma is often discovered as a result of an abnormal retinal light reflex (visible white pupil rather than red) called leukocoria or

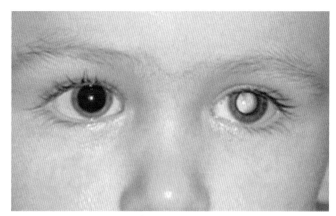

Fig. 35.6 Leukocoria in the left eye, which may indicate retinoblastoma. (Republished with permission of McGraw-Hill Education from Richard P. Ustine, Mindy Ann Smith, Heidi S. Chumley, Camille Sabella, E.J. Mayeaux Jr., Elumalai Appach: The Color Atlas of Pediatrics.)

BOX 35.1 Staging System for Retinoblastoma

Group A
Small tumors (no more than 3 millimeters [mm] across) that are only in the retina and are not near important structures.

Group B
All other tumors (either larger than 3 mm or close to the optic disc or foveola) that are still only in the retina.

Group C
Well-defined tumors with small amounts of spread under the retina or into the vitreous humor.

Group D
Large or poorly defined tumors with widespread vitreous or subretinal seeding.

Group E
The tumor is very large, extends near the front of the eye, is bleeding or causing glaucoma.

Modified from the American Cancer Society. https://www.cancer.org/cancer/retinoblastoma/detection-diagnosis-staging/staging.html Accessed November 6, 2019.

"cat's eye reflex" see Fig. 35.6, which may be noted on a flash photograph or during the pediatrician's routine examination.

An ophthalmologist should examine both eyes thoroughly to document multifocality or bilaterality. Biopsy is typically contraindicated because of the risk of vitreous seeding. Ultrasound scan can be useful to show location and size of tumors. CT scan of the brain and orbit can detect unusual cases with extraocular extension or simultaneous supratentorial-pineal lesions (trilateral retinoblastoma). For evaluation of advanced cases, the CSF may be assessed with lumbar puncture cytology, and a bone marrow biopsy may be indicated. Clinical staging systems have been developed to suggest preferred treatments and predict success rates. The initial system was developed by Reese[24] and correlated tumor size and location with visual preservation. A newer system based on the size of the tumor and spread under or beyond the retina or into the vitreous humor is currently used (Box 35.1).[3]

Treatment Techniques

As mentioned previously, the pediatric ophthalmologist must detail the extent of local disease. With small focal tumors away from the optic disc and macula, photocoagulation, laser hyperthermia, or cryosurgery may result in disease control. Local therapies are used more commonly in conjunction with chemotherapy. In cases with blindness from extensive but unilateral retinoblastoma not involving the optic nerve, enucleation provides excellent control.

External beam radiation has classically been used in cases of bilateral or inoperable unilateral disease. If both eyes are involved, both can be treated with organ-sparing intent, and treatment may preserve vision. It is a technical challenge with external beam therapy to treat the entire retina, which extends anterior to the lateral bony canthus, and still spare the cornea and lens. Modern treatment methods include: (1) a suction cup to displace the anterior globe (pioneered in Europe); (2) 3D/IMRT conformal planning and delivery, especially when tumor is beyond the globe; and (3) conformal proton therapy.

Daily general anesthesia is required, with specialized dosimetry verifying doses in such small-shaped radiation portals. The usual dose is 180 to 200 cGy daily to 4000 to 5000 cGy. Several series report local control and visual preservation ranging from 50% to 100%, depending on the stage.[20,24,25]

If the tumor masses are less extensive, radiation implant plaques can be used. Iodine-125 is the most widely used radionuclide. Doses of 3000 to 4000 cGy over 1 week are delivered, with a cure rate of more than 80% and visual preservation in most patients.[20,26] Implants reduce radiation exposure to bones, contralateral globe, and anterior structures, with a resultant decrease in long-term side effects.

Because retinoblastoma is a small blue cell tumor of neuroectodermal origin, a good response to chemotherapeutic agents is expected. Vincristine, cyclophosphamide, and the platinols have shown good response rates when extraocular or disseminated disease is present. Subsequent trials have involved neoadjuvant chemotherapy with hope of avoiding external radiation therapy or enucleation. This has been successful in 40% to 90% of early-stage cases.[27,28]

Late Effects of Treatment

Long-term sequelae of retinoblastoma therapies include altered growth of the bony orbit, decreased vision, cataract formation, dry eye, and a high risk of a **secondary malignancy** (a new cancer that develops years after treatment of the initial tumor, likely caused by the treatment itself). If enucleation is chosen, the child needs several prosthetic eyes as growth occurs. Because external radiation uses doses of 4000 cGy or more and occurs in children who are young, facial growth likely is impaired. As adults, these patients have small orbits and are narrow between the temples. Cured tumors can leave blind spots, radiation retinitis, dry eyes from decreased lacrimal gland function, and cataracts. However, overall survival rates are high, and visual acuity is often preserved.

NEUROBLASTOMA

Epidemiology

Neuroblastoma is another small, round blue cell tumor derived from cells of neural crest origin. These cells migrate embryologically to form paravertebral sympathetic ganglia, the adrenal medulla, and peripheral nerves. Neuroblastoma-like cells can occur in fetal adrenal glands and are found in approximately 1% of infant autopsies.[29] Interestingly, most of these lesions spontaneously regress, as only about 650 cases of neuroblastoma are diagnosed each year. Neuroblastoma is the most common extracranial solid tumor and the third most common overall. Patients range from newborns to children several years old, with a median age of younger than 17 months.[30]

Like the normal adrenal tissue, neuroblastoma cells can secrete catecholamines including epinephrine, norepinephrine, dopamine, and other substances including vanillylmandelic acid and homovanillic acid, which can be detected in the urine. Some investigators have advocated screening

TABLE 35.4 Key Differences Between Wilms Tumor and Neuroblastoma		
Variable	**Wilms Tumor**	**Neuroblastoma**
Age	Older (3–4 years old)	Younger (<18 months)
Systemic Symptoms	No	Yes
Calcifications	No	Yes
Location	Kidney	Adrenal gland
Crosses midline?	Not typical	May cross
Fixed/immobile?	May be displaced	Fixed/immobile

for neuroblastoma with these urine markers, but screening studies have not shown any impact on survival. Molecular genetic studies have shown loss on the short arm of chromosome 1 in up to 35% of patients and on 11q. Partial gains on chromosome 17q are seen in about 50% of these cases.[31] Surprisingly, neuroblastomas with an excessive or hyperdiploid number of chromosomes yield a better prognosis. N-*myc* is an **oncogene** (a gene that regulates the development and growth of cancer cells) commonly associated with neuroblastoma. This gene is located on the short arm of chromosome 2 and is a promoter of growth. When excessive copies of this gene are present (n-*myc* amplified tumors), aggressive growth and poor survival are typical.[32]

Diagnosis and Staging

Most neuroblastomas occur in the abdomen, typically near the midline with the origin in the adrenal gland (35%) or paraspinal ganglia (32%). Invasion of the spinal canal in a dumbbell fashion from a paravertebral neuroblastoma can cause symptoms of neurologic compromise or even spinal cord compression. Symptoms can include flushing and diarrhea (in response to the vasoactive vanillylmandelic acid and homovanillic acid), abdominal mass, bowel disturbance, and failure to thrive. In infants, a large abdominal mass, liver metastases, or disease in the chest can cause respiratory compromise and necessitate emergency intervention.

Unfortunately, approximately 60% of patients present with metastatic disease. Symptoms of metastatic disease are varied and include fatigue, anemia and bleeding from bone marrow invasion, fever, weight loss, painful bony metastases, blue skin lesions (blueberry muffin sign), and abdominal distention from liver involvement. The most common site of metastatic disease is the bone (50%). Because most neuroblastomas occur in the abdomen, it is important to rule out **Wilms tumor** (childhood embryonal kidney cancer) during workup. In general, patients with neuroblastoma are younger and look sicker than those with a corresponding-sized Wilms tumor. Other key differences can be found in Table 35.4.

The workup for neuroblastoma includes blood work, urine catecholamines, CT of the chest, abdomen, and pelvis, primary tumor biopsy, bone marrow biopsy, echocardiogram (ECG) and multigated acquisition scan, bone scan, and MIBG scintiscan. Abdominal ultrasound and MRI imaging of the primary disease and spine (for paravertebral masses) are increasingly used. Radiographs and CT scans typically reveal calcifications in the mass, which is a classic feature of neuroblastoma. The lungs and liver must be assessed for metastases.

Staging systems have historically evolved based on radiographic and surgical findings. Initially, Evans[33] developed the first prognostic staging system; however, the International Neuroblastoma Staging System (INSS) is now the standard.[3] This system is summarized in Box 35.2. As with other cancers, this staging system relates to prognosis and guides treatment. Neuroblastoma may also be staged using the International Neuroblastoma Risk Group Staging System, which stages disease based on imaging alone.

The INSS designates a special stage, 4S, to infants younger than 1 year old with cancer on one side of the body.[2] This stage is worth noting, as many of these patients have spontaneous regression, and

BOX 35.2   International Staging System for Neuroblastoma

Stage 1: Localized tumor confined to area of origin; complete gross excision, with or without microscopic residual disease; identifiable ipsilateral and contralateral lymph nodes negative microscopically.

   Stage 2A: Unilateral tumor with incomplete gross excision; identifiable ipsilateral and contralateral lymph nodes negative microscopically.

   Stage 2B: Unilateral tumor with complete or incomplete gross excision; with positive ipsilateral regional lymph nodes; identifiable contralateral lymph nodes negative microscopically.

   Stage 3: Tumor infiltrating across the midline with or without regional lymph node involvement; unilateral tumor with contralateral regional lymph node involvement; or midline tumor with bilateral regional lymph node involvement.

   Stage 4: Dissemination of tumor to distant lymph nodes, bone, bone marrow, liver, or other organs (except as defined in stage 4S).

   Stage 4S: Localized primary tumor as defined for stage 1 or 2, with dissemination limited to liver and skin.

Modified from Brodeur GM, Seeger RC, Barrett A, et al. International criteria for diagnosis, staging and response to treatment with neuroblastoma. *J Clin Oncol.* 1988;6:1874–1881.

BOX 35.3   Survival by Children's Oncology Group Risk Group[4] for Neuroblastoma

Low-Risk Group: Children in the low-risk group have a 5-year survival rate that is higher than 95%.

Intermediate-Risk Group: In children in the intermediate-risk group, the 5-year survival rate is around 90% to 95%.

High-Risk Group: The 5-year survival rate in children in the high-risk group is around 40% to 50%.

the cancerous elements turn benign if acute situations can be managed.[34] The age at the time of presentation and risk group are extremely important prognostic indicators. Increasingly, histologic subtypes and molecular genetic markers (especially n-*myc* amplification) are used to predict clinical behavior and direct the aggressiveness of therapy.

Treatment Techniques

The treatment strategy for neuroblastoma is based on risk stratification that considers n-*myc* status, DNA diploidy, age, loss of heterozygosity (LOH), and tumor stage and grade (Box 35.3).[35] Low-risk patients (rare) receive surgery and observation or chemotherapy, depending on the extent of resection. Intermediate-risk patients (rare) with resectable disease receive surgery, chemotherapy, and radiation therapy. Intermediate-risk patients with unresectable disease receive induction chemotherapy followed by surgery. Unfortunately, most patients present with high-risk disease and require aggressive treatment, which includes induction chemotherapy followed by surgical resection, myeloablative chemotherapy, stem cell transplant, radiation therapy, and immunotherapy. In most patients with resection, multiagent chemotherapy has replaced radiation therapy, although radiation maybe used after surgery and chemotherapy to areas of residual disease. Aggressive chemotherapy regimens involving platinum compounds, vincristine, doxorubicin (Adriamycin), etoposide, and cyclophosphamide are frequently indicated.

   Although the behavior of neuroblastoma remains an enigma to most pediatric oncologists, the 5-year overall survival has improved from 25% to 60% since the early 1990s, which reflects a greater understanding of the disease and better chemotherapeutic agents.[36] Unfortunately, patients with advanced disease at presentation are rarely cured.

Radiation therapists may palliatively treat patients who have progressive metastatic disease. Low doses of 1000 cGy may achieve pain relief or regression of soft tissue masses, which are important for short-term quality of life to terminally ill patients and their families.

Late Effects of Treatment

Because patients with neuroblastoma are often infants, the late effects of radiation can be significant. In the acute situation with a newborn, doses of only 500 cGy may be effective with almost no long-term side effects; however, in older patients receiving more than 2000 cGy, the bones and soft tissues of the treated region may have decreased development or asymmetric growth. Radiation exposure to the kidney and liver should be minimized to prevent impaired function. Lung fibrosis can occur with thoracic radiation. The intense doses of multiagent chemotherapy and stem cell transplants used for high-risk neuroblastoma can adversely affect many organ systems. A recent study of long-term survivors of high-risk neuroblastoma shows that the majority have late complications including hearing loss, hypothyroidism, ovarian failure, musculoskeletal abnormalities, and pulmonary dysfunction. However, most complications were considered to be mild to moderate in severity.[37] Although late second malignancies are always a risk after radiation and chemotherapy, the oncogene associated with neuroblastoma does not increase the risk to survivors.

WILMS TUMOR

Epidemiology

Wilms tumor, or nephroblastoma, is a malignant tumor of the kidney that arises from embryonal cells. About 500 cases occur annually in the United States. Most cases of Wilms tumor are solitary lesions, although 6% involve both kidneys and 12% show multifocal involvement within a single kidney.[3] The median age at presentation is 3 to 4 years, and 75% of cases occur by age 5 years. Although the cause of Wilms tumor is unknown, it may arise in the setting of specific genetic disorders. Syndromes associated with a higher risk for developing Wilms tumor include: WAGR syndrome (Wilms, aniridia, genitourinary [GU] malformations, and mental retardation), Beckwith-Wiedemann syndrome, and Denys-Drash syndrome. A genetic abnormality, LOH on chromosomes 1p and 16q, has been described and is associated with poorer outcomes for Wilms.[38] Wilms tumors can contain renal tubular, glomerular, and connective tissue elements. Ten percent to 15% of cases show unfavorable histology. This includes anaplastic Wilms tumor, clear cell sarcoma of the kidney, and rhabdoid tumor of the kidney. These unfavorable histology tumors have lesser cure rates than favorable histology Wilms tumors. Clear cell tumors have a high rate of bone metastases, and rhabdoid tumors are associated with CNS neoplasms.[39]

Multimodal therapy, which includes surgery, radiation therapy, and chemotherapy, is the foundation of modern cancer treatment for many childhood malignancies and has led to dramatic improvements in survival. How the three disciplines coalesced to conquer Wilms tumor is a compelling story that includes two of history's greatest discoveries, x-rays and antibiotics. For more on this intriguing story, go to https://www.ncbi.nlm.nih.gov/pubmed/27305878.

Diagnosis and Staging

Presenting symptoms can include abdominal pain (37%), hypertension because of increased renin production (25%), hematuria, and fever. Wilms tumor typically presents as a painless abdominal mass, which may be noted by the parents bathing or changing the child or by a physician during a routine checkup. Disease tends to grow rapidly,

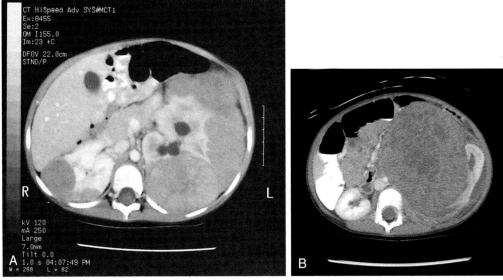

Fig. 35.7 Wilms tumor. (A) Preoperative computed tomographic (CT) scan of a bilateral Wilms tumor in a 3-year-old girl. (B) CT scan of a large left flank mass occupying a large portion of the abdomen.

and symptoms often reflect the pressure put on abdominal organs as a result of the enlarging tumor. Wilms tumors are soft and friable and have a tendency to rupture. Unlike patients with neuroblastoma, children with Wilms tumor do not often appear severely ill despite the large tumor. A differential diagnosis includes neuroblastomas, lymphomas, sarcomas, and liver tumors.

After the physical examination, an abdominal ultrasound scan is usually the first step in a diagnosis. A CT scan of the chest, abdomen, and pelvis is then typically done to assess the extent of disease and evaluate lymph nodes and lungs. It is important to acquire lung images because the lungs are the primary site of metastatic disease. Wilms tumor can be bilateral, therefore the contralateral kidney must be carefully examined (Fig. 35.7). Tumor can invade into or metastasize to the liver and can involve the inferior vena cava. Because these tumors have a high likelihood of rupture, biopsy is typically contraindicated. If a biopsy is performed, the tumor should be accessed through the retroperitoneum and not through the abdomen. Wilms tumor is classified as favorable (90%) or unfavorable/anaplastic (10%), based on histology. Unfavorable histologies include focal anaplasia, diffuse anaplasia, rhabdoid sarcoma, and clear cell sarcoma. These subtypes are associated with more aggressive behavior and frequent metastasis to the brain and bone and require additional imaging such as bone scans and cranial CT scans.

The staging system for Wilms Tumor was originally developed by the National Wilms Tumor Study Group (NWTS) and focused on tumor size, tumor spill or postoperative residua, extent of resection, and metastases. This system is currently used by the COG (cancer.org) (Table 35.5).

Treatment Techniques

In the United States, the removal of the malignant kidney via nephrectomy is nearly always the first step. During surgery, regional lymph nodes are biopsied, and the contralateral kidney is examined for bilaterality. Because of the risk of tumor rupture and spillage into the abdominal cavity, surgery should be performed by a highly qualified pediatric surgeon. Tumors that are judged to be unresectable or pose too great a surgical risk are treated with preoperative chemotherapy, which results in the reduction of the tumor mass and generally renders it resectable.[3] In the first SIOP (International Society of Pediatric

TABLE 35.5	Staging System for Wilms Tumor	
Stage	Percentage	Description
I	40	Tumor limited to the kidney and completely resected
II	20	Tumor beyond kidney but completely resected
III	20	Residual nonhematogenous tumor confined to abdomen. Involved lymph nodes, diffuse tumor spillage, or grossly unresected tumor
IV	10	Hematogenous metastases beyond the abdomen/pelvis (usually lung, liver, bone, or brain)
V	4–8	Bilateral disease at time of diagnosis (stage each site independently)

Oncology) cooperative study, preoperative chemotherapy and subsequent resection reduced intraoperative tumor spill from 32% to 4%.[40] This was verified in SIOP 93-01 when more than 400 patients had an average 60% reduction in tumor size after preoperative chemotherapy.[41] In patients with bilateral disease, a partial resection can be done on the minimally affected side.

Because surgery alone led to cure rates of less than 30% many years ago, Wilms tumor is typically managed using a trimodality approach (surgery, radiation, and chemotherapy), which has greatly increased survival rates. Radiation has been used in the management of Wilms tumor since the 1940s and continues to play an important role, although current clinical trials aim to reduce the indications for radiation therapy. Classically, radiation fields covered the entire tumor bed. If tumor spill occurred, the whole abdomen was treated. Doses higher than 3000 cGy were successful but resulted in significant late effects.[42] Over the years, successive NWTS trials have resulted in refined recommendations. Today, resectable and unilateral (stage I–IV) disease is managed with surgery and adjuvant chemotherapy. Radiation therapy may be indicated in patients with stage III favorable disease and those with unfavorable histology. Unresectable or bilateral (stage V) disease is treated with neoadjuvant chemotherapy followed by surgery and chemoradiation.

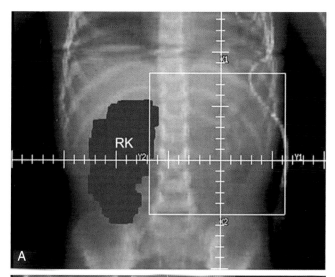

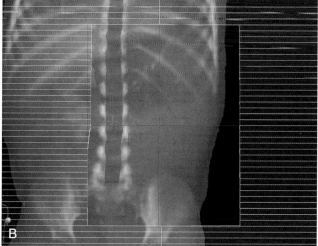

Fig. 35.8 Diagrams of a typical radiation therapy flank field for Wilms tumor treatment. (A) A digitally reconstructed radiograph of the field. (B) A treatment-planning beam's-eye view of the treatment field.

Data from NWTS 3 indicated no significant difference in local control between 1080 and 2000 cGy[43,44]; therefore, a dose of 1080 cGy is used for microscopic residual disease, lymph node metastases, bilateral disease, and pulmonary metastases. All cases of unfavorable histology are treated as high-stage lesions and uniformly irradiated. Known areas of gross residual disease are usually boosted to at least 2000 cGy. In cases that require radiation, radiation therapy should be initiated 9 to 14 days after surgery, as a greater delay is associated with poorer outcomes.

When designing radiation portals, it is important to use preoperative imaging and the surgeon's intraoperative findings. If disease is unilateral, the portal should include the entire width of the vertebral body plus 1 cm contralaterally to ensure both coverage of the paraaortic nodes and homogeneous irradiation of the vertebral bodies to reduce the risk of scoliosis. At the low dose of 1080 cGy, which is the current recommendation, the risk of bony or visceral toxicity (including the remaining kidney) is minimal. Still, it is important to consider minimizing dose to the growth plates of long bones. Fig. 35.8 diagrams a typical radiation therapy flank field for Wilms tumor treatment. The superior and inferior field borders are placed about 1 cm from the preoperative renal tumor volume. The medial border should include the entire width of the thoracic and lumbar vertebral bodies to include lymph nodes and avoid scoliosis (a long-term side effect).[44,45]

Chemotherapy is also an important component of the treatment strategy. Farber[46] first reported the encouraging survival improvement

TABLE 35.6 Long-Term Survival Rates of NWTS-3 and NWTS-4 Patients

Stage	No. of Patients	10-Years Relapse-Free (%)	10-Years Overall Rate (%)
I FH	1582	91	97
II FH	1006	86	93
III FH	1038	84	90
IV FH	592	75	81
V FH	344	65	78
All FH	4562	84	91

FH, Favorable histology; *NWTS,* National Wilms Tumor Study Group protocol study.
Modified from Kalapurakal JA, Dome JS. Wilms' tumor. In: Gunderson LL, Tepper JE, eds. *Clinical Radiation Oncology.* 3rd ed. Philadelphia, PA: Elsevier; 2012.; and from Breslow NE, Ou SS, Beckwith JB, et al. Doxorubicin for favorable histology, stage II–III Wilms tumor: results from the National Wilms Tumor Studies, *Cancer* 2004;101:1072–1080.

associated with Wilms tumor with use of actinomycin-D in 1966. The addition of vincristine and doxorubicin for advanced stages led to cure rates of 80% to 100% in later NWTS studies.

Long-term survival rates for Wilms tumor are excellent; about 85% to 90% of patients with favorable histology can be cured. Even patients with metastatic disease can be cured more than 70% of the time (see Table 35.6).[43,44] Outcomes for patients with unfavorable histology are lower. Because it is challenging to salvage a failure, increased importance is placed on the initial course of treatment. Patients with late pulmonary metastases can often be managed with chemotherapy, lung irradiation, and lung resections. With the high overall cure rates, the present aim of studies is to reduce late toxicity and find more successful multidisciplinary combinations for patients who have advanced disease and unfavorable histology.

Late Effects of Treatment

Historically, when doses of 3000 to 4000 cGy of orthovoltage radiation were used, atrophy of soft tissues on the treated side and scoliosis were common. With technique and dose modification, such late effects should rarely occur. For the treatment of pulmonary metastases, doses must be kept below 1500 cGy to prevent diffuse lung fibrosis. If thoracic radiation is needed for a prepubescent female, breast development can be impaired. High doses of actinomycin-D have resulted in liver damage. Because these children go through life with only one kidney, any urinary tract symptoms must be addressed quickly to prevent infections, stones, or other diseases from damaging the remaining kidney.

Neuroblastoma, Wilms tumor of the kidney, sarcomas, and lymphomas can all present as abdominal masses in children. Their staging, treatments, and prognosis are different, so accurate diagnosis must occur initially. Although radiation is now used less often than in decades past, it can still play a pivotal role with residual disease after surgery and chemotherapy. Cure is still possible even with metastatic disease.

SOFT TISSUE SARCOMAS

Epidemiology

Soft tissue sarcomas arise from mesenchymal tissues and can occur anywhere in the body. A wide variety of histologic appearances can be seen, but **rhabdomyosarcoma** (RMS), a malignant tumor of striated muscle origin, constitutes about 40% of cases in children.[47] There are distinct histologic variants of RMS, including embryonal (most common) and alveolar. Embryonal RMS typically occurs in the head and

TABLE 35.7 Intergroup Rhabdomyosarcoma Study Staging Systems

Clinical System	TGNM System
I. Localized, completely resected	**TUMOR**
II. Grossly resected with microscopic residue or involved lymph nodes	T_1: Confined to site origin T_2: Extension to surrounding tissues a. <5 cm b. ≥5 cm
III. Gross residual tumor	**HISTOLOGY**
IV. Distant metastases	G_1: Favorable: embryonal, undifferentiated, mixed G_2: Unfavorable; alveolar
	NODES
	N_0: Not clinically involved N_1: Clinically involved by tumor
	METASTASES
	M_0: No distant metastases M_1: Metastatic disease at time of diagnosis

TGNM, Tumor, grade, node, metastasis.
Modified from Wexler LH, Meyer WH, Helman LJ: Rhabdomyosarcoma. In: Pizzo PA, Poplack DG, eds. *Principles and Practice of Pediatric Oncology.* 6th ed. Philadelphia, PA: Lippincott Williams and Wilkins; 2011.

neck or GU region and presents in younger patients. Alveolar RMS is less common than embryonal and typically occurs in the legs, chest, abdomen, and genital/anal region. The alveolar variant carries a worse prognosis and presents during the teenage years. Alveolar RMS is often characterized by translocations on chromosome 13. Familial soft tissue sarcoma cases may be related to the *p53* oncogene mutation. About 75% of soft tissue sarcomas occur before the age of 10 years. The most common sites of disease are the head and neck area (34%), abdomen (25%), GU region (23%), and extremities and trunk (17%).[48,49]

Diagnosis and Staging

The presenting symptoms of soft tissue sarcomas depend on the area of involvement. A painless mass can enlarge relatively asymptomatically in an extremity, whereas a small mass in the orbit can cause pain, tearing, and outward displacement of the globe, known as proptosis. The GU occurrences in the prostate and bladder in males cause urinary difficulties. A voluminous, exophytic mass that extrudes from the vagina in young girls has been called sarcoma botryoides because of its resemblance to clusters of grapes.

The staging of RMSs and other soft tissue sarcomas has historically considered size, degree of surgery, nodal involvement, and metastases. The latter are most likely to occur in the lung and bone marrow. The Intergroup Rhabdomyosarcoma Study Group (IRSG) first developed a clinical grouping system based on surgical findings, but some now favor the tumor, grade, node, histology, metastasis (TGNM) system (Table 35.7). After the histologic diagnosis is obtained from an incisional biopsy, staging includes a physical examination and ultrasound, CT, or MRI scan to determine the tumor's size and involvement of adjacent structures. A bone marrow biopsy and chest CT scan are done to detect metastases. The stage and histology dictate the treatment regimen in IRSG and other international studies. Metastatic disease is extremely rare with orbital presentation but may be present in about 25% of patients who have tumors in the extremities and trunk.[39]

Treatment Techniques

Given the propensity of these tumors for local recurrence and regional and distant spread, a comprehensive treatment plan must be developed.

This often includes surgery, chemotherapy, and radiotherapy. After the workup and staging, the surgical possibilities must be assessed. The first choice, if possible, is the complete removal of the mass with appropriate margins without the destruction of precious anatomy. The initial IRSG study proved that small, fully resected lesions have good curability without additional treatment. Complete resection with negative margins is not always possible, nor advisable. In more advanced cases, the local relapse rate was extremely high with surgery alone. The original approach for removing of the entire organ or extremity is no longer necessary because of multidisciplinary treatment including chemotherapy and radiation. The removal of a child's eye or GU structures is generally not preferred and has led to organ-sparing treatments with chemotherapy and radiation.

Radiation improves local control and organ preservation in all RMS groups except small and fully excised lesions. Fortunately, the frequently unresectable tumors of the orbit and pelvis are usually the more favorable embryonal histology. Originally, the margins of radiation fields included the entire muscular compartment. More recently, protocol guidelines have used margins of as little as 1 cm on prechemotherapy tumor volumes in an effort to spare critical healthy tissues. In critical areas such as the orbit, treatment planning and delivery, IMRT, or protons can spare the contralateral eye, facial bones, optic chiasm, and most brain tissues. In the pelvis or along extremities, the growth plates of the long bones must be shielded. With the routine use of chemotherapy, the bone marrow in the pelvic wings should be spared, if possible. In general, the prechemotherapy tumor volume defines the gross tumor volume, and treatment includes a 1-cm margin. IRS-IV included hyperfractionated radiation without advantageous results.[50] Standard doses of 180 cGy/day are used, ranging from a total of 3600 cGy for microscopic residual disease, 41.4 Gy for lymph node disease, and up to 5040 cGy for gross disease.

Chemotherapy was initially used only for metastatic disease, but its use after surgery is common today. IRS studies showed vincristine, actinomycin-D, and Cytoxan to be effective agents, and these are commonly used today. Newer agents are being investigated in current trials. With good tumor reduction, some inoperable cancers can be resected or radiation fields greatly reduced. Surgery or radiation therapy is now performed for local control within the first 3 months of the treatment regimen because resistant clones of cells can lead to tumor growth and lost opportunities. The tumor's histology, stage, and location affect survival rates (Table 35.8). Although the survival rate for patients with orbital lesions is more than 90%, patients with metastatic disease still fare poorly, with survival rates of 10% to 35%.[35] Overall, in IRS-IV, the 3-year failure-free survival rate was 77%.[51]

Late Effects of Treatment

The long-term sequelae of RMS and other soft tissue sarcoma treatment depend on the tumor's location and treatment modality. Amputation and **pelvic exenteration** (a radical surgical treatment that removes all organs from the pelvic cavity) are generally reserved for the salvaging of organ-sparing treatment failures. However, some patients' families may prefer bladder removal rather than the long-term effects of chemoradiation on their young child's reproductive structures. With the high radiation doses, bone and soft tissue growth is affected unless the growth plates of bones can be excluded. In the head and neck region, cosmetic changes may necessitate reconstructive surgery. If invasion of the cranial contents occurs, necessitating CNS radiation to 3000 cGy or more, the survivor may have development of some of the side effects noted in the brain tumor section. Dryness of the treated eye or retinal damage from chemotherapy and radiation sometimes necessitates enucleation, even if the sarcoma is cured. The appropriate use of brachytherapy implants in select cases can spare many of the surrounding healthy tissues from damage.

TABLE 35.8 Actuarial Survival Rates at 3 Years: Results of the Intergroup Rhabdomyosarcoma Studies I, II, and III

Prognostic Factors	IRS I (%)	IRS II (%)	IRS III, 5 yr (%)
Clinical Group			
I	79	88	93
II	68	77	80–89
III	42	68	70
IV	18	32	30
Histologic Type			
Embryonal	—	69	75
Alveolar	—	56	70
Other	—	66	—
Primary Site			
Orbit	91	93	91
GU (mainly group III)	—	64	—
Trunk and extremity	53	57	—
Retroperitoneum and pelvis	39	46	—

GU, Genitourinary; IRS, Intergroup Rhabdomyosarcoma Study Group.
Modified from Wexler LH, Meyer WH, Helman LJ. Rhabdomyo-sarcoma. In: Pizzo PA, Poplack DG, eds. *Principles and Practice of Pediatric Oncology.* 6th ed. Philadelphia, PA: Lippincott Williams and Wilkins; 2011.

TABLE 35.9 Five-Year Survival Trends for Cancers in Children Ages 0 to 14 Years

Diagnosis	Survival Rate (%) for 1960–1963	Survival Rate (%) for 1974–1976	Survival Rate (%) for 1996–2003	Survival Rate (%) for 2003–2009
Acute lymphocytic leukemia	4	52	85	89
Brain tumor	35	53	70	72
Neuroblastoma	25	52	66	78
Wilms tumor	33	74	92	90
Hodgkin disease	52	79	95	97
All sites	28	55	80	82

Modified from Parker SL, Tong T, Bolden S, et al. Cancer statistics, 1996. *CA Cancer J Clin* 1996;46:5-27; and U.S. Government SEER cancer incidence data. National Cancer Institute website. SEER.cancer.gov. Accessed January 20, 2014.

Chemotherapeutic agents can cause acute and chronic neurologic, kidney, heart, and liver damage. The risk of treatment-induced secondary malignancies is present for many years. As survivors grow to adulthood, fertility is questionable after chemotherapy and highly unlikely for those receiving pelvic radiation.

The occurrence of a second malignancy as a result of treatment for a childhood cancer is always a risk. Because patients with childhood cancer have an overall very good survival rate (Table 35.9) and tend to live longer as compared with other cancer survivors, the

TABLE 35.10 Results of the 2010 Childhood Cancer Survivor Study of Patients With a Second Malignancies

Second Neoplasms	No. of Patients
ALL	346
AML	29
Other leukemia	13
Astrocytoma	85
Medulloblastoma or PNET	47
Other CNS	31
Hodgkin lymphoma	453
Non-Hodgkin lymphoma	82
Kidney	51
Neuroblastoma	45
Soft tissue sarcoma	112
Ewing sarcoma	49
Osteosarcoma	55
Other bone	4
Total	1402

Among a total of 14,359 patients treated between 1970 and 1986 and reviewed 30 years after a childhood cancer diagnosis, 1402 patients developed one or more neoplasm.
ALL, Acute lymphoblastic leukemia; *AML,* acute myeloid leukemia; *CNS,* central nervous system; *PNET,* primitive neuroectodermal tumor.
Modified from Friedman DL, Whitton J, Leisenring W, et al. Subsequent neoplasms in 5-year survivors of childhood cancer; the childhood cancer survivor study. *J Natl Cancer Inst.* 2010;102(14):1083–1095.

risk of development of a second primary may be higher. Survival of childhood cancer has a direct impact on the quality and quantity of life. Friedman and colleagues[52] analyzed the rate and type of subsequent neoplasms in 5-year survivors of childhood cancers. In the childhood cancer survivor study, the researchers reviewed a total of 14,359 5-year survivors treated between 1970 and 1986 and found a total of 1402 patients (7.9% rate) that had development of a second primary (excluding nonmelanoma skin cancer). Table 35.10 shows the distribution of second malignancies among 14 different pathologies, of which Hodgkin lymphoma (*n* = 453), acute lymphoblastic leukemia (ALL) (*n* = 346), and soft tissue sarcoma (*n* = 112) were the most common sites.

MISCELLANEOUS CHILDHOOD TUMORS

Germ Cell Tumors

Germ cell tumors are cancers derived from the germ cells. Germ cells normally occur within the gonads (ovaries and testis) but may originate outside the gonads. Because germ cells follow a midline path through the body after development and descend into the pelvis, extragonadal germ cell tumors typically occur in the midline. CNS germ cell tumors are discussed in the brain tumor section of this chapter. Sacrococcygeal teratomas often occur in newborns. Most of these tumors are histologically benign and are almost always cured with surgery.

Ovarian and testicular tumors that occur in adolescents differentiate along seminoma, dysgerminoma, or nonseminomatous lines. The latter group includes embryonal carcinoma, choriocarcinoma, and yolk sac tumors. The nonseminomatous tumors often produce alpha-fetoprotein or human chorionic gonadotropin, which can be used as chemical markers for response to therapy. Surgical removal of the testicles or ovaries is done first and is often curative in stage I disease. For nonseminomatous cancers, chemotherapy with regimens containing cisplatin, bleomycin, etoposide, and vinblastine has led to a high rate of success.[53]

For testicular seminoma seen mostly in older adolescents and young adults, radical orchiectomy and CT staging of the draining pelvic and paraaortic nodes are performed. Historically, moderate doses of radiation in the 2000 cGy to 2500 cGy range have been used to prevent pelvic and paraaortic nodal relapse. Cure rates overall are close to 100%.

Liver Tumors

Liver tumors appear as right upper quadrant abdominal masses, much like Wilms tumor or neuroblastoma. Ultrasound or CT scanning can usually determine the organ of origin. Benign vascular or fetal remnant tumors can be observed if they are small, or, if necessary because of their large size, they can be resected with excellent results. Hepatoblastoma is a malignancy that usually occurs in patients younger than 2 years. Hepatocellular carcinoma occurs in the second decade of life and can be multifocal. Alpha-fetoprotein can be elevated in both hepatic malignancies.[54]

Primary surgical resection is the goal. If this is not possible or postoperative residua are present, chemotherapy with doxorubicin and cisplatin is often used. Radiation has shown some good response but is rarely used except for palliation.

Hematologic Diseases

Leukemia. ALL is the most common childhood cancer. Patients need extensive chemotherapy regimens for 2 years. Radiation can be used for CNS or testicular involvement because those sites have diminished chemotherapy penetration. Doses of 1200 to 1800 cGy, along with systemic and intrathecal chemotherapy, dramatically reduce CNS relapse rates in patients at high risk.[55] Total body radiation is often given as part of the bone marrow transplant preparatory regimen in relapse patients. This requires very specialized facilities, techniques, and dosimetry. See Chapter 26, "Leukemias and Lymphomas" for more information.

Langerhans Cell Histiocytosis. This is a spectrum of diseases that involves abnormal proliferation of the immune system's histiocytic Langerhans cells. Infants can have multifocal visceral disease that involves the lung, skin, liver, and bone marrow and creates a life-threatening condition known as Letterer-Siwe syndrome. More commonly, bones can be involved with a lytic lesion referred to as an *eosinophilic granuloma*. Individual histiocytosis lesions may vary over time and occasionally spontaneously regress. Focal bony lesions can be treated via surgical curettage with success. If an impending fracture is a concern or the lesion is in a surgically unresectable region such as the base of skull or spinal column, low doses of radiation are usually effective. Although no direct dose-response curve has been substantiated, doses from 400 to 1200 cGy can be effective. Steroids, vinblastine, or cyclophosphamide can be used as well.

Hodgkin Lymphoma. In children, Hodgkin lymphoma is almost always treated with chemotherapy initially. Increasingly, risk and response-adapted doses are being used. Sites of original bulk disease are now treated with low-dose involved field radiation (1500 to 2500 cGy) after chemotherapy to reduce recurrence. High cure rates are being achieved with fewer long-term effects.[56] Second malignancy

risks are significant in long-term survivors.[57] Refer to the Hodgkin disease section in this text for more detailed information.

Nasopharynx

Male adolescents may have development of nasopharyngeal angiofibromas, which are highly vascular and can erode bone. Usually, vascular embolization and surgical resection are used to manage these lesions. Moderate doses of radiation (such as 3000 cGy) can control relapses or unresectable lesions.[58]

Undifferentiated nasopharyngeal carcinomas can occur in children and require high-dose radiation, as they do in adults. Recently, chemotherapy has been used to reduce radiation fields and doses. High cure rates can be achieved, but long-term dry mouth and dental problems are of concern.[59]

Thyroid

Benign and malignant thyroid tumors can arise in adolescents (more often in girls). These tumors are surgically approached, and even lymph node metastases do not imply a bad prognosis. External radiation is rarely used, but iodine-131 can be helpful for thyroid ablation or treatment of metastatic lesions.

Keloids

Keloids (excess scar formation after cutaneous injury) are a benign condition; however, they can be bothersome and cosmetically disfiguring for young people. Keloids can occur on any part of the body, but they typically occur on the earlobes (after ear piercing), shoulders, chest, and back.[60] If repeated resections and corticosteroid injections are not successful in managing the condition, the best control is obtained via resection, followed immediately (within 72 hours) by low-dose radiation (900 to 1200 cGy in 3 fractions).[61] Low-energy electrons are typically used, and bolus may be added to ensure adequate surface dose.

Kaposi Sarcoma

Unfortunately, the human immunodeficiency virus infection epidemic has led to the occurrence of Kaposi sarcoma of the skin in children. Focal painful or disfiguring lesions can be palliated with single doses of 700 cGy, although more lasting results are obtained with a short course to 2000 cGy.[62]

PALLIATIVE RADIATION

Although the goal is to cure pediatric malignancies, **palliative** treatments are sometimes necessary to relieve symptoms. Mediastinal malignancies may cause airway or vascular compromise. Spinal cord compression at the time of presentation or late in the course of the illness demands immediate treatment to reduce pain and avoid paralysis. Painful bone metastases can be treated to reduce analgesic needs.

The palliative needs of children in the final stages of cancer must be addressed carefully and compassionately. The goal of such treatments is much different than the usual curative protocols. The attempt must be made to relieve symptoms quickly with a minimal number of treatments to limit the invasion of the family's remaining time together. The successful treatment of painful or disfiguring masses can reduce the need for narcotics or hospitalization and improve cosmetics and quality of life during precious final days or weeks. In these instances, immobilization and simulation techniques are altered in deference to the comfort of the child. Frequently, high daily doses are used for rapid palliation when long-term effects are not of concern.[63] Although this is a difficult time for radiation staff members, such palliative efforts in times of great need are of immeasurable importance to the children and their families. End-of-life care is increasingly being addressed by trained pediatric specialists.

ROLE OF THE RADIATION THERAPIST

Almost all patients in radiation oncology centers are adults, and it is often challenging for staff to address the personal needs of pediatric patients and their families and perform the technically challenging procedures that may be required. It is important for radiation therapists to modify their workflow to accommodate these patients. For patients requiring general anesthesia, treatment position and technique may need to be altered for anesthetic safety. Close cooperation among radiation therapists, nurses, and anesthesia staff members is necessary for patient positioning and visibility of monitors. Allowance of adequate time in the schedule is important, as these complex procedures are often lengthy, sometimes up to an hour. Departments typically treat pediatric patients in the early morning to reduce disruption of the child's feeding patterns and avoid other treatment day conflicts. Therapists often must juggle an already busy schedule of adults, but most patients are willing to change in deference to children and their families.

As mentioned previously, many pediatric patients are on a clinical trial, which requires careful documentation of treatment setups, daily doses, and quality assurance. Clear instructions between the radiation therapist on the CT simulator and treatment machine are essential. Digital images of patient positioning, verification of initial portal images, and dose calculations are usually sent for immediate review by national clinical research groups. Careful adherence to protocol guidelines reflects positively on the quality of a radiation oncology department.

The psychosocial elements of pediatric oncology can be immense. It is important that radiation therapists modify their approach and communication when interacting with pediatric patients. Communicating to pediatric patients and their families requires a much different approach than with adults[64] and should follow age-specific guidelines. Box 35.4 provides some helpful tips when communicating with children of all ages.

Children often evoke sympathy and compassion from everyone involved; however, it is important to provide behavioral limits and structure to ensure quality treatments. Rewards such as stickers or toys should not be used daily, but therapists may be the best judges of when a difficult or sick child needs an uplifting gift. Radiation therapists should strive to be sensitive to the personal, spiritual, financial, and professional challenges families face when managing a sick child. When children with terminal cancer come for palliation,

Box 35.4   Pediatric Communication Tips

Infants and Toddlers (0–2): Encourage use of security object from home (blanket, stuffed animal, etc.) if possible. Avoid overstimulation by speaking softly, darkening the room, and minimizing the number of people involved. Provide consistency. Use diversionary items during procedure. Watch for engagement/disengagement cues. Allow parental involvement, if possible.

Preschoolers (3–6): Encourage patient participation. Give expectations in concrete terms. Provide simple choices and positive reinforcement. Allow the child to verbalize fears and concerns. Clarify misconceptions before the procedure. Explain each step in sensory terms. Provide limits and structure.

School-Aged (7–12): Explain what you are doing when you are doing it. Allow the child to help in his/her care. Incorporate familiar routines. Allow time for questions and suggest ways of coping during procedures.

Adolescents (13–18): Allow access to same-sex medical staff, if possible. Respect privacy. Explain procedures using correct terminology. Involve them in decision-making.

Other Tips: Avoid language that creates fear (replace "shooting an x-ray" with "taking a picture," for example). Never frown at an image or during a procedure. Provide a safe space.

it is an especially difficult time. For the radiation therapist, the treatment of children is demanding and often heart-wrenching; however, the value of their technical expertise and compassion cannot be overstated.

SUMMARY

- A summary of radiation treatment for childhood cancers can be found in Table 35.1.
- The multidisciplinary protocol approach to pediatric oncology is always a learning experience. This strategy has led to dramatic increases in cure rates for childhood cancers over the past 40 years to reach an overall survival rate of over 70% (see Table 35.7).
- Numerous late side effects must be considered in pediatric cases.
- In addition to organ toxicities and risk of second malignancies, childhood cancer survivors have psychologic scars. Social, employment, and insurance discrimination may exist throughout adulthood.
- The COG not only directs clinical trials and research but also acts as an advocate for survivors of childhood cancer.

▮ REVIEW QUESTIONS

The answers to the Review Questions can be found by logging on to our website at: http://evolve.elsevier.com/Washington/principles

1. A tumor that does *not* spread through the entire central nervous system is a(n):
   a. Medulloblastoma.
   b. Craniopharyngioma.
   c. Ependymoma.
   d. CNS germ cell tumor.
2. Anatomically, the radiation treatment area most common for Wilms tumor is the:
   a. Head and neck.
   b. Brain.
   c. Thorax.
   d. Abdomen.
3. The factor not related to survival in neuroblastoma cases is:
   a. Age.
   b. Stage.
   c. n-*Myc* amplification.
   d. Male gender.
4. The retinoblastoma gene is a(n):
   a. Tumor promoter.
   b. Tumor suppressor.
   c. Active haploid.
   d. Inactive haploid.
5. The present protocol dose for occult Wilms tumor is approximately:
   a. 1000 cGy.
   b. 2000 cGy.
   c. 4000 cGy.
   d. 6000 cGy.

6. The tolerance of the kidney is about:
   a. 100 cGy.
   b. 900 cGy.
   c. 1500 cGy.
   d. 3000 cGy.
7. The most likely second malignant neoplasm after radiation for retinoblastoma is:
   a. Leukemia.
   b. Lung cancer.
   c. Lymphoma.
   d. Osteosarcoma.
8. Which of the following has the highest incidence in children?
   a. Retinoblastoma.
   b. Neuroblastoma.
   c. ALL.
   d. Wilms tumor.
9. CSI is usually administered for treatment of:
   a. Retinoblastoma.
   b. Neuroblastoma.
   c. Leukemia.
   d. Medulloblastoma.
10. The role of the radiation therapist involved with pediatric cancers includes:
   a. Working with treatment techniques that may be altered for general anesthesia.
   b. Concern for psychosocial elements of the patient and family.
   c. Monitoring PSA values.
   d. Both A and B.

QUESTIONS TO PONDER

1. List examples of chromosome and gene abnormalities associated with pediatric cancer.
2. Why is shifting the junction between the brain and spinal fields important during CSI?
3. Detail some technical considerations for the simulation and treatment of CSI cases.
4. Note possible long-term effects of high-dose brain radiation and discuss methods to reduce such late effects.
5. What organ-sparing techniques are possible by combining chemotherapy, radiation, and surgery for solid tumors?
6. What types of counseling and advice are needed for long-term survivors of childhood cancer?
7. How much have childhood cancer cure rates improved over the past four decades?

REFERENCES

1. Childhood cancers. National cancer Institute website. https://www.cancer.gov/types/childhood-cancers; 2018. Accessed January 20, 2019.
2. Cancer in children. American cancer Society website. Accessed https://www.cancer.org/cancer/cancer-in-children.html; 2018. Accessed January 20, 2019.
3. Gunderson LL, Tepper JE, eds. *Clinical Radiation Oncology*. 3rd ed. Philadelphia, PA: Elsevier; 2012.
4. Halperin EC, Wazer DE, Perez CA, Brady LW, eds. *Perez and Brady's Principles and Practice of Radiation Oncology*. 6th ed. Philadelphia, PA: Lippincott Williams & Wilkins; 2013.
5. Duffner PK, Horowitz ME, Krischer JP, et al. Postoperative chemotherapy and delayed radiation in children less than 3 years of age with malignant brain tumors. *N Engl J Med*. 1993;328:1725–1731.
6. Garvey M, Packer RJ. An integrated approach to the treatment of chiasmatic-hypothalamic gliomas. *J Neuro Oncol*. 1996;28:167–183.
7. Packer RJ, et al. Pediatric tumors. In: Halperin EC, Wazer DE, Perez CA, Brady LW, eds. *Perez and Brady's Principles and Practice of Radiation Oncology*. 6th ed. Philadelphia, PA: Lippincott Williams & Wilkins; 2013.
8. Merchant TE, LI C, Kun LE, et al. Conformal radiotherapy after surgery for paediatric ependymoma: a prospective study. *Lancet Oncol*. 2009;10(3):258–266.
9. Young JA, Eslinger P, Galloway M. Radiation treatment for the child with cancer. *Issues Comp Pediatr Nurs*. 1989;12:159–169.
10. Chang CH, Housepian EM, Herbert C. An operative staging system and a megavoltage radiotherapeutic technique for cerebellar medulloblastoma. *Radiology*. 1969;93:1351–1359.
11. Patterson E, Farr RF. Cerebellar medulloblastoma: treatment by irradiation of the whole central nervous system. *Acta Radiol*. 1953;39:323–336.
12. Haas-Kogan DA, Barani IJ, Hayden MG, et al. Pediatric central nervous system tumors. In: Hoppe RT, Phillips TL, Roach M, eds. *Leibel and Phillips Textbook of Radiation Oncology*. 3rd ed. Philadelphia, PA: Elsevier Saunders; 2010.
13. Packer RJ, Gajjar A, Vezina G, et al. Phase III study of craniospinal radiation therapy followed by adjuvant chemotherapy for newly diagnosed average-risk medulloblastoma. *J Clin Oncol*. 2006;24:4202–4208.
14. Packer RJ, Goldwein J, Nicholson HS, et al. Treatment of children with medulloblastoma with reduced craniospinal radiation and adjuvant chemotherapy: a Children's Cancer Group study. *J Clin Oncol*. 1999;17:2127–2136.
15. Johnson K, Cullen J, Barnholtz-Sloan J, et al. Childhood brain tumor epidemiology: a brain tumor epidemiology consortium review. *Cancer Epidemiol Biomarkers Prev*. 2014;23(12):2716–2736.
16. Baranzelli MC, et al. Nonmetastatic intracranial germinoma: the experience of the French Society of pediatric oncology. *Int J Radiat Biol Oncol Phys*. 1999;43:783–788.
17. Shibamoto Y, Sasai K, Oya N, et al. Intracranial germonoma: radiation therapy with tumor volume based dose selection. *Radiology*. 2001;218:452–456.
18. Flickinger JC, Kondziolka D, Lunsford LD. Radiosurgery of benign lesions. *Semin Radiat Oncol*. 1995;5:220–224.
19. Garwicz S, Anderson H, Olsen JH, et al. Second malignant neoplasms after cancer in childhood and adolescence: a population-based case control study in the 5 Nordic countries. *Int J Cancer*. 2000;88:672–678.
20. Rodriguez-Galindo C, Buchsbaum JC, Retinoblastoma. In: Gunderson LL, Tepper JE, eds. *Clinical Radiation Oncology*. 3rd ed. Philadelphia, PA: Elsevier; 2012.
21. Dryja TP, Cavenee W, White R, et al. Homozygosity of chromosome 13 in retinoblastoma. *N Engl J Med*. 1984;310:550–553.
22. Weinberg RA. The retinoblastoma gene and gene product. *Cancer Surv*. 1992;12:43–57.
23. Abramson DH. Retinoblastoma: diagnosis and management. *CA Cancer J Clin*. 1982;32:130–140.
24. Reese A. *Tumors of the Eye*. Hagerstown, MD: Harper and Row; 1976.
25. Schipper JJ, Tan KE, Von Peperzeel HA. Treatment of retinoblastoma by precision megavoltage radiation therapy. *Radiother Oncol*. 1985;3:117–132.
26. Shields CL, Shields JA, Cater J, et al. Plaque radiotherapy for retinoblastoma: long term control and treatment complications in 208 tumors. *Ophthalmology*. 2001;108:2116–2121.
27. Abramson DH, Beaverson KL, Chang ST, et al. Outcome following initial external beam radiotherapy in patients with Reese-Ellsworth group IV retinoblastoma. *Arch Ophthal*. 2004;122:1316–1333.

28. Friedman DL, Himelstein B, Shields CL, et al. Chemoreduction and local ophthalmologic therapy for intraocular retinoblastoma. *J Clin Oncol.* 2000;18:12–17.

29. Guin GH, Gilbert EF, Jones B. Incidental neuroblastoma in infants. *Am J Clin Pathol.* 1969;51(1):126–136.

30. Wolden S. Neuroblastoma. In: Gunderson LL, Tepper JE, eds. *Clinical Radiation Oncology.* 3rd ed. Philadelphia, PA: Elsevier; 2012.

31. Maris JM, Matthay KK. Molecular biology of neuroblastoma. *J Clin Oncol.* 1999;17(7):2264–2279.

32. Brodeur GM, Seeger RC. Gene amplification in human neuroblastomas: basic mechanisms and clinical implications. *Cancer Genet Cytogenet.* 1986;19:101–111.

33. Evans AE. Staging and treatment of neuroblastoma. *Cancer.* 1980;45:1799–1802.

34. D'Angio GJ, Evans A, Koop CE. Special pattern of widespread neuroblastoma with a favorable prognosis. *Lancet.* 1971;1:1046.

35. American Cancer Society (website). http://acs.org. Accessed January 20, 2019.

36. Pinto N, Applebaum M, Volchenboum S, et al. Advances in risk classification and treatment strategies for neuroblastoma. *J Clin Oncol.* 2015;33(27):3008–3017.

37. Laverdiere C, Cheung NK, Kushner BH, et al. Long-term complications in survivors of advanced stage neuroblastoma. *Pediatr Blood Cancer.* 2005;45:324–332.

38. Grundy PE, Breslow NE, Li S, et al. Loss of heterozygosity for chromosomes 1p and 16q is an adverse prognostic factor in favorable histology Wilms' tumor: a report from the National Wilms Tumor Study Group. *J Clin Oncol.* 2005;23:7312–7321.

39. Breneman JC, Lyden E, Pappo AS, et al. Prognostic factors and clinical outcomes in children with metastatic rhabdomyosarcoma: a report from the IRS IV. *J Clin Oncol.* 2003;21:78–84.

40. Lemere J, Voute PA, Tournade MF, et al. Effectiveness of preoperative chemotherapy in Wilms tumor: results of SIOP clinical trials. *J Clin Oncol.* 1983;1:604–610.

41. Graf N, Tournade MF, de Kraker J. The role of preoperative chemotherapy in the management of Wilms' tumor: the SIOP studies. *Urol Clin North Am.* 2000;27:443–454.

42. D'Angio GJ, Tefft M, Breslow N, et al. Radiation therapy of Wilms tumor: results according to dose, field, post-operative timing, and histology. *Int J Radiat Biol Oncol Phys.* 1978;4:769–780.

43. Breslow NE, Ou SS, Beckwith JB, et al. Doxorubicin for favorable histology, stage II–III Wilms' tumor: results from the national Wilms' tumor studies. *Cancer.* 2004;101:1072–1080.

44. Kalapurakal JA, Dome JS. Wilms' tumor. In: Gunderson LL, Tepper JE, eds. *Clinical Radiation Oncology.* 3rd ed. Philadelphia, PA: Elsevier; 2012.

45. Taylor RE. Paediatric oncology. In: Symonds P, Deehan C, Mills JA, et al., eds. *Walter and Miller's Textbook of Radiotherapy; Radiation Physics, Therapy and Oncology.* 8th ed. London, UK: Elsevier Churchill Livingstone; 2020.

46. Farber S. Chemotherapy in the treatment of leukemia and Wilms tumor. *J Am Med Assoc.* 1966;138:826.

47. Gurney JG, Severson RK, Davis S, et al. Incidence of cancer in children in the United States. *Cancer.* 1995;75:2186–2195.

48. Haas-Kogan DA, Farmer DL, Wharam MD. Pediatric bone and soft tissue tumors. In: Hoppe RT, Phillips TL, Roach M, eds. *Leibel and Phillips Textbook of Radiation Oncology.* 3rd ed. Philadelphia, PA: Elsevier Saunders; 2010.

49. Schwartzman E, Chantada G, Fandiño A, et al. Results of a stage based protocol for the treatment of retinoblastoma. *J Clin Oncol.* 1996;14:1532–1536.

50. Donaldson SS, Meza J, Breneman JC, et al. Results from the IRS-IV trial of hyperfractionated radiotherapy in children with rhabdomyosarcoma: a report from the IRSG. *Int J Radiat Oncol Biol Phys.* 2001;51:718–728.

51. Crist WM, Anderson JR, Meza JL, et al. Intergroup Rhabdomyosarcoma Group IV: results for patients with nonmetastatic disease. *J Clin Oncol.* 2001;19:3091–3102.

52. Friedman DL, Whitton J, Leisenring W, et al. Subsequent neoplasms in 5-year survivors of childhood cancer; the childhood cancer survivor study. *J Natl Cancer Inst.* 2010;102(14):1083–1095.

53. Williams S, Birch R, Einhorn LH, et al. Treatment of disseminated germ cell tumors with cisplatin, bleomycin and either vinblastine or etoposide. *N Engl J Med.* 1987;316:1435–1440.

54. Fraumeni JF, Miller RW, Hill JA. Primary carcinoma of the liver in childhood: an epidemiologic study. *J Natl Cancer Inst.* 1968;40:1087–1099.

55. Waber DP, et al. Excellent therapeutic efficacy and minimal late neurotoxicity in children treated with 18 Gray of cranial radiation therapy for high risk acute lymphoblastic leukemia: a 7 year follow-up study of the Dana Farber Cancer Institute Consortium Protocol 87-01. *Cancer.* 2001;92:15–22.

56. Sieber M, et al. Two cycles ABVD plus extended field radiotherapy is superior to radiotherapy alone in early stage Hodgkin's disease: results of the German Hodgkin's Lymphoma Study Group Trial HD7. *Blood.* 2002;100:A341.

57. Ng AK, Bernardo MV, Weller E, et al. Second malignancy after Hodgkin's disease treated with radiation therapy with or without chemotherapy: long term risks and risk factors. *Blood.* 2002;100:1989–1996.

58. Cummings BJ, Blend R. Primary radiation therapy for juvenile nasopharyngeal angiofibroma. *The Laryngoscope.* 1984;94:1599–1605.

59. Wolden SL, Steinherz PG, Kraus DH, et al. Improved long term survival with combined modality therapy for pediatric nasopharynx cancer. *Int J Radiat Biol Oncol Phys.* 2000;46:859–864.

60. Young Lee S, Park J. Postoperative electron beam radiotherapy for keloids: treatment outcome and factors associated with occurrence and recurrence. *Ann Dermatol.* 2015;27(1):53–58.

61. Stevens KR Jr. The soft tissue. In: Moss WT, Cox JD, eds. *Radiation Oncology: Rationale, Techniques, Results.* 6th ed. St. Louis, MO: Mosby; 1989.

62. Cooper JS, Fried PR. Defining the role of radiotherapy for epidemic Kaposi's sarcoma. *Int J Radiat Oncol Biol Phys.* 1987;13:35–39.

63. Rudoler S, et al. Patterns of presentation, treatment, and outcome of children referred for emergent/urgent therapeutic irradiation. In: *Evolving Role of Radiation in Pediatric Oncology Conference*, Philadelphia, PA; 1995.

64. Purvis JA. The challenge of communicating with pediatric patients. American Academy of Orthopaedic Surgeons website https://www.aaos.org/search/?srchtext=the+challenge+of+communication+with+pediatric+patients Accessed November 6 2019.

36

Skin Cancers and Melanoma

Charles M. Washington

OBJECTIVES

- Describe the epidemiologic factors of skin cancers.
- Identify, list, and describe the etiologic factors that may be responsible for inducing skin cancers.
- Describe the common symptoms produced by skin and melanoma malignancies.
- Review the methods of skin cancer detection and diagnosis.
- List the varying histologic types of skin tumors.
- Describe the diagnostic procedures used to workup and stage skin cancers.
- Describe the clinical presentation system used for cutaneous squamous cell, Merkel cell, and melanoma variations of skin cancers.
- Describe the common routes of spread for skin tumors.
- Differentiate between histologic grading and staging.
- Describe the anatomy and physiology of the skin.

- Identify skin tumor treatment options.
- Discuss the rationale for treatment about treatment choice, histologic type, and stage of skin cancers.
- Describe the treatment methods available for skin cancers.
- Describe the differing types of radiation treatments that can be used for skin cancer.
- Discuss the expected radiation reactions for the area based on time-dose-fractionation schemes.
- Describe the instructions that should be given to a patient about skin care, expected reactions, and dietary advice.
- Discuss the rationale for use of multimodality treatments in managing skin cancers.
- Discuss survival statistics and prognosis for various stages of skin cancers.

OUTLINE

KEY TERMS

Actinic (solar) keratosis
Basal cell carcinoma
Cutaneous squamous cell carcinoma
Dermis
Desquamation
Epidermis
Erythema
Hyperthermia
Keratin
Keratinocytes
Keratoacanthoma

Melanin
Melanocytes
Merkel cell carcinoma
Mohs surgery
Mycosis fungoides
Squamous cell carcinoma
Subcutaneous layer
Telangiectasia
Ultraviolet protection factor
Xeroderma pigmentosum

Throughout a lifetime, the skin, one of the most visible as well as vulnerable organs of the body, is subjected to many external influences, including cold, heat, friction, ultraviolet (UV) light, pressure, and chemicals. As a result, the skin is especially susceptible to trauma, infection, and disease.

This chapter focuses on the cancers that present in the skin. Before 2010, skin cancers were classified as melanoma and nonmelanoma skin cancers (NMSCs), with squamous cell carcinomas (SCCs) and basal cell carcinomas (BCCs) making up the latter. In some cases, that terminology is still used. However, in 2010, a revised classification system was adopted, and the staging system used to describe the degree of tumor presentation evolved. NMSCs include more than 80 types of skin malignancies that range from those that are rare but offer a poor prognosis (like Merkel cell) to those that are much more common and clinically favorable in comparison (like BCC and SCC)[1]; **cutaneous SCC** (cSCC) embraces those noted cancers. BCC, which uses the same staging system as the cSCCs, is also described in this chapter, along with SCC and melanoma. The staging systems of cSCCs, Merkel cell carcinoma, and melanoma are presented as well.

SKIN CANCERS AND MELANOMA

Epidemiology

Cancer of the skin is the most common form of malignancy in humans.[2,3] The incidence of skin cancers is estimated as being higher than all other types of cancer combined, including breast, prostate, lung, and colon.[3] In the United States, the incidence of NMSC, a term used to describe basal and SCCs, approaches that of all noncutaneous cancers combined. NMSC represents one-third of all cancers, and its incidence is expected to rise into the year 2040, with cSCC representing 20% of all NMSCs.[4] The total number and incidence rate of NMSCs cannot be estimated precisely because reporting to cancer registries is not required.[5,6] More than 5.4 million cases of NMSC were treated in over 3.3 million people in the United States in 2012, the most recent year new statistics were available.[6] The reason for such a large range of estimates is that many early skin cancer lesions are easily treated by primary physicians and dermatologists and are therefore not reported to the various cancer-tracking agencies.

In contrast, the melanoma incidence rate has increased faster than that of any other cancer.

Malignant melanoma is the deadliest form of skin cancer; on an annual basis, it is the fifth most common cancer and is on the rise, with an estimated 91,000 new cases and 9300 deaths from the disease each year.[7] Fig. 36.1 shows the estimated new melanoma cases per year. Unfortunately, the incidence rate of skin cancer is rising and continues to grow throughout the world. More young people continue to be affected; a few theories that might account for this trend are as follows:

1. Tanning continues to be fashionable. Crowded beaches and the proliferation of tanning salons seem to indicate people remain interested in that look.
2. Clothing trends, inclusive of everyday fashions and swimwear, have become more liberal, which allow for more skin to be exposed to the sun's rays.

In contrast to the increasing rates of incidence, the skin cancer death rates have stayed virtually the same over the past 15 years. Melanoma is 20 times more common in whites than in African Americans. Overall, the lifetime risk of getting melanoma is about 2.6% (1 in 38) for whites, 0.1% (1 in 1,000) for blacks, and 0.58% (1 in 172) for Hispanics.[8] The squamous cell and basal cell skin cancers, however, have experienced a decrease in death rate. The fact that death rates are so low and declining in these cancers is good news, but the comparatively higher death rates for melanomas and Merkel cell carcinomas raise some concern.

Melanomas are much more lethal than their nonmelanoma counterparts. An estimated 7,230 people (4,740 males and 2,490 females) are expected to die of melanoma each year.[8] Although melanoma mortality continues to steadily increase, multiple studies have concluded that the mortality rate has not increased as fast as the incidence rate.[9]

Some individuals are more prone to skin cancer than others. Tendencies for people to have development of skin cancers and melanomas can be grouped into four main categories: geographic location, skin type, multiplicity, and gender.

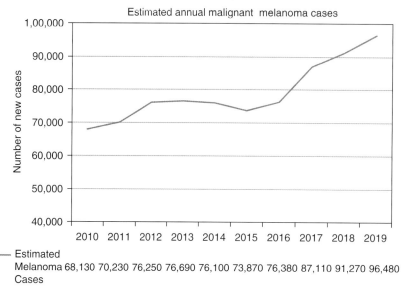

	2010	2011	2012	2013	2014	2015	2016	2017	2018	2019
Estimated Melanoma Cases	68,130	70,230	76,250	76,690	76,100	73,870	76,380	87,110	91,270	96,480

Fig. 36.1 Estimated new melanoma cases per year in the United States. (From American Cancer Society: 2010-2019 Cancer facts and figures. http://www.cancer.org/research/cancerfactsstatistics/index. Accessed February 9, 2019.)

Geographic Location

People who live near the equator have a high chance of development of skin cancer because the sun's rays are more intense and direct. At latitudes away from the equator, the sun's rays are more angled, decreasing the intensity. This angulation causes the rays to travel through more of the atmosphere and allows for the absorption of more harmful rays in areas farther away from the equator than those at the equator itself. Fig. 36.2 depicts the atmospheric phenomenon described.

Skin Type

Individuals with fair skin complexions are more likely to develop skin cancer than those with dark skin.[10] Especially susceptible are albinos, people with freckles or light-colored eyes, and people with xeroderma pigmentosum (a genetic condition caused by a defect in mechanisms that repair DNA damage caused by UV light, characterized by the development of pigment abnormalities and multiple skin cancers in body areas exposed to the sun). These people also tend to tan poorly and burn easily.

People with dark skin have greater quantities of melanin (a natural protective substance that gives color to the skin, hair, and iris of the eye) in their skin, which gives them more protection from the UV rays of the sun. This does not mean that dark-skinned individuals are free of skin cancers, but they get them less often and in more unusual places, such as on the palm of the hand, on the sole of the foot, or in the mucous membranes. Among Black and Asian populations, squamous cell was the most commonly diagnosed skin cancer, whereas BCC was the most common skin cancer in Hispanics.[11]

Multiplicity. Prior skin cancer occurrence increases the odds that a second primary skin cancer will develop. Reasons for this may include the following: (1) other areas of the skin may have been exposed to the same carcinogens that caused the initial skin cancer, and (2) the individual may have a weakness in the immune system that hinders the ability to naturally fight off skin cancers.

A previous melanoma of the skin increases the risk of another primary melanoma. A diagnosis of high-risk primary melanoma offers a teachable moment for some patients, as it points them toward adopting lasting improvements in sun protection. A proportion of patients appear to persist with inadequate sun protection: more commonly, they are males, current smokers, those with lower education, those with some tanning ability, or those not performing skin self-examination.[12] Patients with a history of multiple melanomas whose sunscreen use was inadequate on follow-up had a significantly higher risk of another melanoma primary. As such, targeted education to reduce risk of further primary disease should encourage increased sun protection counseling to melanoma survivors.[12]

Gender. The American Cancer Society reports that men are more likely than women to have basal and squamous cell cancers of the skin; this is thought to be due mainly to increased sun exposure.[13] Overall, melanoma incidence rates are higher in women than in men before age 50 years, but by age 65 years, rates in men are double those in women, and by age 80 years, they are triple. This pattern reflects age and sex differences in occupational and recreational exposure to UV radiation (including the use of indoor tanning) and perhaps early detection practices and use of healthcare.[14] This trend seems to be related to skin care habit differences between the genders rather than genetics.

Etiology

Many factors are directly and indirectly responsible for the development of the various forms of skin cancer, but the major cause is exposure to UV light.

Ultraviolet Light. The American Cancer Society estimates that approximately 90% of all skin cancers would be prevented if people protected their skin from the sun's rays.[15,16] The risk of development of melanoma increases after five or more blistering sunburns during adolescence.[17] At greatest risk for development of a melanoma is the person who primarily stays indoors and receives occasional intense sun exposure. In contrast, people who spend most of the time in the sun (e.g., farmers, construction workers) are most apt to develop BCCs or SCCs.

Sunlight contains two types of UV rays that are harmful to the skin: UVA and UVB.[17] UVB is thought to cause cancer by damaging DNA and its repair systems, which results in mutations that may lead to cancer. It is also thought to play a role in cellular immunity by impairing T-cell function and increasing suppressor T-cell numbers.

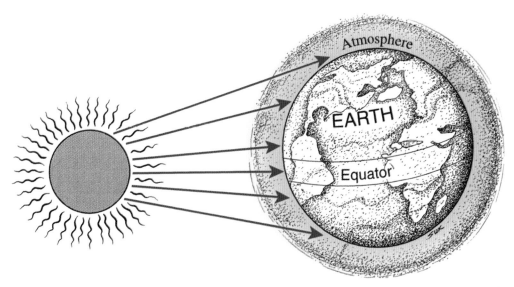

Fig. 36.2 Areas near the equator receive more direct sunlight than areas closer to the poles. Note the way the angled rays near the poles are filtered through larger amounts of the atmosphere before they reach the earth.

Tanning salons have marketed their product as safe for everyone by stating that their machines only put out ultraviolet A (UVA) rays and filter out UVB radiation, which is the most damaging to the skin. However, a 2018 study reported in Cancer Causes & Control found that given the large number of skin cancer cases attributable to indoor tanning, these findings highlight a major public health issue.[18]

Indoor tanning is noted as being a World Health Organization group 1 carcinogen[19] associated with melanoma and nonmelanoma skin cancer (NMSC).[18] Studies have linked indoor tanning practices to an increasing number of cases melanoma and NMSC in Europe and the United States.[18,20,21] The risk of all types of skin cancer is highest in those exposed at young ages, which suggests a susceptibility period in early life. Indoor tanning has even been banned in several locations, including Brazil in 2011 and Australia in 2015.[22] Researchers point to tanning beds and their accompanying UV radiation as a likely culprit, particularly with regard to the high rate of skin cancer in younger age groups. Canada, the United States, Australia, several European countries including France and Germany, and several South American countries including Chile have enforceable indoor tanning legislation that establish conditions of use in response to the increase in carcinogenic potential.[22]

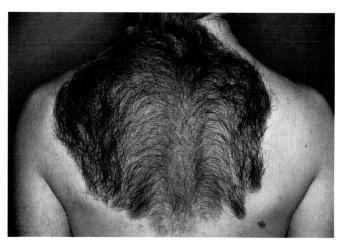

Fig. 36.3 This child with a giant hairy nevus has approximately an 8% chance of development of a melanoma within the first 15 years of life. Because of the high risk, this lesion will be removed in a series of prophylactic surgical procedures. (From James WD, Elston D, Treat JR, et al. *Andrews' Diseases of the Skin: Clinical Dermatology.* 13th ed. Philadelphia, PA: Elsevier; 2020.)

Studies have shown that the stratum corneum absorbs UVB (see the Anatomy and Physiology section in this chapter), whereas 50% of UVA radiation is able to penetrate to the highly mitotic basal layer of the skin, where the potential for malignant changes and premature aging of the skin exists.[23]

Like many other cancers, skin cancer is a disease of aging. Most skin cancers appear after age 50 years, but the damaging effects of the sun's rays are accumulated over a lifetime. Although this is true, skin cancers can develop in infants, children, and young adults, especially those with high risk factors (e.g., xeroderma pigmentosum, giant hairy nevi).

Other Factors Associated With Skin Cancers Other Than Melanoma. Other factors that contribute to NMSCs include exposure to arsenic (an element used in medicines and poisons) and therapeutic or occupational exposure to radiation. Irradiation, particularly if experienced early in life, increases the long-term risk of both basal and SCC of the skin.[19] For basal cell, early exposure to radiation treatment was a risk factor mostly among those without a history of severe sunburns; with SCC, radiation treatment was a risk factor mostly for those with a sun-sensitive skin type.[24]

Besides xeroderma pigmentosum, another genetic condition associated with the formation of BCCs is called basal cell nevus syndrome (a genetically linked condition that appears during the late teen years). Symptoms include multiple BCCs of the skin, cysts of the jaw bones, pitting of the palms and soles, and skeletal anomalies (particularly of the ribs).[25]

SCCs of the skin have also been associated with the following[26-28]:
- Excessive sun exposure.
- Human papillomavirus infection.
- Weakened immune system.
- Rare genetic disorders.
- A personal history of precancerous or cancerous skin lesions.
- Scars or chronic inflammatory conditions.
- Hydrocarbons derived from coal and petroleum.
- Areas of chronic drainage (e.g., fistulas, sinuses).

Smoking is a proven cause of SCC of the lip. It has also been linked to the development of squamous cell skin cancer in other anatomic areas. However, whether cigarette smoke acts directly as a skin carcinogen or has an adverse effect on the immune system, inhibiting the body's ability to defend itself from cancer, is not known.[28]

Other Factors Associated With Melanoma Skin Cancers. Melanomas develop from melanocytes (the skin cells that produce melanin), which grow in clusters to form a mole, or nevus. Moles can be broadly classified according to when they are acquired: congenital melanocytic nevi (those present at birth) and common acquired nevi (those that develop later in life).

Congenital melanocytic nevi can be classified into three sizes: small (less than 1.5 cm in diameter), medium (1.5–19.9 cm in diameter), and large (≥20 cm in diameter).[29] Large nevi (Fig. 36.3) are accompanied by a small risk of development of melanoma compared with a 1% risk in the general population. Some surgeons believe that these moles should be removed prophylactically before malignant changes can occur. Prophylactic removal of small and medium lesions should be made individually because the chance of malignant change in them is small.

Melanocytic nevi can be grouped into three main categories: junctional, compound, and intradermal. Junctional nevi tend to be small (usually <6 mm), well-circumscribed, flat lesions with smooth surfaces that are uniformly brown or black and circular. The melanocyte clusters in junctional nevi are found above the basement layer. Compound nevi contain melanocyte clusters in the dermis and epidermis. They appear as small, well-circumscribed, slightly raised papules that often contain excess hair. The surface is rough, and color ranges from tan to brown throughout. Over time, these lesions may take on a nodular appearance. Intradermal nevi are small, well-circumscribed, dome-shaped lesions that range from flesh to brown. They, too, may contain excess hair. Melanocytic clusters are found only in the dermal layer in these moles.[30]

The propensity of a mole to develop into a melanoma is related to the location of the melanocytic clusters found in the moles. Intradermal nevi rarely transform into melanomas; the likelihood of junctional and compound nevi transforming into melanomas is far greater. One theory for this pattern is that melanocytes located in the dermis do not receive as much UV exposure because they are located deep in the skin. Melanocytes in junctional and compound nevi are closer to the skin's surface and receive higher amounts of melanoma-inducing UV radiation.

Dysplastic nevi, also known as atypical moles, are acquired pigmented lesions of the skin that have one or more of the clinical features of melanoma: asymmetry, border irregularity, color variation, or a diameter greater than 6 mm.[30] Dysplastic nevi are precursor lesions for melanoma and so should be considered important primarily because of their association with an increased risk for melanoma.[31]

The number of moles a person has also influences the chances of acquiring melanoma. People with many moles or dysplastic nevi have a higher risk of developing melanoma. Photographing these moles and monitoring them becomes important in ensuring that any changes are realized early.

People with a family history of melanoma have an eightfold increase in their chances of acquiring the disease.[32] Several studies have pinpointed to a region on the short arm of chromosome 9 (9p) as one involved in the early-stage development of melanoma tumors. Genetic material from this area is thought to play a vital role in the suppression of tumor formation. Without this material, a person may be more susceptible to tumor formation because one of the normal defense mechanisms may be missing. Other chromosomal abnormalities associated with melanomas can be found on chromosomes 1, 6, 7, 11, and 19.[33]

Some families are affected with an inherited familial atypical mole and melanoma syndrome, also known as dysplastic nevus syndrome. The syndrome is defined by: (1) occurrence of melanoma in one or more first-degree or second-degree relatives; (2) a large number of moles (often 50+), some of which are atypical and often variable in size; and (3) moles that have certain distinct histologic features. Persons with this syndrome have a markedly increased risk of development of melanoma. These patients need close monitoring because of the high risks involved. This syndrome has also been described in the nonfamilial setting.[30]

Anatomy and Physiology

The skin is the largest organ of the body; it covers about 17 to 20 ft^2 on the average person. The skin provides many functions:

- It regulates body temperature through perspiration (as perspiration evaporates, it carries heat away from the body) and blood flow through vessels located in the dermis (the skin allows heat carried by the blood to radiate off its surface).
- It acts as a barrier between the external environment and the body, offering protection against factors such as trauma, UV light, and bacterial invasion.
- It participates in the production of vitamin D, which is vital to the process that enables the body to absorb and use calcium in the gastrointestinal tract.
- It provides receptors for external stimuli such as heat, cold, pressure, and touch, allowing the body to be aware of its environment.

Vitamin D is often referred to as the "sunshine vitamin" because the body manufactures vitamin D after being exposed to the sun.[34] Vitamin D is important in the body's absorption of calcium, and it also helps the body keep the right amount of calcium and phosphorus in the blood. Ten to 15 minutes of natural sunlight three times a week is more than enough to keep up with the body's requirements. Vitamin D can also be found in most dairy products, such as milk and cheese, and in fish, oysters, and many fortified cereals.[34]

The skin is an example of an epithelial membrane, a connective tissue covered by a layer of epithelial tissue. The connective tissue layer in the skin is called the dermis; the epithelial layer is called the epidermis (Fig. 36.4). These layers are held together by an intermediate layer called the basement membrane.[35,36]

The dermis is the deeper layer of the skin composed of connective tissue that contains blood and lymphatic vessels, nerves and nerve endings, sweat glands, sebaceous glands, and hair follicles. It contains mainly elastic and collagen fibers that allow for the flexibility and strength of the skin. The upper 20% of the dermis is referred to as the papillary layer and contains dermal papillae, ridges that are responsible for the formation of fingerprints. The lower level of the dermis is the reticular layer and contains many accessory structures of the skin, such as: hair follicles, sebaceous (oil) and sudoriferous (sweat) glands and their ducts, nerve endings, blood vessels, and sensory receptors such as laminated (Pacinian) corpuscles that respond to heavy pressure.[35,36]

A subcutaneous layer that contains nerves, blood vessels, adipose (fat) tissue, and areolar connective tissue lies beneath the dermis. Because the epidermis is avascular, the blood vessels of the dermis and subcutaneous layer are responsible for the nutritional status of the epidermis.

The epidermis is the extremely thin outer layer of the skin, composed of four to five layers (depending on its location). These layers are as follows, from deepest to most superficial[36]:

1. **Stratum basale (base layer).** This is the basal layer that contains stem cells capable of producing keratinocytes (stratified epithelial cells, which comprise most of the epidermal cells of the skin and provide a barrier between the host and the environment and prevent the entry of toxic substances from the environment and the loss of important constituents from the host) and cells that give rise to glands and hair follicles. This layer also contains melanocytes, cells with branching processes that produce the pigment melanin. In hairless skin, a third type of cell, Merkel cells, can also be found. Together with a flattened portion of a neuron called a tactile (Merkel disc), Merkel cells function in the sensation of touch. Tumors of the Merkel cells do occur, and when they do, they are often lethal.

2. **Stratum spinosum (spiny layer).** This layer contains rows of keratinocytes, which have a spiny appearance microscopically. Branches from the melanocytes reach into this layer and allow the keratinocytes to absorb the protective pigment melanin via exocytosis.

3. **Stratum granulosum (granular layer).** This layer contains three to five rows of somewhat flattened cells. The keratinocytes begin to produce a substance called keratohyalin, which is a precursor to a waterproof protein called keratin.

4. **Stratum lucidum (clear layer).** This layer is normally found only in areas in which thick skin is present (soles and palms) and contains three to five rows of clear, flat cells that contain eleidin, another keratin precursor.

5. **Stratum corneum (horny layer).** This layer forms the skin surface and contains thicker rows of flat, dead, scaly (squamous) cells that are filled with keratin and have lost all their internal organelles, including nuclei. The lower layers of cells are closely packed and adhere to each other, whereas the upper layers of cells are loosely packed and continually flake away from the surface.

The stratum basale and stratum spinosum together are sometimes called the stratum germinativum or growth layer.

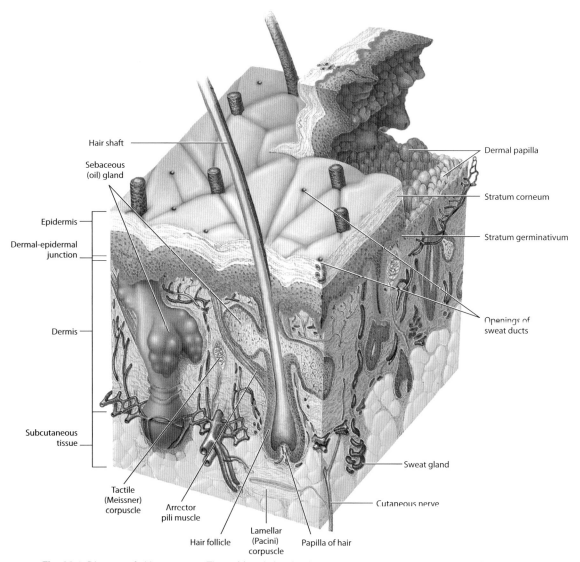

Fig. 36.4 Diagram of skin structure. The epidermis is raised at one corner to reveal the papillae of the dermis. (From Thibodeau GA, Patton KT: *The human body in health & disease*, ed 7, St. Louis, 2018, Mosby, Copyright Elsevier (2018).)

The outer, protective layer of the skin is composed of dead cells filled with keratin. Each day, millions of these cells are sloughed off and continually replaced by cells from the lower layers of the epidermis. Germ cells in the stratum basale give rise to keratinocytes, which go through a process called keratinization as they are pushed toward the surface by new cells. As the cells are relocated, they accumulate keratin to the point that the cells can no longer function, flatten out, and die. The mature keratinocytes serve their protective function and are eventually shed from the surface of the skin. The time necessary for the cell to travel from the germ layer to the surface is approximately 2 to 4 weeks. This cycle continually repeats itself.

Melanin is a pigment that serves a protective function of the skin. It is produced by the melanocytes and absorbed by the keratinocytes in the stratum spinosum layer of the epidermis. UV light damages the keratinocytes by inhibiting synthesis of DNA and RNA (genetic material in the cell), which leads to cell dysfunction

or death. The melanin absorbed by the keratinocytes is placed in the cell so that it lies between the skin surface and nucleus of the cell, thus protecting it from the sun's rays like an umbrella (Fig. 36.5).

Melanin is one of the pigments responsible for differences in skin color among individuals. The more melanin a person's skin contains, the darker his or her skin will be. The number of melanocytes is about the same in all races. Differences in skin darkness are attributed to the amount of melanin that the melanocytes produce. The systemic release of melanocyte-stimulating hormone from the anterior pituitary gland controls overall skin darkness. The more melanocyte-stimulating hormone released by the pituitary, the more melanin the melanocytes produce and the darker the person's skin is.[37] Variations in skin darkness can occur in localized areas of the body because of exposure to UV light. Brief exposure to UV light causes melanin already present in the epidermis to darken considerably, whereas long-term exposure causes melanocytes to increase

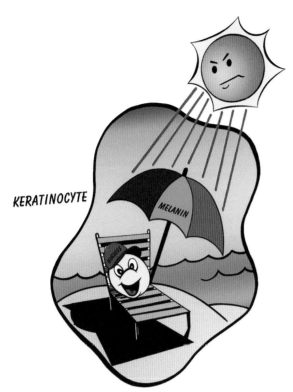

Fig. 36.5 This cartoon depicts the way melanin is strategically placed inside the keratinocyte between the nucleus and sun's rays, protecting it from ultraviolet radiation.

melanin production. Both processes result in darker or tanned skin. A tan is a response by the body to damage caused by UV light. In the absence of UV stimulation, melanocytes decrease melanin production to normal levels, and the skin returns to a normal color.[23]

Skin cancers can be classified according to the cell of the skin from which they originate. Melanoma, one of the more lethal forms of skin cancer (perhaps second only to Merkel cell carcinoma), arises from the melanocytes located in the stratum basale. The most common sites for melanoma are the legs of women and the trunk and face of men. Melanomas can also arise in other areas of the body, such as the uvea of the eye (choroid, iris, or ciliary body) and the mucosal surfaces of the aerodigestive and genitourinary tracts.

BCC, a slow-growing form of skin cancer that does not tend to metastasize, and arises from the stem cells of the stratum basale. It is the most prevalent cancer in humans and, if left untreated, can cause extensive damage.

SCC, a faster-growing cancer than the basal cell type with a higher propensity for metastasis, arises from the more mature keratinocytes of the upper layers of the epidermis. This type of NMSC can arise anywhere on the body but is especially common on sun-exposed areas, such as the head, neck, face, arms, and hands.

Merkel cell carcinoma is a rare tumor thought to arise from Merkel (tactile) cells. It is known for high rates of recurrence after surgical excision, frequent involvement of regional lymph nodes, and distant metastasis that can lead to death. These tumors are structurally like small cell carcinomas and appear as firm, nontender, pink-red nodular lesions with an intact epidermis.[38] These types of cancers are often treated with a combination of chemotherapy and radiation therapy or surgery. Merkel cell carcinoma has evolved in its distinction from other skin cancers and has specific staging criteria and clinical treatment pathways, inclusive of the National Comprehensive Cancer Network guidelines that outline current treatment methods.

Other types of cancers can arise in the skin but are not covered in detail in this chapter. These include but are not limited to the following[39]:

1. **Adenocarcinoma** of the sebaceous and sudoriferous glands. This type of cancer arises in the dermal layer of the skin and is a slow-growing lesion capable of metastasis. It tends to be radioresistant; therefore surgery is the treatment of choice.
2. **Cutaneous lymphoma,** including mycosis fungoides. This disease of lymphocytes can resemble eczema or other inflammatory conditions and tends to remain localized to the skin for long periods. Total skin electron beam radiation therapy has been used to control early stages of the disease. Systemic therapy and total skin electron beam therapy can provide benefit in later disease stages.
3. **Kaposi sarcoma.** This is a slow-growing tumor thought to arise from vascular tissue. The associated nodular purple lesions are often multifocal and common in individuals affected with acquired immunodeficiency syndrome (AIDS) and those of Mediterranean origins. Surgical excision and radiation therapy are viable options for management of localized disease, and systemic therapy can be used for widespread disease.
4. Patients with immunocompromised conditions (including those with AIDS) can harbor an aggressive variant of this disease. Although associated lesions are radiosensitive, patients who acquire it may have a poor prognosis and may be best treated systemically with chemotherapy. Radiation therapy is used to palliate local areas.

> The National Comprehensive Cancer Network (NCCN) is a nonprofit alliance of renowned cancer centers from around the world that strives to improve cancer care by way of defining and sharing guidelines that help define the standard of care for different cancers. Guidelines produced by the NCCN are often cited as clinical practice expands its boundaries. Continued quality improvement and effectiveness of treatment are core goals of the group, and through them, patients benefit from better care.

Clinical Presentation

Although skin cancers and melanomas occur in a wide variety of shapes, sizes, and appearances, similarities exist that facilitate lesion classification. The following is a discussion concerning the tumors seen most often and premalignant growths that may precede them.

Nonmelanoma Precursors and Characteristics. Premalignant lesions are those that, if left untreated or not closely monitored, can develop into cancer. SCCs tend to arise more often from precursor lesions compared with BCCs.[40] The following is a nonexhaustive list of precancerous lesions for nonmelanomas[41]:

1. Actinic (solar) keratoses. These warty lesions or areas of red, scaly patches occur on the sun-exposed skin of the face or hands of older, light-skinned individuals (Fig. 36.6).
2. **Arsenical keratoses.** These multiple, hard, corn-like masses on the palms of hands or soles of feet result from long-term arsenic ingestion.
3. **Bowen disease.** This precancerous dermatosis or carcinoma in situ is characterized by the development of pink or brown papules covered with a thickened, horny layer (Fig. 36.7).
4. Keratoacanthoma. This rapid-growing lesion can appear suddenly as a dome-shaped mass on a sun-exposed area (Fig. 36.8). Microscopically, the nodules are composed of well-differentiated squamous epithelia with a necrotic center or central keratin mass. They can be difficult to distinguish from squamous cell cancer and usually resolve themselves if left untreated.

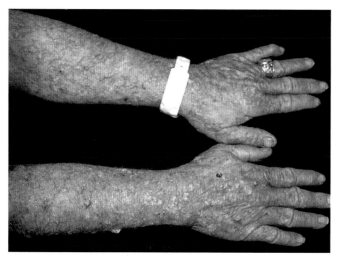

Fig. 36.6 Actinic keratosis. (From James WD, et al: *Andrews' Diseases of the Skin: Clinical Dermatology*. 13th ed. Philadelphia, PA: Elsevier; 2020.)

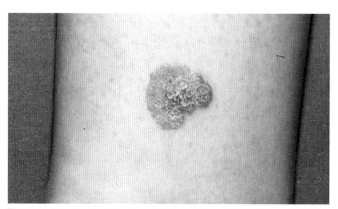

Fig.36.7 Bowen disease. (From Ralston SH, et al. *Davidson's Principles and Practice of Medicine*. 23rd ed. London, UK: Elsevier Ltd.; 2018.)

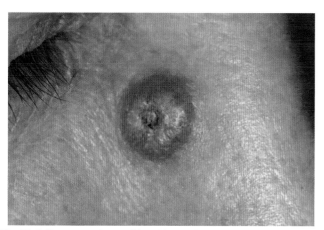

Fig. 36.8 Keratoacanthoma. (From Neville BW, et al. *Color Atlas of Oral and Maxillofacial Diseases*. Philadelphia, PA: Elsevier; 2019.)

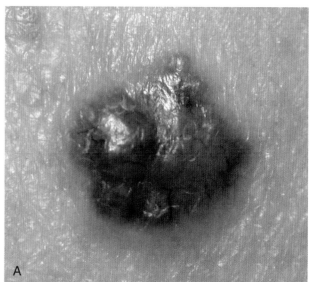

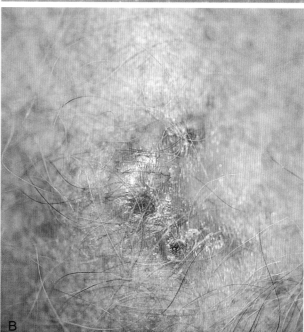

Fig. 36.9 (A and B) Examples of basal cell carcinomas. (From James WD, et al. *Andrews' Diseases of the Skin: Clinical Dermatology*. 13th ed. Philadelphia, PA: Elsevier; 2020.)

head, and neck. Other symptoms that possibly indicate a BCC or SCC include a sore that takes longer than 3 weeks to heal, a recurrent red patch that may itch or be tender, and a wart that bleeds or scabs. Some BCCs may contain melanin, which causes the lesion to appear black and resemble a melanoma. In general, any new growths that persist or change in appearance should be reported to a physician.

Melanoma Precursors and Characteristics. Introduced in the mid-1980s, the ABCD clinical rule assesses the following:

A, *Asymmetry.* Melanomas tend to be asymmetric; most benign moles tend to be symmetric.

B, *Border.* Melanomas tend to have notched, uneven borders; most benign moles tend to possess clearly defined, smooth borders.

C, *Color.* Melanomas can contain different shades of black, brown, or tan; benign moles tend to be uniformly tan or brown.

Squamous and BCCs have a multitude of appearances (Figs. 36.9 and 36.10). BCCs tend to arise as smooth, red, or milky lumps and have a pearly border and multiple telangiectasia (tiny blood vessels visible on the skin's surface). BCCs can be shiny or pale. About 80% of BCCs occur on the head and neck.[42] SCCs tend to have a scaly, crusty, slightly elevated lesion that may have a cutaneous horn and often present on the sun exposed areas of the body such as the arms,

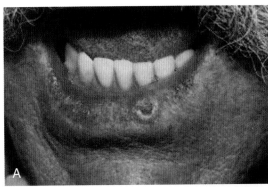

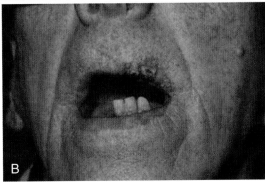

Fig. 36.10 (A) and (B) Examples of squamous cell carcinomas. (From White GM, Cox NH [eds.]: *Diseases of the skin, a color atlas and text,* ed 2, St Louis, 2006, Mosby. Copyright Elsevier (2006).)

D, Diameter. Most melanomas have a diameter greater than 6 mm; most benign moles tend to be less than 6 mm in diameter (about the size of a pencil eraser).[43,44]

Although the ABCD assessment rule has significantly helped clinicians recognize melanoma earlier and encouraged patients to seek medical advice earlier, it is not usually sufficient to uncover melanoma in situ; when the natural asymmetry of melanoma becomes visible to the naked eye, it is likely that the tumor has already invaded the dermis.[43] Fig. 36.11 demonstrates these presentation aspects.

In addition to the ABCDs, the following changes in the appearance of a mole should be monitored as possible signs of melanoma:

1. Change in *color:* red, white, or blue areas in addition to black and tan.
2. Change in *surface:* scaly, flaky, bleeding, or oozing moles or a sore that does not heal.
3. Change in *texture:* hard, lumpy, or elevated moles.
4. Change in *surrounding skin:* spread of pigmentation, swelling, or redness to surrounding skin.
5. Change in *sensation:* unusual pain or tenderness in a mole.
6. Change in *previously normal skin:* pigmented areas that arise in previously normal skin.[43]

A few pigmented lesions of the skin are benign, but these can be difficult to distinguish from melanoma. They are as follows:

1. **Simple lentigo.** This small (1-mm to 5-mm), brown to black macule is round with sharply defined edges, and the surface is flat, like a freckle. Thought to be the precursor to the common mole, some simple lentigines are clinically indistinguishable from junctional nevi.
2. **Solar lentigo.** This small to medium, flat, lightly pigmented macule is better known as a liver spot. It is especially common in older white people on areas of the skin chronically exposed to the sun.
3. **Seborrheic keratoses.** These round or ovoid, wartlike papules range from a few to several millimeters. These growths tend to be

raised (often with a warty, "stuck-on" appearance) and composed of proliferating epidermal cells, especially of the basal type.
4. **Others.** Some common moles may be difficult to distinguish from melanoma. For a description of common moles, see the section on Etiology.

Although all these lesions tend to be benign, they should be monitored for signs of malignant change. Questionable lesions should be biopsied and analyzed to rule out malignancy.

Detection and Diagnosis

The skin lends itself easily to self-inspection and cancer detection. If people were educated on the way to detect skin cancer and took the time to inspect themselves, skin cancer could be found at an early stage and therefore be easily treatable. The following are some of the methods used to detect and diagnose skin cancer.

Everyone should inspect the total surface area of the skin monthly for signs of cancer (Box 36.1). Individuals at high risk should have photographs of the skin taken to document existing moles to which they can refer when questions arise concerning factors such as the size, color, and shape of moles. Body charts that indicate the locations and sizes of moles may also be useful.

Inspections should take place in well-lit areas. Familiarity with existing moles, freckles, and blemishes is important so that newly pigmented areas or blemishes can be distinguished from older ones. When surveying the skin, individuals should consider the ABCD rules. In addition, people should watch for sores that do not heal or other areas of unexplained changes in the skin.

Any unusual changes should be brought to the attention of a physician. The earlier skin cancer is detected, the better the chance it will be cured. People who find unusual lesions must not let their fears of pain, cost, or disfigurement get in the way of seeking a proper diagnosis and treatment. Skin cancer is not something that goes away by itself.

A routine physical examination should include a thorough inspection of the skin's surface by the physician. Physicians must be knowledgeable in distinguishing between benign and malignant conditions; and regional lymph nodes should be inspected for signs or symptoms of metastasis. Also, a family history should be acquired to determine whether a person is at higher risk for development of melanoma because a family member previously had the disease. Patients with a family history of melanoma should be monitored closely.

Individuals should have a biopsy performed for unusual or suspicious lesions. Depending on the size and location of the lesion, the biopsy may be incisional (only a portion of the lesion is removed for tissue diagnosis, usually reserved for large lesions) or excisional (entire lesion is removed). Excisional biopsies (including punch, saucerization, or elliptic incision) may be indicated for suspected SCCs or melanomas to ascertain the depth of the tumor's penetration and should include a portion of the underlying subcutaneous fat for accurate microstaging. A shave or curettage may be adequate for diagnosis of BCC, but is not recommended for lesions suspected to be melanoma.[45,46]

To the naked eye, some lesions are difficult to define as malignant or nonmalignant without a biopsy. A relatively new technique in the diagnosis of melanomas is in vivo (in tissue) epiluminescence microscopy (ELM), or dermatoscopy. ELM is a noninvasive procedure that allows physicians to differentiate between benign and malignant lesions while they are in the early phases of development and have not yet begun to exhibit the features displayed by later melanomatous lesions. The procedure uses a dermatoscope, which resembles an ophthalmoscope. Mineral oil is placed on the surface of the lesion to cause the stratum corneum to become almost invisible and to facilitate the examination of the epidermis, particularly the dermal-epidermal junction. ELM

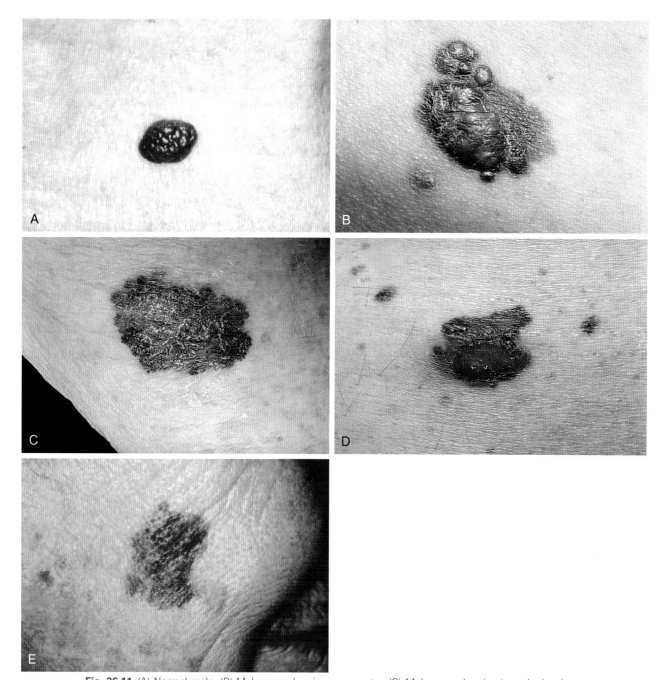

Fig. 36.11 (A) Normal mole. (B) Melanoma showing asymmetry. (C) Melanoma showing irregular borders. (D) Melanoma showing uneven color. (E) Melanoma showing a large diameter. (A and E, Courtesy the National Cancer Institute. B, C, and D, From Callen JP, et al. *Color Atlas of Dermatology.* 2nd ed. Philadelphia, PA: Saunders; 2000.)

images can be digitized by primary care physicians and exported to ELM experts via the internet for quick analysis.[47] Digitized ELM images can also be fed into computers run with specially designed software. These programs evaluate lesions based on factors such as shape, size, color, and border and attempt to make an objective analysis on a previously subjective science.

A dermatologist should be able to identify a type of lesion just by its appearance. Based on this information, the dermatologist should also have a good idea concerning the metastatic potential of the lesion. Again, BCCs have an extremely small chance of metastasis, SCCs have a slightly higher chance, and melanomas have the highest chance of all the common skin cancers.

If the physician suspects that a patient may have an advanced SCC or melanoma, an evaluation for metastasis should be conducted. This evaluation should include the following:

- Physical examination of the patient to find evidence of lymphadenopathy, secondary lesions of the skin, or second primaries
- Evaluation of motor skills to detect possible nerve or brain involvement
- Chest x-ray examination to rule out lung metastasis
- Liver function tests to rule out liver involvement
- Evaluation of alkaline phosphatase levels and bone scan if patient reports bone pain
- Complete blood counts to detect anemias that may be the result of gastrointestinal bleeding caused by metastasis

- A simple skin self-examination performed monthly can aid in the early detection of cancer. The best time to do this self-examination is after a shower or bath in a well-lit room with a full-length and handheld mirror. During the first examination, it is best to begin by noting the location of birthmarks, moles, and blemishes and what they *usually* look like. Check for anything new: a change in the size, texture, or color of a mole or a sore that does not heal.

Examination While Standing
- Check your face, ears, neck, chest, and stomach. Women will need to lift their breasts to check the skin underneath.
- Check **all** areas, including the back, the scalp, between the buttocks, and the genital area.
- Look at the front and back of your body in the mirror; then raise your arms and look at the left and right sides.
- Bend your elbows and look carefully at your palms, fingers, and fingernails; forearms, including the undersides; and the upper arms.
- Examine the back and front of your legs.

Examination While Sitting
- Closely examine your thighs, shins, and feet, including the tops, soles, toes, toenails, and the spaces between the toes.
- Look at the face, neck, and scalp. Use a comb or a blow dryer to move hair to visualize the scalp.

Modified from the American Cancer Society. Skin exams: checking your own skin. https://www.cancer.org/cancer/skin-cancer/prevention-and-early-detection/skin-exams.html. Accessed February 23, 2019.

- Biopsy of regional lymph nodes to compare the number of lymph nodes positive for tumor with the total number of nodes in the biopsy

Computed tomography (CT) and magnetic resonance imaging (MRI) examinations are employed more frequently when signs and symptoms point to locally advanced or metastatic disease. Because melanoma can spread to virtually any part of the body, CT scans (with or without positron emission tomography [PET]) of the neck, chest, abdomen, and pelvis may be ordered to rule out involvement of the lymph nodes, lung, liver, bowel, adrenals, and subcutaneous skin. MRI is often used to assess the brain for potential metastases.

Pathology and Staging

Melanoma. After it has been removed, the biopsy specimen is sent to a pathologist who examines it microscopically and provides information that is used to diagnose, stage, and develop a prognosis for the patient. Essential to a pathology report for melanoma include the diagnosis (whether the biopsy specimen indicates cancer), the thickness of the tumor, and the status of the margins (whether tumor cells are present on the edges of the biopsy specimen). If cancer is diagnosed, additional information may include the following:
- Specific cancer subtype
- Depth of tumor penetration
- Degree of mitotic activity (reproductive rate of cells)
- Growth pattern (radial versus lateral)
- Level of host response (number of lymphocytes present in or around the tumor)
- Presence, if any, of tumor ulceration, tumor regression, or satellitosis (lymphatic extensions of the tumor that result in small lesions adjacent to the primary)

Melanomas can be classified according to their growth patterns, and histologic appearances can be grouped into the following four major categories[48]:
1. *Superficial spreading melanomas (SSMs)*, also called radial spreading melanomas, are the most common melanoma subtype, accounting for approximately 70% of all lesions. They generally arise on any anatomic site as preexisting lesions that evolve over several years and have a radial (horizontal) growth pattern. The periphery of these deeply pigmented lesions is often notched or irregular, and colors in the tumors can vary from brown, black, red, pink, or white. Partial regression of the tumor is common. As time passes, the tumor tends to grow more vertically, which results in a more elevated, irregular surface.
2. *Nodular melanomas (NMs)* account for approximately 15% of all lesions and can also occur on any anatomic site. They are twice as common in men as in women. Lesions tend to be raised throughout and vary in color from dark brown, blue, or blue-black. Some lesions may not contain any pigment at all (amelanotic). These tumors are particularly lethal because they lack a radial growth phase, which makes an early diagnosis difficult. They tend to invade early and frequently and show ulceration when advanced.
3. *Lentigo maligna melanomas (LMMs)*, also called Hutchinson freckles, account for approximately 5% of all lesions and tend to occur in chronically sun-exposed skin of older white people, especially females. LMM begins with a relatively benign radial growth phase that may last for decades before it enters its vertical growth phase. The appearance of an LMM is similar to that of an SMM but lacks the red hues and has minimal elevation during its vertical growth phase.
4. *Acral lentiginous melanomas (ALMs)* account for approximately 10% of all lesions and are found mainly on the palms, soles, nail beds, or mucous membranes. The ALM is the most common form of melanoma in blacks and Asians and has a tan or brown flat stain on the palms or soles. An ALM can also appear as a brown to black discoloration under the nail bed and is often mistaken for a fungal infection.

Because melanocytes are found in the basal layer of the epidermis, melanoma formation takes place in this area. Most melanomas begin their development with a radial (horizontal) growth phase (Fig. 36.12), during which abnormal melanocytes form nests along the basal layer. Later, some of the melanocytes begin to migrate into and form nests in the upper layers of the epidermis. The horizontal phase can last up to 15 years in instances of SSM and 5 years in instances of LMM, or it may be an extremely short (or nonexistent) period in instances of NM.

The second phase of development is the vertical growth phase. During this phase, melanocytes descend across the basal lamina and into the dermis. During this phase, nodules may also become raised on the skin's surface. After invasion into the dermis has taken place, inflammatory cells arrive to defend the body from foreign invaders. If these cells are successful, a spontaneous regression may take place. If they are not successful, the melanoma grows deeper into the dermis and may involve the blood and lymphatic vessels, thus possibly helping the melanoma spread to regional lymph nodes or virtually any organ of the body.[49]

Drs. Wallace Clark and Alexander Breslow developed a microstaging system for melanomas. Both systems are basically indirect measures of tumor volume. Clark's system categorizes melanomas based on their level of invasion through the epidermis and layers of the dermis. Clark's levels (Fig. 36.13) may indicate the potential for metastasis because the access of tumor cells to lymphatic and vascular structures

Melanoma staging is critical in facilitating communication between patients and the care team, assisting in the clinical treatment decision-making process.[52,53] The AJCC updated its assessment system for melanoma of the skin to changes since the manual's 7th edition; the tumor node metastasis (TNM) system has been modified to consider these changes. Familiar to most radiation oncology professionals, this system for melanoma assesses primary tumor thickness, regional node status, and distant metastatic sites as follows[1]:

Melanoma: Primary Tumor (T)

T Category	Thickness	Ulceration Status
TX (Primary tumor cannot be assessed)	Not applicable	Not applicable
T0 (No evidence of primary tumor)	Not applicable	Not applicable
Tis (Melanoma in situ)	Not applicable	Not applicable
T1	<1.0 mm	Unknown or unspecified
T1a	<0.8 mm	Without ulceration
I1b	<0.8mm	With ulceration
	0.8–1.0 mm	With or without ulceration
T2	>1.0–2.0 mm	Unknown or unspecified
T2a	>1.0–2.0 mm	Without ulceration
T2b	>1.0–2.0 mm	With ulceration
T3	>2.0–4.0 mm	Unknown or unspecified
T3a	>2.0–4.0 mm	Without ulceration
T3b	>2.0–4.0 mm	With ulceration
T4	>4.0 mm	Unknown or unspecified
T4a	>4.0 mm	Without ulceration
T4b	>4.0 mm	With ulceration

Melanoma: Regional Lymph Nodes (N)

N Category	Number of Tumor-Involved Regional Lymph Nodes	Presence of In-Transit, Satellite, and/or Microsatellite Metastasis
NX	Regional lymph nodes cannot be assessed Exception: pathological N category is not required for T1 melanoma, use cN	No
N0	No regional metastasis detected	No
N1	One tumor involved node or in-transit, satellite, and/or microsatellite metastases with no tumor-involved nodes	
N1a	One clinically occult	No
N1b	One clinically detected	No
N1c	No regional lymph node disease	Yes
N2	Two or three tumor-involved node or in-transit, satellite, and/or microsatellite metastases with no tumor-involved nodes	

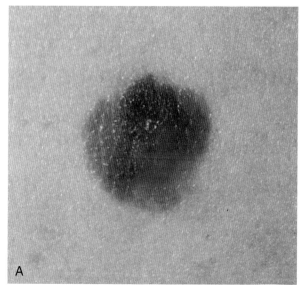

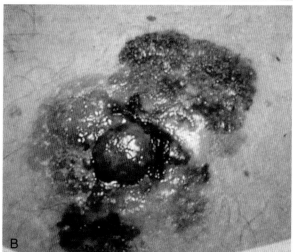

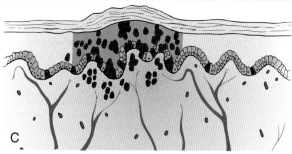

Fig. 36.12 Melanomas: A and B indicate superficial view depicting initial horizontal growth pattern. Image C shows a cross section of a superficial spreading melanoma showing the vertical phase indicative of most late melanomas.

are assessable. Also, the extent of invasion may indicate the tumor's progression from relatively harmless radial growth to more aggressive vertical growth.[49]

Breslow's system historically categorizes melanomas based on tumor thickness from the top of the granular layer of the epidermis or, if the primary tumor is ulcerated, from the ulcer surface to the deepest identifiable melanoma cell, as measured by an ocular micrometer.[50] The revised 2017 American Joint Committee on Cancer (AJCC) staging classification system is the current classification system of choice.[51]

N Category	Number of Tumor-Involved Regional Lymph Nodes	Presence of In-Transit, Satellite, and/or Microsatellite Metastasis
N2a	Two or three clinically occult	No
N2b	Two or three, of which one was clinically detected	No
N2c	One clinically occult or clinically detected	Yes
N3	Four or more tumor-involved node or in-transit, satellite, and/or microsatellite metastases with no tumor-involved nodes	
N3a	Four or more clinically occult	No
N3b	Four or more, of which one was clinically detected, or presence of any matted nodes	No
N3c	Two or more clinically occult or clinically detected, and/or presence of any number of matted nodes	Yes

M Category	Anatomic Site	LDH Level (lactate dehydrogenase)
M0	No evidence of distant metastasis	Not applicable
M1		See below
M1a	Metastasis to skin, subcutaneous tissues, or distant lymph nodes	Not recorded or unspecified
M1a(0)		Not elevated
M1a(1)		Elevated
M1b	Distant metastasis to lung with or without M1a sites of disease	Not recorded or unspecified
M1b(0)		Not elevated
M1b(1)		Elevated
M1c	Distant metastasis to noncentral nervous system (CNS) visceral sites with or without M1a or M1b sites of disease	Not recorded or unspecified
M1c(0)		Not elevated
M1c(1)		Elevated
M1d	Distant metastasis to CNS visceral sites with or without M1a, M1b, or M1c sites of disease	Not recorded or unspecified
M1d(0)		Normal
M1d(1)		Elevated

After a tumor has been classified according to the TNM system, it is typically organized into specific stages. Stage groupings allow healthcare workers to categorize patients with similar disease patterns to assist the care team in treatment planning, facilitation of information exchange, indicate disease spread risk and prognosis, and help evaluate treatment results. In assessment of metastatic spread potential, stage I tumors have a low risk, stage II through IIIA have an intermediate risk, stage IIIB have a high risk, and stage IIIC and IV have a very high risk.[9] The presence of melanoma ulceration upstages the prognosis of stages I to III. The clinical anatomic stage/prognostic groupings that relate TNM and are staged as follows[1]:

The Clinical Stage Is	When T Is	And N Is	And M Is
0	Tis	N0	M0
IA	T1a	N0	M0
IB	T1b	N0	M0
	T2a	N0	M0
IIA	T2b	N0	M0
	T3a	N0	M0
IIB	T3b	N0	M0
	T4a	N0	M0
IIC	T4b	N0	M0
III	Any T, Tis	≥N1	M0
IV	Any T	Any N	M1

Survival rates for patients with an ulcerated melanoma are proportionately lower than those with a nonulcerated melanoma of the same T category but similar to those for patients with a nonulcerated melanoma of the next higher T category.[1]

The two most significant characteristics of the primary melanoma are tumor thickness and ulceration. Other significant prognostic factors are age, site of the primary melanoma, level of invasion, and gender, as noted in the following list:

1. *Tumor thickness.* Thicker tumors yield a poorer prognosis.
2. *Ulceration.* Ulcerated tumors have a worse prognosis than nonulcerated tumors.
3. *Age.* The prognosis for older patients is worse than that for younger patients.
4. *Location of primary tumor.* Tumors located on the extremities, excluding the feet, have a better prognosis than do tumors on the head and neck, which have a better prognosis than a tumor found on the trunk.
5. *Depth of invasion.* The deeper the level of penetration, the poorer is the prognosis.
6. *Gender.* All things being equal, women have a higher survival advantage over men when the disease is found before it has metastasized.

Because the epidermis does not contain any blood vessels or lymphatics, NMSCs confined to that area have virtually no chance of spreading other than via direct extension. After a tumor invades the superficial lymphatic plexus of the dermis, it can spread in any direction from the tumor. Because melanomas can occur on a multitude of different locations throughout the body, the care team must be aware of the lymphatic drainage patterns of the specific area where the melanoma is found. For example, a melanoma found on the shoulder affects different regional nodes than a melanoma found on a lower extremity. The following are areas of the body and the regional nodes that may be affected if a melanoma has developed there[1]:

- Head and neck: Ipsilateral preauricular, submandibular, cervical, and supraclavicular nodes
- Trunk: Ipsilateral axillary or inguinal lymph nodes
- Arm: Ipsilateral epitrochlear and axillary lymph nodes
- Leg: Ipsilateral popliteal and inguinal lymph nodes

Level of invasion

I   II   III   IV   V

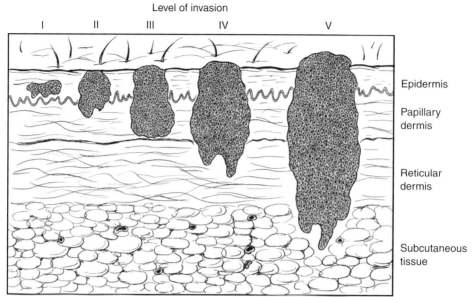

Epidermis

Papillary
dermis

Reticular
dermis

Subcutaneous
tissue

Fig. 36.13 Schematic relating Clark's levels to the layer of the skin through which the tumor has penetrated. (From Rigel DS, et al. *Cancer of the Skin*. 2nd ed. Philadelphia, PA: Saunders; 2011.)

Some melanomas do not fit into specific drainage categories but rather between drainage areas. In those cases, regions on both sides of the area that contains the tumor must be considered potential drainage sites. Procedures have been developed to aid physicians in determining the actual lymphatic flow patterns from the primary melanoma site. *Lymphoscintigraphy* uses a radioactive isotope that is injected in the primary melanoma site. The isotope then filters through the lymphatic channels that drain the tumor, and the patient is scanned to determine which lymph node stations could potentially harbor malignant cells. Another procedure, *Intraoperative lymphatic mapping*, uses special dyes that are injected into the primary tumor. As these dyes are transported through the lymphatic channels, they stain the tissues that they contact. During surgery, the physician can identify the draining lymphatics and follow them to the lymph node closest to the tumor, or the sentinel node.

Sentinel lymph node mapping has evolved from the knowledge that tumors drain in a logical pattern through the lymphatic system. A sentinel lymph node is defined as the first lymph node to receive lymphatic drainage from a tumor. During a sentinel lymph node mapping procedure, blue dye is injected into the tumor site, which indicates the most likely route of lymphatic drainage from the tumor. This allows the surgeons to then go in and remove and biopsy only the first lymph nodes that would be affected from the tumor, saving the patient from a nodal basin dissection, which often causes lymphedema.

The most likely site of early metastases, the sentinel node, is removed and analyzed to determine whether it contains malignant cells.[49]

Melanomas can spread to virtually any organ of the body and tend to spread in the following order: (1) direct extension of the primary, including invasion into the subcutaneous tissues; (2) regional lymphatics; (3) distant skin and subcutaneous tissues; (4) lung; and (5) liver, bone, and brain.

Cutaneous Squamous Cell and Basal Cell Carcinomas. cSCCs can take on a variety of appearances. As mentioned previously, they can

be scaly, slightly ulcerated, or nodular. Occasionally, tumors contain characteristics of BCC and squamous cell cancer.

A verrucous variety of SCC has been described as an indolent, well-differentiated cSCC that grows slowly as cauliflower-like lesion and may be associated with human papilloma virus. Tumor locations associated with poor outcomes include the ear, cheek, lips, temple, and anogenital region.[54]

SCCs have a higher propensity to metastasize than BCCs. This tendency is based on a variety of factors, including the following:
1. *Differentiation.* Poorly differentiated lesions have a higher propensity to metastasize than well-differentiated lesions.
2. *Etiology.* Tumors that develop in patients with immunosuppression or in areas of chronic inflammation, scar tissue, and radiation dermatitis have higher rates of metastasis compared with tumors that develop in sun-exposed areas.
3. *Size and invasion.* Tumors greater than 1 cm in size and more than 2 mm deep have a higher propensity for metastasis, even in sun-exposed areas.

Most studies report a small rate of metastasis from squamous cell skin cancer, but patients with high risk factors can have up to a one-third chance of development of metastasis. Regional lymph nodes are affected most of the time in metastatic cases, with possible involvement of liver, bone, brain, and especially lung.[55]

Because cSCC can occur anywhere on the skin's surface, multiple lymphatic regions may be affected. Lymphatic drainage patterns for these are the same as those for melanomas.

As for BCC, the five main subtypes are as follows[47,56]:
1. *Nodular* BCC is the most common type, accounting for 50% to 80% of presenting lesions. Found mainly on the head and neck, lesions are generally smooth, shiny, translucent and accompanied by telangiectasis. Borders are commonly rolled. Ulceration is common, and lesions may be pigmented.
2. *Superficial* BCC account for 10% to 30% of the lesions seen; they are found mainly on the trunk and appear as well-circumscribed red plaques or scaly patches, which may develop areas of translucent papules as they spread over the skin's surface. These lesions may also develop areas of pigmentation.

3. *Fibroepithelial* BCC are an uncommon, indolent subtype commonly found on the trunk. They are commonly skin-colored or red sessile plaques or stalked polyp,

4. *Infundibulocystic* BCC present as well-circumscribed, pearly papules.

5. *Morphea-form*, or *sclerosing*, BCC frequently appears as a scar-like lesion, often with indistinct margins. This type of lesion is uncommon, is found mainly on the head and neck, and is often aggressive with recurrence after treatment.

Although BCCs do not tend to metastasize, they are capable of extensive local invasion and destruction. They commonly follow the path of least resistance, although they have been known to destroy bone and cartilage if left untreated. However, rare cases of metastatic BCC have been reported. Perineural invasion indicates an aggressive variant that demonstrates increased metastatic and locoregional recurrence rates.[56] Regional lymph nodes are usually involved, but the involvement of liver, lung, and bone has been reported.

Although the last edition of this text cited the 7th edition of the AJCC staging manual, the most recent revision, the 8th edition, does not include a cSCC staging system. That edition does include cSCC information for head and neck malignancies; however, that system does not directly apply to nonhead and neck lesions.[54] For perspective, tumor staging for cSCC has been based on diameter, depth of invasion, and presence of perineural invasion; it is reasonable to believe that prognostic discussion on cSCC would still include these components.

BCC and squamous cell cancer of the skin are not reportable diseases. As such, physicians are not responsible for maintaining accurate records concerning factors such as incidence and survival. Therefore a strong database does not exist for calculating survival rates stage by stage. Although the overall survival rate is not known, early nonmelanoma lesions are very curable, with surgical excision being maintained as the gold standard for disease management.[54]

As noted previously, Merkel cell carcinoma is a relatively rare but potentially aggressive primary cutaneous neuroendocrine disease that has a mortality rate that is twice that observed in melanoma.[8] UV radiation and immunosuppression are likely predisposing factors, and like other skin cancers, Merkel cell carcinoma oftentimes manifests in sun-exposed areas.[1] Its behavior is unique in comparison to SCC and BCC, so a unique staging system is appropriate. Although multiple staging systems are in use for Merkel cell carcinoma, the AJCC system is commonly cited, as it is based on data from extensive National Cancer Database information and extensive literature review.[1,51] The following Merkel cell clinical staging is reported in the *AJCC Cancer Staging Manual*, 8th Edition.[1]

Merkel Cell Carcinoma: Primary Tumor (T)

T Category	T Criteria
TX	Primary tumor cannot be assessed
T0	No evidence of primary tumor
Tis	In situ primary tumor
T1	Less than or equal to 2 cm maximum tumor diameter
T2	Greater than 2 cm but not more than 5 cm maximum tumor diameter
T3	Over 5 cm maximum tumor diameter
T4	Primary tumor invades bone, muscle, fascia, or cartilage

Merkel Cell Carcinoma: Regional Lymph Nodes: Clinical (N)

N Category	N Criteria
NX	Regional lymph nodes cannot be clinically assessed
N0	No regional lymph node metastasis detected on clinical and/or radiologic examination
N1	Metastasis in regional lymph node(s)
N2	In-transit metastasis (discontinuous from primary tumor: located between the primary lesion and the draining lymph nodal basin, or distal to the primary lesion) without lymph node metastasis
N3	In-transit metastasis (discontinuous from primary tumor: located between the primary lesion and the draining lymph nodal basin, or distal to the primary lesion) with lymph node metastasis

Merkel Cell Carcinoma: Distant Metastasis: Clinical (M)

M Category	M Criteria
M0	No distant metastasis detected on clinical and/or radiographic examination
M1	Distant metastasis detected on clinical and/or radiologic examination
M1a	Metastasis to distant skin, distant subcutaneous tissues, or distant lymph nodes
M1b	Metastasis to lung
M1c	Metastasis to all other visceral sites

After a Merkel cell tumor has been classified according to the TNM system, it can be organized into specific stages. As seen earlier, stage groupings allow healthcare workers to categorize patients with similar disease patterns to assist the care team in treatment planning, facilitate information exchange, indicate disease spread risk and prognosis, and help evaluate treatment results. The clinical anatomic stage/prognostic groupings that relate TNM and stages for Merkel cell are as follows[1]:

The Clinical Stage Is	When T Is	And N Is	And M Is
0	Tis	N0	M0
I	T1	N0	M0
IIA	T2	N0	M0
	T3	N0	M0
IIB	T4	N0	M0
III	T0–4	N1–3	M0
IV	T0–4	Any N	M1

Treatment Techniques

Melanoma. Wide local excision has been the mainstay in the treatment of primary melanoma and typically consists of en bloc removal of the intact tumor or biopsy site with a margin of normal-appearing skin and underlying subcutaneous tissue.[16] Chemotherapy, immunotherapy, and biochemotherapy are often used as a treatment for melanomas that have metastasized.[9,57] The role of radiation therapy may be limited to the palliative treatment of metastatic disease sites. Melanoma has a reputation for being a radioresistant tumor, but radiation therapy has been a successful adjuvant to surgery and as the primary treatment modality in selected tumors and tumor sites.

Although surgery is currently the accepted form of curative therapy for melanoma, controversy exists concerning surgical margins and the use of prophylactic lymph node removal to help prevent the occurrence of metastasis.[9] Although early retrospective data suggested less sensitivity to radiation delivered at a conventional dose rate per fraction, current thinking suggests that melanoma cells are radio-responsive if adequate total doses are delivered.

Until the late 1970s, wide local excisions with 5-cm margins of normal skin surrounding the tumor were routine, sometimes creating large defects that necessitated skin grafts to close the wound. The two reasons for the use of these wide margins are: a field effect surrounding tumors with a radial growth phase and the possibility for small groups of melanoma cells arising near the main tumor mass. The evolution and collection of data from well-designed clinical trials have allowed for the development of a set of surgical guidelines that are safe, well tolerated, and associated with acceptable locoregional recurrence rates.[58] Recent studies, however, indicate that wide margins are not always necessary. The thickness of the tumor, site of the tumor, and potential morbidity of the operation should determine the margin size around the primary. Strategies that rely on lesser margins of excision, including approaches that rely solely on the pathologist's report of a tumor-free biopsy site margin, offer little savings of morbidity yet risk higher rates of local recurrence.[58] The decision to use wider margins should be based on the chance of local recurrence, because no clear evidence exists to prove that larger margins increases the likelihood of survival.[58] In all excisions, surgical margins should include subcutaneous tissue down to the fascia and should show no involvement of the tumor.

Biopsies of questionable lesions often encompass a 0.5-cm margin around the tumor. If, at the time of the pathologic examination, the lesion is found to be a melanoma beyond the in situ stage, the surgeon must go back and create the proper margins. In the case of subungual lesions (found beneath the nail beds), all but the earliest lesions are treated with the amputation of the complete digit.

Although a tumor may be removed with clear margins, a few stray cells that can lead to recurrence or metastasis may be left behind. This is the area in which chemotherapy and immunotherapy play a role. These agents hopefully destroy stray cells before they can reseed. (Specifics concerning chemotherapy and immunotherapy are discussed in the section on metastatic disease.) Patients with proven lymph node metastasis should undergo a complete excision of regional lymph nodes, with removal of as much of the soft tissue and its associated lymphatics as possible between the tumor site and the regional lymph nodes. When high-risk factors are present, adjuvant radiation therapy can be used to reduce the likelihood of regional recurrence. Even with such treatment, the risk of distant metastasis is considerable, which makes sentinel node assessment or ultrasound-guided fine-needle aspiration cytology important assessment tools.[59]

When bulky or numerous local melanoma recurrences or in-transit melanoma metastases develop in a limb, simple local treatment modalities, such as excision, cryotherapy, or laser ablation, are likely to be ineffective or simply not possible.[60] Patients who have melanomas on an extremity have been treated with isolated limb perfusion. With this technique, the extremity is isolated with a tourniquet while the blood in the limb circulates through a heart-lung machine to isolate the blood flow. Because this blood is isolated from the rest of the body, large doses of chemotherapy can be introduced and circulated through the limb, with delivery of high doses locally. The procedure is a single-delivery operation, which is different than conventional fractionated systemic chemotherapy. This procedure has also been performed with hyperthermia, a process of increasing the temperature of an area in conjunction with radiation in effort to increase cell kill.

For patients who have distant metastasis, obtaining a cure is challenging. Most therapeutic options available are for symptom relief and the prolongation of life. Surgery can be used to remove local recurrences and localized metastatic areas, such as nonregional lymph nodes, distant skin lesions, and subcutaneous metastases. Because surgery of this type is palliative, it is normally performed on patients whose quality of life may be enhanced with few side effects. Radiation therapy can also be used for palliation. It can be used to relieve symptoms caused by skin, soft tissue, bone, brain, and spinal cord metastases.

Cytotoxic chemotherapy has been successful in producing remission in some patients, but its use in the treatment of melanoma is largely palliative. Dacarbazine as a single agent is the drug of choice, although nitrosoureas and vinca alkaloids have also been used. Tumors of the skin, lymph nodes, and soft tissues respond better to drugs than do visceral metastases.[61] Unfortunately, the response rate is low and lasts an average of 4 to 6 months.[61] The challenge with cytotoxic regimens is their lack of tumor specificity. They affect the surrounding tissue as much as they do the tumor and cause serious complications when administered in large doses. Through the study of the biochemical properties and behavior of melanomas, the addition of cytokines (immune system mediators) to a chemotherapeutic regimen improves the outcome of metastatic melanoma by increasing the time to progression of the disease.[62]

Recent gains in the understanding of the molecular aberrations in melanoma lead to the development of targeted therapies, specific for common genetic mutations in metastatic melanoma. For example, vemurafenib is a medicine that inhibits an abnormal cell signaling pathway in some types of melanoma (those bearing the genetic mutation BRAF V600E) and can prolong survival in patients with this type of melanoma. Although responses to treatment can be rapid and clinically significant, resistance to these medicines often develops, and an alternative therapy is frequently necessary.[61]

Immunotherapy also plays a role in metastatic melanoma treatment. Melanomas have a history of spontaneous regression in which the body is somehow able to fend off the disease with its own natural defenses. Basically, immunotherapy attempts to take advantage of this phenomenon and bolster the body's immune system so that it can fight off the melanoma on its own. Research has found that use of an immune checkpoint inhibiting antibody (nivolumnab and ipilimumab) can prolong survival in patients with metastatic melanoma and produce a cure in a small number.[7]

Immunotherapy is now the fourth pillar of cancer therapy, along with surgery, radiation, and traditional chemotherapy. Enthusiasm for immunotherapy has increased because of, in part, data showing that it consistently improves overall survival in select patients with historically refractory cancers.[63] Types of immunotherapy include:

1. Immune checkpoint inhibitors: Block the ability of immune checkpoint proteins to limit the strength and duration of immune responses

2. Adoptive cellular therapy: Transfer of cells with antitumor properties into the tumor-bearing host to directly or indirectly cause tumor regression

3. Therapeutic antibodies: Antibodies produced in the laboratory that destroy cancer cells by design

4. Cancer treatment vaccines: Vaccines created from the patient's own tumor cells that are designed to treat tumors by strengthening the body's natural defenses

5. Immune system modulators: Uses proteins to regulate or modulate the immune system to enhance the body's immune response against cancer (i.e., cytokines and growth factors)

Other agents used to promote a general immune response are interferons and interleukins. Interferons are special proteins that activate and enhance the tumor-killing ability of monocytes and produce chemicals toxic to cells. Interferons tend to be toxic to the patient and are not often used in single-agent therapy. Interleukins are substances that act as costimulators and intensifiers of immune responses.[64]

Cutaneous Squamous Cell Carcinoma and Basal Cell Carcinoma.

Patients with basal cell or SCCs of the skin have several treatment options. The technique selected depends on factors such as previous methods of treatment (if any), the location on the body, the risk of recurrence and metastasis, and the volume of tissue invasion. The main goal of treatment is eradication of the tumor, followed by good functional and cosmetic results. In instances in which cure rates are similar but the functional or cosmetic results differ, the modality that offers better functional or cosmetic results should be used. If control rates are similar and functional or cosmetic results are similar or unimportant, the most cost-effective or quickest treatment method should be chosen.[65]

Surgery can be performed to remove NMSCs from areas where scarring is acceptable and patients want expedient results. Often, the original excisional biopsy contains all the tumor with acceptable margins, and no further treatment is needed. Otherwise, the surgeon may have to operate on the site a second time to ensure that safe margins around the tumor have been created. Although a uniform recommendation does not exist concerning the size of margins, many surgeons use 3-mm to 5-mm margins for small, low-risk lesions and a larger margin for larger or high-risk tumors.

For large, salvageable, eroding tumors, extensive surgery may be needed to remove not only the tumor but also additional tissue that may have been invaded, such as bone or muscle tissue. Such intervention may include the use of skin grafts or prosthetic devices.[48]

A more precise type of surgery, referred to as Mohs surgery (developed by Dr. Fredric Mohs at the University of Wisconsin), is used in areas where normal tissue sparing is important, in areas of known or at high risk of cancer recurrence, in areas where the extent of the cancer is unknown, or in instances of aggressive, rapidly growing tumors.[66,67] Mohs, or microscopic, surgery is different from conventional surgery in that the tumor is completely mapped out through the examination of each piece of removed tissue to determine the presence and extent of any tumor at the margins. Through the removal of only tissue that contains a tumor, a major amount of tissue is preserved versus conventional surgery.

Mohs surgery is the preferred surgical technique for high-risk cSCCs because it allows intraoperational analysis of the entire excision margin.[66-68] This surgery is performed on an outpatient basis with a local anesthetic. Tissue is removed one layer at a time and examined under a microscope. From the microscopic sample, the surgeon knows where to obtain the next sample. This process repeats itself until the tumor is excised completely. The wound is then stitched or allowed to heal on its own. Of all therapeutic modalities, Mohs surgery has the greatest success rate.[66-68]

One reason that Mohs surgery has not replaced conventional surgery in the treatment of NMSCs is that it is a time-consuming and expensive process. Cancers that are not viewed as problematic are treated almost as effectively and more inexpensively with conventional surgery.

Curettage and electrodesiccation are often used to treat BCC and early SCC. With local anesthesia, the cancer is scooped out with a curette, an instrument in the form of a loop, ring, or scoop with sharpened edges. The destruction of any remaining tumor cells and stoppage of bleeding is carried out through a process called electrodesiccation, which uses a probe emitting a high-frequency electric current to destroy tissue and cauterize blood vessels. The advantage of this method, also known as electrosurgery, is that it often leaves a white scar, which is less noticeable on people with fair skin.

Another method of treatment of early nonmelanoma skin lesions is cryosurgery, in which liquid nitrogen or carbon dioxide is applied to a lesion, lowering its temperature to around −50°C and thereby freezing and killing the abnormal cells. This procedure may have to be repeated once or twice to eliminate the tumor. Again, a white scar is generally formed as a result. Although cryosurgery is convenient and relatively inexpensive, it provides no significant therapeutic or cosmetic advantages over other treatment modalities, and thus its use for skin cancer should be considered largely historic.

Lasers (light amplification by stimulated emission of radiation) can also be used to treat early BCCs and in situ SCCs. Lasers use highly focused beams of light that can destroy areas of a tumor with pinpoint accuracy while preserving the surrounding healthy tissue. Advantages of laser surgery include little blood loss or pain because the blood vessels and nerves are instantly sealed. In addition, laser surgery provides faster healing than conventional surgery.

Radiation therapy is used on BCC and SCC located in places of functional or cosmetic significance, such as the eyelids, lips, nose, face, and ears. It is also used on tumors in which surgical removal is difficult or in areas of recurrence. The major advantage of radiation therapy is healthy tissue sparing. Disadvantages include its cost, number of treatment fractions, and late skin changes in the treatment area. Doses and fractionation schedules should be carefully planned to avoid these late effects, which could include scarring, necrosis, and chronic radiation dermatitis.[3]

Finally, early NMSCs can be treated with topical therapy in the form of a solution or cream. Examples of topical therapies include 5-fluorouracil (a chemotherapy) and imiquimod (an immunotherapy). Application of topical therapy to the affected area daily for several weeks causes the area to become inflamed and irritated during treatment, but scarring does not usually result.[69]

In photodynamic therapy, a photosensitizing agent is injected into the body and absorbed by all cells. The agent is quickly discharged from healthy cells but is retained longer by cancer cells. Light from a laser is directed on the tumor area and causes a reaction within the cells that contain the photosensitizing agent that destroys the cell.[24,70]

Radiation Therapy

Cutaneous Squamous Cell Carcinoma and Basal Cell Carcinoma.

Radiation therapy is effective in the treatment of cSCC and BCCs, especially in the treatment of small tumors in which functional or cosmetic results are important or in areas of extensive disease where the primary tumor and affected lymph nodes can be included in the radiation field. Because most skin lesions tend to be superficially located, electrons and kilovoltage x-rays are often used in their treatment. Megavoltage x-rays are rarely used in the treatment of skin cancers but may be used with or without electrons for special circumstances, such as scalp lesions or tumors that are deeply infiltrating.[3] Also, intensity-modulated radiation therapy may be used for some skin lesions, particularly when the area is near critical structures or needs retreatment. This therapy allows for the delivery of higher overall photon radiation doses while limiting doses to sensitive areas.

Brachytherapy, including temporary implants or superficial applicators with iridium-192, cesium-137, or electronic sources and permanent implants with gold seeds, has produced good curative and cosmetic results.[2,3] As with all forms of brachytherapy, the advantage of this modality in skin cancer is the ability to deliver high doses of radiation while minimizing irradiation of surrounding healthy tissues. There are possible disadvantages in the use of brachytherapy for skin cancer: cost, trauma, and length of stay required for the procedure; radiation exposure to personnel; uncertain dose distribution; and risk associated with anesthesia.[71] Electronic skin surface brachytherapy continues to develop as a modality that may help minimize some of these challenges. To date, short-term efficacy shows promise as a potential alternative to surgery or other radiation therapy options in select patients.[71]

Radiation therapy is often used to treat lesions on the lips, nose, eyelids, face, and ears because they are highly visible and cosmetic results are important. The choice between treatment with kilovoltage x-rays and electrons comes down to the size of the treatment volume, depth of the lesion, underlying anatomic structures, physician preference, and equipment availability. Modern radiation therapy departments have linear accelerators capable of producing a wide range of electrons with energies from 3 to 4 MeV to more than 20 MeV; kilovoltage machines dedicated to therapy fell out of favor for many years but are being used more frequently now.

Each modality has advantages and disadvantages that can be compared with the following five main categories:
1. **Field size.** For the treatment of areas adjacent to critical structures, such as the eye, kilovoltage x-rays allow the target volume to be covered with a smaller field size compared with that of a field producing similar effects near the skin surface using electrons. Because of its physical properties, the electron field must be opened considerably to cover the same area of interest as the kilovoltage machines. One solution to help minimize this problem with electrons is to increase the field size and use tertiary collimation on the skin's surface.
2. **Depth of maximum dose (D_{max}).** A substantial surface is required to effectively treat skin cancers with radiation therapy.[2] The characteristics of the radiation beam must be known for each specific setup to ensure that the skin surface is receiving the correct dose. This is relatively easy with low-energy x-rays because D_{max} is always at the surface regardless of field size or collimation technique. The D_{max} of electrons, in contrast, is a function of field size, location of secondary collimation, and surface contour. Because the D_{max} of electron beams is a function of energy and is usually found at a depth beneath the skin's surface, bolus material of appropriate thickness is often used to bring the dose toward the surface.
3. **Deep-tissue dose.** A characteristic of electrons is their rapid falloff; they penetrate the tissue to a certain point and dissipate, which allows for the sparing of some of the underlying tissues. Kilovoltage x-rays penetrate deeper, however, and affect a greater

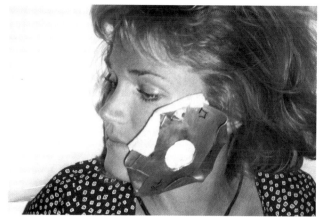

Fig. 36.14 Blocking material for orthovoltage equipment often consists of a thin strip of lead shielding that rests directly on the patient's skin.

volume of underlying tissue. Megavoltage x-rays go even deeper and may not be the optimal choice for treating superficial skin lesions.
4. **Differential bone absorption.** Gram for gram, the absorbed dose is higher in bone and cartilage than in soft tissue with the use of kilovoltage x-rays. This can result in underlying bone and cartilage receiving higher doses than the dose at D_{max}. No significant difference exists between bone and soft tissue doses for electrons used in clinical practice.

Both electron and orthovoltage treatments use various applicator cones to collimate the treatment field, although the shielding cutouts for each type of beam are manufactured by different processes. In electron therapy, departments still manufacture custom cutouts by using low-melting-point alloys like Cerrobend. These cutouts outline the field and protect healthy tissues as the radiation oncologist outlines. Historically, custom cutouts were preceded by the use of a series of layered lead strips to produce the desired outline. These strips rested on the lower portion of the cone and were commonly taped into position. Orthovoltage treatment requires a different type of blocking scheme. Instead of being attached to the machine, the blocking material typically rests on the patient's skin (Fig. 36.14). Because lead is a soft metal, it can be formed into thin sheets that are somewhat pliable. These sheets can be contoured to the patient's anatomy, and holes can be cut into the sheets, creating the field through which the radiation passes. This type of blocking scheme can also be used as tertiary shielding in electron beam therapy.

Radiation fields for skin cancer management should include a margin (1.5–2 cm) completely surrounding the tumor to cover possible microscopic extension (clinical target volume). A 0.5-cm margin may be adequate for small, superficial BCCs. Tumors and their full margins should receive most of the dose, with a boost field that encompasses the gross tumor to deliver the full dose to the tumor. In doing so, the amount of healthy tissue treated is reduced, and the cosmetic effect is improved. Although surgery accounts for the major means of management for most NMSCs, radiation therapy still plays a role, with doses varying according to the size and penetration of the tumor and differing from institution to institution.

Rapid fractionation schemes may be used in areas where late cosmetic results are not important or in instances in which transportation to and from the treatment site is difficult for the patient. Fraction size is the dominant factor in producing adverse reactions in late-responding healthy tissue (the higher the daily dose, the greater the likelihood of adverse late effects).[40]

Depending on the area to be treated and type of radiation used, special considerations exist, including the following:

- Carcinomas of the skin overlying the pinna of the ear or nasal cartilages necessitate special care in dose fractionation. Poorly designed treatment regimens can result in painful chondritis, which may necessitate excision.[72]
- Bolus may be used with electron therapy to fill in gaps on uneven surfaces, maximize the surface dose, or reduce the underlying tissue dose.
- Lip: Cancers that cross the vermilion border of the lip have a higher risk of nodal metastasis, possibly indicating the need for prophylactic neck irradiation. From a historical perspective (still useful in cases today), in the designing of a radiation field for the lip, a lead shield may be created to protect the teeth and gums. Paraffin wax on the outside of the shield helps prevent electron backscatter, reducing the dose to the buccal mucosa.
- Nose: Radiation treatments for skin cancers that involve the nose should also include a wax-coated lead strip in the nostril to help protect the nasal septum. For more invasive lesions, tissue-equivalent material should be inserted into the nostril to remove the air gap and create a more uniform dose to the deeper tissues.
- Eye: For the treatment of carcinomas of the eyelid with radiation, the lens and cornea of the eye should be protected with an appropriately sized eye shield. Small-to-medium internal shields can be placed between the eyelid and eye, whereas larger external shields can be used to cover the eyelid.[73] A thin film of antibacterial ointment can be applied to the inside of the shield before insertion to aid in the prevention of infection and help protect against scratching of the lens. Concern about the increase in lid dose from backscatter is avoidable by coating the outer surface of the shield with a low-atomic-number material. Eye shields should be disinfected and/or sterilized between treatments, especially if used with multiple patients.
- Ear: In the treatment of skin cancers of the ear with radiation, special attention to treatment planning is needed to limit radiation-induced hearing challenges. Because of the unique and varied shape of the external ear and depending on the location and extent of the tumor, bolus material may be necessary to "flatten" the surface of the ear or get rid of the air gap behind the external ear in tumors that involve the base of the auricle.

Melanoma. Traditionally, melanoma has been considered a radioresistant tumor when treated with conventional dose fraction sizes; radiation therapy was reserved mainly for the treatment of metastases. Recently, however, the role of radiation therapy has expanded to that of an adjuvant and, in some instances, the primary treatment modality.

Researchers long speculated that treatment results improve with the use of larger fractions. Because of the initial shoulder of the cell survival curve of melanoma cells exposed to radiation, standard fraction sizes of 180 to 200 cGy were thought to be ineffective. Larger doses per fraction were thought to be necessary to overcome the apparent repair processes that melanoma cells seem to possess.[74] However, randomized clinical trials have confirmed that there is no difference in the response of melanoma when treated with conventional and large dose-fraction sizes. Radiation therapy as the primary treatment modality may be limited to large facial melanoma in situ (lentigo maligna) for which wide surgical resection necessitates extensive reconstruction.

One of the problems physicians face in the treatment of patients with melanoma with bad prognostic features (i.e., neurotropic primary tumor, multiple lymph nodes with melanoma, melanoma that extends outside of lymph nodes) is local recurrence or regional relapse after

wide local excision, with or without lymph node dissection. The aim of adjuvant radiotherapy is to reduce the morbidity associated with local-regional recurrences such as ulceration, disfigurement, and pressure symptoms.

The role of radiation therapy is greatest in the treatment of metastatic or recurrent disease. The role of megavoltage x-rays is also increased as deeper levels of tissue become involved or major organs become affected. Hypofractionation should be used to treat cutaneous, subcutaneous, lymph node, or visceral metastases in small treatment volumes or in areas in which late effects are irrelevant. When affected lymphatics or organs require large treatment volumes or when late effects may be detrimental, lower daily doses may be used up to healthy tissue tolerance. The therapeutic outcome is based primarily on the tumor size and total effective dose of radiation delivered.[75]

Side Effects. A major difference between megavoltage x-ray treatment of internal structures and kilovoltage x-ray or megavoltage-electron treatment of skin lesions is the location of the D_{max}. For the treatment of internal structures, the D_{max} located at least 0.5 cm beneath the skin surface is preferable for maintaining the skin-sparing effect (i.e., if the maximum dosage of radiation is absorbed beneath the skin, the epidermal layer receives a much smaller percentage of radiation and produces fewer side effects as a result). For the treatment of skin cancers, just the opposite should occur. Maximum doses should be applied at or near the skin surface where tumors are located, whereas underlying tissues are spared. As a result, skin reactions can be expected to be worse during the treatment of primary skin cancers than during the properly planned treatment of internal structures.

Radiation reactions can be divided into acute (early) or chronic (late) changes. The severity of the reaction depends on the volume, dose, and protraction of the treatment. High doses to large volumes in short amounts of time result in more severe reactions than low doses to small volumes over long periods.

Early reactions that can be expected during radiation treatment for skin cancers include the following:

- Erythema (inflammatory redness of the skin) is usually the first sign of the effects of irradiation. This condition is caused by the swelling of the capillaries of the dermal layer, which increases the blood flow to the skin.[72]
- Pigmentary changes (hypopigmentation or hyperpigmentation) is caused by the increased production of melanin by the melanocytes, which causes the skin to become darker, or the destruction of melanocytes, which causes the skin to lose its pigment. The melanocytes respond to relatively low doses of x-rays and electrons the same way that they do to UV rays and try to protect the young epithelial cells in the same fashion.
- Dry desquamation, or shedding of the epidermis, appears at intermediate doses of radiation. The radiation affects the sensitive basal cells, and although not all are killed, enough are compromised that the basal layer has a hard time replacing the cells naturally sloughed off. The result is an abnormal thinning of the epithelial layer.[72]
- Moist desquamation appears at the high dose levels necessary to control skin cancer. Because of these high doses, nearly all the cells of the basal layer are destroyed. After the cells of the epidermis have gone through their normal cycle, no cells from the germinal layer exist to replace them. The dermis then becomes exposed and begins producing a serous oozing from its surface. The epidermis is thought to be ultimately repopulated from more radioresistant cells that surround hair follicles or sweat glands.
- Temporary hair loss (alopecia) appears after moderate doses of radiation, around 3 Gy. Higher doses, upward of 5 Gy, may result in permanent hair loss.

- Sebaceous (oil) and sudoriferous (sweat) glands may show decreased or absent function when subjected to curative doses for skin cancer.
- Late reactions that may be expected after a curative course of radiation therapy include skin changes.
- The skin seldom returns to its previous state. Damage to the dermal layer results in some fibrosis, which gives the skin a firmer, rougher appearance. Capillaries are dilated and fewer, which results in telangiectasia. Also, the epithelial layer is thin and more susceptible to injury. Damage to melanocytes results in hypopigmentation and increased sensitivity to the sun.

Prevention

Skin cancer is one of the few malignancies in which one of the primary causes is readily identifiable and preventable. Most skin cancers can be avoided if people take proper precautions against the sun's rays. If people take the time to educate themselves concerning skin cancer prevention and detection and follow through on that knowledge, the trend of rising skin cancer incidence could be reversed.

Exposure to UV light is the main triggering mechanism for skin cancer, so any type of preventive measures stress ways to avoid UV exposure. Sun exposure also causes photoaging of the skin, including processes such as premature freckling, fine wrinkling, and dilation of the capillaries. Irregular pigmentation, commonly referred to as liver spots, often develops during later years in photo-damaged skin.

The ozone layer is the portion of the atmosphere that protects the earth from harmful UV rays. In recent years, this natural defense mechanism has been under attack by synthetic substances, such as chlorofluorocarbons, automobile exhaust, and other agents. The National Aeronautics and Space Administration estimates a 2% increase in UV radiation for every 1% loss of the ozone layer.[76] Efforts are under way by many governments throughout the world to limit the release of these destructive agents into the atmosphere. Through the preservation of the ozone layer, the amount of UV light that reaches the earth's surface can be limited.

With or without a healthy ozone layer, plenty of UV light reaches the planet's surface and is a potential cause of skin cancer. Not all sun exposure is bad, however. The human body needs sunlight to aid in the production of vitamin D, which is essential for calcium absorption in the intestines and may help protect against certain types of cancer. Not much sun exposure is needed; only about 5 minutes a day is necessary to produce sufficient amounts of vitamin D.

The following are some potential UV light sources about which people should be aware:

- *Strong sun.* Avoid exposure to the sun between 10:00 AM and 2:00 PM because the rays are directly overhead and are considered strongest during this time. In the continental United States, the UV intensity is reduced by half at 3 hours before and 3 hours after peak exposure time. The peak exposure time is noon during standard time and 1:00 PM during daylight saving time. One way to judge the amount of UV exposure is by looking at a person's shadow. The longer the shadow, the lower is the intensity of the UV rays. The shorter the shadow, the greater is the intensity.
- *Reflected light.* Snow, sand, water, and cement are capable of reflecting UV light. Added to the direct rays of the sun, the reflective rays can increase overall exposure rates. Even people who wear hats or sit under umbrellas must be aware of the exposure risks of reflected light.
- *Cloudy skies.* UV rays can penetrate through clouds. Depending on cloud conditions, between 20% and 80% of UV rays still reach the ground. Proper precautions are needed even on cloudy days.

- *Fluorescent lights.* Fluorescent lights emit small amounts of UVA radiation, potentially boosting a desk worker's annual exposure.
- *Tanning lamps.* Although most tanning salons and tanning equipment manufacturers want the public to believe that tanning beds are safe, most emit UVA rays capable of skin injury, including skin cancer, premature skin aging, blood vessel damage, and immune system effects. A tan is the body's natural response to damage caused by UV light, whether that light is made by humans or nature.

Protective measures must be undertaken if UV exposure cannot be limited. Slacks, long-sleeved shirts, hats, and visors offer excellent protection from UV light. Care must be taken to protect areas of the skin not directly covered by the various articles. These areas include the ears, the top of the feet, and the back of the knees.

Sunscreens are effective in protecting against UV exposure. The blocking ability of sunscreens is indicated by its sun protection factor (SPF), which tells how long a person can stay in the sun with protection versus without protection before a sunburn develops. For example, a sunscreen with an SPF of 30 enables a person wearing it to stay in the sun 30 times longer than if the person were wearing no sunscreen.[17]

Sunscreens contain different ingredients to protect against UVA and UVB rays. Agents that can block both types of rays are referred to as broad spectrum sunscreens. The use of sunscreens and their role in the prevention of skin cancers is controversial. Some investigators think that although the protective capacity of sunscreens against UVB is good, the protective capacity against UVA is lacking.

Some people think that the use of sunscreens may be counterproductive. They theorize that people who use sunscreens can stay out in the sun for longer periods than without sunscreen because the UVB rays are being effectively blocked. With a minimum number of UVB rays available to cause the skin to feel burned, people can stay in the sun for longer periods. Because sunscreens are not as effective in blocking UVA, people are being exposed to higher levels of UVA than before sunscreens were developed. Increased UVA exposure can promote previous UVB damage or cause other types of damage on its own.

One of the most powerful weapons to fight skin cancers is sun avoidance through the combination of protective clothing and sunscreens. Protective clothing contain a UPF rating. UPF stands for **UV protection factor** and is the amount of UV radiation that a fabric blocks.

After 40 years of investment to reduce the impact of melanoma, there is evidence to suggest that reducing melanoma incidence through evidence-based prevention and early detection interventions not only reduces the risk of melanoma but also is cost effective. The evidence cites several governmental reports from the United States (US Department of Health and Human Services), the United Kingdom (National Institute for Health and Clinical Excellence), and Australia (Department of Health) that provide cited guidance toward evidence-based best practice in skin cancer prevention.[77] Making the necessary investment to reduce the growing trend now has the potential to significantly reduce the human and financial burden of melanoma.[77]

In 1994, the National Weather Service, the US Environmental Protection Agency, and the Centers for Disease Control and Prevention introduced the UV index to inform the public about the type of UV conditions to expect so that proper precautions could be taken. Currently, the index offers forecasts of the likely exposure to UV radiation for a specific location during the peak hour of sunlight around noon. The UV index ranges from 0 to 15; the higher the number, the more intense is the sun intensity. Although there is no direct link between SPF and the UV index, the UV index can inform us what level of protection we should consider using. The index uses a set of four skin-type categories into which the public is divided based on the normal color

TABLE 36.1	**The Four Skin Phototypes**	
Skin Phototypes	**Skin Color in Unexposed Area**	**Tanning History**
Never tans, always burns	Pale or milky white; alabaster	Develops red sunburn; painful swelling occurs; skin peels
Sometimes tans, usually burns	Very light brown; sometimes freckles	Usually burns; pink or red coloring appears; can gradually develop light brown tan
Usually tans, sometimes burns	Light tan, brown, or olive; distinctively pigmented	Infrequently burns; shows moderately rapid tanning response
Always tans, rarely burns	Brown, dark brown, or black	Rarely burns; shows very rapid tanning response

From the classic Fitzpatrick Skin Classification Scale.

of the person's skin and its propensity for sunburn. These phototypes are described in Table 36.1.

In addition to analyzing primary protection against UV rays, the National Cancer Institute is researching chemoprevention of NMSC. Chemoprevention is the use of natural and synthetic substances to prevent cancer. High doses of vitamin A, beta carotene, and isotretinoin (a synthetic form of vitamin A) may help individuals who lack natural defenses (persons with albinism and xeroderma pigmentosum) to fight skin cancer.

Helping people to realize the dangers of overexposure to the sun and the importance of early detection remains a major hurdle in skin cancer prevention. Young people especially feel invulnerable to the damaging and aging effects of the sun. To many, the short-term gratification a tan provides outweighs the seemingly small risks of the sun exposure that provides it. They think that skin cancer is for old people. In a way, they are correct because skin cancer usually shows up as people grow older. However, they do not realize that the cause of skin cancer is overexposure to the sun during a person's younger years.

Mass media campaigns, educational posters, and brochures are aimed at educating the public concerning the dangers of sun exposure and the importance of early screening and detection. Healthcare institutions are trying to help by providing skin cancer screenings as a part of public healthcare fairs. Again, rising skin cancer rates can be reversed if people become educated on the prevention and detection of skin cancers and incorporate the recommendations.

Role of the Radiation Therapist

The radiation therapist plays a prominent role in the management of patients with skin cancer treated with ionizing radiation. Patient education, technical expertise, assessment, and therapeutic communication are as important for the therapist to pay attention to as in the treatment of any other cancer patient. The radiation therapist typically blends their technical and psychosocial skills to achieve the best possible patient outcome.

The radiation therapist reiterates the physician instructions for the patient undergoing treatment, particularly the management of sensitive and injured skin during treatment. As they note changes in the integrity of skin treated, that information can be relayed to the appropriate member of the patient care team so that any issues or problems are addressed on notice.

It is not uncommon for patients to need reminding about cleaning treatment areas on their skin. This being the case, the daily interactions that the radiation therapist has with the patient serve as a unique opportunity to remind them about such things as treatment field management and skin care and to assess how the patient is coping with treatment, both mentally and physically.

Technical skills and treatment delivery competencies in skin cancer treatment are paramount in the radiation therapist's role. Seeing the patient each day and delivering potentially dangerous doses of radiation require great attention to detail and careful consideration of each

step of treatment. This end provider of care is the link to successful delivery of a planned course of therapy; the best plan delivered incorrectly does not serve the patient well.

Case I

Recurrent cutaneous squamous cell carcinoma. A 75-year-old man presents with recurrent cSCC of the left scalp. The patient originally noticed a blister that appeared at the left crown of his left scalp. It was biopsied and showed a keratoacanthoma (a rapidly growing skin cancer that usually appears as a volcano-like bump on the sun-exposed skin). Subsequent to the biopsy, the patient began to note nodules arising at the biopsy edges. The lesion was resected and showed cSCC, 5.1 mm in thickness, with positive margins. It was further resected approximately 2 weeks later; that resection showed 2.5 mm of additional disease with, again, a positive margin. After a month, the patient had a Mohs surgery performed. Negative margins were noted after several surgical stages were performed with the wound extending to the periosteum of the underlying bone. After this, the patient was referred for adjuvant radiation therapy, where he completed 5800 cGy with 6-MeV electrons to the left scalp with 1-cm bolus. Subsequent healing and reactions to treatment were unremarkable.

Several weeks after completing the initial course of radiation therapy, the patient noticed a left parotid swelling, which rapidly grew to more than 1 cm. A PET scan was done and showed a PET-avid left parotid mass more than 3 cm. In addition, a 1.4 cm × 0.9 cm left temporal cutaneous lesion was mildly PET avid. An MRI of the neck showed a 3.5 cm × 3.1 cm × 3.7 cm mass located deep in the left parotid.

The patient had definitive surgery and a left parotidectomy and selective neck dissection with a free-flap reconstruction taken from the right anterolateral thigh. Metastatic cSCC was noted in the subcutaneous soft tissue with close margins. No lymphovascular invasion or perineural invasion were noted. Follow-up treatment was recommended.

There was a long discussion with the patient regarding the natural history and staging of cSCCs, and there was substantial concern regarding the rapid recurrence of his illness after his definitive surgery. The plan was to deliver adjuvant radiation therapy combined with cetuximab chemotherapy to assist in improving local and regional control of the disease. In addition, the patient was referred for dental evaluation, speech evaluation, and audiology and baseline ophthalmology evaluation.

The patient was simulated with a PET-CT simulator to reassess for distant or persistent locoregional disease. Intravenous contrast (100 mL of Omnipaque) was used to enhance visualization. The patient was positioned supine, with his arms by his sides, on a standard headrest. A wire was placed on the inferior border of the previous radiation field to ensure that it was visualized for planning. A custom 5-mm bolus was formed and taped on the left side of the face over the clinical target volume and extended inferiorly to the skin graft, inferiorly to the Mohs surgical deficit, and posteriorly behind the left ear to cover the inferior deep cervical lymph node chain to bring the overall dose more superficially to address potential extracapsular extension. A custom thermoplastic mask was formed over the bolus for immobilization. The nose was exposed from the mask to further facilitate breathing. An angle sponge was placed under the patient's knees for comfort.

The treatment was delivered at 200 cGy per day, 5 days per week, over a 7-week period with intensity-modulated radiation therapy to the areas of gross disease, including the left temple, left parotid bed, and cervical and retroauricular lymphatics. A total of 60 Gy was delivered in 30 fractions with a cone-down boost to 70 Gy for an additional 5 fractions.

The patient tolerated the treatment well; the radiation therapist team facilitated the daily needs of the patient, referring them to nursing as needed during the course of treatment. During treatment, the patient was advised to use Aquaphor ointment twice a day for skin management along with saltwater oral rinses four times a day. Near the end of treatment, the left ear had some minor exudate draining, with some faint erythema. There were no additional reactions at the end of treatment.

SUMMARY

- Skin cancer represents the most commonly diagnosed malignancy, surpassing lung, breast, colorectal, and prostate cancer.
- More than 1 million Americans are diagnosed with skin cancer each year, yet many of these malignancies could have been prevented through the avoidance of prolonged exposure to the sun.
- BCC is usually easily treated with surgery or radiation therapy and is unlikely to metastasize if managed early.

- Melanoma is a very lethal skin cancer, along with Merkel cell carcinoma, and must be taken very seriously.
- The only way to change the upward trend in the incidence of skin cancer is through education of the dangers of sun exposure and stressing the importance of skin cancer screening.

REVIEW QUESTIONS

The answers to the Review Questions can be found by logging on to our website at: http://evolve.elsevier.com/Washington/principles

1. The main triggering mechanism for skin cancer is:
   a. Exposure to UV light.
   b. Therapeutic radiation exposure.
   c. Chronic heat exposure.
   d. Traumatic exposure.
2. The layer of the epidermis that contains cells that are most sensitive to radiation is the:
   a. Stratum basale.
   b. Stratum granulosum.
   c. Stratum lucidum.
   d. Stratum corneum.
3. The disease that is occasionally treated with total skin irradiation with electrons is:
   a. Kaposi sarcoma.
   b. Melanoma.
   c. Mycosis fungoides.
   d. Glandular adenocarcinoma.
4. The layers of the skin, starting with the most superficial to the deepest, are:
   I. Subcutaneous layer.
   II. Epidermis.
   III. Dermis.
   IV. Basement layer.
   a. I, III, IV, II.
   b. II, IV, III, I.
   c. II, III, I, IV.
   d. IV, I, III, II.
5. Melanocytes are found in the _____ layer of the skin stratum.
   a. Basale.
   b. Granulosum.

   c. Spinosum.
   d. Corneum.
6. The treatment of choice for most melanoma skin cancers is:
   a. Surgery.
   b. Isolated limb perfusion.
   c. Chemotherapy.
   d. Radiation therapy.
7. The technique in which the tumor is removed and examined one layer at a time is:
   a. Curettage and electrodesiccation.
   b. Mohs surgery.
   c. Cryosurgery.
   d. Laser surgery.
8. Tanning of the skin in the treated area after a course of radiation therapy is caused by:
   a. Damage to the basal layer.
   b. Increased vascularity of the epidermis.
   c. Stimulation of the melanocytes.
   d. Inflammation of the dermis.
9. With the use of shielding to protect the eye during irradiation, backscatter can be minimized by:
   a. Using a shield composed of Cerrobend.
   b. Using a shield at least 1.7 mm in thickness.
   c. Using a larger-diameter shield.
   d. Coating the outer surface of the shield with a low atomic number material, such as wax.
10. The use of kilovoltage x-rays allows the target volume to be covered with a smaller field size compared with a field that produces similar effects near the skin through the use of electrons.
    a. True.
    b. False.

QUESTIONS TO PONDER

1. Describe the latest trends in the rates of incidence and rates of death in nonmelanoma and melanoma skin cancers.
2. Analyze circumstances that render individuals more susceptible to the development of skin cancer.
3. Contrast the microstaging systems for melanoma developed by Drs. Wallace Clark and Alexander Breslow.

4. Describe and outline the prognostic factors for melanomas.
5. Compare the current methods of radiation oncology treatment regimens commonly used in the management of skin cancer. Note any advantages or disadvantages and the circumstances that justify your thoughts.

REFERENCES

1. American Joint Committee on Cancer. *AJCC Cancer Staging Manual.* AJCC: Chicago, Il; 2017.

2. Pashazadeh A, Boese A, Friebe M. Radiation therapy techniques in the treatment of skin cancer: an overview of the current status and outlook. *J Dermatolog Treat.* 2019;30(8):831–839.

3. Rong Y, Zuo L, Shang L, Bazan JG. Radiotherapy treatment for nonmelanoma skin cancer. *Expert Rev Anticancer Ther.* 2015;15:765–776.

4. Burton KA, Ashack KA, Khachemoune A. Cutaneous squamous cell carcinoma: a review of high-risk and metastatic disease. *Am J Clin Dermatol.* 2016;17:491–508.

5. National Cancer Institute. PDQ skin cancer treatment; 2018. https://www.cancer.gov/types/skin/hp/skin-treatment-pdq. Accessed March 1, 2019.

6. Rogers HW, Weinstock MA, Feldman SR, Coldiron BM. Incidence estimate of nonmelanoma skin cancer (keratinocyte carcinomas) in the U.S. population, 2012. *JAMA Dermatol.* 2015;151:1081–1086.

7. Carreau NA, Pavlick AC. Nivolumab and ipilimumab: immunotherapy for treatment of malignant melanoma. *Future Oncol.* 2018;15:349–358.

8. American Cancer Society. Key statistics for melanoma skin cancer; 2018. https://www.cancer.org/content/dam/CRC/PDF/Public/8823.00.pdf. Accessed March 1, 2019.

9. Gardner LJ, Strunck JL, Wu YP, Grossman D. Current controversies in early-stage melanoma: questions on incidence, screening, and histologic regression. *J Am Acad Dermatol.* 2019;80:1–12.

10. Miller SJ, Alam M, Andersen J, et al. Basal cell and squamous cell skin cancers. *J Natl Compr Canc Netw.* 2010;8:836–864.

11. Nadhan KS, Chung CL, Buchanan EM, et al. Risk factors for keratinocyte carcinoma skin cancer in nonwhite individuals: a retrospective analysis. *J Am Acad Dermatol.* 2019;81(2):373–378.

12. von Schuckmann LA, Wilson LF, Hughes MCB, et al. Sun protection behavior after diagnosis of high-risk primary melanoma and risk of a subsequent primary. *J Am Acad Dermatol.* 2019;80:139–148. e4.

13. American Cancer Society. Basal and squamous cell skin cancer risk factors; 2019. https://www.cancer.org/cancer/basal-and-squamous-cell-skin-cancer/causes-risks-prevention/risk-factors.html. Accessed March 17, 2019.

14. American Cancer Society. Cancer facts and figures 2019; 2019. https://www.cancer.org/content/dam/cancer-org/research/cancer-facts-and-statistics/annual-cancer-facts-and-figures/2019/cancer-facts-and-figures-2019.pdf. Accessed March 12, 2019.

15. American Cancer Society. Cancer immunotherapy. 2016. http://www.cancer.org/treatment/treatmentsandsideeffects/treatmenttypes/immunotherapy/immunotherapy-immune-system. Accessed February 11, 2019.

16. American Cancer Society. Can melanoma skin cancer be prevented? http://www.cancer.org/cancer/skincancer-melanoma/detailedguide/melanoma-skin-cancer-prevention; 2016. Accessed February 11, 2019.

17. Skin Cancer Foundation. Preventing and treating sunburn; 2019. http://www.skincancer.org/prevention/sunburn/facts-about-sunburn-and-skin-cancer. Accessed February 12, 2019.

18. O'Sullivan DE, Hillier TW, Brenner DR, Peters CE, King WD. Indoor tanning and the risk of developing non-cutaneous cancers: a systematic review and meta-analysis. *Cancer Causes Control.* 2018;29(10):937–950.

19. El Ghissassi F, Baan R, Straif K, et al. A review of human carcinogens—part D: radiation. *Lancet Oncol.* 2009;10:751–752.

20. Wehner MR, Shive ML, Chren MM, Han J, Qureshi AA, Linos EJB. Indoor tanning and non-melanoma skin cancer: systematic review and meta-analysis. *BMJ.* 2012;345:e5909.

21. Cornelius L, Winfred A. *A Dangerous Combination for Youths–Indoor Tanning and Skin Cancer.* Mental Health; 2018. https://publichealth.wustl.edu/a-dangerous-combination-for-youths-indoor-tanning-and-skin-cancer/. Accessed October 30, 2019.

22. Reimann J, McWhirter JE, Papadopoulos A, Dewey C. A systematic review of compliance with indoor tanning legislation. *BMC Public Health.* 2018;18:1096.

23. Barnard IRM, Tierney P, Campbell CL, et al. Quantifying direct DNA damage in the basal layer of skin exposed to UV radiation from sunbeds. *Photochem Photobiol.* 2018;94:1017–1025.

24. Jalalat S, Agoris C, Fenske NA, Cherpelis B. Management of non-melanoma skin cancers: basal cell carcinoma, squamous cell carcinoma. In: *Melanoma.* New York, NY: Springer; 2018:591–604.

25. American Cancer Society. *Cancer Prevention and Early Detection Facts & Figures 2017–2018.* Atlanta, GA: American Cancer Society; 2017.

26. Mayo Foundation for Medical Education and Research. Squamous cell carcinoma of the skin; 2018. https://www.mayoclinic.org/diseases-conditions/squamous-cell-carcinoma/symptoms-causes/syc-20352480. Accessed March 19, 2019.

27. Faust H, Andersson K, Luostarinen T, Gislefoss RE, Dillner J. Cutaneous human papillomaviruses and squamous cell carcinoma of the skin: nested case–control study. *Cancer Epidemiol Biomarkers Prev.* 2016;25:721–724.

28. Green AC, Olsen C. Cutaneous squamous cell carcinoma: an epidemiological review. *Br J Dermatol.* 2017;177:373–381.

29. Kinsler V, O'hare P, Bulstrode N, et al. Melanoma in congenital melanocytic naevi. *Br J Dermatol.* 2017;176:1131–1143.

30. O'connor KM, Chien AJ. Management of melanocytic lesions in the primary care setting. *Mayo Clin Proc.* 2008;83(2):208–213.

31. Goldstein AM, Tucker MA. Dysplastic nevi and melanoma. *Cancer Epidemiol Biomarkers Prev.* 2013;22(4):528–532.

32. Rhodes AR, Weinstock MA, Fitzpatrick TB, Mihm MC, Sober AJ. Risk factors for cutaneous melanoma: a practical method of recognizing predisposed individuals. *JAMA.* 1987;258:3146–3154.

33. Gerami P. Primary cutaneous melanocytic neoplasms. In: *Melanoma.* ; 2018:1–28.

34. U.S. National Library of Medicine. Vitamin D; 2019. http://www.nlm.nih.gov/medlineplus/ency/article/002405.htm. Accessed March 19, 2019.

35. Dehdashtian A, Stringer TP, Warren AJ, Mu EW, Amirlak B, Shahabi L. *Anatomy and Physiology of the Skin. Melanoma.* New York, NY; Springer; 2018:15–26.

36. Patton KT, Thibodeau GA. *Mosby's Handbook of Anatomy & Physiology.* St. Louis, MO: Elsevier Health Sciences; 2013.

37. Abdel-Malek ZA. *Melanotropin Effects on Pigment Cell Proliferation.* CRC Press, New York; 2018.

38. Del Marmol V, Lebbé C. New perspectives in Merkel cell carcinoma. *Curr Opin Oncol.* 2019;31:72–83.

39. Kim EJ, Hess S, Richardson SK, et al. Immunopathogenesis and therapy of cutaneous T cell lymphoma. *J Clin Invest.* 2005;115:798–812.

40. Symonds PR, Deehan C, Meredith C, Mills JA. *Walter and Miller's Textbook of Radiotherapy: Radiation Physics, Therapy and Oncology.* St. Louis, MO: Elsevier Health Sciences; 2012.

41. Ferrandiz C, Malvehy J, Guillen C, Ferrandiz-Pulido C, Fernández-Figueras M. Precancerous skin lesions. *Actas Dermosifiliogr.* 2017;108:31–41.

42. Feller L, Khammissa R, Kramer B, Altini M, Lemmer J. Basal cell carcinoma, squamous cell carcinoma and melanoma of the head and face. *Head Face Med.* 2016;12:11.

43. Russo T, Lallas A, Brancaccio G, Piccolo V, Alfano R, Argenziano G. No one should die of melanoma: time for this vision to be realized? *Dermatol Pract Concept.* 2019;9:1.

44. Marks JG, Miller JJ. *Lookingbill and Marks' Principles of Dermatology.* St. Louis, MO: Elsevier Health Sciences; 2017.

45. Namin AW, Cornell GE, Thombs LA, Zitsch RP III. Patterns of recurrence and retreatment outcomes among clinical stage I and II head and neck melanoma patients. *Head Neck.* 2019;41(5):1304–1311.

46. Srivastava A, Srivastava P, Pant A. molecular diagnostics in melanoma: an update. In: *Molecular Diagnostics in Cancer Patients.* New York, NY: Springer; 2019:73–88.

47. Cameron MC, Lee E, Hibler BP, et al. Basal cell carcinoma: contemporary approaches to diagnosis, treatment, and prevention. *J Am Acad Dermatol.* 2019;80:321–339.

48. Casciato DA. *Manual of Clinical Oncology.* 7th ed. Philadelphia, PA: Lippincott, Williams & Wilkins; 2012.

49. Harrell MI, Iritani BM, Ruddell A. Tumor-induced sentinel lymph node lymphangiogenesis and increased lymph flow precede melanoma metastasis. *Am J Pathol.* 2007;170:774–786.

50. Breslow A. Thickness, cross-sectional areas and depth of invasion in the prognosis of cutaneous melanoma. *Ann Surg.* 1970;172:902.

51. Amin MB, Greene FL, Edge SB, et al. The eighth edition AJCC Cancer Staging Manual: continuing to build a bridge from a population-based to a more "personalized" approach to cancer staging. *CA Cancer J Clin.* 2017;67:93–99.

52. Gershenwald JE, Scolyer RA. Melanoma staging: American Joint Committee on Cancer (AJCC) and beyond. *Ann Surg Oncol.* 2018;25:2105–2110.

53. Gershenwald JE, Scolyer RA, Hess KR, et al. Melanoma staging: evidence-based changes in the American Joint Committee on Cancer eighth edition cancer staging manual. *CA Cancer J Clin.* 2017;67:472–492.

54. Kabir S, Schmults CD, Ruiz ES. A review of cutaneous squamous cell carcinoma epidemiology, diagnosis, and management. *Int J Cancer Manag.* 2018;11(1):e60846.

55. Halperin EC, Brady LW, Perez CA, Wazer DE. *Perez & Brady's Principles and Practice of Radiation Oncology.* Philadelphia, PA: Lippincott Williams & Wilkins; 2013.

56. Cameron MC, Lee E, Hibler BP, et al. Basal cell carcinoma: epidemiology; pathophysiology; clinical and histological subtypes; and disease associations. *J Am Acad Dermatol.* 2019;80:303–317.

57. Coit DG, Thompson JA, Algazi A, et al. Melanoma, version 2.2016, NCCN clinical practice guidelines in oncology. *J Natl Compr Canc Netw.* 2016;14:450–473.

58. Riker AI, Rajo MA, Lambert SL, Lam JS. Current surgical management of primary cutaneous melanoma. In: *Melanoma.* New York, NY: Springer; 2018:313–322.

59. Murtha TD, Han G, Han D. Predictors for use of sentinel node biopsy and the association with improved survival in melanoma patients who have nodal staging. *Ann Surg Oncol.* 2018;25:903–911.

60. Kroon HM, Thompson JF. Isolated limb infusion and isolated limb perfusion for melanoma: can the outcomes of these procedures be compared? *Ann Surg Oncol.* 2019;26:8–9.

61. Chapman PB, Hauschild A, Robert C, et al. Improved survival with vemurafenib in melanoma with BRAF V600E mutation. *N Engl J Med.* 2011;364:2507–2516.

62. Hung C-Y, Chang JW-C. Chemotherapy and biochemotherapy for melanoma. In: *Melanoma.* Springer, New York, NY; 2018:525–531.

63. McCune JS. Rapid advances in immunotherapy to treat cancer. *Clin Pharmacol Ther.* 2018;103:540–544.

64. Ferreira VL, Borba HHL, Bonetti ADF, Leonart L, Pontarolo R. Cytokines and interferons: types and functions. In: *Autoantibodies and Cytokines.* IntechOpen: London, UK; 2018.

65. Matthews A, Rhee B, Neuburg JS, Burzynski ML, Nattinger AB. Development of the facial skin care index: a health-related outcomes index for skin cancer patients. *Dermatol Surg.* 2006;32:924–934.

66. Rowe DE, Carroll RJ, Day CL Jr. Mohs surgery is the treatment of choice for recurrent (previously treated) basal cell carcinoma. *J Dermatol Surg Oncol.* 1989;15:424–431.

67. Cohen DK, Goldberg DJ. Mohs micrographic surgery: past, present, and future. *Dermatol Surg.* 2019;45:329–339.

68. Marrazzo G, Zitelli JA, Brodland D. Clinical outcomes in high-risk squamous cell carcinoma patients treated with Mohs micrographic surgery alone. *J Am Acad Dermatol.* 2019;80:633–638.

69. Paul SP. Topical treatment of skin cancers and the risks of 'fighting fire with fire'. In: *Clinical Cases in Skin Cancer Surgery and Treatment.* New York, NY: Springer; 2016:115–125.

70. Jerjes W, Hamdoon Z, Hopper C. Photodynamic therapy in the management of basal cell carcinoma: retrospective evaluation of outcome. *Photodiagnosis Photodyn Ther.* 2017;19:22–27.

71. Ota K, Adar T, Dover L, Khachemoune A. The reemergence of brachytherapy as treatment for non-melanoma skin cancer. *J Dermatolog Treat.* 2018;29:170–175.

72. Cox JD, Ang KK. *Radiation Oncology E-Book: Rationale, Technique, Results.* St. Louis, MO: Elsevier Health Sciences; 2009.

73. Vu K, Tai P, SK Au J. Radiotherapy for non-melanoma skin cancer. *Curr Cancer Ther Rev.* 2016;12:110–123.

74. Ang KK, Peters LJ, Weber RS, et al. Postoperative radiotherapy for cutaneous melanoma of the head and neck region. *Int J Radiat Oncol Biol Phys.* 1994;30:795–798.

75. DeVita VT, Lawrence TS, Rosenberg SA. *Cancer of the Skin: Cancer: Principles and Practice of Oncology.* Philadelphia, Lippincott Williams & Wilkins; 2015.

76. Thomas JM, Giblin V. Cure of cutaneous melanoma. *BMJ.* 2006;332:987–988.

77. Sinclair C, Wilson LF, Olsen C, Nicholson A. Prevention of cutaneous malignant melanoma. In: *Melanoma.* Springer; 2018:1–16.

abdominoperineal resection: Anterior incision into the abdominal wall, with the construction of a colostomy followed by a perineal incision to remove the rectum and anus and draining lymphatics.

ablation: Surgical excision or amputation of any part of the body.

absorbed dose: Energy absorbed per unit mass of any material; units are the centigray or rad.

abstracting: Gathering data for measuring and evaluating patterns of care and outcomes among the general population. In oncology centers, this is done on an ongoing basis with a tumor registry system.

accelerated fractionation: Technique in which the overall treatment time is shortened through the use of doses per fraction less than conventional doses.

accelerated hyperfractionation: Technique in which there are more treatment days than accelerated fractionation. Total dose (cGy) of primary radiation is more than conventional fractionation, hyperfractionation, or accelerated fractionation.

accelerator structure: Structure resembles a length of pipe and is the basic element of the linear accelerator. Accelerator structure allows electrons produced from a hot cathode to gain energy until they exit the far end of the copper tube.

accreditation: Process of voluntary external peer review in which a nongovernmental agency grants public recognition to an institution or specialized program of study that meets specific qualifications.

achalasia: Loss of the normal peristaltic activity of the lower two-thirds of the esophagus, resulting in dilation of the esophagus. This is a risk factor for the development of esophageal cancer.

acromegaly: Enlarged extremities.

actinic keratosis: Warty lesion with areas of red, scaly patches occurring on the sun-exposed skin of the face or hands of older, light-skinned individuals.

action levels: Tolerance levels set for a procedure that, when they fall outside the allowed deviation, will bring about actions to return values back to compliance.

ADCZ: Combination of the following drugs: doxorubicin, dacarbazine, cisplatin, and vincristine, which are commonly used in chemotherapy.

ADDIE model: Model is a step-by-step approach in which the Analysis, Design, Development, Implementation, and Evaluation can be used in creating an educational tool for patients or students.

adenocarcinoma: Epithelial cells that are glandular. An example is the tissue lining the stomach. A tumor originating in the cells of this lining is called *adenocarcinoma of the stomach.*

adenohypophysis: Anterior lobe of the pituitary.

adenomas: Benign tumor originating in glandular epithelial tissue.

adjacent: Refers to the length of the side of the right triangle that is close, or adjacent, to the specified angle.

adjuvant therapy: Use of one form of treatment in addition to another treatment.

advance directives: Legal documents (such as a living will) signed by a competent person to provide guidance for medical and healthcare decisions (e.g., the termination of life support or organ donation) in the event the person becomes incompetent to make such decisions.

advocate: Supporter who can act as a promotor and/or friend. Advocate assists patients by ensuring that their needs are fulfilled and their rights enforced.

affective: Content that may be verbal or nonverbal and comprises feelings, attitudes, and behaviors.

afferent lymphatic vessel: Lymphatic vessels that flow into a lymph node. There are more afferent vessels than efferent vessels associated with each lymph node, which are designed to increase the pressure and slow the flow of lymph out of the node.

afterloading: System that was developed to allow low-dose-rate (LDR) brachytherapy devices known as *applicators* to be inserted into the treatment area first, then loaded with a radioactive source quickly and safely. In this way, dose to personnel is kept to a minimum.

agreement state: State that enters into an agreement with the Nuclear Regulatory Commission to assume the responsibility of enforcing regulations for ionizing radiation.

akimbo: Supine position in which the arms are bent by the side.

ALARA: Abbreviation for *as low as reasonably achievable.*

algebraic equation: Mathematical formula that describes a physical phenomenon based on the interaction of several factors or variables.

algorithms: A finite set of instructions used by computers to compute a desired result.

allergic reaction: Reaction resulting from an immunologic response to a drug to which the patient has already been sensitized.

alopecia: Hair loss. Partial or complete lack of hair.

Alpha Cradle: Trade name for an immobilization device created from a Styrofoam shell and foaming agents.

alpha particle: High-linear energy transfer (LET) particulate radiation, positively charged, which consists of two protons and two neutrons; emitted during nuclear decay.

amenorrhea: The absence of menstruation.

American Association of Physicists in Medicine (AAPM): Association of physicists with a mission to advance the science, education, and professional practice of the medical physicist.

American College of Radiology: Professional medical association composed of diagnostic radiologists, radiation oncologists, interventional radiologists, nuclear medicine physicians, and medical physicists.

American Joint Committee on Cancer (AJCC): Classification and anatomic staging system.

American National Standards Institute (ANSI): Institute that seeks to provide standardization of interfaces and data sources by outlining industry-specific requirements.

American Registry of Radiologic Technologists (ARRT): World's largest credentialing body, which tests and certifies radiologic technologists and the radiation therapist for practice in the United States.

American Society of Radiologic Technologists (ASRT): Mission of the ASRT is to foster the professional growth of radiologic technologists and radiation therapists by expanding knowledge through education, research, and analysis.

analytical model: Also referred to as an *engineering model.* Identifies the caregiver as a scientist dealing only in facts and does not consider the human aspect of the patient.

anaphylactic shock: Severe reaction (marked by respiratory arrest and vascular shock) to a sensitizing substance such as insect stings, contrast media, and other drugs.

anaplastic: Pathologic description of cells, describing a loss of differentiation and more primitive appearance.

anatomic position: Position in which the subject stands upright, arms straight down by the sides of the body with palms facing forward.

anemia: Decrease in the peripheral red cell count.

anesthetic: Agent that produces complete or partial loss of sensation with or without loss of consciousness.

aneuploid: Condition in which the cells have an abnormal number of chromosomes.

Ann Arbor staging system: Classification system used for non-Hodgkin's lymphomas and Hodgkin's disease.

anode: Positive part of the x-ray tube that becomes a target for the source of electrons (the cathode).

anorexia: Loss of appetite resulting in weight loss.

ANSI: *See* American National Standards Institute (ANSI).

anterior: Relates to anatomy nearer to the front of the body.

anterior resection: Abdominal incision to remove an affected portion of the bowel with the margin plus the adjacent lymphatics.

antibody: Protein substance manufactured by the immune system's plasma cells in a defensive response to the presence of a specific antigen.

antigen: Substance or pathogen that is viewed as foreign by a person's immune system and induces the formation of antibodies.

anxiety: Response to a perceived threat at an emotional level with an increased level of arousal associated with vague, unpleasant, and uneasy feelings.

apertures: A metal block containing a hole through which the radiation (photon or proton) beam passes. Each portal for each patient requires a custom-made aperture. The shape of the hole is the approximate shape of the target being treated by the proton beam.

apoptosis: Programmed cell death.

application service providers (ASP): Provider who maintains computer servers. Web-based electronic medical records (EMR) use the internet to gain controlled access to servers maintained by application service providers. Applications and data are stored off-site and maintained by the EMR provider.

applied dose: *See* Given Dose (GD). *See also* Dose Maximum (D_{max}).

Aquaplast: Trade name for a thermoplastic that is frequently used as an immobilization device.

articular cartilage: Thin layer of hyaline cartilage covering the joint surface of the epiphyses.

artifact: Unwanted image abnormalities, such as blurring, star, and beam-hardening artifacts that can be caused by patient motion, anatomy, design of the scanner, or system failure.

array processors: The array processor takes the raw data from the computed tomography (CT) detector measurements and reconstructs the data by performing simultaneous calculations.

asepsis: Condition free from germs.

ASP: *See* Application Service Providers (ASP).

assault: Threat of touching in an injurious way.

assessment: Information obtained through a continuous, systematic assessment allows the healthcare provider to (1) determine the nature of a problem, (2) select an intervention for that problem, and (3) evaluate the effectiveness of the intervention.

astrocytoma: Central nervous system tumor originating from the nonneuronal supporting cells. It can be low grade or anaplastic.

asymmetric collimation: Process using collimators in which the blade pairs are capable of independent movement.

asymptomatic: Absence of symptoms. Patient who does not have or experience symptoms is asymptomatic.

atlas: First cervical vertebral (C-1) body with the specialized function of supporting the skull and allowing it to turn.

atom: Smallest unit of an element that retains the properties of that element.

atomic mass unit (amu): Quantity that describes the very small masses of subatomic particles. Mass of an atom of carbon 12 is exactly 12.000 amu.

attenuation: Removal of photons and electrons from a radiation beam by scatter or absorption as it travels through a medium.

attributable risk: Risk that can be linked to a specific disease.

atypical hyperplasia: Proliferation of unusual-appearing cells in a normal tissue arrangement.

Auer rods: Structures in the cytoplasm of myeloblasts, myelocytes, and monoblasts.

autoclave: Device used for sterilization by steam under pressure.

autonomy: Quality or state of being self-governing; self-directing freedom, especially moral independence.

axial: Anatomical term used to describe the body in the transverse plane.

axillary lymph nodes: Primary deep lymphatic drainage of the breast. Between 10 and 40 lymph nodes are in each axilla. These can be divided into three major sections (levels I, II, and III) based on location in relation with the pectoralis minor muscle and the sequential drainage patterns.

axillary lymphatic pathway (principal pathway): Comes from trunks of the upper and lower half of the breast and moves toward the underarm.

B symptoms: Group of symptoms (fevers, night sweats, weight loss) associated with lymphomas.

backscatter factor: Ratio of the dose rate with a scattering medium (water or phantom) to the dose rate at the same point without a scattering medium (air).

backup timer setting: Backup timer device refers to a safety device that will stop the treatment if the primary timer device fails.

barium sulfate: Heavy metal salt; the most commonly used contrast agent for examinations of the gastrointestinal tract.

Barrett esophagus: Condition in which the distal esophagus is lined with a columnar epithelium rather than a stratified squamous epithelium. It usually occurs as a result of gastroesophageal reflux.

basal cell carcinoma: Slow-growing, locally invasive, but rarely metastasizing neoplasm derived from basal cells of the epidermis or hair follicles.

base: Special number (e = 2.718272...) discovered by Euler, a mathematician.

baseline study: Initial study performed so that future studies can be compared with the original values.

battery: Touching of a person without permission.

beam-flattening filter: Located on the carousel within the head of the linear accelerator. This high-density metal filter shapes the x-ray beam in its cross-sectional dimension, providing a more even dose distribution across the radiation field.

beamlet: Small photon intensity element, also referred to as a bixel, used to subdivide an intensity-modulated radiation therapy (IMRT) beam for calculation purposes.

beam modifiers: Devices that change treatment field shape or radiation distribution at depth.

beam optimization: The culmination of the radiation treatment planning process that offers the best beam arrangements and beam energies to produce the planned and intended treatment.

beam sculpting: Producing a beam shape consistent with the three-dimensional volume of the tumor. Usually used with intensity-modulated radiation therapy (IMRT).

beam-specific PTV (bsPTV): Process created by modifying the ray tracing to account for potential misalignments because of setup error or organ motion.

beam's-eye views (BEVs): Visualization perspective that is "end-on" or positioned as if looking at a volume from the source or radiation. Made possible from collected computed tomography (CT) data, this perspective is essential in three-dimensional planning.

becquerel (Bq): A Standard International (SI) unit of radioactivity that equals 1 disintegration per second.

behavior: (or quality/safety behavior) is one of the following:
- Quick fixing: This behavior consists of detection and correction of defects often accompanied by a discussion or description – most often in the form of a complaint – of the problem to coworkers and the immediate manager, but without formal reporting of defects.
- Initiating: This behavior involves formal reporting of defects and the initiation of an improvement effort to improve the system.
- Conforming: This behavior is characterized by compliance with standard procedures and processes under the conditions of a system free of defects.
- Expediting: This type of behavior describes noncompliant procedures performed to complete the work under the conditions of a system free of defects.
- Enhancing: Enhancing behavior is seen in efforts to make long-lasting system improvements with regard to work efficiency, effectiveness, or patient safety, although the system is not overtly defective.

bending magnet: Used in high-energy linear accelerators to bend the electron stream within the head of the gantry, sometimes at right angles.

beneficence: Doing or producing of good; acts of kindness and charity.

benign: Tumors that are generally well differentiated and do not metastasize or invade surrounding normal tissue. Benign tumors are often encapsulated and slow growing.

benign prostatic hypertrophy (BPH): Enlargement of the prostate gland common in men older than 50 years. It generally causes a narrowing of the urethra.

bimodal: Occurring with two peaks of incidence. With Hodgkin's disease, the disease occurs with greater frequency during the young adult years and then again in the fifth or sixth decade of life.

binding energy: The amount of energy required to remove that electron from the atom. The electron binding energy has a negative value and is usually measured in kilo electron volts (keV).

biological effective dose (BED): In fractionated radiation therapy, the quantity by which the different fractionation regimens are compared.

biometric technology: Form of password security, such as fingerprint or retinal scanning.

biopsy: Surgical removal of a small tissue sample from a solid tumor to determine the pathology for the diagnosis of disease.

bite block: Object placed between the patient's teeth to assist in immobilization and to position the tongue. Positioning device made of cork, Aquaplast pellets, or dental wax that may also be used with a mask to position the chin and move the tongue out of the treatment area.

bitemporal hemianopsia: Loss of peripheral vision, sometimes caused by pituitary adenoma.

blocked field size: Equivalent rectangular field dimensions of the open treated area within the collimator field dimensions, often defined by multileaf collimator position.

blood-brain barrier (BBB): Barrier system that hinders the penetration of some substances into the brain and cerebrospinal fluid. The BBB exists between the vascular system and brain.

body cavities: Spaces within the body that contain internal organs.

body habitus: Physique of the human body. Internal anatomy of a person varies with the physique. Four standard body habiti are hypersthenic, sthenic, hyposthenic, and asthenic.

Bohr atom: Bohr atom model states that the electrons surrounding the nucleus exists only in certain energy states or orbits, and when an electron moves from one orbit to another, it must gain or lose energy. This model is sometimes replaced with complex quantum mechanical models of the atom, but it is still an excellent way to derive a mental picture of the atom's structure.

bolus: Tissue =0equivalent material that is usually placed on the patient to increase the skin dose and/or even out irregular contours in the patient.

boost fields: Fields that are used to deliver a high dose to a small volume. With boost fields, the radiation dose is generally delivered to the gross tumor volume only, excluding regional lymph nodes and organs at risk (OARs).

Bowen disease: Precancerous dermatosis or form of intraepidermal carcinoma characterized by the development of pink or brown papules covered with a thickened, horny layer.

brachytherapy: Radiation treatment at a short distance accomplished by inserting radioactive sources directly into or near the tumor site.

Bragg peak: Sharp increase in the dose distribution curve of a charged particle, such as protons, at a particular depth.

breast conserving therapy: Breast conserving surgery followed by adjuvant radiation therapy. For patients with early-stage breast cancer, breast conserving therapy has been shown to provide the survival equivalent of mastectomy with a low rate of recurrence in the treated breast in multiple randomized studies with long-term follow-up.

bremsstrahlung: German term for "braking" radiation, which is a common reaction between an electron and target material inside the x-ray tube.

bronchogenic carcinoma: Cancer of the lung that arises in the anatomy of the bronchial tree.

bronchoscope: Long flexible tube used in the diagnosis and management of lung cancer, and is used to examine the bronchial tree, to obtain a specimen for biopsy, or, in some cases, to remove a foreign body.

Brown-Séquard syndrome: A radiation-induced cord transection, which results in paralysis, numbness, and loss of bladder and bowel functions. The extent and nature of loss is dependent on the spinal cord level involved in the damage.

buildup region: Region between the skin surface and the depth of D_{max}. Build-up region is a characteristic of megavoltage irradiation. In this region, the dose increases with depth until it reaches a maximum at the depth of D_{max}. The higher the x-ray energy, the greater the buildup region.

bulbous urethra: Dilated proximal portion of the anterior urethra.

burnout: A reaction to chronic, job-related stress characterized by physical, emotional, and mental exhaustion that results from conditions of work, job strain, worker strain, and defensive coping.

cachexia: State of general ill health and malnutrition with early satiety; electrolyte and water imbalances; and progressive loss of body weight, fat, and muscle.

caliper: Graduated ruled instrument with one sliding leg and one that is stationary is used to figure out the thickness of the patient's tissue.

calvaria: Part of the skull that protects the brain.

cancer rehabilitation: A process that assists the cancer patient to obtain maximal physical, social, psychological, and vocational functioning within the limits created by the disease and its resulting treatment.

carcinomas: Tumors that originate from the epithelium and include all tissues that cover a surface or line a cavity.

carcinoma in situ: Malignant changes at the cellular level in epithelial tissues without extension beyond the basement membrane.

carina: Area in which the trachea divides into two branches at the level of T-4/5.

carrier: Person who carries a specific pathogen but is free of signs or symptoms of the disease and yet is capable of spreading the disease.

case manager: Member of the healthcare team who is assigned to manage the continuum of care for the patient.

cassette: Cassette provides the light-tight conditions necessary for x-ray film, photostimulable plates, and intensifying screens to work properly.

cathode: One of the electrodes found in the x-ray tube that represents the negative side of the tube.

cell cycle: Sequence of recurring biochemical and morphologic events observed in a population of reproducing cells.

cellular differentiation: A stem cell that undergoes mitosis and divides into daughter cells. It is the degree to which a cell resembles its cell of origin in morphology and function.

centigray: Unit of energy absorbed per unit mass of any material. 100 cGy = 1 Gy.

cerebellum: Part of the brain that plays a role in the coordination of voluntary muscular movements located in the occipital region.

cerebrospinal fluid (CSF): Fluid that flows through and protects the brain and spinal canal.

cerebrum: Largest part of the brain, consisting of two hemispheres.

Cerrobend: A form of Lipowitz metal used for designing custom shielding blocks and electron cutouts and consists of 50.0% bismuth, 26.7% lead, 13.3% tin, and 10.0% cadmium.

certification: Process by which a government or nongovernment agency or association grants authority to an individual who has met predetermined qualifications to use a specific title.

cervical cancer: Slowly progressive disease of the distal uterus, with the earliest phase (noninvasive carcinoma in situ) occurring approximately 10 years earlier than invasive cancer.

cervix: Part of the uterus that protrudes into the cavity of the vagina.

cesium: Radioactive isotope with a half-life of 30 years that was commonly used as a low-dose brachytherapy source.

characteristic radiation: Within the x-ray tube, radiation that is created by the direct interaction of cathode electrons with inner-shell electrons of the target material.

chemical name: Identifies the actual chemical structure of the specific drug.

chemotherapeutic agents: Cytotoxic drugs that are classified by their action on the cell or their source.

chemotherapy: Use of chemical agents to induce specific effects on disease.

chief complaint: Patient's reason for visiting with the clinician. Chief complaint is recorded by the clinician.

childhood cancer: Incidence of malignancies in people less than 18 years old.

chromophobe: Refers to histological structures of tissue that do not take up colored dye and, thus, appear more pale under the microscope.

chromosomes: Gene-bearing protein structures in the nuclei of animal cells.

chronic ulcerative colitis: Extensive inflammation and ulceration of the bowel wall resulting in bloody mucoid diarrhea several times a day, associated with an increased risk of colorectal cancer.

circulator: One of four major components housed in the drive stand, which prevents backflow of microwave power.

civil law: Law that governs relationships between individuals.

Clarkson integration or Clarkson technique: Method used to calculate the dose in an irregularly shaped field.

clinical target volume (CTV): Visible (imaged) or palpable tumor plus any margin of subclinical disease that needs to be eliminated through the treatment planning and delivery process.

cobalt-60: Radioactive isotope with a half-life of 5.26 years that is used as a source for external-beam radiation therapy.

Code of Ethics: Serves as a guide by which radiation therapist may evaluate their professional conduct as it relates to patients, healthcare consumers, employers, colleagues, and other members of the healthcare team.

cognitive: Pertaining to an individual's basic reasoning processes.

cold thyroid nodule: Nodule having no uptake.

collegial model: Cooperative method of pursuing health care for the provider and patient. It involves sharing, trust, and consideration of common goals.

collimation: process controlling radiation field spread with a lead diaphragm, tube, or cone.

collimator: Arrangement of shielding material designed to define the "x" and "y" dimensions of the beam of radiation.

collimator field size: Unblocked or open field size as defined by the collimator setting and projected at the reference distance, usually the isocenter of the linear accelerator.

colonization: Presence of an agent that is infectious but does not initiate an immune response.

colostomy: Surgical construction of an artificial excretory opening from the colon on the surface of the abdominal wall.

combination chemotherapy: Selection of drugs that act on the cell during different phases of the cell cycle, increasing the cell killing potential. In addition, drugs with known toxicities are used for maximum effectiveness, resulting in fewer side effects.

common iliac nodes: Nodes that lie at the bifurcation of the abdominal aorta at the level of L4. These nodes directly drain the urinary bladder, prostate, cervix, and vagina.

communication: Ability to transfer concrete and abstract information from one person to another person or a group of people while keeping the same meaning. Communication can be verbal, nonverbal, or a combination of the two techniques.

compensator: Beam modifier that changes radiation output relative to loss of attenuation over a changing patient contour.

compensatory vertebral curves: Specific sections of the curvature of the vertebral column that form after birth because of the development of muscles as an infant grows. Cervical and lumbar curves are compensatory curves.

complex immobilization devices: Individualized devices that restrict patient movement and ensure reproducibility in positioning.

Compton scattering: Produced when an x-ray photon interacts with an outer-shell orbital electron with sufficient energy to eject it from orbit and alter its own path.

computer-based patient record (CPR): Electronic patient record stored digitally.

computerized physician online order entry (CPOE): Method of online management of medical orders, such as laboratory orders, radiology exams, and medications for the computerized tracking and documentation process related to the electronic medical record.

computer tomography dose index (CTDI): With CT scanners, there are several ways that dose or exposure is represented. CTDI is a normalized value that is computed from measurements on a standard phantom, displayed in milligray.

concomitant: Situation in which two types of treatment take place at the same time.

cone-beam computed tomography (CBCT): A form of CT using wider x-ray beam angles for scanning, thus yielding the ability to scan a much larger volume within one rotation. It differs from fan beam CT in that the CT detector is an area detector. At certain degree intervals during the rotation of the gantry, single projection images are acquired. Net result is a three-dimensional reconstruction data set, which can project images in three orthogonal planes (axial, sagittal, and coronal).

confidentiality: Principle that relates to the knowledge that information revealed by a patient to a healthcare provider, or information that is learned in the course of a healthcare provider performing her/his duties, is private and should be held in confidence.

conformal radiation therapy (CRT): Therapy that, with the use of three-dimensional treatment planning, allows the delivery of higher tumor doses to selected target volumes without increasing treatment morbidity.

consequentialism (the theory of utility): Evaluates an activity by weighing the good against the bad or the way a person can provide the greatest good for the greatest number.

Consumer Assurance of Radiologic Excellence (CARE) bill: The Consumer Assurance of Radiologic Excellence bill would require those who perform medical imaging and radiation therapy procedures to meet minimum federal education and credentialing standards.

contact therapy unit: Machine that operates at potentials of 40 to 50 kV and uses an extremely short source-skin distance.

content specifications: Document outlines the specific topics with corresponding number of questions that may appear on the ARRT certification examination.

continuous quality improvement (CQI): A set of philosophies, methods, and tools for continuously quality improvement efforts. Lean and Six-Sigma are examples of CQI programs.

contour: Reproduction of an external body shape, usually taken through the transverse plane of the treatment beam.

contour corrections: Corrections for beam incidence onto surfaces other than flat surfaces and for angles of incidence other than 90 degrees ("normal" incidence). Also called *obliquity corrections*.

contractual model: Model that maintains a business relationship between the provider and patient; a sharing of information and responsibility.

contraindications: A condition or reason to not administer a particular medical treatment.

contralateral: Opposite side of the body.

contrast: Image contrast has been described as the tonal range of densities from black to white or the number of shades of gray in the image.

contrast media: High-density substances used radiographically to visualize internal anatomy for imaging.

convalescence: Period of recovery after an illness.

conventional fractionation: Fractionation in which the total dose of radiation is typically divided into 180- or 200-cGy increments and delivered once a day, 5 days a week.

coping strategies: Every patient brings a history of coping strategies to the cancer experience. Patients use whatever has worked for them in the past in managing their anxiety.

coplanar: Geometrical principle describing two radiation fields configured in such a way that the beam edges lie in the same plane. (Central ray is not parallel opposed.)

coronal plane: Perpendicular (at right angles) to the sagittal plane and vertically divides the body into anterior and posterior sections.

corpora cavernosa: One of the basic structural components of the penis that is encased in a dense fascia (Buck fascia), which is separated from the skin by a layer of loose connective tissue.

corpus spongiosum: One of two basic structural components of the penis.

cortex: Outer portion of a structure as in the adrenal gland. Inner portion of the adrenal gland is the medulla.

cosine: One of three of the most common functions associated with the right triangle. The other two functions are the sine and tangent.

covenant model: Model that deals with an understanding between the patient and healthcare provider and is based on traditional values and goals.

CR: Computed radiography or digital radiography (DR). It has served as a transition between film-based image receptors and digital imaging.

craniospinal irradiation (CSI): Complex irradiation of all central nervous system and cerebrospinal fluid regions from behind the eye down to the midsacrum for treatment of medulloblastoma and other cerebrospinal fluid seeding tumors.

Crew Resource Management (CRM): A training program focused on culture, teamwork, communication, and inevitability of errors and ways to avoid, trap, and mitigate hazards before they lead to serious or catastrophic harm.

critical structures: Normal tissue or vital organs whose radiation tolerance limits the deliverable dose.

critical thinking: Cognitive process that allows mastery of theory and uses practical experiences. Critical thinking incorporates the use of cognitive, affective, and psychomotor domains.

cryotherapy: Use of cold temperatures to treat a disease.

cryptorchidism: Undescended testes.

computed tomography (CT) imaging: Cross-sectional information provided by CT scanning contributes considerable information to the radiation oncologist in four major areas: diagnosis, tumor, and normal tissue localization; tissue density data for dose calculations; and follow-up treatment monitoring.

computed tomography (CT) simulator: Computed tomography scanner equipped with software that can provide information needed to design the patient's treatment parameters.

cultural competency: A set of congruent behaviors, attitudes, and policies that come together in a system or agency or among professionals that enables effective work in cross-cultural situations.

culture of safety: A set of values, beliefs, and artifacts allowing workers feel comfortable in raising concerns about safety, efficiency, quality, reliability, value, etc., without concern of retaliation or reprimand.

cumulative effect: Effect that develops if the body is unable to detoxify and excrete a drug quickly enough or if too large a dose is taken.

Curie (Ci): Historical unit of radioactivity that equals 3.7×10^{10} Bq.

curriculum: Body of courses and formally established learning experiences presenting the knowledge, principles, values, and skills that are the intended consequences of a program's formal education.

customer: Person who is not employed by the particular institution or hospital with whom employees come in contact.

cutaneous squamous cell carcinoma (cSCC): Cancer that manifests in the epithelial cells of the skin. These cells comprise the epidermis of the skin, and this cancer is one of the major forms of skin cancer.

cyclotron: Charged particle accelerator used mainly for nuclear research and more recently for generating proton and neutron beams.

cystectomy: Surgical removal of the bladder.

cytoplasm: All the cellular protoplasm except the nucleus and its contents. It consists of a watery fluid (cytosol) in which numerous organelles are suspended.

cytotoxic: Ability to kill cancer cells. Cytotoxic drugs are used to destroy cells of the primary tumor and those that may be circulating through the body.

CYVADIC: Chemotherapy program that consists of the combination of the following drugs: cyclophosphamide (Cytoxan), vincristine, doxorubicin (Adriamycin), and dacarbazine. CYVADIC is one of the most used drug programs in chemotherapy.

daily treatment record: Document recording the actual treatment delivery.

Data Acquisition System (DAS): A system that serves three functions: the transmitted radiation beam is measured, measurements are encoded to binary, and the binary data is transmitted to the computer.

data mining: Combination of computer science and statistics. Creates processes for the extraction of implicit, previously unknown, potentially useful information. It uses many different statistical and nonstatistical methods and compliments contemporary methods for exploring large quantities of data.

debulking surgery: Surgical procedure used to reduce tumor size, reduce tumor burden, and increase the opportunity to obtain a pathologic diagnosis.

decay constant: Total number of atoms that decay per unit time.

definitive: Course of radiation therapy in which the objective is to cure by eradication of the disease.

de novo: Latin term that means "anew."

densitometer: Special device that measures the degree of blackening on the film.

density: Degree of darkening on the image.

deontology: One of three ethical theories. Deontology uses formal rules of right and wrong for reasoning and problem-solving.

deoxyribonucleic acid (DNA): Large, double-stranded nucleic acid molecule that carries the genetic material of the cell on the chromosomes. This genetic information is composed of a sequence of nitrogen bases and molecular subunits.

depression: Perceived loss of self-esteem resulting in a cluster of affective behavioral (e.g., change in appetite, sleep disturbances, lack of energy, withdrawal, and dependency) and cognitive (e.g., decreased ability to concentrate, indecisiveness, and suicidal ideas) responses.

depth: Distance beneath the patient's skin to the point of calculation.

dermis: Deeper layer of the skin composed of connective tissue that contains blood and lymphatic vessels, nerves and nerve endings, sweat glands, and hair follicles.

desquamation: Acute effect of irradiation characterized by shedding of the epidermis.

detectors: Solid-state detectors in a computed tomography (CT) scanner are designed to convert radiation to light.

diaphysis: Shaft or long axis of the bone.

Digital Imaging and Communications in Medicine (DICOM): Standards produced by a joint committee of the National Electrical Manufacturers Association (NEMA) and the American College of Radiology (ACR) and affiliated with several international agencies. This committee was formed to provide communication standards for sharing image information regardless of manufacturer and has included radiation therapy treatment information. This facilitates the use of picture archival and communications systems (PACS) and allows diagnostic images to be widely distributed.

digitally reconstructed radiograph (DRR): Based on acquired computed tomography (CT) information, these are images that render a beam's-eye-view display of the treatment field anatomy and areas of treatment interest. These images resemble conventional radiographs.

distal blocking: Technique that adds thickness to a compensator to achieve additional sparing of a critical structure distal to the tumor volume; sometimes used with proton therapy.

dimensional analysis: Process that involves assessment of units of measure used in calculating some scientific quantity. This practice involves canceling of common units in an effort to leave the specified unit.

diplopia: Double vision.

direct proportionality: Relationship between measurable quantities and factors; as one increases, the other increases and vice versa.

divergence: Divergence is the spreading out of the beam of radiation. Farther from the source, the more the beam has spread.

D_{max}: *See* Dose Maximum (D_{max}).

D_o: Graphic representation of the cell's radiosensitivity.

doctrine of foreseeability: Principle of law that holds a person liable for all consequences of any negligent acts to another individual to whom a duty is owed and should have been reasonably foreseen under the circumstances.

doctrine of personal liability: Doctrine stating that all persons are liable for their own negligent conduct.

doctrine of *res ipsa loquitur* ("the thing speaks for itself"): Doctrine that is an accepted substitute for the medical expert, requiring the defendant to explain an incident and convince the court that no negligence was involved.

doctrine of respondent superior: Legal doctrine that holds an employer liable for negligent acts of employees occurring while he or she is carrying out his or her orders or otherwise serving his or her interests.

domain: Group of job activities related on the basis of required skills and knowledge.

dose calculation matrix: Grid of points at which dose is computed and subsequently displayed.

dose clouds: Defined area of accumulated dose deposited in tissue that represents uniform, homogeneous dose distribution.

dose distributions: Spatial representations of the magnitude of the dose produced by a source of radiation. They describe the variation of dose with position within an irradiated volume.

dose equivalent: Product of the absorbed dose and a quality factor (QF), which takes into account the biologic effects of different types of radiation on humans; units are the rem (1 rem = 1 rad × QF) or sievert (1 Sv = 1 Gy × QF). 1 Sv = 100 rem.

dose escalation: Refers to the delivery of higher than traditional doses to a treatment volume.

dose maximum (D_{max}): The depth of maximum buildup, in which 100% of the dose is deposited beneath the skin. Depth at which electronic equilibrium occurs for photon beams. This is also the depth of maximum absorbed dose and ionization, for photons, from a single treatment field. Depth of maximum ionization and maximum absorbed dose are usually not the same depth for electrons. *See also* Given Dose (GD).

dose rate: Also known as *output*, the dose rate of a treatment machine is the amount of radiation exposure produced by a treatment machine or source as specified at a reference field size and at a specified reference distance.

dose-volume histogram (DVH): Plot of target or normal structure volume as a function of dose.

dosimetrist: Radiation therapy practitioner responsible for production of the patient's treatment plan and any associated quality assurance components.

D_q: This parameter represents the dose at which survival becomes exponential, meaning that below this threshold dose, there appears to be no effect on cell death.

drop metastases: Secondary tumors that occur via the cerebrospinal fluid.

droplet nuclei: Residual remains of airborne pathogens after the evaporation of moisture.

DRR: *See* Digitally Reconstructed Radiograph (DRR).

drug: Any substance that alters physiologic function, with the potential for affecting health.

drug interactions: Mutual or reciprocal action or influence between drugs and/or food that can create positive or negative effects in the body.

ductal carcinoma in situ (DCIS):   DCIS is carcinoma confined to a preexisting duct system of the breast without penetration of the basement membrane and invasion of surrounding tissues on microscopic examination. DCIS can be characterized by its architectural patterns and nuclear grade. It represents approximately 21% of all breast cancers.

durability power of attorney: Legal document that allows an individual to designate anyone willing, 18 years of age or older, to be their surrogate and make decisions in matters of healthcare.

dynamic wedge: Use of a moving collimator jaw (X1, X2, Y1, Y2) to produce a wedged isodose distribution. (Also called a *virtual wedge*, used for computerized shaping of isodose curves within the treatment field.)

dysphagia: Difficulty in swallowing. Sensation of food sticking in the throat.

Dysplasia: The enlargement of an organ or tissue by the proliferation of cells of an abnormal type, as a developmental disorder or an early stage in the development of cancer.

dysplopia: Double vision.

dyspnea: Difficult, labored, or uncomfortable breathing.

ecchymoses: Escape of blood into the tissues, causing large, blotchy areas of discoloration.

edema: Excessive accumulation of fluid in a tissue, producing swelling.

edge effect: A particle beam passing through the edge of an immobilization device or boundary, that is, table edge or head holder device. The particle beam range can be significantly impacted when the patient is shifted relative to this edge if a beam passes through it. Setup differences relative to these edges not only affect the range but also the heterogeneity of the dose around the edge.

effective field size (EFS):   Another term for blocked field size (BFS). Effective field size is the equivalent rectangular field dimensions of the open or treated area within the collimator field dimensions. Effective field size is the actual blocked area treated.

efferent lymphatic vessels: Lymphatic vessels that flow out of the hilum of a lymph node.

elapsed days: Total time over which radiation treatment is delivered (protracted).

electrical charge: Measure of how strongly the particle is attracted to an electrical field and can be either positive or negative.

electrocautery: Instrument for directing a high-frequency current through a local tissue area.

electron binding energy: Amount of energy required to remove an electron from its orbit in an atom.

electron density: Number of electrons per unit mass.

electron gun: Responsible for producing electrons and injecting them into the accelerator structure.

electron shields: "Cutouts" that collimate and shape the electron treatment field.

electronic medical record (EMR):   Computerized account chronicling the care process story of a patient from presentation through their diagnosis and treatment.

electronic prescribing (e-Prescribing or eRx):   A fast, efficient way to write or reorder and transmit prescriptions using an electronic system that provides guided dose algorithms to assist providers.

electronic portal imaging device (EPID):   System producing near real-time portal images on a computer screen for evaluation. Most electronic portal-imaging systems are lightweight and come with a retracted arm along the gantry's axis. Arm may be equipped with Amorphous Silicon (aSi) imaging technology, which provides a quick and accurate comparison of its images with reference images.

electrons: Negatively charged subatomic particles that can be accelerated by a variety of machines or are emitted from decaying isotopes and used for external beam treatment and brachytherapy.

emotional intelligence: The ability of a person to perceive, evaluate, understand, and control emotions in self as well as others.

empathy: Identifying with the feelings, thoughts, or experiences of another person.

en bloc: French term meaning "in one block." In surgical cancer care it means "in one specimen."

end-of-life care: When the oncology medical professionals have determined that the therapeutic interventions have ceased to work and cancer control is not sustainable, then end-of-life care may be initiated.

endocavitary radiation therapy: Sphincter-sparing procedure in which the radiation treatment is delivered by a 50-kVp contact unit inserted into the rectum.

endometrial cancer: Cancer of the endometrium or uterus.

endophytic pattern: Growth pattern that invades within the lamina propria and submucosa.

endoplasmic reticulum: Continuous membrane in the cellular cytoplasm containing the ribosomes.

engineering model: Model that identifies the caregiver as a scientist dealing only in facts and does not consider the human aspect of the patient.

ependymoma: Tumors arising from the ependymal cells lining the brain ventricles and central spinal canal. They may be low or high grade.

epidemiology: Study of defining the distribution and determinants causing disease and injury in human populations.

epidermis: Extremely thin outer layer of the skin composed of four or five distinct layers of cells.

epiphyseal line: Cartilage at the junction of the diaphysis and epiphysis in young bones that serves as a growth area for long-bone lengthening.

epiphyses: Knoblike portions of a long bone made up of spongy bone. It is located at either end of a long bone.

epistaxis: Nosebleed.

equivalent square: Square field that has the same percentage depth dose and output of a rectangular field. This method takes different rectangular field sizes and compares them to square fields that demonstrate the same measurable scattering and attenuation characteristics.

erythema: Acute radiation effect, manifested by redness and inflammation of the skin or mucous membranes, is affected by capillary congestion, caused by dilation of the superficial capillaries.

erythroplasia: Reddened, velvetlike patches on the mucous membranes.

esophagitis: Inflammation of the esophagus. Patients complain of substernal pain and food sticking. Esophagitis may begin after 2 weeks of radiation therapy and continues for 2 to 4 weeks after treatment with conventional fractionation.

ethics: Discipline dealing with what is good and bad, with a concern for moral duty and obligations; a set of moral principles or values; a theory or system of moral values; the principles of conduct governing an individual or professional group.

etiology: Study of the causes of disease.

event: *See also* safety event. Any of the following: (1) An incident that reaches the patient with (accident) or without harm; (2) a near miss, which is an incident that comes close to reaching the patient but is caught and corrected beforehand; or 3) an unsafe condition, which is any condition that increases the probability of an incident reaching the patient.

evidence-based care: Practitioners commonly base clinical decision-making on their knowledge and experience, patient preference, and clinical circumstances. Evidence-based care combines this information with scientific evidence.

excisional biopsy: Removal of the entire tumor by cutting it out so that a diagnosis can be made.

excretion: The elimination of drugs and their by-products from the body.

exenteration (pelvic):   Radical removal of most or all pelvic organs.

exfoliative cytology: Exfoliative cytology is the study of single cells obtained from various surfaces or secretions shed by the tumor.

exit dose: Term used for the dose at the exit surface of the patient or to a depth that is the equivalent of the depth of D_{max}.

exophthalmos: Abnormal protrusion of the eyeball.

exophytic: Tumors that project out from an epithelial surface.

exponent: Exponent, or "power," is a shorthand notation that represents the multiplication of a number by itself a given number of times.

exposure:　Amount of ionization produced by photons in air per unit mass of air; units are the roentgen (R) or Coulomb per kilogram (C/kg). 1 R = 2.58 × 10^{-4} C/kg.

extended-field irradiation:　Extended distance setup occurs when the setup source-skin distance (SSD) is greater than the reference SSD.

external auditory meatus (EAM):　The ear canal that connects the outer and middle ear.

extrapolation number (n):　Part of a graphic representation of a cell-survival curve, determined by extrapolating the linear portion of the curve back until it intersects the *y*-axis.

extravasation:　Accidental leakage into the surrounding tissues; a discharge or escape (e.g., of blood) from a vessel into the tissues.

false imprisonment:　Intentional confinement without authorization by a person who physically constricts another with force, threat of force, or confining clothing or structures.

false positive/false negative:　Screening tests may yield false-positive or false-negative readings. False-positive reading indicates disease when in reality none is present. False-negative reading is the reverse; the test indicates no disease when, in fact, the disease is present.

familial adenomatous polyps (FAP):　Hereditary disease in which the entire large bowel is studded with polyps. If left untreated, the patient develops a cancer of the large bowel.

feathering:　Migration of a gap between treatment fields through the treatment course.

fibrosarcoma:　Soft tissue sarcoma (STS) derived from collagen-producing fibroblasts. *See also* Soft Tissue Sarcoma (STS).

fibrosis:　Abnormal formation of fibrous tissue caused by alterations in the structure and function of blood vessels.

fiducial marker:　Fiducial markers may include natural anatomy or be artificial markers placed internally or at the skin surface or fixed external to the patient to document location through various imaging modalities.

field of view:　Smaller than the computed tomography (CT) aperture of the gantry, this is where the patient's anatomy will be visible in the scanning window.

field size:　Dimensions of a treatment field at the isocenter (usually represented by width ¥ length).

filament:　Small coil of wire made of thoriated tungsten, which has an extremely high melting point (3380°C).

file server:　Central computer where the database and program executables reside.

film speed:　Reciprocal of the exposure in roentgens needed to produce a density of 1.0.

filtered back projection:　Commonly used method of reconstructing computed tomography (CT) data. It is also called the *summation method*.

flat-panel detectors:　Imaging device that uses amorphous silicon and solid-state integrated circuit technology to produce images with quality far superior to conventional film-screen combinations.

flatness:　Difference between the maximum and minimum intensity of the central 80% of the beam profile and specifying this difference as a percentage of the central axis intensity. Degree of evenness of dose across a beam profile.

fluence pattern:　Refers to an intensity pattern of the intensity-modulated radiation therapy (IMRT) beam. This may be described as the sequence and progression of dose delivered per beam, as a product of several segments.

fluorine-18 fluorodeoxyglucose (FDG):　An analog of glucose that is currently the most common agent used in positron emission tomography (PET) imaging.

fluoroscopy-based simulation:　Conventional simulation, also referred to as fluoroscopy-based simulation, implies the use of a piece of x-ray equipment capable of the same mechanical movements of a treatment unit.

focal spot:　Section of the target at which radiation is produced.

focusing cup:　Small oval depression in the cathode assembly.

fomite:　Any inanimate object (vehicle) involved in the transmission of disease.

Food and Drug Administration:　A governmental agency of the U.S. Department of Health and Human Services that is responsible for protecting and promoting public health through the regulation and supervision of food safety, tobacco products, dietary supplements, prescription and over-the-counter pharmaceutical drugs (medications), vaccines, biopharmaceuticals, blood transfusions, medical devices, electromagnetic radiation emitting devices (ERED), cosmetics, and veterinary products.

forward planning:　Process of entering dose-altering parameters and beam modifiers into the treatment plan by the planner.

four-dimensional (4D):　Uses three-dimensional treatment planning + time.

fractionation:　Radiation therapy treatments given in daily fractions (segments) over an extended period of time, sometimes up to 6 to 8 weeks.

free radical:　Atom or atom group in a highly reactive transient state that is carrying an unpaired electron with no charge.

free space:　Term used for dosimetry measurements using a buildup cap or miniphantom.

French Federation of Cancer Centers Sarcoma Group (FNCLCC):　Tumor grading system that is used to predict the extent of tumors.

frequency of the wave:　Represented by the Greek letter ν (read as nu), the number of times that the wave oscillates or cycles per second and is measured in units of cycles per second.

friable tumors:　Tumors that are easily broken or pulverized.

functional subunits (FSUs):　Many tissues can be thought of as consisting of discrete functional subunits.

gadolinium:　Non-iodine-based intravenous contrast agent used for computed tomography and magnetic resonance imaging scans. Gadolinium helps differentiate between edema and a tumor.

galactorrhea:　The discharge of milk when not pregnant or breastfeeding.

gamma rays:　Electromagnetic radiation emitted from decaying isotopes, used in brachytherapy. This high-energy electromagnetic radiation has no mass and no charge emitted during nuclear decay.

gantry:　On a conventional simulator, it is a mechanical C-shaped device that supports the x-ray tube and collimator device at one end. On a computed tomography (CT) scanner, it is the circular ring housing the x-ray tube and solid-state detectors. On a linear accelerator, it is responsible primarily for directing the photon (x-ray) or electron beam at a patient's tumor.

gap:　Distance between the borders of two adjacent fields. Gap is usually measured on the patient's skin. Skin gap is usually calculated to verify the depth at which the two adjacent fields abut.

Gardner syndrome:　Inherited disorder (similar to familial adenomatous polyps) consisting of adenomatous polyposis of the large bowel, upper gastrointestinal polyps, lipomas, fibromas, and other tumors. This condition is associated with an increased risk in the development of colorectal cancer.

gated treatments:　Radiation treatment where the beam is turned "on" when the target is within the treatment volume and turned "off" when the target is outside the target volume. Length of time required deliver the treatment will increase significantly.

Geiger Muller Detector:　Instrument used to measure ionizing radiation.

generic name:　Drug name coined by the original manufacturer.

genome:　Complete complement of hereditary factors as found on a haploid distribution of chromosomes.

germ cell tumors:　Tumors developing from embryologic nests of tissue located throughout the body, from the brain down to the ovaries and testes.

germ theory:　Hypothesis that microorganisms cause disease.

given dose (GD):　The dose delivered at the depth of maximum equilibrium (D$_{max}$) through a single treatment field. Also known as *applied dose* or *D$_{max}$ dose*.

Golgi apparatus:　Cytoplasmic organelle consisting of flattened membranes that modify, store, and route products of the endoplasmic reticulum.

good catch:　A good catch system is a way to allow department members to quickly report into the system various issues they notice during the course of their day.

grade:　Grade of a tumor provides information about its biological aggressiveness and is based on the degree of cell differentiation. For some tumors, such as a high-grade astrocytoma, grade is the most important prognostic indicator.

gradient:　Change in position with the rate of change of a value (dose).

gray:　A measurement of absorbed dose.

Grenz ray: Low-energy x-ray in the range of 10 to 15 kV.

gross tumor volume (GTV): Gross palpable or visible tumor.

ground state: Minimum amount of energy needed to keep the atom together.

half-life: Time period in which the activity decays to one-half of the original value. It is the essential value to employ the decay formula for a particular isotope.

half-value layer: Thickness of absorbing material necessary to reduce the x-ray intensity to half its original value.

healthcare quality: The degree to which health services for individuals and populations increase the likelihood of desired health outcomes and are consistent with current professional knowledge.

Health Insurance Portability and Accountability Act (HIPAA): Congress passed HIPAA in 1996. HIPAA guidelines and regulations require security precautions not only to restrict access but also to keep records of who is accessing information.

Health Level 7, Inc. (HL7): ANSI-accredited organization that develops standards for exchanging clinical and administrative data. Specifically, HL7 defines standards for "the exchange, management and integration of data that supports clinical patient care and the management, delivery and evaluation of healthcare services." HL7 interfaces allow sharing of information available used across the entire healthcare facility.

heat units: Capacity of the anode and x-ray tube housing to store thermal energy.

helical computed tomography (CT): Also referred to as spiral CT. Patient is positioned at a fixed point, and, while the x-ray tube is rotating, the patient moves into the aperture to create a scan pattern that resembles a "slinky" or coiled spring.

hematochezia: Patients with rectal cancer usually have rectal bleeding. This may be bright red blood on the toilet paper or mixed in or on the stool.

hematuria: Common symptom of bladder and kidney tumors with an abnormal presence of blood in the urine.

hemiglossectomy: Surgical removal of half the tongue.

hereditary nonpolyposis: Colorectal syndrome. Frequent occurrence of colorectal cancer in families without adenomatous polyposis. This syndrome is associated with an increased risk of developing a second malignancy of the colon and adenocarcinomas of the breast, ovary, endometrium, and pancreas.

heterogeneity corrections: Corrections that account for the presence of irradiated media other than water.

high dose rate (HDR): Brachytherapy treatment at a dose rate that exceeds 12 Gy/hr.

high osmolality: High number of particles in solution.

high-reliability organization (HRO): Organizations that successfully manage their risks over prolonged time periods.

hilum: Area of an organ where blood, lymphatic vessels, and nerves enter and exit.

hinge angle: Measure of the angle between central rays of two intersecting treatment beams. If a lateral and anteroposterior beam intersect at the isocenter, the hinge angle would be 90 degrees.

HIPAA: *See* Health Insurance Portability and Accountability Act (HIPAA).

histiocyte: Phagocytic cell found in loose connective tissue.

histiocytosis X: Spectrum of diseases caused by abnormal proliferation of a variety of immune cells affecting single or multiple organs.

history and physical: Initial presentation and plan for assessment and treatment that becomes part of the patient's medical record.

history of present illness: Clinician records, through conversation with the patient, a history of the present illness, and this becomes part of the patient's medical record.

HL7: *See* Health Level 7, Inc. (HL7).

homogeneous radiation beam: Producing a homogeneous beam attempts to deliver the same dose throughout a defined volume of tissue through multiple treatment angles and beam intensities.

homeostasis: Cells that maintain themselves in the range of normal function, in a state of equilibrium.

Horner syndrome: Condition caused by paralysis of the cervical sympathetic nerves. It may cause sinking in of the eyeball, ptosis of the upper eyelid, slight elevation of the lower lid, constriction of the pupil, and flushing of the affected side of the face.

hospice: Program that provides care for patients who have limited life expectancy. Care is provided in the patient's home or a hospital setting.

hot thyroid nodule: Nodule having a radionuclide uptake much higher than the rest of the thyroid gland.

Hounsfield units: Also called *computed tomography (CT) numbers*, which range from +1000 to −1000. Hounsfield units represent various tissue densities and linear attenuation coefficients.

human error (or error): Slips, lapses, and mistakes are all considered forms of error. For example:
- Slip: actively doing something unintended, and the unintended nature is observable (e.g., inadvertently writing the prescription incorrectly).
- Lapse: failing to do something that was intended to be done. Often not observable (e.g., failing to write the prescription).
- Mistakes: purposeful actions (perhaps done flawlessly) that were based on incorrect knowledge or judgment (e.g., prescribing radiation for a patient in a situation where it is not supported by the data).

human factors engineering: An engineering knowledge domain that covers three major areas:(1) physical ergonomics concerned with physical activity, (2) cognitive (or information processing) ergonomics concerned with mental processes, and (3) organizational ergonomics

(also called macroergonomics) concerned with sociotechnical system design.

hyperfractionation: Fractional doses smaller than conventional, delivered two or three times daily to achieve an increase in the total dose in the same overall time.

hyperparathyroidism: Condition caused by a tumor in the parathyroid, in which calcium is leaked from the bones, resulting in softening and deformity as the mineral salts are replaced by fibrous connective tissue.

hyperpigmentation: Excessive coloration to the skin.

hyperplasia: The enlargement of an organ or tissue caused by an increase in the reproduction rate of its cells, often as an initial stage in the development of cancer.

hyperthermia: A process of increasing the temperature of an area in conjunction with radiation in effort to increase cell kill.

hyperthyroidism: Hyperactivity of the thyroid gland.

hypertrophic pulmonary osteoarthropathy: Frequently seen phenomenon associated with lung cancer, which is manifested by clubbing of the distal phalanges of the fingers.

Hypophysis: Pituitary gland.

hypotenuse: Length of the longest side of the triangle.

hypothesis: Prediction of the relationship between certain variables.

hypothyroidism: Underactivity of the thyroid gland.

Hypovolemia: State of decreased blood volume; this can occur with dehydration or bleeding.

iatrogenic: Disease or illness created as a result of the treatment or diagnosis of another condition.

ICRU: International Commission on Radiation Units and Measurements.

idiosyncratic response (effects): Inexplicable and unpredictable symptoms caused by a genetic defect in the patient.

image fusion: Process of combining images from different modalities with a computed tomography (CT) image. Properly fused images combine the enhanced imaging capabilities of magnetic resonance imaging (MRI) and/or positron emission tomography (PET) with the spatial accuracy of CT. Anatomy can be defined on any of the image data sets and can then be displayed on the CT image.

image-guided radiation therapy (IGRT): It may be used in a variety of forms, including EPID, an in-room computed tomography (CT) scanner, kV cone-beam computed tomography, MV cone-beam computed tomography, ultrasound, and others. Rational for IGRT is to image the patient just before treatment and compare the position of external setup marks and internal anatomy to the treatment plan.

image intensifier: It is a useful tool during fluoroscopy because it converts an x-ray image into a light image.

image matrix: Images seen on the monitor are a display of cells in rows and columns, which is called the *image matrix*. Matrix size can be selected. However, 512 × 512 is commonly used in computed tomography (CT).

image registration: Process where the images of the patient are with respect to the isocenter of the accelerator.

immobilization: Process of ensuring that a patient does not move out of treatment position, thus allowing for reproducibility and accuracy in treatment.

immobilization device: Device that assists in reproducing the treatment position while restricting movement (i.e., casts, masks, or bite blocks).

immune serum globulin: Serum-containing antibody; a form of artificial immunity.

immunity: Ability of the body to defend itself against infectious organisms, foreign bodies, and cancer cells.

immunoglobulin: System of closely related, although not identical, proteins capable of acting as antibodies. Humans have five main types.

immunotherapy: The goal of immunotherapy is to amplify the body's own disease-fighting system to destroy the cancer.

impotence: Significant side effect associated with the treatment of prostate cancer in which the adult male is unable to obtain an erection or ejaculate after achieving an erection.

improvement cycles: Such a system supported by reliable methods and tools ensures that improvements made to the process can be sustained over time.

incidence: Occurrence of a particular disease over a period of time in relationship to the entire population.

incident: Any happening not consistent with the routine operation of the hospital or routine care of a particular patient.

incisional biopsy: Act of cutting into tissue to remove part of the tumor so that a diagnosis can be made.

incubation: Time interval between exposure to infection and the appearance of the first sign or symptom characteristic of the disease.

indexing: Allows for increased accuracy in treatment setup reproducibility from simulation to treatment delivery and through multiple treatments over the course of daily radiation therapy delivery.

indolent: A disease condition that causes little or no pain.

induration: Process of becoming hard and firm in soft tissues.

inferior: Toward the feet (opposite of superior).

infiltration: Swelling around the injection site accompanied by cool, pale skin and possibly hard patches or localized pain.

inflammatory response: The inflammatory response is a complex, immunochemical reaction initiated by normal cells that have been injured or damaged.

information flow: Process between multiple databases and primary information generating systems networking an essential part of accurate treatment delivery in radiation oncology.

information system department: Department that may employ several computer specialists in areas ranging from hardware to network to application support for managing the array of requirements, from running the

computer system to ensuring that it is employed efficiently by clinicians and staff.

informed consent: Assurance that the purpose, benefit, risk, and any alternative options have been explained and understood and a disclaimer (which will not always hold up in court) releasing the caregiver and facility from liability if complications develop or the treatment fail.

infundibulum: Stalklike structure that attaches the pituitary to the hypothalamus.

in situ: An early form of cancer defined by the absence of invasion.

intensity-modulated proton therapy (IMPT): Proton treatment delivery process that delivers protons as discrete spots throughout the tumor.

intensity-modulated radiation therapy (IMRT): Therapy that delivers nonuniform exposure across the radiation field using a variety of techniques and equipment.

interdisciplinary: All the disciplines cooperating in the management of the disease process, as in the cancer management team.

interferons: Naturally occurring body proteins capable of killing or slowing the growth of cancer cells.

interfraction: Changes occurring between treatment sessions.

interfraction motion: This is the change in target position from one fraction to another.

interfraction uncertainties: Variations in setup that exist between each setup (e.g., inaccuracies in positioning, variations in machine characteristics, patient differences).

interlocks: Safety switches blocking or terminating radiation production.

interstitial: Placement of radioactive implant into a tissue directly.

internal mammary lymph nodes: Lymph nodes located in the parasternal space, embedded in fat in the intercostal spaces, and running alongside the corresponding artery and vein. Most internal mammary nodes are in the first, second, and third intercostal spaces.

internal mammary lymphatic pathway: Lymphatic chain that runs toward the midline and passes through the pectoralis major and intercostal muscles close to the body of the sternum (T4 to T9).

internal radiation therapy: A form of treatment in which a source of radiation is put inside the body. Brachytherapy is a form of internal radiation therapy in which the radiation source is a solid in the form of seeds, ribbons, or capsules, which are placed in a patient's body in or near the cancer cells.

International Standards Organization (ISO): Organization that accredits various specialty organizations that produce standards for industry-specific requirements.

interpolation: To estimate values between two measured, known values. Mathematical process used in radiation therapy in which unlisted values in tables can be derived.

internal target volume: Indicates the clinical target volume (CTV) plus the internal margin that accounts for tumor motion.

interprofessional: Because *inter* means between, among, and mutually, the interprofessional approach to patient care may be defined as involving practitioners from different professional backgrounds delivering services and coordinating care programs to achieve different and often disparate service client needs.

interstitial brachytherapy: Treatment technique that is characterized by the placement of radioactive sources directly into a tumor or tumor bed. Interstitial implants can be either permanent or temporary.

interstitial radiation therapy: Insertion of radioactive sources into the tissue to treat the disease.

intracavitary brachytherapy: Radioactive sources are placed within a body cavity for treatment. This type of brachytherapy has been the mainstay in treatment of cervical cancer for more than 50 years.

intradermal: Shallow injection between the layers of the skin.

intrafraction motion: Changes or motion during the treatment administration.

intrafraction uncertainties: The variations that occur within a fraction; organ motion.

intrahypophyseal tumors: Pituitary tumor that stays in the pituitary gland.

intraluminal brachytherapy: Places sources of radiation within body tubes such as the esophagus, uterus, trachea, bronchus, and rectum. Many high-dose-rate applications are performed for intraluminal applications.

intramuscular (IM): Administrative route for drugs. It is used for large amounts or quick effects.

intraoperative radiation therapy (IORT): Radiation technique in which a single dose of 10 to 20 Gy is delivered directly to the tumor bed with electrons or photons. Tumor bed has been surgically exposed, allowing critical normal structures to be shielded or displaced out of the radiation beam.

intrasellar lesions: Pituitary tumors that grow within the confines of the sella turcica.

intrathecal: Injection that requires drugs to be instilled into the vertebral space containing cerebrospinal fluid.

intravenous (IV): Injection directly into the bloodstream providing an immediate effect.

intravenous pyelogram (IVP): Radiographic procedure using contrast media to outline the kidneys, ureters, and bladder.

invasion of privacy: Revealing confidential information or improperly and unnecessarily exposing a patient's body.

inverse planning: Treatment planning in which the clinical objectives are specified mathematically and computer software is used to determine the best beam parameters (mainly intensity-modulated radiation therapy [IMRT] beamlet weighting) that will lead to the desired dose distribution.

inverse proportionality: Relationship between measurable quantities and factors in that as one increases, the other decreases, and vice versa.

inverse square law: Mathematical relationship that describes the change in beam intensity as the distance from the source changes, where intensity is inversely proportional to the distance squared.

inverted Y: A defined area of irradiation below the diaphragm, covering the spleen, extending down the midline, and branching inferiorly to form tails across the inguinal areas.

involved field radiation: Radiation that includes only the affected lymph node region such as the supraclavicular, ipsilateral cervical, or the inguinal nodes.

ionic contrast media: Contrast having high osmolality or a high number of particles in isolation. A large amount of iodine provides greater contrast but also increases toxicity and viscosity.

ionizing radiation: Radiation with sufficient energy to separate an electron from its atom.

ipsilateral: Refers to a body component on the same side of the body.

iridium: Radioactive isotope with a half-life of 74 days. It is used in wire form for interstitial brachytherapy.

irradiated volume: Volume of tissue receiving a significant dose (e.g., >50%) of the specified target dose.

ISO: *See* International Standards Organization (ISO).

isocenter: Point of intersection of the three axes of rotation (gantry, collimator, and base of couch) of the treatment unit.

isocentric technique: Approach to three-dimensional treatment using multiple imaging modalities, including fluoroscopy, computed tomography (CT), magnetic resonance imaging (MRI), positron emission tomography (PET), single-photon emission computed tomography (SPECT), and ultrasound, planning where the isocenter is placed in or near the target volume.

isodose distributions: Two-dimensional spatial representations of dose.

isodose lines: Lines connecting points of equivalent relative radiation dose.

isthmus: Connects the lobes of the thyroid gland.

iteration: Refers to a repetitious process, which follows a sequence of instructions in a computer program, making slight adjustments in each treatment plan until the best result is achieved. It is usually used with intensity-modulated radiation therapy (IMRT).

iterative reconstruction: Techniques that reduce the noise and artifacts present in a computed tomography (CT) reconstructed image.

Joint Review Committee on Education in Radiologic Technology (JRCERT): Purpose of the JRCERT is to promote excellence in education and enhances quality and safety of patient care through the accreditation of educational programs.

jugulodigastric: Group of high neck nodes below the mastoid tip and near the angle of the mandible.

justice: Quality of being just, impartial, or fair; treatment that is fair or adequate.

Karnofsky performance scale (KPS): Scale that measures the neurologic and functional status. KPS allows measuring of the quantity and quality of neurologic defects. Scale ranges from 1 to 100.

keratin: Extremely tough and waterproof protein substance in hair, nails, and other tissue.

keratinocyte: Any one of the cells in the skin that synthesizes keratin.

keratoacanthoma: Papular lesion filled with a keratin plug that can resemble squamous cell carcinoma. It is benign and usually subsides spontaneously within 6 months.

keratosis: Lesion on the epidermis marked by the presence of a circumcised overgrowth of the horny layer.

kilovoltage (kV) imaging: An imaging device which consist of a flat panel detector and simple x-ray tube has become very useful in improving the application of radiation therapy dose delivery.

kilovoltage units: Equipment carrying out external-beam treatment by using x-rays generated at voltages up to 500 kVp.

kilovolts peak (kVp): Unit of measurement for x-ray voltages (1 kV = 1000 V of electrical potential).

klystron: Equipment that converts kinetic energy to microwave energy in the linear accelerator.

kwashiorkor: Protein malnutrition that includes an adequate intake of carbohydrates and fats but an inadequate intake of protein.

kyphosis: Excessive curvature of the vertebral column that is convex posteriorly.

LAN: *See* Local Area Network (LAN).

lasers: Each positional laser projects a small red or green beam of light toward the patient during the simulation or treatment process. This provides the therapist several external reference points in relationship to the position of the isocenter.

latent period: Time between the exposure and incidence of an abnormality.

lateral: Toward one side or the other.

law: Primarily concerned with the good of a society as a functioning unit.

law of Bergonié and Tribondeau: Law stating that ionizing radiation is more effective against cells that (1) are actively mitotic, (2) are undifferentiated, and (3) have a long mitotic future.

LD$_{50/30}$: Lethal effect of acute whole-body exposure in which 50% of the total population exposed is affected in 30 days.

leakage radiation: The amount of radiation that is transmitted through the head treatment units that adds to the absorbed dose in patients.

legal concepts: Sum of artificial rules and regulations by which society is governed in any formal and legally binding manner.

legal ethics: Study of the law mandating certain acts and forbidding others under penalty of criminal sanction.

leiomyosarcoma: Soft tissue sarcoma (STS) arising from smooth muscle. *See also* Soft Tissue Sarcoma (STS).

leukoencephalopathy: Widespread demyelinating lesions of the brain, brainstem, and cerebellum.

leukopenia: Abnormal decrease in the white blood cell count, usually below 5000 cells per mm^3.

leukoplakia: Small, white raised patches on the mucous membrane.

L'hermitte's syndrome: Pain resembling sudden electric shock throughout the body. It is produced by flexing of the neck or some cervical trauma.

libel: Written defamation of character.

licensure: Process by which an agency or government grants permission to an individual to work in a specific occupation after finding that the individual has attained the minimal degree of competency to ensure the health and safety of the public.

life experiences: Life experiences can be described as information gathered through a normal day's activity that is useful to enhance an existing cognitive knowledge base.

light cast: Fiberglass tape that contains resin, which can be molded around a patient. When exposed to ultraviolet light, it hardens, creating a rigid immobilization device.

limb-sparing surgery (LSS): Radical or wide en bloc resection for soft tissue masses that requires a 1- to 3-cm normal tissue margin that allows the limb and extremity to remain intact (avoids amputation). Also called *limb salvage surgery*.

linear accelerator: Radiation therapy treatment unit that accelerates electrons and produces x-rays or electrons for treatment.

linear energy transfer (LET): Average energy deposited per unit path length to a medium by ionizing radiation as it passes through that medium. An average value calculated by dividing the energy deposited in keV by the distance traveled in micrometers (μm or 10^{-6} meters).

linear interpolation: Process of calculating unknown values from known values.

liposarcoma: Soft tissue sarcoma (STS) arising from fat. *See also* Soft Tissue Sarcoma (STS).

living will: Purpose of the living will is to allow the competent adult to provide direction to healthcare providers concerning their choice of treatment under certain conditions, should the individual no longer be competent, by reason of illness or other infirmity, to make those decisions.

localization: Geometrical definition of the tumor and anatomic structures using surface and/or fiducial marks for reference.

logarithm: Inverse or exponential notation. Exponent that indicated the power to which a number is raised to produce a given number.

low-contrast resolution: Refers to the ability to see differences in objects that are of similar shades of gray in tissue.

low-dose-rate (LDR) brachytherapy: Treatment at a dose rate of less than 2 Gy/hr.

low osmolality: Refers to contrast agents in which the iodides remain intact instead of splitting, and therefore they agitate the cells less.

lymph: Excessive tissue fluid consisting mostly of water and plasma proteins from capillaries.

lymphatic system: Consists of lymphatic vessels, lymphatic organs, and the fluid that circulates through it, called *lymph*.

lymphovascular invasion: Lymphovascular invasion (LVI) refers to the invasion of lymphatic spaces, blood vessels, or both by tumor emboli.

lysosome: Membranous sac containing hydrolytic enzymes and found in the cellular cytoplasm. It functions in intracellular digestion.

lytic: Pertaining to the destruction of cells.

magnetic resonance imaging (MRI): Diagnostic, nonionizing means of visualizing internal anatomy through noninvasive means. Imaging is based on the magnetic properties of the hydrogen nuclei.

magnetron: A special type of electron tubes that are used to provide microwave power to accelerate electrons in a linear accelerator.

MAID: Chemotherapy drug programs consisting of the following drugs: methotrexate, doxorubicin, ifosfamide, and dacarbazine.

malignant: Tumors that are malignant often invade and destroy normal surrounding tissue and, if left untreated, can cause the death of the host.

malignant fibrous histiocytoma (MFH): Deep STS tumor showing partial fibroblastic and histiocytic differentiation with a variable pattern and giant cells.

malignant melanoma: Most lethal form of skin cancer, which arises from the melanocytes found in the stratum basale of the epidermis.

mammographically occult breast cancer: Breast cancer not detected by mammogram. Mammography can miss 10% to 15% of breast cancers, especially in women with dense breasts. This is often because of radiographic overlap between glandular tissue and tumor, rendering the tumor difficult to discern.

mantle field: Radiation field that treats the lymph nodes superior to the diaphragm, sometimes used to treat lymphomas.

Mantoux tuberculin skin test: Purified protein derivative (PPD) of tuberculin used in skin tests to show if a person has ever been "infected" by tuberculosis (TB) germs.

marasmus: Calorie malnutrition that is observed in patients who are slender or slightly underweight and characterized by weight loss of 7% to 10% and fat and muscle depletion.

mass equivalence: Measure of the mass of photons used to help explain related physical characteristics.

mass stopping power: Sum of all energy losses. This includes both losses caused by collisions of electrons with atomic electrons and radiation losses or bremsstrahlung production.

mastectomy: The complete surgical resection of breast tissue.

mastoid process: Extension of the mastoid temporal bone at the level of the earlobe.

matrix computed tomography (CT): Images seen on the screen are a display of cells in rows and column.

Mayneord factor: Used to convert the percentage depth dose at the reference distance to the percentage depth dose at a nonreference distance. This would occur, for example, at extended distance setups.

mean life: Average lifetime for the decay of radioactive atoms.

medial: Toward the midline of the body.

median sagittal plane: Also called the *midsagittal plane*, divides the body into two symmetric right and left sides. There is only one median sagittal plane.

mediastinoscopy: Small flexible tube frequently used for the evaluation of the superior mediastinal extent of disease.

mediastinum: Tissue and organs separating the lungs. Mediastinum contains the heart and its large vessels, trachea, esophagus, thymus, lymph nodes, and other structures.

medical dosimetrist: Radiation therapy practitioner responsible for production of the patient's treatment plan and any associated quality assurance components.

medical informatics: Organization, analysis, management, and use of information in healthcare and the electronic medical record.

medical information systems: Medical information system departments may employ several specialists in areas ranging from system analysts to hardware and network specialists.

medical physicist: Oversees all treatment planning and radiation safety programs and is involved with clinical physics procedures.

medical record: All components used to document chronologically the care and treatment rendered to a patient.

medication: Drug administered for its therapeutic effects.

medulla: Inner portion of the adrenal gland.

medullary: Cavity within the bone that contains fats or yellow bone marrow.

medulloblastoma: Highly malignant pediatric cerebellar tumor usually arising in the midline with the propensity to spread via the cerebrospinal fluid.

melanin: Pigment that gives color to the skin and hair and serves as protection from ultraviolet light.

melanocyte: Melanin-forming cell found in the stratum basale layer of the epidermis.

melanoma: Dark pigmented malignant tumor arising from the skin.

menarche: Beginning of a woman's first menstrual period.

menopause: End of a woman's menstrual activity.

menorrhagia: Pain during menstruation.

Merkel cell carcinoma (MCC): A relatively rare but potentially aggressive primary cutaneous neuroendocrine disease that has a mortality rate twice that observed in melanoma.

mesothelioma: Malignant tumors that develop in the mesothelial lining, the pleura, and possibly the pericardium.

metabolism: Process by which the body alters the chemical composition of a substance.

metastases: Spread of cancer beyond the primary site.

metastasize: Process of tumors spreading to a site in the body distant from the primary site.

meterset: units measuring exposure produced by a treatment machine, usually Monitor Units (MU) or time

microwaves: Similar to ordinary radio waves but have frequencies thousands of times higher. Microwave frequencies needed for linear accelerator operation are about 3 billion cycles per second (3000 MHz).

milliamperes (mA): Units of measurement for x-ray currents in which the ampere (Å) is a measure of electrical current.

MIP: Maximum-intensity projection.

mitochondria: Cytoplasmic organelle serving as the site of cellular respirations and energy production.

mitosis: Cell division involving the nucleus and cell body.

Mohs surgery: Surgical method in which the tumor (usually a skin tumor) is removed one layer at a time and examined microscopically.

monitor unit (MU): Unit of output measure used for linear accelerators. Accelerators are calibrated so that 1 MU delivers 1 cGy for a standard, reference field size at a standard reference depth at a standard source-to-calibration point.

monoclonal antibody: Antibody derived from hybridoma cells that can be used to identify tumor antigens.

moral ethics: Study of right and wrong as it relates to conscience, God, a higher being, or a person's logical rationalization.

morphology: Glandular pattern, distribution of glands, and stromal invasion of the tumor.

multicentric: Arising from many foci and having multiple originations.

multidisciplinary: Use of several disciplines at the same time. Having two or more modalities in a combined effort to treat a disease process.

multileaf collimator (MLC): Distinct part of the linear accelerator that allows treatment field shaping and blocking through the use of motorized leaves in the head of the machine. Usually made of tungsten, these metal collimator rods slide into place to form the desired field shape by projecting 0.25 cm to 1 cm beam widths per rod as measured at isocenter.

mutation: Change; transformation.

mycosis fungoides: Chronic, progressive lymphoma arising in the skin. Initially, the disease stimulates eczema or other inflammatory dermatoses. In advanced cases, ulcerated tumors and infiltrations of lymph nodes may occur.

myelosuppression: Reduction in bone marrow function.

nadir: Lowest point and the time of greatest depression of blood values, before levels begin to rise again.

nasion: Center depression at the base of the nose.

natural background radiation: The amount of ionizing radiation that is present in our everyday surroundings.

natural history: Normal progression of a tumor without treatment.

near miss: An event, circumstance, or incident that did not occur and was identified before treatment delivery.

necrosis: Death or disintegration of a cell or tissue caused by disease or injury.

NED (no evidence of disease):   At the time of patient follow-up examination, there is no residual cancer noted.

negligence: Neglect or omission of reasonable care or caution.

Neoplasia: New growth.

network: System of independent, interconnected computers or terminals communicating with one another over a shared medium, consisting of hardware and communication protocols.

neuroblastoma: Cancer of neural crest tissues (small blue round cells), usually adrenal medulla or spinal ganglia, with frequent metastases.

neurofibromatosis (von Recklinghausen disease):   Small, discrete pigmented skin lesions (e.g., cafe au lait spots, pigmented nevi) that develop into multiple neurofibromas along the course of peripheral nerves; may undergo malignant transformation.

neurohypophysis: Posterior lobe of the pituitary.

neutrons: Neutral subatomic particles found in the nucleus of an atom.

nevus: Benign, localized cluster of melanocytes arising in the skin, usually early in life.

node of Rouvière: One of the lateral retropharyngeal lymph nodes located between the pharynx and the prevertebral fascia. They receive lymph from the nasopharynx and the auditory mode tube. Also called the *lateral retropharyngeal node.*

noise: This is the grainy appearance of an image.

nonionic contrast media: Contrast having low osmolality. Iodides remain intact instead of splitting; therefore they agitate the cells less. These agents are equally effective but cost much more than ionic agents.

nonmaleficence: Not doing wrong or harm to an individual.

nonuniform scanning: Heterogeneous delivery across targeted volume with scanning beam. Also called IMPT because it shares similar optimization techniques with its photon counterpart.

normalization (of dose):   The presentation of a radiation treatment plan.

nosocomial: Infection acquired in a hospital.

nozzle: The component on a proton therapy unit closest to the patient that contains components to focus and shape the proton beam.

nuclear binding energy: Total amount of energy that it takes to hold a nucleus together and is measured in MeV (10^6 electron volts).

nuclear energy level: High-energy states of the atom.

nuclear force: Major force that holds the nucleus of an atom together.

nuclear medicine: Branch of medicine that uses radioisotopes in the diagnosis and treatment of disease.

nuclear membrane: Membranous envelope enclosing the nucleus and separating it from the cytoplasm.

Nuclear Regulatory Commission: Independent agency of the U.S. government that is charged with overseeing reactor safety and security, reactor licensing and renewal, radioactive material safety, and spent fuel management.

nucleoli: Rounded internuclear organelle serving as the site of construction of the ribosomes.

nucleoside: Compound composed of a nitrogenous base and a five-carbon sugar. With the addition of a phosphate group, a nucleoside becomes a nucleotide.

nucleotide: Compound composed of a nitrogenous base, five-carbon sugar, and phosphate group. Basic building blocks of the nucleic acids RNA and DNA.

nucleus: Conspicuous cytoplasmic organelle containing most of the genetic material (a small amount is located in the mitochondria) and nucleolus.

nulliparity: The state of a female that has never borne a child.

objectives: The required behaviors needed to achieve the desired results, including the knowledge, skills, and attitudes the student or patient will learn.

obliquity corrections: *See* Contour Corrections.

Occupational Safety and Health Administration (OSHA):   Administrative regulatory agency requiring employers to ensure the safety of workers.

odontalgia: Toothache.

odynophagia: Painful swelling.

on-board imaging (OBI):   The software and hardware requirements of a linear accelerator that provide the user daily image verification capabilities.

oncogene: Gene that regulates the development and growth of cancerous tissues.

Oncology Information System (OIS):   Computer systems facilitating the flow of information between administrative functions and medical equipment.

oophorectomy: Surgical removal of the ovaries.

oophoropexy: Fixation of the ovaries behind the uterus.

opposite: Length of the side of the right triangle that is opposite the specified angle in equations.

optical distance indicator (ODI):   Sometimes called a *rangefinder,* it projects a scale onto the patient's skin, which corresponds to the source-skin distance (SSD) used during the simulation or treatment process.

optimal contrast: When technical factors (kVp and mAs) are selected that maximize the rate of differential absorption between body parts of varying tissue density and effective atomic number.

optically stimulated luminescence: A method for measuring doses from ionizing radiation.

optimization: Procedure to make a system as effective as possible.

organ at risk (OAR):   Normal tissues (critical structures) in which sensitivity to radiation damage may influence treatment planning and/or the delivery of a prescribed dose of radiation.

organ segmentation: Process of identifying structures, target volumes or normal tissues, by creating contours around them.

organelle: One of many membrane-bound particles suspended in the cytoplasm of cells and having specialized functional characteristics.

orthogonal: Two images taken 90 degrees apart. They may be required for treatment planning purposes to define the location and relationship of various anatomic structures relative to the field's isocenter.

orthopnea: Difficulty breathing except in an upright position.

orthovoltage therapy: Treatments using x-rays produced at potentials ranging from 150 to 500 kV.

osmolality: Property of a solution that depends on the concentration of the solute per unit of solvent.

osseous: Composed of bone or resembling bone; bony.

osteoblastic: Bone forming cells.

osteomyelitis.   Infection of bone and marrow caused by the growth of germs in the bone. Infection may reach the bone through the bloodstream or by direct injury.

otalgia: Earache.

outcomes: Result of the performance, or lack of performance, of a process.

output: Referred to as the *dose rate of the machine.* Dose rate should be specified for field size, distance, and medium.

output factor: Ratio of the dose rate of a given field size to the dose rate of the reference field size.

ovarian cancer: Cancer of the ovaries.

oxygen enhancement ratio (OER):   Magnitude of the oxygen effect on cell death is termed the OER, which compares the response of cells with radiation in the presence and absence of oxygen.

PACS: Picture archiving and communication system that is used to store digital medical images.

Paget disease: Disease characterized by excessive and abnormal bone reabsorption and formation. It may affect any part of the skeletal system but primarily strikes the spine, pelvis, femur, and skull.

palliation: Noncurative treatment to relieve pain and suffering when the disease has reached the stage at which a cure is no longer possible.

palliative care: This is the delivery of interventions aimed at relieving symptoms and side effects of the disease and of the treatment and improving quality of life for the patient.

palpation: Use of touch to acquire information about the patient. Physician palpates the patient by using the tips of the fingers.

Pancoast tumor: Malignant superior sulcus tumor in the apex of the lung with clinical symptoms that include (1) pain around the shoulder and down the arm, (2) atrophy of the muscles of the hand, (3) Homer syndrome caused by involvement of the brachial plexus, and (4) bone erosion of the ribs and sometimes vertebrae.

Papanicolaou smear (Pap smear):   Procedure to test for cervical cancer in women. A Pap smear involves collecting cells from the cervix to test for changes in the cervical cells.

papilledema: Swelling of the optic disc, usually associated with increased intracranial pressure.

paraaortic field: Radiation field that treats the subdiaphragmatic nodes.

paraaortic nodes: Inferior to the cisterna chyli, which is the beginning of the thoracic duct. These nodes run adjacent to the abdominal aorta from T12 to L4.

parallel-opposed field set: Two treatment fields share common central axes, 180 degrees apart.

parallel response tissues: High-dose region of a serial-tissue DVH is of particular importance. Overall function of organs consisting of parallel response tissues is affected by the injury of a number of elements of that organ above a certain minimum "reserve."

parametrium: Tissues lateral to and around the uterus.

paranasal sinuses: Air spaces in the skull, lined by mucous membranes, that reduce the weight of the skull and give the voice resonance. Four paranasal sinuses are the ethmoid, maxillary, sphenoid, and frontal.

paraneoplastic syndrome: Collective term for disorders arising from metabolic effects of cancer on tissues remote from the tumor. Such disorders may appear as endocrine, hematologic, or neuromuscular disorders.

parenteral: Medication bypassing the gastrointestinal tract. Taken literally, this would include the topical and some mucous membrane routes, but the word has come colloquially to mean "by injection."

parity: Viable pregnancy (500-g birth weight or 20-week gestation), regardless of the outcome.

partial breast irradiation: Adjuvant radiation after breast conserving surgery delivered to the lumpectomy cavity with a margin as opposed to whole breast irradiation.

particle therapy: A form of external beam therapy using particles that are accelerated to high energies. The most common particles used therapeutically are protons and carbon, but others such as neutrons, helium, neon, and silicon have been used.

passively scattered protons (PSPT):   A beam that is spread out by placing scattering material into the path of the protons. A single scattering device broadens the beam sufficiently for treatments requiring small fields.

patch planning: Treatment planning process that uses two beams to treat the tumor, each beam treating a partial volume of the tumor.

pathogenicity: Ability of an infectious agent to cause disease.

patient couch: Treatment couch, sometimes mounted on a turntable, allows rotation about a fixed axis that passes through the isocenter.

patient navigators: Designated individuals who provide personal guidance with medical, social, and financial services to patients as they move through the healthcare system.

patient positioning aids: Devices that place the patient in a particular position for treatment but do not ensure that the patient does not move.

patient safety incident: An event or circumstance that could have resulted, or did result, in unnecessary harm to a patient.

patient support assembly (PSA):   Also called a *couch* or *table*, it allows the tabletop its mobility, permitting the precise and exact positioning of the isocenter during simulation or treatment.

PDSA: This is an improvement cycle based on Plan (P)-Do (D)-Study (S)-Act (A) phases. Safety rounds. A method for the departmental leaders to speak with front-line employees about ways to make their work areas safer and more efficient.

peak scatter factor: Peak scatter factor is a backscatter factor sometimes normalized to a reference field size, usually 10×10 cm, for energies of 4 MV and above.

PEG tube: A percutaneous endoscopic gastrostomy tube, which is used for patients who experience significant weight loss as a result of radiation treatment side effects.

pelvic exenteration: A radical surgical treatment that removes all organs from a person's pelvic cavity.

pelvic inlet: Upper entrance into the pelvis, bordered by the sacral promontory, medial pelvic sidewalls, and pubic bones.

pencil beam scanning protons (PBS):   Proton delivery system that delivers a single, narrow proton beam, which may be less than a millimeter in diameter, that is magnetically swept across the tumor, depositing radiation like a painter's brush, without the need to construct beam-shaping devices.

pendant: Set of handheld local controls suspended from the ceiling or attached to the treatment couch that mimic those of the treatment unit.

penumbra: Area or region at the beam's edge where the radiation intensity falls to 0.

percentage depth dose (PDD):   Ratio, expressed as a percentage, of the absorbed dose at a given depth to the absorbed dose at a fixed reference depth, usually D_{max}.

periosteum: Glistening white, double-layered membrane covering the outer surface of the diaphysis.

peritoneal cytology: Pathologic examination of cells obtained from the fluid surrounding the abdominal wall and its contained viscera.

peritoneal seeding: Shedding or sloughing of tumor cells into the abdominal (peritoneal) cavity.

peroxisome: Intracellular enzyme-containing body that participates in the metabolic oxidation of various substrates.

petechiae: Minute red spots caused by the escape of small amounts of blood.

Peyer's patches: Extra lymphatic tissue located within the submucosal layer in the distal ileum.

pharmacodynamics: Way drugs affect the body.

pharmacokinetics: Way drugs travel through the body to their receptor sites.

pharmacology: Science of drugs and their sources, chemistry, and actions.

pharynx: Membranous tube that extends from the base of skull to the esophagus and connects the oral and nasal cavities with the larynx and esophagus.

phase I, II, III studies: Series of studies performed to assess the risk, benefits, and effects of proposed treatment options. Phase I study is the first step in testing a new treatment in humans, assessing the best way to give a new treatment and the best dose. Dose is usually increased a little at a time to find the highest dose that does not cause harmful side effects. Phase II study tests whether a new treatment has an appropriate tumoricidal effect against certain cancers. Phase III study compares the results of people taking a new treatment with the results of people taking the standard treatment to prove the safety and efficacy of a new treatment.

phlebitis: Inflammation of a vein.

photoelectric effect: Interaction, sometimes described as true absorption, occurs when the incident photon penetrates deep into the atom and ejects an inner-shell electron from orbit.

photon: Small packet of electromagnetic energy (e.g., radio waves, visible light, and x-rays and gamma rays).

photostimulable plate: Method using x-ray detectors that convert x-rays to a digital image. Flat plate contains a layer of phosphor material, which, when exposed to x-rays, stores the latent image as a distribution of electron charges.

photo timing: Form of automatic exposure control (AEC) in which one or more ionization cells automatically stop the exposure during the creation of a simulation image.

pigmentation: Coloration of the skin caused by the presence or absence of melanin.

pitch: Used in spiral computed tomography (CT), it is determined by the couch movement in the longitudinal direction during one rotation of the gantry, divided by the slice thickness.

pixels: Small, discrete elements that make up an image.

Plan-Do-Check-Act (Plan-Do-Study-Act):   A quality improvement model used in industry and healthcare promoting small changes, done rapidly for incremental improvement of a process.

planning target volume (PTV):   Volume that indicates the clinical target volume (CTV) plus margins for geometric uncertainties, such as patient motion, beam penumbra, and treatment setup differences.

ploidy: Number of chromosome sets in a cell. (Haploid cells have one set, and diploid cells have two sets.)

Plummer-Vinson syndrome: Iron-deficiency anemia characterized by esophageal webs and atrophic glossitis. It predisposes an individual to the development of esophageal cancer.

pluripotent: Pertaining to an embryonic cell that can form different kinds of cells.

point A: The original point A concept of the Manchester System defined the measurement point as 2 cm lateral to the central canal of the uterus and 2 cm up from the mucous membrane of the lateral fornix, in the axis of the uterus.

point B: A reference point that lies 3 cm lateral to point A and is used as a means of evaluating pelvic wall dosage.

polypeptide: Chain of many amino acids linked by peptide bonds. Polypeptides are the subunits of proteins.

polyurethane mold: Immobilization-repositioning device in which polyurethane (a synthetic rubber polymer) foam hardens and shapes to the patient's body build.

portal verification: Documentation of treatment portals through radiographic images or electronic portal imaging devices.

positioning aids: Devices designed to place the patient in a particular position for treatment. There is generally very little structure in these device s to ensure that the patient does not move.

positioning lasers: Lasers that project a small red or green beam of light toward the patient during the simulation process. These lasers provide the therapist several external reference points in relationship to the position of the isocenter.

positron emission tomography (PET):   Nuclear medicine procedure that has become useful in oncology to examine the biochemical or physiological (functional) aspects of a tumor. This diagnostic tool is useful in determining the physiology of the organ in question. Beneficial diagnostic tool that may be useful in determining differences between necrosis and malignancy, which are associated with areas of high metabolism.

positrons: Positively charged electrons.

practice standards: Authoritative statements established by the profession for judging the quality of practice, service, and education.

premalignant: Physiologic characteristics of predisposing factors that may lead to malignancy.

prevention: Effective strategy for saving lives lost from cancer and diminishing suffering. Prevention includes measures that stop cancer from developing.

priestly model: Model that provides the caregiver with a godlike, paternalist attitude by making decisions for the patient and not with the patient.

primary site compartment: Natural anatomic boundaries surrounding the soft tissue sarcoma primary. It is composed of common fascia plane(s) of muscles, bone, joint, skin, subcutaneous tissues, and major neurovascular structures.

primary tumor: Main, or initial, source of malignant or benign tumor location, without reference to secondary sites of spread.

primary vertebral curves: Vertebral curves that are developed in utero as the fetus develops in the C-shaped fetal position, and they are present at birth.

profile: Description of radiation intensity as a function of position across the beam at a given depth.

progenitor: Originator or precursor.

prognosis: Estimation of life expectancy.

projection: That part of the computed tomography (CT) beam that falls on one detector is called a *ray*. One complete translation of rays is called a *view*, which generates a profile or projection that are then created and stored in digital form.

proliferation: Rapid and repeated reproduction of a new part (e.g., through cell division).

proportion: Two ratios that are equal. Proportion can also be an equation relating two ratios.

prospective study: Study in which the theory of the cause of a condition or disease is tested by examining those who have a particular characteristic or trait. Population to be examined is selected in the beginning of the study.

prostate: Walnut-shaped organ that surrounds the male urethra, located between the base of the bladder and urogenital diaphragm.

prostate gland: Gland that surrounds the male urethra between the base of the bladder and the urogenital diaphragm.

prostate-specific antigen (PSA):   Glycoprotein that is produced by epithelial cells in the prostate. Serum PSA level has been roughly correlated with prostate tumor volume.

prostatic hypertrophy: Enlargement of the prostate gland, leading to narrowing of the urethra.

protein: Complex biologic compound composed of amino acids. Linked together in a determined, three-dimensional sequence, 20 different amino acids are commonly found in proteins.

protein kinases: An enzyme that modifies other proteins by chemically adding phosphate.

protocols: Specified treatment regimen. It describes the specifics of the type of treatment, the time schedule of the treatment, the total dose of the treatment, and specific areas to be included in the treatment.

proton: Subatomic particle, located in the nucleus, with a positive charge.

protraction: Time over which total dose is to be delivered.

programmatic accreditation: Radiation therapy student's assurance the program meets the minimum professional curriculum developed by the ASRT.

pseudocapsule: Soft tissue sarcomas that are surrounded by compressed normal tissue, reactive inflammation, and fibrosis to give the gross anatomic appearance of a capsule.

psychosocial: Psychological support of the patient during the course of disease, with the recognition that social aspects of the treatment and disease prognosis may require special care.

purpura: Blotchiness and red spots caused by petechiae and ecchymoses.

quality: The totality of features and characteristics of a radiation therapy process that bear on its ability to satisfy stated or implied needs of the patient.

quality assessment: Systematic quality analysis and review of patient care data.

quality assurance (QA):   Systematic monitoring of the quality and appropriateness of patient care with an emphasis on performance levels.

quality assurance (QA) program: Series of activities and documentation performed with the goal of optimizing patient care.

quality audit: Review of the radiation therapy process that is routinely and continuously measured, the results analyzed, and corrective action taken as required to ensure quality patient care.

quality control (QC):   Component of quality assurance used in reference to the mechanical and geometrical tests of the radiation therapy equipment.

quality improvement (QI):   Continuous improvement of healthcare services through the systematic evaluation of processes.

quality indicator: Measurement tool used to evaluate an organization's performance.

quality management (QM):   Systems and processes used for decision-making related to reliable functioning of continuous quality improvement (CQI), quality assurance (QA) and quality control (QC).

quality of life: Person's subjective sense of well-being derived from current experience of life as a whole.

QUANTEC: Quantitative analyses of normal tissue effects in the clinic assesses normal tissue responses to ionizing radiation based on modern dose distributions calculations. Updates the 1991 Emani tolerance tables.

radiation necrosis: Tissue death resulting from the effects of radiation.

radiation oncologist: Physician who reviews the medical findings with the patient and discusses treatment options and the benefits of radiation therapy as well as the possible side effects.

radiation oncology QI team: Group committed to quality improvement and includes radiation oncologists, medial physicists, radiation therapists, medical dosimetrists, nurses, engineers, and other support staff.

radiation oncology team: Group consisting of all staff employees in radiation oncology who come in contact with the patient and/or family members throughout the course of radiation treatments.

radiation pneumonitis: Inflammation of the lung tissue.

radiation therapist: Medical practitioner on the radiation oncology team who sees the patient daily and is responsible for performing simulation, treatment delivery, and daily assessment of patient tolerance to treatment.

radiation therapy domain: Confines of the radiation therapy department and the socialization that takes place inside.

radiation therapy prescription: Legal document written by a radiation oncologist that provides the therapist with the information required to deliver the appropriate radiation treatment. It defines the treatment volume, intended tumor dose, number of treatments, dose per treatment, and frequency of treatment.

radical resection: Surgical removal of structures.

radioactive decay: Process of unstable nuclei emitting radiation.

radioactivity: Emission of energy in the form of electromagnetic radiation or energetic particles.

radiographic contrast: Element of imaging that provides visual evidence of the differential absorption rates of various body tissues. Radiographic contrast has been described as the tonal range of densities from black to white or the number of shades of gray in the radiograph.

radiographic density: Degree of darkening on the film. Radiograph of high density is dark, and a radiograph of low density is light.

radiolysis: Initial event in the radiolysis (splitting) of water involves the ionization of a water molecule, thus producing a water ion.

radiopaque marker: Material with a high atomic number used to document structures radiographically.

radioprotectors: Certain chemicals and drugs that diminish the response of cells to radiation.

radiosensitizers: Chemicals and drugs that help enhance the lethal effects of radiation.

random error: Variation in individual treatment setup.

randomization: Method by which patients are blindly assigned to participate in specific portions of a protocol called an *arm*. Use of randomization ensures an equitable distribution of patients in each arm without prejudices that can later be blamed for unfair patient selection and can be detrimental to the outcome of the trial.

randomize: To make random for scientific experimentation.

range modulator wheel (RMW): Device used to create the spread-out Bragg peak (SOBP) so that the maximum energy can treat the entire tumor from the most distal edge to the most proximal edge.

range uncertainty: Inherent variations in the defined range depth of a proton beam energy.

ratio: Mathematical comparison of two numbers, values, or terms that denotes a relationship between the two.

recombinant deoxyribonucleic acid (DNA): DNA molecule in which rearrangement of the genes has been artificially induced.

recombinant DNA technology (genetic engineering): Techniques that facilitate the manipulation and duplication of pieces of DNA.

reconstructed field of view: Diameter or the area of a computed tomography (CT) scan that is displayed on the computer. It should be large enough to display the entire contour of the patient.

reconstruction: The process in which the computed tomography (CT) computer analyzes and processes the information received from the detectors and displays it on a TV monitor.

Reed-Sternberg cell: Giant multinucleated connective tissue cell that is characteristic of Hodgkin disease.

reflective listening: Healthcare workers can reflect the specific content or implied feelings of their nonverbal observations or communication they feel has been omitted or emphasized.

regeneration: Repair, regrowth, or restoration of a part (as tissue).

regional accreditation: Agencies that serve select regions of the United States.

regulatory: Requirements for limits of exposure to radiation for various groups.

regulatory agency: Agencies authorized by Congress to establish mandates and regulations that explain the technical, operational, and legal details necessary to implement laws.

relative biologic effectiveness (RBE): The ratio of biological effectiveness of one type of ionizing radiation relative to another, given the same amount of absorbed energy. RBE equals dose from a 250-keV x-ray divided by dose from test radiation to produce the same biologic effect.

relative stopping power (RSP): The retarding force acting on charged particles because of interaction with matter, resulting in loss of particle energy.

remote afterloading: Afterloading using a treatment unit controlled from outside the treatment vault.

repainting: The process of delivering a fraction in portions of the fractional dose multiple times throughout the treatment volume.

reproductive failure: Decrease in the reproductive integrity or the ability of a cell to undergo an infinite number of divisions after radiation.

respiratory cycle: Healthy adult at rest breathes in and out, one respiratory cycle, about 12 to 16 times per minute, or approximately 1 cycle every 4 seconds.

rest mass: Mass (weight) of the particle when it is not moving.

restricted mass stopping power: Refinement of the total mass stopping power. Restricted mass collisional stopping power better describes the absorbed dose by accounting for energy transferred by delta rays.

retinoblastoma: Primitive neuroectodermal tumor of the retina that may be inherited. It usually occurs in children younger than 4 years.

retrospective studies: Studies that review information from a group of patients treated in the past are retrospective.

review of systems: Includes the patient's description of the signs and symptoms that lead the patient to present to the doctor, including subjective report of overall feelings of wellness.

rhabdomyosarcoma (RMS): Malignancy of skeletal muscle origin that can occur in many areas of the body and disseminates early. Soft tissue sarcoma (STS) arising from striated muscle. *See also* Soft Tissue Sarcoma (STS).

ribosome: Organelle constructed in the nucleolus and concerned with protein synthesis in the cytoplasm.

right angle: Three-sided polygon on which one corner measures 90 degrees.

right lymphatic duct: Serves only the right arm and right side of the head and neck and drains into the right subclavian vein. This duct is about 1 to 2 cm in length.

risk: Product of the probability of occurrence of error and the severity of that error.

risk management: Process of avoiding or controlling the risk of financial loss to the staff members and hospital or medical center.

RND: The radical neck dissection.

robotic Couch: A patient support system used in a treatment delivery suite that provides additional degrees of precision for patients undergoing radiation therapy.

robust analysis: A system that is commonly performed on cases that may have a large degree of uncertainty. This analysis is performed by scaling the computed tomography (CT) number to conversion curves by the same degree of expected range uncertainty.

robust optimization: A treatment planning approach to minimizing uncertainties for passive beam scattering systems.

role fidelity: Principle that reminds healthcare professionals that they must be faithful to their role in the healthcare environment.

room's-eye view: Image rendering technique that demonstrates the geometric relationship of the treatment machine to the patient. This view may also help prevent possible orientations of the beam that could result in collisions with the patient.

Rouvier's node: Node located just inferior to the base of the skull and medial to the internal carotid artery.

safety mindfulness: A worker's broad awareness of, and appreciation for, the potential presence of latent failures pathways, the risk of active failures pathways, and the critical role that they play in improving their (and the broader system's) overall safety and performance.

sarcoma: Tumors arising from mesenchymal cells or connective tissue.

Salpingo-oophorectomy: The removal of an ovary together with the Fallopian tube.

SBRT: Stereotactic body radiation therapy.

scan field of view: Area for which projection data is collected for a computed tomography (CT) scan is determined by the scan field of view. It helps to position the patient in the center of the CT bore so the patient's contour is not cut off laterally and is centered in the scan field of view.

scanning beams: Narrow "pencil beam" of electrons is scanned by magnetic fields across the treatment area. This constantly moving pencil beam distributes the dose evenly throughout the field.

scatter air ratio (SAR): Ratio of the scattered dose at a given point to the dose in free space at the same point.

scattering: Produced when an x-ray photon interacts with an outer-shell orbital electron with sufficient energy to eject it from orbit and alter its own path.

scattering foil: Most common method of producing an electron beam wide enough for clinical use is to use a scattering foil. Scattering foil is a thin sheet of a material that has a high Z number placed in the path of the "pencil beam" of electrons. Second scattering foil may be added to create a "dual scattering foil" arrangement. First scattering foil is used to widen the beam; the second is used to improve the flatness of the beam.

schwannoma: Nonencapsulated tumor resulting from disorderly proliferation of Schwann cells that includes portions of nerve fibers; typically undergoes formation to malignant schwannomas.

scientific notation: Special use of exponents that uses base 10 notation. It is used to represent either very large or very small numbers.

scientific revival: Intellectual resurgence of the sixteenth century.

scintillation detector: An electronic device that is used to measure radiation. The device is used in applications such as finding lost or misplaced sources and detecting the presence of low levels of contamination.

scope of practice: This describes the procedures, actions, and processes that a healthcare practitioner is permitted to undertake in keeping with the terms of his or her professional license.

screening: Selecting appropriate tests and studies to check for disease.

secondary vertebral curves (compensatory vertebral curves): Vertebral curves that develop after birth as the child learns to sit up and walk. Muscular development and coordination influence the rate of secondary curvature development.

second malignant neoplasm (SMN): Cancer developing years after the treatment of an initial tumor related to genetics and previous carcinogenic chemotherapy and radiation.

segment: Refers to the shape that the mechanical aperture multileaf collimator (MLC) creates during part of the total intensity-modulated radiation therapy (IMRT) dose delivered.

seminoma: Most common malignant testicular tumor.

sensitive test: A 100% sensitive test will give 0% false negative for detecting tumors.

sensitivity: Ability of a test to give a true, positive result.

sentinel node: Primary drainage lymph node of a specific anatomic area. For example, the sentinel node for the breast is most commonly located near the axilla.

separation: Measurement of the thickness of a patient along the central axis or at any other specified point within the irradiated volume.

serial response tissues: Tissues in organs that can be affected by the incapacitation of only one element. Spinal cord is such an organ. High-dose region of a serial-tissue dose-volume histogram (DVH) is of particular importance.

shelling: Surgical procedure that removes the primary tumor and its pseudocapsule, giving it the gross appearance of having removed all viable tumor.

shielding: Material that is used to limit the exposure to ionizing radiation.

shrinking fields: Technique that reduces the treated field area one or more times during the course of treatment in response to a tumor that reduces in size and/or the need to limit doses to normal structures.

Sievert: The SI unit of ionizing radiation dose.

significant figures: Number of figures in a measurement or calculation that are known with some degree of reliability. For example, the number 10.2 is said to have 3 significant figures. Number 10.20 is said to have 4 significant figures.

simple immobilization devices: Devices that restrict movement but require a patient's voluntary cooperation.

simulation: Process carried out by the radiation therapist under the supervision of the radiation oncologist. It is part of the treatment planning procedure, which delineates the treatment fields and constructs any necessary immobilization or treatment devices.

sine: One of three most common functions associated with the right triangle. Other two are the cosine and tangent. Sine of the angle is the ratio opposite the hypotenuse.

situational awareness: A hypothetical construct that represents the perception, comprehension, and projection of the system elements, their meaning, and their status in the environment within its volume of time and space.

Six Sigma process improvement method: Focuses on improving the process through precision and accuracy with the elimination of defects in the process. It was originally formulated by Bill Smith for the Motorola Corporation in 1986.

skin sparing: Property of megavoltage irradiation where the maximum dose occurs at some depth beneath the skin surface.

skin squames: Superficial skin cells that serve as vehicles for airborne pathogens.

skip metastasis: Situation that may occur where lymph nodes in a higher level may be involved while the nodes in the lower level(s) are negative for tumor.

slander: Oral defamation of character.

slice increment: This a computed tomography (CT) reconstruction parameter that determines the distance between the center of CT slices.

slice thickness: This is a computed tomography (CT) reconstruction parameter that determines the thickness of reconstructed images.

sliding window: Intensity-modulated radiation therapy (IMRT) technique describing the movement of the multileaf collimator (MLC) from one side of the field to the other within a narrow opening while the beam is on. See segmental MLC (SMLC).

slip ring: Computed tomography (CT) x-ray tube and detector can continue to rotate around the patient without concern of cables becoming tangled because of slip rings, which are metal strips carrying electronic signals and power that is swept up by special metal brushes.

smearing: Process that modifies the compensator design to take into account internal motion of the tumor and setup uncertainties.

SOAP note: Initial presentation and plan for assessment and treatment described in the history and physical (H&P) may be referred to as a "SOAP note." The acronym, SOAP, is described as follows: Subjective findings as reported by the patient; Objective or observations of the clinician, including vital signs and physical examination; Assessment of the disease or condition; and Plan for further examination and/or treatment. This information becomes part of the patient's medical record.

soft tissue sarcoma (STS): Malignant tumor arising primarily, but not exclusively, from mesenchymal connective tissues. *See also* Liposarcoma, Leiomyosarcoma, Rhabdomyosarcoma (RMS), and Fibrosarcoma, which are all types of sarcomas.

somatic cells: Nonreproductive cells

spondylolisthesis: An abnormal forward displacement of a vertebra that commonly occurs in the lumbar spine. This occurrence can cause narrowing of the spinal canal and result in subsequent symptoms associated with nerve impingement.

segmental MLC (SMLC): Refers to an intensity-modulated radiation therapy (IMRT) technique describing the sequence of leaves moving for repositioning, then coming to rest while the beam is delivered in multiple segments at each gantry angle.

source-axis distance (SAD): Distance from the source of radiation to the axis of rotation of the treatment unit.

source-skin distance (OOD): Distance from the source of radiation to the patient's skin.

spatial resolution: Refers to the clarity or the measure of detail in a computed tomography (CT) image.

specific activity: Activity per unit mass of a radioactive material (Ci/g). Specific activity dictates the total activity that a small source can have.

specific test: Test for detecting tumors, a 99% specific test gives 1% false-positive results.

specificity: Ability of the test to obtain a true-negative result.

SPECT: Single-photon emission computed tomography

spiral computed tomography (CT): Also referred to as *helical CT*. Patient is positioned at a fixed point, and, while the x-ray tube is rotating, the patient moves into the aperture to create a scan pattern that resembles a "slinky" or coiled spring.

Spread-out Bragg peak (SOBP): The sum of several individual Bragg peaks at staggered depths. This provides a useful beam over a greater range in the patient.

squamous cell carcinoma: Cancer originating in epithelial tissue from cells that are squamous (single or multiple layers) in size and shape. Examples include lung cancer and skin cancer.

staging: Cancer is "staged" after a histologic diagnosis is made. Staging helps determine the anatomic extent of the disease. Treatment decisions are based on the histologic diagnosis and extent of the disease.

stand: Drive stand appears as a large, rectangular cabinet, at least as large as the gantry. As its name indicates, the drive stand is a stand containing the apparatus that drives the linear accelerator.

standard precautions: Precautions that should be followed because of potential contact with body fluids. These precautions include wearing gloves, a mask, and protective eyewear; properly handling needles; and disposing of used equipment into containers for biohazardous material.

standard work procedures: Highly specified step-by-step instruction on how to perform tasks.

step and shoot: *See* segmental multileaf collimator (SMLC).

stereoscopic images: Two images from different angles focused on the same point.

stereotactic ablative radiotherapy (SABR; SBRT): A type of radiation therapy in which a few very high doses of radiation are delivered to small, well-defined tumors.

stereotactic radiosurgery (SRS): Use of a high-energy photon beam with multiple ports of entry convergent on the target volume.

stomatitis: Inflammation of the mouth.

stratified: Segregate populations according to certain specific characteristics.

striae: Lines or bands elevated above or depressed below surrounding tissue.

stridor: Harsh, rasping breath.

subcutaneous: Tissue just below the skin.

subcutaneous injection: A 45- or 90-degree injection into the subcutaneous tissue just below the skin.

subcutaneous layer: Layer of areolar connective tissue and adipose tissue that lies beneath the dermis that contains nerves and blood vessels.

superficial therapy: Treatment with x-rays produced at potentials ranging from 50 to 150 kV.

superior vena cava syndrome: Edema of the face, neck, or upper arms resulting from increased venous pressures caused by compression of the superior vena cava. It is most commonly caused by a metastatic, mediastinal tumor in lung cancer.

supraclavicular fossa: Where the supraclavicular lymph nodes are located; it is a space defined by the omohyoid muscle and tendon laterally and superiorly, the internal jugular vein medially, and the clavicle and subclavian vein inferiorly. The supraclavicular lymph nodes not only provide drainage for the internal mammary lymph node and axillary lymph node chains, but small number of breast tumors, especially centrally located tumors, may have direct drainage to the supraclavicular nodes.

suprasternal notch (SSN): Depression in the manubrium, which occurs at the level of T2 and articulates with the medial ends of the clavicles.

Surveillance, Epidemiology, and End Results (SEER) program: Program initiated in 1973 to collect data in an effort to determine the epidemiology and etiology of cancer.

symmetry: Maximum point-to-point difference in the central 80% of the profile.

synchrotron: Accelerator used in the production of proton beams and is characterized by having a continuously variable energy.

synergistic: Body organ, medicine, or substance that cooperates with another or others to produce a total effect greater than the sum of the individual elements.

systemic error: Variation in the translation of the treatment setup from the simulator to the treatment unit.

systemic treatment: Killing cells of the primary tumor and those that may be circulating through the body.

tabletop: Part of the treatment couch on which a patient is positioned during treatment or simulation; may be called a *treatment couch* or *patient tabletop.*

tandem and ovoid: An apparatus that is used to insert brachytherapy sources for gynecologic cancers, such as endometrial cancer or cervical cancer. The tandem is a long, narrow tube that inserts into the opening of the cervix *(cervical os)* into the uterus, and it holds radioactive sources and is used in the treatment of gynecologic tumors. The ovoids, also called *colpostats,* are oval-shaped applicators that insert into the lateral fornices of the vagina and accommodate radioactive sources and shielding material.

tangent: Tangent of the angle is equal to the length of the opposite side divided by the length of the adjacent side.

target volume: Area of a known and presumed tumor.

TD$_{5/5}$: Dose of radiation that is expected to produce a 5% complication rate within 5 years.

TD$_{50/5}$: Dose of radiation that is expected to produce a 50% complication rate within 5 years.

telangiectasia: Dilation of the surface blood vessels caused by the loss of capillary tone, resulting in a fine spider-vein appearance on the skin surface.

teleology: Also called *consequentialism,* an ethical theory where the consequences of an act or action should be the major focus when deciding how to solve an ethical problem.

teletherapy: Treatment at a distance, including cobalt-60 treatment.

temporal resolution: The ability to freeze or decrease motion of the scanned object, especially in four-dimensional computed tomography (CT) simulation.

tenesmus: Ineffective and painful straining during a bowel movement.

tensile strength: Resistance in lengthwise stress, measured in weight per unit area.

The Joint Commission (TJC): An independent, not-for-profit organization dedicated to improving quality of care in organized healthcare settings. It is the accrediting body for healthcare organizations.

therapeutic relationship: Genuine collaborative effort between the patient and healthcare provider. This requires good reflective listening skills and paying careful attention to all the cues. In addition, these cues need to be interpreted in the context of the patient's values, beliefs, and culture to be truly meaningful and helpful in treating and respecting the uniqueness of each cancer patient.

thermionic emission: In an oversimplification, x-rays are produced when a stream of electrons liberated from the cathode is directed across the tube vacuum at extremely high speeds to interact with the anode. These cathode electrons are freed from the tungsten filament atoms in a process called *thermionic emission.*

thermoluminescent dosimeter (TLD): Device for measuring dose. It uses the phenomenon that some solid materials, when irradiated, will subsequently give off light when heated. Amount of light emitted is proportional to the dose delivered to the crystal.

thoracic duct: Located on the left side of the body, the thoracic duct is typically larger than the right lymphatic duct. It serves the lower extremities, abdomen, left arm, and left side of the head and neck and drains into the left subclavian vein. This duct is about 35 to 45 cm in length and begins in front of the second lumbar vertebra (L2) called the *cisterna chyli.*

three-dimensional conformal radiation therapy (3DCRT): Three-dimensional image visualization and treatment-planning tools are used to conform isodose distributions to target volumes while excluding normal tissues as much as possible.

three-point setup: Three marks placed on a patient to define the isocenter. It is used to triangulate the patient's position and level the patient daily to ensure reproducibility and consistency of the setup and treatment delivery.

thrombocytopenia: Abnormal decrease in the number of platelets.

time-out: Use of standardized approach to help review most crucial aspects of a radiation treatment delivery process.

tissue absorption factor: Beam of radiation gives up energy as it travels through the body. The more tissue the beam traverses, the more it is attenuated (absorbed). There are a number of different methods for measuring the attenuation of the beam as it travels through tissue; these are percentage depth dose, tissue-air ratio, tissue-phantom ratio, and tissue-maximum ratio. First method used was percentage depth dose.

tissue-air ratio: Ratio of the absorbed dose at a given depth in phantom to the absorbed dose at the same point in free space.

tissue maximum ratio: Ratio of the absorbed dose at a given depth in phantom to the absorbed dose at the same point at the level of D_{max} in phantom.

tissue-phantom ratio: Ratio of the absorbed dose at a given depth in phantom to the absorbed dose at the same point at a reference depth in phantom. If the reference depth is chosen to be the depth of D_{max}, then the tissue-phantom ratio is called the *tissue-maximum ratio.*

titers: Measurement of the number of specific antibodies in a person's body or blood specimen.

tolerance: Body's adaptation to a particular drug and requirement of ever greater doses to achieve the desired effect.

TomoTherapy: A treatment unit where the linear accelerator rotates continuously while the treatment couch moves through the gantry bore producing a spiral treatment beam.

tort law: Type of law that governs rights between individuals in noncriminal actions. This law deals with violations of civil as opposed to criminal law.

total quality management (TQM): Professional performance standards that define activities in the areas of education, interpersonal relationships, personal and professional self-assessment, and ethical behavior.

TPS: Toyota Production System, or "Lean."

transcription: Process resulting in the transfer of genetic information from a molecule of DNA to a molecule of RNA.

transfer: Understanding of a subject matter to a depth that allows transfer of knowledge from one event to deal with another event. Ability to use knowledge in more than one setting. Use of preexisting knowledge to problem-solve.

transformational leadership: This focuses on the relationship between the leader and follower. It is concerned with motivating and inspiring followers to do more than expected.

translation: Process resulting in the construction of a polypeptide in accordance with genetic information contained in a molecule of RNA.

transmission factor: Any device placed in the path of the radiation beam will attenuate the beam.

transmission filters: Filters that allow the transmission of a predetermined percentage of the treatment beam.

transpectoral lymphatic pathway: Lymphatic pathway that passes through the pectoralis major muscle and provides efferent drainage to the supraclavicular and infraclavicular fossa nodes.

transurethral resection (TURP): Surgical procedure of the prostate performed through the urethra.

treatment console: Operating center where timers and system-monitoring indicators are displayed.

treatment couch: Part of the linear accelerator, the treatment couch is the area on which patients are positioned to receive their radiation treatment. Some treatment couches provide 6 degrees of freedom to better enable patient positioning and treatment delivery.

treatment field (portal): Volume exposed to radiation from a single radiation beam.

treatment planning: Process by which dose delivery is optimized for a given patient and clinical situation.

treatment record: Documents the delivery of treatments, recording fractional and cumulative doses, machine settings, verification imaging; and the ordering and implementation of prescribed changes.

treatment technique: Defined method by which a treatment is delivered to the patient.

treatment verification: Process using images of each treatment field and comparing them to a digitally reconstructed radiograph (DRR) from the initial simulation procedure to determine the accuracy of the treatment plan.

treatment volume: Generally larger than the target volume, the treatment volume encompasses the additional margins around the target volume to allow for limitations of the treatment technique.

triangulation: Treatment isocenter is located relative to three setup coordinates on the patient's surface or on the equipment fixed relative to their anatomy.

trigone: Portion of the bladder (shaped like a triangle) formed by the openings of the two ureters and orifice of the urethra.

triple negative breast cancers: Cancers with absent expression of estrogen receptor (ER), progesterone receptor (PR), and human epidermal growth factor type 2 (HER2) have poorer prognoses compared with patients with other breast cancer subtypes with receptor expressions. Triple-negative breast cancer behaves more aggressively than other types of breast cancer, and there is a lack of targeted treatment available for triple-negative breast cancer.

TTL: Transactional-transformational leadership.

tuberculin skin test (Mantoux test): Intradermal injection of purified protein derivative (PPD) or tuberculin used to test for exposure to tuberculosis.

tumor localization: Usually involves the use of a computed tomography (CT) simulator in determining the extent of the tumor and location of critical structures.

tumor board: Cancer specialists who work together to review information about newly diagnosed tumors and devise effective treatment plans.

tumor grade: Tumor grade is a specification that describes the apparent microscopic aggressiveness of the cancer as determined by cytologic and morphologic criteria.

tumor registry: Database tracking mechanism for cancer incidence, characteristics, management, and results in cancer treatment facilities for patients diagnosed with cancer.

tumor staging: Means of defining the tumor size and extension at the time of diagnosis. Tumor staging provides a means of communication about tumors, helps in determining the best treatment, aids in predicting prognosis, and provides a means for continuing research.

tumoricidal dose: Dose high enough to eradicate the tumor.

Tumor suppressor gene: Gene whose presence and proper function produces normal cellular growth and division. Absence or inactivation of such a gene leads to uncontrolled growth or neoplasia.

ulceration: Rare, late radiation reaction exhibited by an open sore on the skin or mucous membrane. It is caused by the shedding of dead tissue.

ultrasound: Imaging that involves high frequency sound waves sent into the body. Echo waves as the sound bounces back from various tissue interfaces are recorded.

ultraviolet protection factor (UVP): The amount of ultraviolet radiation that a fabric or protective clothing blocks.

uniform scanning: Homogeneous delivery across targeted volume with scanning beam.

universal precautions: Method of infection control in which any human blood or body fluid is treated as if it were known to be infectious.

urticaria: Hives.

user interface (UI): Part of the electronic medical record that refers to the graphical, textual, and auditory information the program presents to the user, and the input methods the user employs to control the program.

Vac-Lok: Trade name for an immobilization device that consists of a cushion and a vacuum compression pump.

vacuole: Membrane-bound cavity in the cytoplasm of a cell having a variety of storage, secretory, and metabolic functions.

vaginal cancer: Malignancy that arises in the vagina and does not extend to the vulva or cervix. Vaginal cancer is a rare disease that accounts for approximately 2% of all gynecologic cancers.

vaginal cylinder implant: Domed-ended tubular brachytherapy device used to give even dose distribution to the apex or entire vaginal surface. This resembles a candle with a central hollow canal for later afterloading.

vaginal stenosis: A narrowing of the vagina, often accompanied with dryness, loss of elasticity and resilience, and scar tissue.

Van de Graaff generator: Electrostatic accelerator designed to accelerate charged particles. In radiation therapy procedures, the unit produces high-energy x-rays typically at 2 MeV.

vector: Animal, usually an arthropod, that carries and transmits a pathogen capable of causing disease.

venipuncture: Puncture of a vein.

ventricles: Cavities that form a communication network with each other, the center canal of the spinal cord, and the subarachnoid space. They are filled with cerebrospinal fluid (CSF).

veracity: Truthfulness within the realm of healthcare practice.

verification: Final check that each of the planned treatment beams does cover the tumor or target volume and does not irradiate normal tissue structures.

virtue ethics: Use of practical wisdom for emotional and intellectual problem-solving.

virulence: Relative power of a pathogen to cause disease. Severity expressed in terms of morbidity and mortality.

vital signs: Information such as blood pressure, pulse, and respiration that may be gathered along with a chief complaint at the patient's initial encounter with a nurse or other clinical specialist.

voxel: Volume elements.

vulva: Female external genitalia composed of the mons veneris, labia majora, labia minora, vestibule of the vagina, and vestibular glands.

vulvar cancer: Cancer of the outermost portion of the gynecologic tract. Vulvar cancer patients usually have a subcutaneous lump or mass. Patients with more advanced disease have an ulcerative exophytic mass.

Waldeyer ring: Ring of tonsillar tissue that encircles the nasopharynx and oropharynx: two palatine tonsils, lingual, and pharyngeal tonsils.

WAN: *See* Wide Area Network (WAN).

warm thyroid nodule: Nodule having a slightly higher concentration than the rest of the thyroid gland.

water-equivalent thickness (WET): The thickness of water that is equivalent to the thickness between the patient's skin surface and the distal surface of the target.

waveguide: Hollow, tubelike structure within the linear accelerator that is used to transfer microwave power to the accelerator structure.

wavelength of the wave: Physical distance between peaks of the wave.

wave-particle duality: Photons exhibit the characteristics of a particle at times and the characteristics of a wave at other times.

wedge: Beam modifier that changes. Angle is defined relative to the horizontal plane at depth.

wedge angle: Angle between the slanted isodose line and a line perpendicular to the central axis of the beam.

wedge filter: Tool that modifies the isodose distribution of a beam to correct for oblique incidence or tissue inhomogeneities by progressively decreasing beam intensity across the field irradiated.

wide resection: Surgical procedure for soft tissue carcinoma. Procedure involves a wide en bloc excision for limb salvage and/or wide through-bone amputation.

Wilms tumor: Childhood embryonal kidney cancer.

window level: Represents the central Hounsfield unit of all the computed tomography (CT) numbers within the window width.

window width: Range of numbers displayed or the contrast on a computed tomography (CT) image.

windowing: Technique allows the radiation therapist to change the appearance of the image after it has been acquired by the computed tomography (CT) scanner. Two characteristics of the window are window level and window width.

wipe test: Test done to evaluate the contamination or leakage of a sealed radioactive source.

workload: A hypothetical construct that represents the overall cost incurred by a human operator to achieve a particular level of performance.

xeroderma pigmentosum: Rare disease of the skin starting in childhood and marked by disseminated pigment discolorations, ulcers, cutaneous and muscular atrophy, and death.

x-ray: Electromagnetic radiation that is produced when a fast electron stream hits a target. Synergy of the resultant x-ray beam increases with the voltage that accelerates the electrons.

x-ray generator: Generator that provides radiographic and fluoroscopic control of the simulator through the selection of various exposure factors, which include focal spot, mAs, kVp, and time.

4D CT: Four-dimensional computed tomography incorporating motion.

INDEX

Note: Page numbers followed by "f" indicates figures, "t" indicates tables, and "b" indicates boxes.